W9-DCH-107

Psychiatry Update and Board Preparation

Psychiatry Update and Board Preparation

EDITORS

THEODORE A. STERN, M.D.
Chief, The Avery D. Weisman, M.D., Psychiatry Consultation Service
Massachusetts General Hospital
Associate Professor of Psychiatry, Harvard Medical School
Boston, Massachusetts

JOHN B. HERMAN, M.D.
Director, Adult Psychiatry Residency Training Program
Director, Continuing Education Division, Department of Psychiatry
Massachusetts General Hospital
Assistant Professor of Psychiatry, Harvard Medical School
Boston, Massachusetts

McGraw-Hill
Health Professions Division

New York St. Louis San Francisco Auckland Bogotá Caracas Lisbon
London Madrid Mexico City Milan Montreal New Delhi San Juan
Singapore Sydney Tokyo Toronto

McGraw-Hill

A Division of The **McGraw·Hill** *Companies*

PSYCHIATRY UPDATE AND BOARD PREPARATION

Copyright © 2000 by The McGraw-Hill Companies, Inc. All rights reserved. Printed in the United States of America. Except as permitted under the United States Copyright Act of 1976, no part of this publication may be reproduced or distributed in any form or by any means, or stored in a data base or retrieval system, without the prior written permission of the publisher.

23456789 MALMAL 03 02 01 00

ISBN 0-07-135435-2

This book was set in Times Roman by Keyword Publishing Services.
The editors were Michael Medina and Susan Noujaim.
The production supervisor was Catherine Saggese.
Project management was performed by Keyword Publishing Services.
The cover designer was Marlisa Clapp.
The index was prepared by Jerry Ralya.

Malloy Lithographing was printer and binder.

This book is printed on acid-free paper.

Cataloging-in Publication-Data is on file for this title at the Library of Congress.

To life-long learners everywhere, and especially to those hard-working and hard-learning course participants who, for 25 years, have held us true to the mission: speak straight and teach clearly.

T.A.S.
J.B.H.

... and to my son, Tommy, whose ability to learn, and whose sense of humor, has been a joy to behold.

T.A.S.

Contents

Contributors

Robert S. Abernethy III, M.D. [58]
Psychiatrist
Massachusetts General Hospital
Instructor in Psychiatry
Harvard Medical School
Boston, Massachusetts

Annah N. Abrams, M.D. [4, 5]
Clinical Assistant in Psychiatry
Massachusetts General Hospital
Instructor in Psychiatry
Harvard Medical School
Boston, Massachusetts

Schahram Akbarian, Ph.D., M.D. [41, 42]
Clinical Assistant in Psychiatry
Massachusetts General Hospital
Instructor in Psychiatry
Harvard Medical School
Boston, Massachusetts

Anne W. Alonso, Ph.D. [62]
Psychologist, Department of Psychiatry
Massachusetts General Hospital
Director, Center for Psychoanalytic Studies and the Center
for Group Therapy
Professor of Psychology, Department of Psychiatry
Harvard Medical School
Boston, Massachusetts

Menekse Alpay, M.D. [33, 40]
Clinical Assistant in Psychiatry
Massachusetts General Hospital
Instructor in Psychiatry
Harvard Medical School
Boston, Massachusetts

Jonathan E. Alpert, Ph.D., M.D. [51]
Assistant Psychiatrist and Associate Director,
Depression Clinical and Research Program
Massachusetts General Hospital
Assistant Professor of Psychiatry
Harvard Medical School
Boston, Massachusetts

Lee Baer, Ph.D. [67]
Psychologist and Director of Research
Obsessive Compulsive Disorders Clinic
Massachusetts General Hospital
Associate Professor of Psychology
Harvard Medical School
Boston, Massachusetts

B. J. Beck, M.S.N., M.D. [9, 75, 79, 80]
Clinical Assistant in Psychiatry
Massachusetts General Hospital
Medical Director, Mental Health/Social Services
East Boston Neighborhood Health Center
Clinical Instructor in Psychiatry
Harvard Medical School
Boston, Massachusetts

Anne E. Becker, M.D., Ph.D. [21]
Clinical Assistant in Psychiatry
Massachusetts General Hospital
Assistant Professor of Psychiatry and Medical Anthropology,
Departments of Psychiatry and Social Medicine
Director of Research,
Harvard Eating Disorders Center
Harvard Medical School
Boston, Massachusetts

Eugene V. Beresin, M.D. [2]
Psychiatrist
Massachusetts General Hospital
Director of Child and Adolescent Psychiatry Residency
Training,
Massachusetts General Hospital and McLean Hospital
Associate Professor of Psychiatry
Harvard Medical School
Boston, Massachusetts

Mark A. Blais, Psy.D. [31, 32, 59]
Assistant Psychologist
Massachusetts General Hospital
Assistant Professor of Psychology, Department of Psychiatry
Harvard Medical School
Boston, Massachusetts

Jeff Q. Bostic, M.D., Ed.D. [1]
Clinical Associate in Psychiatry
Massachusetts General Hospital
Clinical Instructor in Psychiatry
Harvard Medical School
Boston, Massachusetts

Cristina M. Brusco, M.D. [17]
Clinical Assistant in Psychiatry
Massachusetts General Hospital
Clinical Fellow in Psychiatry
Harvard Medical School
Boston, Massachusetts

Ned H. Cassem, M.D., Ph.L., S.J. [40, 52, 70, 72]
Psychiatrist and Chief,
Department of Psychiatry
Massachusetts General Hospital
Professor of Psychiatry
Harvard Medical School
Boston, Massachusetts

M. Cornelia Cremens, M.D. [65]
Assistant Psychiatrist and Geriatric Psychiatrist,
Beacon Hill Senior Health Practice
Massachusetts General Hospital
Instructor in Psychiatry and Medicine
Harvard Medical School
Boston, Massachusetts

Darin D. Dougherty, M.D. [29]
Clinical Assistant in Psychiatry
Massachusetts General Hospital
Instructor in Psychiatry
Harvard Medical School
Boston, Massachusetts

William E. Falk, M.D. [7]
Psychiatrist and Director,
Geriatric Psychopharmacology,
Clinical Psychopharmacology Unit
Massachusetts General Hospital
Assistant Professor of Psychiatry
Harvard Medical School
Boston, Massachusetts

Maurizio Fava, M.D. [30, 46]
Psychiatrist and Director,
Depression Clinical and Research Program
Massachusetts General Hospital
Associate Professor of Psychiatry
Harvard Medical School
Boston, Massachusetts

John K. Findley, M.D. [73]
3rd Year Resident in Psychiatry
Massachusetts General Hospital
Clinical Fellow in Psychiatry
Harvard Medical School
Boston, Massachusetts

Anne K. Fishel, Ph.D. [60]
Clinical Associate in Psychology,
Director, Couples Therapy Training
Massachusetts General Hospital
Clinical Instructor in Psychology,
Department of Psychiatry
Harvard Medical School
Boston, Massachusetts

Jean A. Frazier, M.D. [5]
Assistant in Psychiatry and Director,
Psychotic Disorders Program for Children and Adolescents
Massachusetts General Hospital and McLean Hospital
Assistant Professor of Psychiatry
Harvard Medical School
Boston, Massachusetts

Edith S. Geringer, M.D. [17, 79]
Psychiatrist and Co-Director,
Primary Care Psychiatry Unit
Massachusetts General Hospital
Instructor in Psychiatry
Harvard Medical School
Boston, Massachusetts

S. Nassir Ghaemi, M.D. [14, 48]
Assistant in Psychiatry and Assistant Director,
Harvard Bipolar Research Program
Massachusetts General Hospital
Assistant Professor of Psychiatry
Harvard Medical School
Boston, Massachusetts

Donald C. Goff, M.D. [12, 45, 74]
Psychiatrist and Director,
Psychotic Disorders Program
Massachusetts General Hospital
Associate Professor of Psychiatry
Harvard Medical School
Boston, Massachusetts

Lee E. Goldstein, M.D., Ph.D. [65]
Clinical Assistant in Psychiatry
Massachusetts General Hospital
Instructor in Psychiatry
Harvard Medical School
Boston, Massachusetts

Gary L. Gottlieb, M.D., M.B.A. [65, 81]
Psychiatrist and Chairman, Partners Psychiatry and Mental Health System
Partners HealthCare System
Professor of Psychiatry
Harvard Medical School
Boston, Massachusetts

Donna B. Greenberg, M.D. [71]
Psychiatrist and Director,
Medical Student Education, Department of Psychiatry
Massachusetts General Hospital
Associate Professor of Psychiatry
Harvard Medical School
Boston, Massachusetts

James L. Griffith, M.D. [61]
Director, Residency Training Program
Department of Psychiatry and Behavioral Sciences
George Washington University Medical Center
Washington, D.C.

James E. Groves, M.D. [59]
Psychiatrist
Massachusetts General Hospital
Associate Clinical Professor of Psychiatry
Harvard Medical School
Boston, Massachusetts

Stephan Heckers, M.D. [6, 34, 36, 43]
Clinical Associate in Psychiatry
Assistant Director of Psychiatric Neuroimaging Research
Massachusetts General Hospital
Assistant Professor of Psychiatry
Harvard Medical School
Boston, Massachusetts

David C. Henderson, M.D. [12, 45, 78]
Assistant Psychiatrist
Massachusetts General Hospital
Director, Clozapine Clinic
Freedom Trail Clinic
Assistant Professor of Psychiatry
Harvard Medical School
Boston, Massachusetts

John B. Herman, M.D. [57]
Psychiatrist and Director, Adult Psychiatry Residency
Training Program
Director, Continuing Education Division, Department of
Psychiatry
Massachusetts General Hospital
Assistant Professor of Psychiatry
Harvard Medical School
Boston, Massachusetts

Dan V. Iosifescu, M.D. [15, 44]
4th Year Resident in Psychiatry
Massachusetts General Hospital
Clinical Fellow in Psychiatry
Harvard Medical School
Boston, Massachusetts

Robert W. Irvin, M.D. [77]
Clinical Assistant in Psychiatry
McLean Hospital
Instructor in Psychiatry
Harvard Medical School
Boston, Massachusetts

Joshua A. Israel, M.D. [46]
4th Year Resident in Psychiatry
Massachusetts General Hospital
Clinical Fellow in Psychiatry
Harvard Medical School
Boston, Massachusetts

Michael S. Jellinek, M.D. [81]
Psychiatrist and Chief, Child Psychiatry Service
Senior Vice-President for Administration
Massachusetts General Hospital
Professor of Psychiatry and Pediatrics
Harvard Medical School
Boston, Massachusetts

John N. Julian, M.D. [8]
Clinical Assistant in Psychiatry
Massachusetts General Hospital
Clinical Instructor in Psychiatry
Harvard Medical School
Boston, Massachusetts

Ali Kazim, M.D. [76]
Clinical Fellow in Psychiatry
Massachusetts General Hospital
Clinical Fellow in Psychiatry
Harvard Medical School
Boston, Massachusetts

M. Elyce Kearns, M.D., M.P.H. [3]
Assistant in Psychiatry
Massachusetts General Hospital
Instructor in Psychiatry
Harvard Medical School
Boston, Massachusetts

Shahram Khosbin [37, 38]
Neurologist,
Brigham and Women's Hospital
Associate Professor of Neurology
Harvard Medical School
Boston, Massachusetts

Helen G. Kim, M.D. [26, 71]
4th Year Resident in Psychiatry
Massachusetts General Hospital
Clinical Fellow in Medicine
Harvard Medical School
Boston, Massachusetts

Sara I. Kulleseid, M.D. [64]
Clinical Assistant in Psychiatry
Massachusetts General Hospital
Instructor in Psychiatry
Harvard Medical School
Boston, Massachusetts

Bandy X. Lee, M.D. [82]
4th Year Resident in Psychiatry
Massachusetts General Hospital
Clinical Fellow in Psychiatry
Harvard Medical School
Boston, Massachusetts

Carl D. Marci, M.D. [81]
3rd Year Resident in Psychiatry
Massachusetts General Hospital
Clinical Fellow in Psychiatry
Harvard Medical School
Boston, Massachusetts

John D. Matthews, M.D. [11, 13, 63]
Assistant Psychiatrist and Director,
Inpatient Psychiatry Service
Massachusetts General Hospital
Assistant Professor of Psychiatry
Harvard Medical School
Boston, Massachusetts

Dominic J. Maxwell, M.D. [57]
4th Year Resident in Psychiatry
Massachusetts General Hospital
Clinical Fellow in Psychiatry
Harvard Medical School
Boston, Massachusetts

Edward Messner, M.D. [82]
Psychiatrist
Massachusetts General Hospital
Associate Clinical Professor of Psychiatry
Harvard Medical School
Boston, Massachusetts

David Mischoulon, Ph.D., M.D. [30, 53]
Assistant in Psychiatry
Massachusetts General Hospital
Instructor in Psychiatry
Harvard Medical School
Boston, Massachusetts

Andrew A. Nierenberg, M.D. [53]
Psychiatrist and Associate Director,
Depression Clinical and Research Program
Massachusetts General Hospital
Associate Professor of Psychiatry
Harvard Medical School
Boston, Massachusetts

Dennis K. Norman, Ed.D. [32]
Psychologist and Chief of Psychology
Massachusetts General Hospital
Associate Professor of Psychology, Department of Psychiatry
Harvard Medical School
Boston, Massachusetts

Edward R. Norris, M.D. [39, 52]
4th Year Resident in Psychiatry
Massachusetts General Hospital
Clinical Fellow in Medicine
Harvard Medical School
Boston, Massachusetts

Sheila M. O'Keefe, Ed.D. [31]
Assistant in Psychology
Massachusetts General Hospital
Instructor in Psychology, Department of Psychiatry
Harvard Medical School
Boston, Massachusetts

Rafael D. Ornstein, M.D. [16, 19]
Assistant in Psychiatry
Massachusetts General Hospital
Instructor in Psychiatry
Harvard Medical School
Boston, Massachusetts

Lawrence Park, M.D. [33]
4th Year Resident in Psychiatry
Massachusetts General Hospital
Clinical Fellow in Psychiatry
Harvard Medical School
Boston, Massachusetts

Roy H. Perlis, M.D. [7, 54]
3rd Year Resident in Psychiatry
Massachusetts General Hospital
Clinical Fellow in Psychiatry
Harvard Medical School
Boston, Massachusetts

Mark H. Pollack, M.D. [15, 44]
Psychiatrist and Director,
Anxiety Disorders Program
Clinical Psychopharmacology and Behavior Therapy Unit
Massachusetts General Hospital
Associate Professor of Psychiatry
Harvard Medical School
Boston, Massachusetts

Alicia D. Powell, M.D. [24, 74]
Clinical Assistant in Psychiatry
Massachusetts General Hospital
Instructor in Psychiatry
Harvard Medical School
Boston, Massachusetts

Jefferson B. Prince, M.D. [50]
Clinical Assistant in Psychiatry
Massachusetts General Hospital
Director, Child Psychiatry
North Shore Medical Center
Salem, Massachusetts
Instructor in Psychiatry
Harvard Medical School
Boston, Massachusetts

John Querques, M.D. [27, 70]
Graduate Assistant in Psychiatry
Massachusetts General Hospital
Clinical Fellow in Psychiatry
Harvard Medical School
Boston, Massachusetts

Paula K. Rauch, M.D. [4]
Associate Psychiatrist and Director,
Pediatric Consultation Liaison Service
Massachusetts General Hospital
Assistant Professor of Psychiatry
Harvard Medical School
Boston, Massachusetts

Scott L. Rauch, M.D. [29, 83]
Associate Psychiatrist and Director,
Psychiatric Neuroimaging Research,
Departments of Psychiatry and Radiology
Massachusetts General Hospital
Associate Professor of Psychiatry
Harvard Medical School
Boston, Massachusetts

Brad H. Reddick, M.D. [28, 72]
4th Year Resident in Psychiatry
Massachusetts General Hospital
Clinical Fellow in Psychiatry
Harvard Medical School
Boston, Massachusetts

John A. Renner Jr., M.D. [10]
Associate Psychiatrist
Massachusetts General Hospital
Chief, Substance Abuse Treatment Program and Associate
Chief, Psychiatry Service,
Veterans Administration Medical Center,
Boston, Massachusetts
Associate Professor of Psychiatry
Boston University School of Medicine
Clinical Instructor in Psychiatry
Harvard Medical School
Boston, Massachusetts

Gary S. Sachs, M.D. [49]
Associate Psychiatrist and Director,
Harvard Bipolar Research Program
Massachusetts General Hospital
Assistant Professor of Psychiatry
Harvard Medical School
Boston, Massachusetts

Martin A. Samuels, M.D. [35, 39, 41, 42]
Senior Consultant
Massachusetts General Hospital
Chairman, Department of Neurology,
Brigham and Women's Hospital
Professor of Neurology
Harvard Medical School
Boston, Massachusetts

Kathy M. Sanders, M.D. [23, 77]
Associate Psychiatrist and Director,
Acute Psychiatry Service, Emergency Department
Massachusetts General Hospital
Assistant Professor of Psychiatry
Harvard Medical School
Boston, Massachusetts

Adam J. Savitz, Ph.D., M.D. [49]
Assistant in Psychiatry
Massachusetts General Hospital
Instructor in Psychiatry
Harvard Medical School
Boston, Massachusetts

Steven C. Schlozman, M.D. [19, 58]
6th Year Resident in Psychiatry
Massachusetts General Hospital
Clinical Fellow in Psychiatry
Harvard Medical School
Boston, Massachusetts

Ronald Schouten, M.D., J.D. [55, 56, 69]
Psychiatrist and Director,
Law and Psychiatry Service
Massachusetts General Hospital
Assistant Professor of Psychiatry
Harvard Medical School
Boston, Massachusetts

Linda C. Shafer, M.D. [20]
Psychiatrist and Director,
Sexual Dysfunction Section, Outpatient Psychiatry
Massachusetts General Hospital
Instructor in Psychiatry
Harvard Medical School
Boston, Massachusetts

Lois S. Slovik, M.D. [61]
Psychiatrist
Director, Family Therapy Training
Massachusetts General Hospital
Assistant Clinical Professor of Psychiatry
Harvard Medical School
Boston, Massachusetts

Patrick Smallwood, M.D. [22, 25]
Assistant in Psychiatry
Massachusetts General Hospital
Instructor in Psychiatry
Harvard Medical School
Boston, Massachusetts

Jordan W. Smoller, M.D., M.S. [68]
Assistant in Psychiatry
Massachusetts General Hospital
Instructor in Psychiatry
Harvard Medical School
Boston, Massachusetts

Theodore A. Stern, M.D. [18, 22, 28, 54, 70]
Psychiatrist and Chief,
The Avery D. Weisman, M.D. Psychiatry Consultation
Service
Massachusetts General Hospital
Associate Professor of Psychiatry
Harvard Medical School
Boston, Massachusetts

Paul Summergrad, M.D. [81]
Psychiatrist and Director,
Psychiatry Network
Partners HealthCare System, Inc.
Massachusetts General Hospital
Associate Professor of Psychiatry
Harvard Medical School
Boston, Massachusetts

Owen S. Surman, M.D. [64, 73]
Psychiatrist and Psychiatric Consultant for the Transplant
Unit
Massachusetts General Hospital
Associate Professor of Psychiatry
Harvard Medical School
Boston, Massachusetts

Adele C. Viguera [18, 26]
Assistant in Psychiatry,
Associate Director, Perinatal Psychiatry Program
Massachusetts General Hospital
Instructor in Psychiatry
Harvard Medical School
Boston, Massachusetts

Anthony P. Weiss, M.D. [35, 47]
4th Year Resident in Psychiatry
Massachusetts General Hospital
Clinical Fellow in Psychiatry
Harvard Medical School
Boston, Massachusetts

Charles A. Welch, M.D. [47]
Psychiatrist and Director,
Somatic Therapies Consultation Service
Massachusetts General Hospital
Instructor in Psychiatry
Harvard Medical School
Boston, Massachusetts

Candace White, M.Ed. [68]
Massachusetts General Hospital
Harvard Medical School
Boston, Massachusetts

Jonathan L. Worth, M.D. [27]
Psychiatrist and Director, Robert B. Andrews (HIV
Psychiatry) Unit
Massachusetts General Hospital
Instructor in Psychiatry
Harvard Medical School
Boston, Massachusetts

Albert S. Yeung, Sc.D., M.D. [66]
Assistant in Psychiatry,
Staff Member, MGH Depression Clinical and Research
Program
Massachusetts General Hospital
Instructor in Psychiatry
Harvard Medical School
Boston, Massachusetts

Preface

In 1976 Tom Hackett, M.D. (Chief of Psychiatry, MGH, 1975–1988) inspired our department to embark upon a mission which then seemed bold if not quixotic: to offer to a national audience a two-week, comprehensive review of psychiatry. 132 trusting souls attended that first course, launching what was to become America's most respected, academically based postgraduate educational program in psychiatry.

As we have grown in size and reputation through the years, so, too, has the variety and frequency of our courses. Every year over 2,000 clinicians from across the country and around the world return to Boston to study and learn in the rigorous and engrossing atmosphere of the medical classroom.

Our flagship course, *Psychiatry: A Comprehensive Review and Board Preparation*, has graduated over 9,500 participants in the quarter century since its inauguration and has set the standard for our field. Given each year shortly before the American Board of Psychiatry and Neurology Part I examinations, this course has been continuously refined and refreshed to reflect psychiatry's rapidly evolving knowledge base.

Through the years those who have attended our course have urged us to create a companion text (with board-style sample test questions) as a tool to aid in their studies and to serve as a basic reference source in everyday clinical practice. As the ABPN recertification examination approaches its 2004 launch, such requests have increased.

This book represents our response to that encouragement. Like the course itself, its creation has been a team effort, inspired of appreciation for course participants, our partners in life-long learning. 82 authors have created 83 chapters and 400 annotated questions.

Thoroughly indexed, it is designed to allow for quick access to specific areas of inquiry while providing a broad, in-depth review of accepted standards in our field.

T.A.S.
J.B.H.

Acknowledgments

Like our courses, the contents of this highly refined resource were mined from the rich ore of a mountain of collaborators, too massive to recognize by name. Through the years, scores of faculty and friends have contributed lectures, curbside consultations, and course ideas in the effort to improve on the previous years' offerings. Course Directors have included Bill Anderson, M.D., Jon Borus, M.D., Gene Beresin, M.D., Rob Abernethy, M.D., Paula Rauch, M.D., and our current Chief of Psychiatry, Ned Cassem, M.D. Course Coordinators Heidi Mann and Gail Dickson have been the engines driving the entire enterprise from its infancy. Without them we would not have prospered. We are grateful to the able hands at Harvard Medical School's Department of Continuing Education, particularly Norm Shostak, Nancy Bennett, Ph.D., and Steve Goldfinger, M.D. Marlisa Clapp, gifted graphic designer, has brought our courses a new clean "look," and designed the snappy cover to this book. Jim Groves, M.D., designed the round Bullfinch medallion that has become our department's logo. Jerry Ralya, our excellent indexer, dedicated countless hours to our project. Alan Hunt and associates from Keyword Publishing Services Ltd. in Barking, England were intrepid editors and typesetters. At McGraw-Hill we thank Michael Medina, Susan Noujaim, Catherine Saggese, Peter McCurdy, Marty Wonsiewicz, and Joe Hefta (for his help getting this project off the ground) and allowing us to complete this entire book in less than one year. We are also indebted to Laura L. Stephens of the MGH's Office of General Counsel who ably steered us through legal currents. Barbara Burns contributed mightily with administrative, typing, and organizational support, and Cynthia Soreff Mortlock provided substantive assistance with typing of hundreds of questions and answers. To our colleagues and co-authors, who did yeoman's work at a maniacal pace, we owe special thanks.

Psychiatry Update and Board Preparation

SECTION I

Test-Taking Strategies

Chapter 1
Test-Taking Strategies and Combating Test Anxiety

Jeff Q. Bostic

I. Overview

The Board exam is not designed to fail candidates. Instead, it allows candidates to demonstrate that they understand the core terminology and knowledge of psychiatry (Part I), and that they know how to be sensitive to patients as they arrive at a differential diagnosis and plan safe, reasonable treatment (Part II). Each candidate has had at least 4 years of training which should prepare one for this task; the Board Examination aims to assure that candidates have the required skills of an appropriate (not perfect), practicing psychiatrist.

II. Part I (The Written Examination)

A. **Components of the Exam**
The exam is divided into two sessions (or booklets), one in the morning and the second after lunch. The first question booklet covers psychiatry and neurology mixed together and is usually given in the morning session. After lunch, the second question booklet addresses psychiatry. Each question booklet includes approximately 200 questions, and candidates may skip about the test booklets as there are not timed subsections during these two sessions (but candidates cannot return to the morning booklet if they finish the afternoon booklet early). **The examination questions are multiple choice (usually five choices), and the Board has attempted to employ more type A (five choices), matching, and clinical vignette items, and to** *decrease* **the type E items (A = 1, 2, and 3 are correct; B = 1 and 3, C = 2 and 4; D = 4 only; E = all are correct).**
1. **Psychiatry. Approximately 300 items will address fundamental psychiatry knowledge.**
   a. Development and the life cycle
   b. Neurobiological and psychosocial aspects of psychopathology
   c. Diagnostic procedures
   d. Psychiatric disorders and co-morbid disorders
   e. Pharmacological and nonpharmacological treatments
   f. Special topics in psychiatry (suicide, dangerousness, ethics, mental health delivery systems, history of psychiatry, and community, consultation-liaison, emergency, and forensic psychiatry)
2. **Neurology. Approximately 100 mostly multiple-choice (up to five answer choices) items will address neurology knowledge.**
   a. Basic science aspects of neurological disorders (cellular and molecular neurobiology, neuroanatomy, neuropathology, and neurophysiology)
   b. Incidence/risk of neurological disorders
   c. Diagnostic procedures (history, neurological evaluation, neurochemistry, neuroelectrophysiology, neuroradiology, neuropsychological testing)
   d. Clinical evaluation and management of neurological disorders

B. **Preparation**
To become a hurdler, hurdle. To become a test-taker, take tests. Nothing prepares one better to do a task than practice. Taking written tests such as the **PRITE** (Psychiatry Residency in Training Examination), or review tests is helpful, and educational research clarifies that **familiarity with testing format predicts success better than studying longer or harder.** The more the real test-taking situation can be simulated, the more likely success will occur in the real situation.
1. **Study recent (within the past 5 years) textbooks and review articles** which best capture the content of the exam.
2. **Study over a longer time (3 months) with smaller material** (ten pages). This strategy is more effective and also diminishes test anxiety more than studying intensively during a shorter interval (30 pages per night the last month).
3. **Make study plans** known and even "write contracts" with oneself or others (spouses, colleagues) to increase both study time and scores on multiple-choice examinations.
4. **Devise your own multiple-choice questions at varying levels of complexity** to score better on these type of exams. Some questions assess basic facts while others require higher levels of synthesis or analysis.
5. **Construct the same types of multiple-choice questions in other subject areas** (e.g., spouse's work, child's academic courses). This reinforces the metacognitive skills associated with test-taking which generalizes across all subjects.
6. **Take two to three practice examinations in the mornings with the same time constraints as the actual examination;** this optimally simulates the real test-taking situation. The first exam should be taken early in the preparation process (months before the exam), and subsequent tests about 3–4 weeks before the actual exam.

C. Test-Taking Skills

1. **Approach the test systematically**
   a. **Make the setting predictable.** Familiarity with the test site enhances comfort while taking an exam. To **minimize distractions by others or outside noises,** candidates should select a seat toward the middle of a row and closer to the front of the room.
   b. **Scan the entire examination section before beginning;** this improves one's pace and diminishes anxiety.
   c. **Pace yourself. People who finish faster do not score higher than people who finish slower, so proceed at your own pace.** Most people actually answer questions more quickly as the test progresses and as the task becomes more familiar; being behind initially warrants little concern. A pace which allows 5–10 min at the end for review of difficult questions is optimal.

2. **Focus on key words in both item *stems* (i.e., the question) and in *answers*** to clarify the purpose of each question. Determine what is the *important* information or concept being sought in each question.
   a. **Stem options.** Often keywords in the stem provide clues about what is being sought in the answer.
      i. Example: Which of the following medications would be the most appropriate monotherapy for a depressed psychotic patient? (a) fluoxetine, (b) nortriptyline, (c) paroxetine, (d) amoxapine, (e) amitriptyline. Careful reading of the stem indicates that only one medication must address depression and psychosis, but also that no specific diagnosis is provided. Thus, the best answer is (d), since this could be a psychotic patient now depressed as well as a patient with an affective disorder.
   b. **Deductive reasoning strategies are based on choosing the *best* answer to each question.** Similar answers may be present, thereby eliminating multiple answers. Board questions have often employed this strategy in having multiple answers pertaining to symptoms of anticholinergic crisis or neuroleptic malignant syndrome.
      i. Example: The preceding example question illustrates this since choices a and c are both serotonin reuptake inhibitor antidepressants and choices b and e are both tricyclics. Only choice (d) is substantially different from the other choices.
      ii. Example: Rimfodine is used to treat (a) psychiatric disorders complicated by a thought disorder, (b) psychotic disorders, (c) depression with psychotic features, (d) impaired reality testing, or (e) anxiety disorders. Answers (a)–(d) all indicate treatment of psychosis, making (e) the best answer. (No drug named rimfodine exists.)
   c. **Specific determiners, such as "always" or "never," are less likely to be correct than are choices which include words such as "sometimes, often, or rarely."** Still, Board questions may include correct answers with "all" or "never." Similarly, answers with "sometimes," "often," or "may," are more often correct.

   d. **Since many issues in psychiatry remain ambiguous, longer answers with more qualifiers are often correct.**

3. **Avoid making mistakes**
   a. **Circle correct answers on the test booklet and fill them in on the answer sheets to enhance rapid review of items;** preferred strategies include stopping at every tenth item to fill in, or at least checking at every ten items that test book answers correspond to correct answer sheet items.
   b. **For items to be revisited if time permits, circle the entire question in the test book** and make a small line to the left of the number on the answer sheet to allow rapid location of these items.

4. **Increase accuracy levels**
   a. **Change answers.** Even when instructed not to change answers, college students *scored better when they went back and changed answers.* The more rapidly one completes a test, the more reasonable it is to go back and change an answer. In addition, changing answers benefited medical students on multiple-choice exams when they changed their answers because they recalled new information (oftentimes, subsequent test items aided recall useful for earlier items) or reread the question more carefully.

5. **Analyze items perceived as difficult**
   a. **Consider why this particular item is important enough to be on the exam.**
   b. **Return later to difficult items** to allow information from other items to clarify answers and allow the item to be read afresh.
   c. **Since each item counts the same, proceed to simpler items (e.g., matching) rather than spending excessive time trying to reason through one item.**

6. **Guess**
   a. There are no penalties for guessing; at least a 20% chance of guessing the correct answer is preferable to 0% (not filling in anything).
   b. There is no pattern to use when guessing (e.g., always choosing "B"); instead, attempt to eliminate wrong choices to increase the probability of choosing a correct answer.

D. Test Anxiety (Part I)

Among medical students, test anxiety was *positively* related to academic success. **On written exams, test anxiety is most impairing for those who also have *negative mood* (dreading the exam and feeling inadequate for months).** As a result, efforts to both improve optimism toward the exam, and efforts to decrease test anxiety are necessary. **Test anxiety does not usually intensify throughout exams, but rather diminishes from the half-way point.**

1. **Weeks before the examination**
   a. **Engage in relaxation training (deep muscle techniques);** this improves test scores, although it is less effective for reducing "state" anxiety. That is, relaxation techniques are preferred *before* exams rather than during

the exam. If one "freezes up" during the exam, a brief (< 1 min) exercise may be helpful.

b. **Performance improves when an examination is perceived as an opportunity for self-growth and demonstration of knowledge.** Examination performance decreases when the examination is perceived as a *threat* to the individual's aptitude or self-esteem. Accordingly, studying information of one's selected profession should be perceived as valuable and time spent which will improve patient care.

2. **The night before the examination**
   a. Aerobic exercise diminishes test anxiety; **plan *light* aerobic exercise the night before an exam.**
   b. **Studying the night before the examination is not usually helpful; familiarity with the format of the test is preferable.** If studying cannot be avoided, broad review of the major psychiatric diagnoses and treatments is preferred to reading journal articles or review of PRITE examinations.

3. **The morning of the examination**
   a. **Eat a normal breakfast;** this is preferable to eating nothing or to eating something atypical.
   b. **Drink the same amount of caffeine as one normally drinks** (to avoid increased anxiety but also to prevent withdrawal discomfort). No formal research has been conducted on the use of caffeine, alcohol, or nicotine to enhance Board performance. Still, initiating use (or abuse) of a substance is not perceived as beneficial prior to the exam. Similarly, deciding to stop smoking immediately prior to the exam will not diminish anxiety.
   c. Study on the morning of the test makes candidates less confident and more anxious; impairments in test-taking performance exceed any benefits from attempted learning.

4. **During the examination**
   a. Unlike many standardized tests, the items are *not* arranged in order of difficulty. **Candidates should not become demoralized if the first items appear difficult.**
   b. **Focus on the external (task at hand) cues, and selectively ignore internal responses that interfere with task performance** (Sarason, 1983).
   c. **If anxiety becomes overwhelming, use foods or snacks to put one at ease.** Chewing gum improved test performance for anxious college students.
   d. **During breaks, discussion of test items increases anxiety.** Truth does not occur by consensus, and negative effects on confidence outweigh the benefits of any knowledge item clarification.
   e. **Eat lunch with friendly, familiar others (who do not discuss test items).** Greasy or fatty foods may cause tiredness and should be avoided. Similarly, sugar snacks or candy bars are preferred in the afternoon session rather than in morning sessions.

III. Part II (The Oral Examination)

Of the candidates who have passed Part I, 88% will ultimately pass Part II.

A. Components of the Exam

1. **Videotape interview.** The first component is **a 30-min videotape of a patient interview which candidates watch (in a room with usually 10–20 other candidates);** after watching the video each candidate goes into a room to present the case to two or three examiners. The videotapes are excerpts from longer interviews done by non-candidates, and do *not* represent a model for candidates to employ during the live interviews.
   a. **Most candidates perform better on the videotape examination,** where the examination focuses on the candidate's ability to organize and present information; **here they can show how they formulate and plan treatment based on available information.**

2. **Patient interview.** The second component is a "live" interview where each candidate meets and interviews an adult psychiatric patient (inpatient or outpatient) for 30 min, and then presents that case to two or three examiners.
   a. **Essential to the patient examination is to balance the differing agendas of the patient, the examiners, and the candidate during the interview.** Throughout the interview, consideration of this balance helps prevent the candidate from under- or over-controlling the interview and ensures that all parties are treated respectfully.
      i. **The candidate's agenda is to take the information the patient provides and to *start* treatment planning,** mindful of establishing a treatment alliance so that the patient and candidate could work together.
      ii. **The patient's agenda is to tell his or her story to someone who appears compassionate and helpful.** Most importantly, one should show respect for the patient's agenda. This allows the candidate to demonstrate the sensitivity which distinguishes them from other medical professionals. **The most conspicuous deficiency observed in candidates who fail the live patient interview is their inability to follow the affective and informational cues of the patient.** So, it is essential not to allow the candidate agenda (i.e., seeking clinical information to formulate a diagnosis and plan) to dominate the patient's agenda.
      iii. **The Board examiner's agenda is to *impartially* ensure that the candidate is sensitive to the patient's plight, so that a treatment alliance can occur, and that the candidate's plan is safe, and reasonable.** Their job is to focus on the candidate as a clinician and to avoid being biased by personality factors. The specific Part II grading criteria are summarized in Fig. 1-1.

Interview Style

1. Opening and closing — Uses appropriate strategies
2. Informational cues — Follows vs. ignores leads
3. Affect cues — Explores appropriately vs. ignores
4. Communication — Uses adequate language and cultural sensitivity vs. a lack which interferes with obtaining data
5. Questioning technique — Uses open-ended but appropriately structured vs. abrupt forced choice questions
6. Control and direction of interview — Develops a cohesive interview vs. scattered fragmented series of questions

Substance of Interview

7. Presenting problem and history of present illness — Obtains adequate data vs. leaves vague or ambiguous
8. Past history—Family, social, medical, and developmental history — Gathers relevant data at least in a brief form vs. ignores major issues (e.g., child abuse)
9. History of drug and alcohol abuse — Sensitively gathers vs. ignores
10. Assessment of suicidal, homicidal risk — Sensitively explores vs. ignores

Presentation and Discussion

11. Summary — Presents important data concisely and coherently vs. disorganized
12. Mental status examination — Organizes and accurately presents vs. incomplete
13. Emergency issues — Considers suicide, violence, drug and alcohol abuse vs. ignores
14. Workup—additional history, collateral information, test to be ordered — Considers appropriate diagnostic workup vs. demonstrates a lack of rationale
15. Differential diagnosis — Presents pros and cons of pertinent Axis I, II, or III, and chooses an appropriate working diagnoses vs. too narrow or broad a differential
16. Biopsychosocial formulation — Includes all three dimensions of a formulation vs. a unidimensional view
17. Treatment plan — Provides a comprehensive and specific plan for this patient including appropriate use of medication, psychotherapy (justification for type of therapy used), criteria for hospitalization; knows milieu principles and family systems
18. Prognosis — Discusses positive and negative prognostic indicators, including anticipated transference/countertransference

Fig. 1-1. Part II psychiatry grading criteria. Scoring: 1=dangerous or grossly inadequate, 2=fail, 3=conditional, 4=pass, 5=high pass. (From McDermott et al., 1996.)

B. Preparation

1. **Plan a format to organize and present information.** Most candidates devise a comfortable but complete list of categories such as identifying information (**ID**), history of present illness (**HPI**), substance abuse (**SA**), past psychiatric history (**P**), past medical history (**PMHx**), developmental/social history (**D/S**), family history (**FHx**), mental status examination (**MSE**) with appearance, mood, sensorium, intellect, thought (**AMSIT**), formulation (**FORM**), provisional diagnoses (**Dx**), and treatment plan (**Tx**) which includes differential (**DDx**) and procedures/labs/testing to clarify diagnoses (**Test**), biologic treatments (**Rx**), psychotherapies (e.g., individual [**IT**], family [**FT**]) and psychosocial inter- ventions (**PS**) for work, school, or individual quality of life improvement. This is illustrated in Fig. 1-2.

2. **Simulate the interview.** People who practice for the Boards should take turns being the patient and the psychiatrist and have someone (*preferably, a Board examiner or someone who has passed the Boards*) question them about the interview. The "patient" reads about a diagnosis and presents with a disorder(s). The candidate should interview this "patient" *for 30 min* with someone sitting next to them.

3. **Videotape practice interviews and presentations. A very helpful strategy is to videotape practice interviews and discussions of the case.** Candidates are

ID (Identifying information)

HPI (History of present illness)

SA (Substance abuse)

P (Psychiatric history)

PMHx (Past medical history)

D/S (Development/social history)

FHx (Family history)

MSE: (Mental status examination)

    A (Appearance)

    M (Mood)

    S (Sensorium)

    I (Intellect)

    T (Thought)

FORM (Formulation)

DX (Diagnoses)

TX (Treatment plan)

DDx (Differential diagnoses)

Labs/Tests (Labs/tests/procedures to clarify diagnoses)

Rx (Medications, somatic therapies)

IT (Individual therapies)

FT (Family/couples/group therapies)

PS (Psychosocial recommendations)

Fig. 1-2. Sample presentation format. Only the abbreviations (bold) should be written down on the left side of the paper, and then clinical information added in as it emerges during the interview.

invariably amazed at how their appearance on tape (similar to what the examiner sees) diverges from what they thought transpired. This also helps a candidate recognize any idiosyncrasies or "quirks" which might alienate an examiner.

4. **Address cross-cultural factors.** Candidates with impressive ability must be able to communicate that in the current cultural context. **International students who have *integrated social assistance* into their learning have been more successful.** Specifically, foreign candidates have found it help-

ful to consider cultural differences which might impede forming a relationship with a patient, and to talk with someone who has passed the exam about any mannerisms which might disadvantage them while interviewing an American patient.

5. **Attire. Conservative, classic fashion is appropriate for Part II.** Women should wear a business suit or conservative dress. Men should wear shirt and tie, slacks, and a sports coat, or a suit. Consulting with a senior clothing store representative about appropriate apparel for a business interview may be helpful. In addition, John Molloy has written extensively about specific clothing choices effective for interviewing. Mr. Molloy has been criticized by some women for his conservative recommendations (but remember who will be evaluating candidates), and Susan Morem also has written a recent book for women's clothing.

C. Test-Taking Skills for Part II

1. **The videotape interview**

    a. Successful candidates tend to **sit in the middle of the room where the monitors are easily viewable.**

    b. **Candidates may bring *blank* paper and writing instruments, but no audiovisual equipment** (e.g., tape recorder, camcorder) is allowed, and indeed would be cause for invalidation of Part II (Section I [H] 5). **Once seated, candidates may write down a psychiatric interview outline** (see Fig. 1-2) to most easily organize the information from the videotape.

    c. **During the videotape, candidates may fill in information in the appropriate category,** including appearance and mannerisms which fit in the mental status examination.

    d. **At the conclusion of the videotape, candidates will be escorted to individual examining rooms where they should expect to begin with the summary** (see section C.2.e).

    e. After the examination, examiners will take any candidate notes/outlines. These are not "graded" but are discarded to preserve patient confidentiality.

2. **The live patient interview**

    a. **Meeting the examiners.** One or two examiners will meet the candidate in a waiting area. They may not appear friendly, and candidates should not make small talk with them. **Examiners are attempting to remain impartial,** so it is appropriate to simply shake hands, smile, and follow them to the examination room. They may review the time parameters with you before you meet the patient.

    b. **Greeting the patient.** Patients have been prepared for the interview and should know their role, and past research indicates most patients view this as a positive experience, so candidates should not feel guilty or apologize for interviewing them. Still, patients may forget the purpose of the interview, they may be psychotic or despondent, or they may act inappropriately.

Candidates should be prepared to be sensitive to their needs; indeed, if the patient refuses to speak or "goes on a tirade," as has most likely occurred to every candidate during their 4 years of training, candidates should be respectful to the patient rather than attempt to force the patient to answer questions. As in real psychiatric practice, empathizing with the patient's difficulty or frustration may help such patients begin talking about their discomfort or frustration. **Examiners want to know that candidates can *contend* with whatever the patient presents.**

c. **The interview**

   i. It is *not* appropriate for candidates to be familiar (e.g., talk about the weather or comment about clothing), but **it is appropriate for candidates to *clarify* to patients that this interview is to allow the examiners to watch candidates conduct an interview.**

   ii. **After clarifying the purpose of the interview, candidates should follow the format of the psychiatric interview (Chap. 2) by beginning with an open-ended question** (e.g., "Can you help me understand what's led to you getting treatment?") which allows the patient the opportunity to describe, in their own words, their condition. **Examiners want candidates to be able to listen to a patient's story and fit the patient's descriptions into psychiatric categories, rather than observe the candidate ask a list of yes-no questions about diagnoses.** Candidates are expected to clarify whether this is a new problem or an exacerbation of a previous difficulty. Lists of diagnostic symptoms can be appropriately interjected during the history of present illness once a patient describes a major symptom, its onset, duration, and intensity. For example, once the patient indicates that depression (e.g., anxiety or mood swings) is the primary complaint, assessment of diagnostic criteria helps the examiner recognize that the candidate knows how to follow up on presenting symptoms to arrive at a diagnosis. When psychiatric history reveals, for example, substance abuse issues, follow-up with full diagnostic criteria questions again becomes appropriate.

   iii. **While note-taking is allowed** (brief phrases or even single words may help candidates later remember specific details), **candidates will want to demonstrate *listening* to the patient** by exhibiting eye contact (to the patient, not the examiner), by nodding at appropriate intervals, by rephrasing patient descriptions in the patient's own words to show understanding (e.g., "It felt 'horrible' when your neighbor Lynn started moving things in your house."), and by gently interrupting, if necessary, to obtain clarification or more details about a symptom (e.g., "I'm sorry, help me understand your trouble sleeping.").

   iv. **It is critically important for the candidate to follow the patient's cues, both informationally and affec-**

tively. If the patient shows affect, such as tearfulness, **the candidate's capacity to empathize with the patient** (and not avoid the affect) **is as important as any question the candidate will ask during the interview.**

   v. **Candidates should ultimately identify the constellation of patient symptoms so that a working diagnosis might evolve.** This usually requires that the candidate ask some structured but sensitive questions about the symptoms of specific psychiatric disorders.

   ● Some candidates find it helpful to devise or employ mnemonics for the most common diagnoses so that they might more easily recall specific criteria. Several of these mnemonics have been published (e.g., Reeves and Bullen, 1995; Short et al., 1992).

   ● Examiners are *explicitly* directed to check to see whether candidates **sensitively obtain** (vs. ignore) **psychiatric history** (including family, social, medical, and developmental history), **substance abuse history, and, particularly, suicide/homicide risks.** In addition, **candidates must attempt a mini-mental status examination,** and pursue any parts that appear significant (e.g., the patient appears disoriented, so ensure that orientation is specifically evaluated).

d. **Saying good-bye to the patient**

   i. If at all possible, candidates should **ask questions until stopped by examiners** (examiners alert candidates when 5 min remain). Otherwise, it will not be possible for candidates to indicate that if they had had more time, they would have further investigated a topic in greater detail. "Disregarding time limits" is specifically identified as "irregular behavior" and could be cause for invalidation of the Part II. Thus, when time is "called," it would be dangerously inappropriate to question the patient any further.

   ii. **Candidates should acknowledge that the interview is almost over, and ask if there is anything else that would be particularly important to know that has not been talked about.**

   iii. **Patients should be thanked for participating.** *Only if* the patient asks a candidate about the patient's treatment (or can talk *more* with the candidate later), should the candidate clarify that they will discuss this case with these other doctors now. If the patient asks if the candidate will talk with their doctor, candidates should be honest and indicate that will not occur, empathize with the patient's need for understanding, and reiterate that this interview was to examine the candidate.

e. **Summarizing the case**

   i. The examiners may allow the candidate "a moment to collect thoughts." This time is best used to **organize information to present in a coherent format.**

ii. After the examiner takes the patient out of the room, the candidate will be asked to provide impressions. **The candidate's objective is to succinctly summarize the case in an organized presentation.** The case presentation ordinarily begins with identification ("Ms. Jones is a 34-year-old married White female who resides alone in an apartment and now complains of . . ."). The candidate should proceed *succinctly* through the history of present illness, psychiatric history, medical history, developmental/social history, family history, and mental status examination.

iii. The candidate should *expect to be interrupted during the summary, but be prepared to proceed on to the formulation.* If interrupted, candidates should not try to return to the presentation, but rather answer *concisely* whatever question the examiner poses. Examiners will either ask additional questions, or ask the candidate to resume presenting.

iv. **If the patient evades an answer in an area (or if the candidate forgot to ask), the candidate should indicate that if more time had been available, further clarification in that area would have occurred** so that examiners know the candidate *knew* what should be covered in an evaluation.

f. **Formulating the case.** For candidates failing both the live patient and audiovisual components of Part II, an inadequate formulation is the most likely problem.

i. **Integrating the available information and presenting it with a biopsychosocial formulation is essential for all candidates.** This requires description of biological factors (e.g., family history of affective disorders, physical illnesses contributing to symptoms), psychological factors (e.g., how the patient perceives his/her predicament and understands the world), *and* social factors (e.g., work, family, spousal events that impact the illness). All three pieces should be described.

ii. **The formulation should conclude with *provisional diagnoses on axes I, II, and III*.**

iii. **Differential diagnoses *must* be entertained.** While it may seem obvious that a patient has major depressive disorder, it is *essential* candidates discuss this patient could also have bipolar disorder, depression secondary to medical illness/another psychiatric disorder/substance abuse, dysthymia, and/or "double depression." If any indication of a psychotic or anxiety disorder (e.g., obsessive-compulsive disorder [OCD]) were present, the candidate should discuss how they would monitor for the emergence of those symptoms.

iv. Many patients have *comorbid* disorders, so secondary or less severe disorders also warrant consideration.

g. **Planning treatment**

i. **Treatment planning should first include efforts to further clarify the diagnoses, by appropriate testing and by monitoring for additional or more persistent symptoms.** The patient may have taken great pains to conceal a disorder, e.g., OCD or substance abuse, so candidates should clarify that this first interview warrants treatment for the elicited disorder while a treatment alliance may reveal additional diagnoses in need of further intervention.

ii. Candidates should **describe treatment interventions with *both* medication and with psychotherapy.**

● Candidates should **be prepared to *defend* medication and psychotherapy choices;** it is *never helpful to indicate convictions of not prescribing medications or not believing in psychotherapy.*

● Candidates often find it helpful to **prepare (before the examination) single-sentence descriptions of treatment modalities** (e.g., couples therapy, electroconvulsive therapy, tricyclic antidepressants) and another sentence describing appropriate clinical indications for each of these modalities so that these are more easily described and defended during the actual interviews.

● This is *not* the circumstance to demonstrate creativity by recommending unconventional, unproven, or risky treatments.

iii. **Candidates should clarify the appropriate *treatment setting* for the patient.** Whether these treatments could be initiated as an outpatient or require hospitalization is important, and criteria for hospitalization and preferred milieu treatment (e.g., hospital, day programs) should be discussed.

iv. **Family/support system interventions should be described,** particularly emphasizing how resources in vivo can be used to enhance the patient's care.

D. Test Anxiety (Part II)

Over 80% of candidates who pass Part II after failing it previously attribute their initial failure to their "high level of anxiety that interfered with performance" (Rudy et al., 1981). When they pass Part II, candidates indicate that familiarity with the format of the examination and "knowing what to expect" were more important than remediating knowledge deficiencies. **Practicing the oral examination with someone who has passed or is familiar with Part II is encouraged.**

1. **Light exercise and adherence to normal routines** as in Part I remain appropriate.

2. **Medications.** Candidates should discuss these with their physician, and, if determined appropriate, a trial *prior to the exam* is recommended. Candidates should never try any medication *for the first time* at the Board exam.

a. Low doses of beta-blockers, such as propranolol (Drew et al., 1985; Lader, 1988), nadolol (James and Savage, 1984), and atenolol (Liebowitz et al., 1991), appear effective in "performance anxiety" situations (e.g., test-taking).

b. Buspirone has not appeared effective in this situation (Clark and Agras, 1991).

c. Deteriorations in performance have been reported with benzodiazepines, such as diazepam (James and Savage, 1984) and lorazepam (Walsh et al., 1983).

d. Alcohol should never be used before or during any part of the Board exam.

E. Handling Adversity

1. **When the candidate does not know the answer to a question.** This *usually* occurs. Examiners often want to know how a candidate contends with ambiguity. It is appropriate for candidates to indicate they are unsure of the answer, and then indicate how they would find the answer to something they don't know (e.g., refer to a book to find side effects, to a specialist regarding unusual drug interactions). Indicating that one would seek consultation in one's actual practice is reassuring to examiners. Even if the examiner probes the candidate to guess, the guess is made in the context of demonstrating appropriate caution. **Examiners *know* candidates don't know everything; candidates who try to prove otherwise can be perceived as arrogant or dangerous.**

2. **The disastrous patient.** Sometimes patients will leave early in the examination. Although this experience is unusual, it is not unusual for another patient to be brought in. Candidates should *not request a different patient* if difficulties emerge, but **candidates should not feel disadvantaged if a patient leaves and a substitute patient is provided.**

3. **Failing the exam.** Unfortunately, a number of candidates do not pass the Board on their first try. Candidates fare best who remediate any areas of weakness, practice to regain confidence, and retake the exam at the next available opportunity. In order of importance, **candidates who initially failed Part II listed the following factors as most important in their subsequent successful passing of Part II: having taken the exam previously, having different examiners, having decreased anxiety, having studied more, getting feedback from others, having a more appropriate patient, being tested in different areas, having additional clinical experience, having a better examination environment, having additional colleague support, attending a Board review course, getting additional tutoring, and having easier and better travel/hotel arrangements.**

F. Testing Accommodations

1. Applicants with disabilities (including learning disabilities, attention deficit hyperactivity disorder) may complete an Application for Testing Accommodations in the application materials provided by the Board. Generally, the disability must have been formally diagnosed by someone specialized to do thorough evaluations (including appropriate objective testing), present during the previous 3 years, and a rationale must be provided for any accommodation requested.

a. Part I accommodations include (but are not limited to) assistance in completing answer sheets, extended testing time, large print examinations, separate examination rooms, a reader, and use of assistive devices.

b. Part II accommodations include (but are not limited to) infrared headphones during videotaped interviews, and the use of assistive devices.

Suggested Readings

Ball S: Anxiety and test performance. In Spielberger CD, Vagg PR, et al. (eds): *Test Anxiety: Theory, Assessment, and Treatment (Series in Clinical and Community Psychology)*. Washington, DC: Taylor and Francis, 1995:107–113.

Johnson S: *Taking the Anxiety out of Taking Tests: A Step-By-Step Guide*. Oakland, CA: New Harbinger, 1997.

Kaufman DM: *Clinical Neurology for Psychiatrists*, 4th ed. New York: WB Saunders, 1996.

Luckie WR, Smethurst W: *Study Power: Study Skills to Improve Your Learning and Your Grades*. Cambridge, MA: Brookline Books, 1998.

McDermott JF, Streltzer J, Yen Lum K, et al: Pilot study of explicit grading criteria in the American Board of Psychiatry and Neurology. Part II examination. *Am J Psychiatry* 1996; 153:1097–1099.

Molloy JT: *John T. Molloy's New Dress for Success*, 2nd ed. New York: Warner, 1988.

Morem S: *How to Gain the Professional Edge*. New York: Better Books, 1997.

Morrison J, Munoz RA: *Boarding Time: A Psychiatry Candidate's Guide to Part II of the ABPN Examination*, 2nd ed. Washington, DC: American Psychiatric Press, 1996.

Reeves RR, Bullen JA: Mnemonics for ten DSM-IV disorders. *J Nerv Ment Dis* 1995; 183(8):550–551.

Short DD, Workman EA, Morse JH, Turner RL: Mnemonics for eight DSM-III-R disorders. *Hosp Commun Psychiatry* 1992; 43: 642–644.

Zeidner M: *Test Anxiety: The State of the Art*. New York: Plenum, 1998.

Chapter 2
The Psychiatric Interview Examination

Eugene V. Beresin

I. Introduction to the Oral Examination

A. Overview

The Oral Board Examination is the most anxiety-provoking part of the certification process. There are a number of reasons for the stress inherent in this component of the Boards. First, most clinicians are rarely observed doing psychiatric interviews, and certainly not by two examiners. The short time-frame for examination and discussion is quite stressful. There is a great deal of uncertainty about what is expected of the examinee. And most clinicians, even recently graduating residents, have little opportunity to present a succinct history, mental status examination, formulation, differential diagnosis and treatment plan on the spot. The purpose of this chapter is to help clarify the goals and objectives of the psychiatric interview examination, and to provide a framework for preparing for a good performance.

There are two parts to the Oral Examination in General Psychiatry. One is **observation of a videotaped interview,** followed by the requirement to present a case history, differential diagnosis and treatment plan based on what was seen. The second part is an **interview of a real adult patient** followed by a formal presentation. Both examinations are performed in front of two examiners, and the team leader may drop in to ask a question or two. This chapter will focus on the live interview. All of the principles of preparation and presentation are the same for both examinations.

B. Format

The psychiatric interview for the Oral Board Examination consists of a **30-min interview of a live adult patient, followed by a 30-min case presentation and discussion.** The examinee will be introduced to the patient by name. There will be no identifying data, such as whether the patient is an inpatient, partial hospital patient, or ambulatory patient. The examinee will not be given any directions as far as conducting the interview is concerned. **It is up to the examinee to watch the time.** The examiners will inform the candidate when there are 5 min left. Following the interview, there will be a few minutes to collect one's thoughts, and then the examinee will be asked to present the case. It must be kept in mind that this is quite a different interview from a typical office-based or inpatient diagnostic evaluation for psychiatric treatment. **It is similar to an emergency ward visit or a crisis intervention evaluation. It is imperative that one is very familiar with this format.**

C. General Principles

The Interview Examination has three broad areas of concern: skill in gathering information, skill in formulation and differential diagnosis, and skill in therapeutic planning.

1. **Skill in gathering information.** The examiners are looking to see whether the candidate can **establish rapport, follow the patient's lead, ask relevant questions and focus on significant themes in the interview.** The data need to be collected by history-taking, performing a mental status examination, and determining what ancillary sources would be useful to fill in gaps in the history, such as talking with relatives and health care professionals, reviewing medical records, and determining the need for appropriate laboratory and psychological workups, as well as additional consultations.

2. **Skill in formulation and differential diagnosis.** A sound formulation must take into account the **biological, psychological, and sociocultural factors** that are intrinsic to the patient's life. There must be an **accurate interpretation of significant data and awareness of data that could be important but are missing.** The examiner should be able to integrate all significant findings and present a formulation that conveys reasonable clinical hypotheses based on supporting evidence. The formulation should include an assessment of the patient's strengths and maximal level of functioning, as well as the nature and degree of psychopathology.

   The differential diagnosis must be complete and include all pertinent symptoms and signs observed in the interview, as well as those that are reasonable to infer but were not elicited in the interview itself. The latter, of course, should be considered as hypotheses, since they were not obtained in the interview proper. **Consideration should be given to all possible diagnoses, and the examiner should be able to state the pros and cons of each.** Finally, the candidate would come to a reasonable number of working diagnoses for consideration in the treatment planning presentation.

3. **Skill in treatment planning.** The plan for treatment should be based on all data collected and those hypothesized from data missing in the interview. It would evolve from the differential diagnosis, and should consider ancillary means of data collection, such as laboratory tests, psychological tests, and professional consultations. It should include biological, psychological, and social approaches to treatment, and be **framed in a multimodal format. All possible treatment modalities should be considered, stating the relative priorities** for one modality compared with another. If there are contraindications for treatment, they should be proposed. The treatment plan should not at first be based on any particular health care delivery system, such as managed care, but should be an "ideal" treatment model regardless of constraints in the market. The interviewer, however, should be prepared to discuss later the feasibility of the proposed plan, based on limitations in the health care delivery system. Above all, each treatment modality should be passed on sound and specific therapeutic goals. Considerations of efficacy and prognosis should be discussed.

4. **Purpose and criteria for evaluation. The purpose of the clinical interview and presentation is to demonstrate that you are safe.** The age-old standard of care, "physician, do no harm," is the gold standard of the Boards. Now, what does safety entail in such an interview? The best way to think of this is to imagine that the patient you are examining comes into your emergency room or office, and you only have 30 min in which to make a reasonable assessment and plan for follow-up. Naturally, in such a short period of time with a complete stranger and without collateral sources of information, you need to be looking for the most serious problems, and understand that much important clinical and historical information will be lacking. What does such an interview require? First, one needs to **form an alliance** around the situation at hand. The relationship with the patient is the single most important element in an attempt to collect accurate historical and current symptoms. In a clinical setting, the alliance, of course, would be formed around the nature of the crisis. One would naturally attempt to develop rapport and comfort, respecting and listening to the patient. The clinician should elicit present and past data about the current illness, and make differential diagnostic hypotheses based on the data, leading on to a treatment plan. One would want to be sure that, once the patient leaves your presence, you are confident that you have a good idea of the nature of the clinical problems, that the patient is in no imminent danger,

and that your prescription for treatment and follow-up are consistent with the data collected. This lets us all sleep at night. It also is exactly what the Board examiners are looking for.

The examiners are not instructed to grill you, or to shake you up. They are, in fact, instructed to help you perform your best. This does not mean, however, that they will be warm and friendly, or nod their heads as some of your colleagues would were they to watch you perform an examination and hear your discussion. Nor will they prompt you. **They want to see that you are careful, thoughtful, and, most importantly, that your clinical reasoning is based on the data collected, and that it is logical and clinically sound.** The examiners are very interested in **the way you think—the way you organize your clinical approach, and base your clinical hypotheses on the data obtained.** They want to know that you have a logical, coherent, systematic way of organizing data, taking into account possible areas of concern that were not elicited in the interview.

5. **Focus.** Since the examiner only has 30 min and the most important issue is safety, the **primary concern is the present illness: its diagnosis, differential diagnosis, and management.** After you feel comfortable knowing the current clinical situation, then it is important to examine how it relates to the past psychiatric history, medical history, developmental, family, and social history.

6. **Preparation**

   a. **Books to review.** Although examiners are interested in your presentation being supported by a solid knowledge-base, they are not interested in psychiatric facts and figures from the literature. This was tested in the written exam, and, by virtue of passing it, you are qualified for the oral examination. The best study guide is to review the DSM-IV, and memorize the criteria from the Mini DSM-IV. In such a short interview, you will only have time to run though diagnostic criteria. Details of epidemiology, course, comorbidity, etc. are not necessary for review. It may be helpful to read the DSM-IV Casebook to see how data are put together from clinical vignettes. No other "book" study is needed.

   b. **Practice. One important reason for failing the Oral Boards is unfamiliarity with the format and too little practicing.** It is imperative to perform a number of these special interviews in front of one or two colleagues, so you can become comfortable with the time limitation of the interview, the stress of clinical presentation, and performing for an observer. It would be best to find colleagues you do not regularly work with in order to simulate the stress of evaluation by peers who are not your close professional friends. They should make the practice examinations as close to the real thing as possible: use patients unknown to you, and do not give you any feedback until after the interview and discussion.

    c. **Script.** It is essential to prepare and practice a systematic way of handling the interview, and the data for discussion. This amounts to **a model for presenting the psychiatric history, mental status examination, differential diagnosis, and treatment plan.** A script is essential because it represents an outline of clinical categories. If one has this in mind, any gaps in the interview or discussion can be readily discerned, since they will be left out of the conceptual framework. I recommend the standard medical model for history and multiaxial DSM-IV axes for discussion of differential diagnosis. We all knew the medical history by heart. This was, indeed, essential for situations such as having been up all night as an intern and having to present a number of admissions to your attending on "auto-pilot." It was not that long ago that any one of us could rattle off data such as the following: "Chief complaint: This is a 64-year-old married Caucasian female presenting with shortness of breath, three pillow orthopnea, four-plus pitting edema, and palpitations. History of present illness: #1 Cardiac: Mrs. Jones sustained her first myocardial infarction 4 years ago, having complained of progressive angina. She was brought to County General ...." I am sure that any of us in those days could produce an entire medical history, physical examination, laboratory examination, differential diagnosis, and treatment plan with our eyes closed (and sometimes we were half-asleep!). **If some data were missing from the presentation, we knew exactly where they were, because we had a script memorized,** and had practiced it ad nauseam. And, we were all questioned by the attendings on our clinical reasoning. This is exactly the mind- and skill-set needed for excellent performance in the Oral Boards. All too rarely, however, do we continue to make such presentations in psychiatric practice. But this is what is needed for the Boards.

II. The Clinical Interview

A. Doctor–Patient Relationship

As noted above, **the alliance is critical for this examination.** You will be watched for how you make a relationship with the patient from the first encounter. Establishing rapport is a crucial part of safe, effective psychiatric history-taking and care.

1. **Introduce yourself, and explain the nature of the interview,** inviting cooperation. For example, "Hello, my name is Dr. Beresin. Has anyone told you about the nature of this interview? Let me explain. I am taking a clinical examination, and these two doctors watching us are going to see how effective I am in talking with you and understanding your problems. I want to thank you for coming here today. If there is anything you do not feel comfortable talking about, please feel free to tell me, and you do not have to talk about it. We will have 30 min to talk, and at the end I will offer you a chance to ask me any questions you have."

2. **Form an alliance around the task of exploring the current illness.**

3. **Help the patient feel comfortable.** Demonstrate politeness, empathy and concern, responsiveness, and respect. Respond honestly to the patient's questions/comments. **Thank the patient for cooperating.**

4. **Maintain eye contact and avoid using medical/psychiatric jargon.** If you are used to taking notes, this is not a problem, so long as you keep good eye contact and do not look down too much.

B. Conducting the Interview

It is crucial to appreciate that no interview of this nature can be complete—some data will not be obtained. Moreover, the examiner needs to be flexible with different patients. **Remember, if questions are not asked, or data not collected, there is always an opportunity to make up for this in the presentation.**

1. **Begin, after your introduction, with open-ended questions for about 5 min.** It is valuable to see what is most important to the patient, and what his/her associations are. This may give you important clues about diagnosis and/or disposition. In addition, it gives you an opportunity to demonstrate empathic skill, respect, and concern for the patient's priorities. Furthermore, from a psychodynamic standpoint, which is still highly valued by examiners, it gives you a window into the mindset, and the cognitive and affective style of the patient. **After the initial 5 min, start to focus down on specific areas of concern and detailed questions.** For patients who ramble, or are tangential or circumstantial, gentle redirection will be needed.

2. **Focus on the primary concern, the present illness:** symptoms, precipitants, social setting and supports, current and past treatment, and complications.

3. **Listen to the patient.** Follow the patient's leads, be flexible, clarify the patient's use of terms (e.g., patient: "I was really nervous"; examiner: "What do you mean by 'nervous'"?) and deal sensitively with the patient's affective responses.

4. **Collect relevant clinical data, if possible: past psychiatric history (previous disorders, therapies, hospitalizations, medications (their benefits and adverse effects), suicide, homicide, alcohol and drug use, medical history, family history (particularly psychiatric history), development, social history (including marital history, work, and interpersonal relationships).**

5. **Never forget: suicidal and homicidal potential, alcohol and drug use.**

6. **Mental status examination.** A cornerstone of the psychiatric interview is the mental status examination. This should be a core part of the interview (but no more than 5 min), since much of the differential diagnosis will be based on history. The standard "textbook" examination is presented below (see III.A.1).

7. **Cognitive examination.** There is much controversy about whether to perform a formal cognitive examination. It is essential to perform an organized, brief assessment of cognition, such as one outlined below. A more formal, quantifiable examination, such as the **Mini-Mental State Examination,** is highly desirable. This type of highly structured examination **should be performed if there is suspicion of organicity or psychosis, with or without depression.** The Mini-Mental State Exam is outlined in Fig. 2-1. It is brief, efficient, and quantifiable. If a formal cognitive examination is not performed, be able to say why it was not necessary; for example, "I did not perform a formal, quantifiable cognitive examination such as the Mini-Mental State Exam, because the patient was lucid, well oriented, and in his/her normal discussion there was no evidence of a thought disorder, memory, attention, or concentration defect, or impaired judgment." When in doubt, perform the examination.

8. **Always close by asking the patient if he/she has any questions and thanking the patient.**

III. The Case Presentation

A. Format

Begin with a formal, concise, medical presentation, including the categories below. If you don't have data in a particular category, mention it and the material you would have obtained if you had had time. This gives the examiners the important information that you know what data you need in each relevant area.

1. **History and mental status examination**
   a. Chief complaint/identifying data
   b. History of present illness
   c. Past psychiatric history
   d. Past medical history
   e. Family history
   f. Developmental history
   g. Social history
   h. Mental status examination
      i. General appearance and behavior
      ii. Speech
      iii. Affect
      iv. Mood
      v. Perception

vi. Cognition (or Mini-Mental State Examination; Fig. 2-1)
- Level of consciousness
- Orientation
- Attention and concentration
- Memory: recent and remote
- General information
- Calculation
- Abstraction
- Judgment
- Insight

2. **Formulation and differential diagnosis**
3. **Treatment plan**
4. **Prognosis**

B. Presenting the Differential Diagnosis

This is one of the most challenging parts of the presentation. The following are a few tips for a coherent, inclusive biopsychosocial case discussion.

1. **Begin with the descriptive signs and symptoms.** Build your diagnostic possibilities around constellations of specific symptoms. In other words, move from the specific to the generic. Begin with the most likely possibilities and consider the pros and cons of all other possible psychiatric conditions. **It is crucial to mention all categories, even the very unlikely ones.** A core concept for this exam is the following: if you do not mention a diagnostic or treatment category, the examiners must assume that you do not know it exists. Thus it is imperative to **be overinclusive.** I would mention ALL diagnostic categories in each of the DSM-IV Axes, even if some are clearly out of the question.

2. **Use the multiaxial framework as your script for the discussion.**

3. **Always run through the major Axis I diagnoses,** ruling in or out major illnesses, such as schizophrenia, mood disorders, substance-related disorders, anxiety disorders, including each of the subcategories of disorders within each of the major classes. This is best thought of as the "psychiatric biological axis."

4. **Use Axis II to discuss personality traits or disorders and include here a psychodynamic formulation.** Despite our reliance on DSM-IV for psychiatric nosology, good clinical care requires an understanding of the inner world of the patient. Surely, in a 30-min interview, one can hardly make a personality disorder diagnosis, or fully understand the complexity of intrapsychic structure. However, this is a place to discuss your hypotheses on common defense mechanisms, personality trait disturbances, and possible intrapsychic conflicts, all of which may be important in treatment planning and prognosis.

5. **Use Axis III to consider possible medical illness** which may be related as causes or complicating

MINI-MENTAL STATE EXAM

Mean Scores

Dementia	9.7
Depression with impaired cognition	19.0
Uncomplicated depression	25.1
Normals	27.6

Maximum Score	Score	
		Orientation
5	( )	What is the (year) (season) (date) (day) (month)?
5	( )	Where are we (state) (county) (town) (hospital) (floor)?
		Registration
3	( )	Name 3 objects: 1 second to say each. Then ask the patient all 3 after you have said them. Give 1 point for each correct answer. Then repeat them until he/she learns all 3. Count trials and record.
		TRIALS_____
		Attention and Calculation
5	( )	Serial 7s: 1 point for each correct. Stop after 5 answers. Alternatively spell "world" backwards.
		Recall
3	( )	Ask for 3 objects repeated above. Give 1 point for each correct answer.
		Language
2	( )	Name a pencil and watch. (2 points)
1	( )	Repeat the following: "no ifs, ands or buts." (1 point)
3	( )	Follow a 3-stage command: "Take a paper in your right hand, fold it in half, and put it on the floor." (3 points)
1	( )	Read and obey the following: "Close your eyes." (1 point)
1	( )	Write a sentence. Must contain a subject and a verb and be sensible. (1 point)
		Visual-Motor Integrity
1	( )	Copy design (2 intersecting pentagons. All 10 angles must be present and 2 must intersect). (1 point)

Total Score: _____

Assess level of consciousness along a continuum:

Alert	Drowsy	Stupor	Coma

Fig. 2-1. Mini-Mental State Exam. (Adapted from Folstein MF, Folstein SE, McHugh PE: Mini-mental method for grading the cognitive state of patients for the clinician. *J Psychiatr Res* 1975; 12: 189–198. Copyright 1975, Pergamon Press Ltd.)

entities in the clinical picture. **Drug–drug interactions,** allergies, and other medical issues should also be raised here.

6. **Use Axis IV to discuss the social/environmental and cultural dimension,** such as nature of object relations, impact of ethnicity and cultural heritage, sources of precipitants, supports, and life stressors.

7. **Global assessment of functioning (GAF).** It is always useful to attempt to rate an approximate GAF currently and possible highest in the past.

8. **The key to the discussion.** Let the examiners know you have an organized way of **moving from the specific clinical data through the various diagnostic possibilities,** and that you take into account and integrate the biological, psychological, and social/environmental/cultural components of psychiatric health and illness.

9. **An important concept to keep in mind: making the "right" diagnosis is not as crucial as having a systematic approach to obtaining it.** It is always valu-

able to indicate your omissions; e.g. "I would have liked to explore this area further, if I had more time," or "I didn't ask about ..., and this may have helped establish a ... diagnosis."

C. Treatment Plan

Be sure the treatment plan includes multimodal components. Remember that each modality has multiple specific components, and each should be mentioned, even if not appropriate for the case at hand. Start with ancillary procedures that may be necessary either for clarifying the diagnosis or as helping in the treatment process:

1. **Laboratory and ancillary procedures**
   a. Clinical laboratory examination: e.g., CBC (complete blood count), LFTs (liver function tests), EKG (electrocardiogram), BUN (blood urea nitrogen), TFTs (thyroid function tests).
   b. Neuroimaging studies
   c. EEG (electroencephalogram)
   d. Psychological testing: cognitive and projective tests
2. **Biological therapies**
   a. Pharmacotherapy. Include all classes of drug treatment, even if certain agents are not appropriate for the clinical situation. State these as inappropriate and give reasons.
   b. ECT (electroconvulsive therapy)
3. **Psychotherapies.** These should include long- and short-term therapies, depending on the case. Possible categories to include are:
   a. Individual psychodynamic (specify type if possible: e.g., classical, ego psychological, object relations, self-psychology)
   b. Individual supportive
   c. Couples
   d. Family (specify type, if possible: e.g., structural, strategic, systemic, problem-solving)
   e. Cognitive and cognitive-behavioral therapy (specify type, as above: e.g., operant conditioning, dialectical behavior therapy)
   f. Group (homogeneous, heterogeneous, and specify model if possible)
   g. Interpersonal psychotherapy
   h. Relaxation techniques
   i. Hypnosis
   j. Biofeedback
   k. Other miscellaneous therapies as needed: e.g., 12-step programs, psychoeducational groups
4. **Hospital-based treatment**
   a. Inpatient: acute, subacute, chronic
   b. Partial hospital
   c. Residential: e.g., group homes, half-way houses

D. Helpful Tips on the Presentation and Discussion

1. **Interruptions and questions.** Remember to keep your scripts in mind for the history and differential diagnosis. Begin with your formal presentation, as indicated above. The examiners will, at times, interrupt you to ask questions. Do not assume that you have done anything wrong, or that they are questioning your reasoning. There are many reasons examiners ask questions. It is not up to you to figure them out. Try not to get rattled by interruptions. It is most useful to respond to an examiner's questions, then continue where you left off with your scripted presentation (again, a structured script is very reassuring in such situations, particularly if you are answering a difficult question). It is vital first to **demonstrate that you know the basics about psychiatric diagnosis and treatment.** Then, if time permits, and if you see from the nature of their questions that the examiners wish to go into greater depth, you can discuss the fine points, controversial issues, or current research data. For the most part, such detail is beyond the scope, goals, and objectives of this examination.

   If you do not know the answer to a question, do not attempt to guess. Such a response is an indicator that you are not safe. It is important to be comfortable saying: **"I don't know the answer to that question, but I would get assistance by** asking an expert colleague, looking up the topic in ... journal or ... textbook." Making references to specific journals, articles, or texts is useful here. Remember, the examiners do not expect you to know everything, and the hallmark of a safe physician is knowing where to get information and appropriate consultation quickly.

2. **Coping with anxiety.** It is useful in your practice exams to **know what makes you anxious:** which types of patients, which countertransference responses, what kinds of questions from examiners, etc. Once you discern the factors that heighten your anxiety, **practice a desensitization approach,** by making yourself face such situations before the Boards. For example, if you have problems with rambling, tangential patients, who give you vague, spotty clinical data, find as many as possible such patients to interview ahead of time. Beyond desensitization, there are other techniques to reduce anxiety. Deep breathing before the exam or talking to yourself to calm down are useful examples. For some, note-taking in a scripted format helps. For example, dividing your pad into three vertical sections—one for obtained clinical data, one for missing data, and one for diagnostic categories—may help. The most important form of self-reassurance is knowing that you have done many other exams successfully and that you know what works well for you.

   It is not usually a good idea to medicate yourself for such exams in advance unless this has been done repeatedly with success. There are individuals who do better with a tad of propranolol if they tend to develop a peripheral tremor when anxious, or those who use a small dose of lorazepam before testing. However, these methods are, for the most part, unnecessary, and could impair your cognition under stress.

An important method of reducing anxiety is keeping good track of your time. Too often, under pressure, an examinee loses a sense of time and, on hearing there are only 5 min left, needs to do a cognitive examination as well as cover a number of specific questions for one or more diagnostic categories.

3. **Monitor your style under stress.** Each of us has coping mechanisms under pressure. Be sure to appreciate the ways you tend to react to stressful situations. Some examinees become **argumentative, flip or joking, or noncommittal and vague** under examination situations. Practice examinations are the best way to determine how you tend to respond under such conditions. There are rare situations when you disagree with an examiner, or when you know the literature on a particular topic in depth, and could get into a controversial discussion or argument with the examiner. This, of course, is not in your best interests, even if you know you are right. It is best to **avoid power struggles** and proceed with conventional clinical wisdom, avoiding the controversies. An excellent example comes from my own experience taking the Child Boards. I

was discussing the treatment of a young adolescent with a tricyclic antidepressant, and the examiner asked me what I could do in the office, in the absence of a laboratory, to determine if the boy were toxic. I knew he was looking for taking the pulse and orthostatic blood pressure, but I knew there is not necessarily a correlation between anticholinergic adverse effects and blood levels of the drug. I answered that I would take the pulse and blood pressure. This, is, in fact, good clinical practice, and I would do it in my office. However, if I wanted to know if the child was in the toxic range, I would need a blood test and would like an EKG as well. I did not push the issue. It is typically the case that, when an examinee is asked about highly specific or controversial issues, it is a good indication of having passed.

Suggested Readings

Kaplan HI, Sadock BJ: Psychiatric report. In Kaplan HI, Sadock BJ (eds): *Comprehensive Textbook of Psychiatry*, 6th ed. Baltimore: Williams & Wilkins, 1995:531–535.

Silberman SE: Psychiatric interview: settings and techniques. In Tasman A, Kay J, Lieberman JA (eds): *Psychiatry*. Philadelphia: WB Saunders, 1997:19–34.

Strauss GD: The psychiatric interview, history and mental status examination. In Kaplan HI, Sadock BJ (eds): *Comprehensive Textbook of Psychiatry*, 6th ed. Baltimore: Williams & Wilkins, 1995:521–531.

SECTION II

Approach to Psychiatric Diagnosis and Psychiatric Conditions

Chapter 3

The DSM-IV: A Multiaxial System for Psychiatric Diagnosis

M. ELYCE KEARNS

I. Introduction

The *Diagnostic and Statistical Manual of Mental Disorders, Fourth Edition* (**DSM-IV**), published in 1994, is **the official classification system of psychiatric conditions currently in use in the United States.** All mental health professionals use this as a common means for communicating about the more than 300 specific disorders that have been characterized.

DSM-IV diagnostic criteria are used to facilitate communication among mental health and health care professionals, as a common standard for research criteria, and to communicate with third-party payors.

According to the DSM-IV, a **mental disorder is a disorder with significant behavioral or psychological symptoms** associated with present distress (e.g., pain), disability (i.e., impairment in one or more area of function), or with an increased risk of suffering death, pain, disability, or an important loss of freedom. The condition must not be merely an expectable and culturally sanctioned response to a particular event (e.g., the death of a loved one). Independent of its cause, it must be a manifestation of a behavioral, psychological, or biological dysfunction (American Psychiatric Association [APA], 1994, p. xxi).

II. Overview

The **DSM-IV is a descriptive classification system** that presents the clinical features that must be present for the diagnosis of a disorder. It does not address etiology or treatment related to disorders. Criteria have been made specific to increase the reliability of a diagnosis among clinicians (Sadock and Kaplan, 1995). **There are 16 major diagnostic classes and an additional section: "Other Conditions that May Be a Focus of Clinical Attention"** (Table 3-1). The diagnostic classes are listed in order of their priority in differential diagnosis, reflecting the hierarchical nature of the classification system.

The DSM-IV allows multiple diagnoses to be given to an individual who presents with symptoms that meet criteria for more than one disorder. In several situations the differential diagnosis is aided by exclusion criteria:

A. **When a Mental Disorder due to a General Medical Condition or a Substance-Induced Disorder is responsible for the symptoms,** it pre-empts the diagnosis of the corresponding primary disorder with the same symptoms.

B. **When a more pervasive disorder** (e.g., schizophrenia) **has among its defining symptoms** (or associated symptoms) **the defining symptoms of a less pervasive disorder** (e.g., Dysthymic Disorder), **only the more pervasive disorder is diagnosed.**

C. **When there are particularly difficult differential diagnostic boundaries, the phrase "not better accounted for by ..." is included, to indicate that clinical judgment is necessary to determine which diagnosis is most appropriate.** In some cases both diagnoses may be appropriate (APA, 1994, p. 6).

III. The DSM Revision Process

The three-stage revision process from the *Diagnostic and Statistical Manual, Third Edition-Revised* (DSM-III-R) to DSM-IV included: comprehensive and systematic reviews of the published literature, a reanalysis of already-collected data, and extensive issue-focused field trials (APA, 1994, p. xviii).

The United States is under treaty obligation to maintain a terminology that is compatible with the disease classification, International Classification of Disease (ICD), that is used by the World Health Organization (WHO). ICD is in its tenth revision. Although ICD-9 remains in general use currently, the transition to ICD-10 is expected within the next several years. It includes a section of psychiatric diagnoses, "Mental and Behavioral Disorders," which correlate with those in the DSM-IV. Drafts of ICD-10 were reviewed by the DSM work-groups during the process of revision. The outcome was a diagnostic system in use in the United States that has terms and codes compatible with those accepted internationally.

Table 3-1. Other Conditions that May Be a Focus of Clinical Attention

- Psychological Factors Affecting Medical Condition
- Medication-Induced Movement Disorders
- Adverse Effects of Medication not Otherwise Specified
- Relational Problems
- Problems Related to Abuse or Neglect
- Additional Conditions that May Be a Focus of Clinical Attention

---

Several other countries (including China, Japan, and Cuba) are adapting the ICD-10 classification system to their own independent psychiatric classifications (Mezzich, 1995). **DSM-IV also includes an Appendix that addresses cultural formulations and culture-bound syndromes.**

IV. Differences Between the DSM and the ICD

Unlike the DSM, the ICD is a system used worldwide by clinicians in all medical disciplines and specialties to communicate about the characteristics of various disorders. This includes a common mode of diagnosis of mental disorders in which language, culture, and the approach to treatment may vary significantly from one area to another. The ICD system has some diagnoses that account for comorbidity (e.g., depressive conduct disorder), unlike the DSM, in which all diagnoses are separate and comorbidity is accounted for by listing co-occurring disorders separately on each axis (Schwab-Stone and Hart, 1996).

Some terminology has changed in the DSM-IV. The diagnosis of organic mental disorder and the terms "neurasthenia," "psychogenic," and "neurosis" have been eliminated from DSM-IV but remain in some form in the ICD-10. The ICD-10 does not use the term "bipolar II" (Sadock and Kaplan, 1995, p. 691).

ICD-10 uses a three-axis system: Axis I—Clinical Diagnoses; Axis II—Disablements; and Axis III—Contextual Factors. Appendix H in DSM-IV lists the ICD-10 codes that coincide with the DSM-IV diagnoses.

V. The Five Axes

Multiple diagnoses may be present on Axes I, II, and III.

A. **Axis I includes clinical disorders and "Other Conditions that May Be a Focus of Clinical Attention"** (see Table 3-2). There are codes that signify that there is either no diagnosis or that diagnosis is deferred on Axis I until further information is obtained.

B. **Axis II includes personality disorders and mental retardation.** If the principal diagnosis or reason for visit is a diagnosis coded on Axis II, the diagnosis should be labeled as such (see Table 3-3).

C. **Axis III includes general medical conditions** that are outside the "Mental and Behavioral Disorders" chapter of ICD. These diagnoses may have some bearing on the understanding and treatment of an individual's psychiatric condition. If a general medical condition is causing or is related to a psychiatric diagnosis, the diagnosis on Axis I may be "Mental Disorder NOS Due to ..." for which

---

Table 3-2. Axis I: Clinical Disorders: Other Conditions that May Be a Focus of Clinical Attention

- Disorders usually first diagnosed in infancy, childhood, or adolescence (*excluding Mental Retardation, which is diagnosed on Axis II*)
- Delirium, Dementia, and Amnestic and Other Cognitive Disorders
- Mental Disorders due to a General Medical Condition
- Substance-Related Disorders
- Schizophrenia and Other Psychotic Disorders
- Mood Disorders
- Anxiety Disorders
- Somatoform Disorders
- Factitious Disorders
- Dissociative Disorders
- Sexual and Gender Identity Disorders
- Eating Disorders
- Sleep Disorders
- Impulse-Control Disorders not Elsewhere Classified
- Adjustment Disorders
- Other Conditions that may Be a Focus of Clinical Attention

SOURCE: DSM-IV, p. 26.

Table 3-3. Axis II: Personality Disorders and Mental Retardation

- Paranoid Personality Disorder
- Schizoid Personality Disorder
- Schizotypal Personality Disorder
- Antisocial Personality Disorder
- Borderline Personality Disorder
- Histrionic Personality Disorder
- Narcissistic Personality Disorder
- Avoidant Personality Disorder
- Dependent Personality Disorder
- Obsessive-compulsive Personality Disorder
- Personality Disorder Not Otherwise Specified
- Mental Retardation

SOURCE: DSM-IV, p. 27.

---

the medical condition is listed on both Axis I and Axis III (see Table 3-4).

D. **Axis IV describes the psychosocial and environmental problems experienced by the individual.** These may

Table 3-4. Axis III: General Medical Conditions (with ICD-9-CM Codes)

- Infectious and Parasitic Diseases (001–139)
- Neoplasms (140–239)
- Endocrine, Nutritional, and Metabolic Diseases and Immunity Disorders (240–279)
- Diseases of the Blood and Blood-Forming Organs (280–289)
- Diseases of the Nervous System and Sense Organs (320–389)
- Diseases of the Circulatory System (390–459)
- Diseases of the Respiratory System (460–519)
- Diseases of the Digestive System (520–579)
- Diseases of the Genitourinary System (580–629)
- Complications of Pregnancy, Childbirth, and the Puerperium (630–676)
- Diseases of the Skin and Subcutaneous Tissue (680–709)
- Diseases of the Musculoskeletal System and Connective Tissue (710–739)
- Congenital Abnormalities (740–759)
- Certain Conditions Originating in the Perinatal Period (760–779)
- Symptoms, Signs, and Ill-Defined Conditions (780–799)
- Injury and Poisoning (800–999)

SOURCE: DSM-IV, p. 28.

Table 3-5. Axis IV: Psychosocial and Environmental Problems

- Problems with primary support group
- Problems related to the social environment
- Educational problems
- Occupational problems
- Housing problems
- Economic problems
- Problems with access to health care services
- Problems related to interaction with the legal system/ crime
- Other psychosocial and environmental problems

affect the diagnosis, treatment, and prognosis of mental disorders (APA, 1994, p. 29). Typically, factors have been present during the preceding year. Multiple factors may be recorded (see Table 3-5).

E. Axis V involves the numerical assignment of a rank of global assessment of functioning of the individual considering only psychological, social, and occupational function (APA, 1994, p. 30). It is based on a 100-point scale.

VI. Diagnostic Codes

Every diagnosis on Axes I, II, and III has its own distinct numerical code. The codes used in DSM-IV are compatible with those used in ICD-10. Codes are used for medical record-keeping, data collection, and reporting data and research activities.

In addition to the main code given to each diagnosis, **the subtypes of the diagnosis or specifiers as described in the narrative descriptions in DSM-IV are also coded, usually in the first two decimal positions.** This allows increased specificity of the diagnosis.

Subtypes are mutually exclusive. **Specifiers** do not designate mutually exclusive subgroupings. They provide an opportunity to define a more homogeneous subgrouping of individuals with the disorder (APA, 1994, p. 1).

VII. Specifiers

Specific criteria are noted for certain diagnoses in DSM-IV.

A. Severity. Level is based on number of symptoms and functioning.
1. **Mild.** Few, if any, symptoms are present in excess of those required for diagnosis. There is no more than minor impairment in functioning.
2. **Moderate.** Intermediate between mild and severe in terms of symptom presence and impairment of function.
3. **Severe.** Many symptoms in excess of those required for diagnosis or several very severe symptoms are present, or there is marked impairment in functioning.

B. Course
1. **In partial remission.** The individual previously met full criteria for diagnosis and currently has some signs or symptoms.
2. **In full remission.** No signs or symptoms of the disorder remain, but the record should indicate that the disorder was present in the past.
3. **Prior history.** The person is considered to be recovered from the disorder.

C. Principal diagnosis. The disorder was established, after evaluation, to be mainly responsible for the entrance into treatment.

D. Provisional diagnosis. There is "strong presumption" that the person will meet the full criteria for a disorder, but information is currently inadequate.

E. Not otherwise specified (NOS). These terms are used to account for diversity in clinical presentation when the more specific diagnoses do not fit. Each diagnostic category has designated at least one NOS diagnosis.

VIII. Exclusion Criteria and Differential Diagnosis

In addition to listing the criteria that must be met for the diagnosis of a certain disorder, DSM-IV specifies that other disorders should be considered during the diagnostic process. Due to the existence of comorbid conditions and the desirability to establish a differential diagnosis and distinguish the boundaries of diagnoses when symptoms overlap, **the following qualifiers are used.** They serve to clarify when multiple diagnoses should be used.

A. **"Criteria have never been met for ..."**: defines a lifetime hierarchy.

B. **"Criteria are not met for ..."**: defines a cross-sectional hierarchy.

C. **"Does not occur exclusively during the course of ..."**: used to assure that the criteria for the disorder are not met only during the course of another disorder.

D. **"Not due to the direct physiological effects of a substance (e.g., a drug of abuse, a medication) or a general medical condition."** Any condition that is substance-induced or etiologically related to a general medical condition must be ruled out before the disorder can be diagnosed.

E. **"Not better accounted for by ...."** The process of differential diagnosis should include the other disorders mentioned in the criteria, and clinical judgment should be used in differentiating diagnoses that occur on the border (APA, 1994, pp. 5–6).

IX. Areas Addressed in Descriptions of DSM-IV Diagnoses

Topics addressed include:

A. **Diagnostic features**

B. **Subtypes and/or specifiers**

C. **Recording procedures**

D. **Associated features and disorders**
   1. Associated descriptive features and mental disorders
   2. Associated laboratory findings
   3. Associated physical examination findings and general medical conditions

E. **Specific culture, age, and gender features**

F. **Prevalence**

G. **Course**
   1. Age at onset
   2. Mode of onset
   3. Episodic versus continuous course
   4. Single episode versus recurrent

   5. Duration
   6. Progression

H. **Familial pattern**

I. **Differential diagnosis**

X. Algorithms

The DSM-IV has algorithms that were developed to assist clinicians in the process of identifying the presenting symptoms and considering how those symptoms may be reflective of a psychiatric diagnosis. **They aim to guide the clinician's thinking during the decision process for making a differential diagnosis.** The six areas for which they were developed are: Mental Disorders Due to a General Medical Condition; Substance-induced Disorders; Psychotic Disorders; Mood Disorders; Anxiety Disorders; and Somatoform Disorders.

XI. Conclusion

The purpose of the DSM-IV is to enhance communication among mental health clinicians and those who keep track of these disorders on an individual or population-wide basis. In addition, it is used to clarify the thought and decision-making processes about diagnosis when a clinician is faced with an individual presenting with any number of seemingly related or unrelated symptoms. **Keep in mind that symptoms and disorders are classified, not the individual. The DSM-IV does not minimize the importance of clinical judgment.**

Suggested Readings

American Psychiatric Association (APA): *Diagnostic and Statistical Manual of Mental Disorders, Fourth Edition.* Washington, DC: APA, 1994.

Cooper J: On the publication of the *Diagnostic and Statistical Manual of Mental Disorders*: Fourth Edition (DSM-IV). *Br J Psychiatry* 1995; 166:4–8.

Frances AJ, Widiger TA, Pincus HA: The development of DSM-IV. *Arch Gen Psychiatry* 1989; 46:373–375.

Mezzich JE: International perspectives on psychiatric diagnosis. In Kaplan HI, Sadock BJ (eds): *Comprehensive Textbook of Psychiatry*, 6th ed. Baltimore: Williams and Wilkins, 1995:692–703.

Sadock, BJ, Kaplan, HI: Classification of mental disorders. In Kaplan HI and Sadock BJ (eds): *Comprehensive Textbook of Psychiatry*, 6th ed. Baltimore: Williams and Wilkins, 1995:671–692.

Schwab-Stone ME, Hart EL: Systems of psychiatric classification: DSM-IV and ICD-10. In Lewis ML (ed.): *Child and Adolescent Psychiatry: A Comprehensive Textbook*, 2nd ed. Baltimore: Williams and Wilkins, 1996:423–430.

Volkmar FR: Classification in child and adolescent psychiatry: principles and issues. In Lewis ML (ed.): *Child and Adolescent Psychiatry: A Comprehensive Textbook*, 2nd ed. Baltimore: Williams and Wilkins, 1996:417–422.

Chapter 4

Child and Adolescent Development

Annah Abrams and Paula Rauch

I. Introduction

This chapter outlines the normal development of a child, which occurs along a continuum. **Each age group is associated with physical, social, sexual, and cognitive changes.** Pediatricians and child psychiatrists use developmental screening tests to measure (monitor) the developmental tasks a child should achieve by a given age. **Developmental milestones as might appear in a screening test are outlined in Table 4-1.** Theories of child development describe and explain the social, sexual, and cognitive changes that occur for the child. The most often cited theorists in child development include Sigmund Freud, Erik Erikson, and Jean Piaget, who are discussed here. **Table 4-2 gives an overview of each theorist's approach to the development of the child.**

II. Infancy

Infancy begins at birth and lasts until the child is verbal (age 2+ years). During this phase the major emotional milestone is attachment. Attachment is the connection that develops between the infant and the primary caretaker. Bowlby and Mahler are key theorists who **describe the stages of attachment and separation.** Multiple developmental milestones in social, motor, and language skills are met (see Table 4-1).

III. Preschool (ages 2½ to 6 years)

Important aspects of the child's emotional and cognitive development during the preschool phase include egocentricity, magical thinking, and body image anxiety.

A. **Egocentricity** is the child's perception that all life events revolve around him.

B. **Magical thinking** is the creative weaving of reality and fantasy to explain how things occur in the world (**associative logic**).

C. **Body image anxiety** is a result of the child's immature sense of body integrity. The preschooler feels that his whole body is vulnerable when any body part is injured (e.g., my arm is broken, therefore I am broken).

IV. School Age/Latency (ages 6–12 years)

Latency is the **phase of development that is characterized by mastery of skills.** Children are gaining skills in many areas: academic, athletic, artistic, and social. **School and peer groups play a fundamental role** for the child. **Status**

Table 4-1. Developmental Milestones that Might be Used in Screening Tests

Age	Social	Gross motor	Fine motor	Language
6 weeks	Social smile		Follows past midline	Responds to bell
2 months	Recognizes mother	Sits with head steady	Reaches for object	
4 months		Rolls over	Holds a rattle	Coos
6 months		Sits alone	Passes cube hand to hand	Laughs
8–10 months	Stranger anxiety	Stands	Thumb-finger grasp	Dada/mama nonspecific
	Plays peek-a-boo	Creeps		
12 months	Drinks from a cup	Walks		Dada/mama specific
14–18 months	Imitates housework	Throws ball overhand	Four-cube tower	Combines two different words
24 months	Plays interactive games	Rides a tricycle	Eight-cube tower	Knows 50+ words
3 years			Copy a '0'	Gives first and last name
4 years	Dresses with supervision	Hops on one foot	Copy a '+'	Recognizes colors
			Draws man in three parts	
5 years	Dresses alone		Copies a square	

Table 4-2. Theorists' Approach to Child Development

	Cognitive Stages—Piaget	Psychosocial Stages—Erikson	Psychosexual Stages—Freud
Birth to 12 months	Sensorimotor stage	Trust vs. mistrust	Oral
1–2 years		Autonomy vs. shame Doubt	Anal
3–5 years	Preoperational thought	Initiative vs. guilt	Phallic
6–10 years	Concrete operations	Industry vs. inferiority	Latency
11–18 years	Formal operations	Identity vs. role confusion	Adolescence

within the peer group depends on a child's abilities and how they compare with those of his/her peers. During this phase **children develop best friends.** Cognitively, the child is **able to use logical thinking (causal logic)** and appreciate another person's point of view. **The disorders that present during this phase are often related to school performance and peer relationships.**

V. Adolescence (ages 12–18 years)

The emphasis during adolescence **is on autonomy and sexuality.** The adolescent is **struggling to create a sense of identity that is separate from his or her parents.** His/her **emerging identity relies on the peer group** to determine what is "in" and what is "out." **Attractiveness is a key component of self-esteem.** There is tremendous self-consciousness, heightened by the range of maturation at any given age. Adolescents are reaching new levels both cognitively and emotionally. At this stage they are **capable of abstract thinking.**

VI. Theories of Development

A. Bowlby's Attachment Theory

1. **John Bowlby: attachment theory is a reciprocal process of bonding that is based on the care and the relationship that develop between the infant and his primary caregiver.** Attachment is the observable behavior of an infant responding to his caregiver. The infant at 6–8 weeks of age smiles in recognition of the mother and imprints the mother's face as the person to whom he will turn. A mutual connection and admiration has formed between the infant and the mother (caretaker). **The result of this attachment behavior is an infant who feels and is protected by his mother.** Bowlby asserts that attachment evolved to protect helpless infants from potential predators. **The three stages of mother-infant separation are:**
   a. Protest: the infant is separated from the caregiver and cries or calls out.

   b. Despair: the infant gives up hope that the mother will return.

   c. Detachment: the infant has emotionally separated himself from the mother.

2. **Mary Ainsworth created a model to determine the quality and strength of the attachment between the infant and the mother.** The **stranger situation was developed** to observe the infant in increasingly stressful situations. This **seven-step process** follows a sequence of the infant and the mother being together in a room→a stranger enters the room →the mother leaves the room→the infant is left alone with the stranger→the mother returns and the process is repeated. Through these observations, **Ainsworth concluded** that **more than 60% of infants have secure attachments by the age of 24 months.**

B. Mahler's Separation-Individuation Process

Margaret Mahler described the **separation-individuation process** that **occurs between a mother and a child.** This theory is based on behavioral observations. Mahler describes the **first phase as symbiosis (birth to 5 months),** during which the infant does not differentiate from the mother. The **separation-individuation process begins at approximately 5 months of age and follows four stages through the first 3 years of life.**

1. **Differentiation** (5–10 months)
   a. Physical movement away from the mother begins to occur.

   b. The infant begins to explore through play with his/her own body.

   c. Stranger anxiety develops.

2. **Practicing** (10–15 months)
   a. The infant gains physical distance through walking.

   b. Greater exploration occurs.

   c. Separation anxiety occurs.

3. **Rapprochement** (18–24 months)
   a. Self-awareness begins to develop. This increased self-awareness leads to anxiety and conflict.

b. The child wants to stay close to the mother, but also wants to explore.

4. **Consolidation and object constancy** (24–36 months)

a. The child is able to maintain an internal representation of the mother.

b. The child tolerates separations from his mother, knowing that they will be reunited.

C. **Freud's Psychosexual Model of Development**

Sigmund Freud outlined the psychosexual development of the child from a psychoanalytic perspective. According to Freud, **the sexual goal of each stage is to derive pleasure and to relieve pain.** Accordingly, the infant is first soothed by the mother's breast and derives satisfaction orally; hence the first stage is the oral stage. **Freud's psychosexual stages are based on the child's development of sexual drives, body maturation, and nervous system development.**

1. **Oral phase** (birth to 1 year). The infant's urges are focused on feeding and sucking at the breast. This is the source of all the infant's satisfaction and frustration.

2. **Anal phase** (1–3 years). The child's urges are centered on bowel functioning. His/her ability to have control over his/her bodily functions becomes the main issue in the relationship between the child and the caregiver.

3. **Phallic (genital) phase** (3–5 years). The genitals become the child's focus for pleasure and satisfaction. Masturbation is used as a way of releasing tension and leads to anxiety and guilt.

a. **Oedipal complex.** The child falls in love with the parent of the opposite sex. The child wants to have exclusive possession of the parent and wants to eliminate the other parent.

b. **Castration anxiety.** The boy fears that his father will cut off his penis in retaliation for the boy's coveting his mother. This anxiety leads to repression of the sexual desire for the mother.

c. **Penis envy.** A girl's curiosity and desire to have a penis.

d. **Resolution of the Oedipal complex.** The child identifies with the same sex parent and begins to form relationships with same sex peers.

4. **Latency** (6–11 years). Sexual development during this phase is relatively stagnant.

5. **Adolescence** (12–18 years). Genital sexuality develops and proceeds into adulthood.

D. **Erikson's Epigenetic Model of Development**

Erik Erikson presents an **epigenetic model of development from birth to old age.** The epigenetic principle holds that the **eight stages of the life cycle are sequential, each stage relying on the next.** For successful development, a person must complete one stage before moving on to the next stage. If a stage is not completed, the unresolved issues continue to arise and create problems in the subsequent stages. **Each stage addresses cognitive, ego, sexual, social, and societal issues,** and offers positive and negative adaptations. Erikson also emphasizes the importance of adaptation to society.

1. **Basic trust vs. basic mistrust** (birth to 1 year)

a. A sense of basic trust is derived from the attachment that forms between the child and the parent who provides consistent care.

b. Mistrust develops when the child is unable to rely on his or her parent for basic care, which leads to feelings of emptiness and despair.

2. **Autonomy vs. shame and doubt** (1–3 years)

a. The child's sense of self is in part based on his or her ability to control his/her bodily functions (e.g., anal sphincter control).

b. The child is able to explore and briefly separate from the parent without significant distress. The trust developed during the first stage gives the child the freedom to explore.

c. Shame and doubt develop when the child is required to perform, but is unable.

3. **Initiative vs. guilt** (3–6 years)

a. The child takes steps towards establishing a special relationship with the parent of the same sex.

b. Fantasy allows the child to feel both the pleasure and the pride of being powerful and the guilt of having the imagined power to do harm to others.

4. **Industry vs. inferiority** (6–12 years)

a. This stage corresponds to entering school. The main tasks for the child are ones of learning and doing.

b. The child strives for a sense of accomplishment and develops a sense of mastery and control of his environment (i.e., school), avoiding failure at all costs.

c. Feelings of inferiority develop when the child is unable to master all tasks.

d. The child begins to understand that his family is a part of a larger society. Parents are no longer perceived as the only authorities.

5. **Identity vs. role confusion** (12–20 years)

a. Adolescence is a phase of development that combines the potential for significant growth and crisis. Adolescents are at a fragile point of finding themselves at the same time as losing themselves.

b. Multiple physical and social changes occur.

c. Normative crises may evolve into disruptive and pathological behavior, but are not inherently maladaptive.

d. Adolescents must identify within themselves and with the society at large.

6. **Intimacy vs. isolation** (20–40 years)

a. The establishment of a stable love relationship requires that a person have a reasonable sense of self/personal identity.

b. The fear of intimacy may lead one to choose isolation.

c. The mature individual chooses the vulnerable position of intimacy over the loneliness of isolation.

d. These adaptations also extend into one's career aspirations.

7. **Generativity vs. stagnation** (40–65 years)

a. Adults can be generative through child rearing and mentoring in the community, passing along to the next generation what they have learned and achieved.

b. Stagnation occurs when the adult is unable to give to others and remains isolated and self-involved.

8. **Ego integrity vs. despair** (65 years and older)

a. Integrity develops for a person who feels that they have led a fulfilled life and are content with their place in the life cycle.

b. Despair occurs for those who feel that life had no meaning. Death becomes a feared end to an unfulfilled life.

E. **Piaget's Model of Cognitive Development**
Jean Piaget focused on **the cognitive development of the child.** In this model the child follows a continuous pattern of behavior of adapting and responding to the various stimuli in the environment. Piaget describes this behavior as **a schema, a pattern or loop of behavior: stimulus-response-awareness.** The development of the child's cognitive abilities is categorized in **four stages:**

1. **Sensorimotor stage** (birth through 18–24 months)

a. The senses receive a stimulus and the body reacts to it in a stereotyped way.

b. **Object permanency** develops during the second year. The child is able to maintain a mental image of the object. The child will look for a toy where it disappeared.

2. **Preoperational thought—prelogical** (2–6 years)

a. **Symbolic functions develop.**

b. Language development changes the child's ability to interact.

c. **Egocentric thinking** (i.e., the perception that everything revolves around them) occurs. Minimal objectivity is involved.

d. **Magical thinking,** in which reality and fantasy are interwoven to explain the world around them, arises. Unable to use a logical process to explain how and why they know what they know.

e. Moral thought occurs, which is based on something being good or bad.

3. **Concrete operations** (7–11 years)

a. Here, a rational and logical thought process is used.

b. A more conceptual framework is applied to the world.

c. An ability to understand someone else's point of view develops.

d. The **concept of conservation.** The child is able to understand the combination of two variables (e.g., height and width). An example of a beaker experiment is often used: water is placed in two identical beakers

(A and B), then water from beaker B is transferred into a taller, narrower beaker C. The child is asked if the amount of water in beakers A and C is the same or different. A child at this stage of development will understand that the amount of water present in beakers A and C is the same even though the levels in the beakers are different.

4. **Formal operations** (12 + years)

a. During this stage, **abstract thinking, deductive reasoning, and conceptual thinking develop.**

i. **Abstract thinking** is the ability to manipulate ideas and theoretical constructs.

ii. **Deductive reasoning** is the ability to go from the general to the particular.

iii. **Conceptual thinking** is the ability to define concepts or ideas.

F. **Chess and Thomas' Theory of Temperament**
Stella Chess and Alexander Thomas described children as having individual styles that are shaped as the child and the family develop. The temperament of the child **takes into account nine observed behaviors** and **categorizes children as "easy," "difficult," and "slow to warm up."** These behaviors include activity level, rhythmicity, approach or withdrawal response, adaptability to change in the environment, threshold of responsiveness, intensity of any given reaction, mood, degree of distractibility, and persistence in the face of obstacles. They describe children as being active participants in their own development and experience.

G. **Kohlberg's Model of Moral Development**
Lawrence Kohlberg described **three major levels of development** of moral judgment. His theory has been criticized for being culture-bound, middle-class, and male-oriented.

1. Level I: **Premorality (preconventional) morality.** Here, the child follows the rules set forth by his parents. Parents are the authority figures and they establish the standards of punishment and obedience.

2. Level II: **Morality of conventional role-conformity.** The child conforms to the norms of the group in order to gain acceptance and to maintain relationships.

3. Level III: **Morality of self-accepted principles.** The child voluntarily follows rules based on the concept of ethical principles and makes exceptions when they are determined to be appropriate.

H. **Gilligan's Model of Morality**
Carol Gilligan presented a view of the development of morality that includes **alternate pathways to the same moral pinnacle.** She proposed that **girls have a greater sense of connection and concern with relationships than with rules** and meet the highest level of moral development through other routes.

VII. Other Significant Issues During Childhood

A. Divorce
1. Over 1 million children each year are affected by divorce.
2. Marriages end in divorce after an average of 6–7 years.
3. The impact of divorce on children is significant and depends on multiple factors, including the parents' attention to the child and the age of the child. Half of children have difficulties during the first year after divorce. Factors that contribute to an adjustment period longer than 1 year include: parental discord, parental psychiatric illness, and poverty.
4. The impact on family is also significant:
   a. Relationships: the mother is the custodial parent 90% of the time.
   b. Psychiatric: higher rates of depression occur in parents after the divorce.
   c. Financial: women experience significant drops in their disposable income.

B. Child Abuse
1. **Physical abuse** (any inflicted rather than accidental injury) **and child neglect** (the major needs of the child, such as nutrition, shelter, protection, health care, education, and emotional needs, are not met) occur to more than 1 million children in the United States each year. More than 3,000 deaths are caused by child abuse each year.
   a. Risk factors include low birth weight, handicapped (e.g., mental retardation) and behaviorally disordered children.
   b. The abuser is most commonly a parent, often one who was abused in childhood himself or herself.
2. **Sexual abuse.** The engaging of the child in sexual activities that the child can not comprehend, for which the child is developmentally unprepared to give consent for, and/or which violates the social and legal taboos of society.
   a. In the majority of cases the perpetrator is known to the victim and most often is a father, or stepfather/ surrogate father.
   b. The median age of victims is between 9 and 10 years.
   c. Risk factors include physical or sexual abuse history of the perpetrator, substance abuse, impulsivity, sexual deviancy, and violent tendencies.

Suggested Readings

Abrams A, Rauch P: Developmental considerations in critical care medicine. *New Horiz* 1998; 6:321–330.

Bowlby J: *Attachment and Loss, Vol. 1: Attachment.* New York: Basic Books, 1969.

Erikson E: *Childhood and Society*, 2nd ed. New York: WW Norton, 1963.

Gilligan C: *In a Different Voice: Psychological Theory and Women's Development.* Cambridge, MA: Harvard University Press, 1982.

Kohlberg L: *The Psychology of Moral Development: The Nature and Validity of Moral Stages.* San Francisco: Harper and Row, 1984.

Lewis M: Normal growth and development: an overview. In Lewis M (ed.): *Child and Adolescent Psychiatry: A Comprehensive Textbook*, 2nd ed. Baltimore: Williams and Wilkins, 1996.

Mahler MS, Pine F, Bergman A: *The Psychological Birth of the Human Infant: Symbiosis and Individuation.* New York: Basic Books, 1975.

Thomas A, Chess S, Birch HG: *Temperament and Behavior Disorders in Children.* New York: New York University Press, 1968.

Vaughan VC, Litt IF: Growth and development. In Behrman RE (ed.): *Nelson Textbook of Pediatrics*, 14th ed. Philadelphia: WB Saunders, 1992:13–104.

Wallerstein JS, Kelly JB: *Surviving the Breakup: How Children and Parents Cope with Divorce.* New York: Basic Books, 1980.

Chapter 5

Child and Adolescent Disorders

ANNAH ABRAMS AND JEAN FRAZIER

I. Overview

Approximately 10% of the child and adolescent population suffers from psychiatric disorders (Wilens et al., 1998). **When psychiatric illnesses present in childhood, they tend to be more familial and chronic, and to be associated with greater morbidity.** This chapter outlines the disorders of infancy, childhood, and adolescence, and presents them in the diagnostic categories as outlined in the *Diagnostic and Statistical Manual, Fourth Edition* (DSM-IV). In addition, treatment for these childhood-onset psychiatric disorders is addressed.

II. Disruptive Behavioral Disorders

A. Attention Deficit Hyperactivity Disorder (ADHD)
1. **Diagnosis. Attention deficit hyperactivity disorder (ADHD) is the most common psychiatric disorder in children; its prevalence is 3–5% in school-age children (DSM-IV).** It often **presents as a classic triad of inattention, hyperactivity, and impulsivity.** However, some children may be primarily hyperactive and others primarily inattentive.
2. **Symptoms** must include at least six signs of inattention and six signs of hyperactivity–impulsivity for 6 months.
   a. **Symptoms of inattention include:** failure to pay close attention to details, difficulty sustaining attention in tasks or activities, failure to listen when spoken to directly, difficulty organizing tasks, avoidance of activities that require mental effort, losing things necessary for tasks or activities, distractibility, and forgetfulness in daily activities.
   b. **Symptoms of hyperactivity include:** fidgeting with the hands or feet, inability to sit still, running around when it is not appropriate, difficulty engaging in leisure activities quietly, feeling "on the go" or "driven by a motor," and talking excessively.
   c. **Symptoms of impulsivity include:** blurting out answers before questions are completed, having trouble waiting one's turn, and interrupting others.
3. The diagnosis is specified as either combined type, predominately inattentive type, or predominately hyperactive–impulsive type. The pattern of behavior must be more frequent and severe than that observed in other children of the same developmental level. The symptoms of the disorder must be present before the age of 7 years. Many children are diagnosed after this age, but the symptoms often have been present for years prior to the diagnosis. **Impairment must cross situations and must be noted in at least two settings (e.g., school and home).** The symptoms are not exclusively present when another disorder, such as depression, is present.
4. **Prevalence is 3–5% amongst school-age children.** The disorder is **reported to persist into adolescence and adulthood for approximately 50% of those affected. The male to female ratio is 4–9:1,** depending on the type and setting.
5. **Medication is the first line of treatment for ADHD. There is a 70–80% response rate to psychostimulants** (Wilens et al., 1998). The psychostimulants include methylphenidate, dextroamphetamine, magnesium pemoline, and amphetamine sulfate.
   a. **Psychostimulants**
      i. **Methylphenidate (Ritalin)** should be started at 2.5–5 mg/day, and increased if necessary by 2.5–5 mg/day (reaching an optimal dose of 0.3–2 mg/kg/day). **Side effects** include insomnia, decreased appetite, mood disturbance, tics (rare), headache, gastrointestinal distress, and psychosis (rare).
      ii. **Dextroamphetamine (Dexedrine)** is twice as potent as methylphenidate. It has a similar side effect profile to methylphenidate.
      iii. **Magnesium pemoline (Cylert)** has a longer half-life and is dosed differently than methylphenidate and dextroamphetamine. The initial dose is 18.75 mg/day, which is increased by 18.75 mg every few days. The dose range is 1–3 mg/kg/day. Its side effect profile is similar to that of methylphenidate; however, liver toxicity is a concern and, as a result, pemoline is not a first-line treatment. Liver function tests (LFTs) should be checked at baseline and every 3–6 months.
      iv. **Amphetamine sulfate (Adderall)** is a long-acting amphetamine compound.
   b. **Antihypertensive** medications (which are α-agonists) may also be used to treat ADHD, especially if a tic disorder or aggression is present.
      i. **Clonidine** should be initiated at 0.025 mg b.i.d., and may be dosed up to 4–5 μcg/kg/day total. Side effects include sedation, depression, and rebound hypertension.
      ii. **Guanfacine (Tenex)** is similar to clonidine, but less potent and less sedating. It is dosed up to 1–2 mg t.i.d.
   c. **Antidepressants.** Tricyclic antidepressants (TCAs) and bupropion (Wellbutrin) may also be used for the treat-

31

ment of ADHD. TCAs have been shown to be 60–70% effective (Wilens et al., 1998).

B. Conduct Disorder (CD)

1. **Diagnosis. A child with conduct disorder (CD) has a pattern of behavior in which the rights of others or societal norms/rules are violated. Four categories of behavior are described:**

   a. Aggression towards people and animals

   b. Destruction of property

   c. Deceitfulness or theft

   d. Serious violation of rules

2. **The child must have the symptoms of the disorder in the past year and at least one symptom in the past 6 months. Affected children have impairment in social, academic, and occupational functioning.** If the person is over the age of 18 years, he or she may be diagnosed with conduct disorder if the criteria for Antisocial Personality Disorder are not met.

3. **Subclassification:** There are **two subtypes** of the disorder:

   a. **Childhood onset:** at least one criterion must be present prior to the age of 10 years.

   b. **Adolescent onset:** no criteria are present prior to age 10 years.

4. **Prevalence.** There is an **earlier average age of onset for boys** than for girls: ages 10–12 years for boys and 16 years for girls. Prognosis is worse with an earlier onset of the disorder. Prevalence depends on the population sampled; ranges of 6–16% in males and 2–9% in females have been reported.

5. **Treatment. The mainstay of treatment for CD is behavioral therapy.** There are no specific medications for the core symptoms of this disorder. The symptoms of **aggression and agitation may be treated with medications,** including α-agonists, β-blockers, mood stabilizers, and antipsychotics. It is important to assess and treat comorbid conditions.

C. Oppositional Defiant Disorder (ODD)

1. **Diagnosis.** These children have **a pattern of negative, hostile, and defiant behavior** of at least 6 months' duration. The behavior is usually directed at an authority figure (e.g., a parent or teacher). The behavior causes significant distress in social or academic settings. Oppositional Defiant Disorder (ODD) is not diagnosed in the context of a mood or psychotic disorder. ODD cannot be diagnosed if Conduct Disorder (CD) is present.

2. **Prevalence.** Prevalence is reported to be **between 2% and 16%.** Males with the disorder are more prevalent than females prior to puberty; however, after puberty, the male to female ratio equals out. There is a gradual onset of symptoms, usually appearing before the age of 8 years. Approximately 25% of children diagnosed with ODD no longer meet the criteria after several years; others worsen and many are eventually diagnosed with CD.

3. **Treatment.** Treatment for ODD is **behavioral therapy.**

III. Mood Disorders

Mood disorders in children are classified as unipolar or bipolar, with major and minor levels of severity. Juvenile mood disorders tend to be more chronic and more refractory to pharmacologic interventions than adult-onset mood disorders. **The prevalence of these disorders increases with age.** Mood disorders are not classified as childhood disorders in the DSM-IV. For treatment of mood disorders in children see Table 5-1.

A. Major Depression

1. **Diagnosis.** In children, major depression may present with **a sad or irritable mood and/or a loss of interest or pleasure in the child's usual activities.** Child-specific symptoms include **school difficulties, school-refusal, somatic complaints, and aggressive/antisocial behavior patterns.** Physiologic changes, such as **weight change or sleep pattern disruption,** also may be present. Psychotic symptoms may be present in a depressed child.

2. **Prevalence. The prevalence is 0.3% in preschoolers, 1–2% in school-age children, and 5% in adolescents.** There is an equal male to female ratio until adolescence, when the adult pattern of 3:2 female to male emerges.

B. Bipolar Disorder

Mania in children often presents as an extremely irritable or explosive mood with poor psychosocial functioning. Children may exhibit unrestrained high energy, over-talkativeness, racing thoughts, decreased sleep, and increased goal-directed activity. Poor judgment, as manifested by reckless thrill-seeking behavior, may also be present. It is important to differentiate juvenile mania from ADHD, conduct disorder, depression, and psychotic disorders that commonly occur with mania (Wozniak et al., 1995). See Table 5-1 and Chap. 14 for the treatment of Bipolar Disorder.

IV. Anxiety Disorders

Multiple anxiety disorders can be diagnosed during childhood; however, **according to the DSM-IV only Separation Anxiety Disorder is classified as a childhood-onset anxiety disorder.**

A. Separation Anxiety Disorder

1. **Diagnosis.** Separation anxiety is defined as **excessive anxiety that occurs when a child is separated from home or from significant attachment figures.** Such anxiety occurs as **part of normal development in chil-**

dren around the age of 2 years. However, when the symptoms have an onset later during childhood and they become excessive to the point of impairing functioning, a disorder is diagnosed. Afflicted children have excessive anxiety when separated from parents (or other important figures) and excessive worry (about losing someone or about something untoward happening to their primary caretaker).

2. **Prevalence. Symptoms must last at least 4 weeks; the onset must occur before 18 years of age. The prevalence is 4% of school-age children and 1% of adolescence.** It occurs equally in boys and girls.

3. **Treatment.** Treatment includes **cognitive–behavioral therapy** and **medications** (selective serotonin reuptake inhibitors [SSRIs], buspirone, and benzodiazepines).

B. **Obsessive–Compulsive Disorder (OCD)**
   1. **Diagnosis. OCD is manifest by recurrent and distressing ideas (obsessions) that are intrusive in one's thoughts. These may lead to repetitive and purposeful behaviors (compulsions).** Children's thoughts may include fears of contamination, or feelings of self-doubt or guilt. The resulting compulsive behaviors that alleviate the obsessions include checking, counting, hand-washing, and touching.
   2. **Prevalence. The prevalence of the disorder is approximately 1–2%** in the adult population. The disorder often initially presents during childhood and adolescence. Treatment issues are the same as in adults; see Table 5-1 and Chap. 15.

C. **Post-Traumatic Stress Disorder (PTSD)**
   Children with PTSD **experience or witness a traumatic event and develop symptoms of the disorder subsequent to that trauma.** The symptoms of the disorder include **re-experiencing of the event** (e.g., recurrent intrusive recollections or recurrent distressing dreams of the event), **autonomic arousal** (e.g., increased heart rate or blood pressure) and **avoidance of any stimuli associated with the trauma.** For treatment, see Table 5-1 and Chap. 16.

D. **Social Phobia**
   Social phobia involves **a fear of embarrassment in social situations.** Children may exhibit their fears by crying or by staying close to familiar adults. They may appear to be very shy and often are on the periphery in social situations (e.g., not participating on the playground). Unlike adults, children often are unable to avoid the situations that cause the anxiety (e.g., school) and/or are unable to identify the source of the anxiety. The symptoms may interfere with class performance and social activities. The phobia must be present in same age peer group situations and not just with adults. The course depends on the age that it presents. If the onset is in childhood it may lead to a failure to achieve, whereas adolescents may experience a decline in functioning. For treatment, see Table 5-1 and Chap. 15.

E. **Generalized Anxiety Disorder (GAD)**
   The main feature of this disorder **is excessive anxiety and worry present for at least 6 months.** Children tend to worry about their ability to perform. The worries may be focused on school or athletic performance, even when they are not being evaluated. The anxiety also may be focused on catastrophic events (e.g., a hurricane). Frequently, these children are perfectionistic, which causes them to redo tasks and to seek constant reassurance that they have done well. For treatment, see Table 5-1 and Chap. 15.

V. Psychotic Disorders

1. **Diagnosis.** Psychosis may present in childhood (rarely); it refers to **abnormal behavior** that is accompanied by **impaired reality testing.** Psychosis is defined by the presence of positive symptoms, which include **delusions, hallucinations, bizarre behavior, thought disorder,** and negative symptoms of **inattention, anhedonia, avolition, apathy, and alogia** (poverty of speech). **Developmental issues complicate the diagnosis of a child with a psychotic disorder.** Normal children have rich fantasy lives in their preschool and latency years. Therefore, differentiating normal fantasies from delusions can be difficult. In addition, normal preschool and latency age children have speaking patterns that could be described as looseness of associations due to their language and cognitive development. However, if a child is psychotic he or she has extreme degrees of disordered thought. The diagnosis of a psychotic disorder in children should be reserved for those who are consumed with fantasy and who do not recognize how fantasy differs from reality. Children have visual hallucinations more commonly than do adults. These usually occur with auditory hallucinations. In addition, children may have delusions, but they are less fixed in nature than are the delusions in adults.

2. **Prevalence.** Childhood-onset schizophrenia **occurs rarely (in roughly 1/10,000 children)** and develops insidiously over more than 6 months. The male to female ratio ranges from 3:1 to 5:1 (Frazier et al., 1997). The majority of children who present with psychotic symptoms have a primary affective disorder. Afflicted children typically have an acute onset of symptoms (Frazier et al., 1997).

3. **Treatment.** The cornerstone of treatment for psychotic disorders in children is antipsychotic medica-

Table 5-1. Characteristics and Treatment of Child and Adolescent Disorders

Disorder	Main Characteristics	Treatment	
Disruptive Behavior Disorders		*Therapy*	*Medication*
Attention Deficit Hyperactivity Disorder	Inattention, hyperactivity, impulsivity		Stimulants, TCAs, α-agonists, atypical antidepressants
Conduct Disorder	Patterns of aggressive and antisocial behavior	Behavioral therapy	No specific medications for core symptoms; assess and treat comorbid conditions; may treat aggression and agitation with α-agonists, β-blockers, mood stabilizers, and antipsychotics
Oppositional Defiant Disorder	Pattern of negative, hostile, and defiant behavior	As for Conduct Disorder	As for Conduct Disorder
Mood Disorders			
Depression	Sad or irritable mood and/or loss of interest in usual activities; neurovegetative symptoms; age-specific associated features (e.g., school refusal)	Psychotherapy, cognitive–behavioral therapy	SSRIs, TCAs, atypical antidepressants
Bipolar Disorder	Extreme irritability or explosive mood; neurovegetative symptoms as seen in adults	Supportive psychotherapy	Mood stabilizers, antipsychotics (typical and atypical)
Anxiety Disorders			
Separation Anxiety Disorder	Excessive anxiety when a child is separated from caretaker	Cognitive–behavioral therapy	BZDs, buspirone, SSRIs
Obsessive Compulsive Disorder	Recurrent obsessions and compulsions, severe and distressing	Cognitive–behavioral therapy, psychotherapy	Clomipramine, SSRIs
Post-Traumatic Stress Disorder	Trauma followed by hypervigilance, autonomic reactivity, and avoidance	Psychotherapy, dialectical behavioral therapy	α-agonists, SSRIs, BZDs, occasionally antipsychotics
Social Phobia	Fear of embarrassment in social situations	Cognitive–behavioral therapy	
Generalized Anxiety Disorder	Excessive anxiety and worry	Cognitive–behavioral therapy	BZDs, buspirone, SSRIs
Psychotic Disorders	Delusions, hallucinations, bizarre behavior, thought disorder, and negative symptoms (inattention and anhedonia, avolition, apathy, and alogia)		Antipsychotics (typical and atypical)

Table 5-1. (*Continued*)

Disorder	Main Characteristics	Treatment	
Developmental Disorders			
Pervasive Developmental Disorders	Impairment in multiple areas: motor, language, social, and academic	Behavioral therapy; treat comorbid disorder. Important interventions include appropriate school placement, OT/PT, and speech and language therapy	
Autistic Disorder	Same as above	Same as above	
Learning Disorders	Reading, mathematics, written expression	Appropriate school accommodation for the learning disability; tutoring	
Communication Disorders	Expressive and/or receptive language deficits	Appropriate school accommodation; tutoring; speech therapy	
Motor Skills Disorders	Coordination impairment	OT/PT	
Elimination Disorders			
Encopresis	Fecal incontinence	Behavioral therapy	Medical management of constipation and diarrhea
Enuresis	Urinary incontinence	Behavioral therapy (bell and pad conditioning)	TCAs (imipramine), ddAVP
Feeding Disorders			
Pica	Eating of nonnutritional substances	Behavioral therapy	
Rumination Disorder	Rechewing or regurgitation of food		Treatment of medical consequences of disorder
Feeding Disorder of Infancy and Early Childhood	Failure to eat leading to weight loss or failure to gain weight	Infant–parent work, behavorial therapy	
Tic Disorders			
Complex Motor or Vocal Tics	Either motor or vocal tics		α-agonists, antipsychotics
Tourette's	Multiple motor and one or more vocal tics; comorbid with OCD and ADHD		α-agonists, antipsychotics
Other Disorders of Childhood			
Selective Mutism	Does not speak in some social situations, but fluent in others	Psychotherapy, cognitive-behavioral therapy	SSRIs
Reactive Attachment Disorder	Disturbed ability to relate socially	Consistent placement/ caregivers, infant–parent work	

ADHD, Attention Deficit Hyperactivity Disorder; BZD, benzodiazepine; ddAVP, imipramine and vasopressin; OCD, Obsessive–Compulsive Disorder; OT/PT, occupational/physical therapy; SSRI, selective serotonin reuptake inhibitor; TCA, tricyclic antidepressant.

tion. Given the lower risk of tardive dyskinesia associated with atypical neuroleptics, they are now being used as first-line treatment. Adjunctive medications should be used according to the symptoms present (e.g., antidepressants for depression or mood stabilizers for bipolar disorder) and their side effect profiles (e.g., benztropine for parkinsonian symptoms).

VI. Pervasive Developmental Disorders

Children with these disorders have **severe and pervasive impairment, in multiple areas of development.** All of these children require thorough evaluations. Treatment is multidisciplinary and includes behavioral, occupational, speech, and language therapy. These children also require individualized school programs to ensure appropriate placement and expectations. Recognition and treatment of comorbid disorders is important.

A. Autistic Disorder
  1. Children with autism have **impairment with social interaction, communications, and behavior.**
     a. **Impaired social interactions** may present as abnormal gaze, posture, and expression in social interactions. There is a relative lack of peer relationships, emotional reciprocity, and spontaneous seeking of enjoyment.
     b. **Impaired communication** (verbal and social play) may present as a delay or lack of speech, impaired ability to initiate or sustain conversations, repetitive use of language, and inability to play with others.
     c. **Impaired behavior** may present as restricted repetitive and stereotyped patterns of behavior, interests, and activities.
  2. The **onset** of the disorder is **prior to age 3 years.** Prevalence is 2/10,000 to 5/10,000 with **a male to female ratio of 4:1. Approximately 75% of children with autism are mentally retarded.**

B. Asperger's Disorder
  This disorder is similar to autism in terms of abnormal social interactions and restricted repetitive and stereotyped patterns of behavior, interests, and activities. In contrast to Autism, Asperger's syndrome has **no delay in language or in cognitive development.** These individuals also have **no delay in age-appropriate self-care, adaptive behavior (except in social interactions) or curiosity about the environment.** The prevalence is not known, but it appears to be more common in males.

C. Rett's Disorder
  This disorder is similar to autism except that these individuals **function normally through the first 5 months of life.** Beginning between the ages of 5 and 48 months multiple deficits develop, including decreases in the following areas: head growth, hand skills, social engagement, gait and trunk movements, language, and motor skills. This disorder often is associated with severe or profound mental retardation. The prevalence is not known (uncommon) and **has only been reported in females.**

D. Childhood Disintegrative Disorder
  This disorder is similar to autism except that these individuals **develop normally for the first 2 years of life and then experience significant regression in multiple areas.** The losses of previously acquired skills occur between the ages of 2 and 10 years and involve **language, behavior, bowel/bladder control, play and/or motor skills. Abnormal** functioning in **social interactions, communication, and behavior** develop. **This disorder is usually associated with severe mental retardation.** The prevalence is **rare.**

E. Mental Retardation (MR)
  1. **Subaverage general intellectual functioning** based on a standardized intelligence test (IQ) **with** concurrent **impairment in adaptive functioning** in at least two of the following areas: communication, self-care, home living, and social/interpersonal skills. **Subaverage** is defined as a full-scale IQ of less than 70 (i.e., two standard deviations below the mean). **Four diagnostic severity levels of MR** are described:
     a. **Mild** (IQ range of 50—55 to 70). Children with mild MR can develop social and communication skills, and can function relatively normally as adults.
     b. **Moderate** (IQ range of 35–40 to 50–55). Children with moderate MR have limited social awareness. They can be trained to care for most personal needs and to work in sheltered job placements. Moderate supervision is usually required (e.g., as in a group home).
     c. **Severe** (IQ range of 20–25 to 35–40). Children with severe MR have slow and poor motor development. They have limited to no speech and require close supervision.
     d. **Profound** (IQ falls below 20–25). Children with profound MR have poor cognitive and social capacities. Speech is often absent. Constant supervision is needed (e.g., special care setting).
  2. The **onset** of MR must occur **before age 18 years.** Prevalence is 2–3% of the school-aged population. See Chap. 8 for a more complete review of MR.

VII. Learning Disorders

Learning disorders are **associated with below expected abilities in academic achievement in reading, mathematics, and/or writing,** based on the child's chronological age, measured intelligence, and age-appropriate education. **The difference between achievement and IQ must be at least two standard deviations below the mean.** Reading, mathematics, and writing disorders often are comorbid. The disorder is usually diagnosed during or after first grade when reading, math, and writing are being taught in school. Children with learning disorders have a school drop-out rate of 40% (approximately 1.5 times the average). The **prevalence of learning disorders ranges from 2% to 10%,** with approximately 5% of school children in the United States carrying a diagnosis of a Learning Disorder. Treatment involves appropriate school accommodation for the learning disability and tutoring.

A. Reading Disorder

This condition is manifest by a below expected reading achievement accompanied by a decreased ability to recognize words, to comprehend, and/or to read accurately. This disorder was **previously known as dyslexia.** The **prevalence is 4%** of school-age children, with **a male to female ratio of 4:1.**

B. Mathematics Disorder

This disorder involves a lower than expected mathematical ability as demonstrated by decreased skills in understanding, recognizing, copying, and following mathematical terms, symbols, figures, and steps. **The prevalence is 1% and occurs equally in males and females.**

C. Disorder of Written Expression

This condition is manifest by a below expected ability in spelling, punctuation, and grammar. The prevalence is not known. Children with this disorder are often grouped with other learning disorders.

VIII. Communication Disorders

The communication disorders interfere with academic achievement and social communication and usually present during or after first grade. Treatment includes tutoring and appropriate school accommodation usually including speech therapy.

A. Expressive Language Disorder

In this condition, standardized test scores for expressive language are below those for nonverbal intellectual capacity and for receptive language development. The presentation of the disorder depends on the age of the child and may include a **limited amount of speech, a limited range of vocabulary, errors in tense, and an immature language sentence construction.** Two types are known: an **acquired type,** in which impairment occurs after a period of normal development as a result of an insult (e.g., neurological or medical), and a **developmental type,** in which impairment is not associated with a neurological or medical insult. The prevalence for the developmental type is about 3–5%, whereas the acquired type is less common.

B. Mixed Receptive–Expressive Language Disorder

This condition, an Expressive Language Disorder with **receptive language deficit (difficulty understanding words and sentences),** has a prevalence that is less common than expressive language disorder (approximately 3%).

C. Phonological Disorder

Difficulties with phonological disorders occur in **speech production.** The prevalence of moderate to severe symptoms is 2–3% in 6- and 7-year-olds. This decreases to 0.5% by age 17 years.

D. Stuttering

Stuttering is a **disturbance in the normal fluency of speech.** Speech difficulties may include sound repetitions, prolongation, interjections, pauses within words, and word blocking. Stuttering is **often absent in singing.** The disorder begins between the ages of 2 and 7 years with a peak at age 5 years. Almost all cases present before the age of 10 years. The **prevalence is 1% in prepubertal children** with **a male to female ratio of 3:1.** The symptoms often remit in adolescence. There is a familial pattern for the disorder with the risk for a first-degree biological relative developing stuttering at three times the risk of the general population.

IX. Motor Skills Disorder

A. Developmental Coordination Disorder

This is a disorder with an impaired ability to perform daily activities due to a coordination difficulty not accounted for by a medical condition (e.g., cerebral palsy or hemiplegia). These children may be slow to crawl or walk and/or clumsy with fine and gross motor skills. Often this disorder is seen in premature infants. The **prevalence is 6%** in school-age children. The course is variable and may persist into adulthood. These children benefit from occupational and physical therapy.

X. Elimination Disorders

A. Encopresis

This condition is manifest by the repeated passage of feces into inappropriate places (intentional or involuntary); it is not due to a medical condition. This behavior occurs at least **one time per month for 3 months.** Encopresis may occur with or without constipation and overflow incontinence. There are two types of this disorder: **primary (i.e., never toilet-trained) and secondary (i.e., regressed after being toilet-trained). The child must be at least 4 years of age** (chronologically and developmentally). The prevalence is 1% of 5-year-olds. It is more common in boys than in girls. The treatment of encopresis is behavioral therapy. Some children need medical intervention for constipation and diarrhea.

B. Enuresis
1. **Diagnosis. Enuresis is manifest by the repeated voiding of urine into bed or clothes (intentional or involuntary) that is not due to a medical condition.** This occurs at least **two times per week for 3 consecutive months** or causes significant distress or social impairment for the child. Enuresis may be **nocturnal, diurnal, or both.** Like encopresis there are two types of the disorder (primary and secondary). The child must be **at least 5 years of age** (chronologically and developmentally).
2. **Prevalence.** The prevalence varies with age ranging from 7% of 5-year-old boys and 3% of 5-year-old girls to 1% of 18-year-old boys and less than 1% of 18-year-old girls.
3. **Treatment.** Treatment should begin with behavioral therapies. Techniques include **star charts and the bell and pad technique** (i.e., a pad is placed on the bed, when the pad gets wet, the bell goes off). If these methods are not successful, medication is the next step. **Imipramine and vasopressin (ddAVP)** have been shown to be effective. Enuresis may remit spontaneously; it is therefore important not to continue these medications indefinitely.

XI. Feeding and Eating Disorders of Infancy

A. Pica
Pica is the persistent eating of a non-nutritional substance for at least a 1-month period. This behavior is developmentally and culturally inappropriate and is often associated with mental retardation, poverty, and nutritional deficiencies. A medical etiology for the disorder must be ruled out. Behavioral techniques are used for treatment.

B. Rumination Disorder
Rumination disorder involves the repeated regurgitation and rechewing of food occurring for at least 1 month following a period of normal eating. This disorder may be associated with neglect and with developmental delay. The symptoms are not due to a gastrointestinal or medical condition. This disorder develops between the ages of 3 and 12 months. The prevalence is rare. Outcome ranges from spontaneous remission to death secondary to malnutrition (mortality rates as high as 25%). Treatment must address the medical consequences of the illness, such as dehydration and malnutrition, as well as the etiology of the illness, whether it is neglect or developmental delay.

C. Feeding Disorder of Infancy and Early Childhood
A failure to eat leading to an inability to gain weight or a significant loss of weight over a 1-month period characterizes the condition. The symptoms are not due to a medical condition. The disorder must present prior to the age of 6 years, but usually presents during the first year of life. This disorder may be associated with attachment issues and treatment should involve work with the infant–caregiver dyad.

XII. Tic Disorders

A tic is a sudden rapid recurrent nonrhythmic stereotyped motor movement or vocalization. Tics are described as motor (e.g., eye blinking or neck jerking) or vocal (e.g., grunting or snorting) and as **simple or complex.** A complex tic has more purposeful movements or imitative behaviors. **Tics are involuntary movements, but may be voluntarily suppressed.** Anxiety and stress exacerbate tics. During sleep or while doing an absorbing activity (e.g., playing video games) tics are often decreased.

The disorders listed below **occur prior to the age of 18 years.** If the symptoms present after age 18 years, the diagnosis is Tic Disorder, Not Otherwise Specified.

A. Tourette's Disorder
Tourette's disorder is a childhood-onset neuropsychiatric disorder with **multiple motor tics and at least one vocal tic** at some time during the illness, but the motor and vocal tics need not be concurrent. **The tics occur many times a day, usually daily, for at least 1 year** and there is never a tic-free period of more than 3 consecutive months. Impairment occurs in social and/or academic functioning. The tics are not due to the effect of medications (e.g., stimulants) or a medical illness (e.g., chorea). The symptoms often diminish in intensity in adolescence. Tourette's disorder is commonly associated with OCD, ADHD, and anxiety disorders. There is a significant familial association of the disorder with evidence of genetic transmission for vulnerability. Onset occurs before the age of 18 years. The usual age of onset is 7 years with motor tics presenting prior to vocal tics. Prevalence is 4/10,000 to 5/10,000, and is about three times more common in males than females

B. Chronic Motor or Vocal Tic Disorder
This disorder is similar to Tourette's disorder except that children have either motor or vocal tics. This disorder is more common than Tourette's; it occurs in 1–2% of school-age children and is more common in boys. If a person has a history of Tourette's, they can not be diagnosed with this disorder.

C. Transient Tic Disorder
The symptoms of this disorder are single or multiple motor and/or vocal tics. The symptoms occur for at least 4 weeks, but not greater than 12 months and may remit without treatment.

XIII. Other Disorders of Childhood

A. **Selective Mutism**
The child with this disorder will not speak in specific social situations even though their speech is fluent in other settings (usually home). The child usually communicates nonverbally in these settings (e.g., eye contact or head nodding). The diagnosis should not be made if the child is not comfortable with the spoken language (e.g., an immigrant child). The symptoms must be present for at least 1 month. It is associated with anxiety and shyness. The disorder is uncommon and occurs in less than 1% of children. Treatments include psychotherapy, cognitive–behavioral therapy (CBT), and the use of SSRIs.

B. **Reactive Attachment Disorder of Infancy and Early Childhood**
The child with this condition has **a disturbed and developmentally inappropriate ability to relate socially.** There are two types: the **inhibited type** (in which the child fails to initiate or respond to most social interactions) and the **disinhibited type** (in which the child is indiscriminately social as manifested by diffuse attachments). **Pathological child care,** either emotional and/or physical disregard for the child's basic needs or repeated changes in the primary caregiver, often is the etiology of the disorder. The disorder is not accounted for by developmental delay. The symptoms present prior to age 5 years. It is an uncommon disorder. Treatment of reactive attachment disorder includes consistent placement and caregiver and infant dyad work.

C. **Other Significant Issues During Childhood**
1. **Suicide** (see Chap. 54). **Suicide is the third leading cause of death in adolescents behind accidents and homicide.** The death rate for adolescents from suicide is 13/100,000. As with adults, the ratio of males to females for completed suicide is 4:1 and the reverse is true for attempted suicide (i.e., 4:1 female to male). The most common successful means used is firearms for both males and females. Other means include hanging, suffocation, and poisoning/overdose (OD). Risk factors include a previous attempt (25%), substance abuse, chronic illness, depression, psychosis, gender identity issues (homosexuality), and family issues including history of suicide, discord, and psychiatric illness/substance abuse.
2. **Eating disorders. Anorexia** and **bulimia** are reviewed in Chap. 21.

XIV. Child-Specific Pharmacologic Issues

A. Many of the disorders that present during childhood are responsive to medication. However, the use of medications in children is not as well established as it is in adults. The use of medications in children should occur only after completion of a thorough diagnostic evaluation. This process includes a full psychiatric assessment, structured psychiatric interviews and rating forms as indicated, and relevant laboratory studies to rule out underlying medical conditions.

B. **Children often benefit significantly from the initiation of medications for the treatment of psychiatric disorders.** Medication may decrease the symptoms of a disorder, effect a positive change in the social/emotional and behavioral presentation of the child, and optimize the developmental trajectory of the child.

C. **The following basic pharmacologic principles should be considered when medications are used in children.**
1. **Children metabolize most medications more efficiently than adults** and may require two-fold greater weight-corrected doses of medications.
2. **Children may have higher peak plasma concentrations.**
3. **Children may have lower trough plasma concentrations.**

XV. Conclusion

This chapter underscores that psychopathology does occur in children and adolescents and that this inherently involves some degree of developmental deviance. It is important to be able to recognize the disorders and how they present in childhood in order to initiate appropriate therapeutic interventions. The aim of these interventions is to decrease the child's symptoms and to facilitate development.

Suggested Readings

American Psychiatric Association (APA): *Diagnostic and Statistical Manual of Mental Disorders, Fourth Edition.* Washington, DC: American Psychiatric Association, 1994.

Frazier JA: The person with mental retardation. In Nicoli AM (ed.): *The New Harvard Guide to Psychiatry.* Cambridge, MA: Harvard University Press, 1999:660–671.

Frazier JA, Spencer T, Wilens T, et al.: Childhood onset schizophrenia: the prototypic psychotic disorder of childhood. In Dunner DL, Rosenbaum JF (eds): *The Psychiatric Clinics of North America: Annual of Drug Therapy.* Philadelphia: WB Saunders, 1997;4:167–193.

Pfeffer CR: Suicidal behavior in children and adolescents: causes and management. In Lewis M (ed.): *Child and Adolescent*

Psychiatry: A Comprehensive Textbook, 2nd ed. Baltimore: Williams and Wilkins, 1996:666–673.

Wilens T, Spencer TJ, Frazier JA, Biederman J: Child and adolescent psychopharmacology. In Ollendick T, Hersen M (eds): *Handbook of Child Psychopathology*, 3rd ed. New York: Plenum Press, 1998:603–636.

Wozniak J, Biederman J, Kiely K, et al.: Mania-like symptoms suggestive of childhood-onset bipolar disorder in clinically referred children. *J Am Acad Child Adolesc Psychiatry* 1995; 34:867–876.

Chapter 6

Delirium

Stephan Heckers

I. Overview

Delirium is a reversible organic mental disorder whose hallmarks are confusion and an altered level of consciousness. Most cases of delirium have an acute onset. It has, therefore, also been referred to as an *acute confusional state*. **Although delirium is usually reversible within a period of days to weeks, some cases progress to irreversible brain failure.**

II. Epidemiology

A. **The prevalence of delirium in medically and surgically ill patients is 11–16%; its incidence varies between 4% and 31%.** The highest incidence is found in the surgical intensive care unit (ICU), followed by the coronary care unit, and then on medical and surgical wards.

B. **Several risk factors for the development of delirium have been identified:**
   1. **Being elderly.** Delirium tends to develop more frequently in the elderly than in younger patients, most likely as a result of pre-existing medical conditions (including impaired brain function and the frequent administration of numerous medications).
   2. **Having a history of brain damage** (e.g., stroke, dementia), **drug dependency, and acquired immunodeficiency syndrome (AIDS).**
   3. **Having cardiac surgery or being burned.** The prevalence of delirium after cardiac surgery is about 32%. The incidence of delirium in burn patients is approximately 18–30%; it increases with age and with the severity of burns.
   4. Having certain psychosocial and environmental factors, especially sleep deprivation, has not been closely linked to an increased risk of delirium.

C. **Morbidity and Mortality**
   1. **The majority of delirious patients recover without observable sequelae,** but the exact percentage is unknown. Patients in drug withdrawal states may develop seizures. **Some patients fail to recover from the acute confusional state, progress to stupor or coma, and die.**
   2. **Delirium and agitation increase the risk for complications** (e.g., decubiti and aspiration pneumonia) **and tend to prolong the length of hospital stay.** A substantial number of elderly patients who develop delirium as inpatients (22–76% according to differ-

ent studies) die during the hospitalization; **about 25% of delirious hospitalized patients die within 6 months of discharge.**

III. Clinical Features of Confusional States

Three domains (i.e., attention, orientation, and memory) are typically impaired in delirious patients; other features are more variable. Delirium can be diagnosed if the patient shows several features during parts of the evaluation process.

A. **Attention deficits are the *sine qua non* of confusional states.** The patient is easily distracted and cannot maintain his or her focus of attention during a task. Inattention and distractibility are often easily observed, or **can be assessed at the bedside by asking the patient to name the months of the year in reverse order or to repeat several numbers in sequence.**

B. **Memory is typically impaired.** Deficits are readily apparent when the patient is asked to encode new information (e.g., to recall three words) either immediately or after a delay of 5 min. Some patients will be partially or completely amnestic for the delirious episode.

C. **Impaired orientation is the third main feature** of confusional states. Except for lucid intervals, delirious patients are typically disoriented to time and to place, but rarely to person.

D. **Thinking is often altered in acute confusional states.** Some patients are disorganized, irrational, and manifest impaired reasoning, whereas others are grossly impaired with delusions and paranoia.

E. **Poor insight and judgment** about medical treatment often make decision-making impossible.

F. **Altered perception** in the form of **illusions** or, less often, **hallucinations** are seen in some confusional states. **Visual hallucinations are more common than auditory or tactile hallucinations.** Confusional states secondary to sedative-hypnotic withdrawal are more likely to present with hallucinations.

G. **Neurological signs such as tremor, myoclonus, or asterixis** are seen in some types of delirium (e.g., hepatic encephalopathy). Other deficits, such as **impaired constructional ability, word-finding difficulties (dysnomia), or writing disturbances (dysgraphia),** are more generally found. The **clock-drawing**

41

test often provides a rapid screen for the presence and degree of delirium. **Dysgraphia,** easily tested by asking the patient to write a sentence, is a very sensitive, albeit nonspecific, test for delirium.

IV. Differential Diagnosis of Delirium

A. Numerous **organic disturbances** have been **implicated in the etiology of delirium** and fall into **four major categories: primary intracranial disease, systemic diseases that secondarily affect the brain, exogenous toxic agents, and withdrawal from substances** on which the patient has become dependent.

B. **Three steps are important in the differential diagnosis** of delirium: rule out potentially life-threatening causes, rule out harmful effects of prescription or illicit drugs, and be aware of the complete list of conditions, illnesses, and medications that can lead to delirium.

1. **Rule out potentially life-threatening causes. The mnemonic WWHHHIMP can guide the clinician** during the rapid assessment of serious and potentially life-threatening causes of delirium.
   a. Wernicke's encephalopathy is strongly suggested by the triad of confusion, ataxia, and ophthalmoplegia.
   b. Withdrawal states occur after discontinuation of illicit or prescription drug use, even when small dosages are used for short periods of time.
   c. Hypertensive encephalopathy can be assessed with vital signs.
   d. Hypoxia can be assessed with arterial blood gases.
   e. Hypoglycemia can be assessed with a serum glucose level.
   f. Intracranial bleed.
   g. Meningitis and encephalitis almost always produce focal neurological signs as well as headache, loss of consciousness, and seizures.
   h. Poisons that may lead to delirium include pesticides, solvents, or heavy metals.

2. **Rule out the impact of drugs.** Many prescription drugs and several illicitly used drugs cause delirium (Table 6-1). Drug overdose, either accidental or as a result of a suicide attempt, is a frequent cause of delirium in the medical intensive care unit.

3. **Continue the search. When life-threatening causes of delirium and the impact of several specific drugs have been excluded, the clinician will often proceed to empiric treatment of the delirious patient.** However, it is important to continue the search for an underlying cause, which can be found in more than 85% of cases. **Table 6-2 offers the mnemonic "I WATCH DEATH" to organize the differential diagnosis of delirium.** Considering the mortality associated with acute confusional states, the mnemonic is appropriate.

V. Treatment

Treatment of delirium includes specific treatment if the etiology is reasonably clear, and empirical treatment to avoid immediate danger while awaiting clarification of the specific etiology.

A. Specific Treatment of Agitation and Confusion
1. **Maintenance of normal blood pressure, circulation, and blood oxygenation, correction of metabolic derangements, and treatment of local or systemic infections are essential to good medical care. Such treatment averts many mental status changes.**
2. **Treat drug toxicity and drug withdrawal.** Stop the offending drug and find an alternative compound without similar adverse effects. If necessary, antidotes can be administered:
   a. **Naloxone hydrochloride,** 0.4 mg subcutaneously or intravenously, is often used to reverse acute confusional states due to the use of narcotics.
   b. **Normeperidine** (the CNS-stimulating metabolite of meperidine) **toxicity** leads to hallucinations, irritability, myoclonus, and seizures, and might require additional aggressive treatment with barbiturates or benzodiazepines.
   c. **Physostigmine,** 1–2 mg, infused slowly intravenously as a one-time dose or given as a continuous drip, can effectively treat anticholinergic delirium.
   d. Intravenous **verapamil** has been used for the treatment of phencyclidine intoxication.
   e. The benzodiazepine antagonist **flumazenil** has been used to reverse the effects of benzodiazepine excess.

B. **Non-Specific Treatment of Agitation and Confusion Pharmacological intervention, mechanical restraints, and supportive measures (to reorient and calm the patient) are central to the treatment of delirium.**
1. **Pharmacological treatment. Neuroleptics and benzodiazepines are the primary drugs used to manage the agitated and/or confused patient.** If the patient's agitation cannot be controlled by these two classes of medications, narcotics and paralyzing agents can be used as the last resort (Table 6-3).
   a. **Neuroleptics**
      i. **Haloperidol is most often used to treat the agitated, delirious patient.** Other typical neuroleptics (e.g., chlorpromazine, droperidol, thiothixene, and trifluoperazine) can also be used. Haloperidol is approved by the Food and Drug Administration (FDA) for intramuscular and oral use only, but it can be given intravenously. Typically the agitated patient will be given haloperidol at a starting dose of 0.5–5 mg. The elderly and those with known CNS dysfunction (e.g., dementia, stroke) require doses as low as 0.5 mg two to three times per day; doses of 2–5 mg two to four times per day are not uncommon.
      ii. **All neuroleptics predispose to extrapyramidal side effects.** Acute dystonia, especially the life-threat-

Table 6-1. Drugs that Can Cause Delirium

Antibiotic	*Anti-inflammatory*	*Sedative-Hypnotic*
Acyclovir	Adrenocorticotropic hormone	Barbiturates
Amphotericin	Corticosteroids	Glutethimide
Cephalexin	Ibuprofen	Benzodiazepines
Chloroquine	Indomethacin	
Isoniazid	Naproxen	*Sympathomimetic*
Rifampin	Phenylbutazone	Amphetamine
		Phenylephrine
Anticholinergic	*Antineoplastic*	Phenylpropanolamine
Antihistamines	5-Fluorouracil	
Antispasmodics		*Miscellaneous*
Atropine	*Antiparkinson*	Aminophylline
Belladonna alkaloids	Amantadine	Bromides
Benztropine	Carbidopa	Chlorpropamide
Biperiden	Levodopa	Cimetidine
Chlorpheniramine		Disulfiram
Diphenhydramine	*Analgesics*	Drug withdrawal
Phenothiazines	Opiates	– Alcohol
Promethazine	Salicylates	– Barbiturates
Scopolamine	Synthetic narcotics	– Benzodiazepines
Tricyclic antidepressants		Lithium
Trihexyphenidyl	*Cardiac*	Metrizamide
	Beta-blockers	Metronidazole
Anticonvulsant	Propranolol	Podophyllin
Phenobarbital	Clonidine	Propylthiouracil
Phenytoin	Digitalis	Quinacrine
Valproic acid	Disopyramide	Theophylline
	Lidocaine	Timolol ophthalmic
	Mexiletine	
	Methyldopa	
	Quinidine	
	Procainamide	

SOURCE: Adapted from Wise MG, Gray KF: Delirium, dementia, and amnestic disorders. In Hales RE, Yudofsky SC, Talbott JA (eds): *The American Psychiatric Press Textbook of Psychiatry*. Washington, DC: 1994:311–353.

ening **laryngeal dystonia, should be treated promptly** with benztropine mesylate 1–2 mg IV, or diphenhydramine 25–50 mg IV. **Akathisia responds well to reduction of the neuroleptic dose and concomitant administration of a beta-blocker** (e.g., propranolol 10–20 mg two to three times per day) or a benzodiazepine (e.g., diazepam or lorazepam 0.5–1 mg two to three times per day). Parkinsonian side effects occur more often in older individuals and respond to treatment with an anticholinergic agent, which unfortunately can aggravate the acute confusional state.

iii. **High doses of haloperidol have been associated with prolongation of cardiac conduction, leading to QTc increases.** In some patients, particularly in those with pre-existing dilated ventricles and a history of alcohol abuse, *torsades de pointes* arrhythmia has developed.

b. **Benzodiazepines**

i. **Agitation due to panic attacks, generalized anxiety, or fear of being in the ICU** should be treated primarily with a benzodiazepine. Diazepam at a starting dose of 2–5 mg, and lorazepam or clonazepam at a starting dose of 0.5–1 mg, are effective

Table 6-2. Differential diagnosis of delirium ("I WATCH DEATH")

Infectious	Encephalitis, meningitis, syphilis
Withdrawal	Alcohol, barbiturates, sedative-hypnotics
Acute metabolic	Acidosis, alkalosis, electrolyte disturbance, hepatic failure, renal failure
Trauma	Heat stroke, severe burn, postoperative state
CNS pathology	Abscess, hemorrhage, normal pressure hydrocephalus, seizure, stroke, tumor, vasculitis
Hypoxia	Anemia, carbon monoxide poisoning, hypotension, pulmonary/cardiac failure
Deficiencies	Vitamin B12, niacin, thiamine
Endocrinopathies	Hyper- or hypoadrenocortisolism, hyper- or hypoglycemia
Acute vascular	Hypertensive encephalopathy, shock
Toxins or drugs	Medications
Heavy metals	Lead, manganese, mercury

SOURCE: Adapted from Wise MG, Gray KF: Delirium, Dementia, and amnestic disorders. In Hales RE, Yudofsky SC, Talbott JA (eds): *The American Psychiatric Press Textbook of Psychiatry*. Washington, DC: 1994:311–353.

in calming the anxious and agitated patient. In case of panic attacks, maintenance treatment (e.g., with clonazepam 0.5 mg three times per day) is often recommended. Psychotic episodes and manic presentations have also been managed exclusively with clonazepam.

    ii. **Midazolam, a benzodiazepine with a rapid onset of action and an elimination half-life of 1–4 h, has been used successfully in the treatment of agitation.** Intramuscular administration of 2–3 mg of midazolam calms patients within 5–10 min. Continuous infusion of midazolam, with a mean infusion rate of approximately 0.6–6 μg/kg/min, is an effective treatment for severely agitated patients.

    iii. **Many agitated patients benefit from the combined use of a neuroleptic and a benzodiazepine.** Benzodiazepines can cause respiratory depression if large doses are given. All benzodiazepines can lead to clouded consciousness, mimicking the mental status changes seen in acute confusional states.

  c. **Narcotics and nondepolarizing muscle relaxants**

    i. **Morphine sulfate can be used for pain control and to sedate the agitated patient in the ICU.** Parenteral administration leads to a prompt effect that lasts 4–5 h. Respiratory depression and aggravation of confusion are potential adverse effects.

    ii. **Intubation, sedation, and paralysis using metocurine iodide or pancuronium bromide are the final treatment options when other measures fail to control severe agitation.** The cardiovascular effects of metocurine iodide and pancuronium bromide, pulmonary complications associated with intubation, and traction injuries that develop during paralysis are potential adverse effects of this treatment strategy.

2. **Mechanical restraints.** Even when optimally medicated with a neuroleptic and/or a benzodiazepine, the calm but confused patient might still perform dangerous maneuvers. In such situations it is recommended that the patient be placed in mechanical restraints. **The indication should be clearly documented in the medical records and the need for restraints assessed continuously.**

3. **Supportive measures. The confused patient benefits from frequent reorientation to time and place. Adequate lighting can reduce the likelihood of illusionary misperceptions. The presence of a calm and reassuring family member and nursing staff is helpful** for the patient. A "sitter" can also help reduce anxiety. **Education** of the staff, the patient's family, and the patient about the nature of confusion and/or agitation **is calming and therapeutic for all of the parties involved.**

Table 6-3. Drugs Used to Treat Delirium and Agitation

Drug	Route	Onset (min)	Peak effect (min)	Starting dose	Important adverse effects
Neuroleptics					
Haloperidol	IV, IM	5–20	15–45	Degree of agitation:	
	PO	30–60	120–240	Mild: 0.5–2 mg	Cardiac arrhythmia (QTc increased, torsades de pointes)
				Moderate: 5–10 mg	
				Severe: > 10 mg	Extrapyramidal side effects
Droperidol	IV, IM	3–10	15–45	2.5–10 mg	Hypotension
Chlorpromazine	IV, IM	5–40	10–30	25 mg	
Benzodiazepines					
Diazepam	IV	2–5	5–30	2–5 mg	
	PO	10–60	30–180		
Lorazepam	IV, IM	2–20	60–120	1–2 mg	Respiratory depression
	SL	2–20	20–60	0.5–1 mg	May aggravate delirium
	PO	20–60	20–120	0.5–1 mg	
Midazolam	IV, IM	1–2	30–40	0.05–0.15 mg/kg	
Narcotics					Respiratory depression
Morphine sulfate	IV, IM	1–2	20	4–10 mg	May aggravate delirium
Paralytics					
Metocurine iodide	IV	1–4	2–10	0.2–0.4 mg/kg	Hypotension
Pancuronium bromide	IV	0.5–1	5	0.04–0.1 mg/kg	Tachycardia, Hypertension

IV, intravenous; IM, intramuscular; PO, oral; SL, sublingual.

Suggested Readings

Crippen DW: The role of sedation in the ICU patient with pain and agitation. *Crit Care Clin* 1990; 6:369–392.

Heckers S, Tesar GE, Stern TA: Diagnosis and treatment of agitation and delirium in the intensive care unit patient. In Irwin RS, Cerra FB, Rippe JM (eds): *Irwin and Rippe's Intensive Care Medicine*. Philadelphia: Lippincott-Raven; 1999:2383–2393.

Lipowski ZJ: *Delirium: Acute Brain Failure in Man*. Springfield, IL: Charles C Thomas, 1980.

Lipowski ZJ: Delirium (acute confusional states). *J Am Med Assoc* 1988; 258:1789–1792.

Tesar GE, Murray GB, Cassem NH: Use of high-dose intravenous haloperidol in agitated cardiac patients. *J Clin Psychopharmacol* 1985; 5:344–347.

Thompson TL, Thompson WL: Treating postoperative delirium. *Drug Ther* 1983; 13:30–40.

Trzepacz PT, Baker RW, Greenhouse J: A symptom rating scale for delirium. *Psychiatry Res* 1988; 23:89–97.

Chapter 7

Dementia

ROY H. PERLIS AND WILLIAM E. FALK

I. Definition

A. DSM-IV Criteria

The DSM-IV criteria for dementia require the demonstration of **a decline in memory, as well as impairment of at least one other domain of cognitive function:**

1. **Aphasia,** or difficulty with any aspect of language.
2. **Apraxia,** or impaired ability to perform motor tasks despite intact motor function.
3. **Agnosia,** or impaired object recognition despite intact sensory function.
4. **Executive dysfunction,** or difficulty in planning, organizing, sequencing, or abstracting.

B. Qualifiers to the Diagnosis

Several important qualifiers are included in the definition:

1. The condition must represent a **change from baseline** (i.e., patients with mental retardation would not meet the definition unless their cognition deteriorated further).
2. The deficits must be clinically significant in that they **interfere with social or occupational function.**
3. The deficits cannot occur exclusively during an episode of delirium.
4. The condition cannot be accounted for by another Axis I diagnosis such as Major Depression.

C. Age-Associated Memory Impairment

Some decline in cognitive function, known as age-associated memory impairment, may be seen in normal aging, but it does not interfere with work or social abilities and is generally stable over time.

II. Epidemiology

Estimates of the prevalence of dementia vary widely, depending on which set of diagnostic criteria is utilized. Alzheimer's disease, which accounts for up to 70% of cases of dementia, affects some 4 million people in the United States. The cost of providing care for demented patients exceeds $113 billion each year.

A. Demographic Factors

The incidence of dementia increases with age: dementia affects 15–20% of individuals after the age of 65 years, and up to 45% after the age of 80 years. Whereas the etiology of dementia differs somewhat between genders (with higher rates of vascular dementia and lower rates of Alzheimer's disease in men), the overall incidence is equivalent in men and women.

B. Trends

As average life-expectancies increase, the number of demented patients is expected to increase dramatically.

III. Differential Diagnosis

A. Confounding Disorders

As noted above, the diagnostic criteria for dementia require that a number of confounding disorders be ruled out. Chief among these is delirium, which requires a rapid medical and neurologic evaluation (see Chap. 6). Other psychiatric illnesses, including Major Depression, may also resemble dementia. Differences in presentation may be useful in distinguishing delirium or depression from dementia.

Of note, **an underlying diagnosis of dementia may predispose a patient to delirium;** thus, further evaluation is required once the delirium has been treated successfully.

1. **Delirium generally differs from dementia in several important ways:**
   a. **The onset is acute or subacute** (hours to days).
   b. **The course often fluctuates.**
   c. **The level of consciousness, and attention in particular, may be impaired.**
2. **Depression may be difficult to distinguish from dementia, particularly as the two diagnoses are often comorbid.** In addition, depression alone may cause cognitive impairment; in such cases, it may presage Alzheimer's disease by several years. **Certain features favor a diagnosis of depression:**
   a. A better premorbid level of function.
   b. A more acute onset.
   c. Poor motivation and/or prominent negativity on mental status testing. Depressed patients may state that they are unable to perform a particular task. At times, they can succeed at more difficult tasks and fail at easier ones.
   d. A family history that is positive for depression.

B. Reversible Conditions

Establishing a precise etiology (see Table 7-1) whenever possible allows more focused treatment

Table 7-1. Etiology of Dementia

Vascular:
Stroke, chronic subdural hemorrhages, postanoxic injury, diffuse white matter disease

Infectious:
HIV infection, neurosyphilis, progressive multifocal leukoencephalopathy (PMLE), Creutzfeldt-Jakob disease, tuberculosis, sarcoidosis, Whipple's disease

Neoplastic:
Primary versus metastatic carcinoma, paraneoplastic syndrome

Degenerative:
Alzheimer's disease, frontotemporal dementia, dementia with Lewy bodies, Parkinson's disease, progressive supranuclear palsy, multisystem degeneration, amyotrophic lateral sclerosis (ALS), corticobasal degeneration, multiple sclerosis (MS)

Inflammatory:
Vasculitis

Endocrine:
Hypothyroidism, adrenal insufficiency, Cushing's syndrome, hypo/hyperparathyroidism, renal failure, liver failure

Metabolic:
Thiamine deficiency (Wernicke's encephalopathy), vitamin B_{12} deficiency, inherited enzyme defects

Toxins:
Chronic alcoholism, drugs/medication effects, heavy metals, dialysis dementia (aluminum)

Trauma:
Dementia pugilistica

Other:
Normal pressure hydrocephalus (NPH), obstructive hydrocephalus

---

and an accurate estimation of prognosis. Whereas **a reversible cause will be identified in fewer than 15% of cases,** a diagnosis may be comforting to patients and their families, and useful in planning.

IV. Evaluation of the Patient with Suspected Dementia

A. General Approach
History should be obtained from the patient as well as family members or others who have observed the patient; family or other informants should be interviewed separately from the patient. Note that **patients themselves often fail to report deficits, usually because they are unaware of them.**

B. History
1. **Present illness**
   a. **Nature of presentation**
      i. An abrupt or precipitous onset favors a diagnosis of vascular dementia, whereas insidious onset suggests Alzheimer's disease.
      ii. Behavioral symptoms which precede cognitive ones suggest a frontotemporal dementia.
   b. **Course: a stepwise decline is more consistent with a vascular dementia,** whereas a gradual deterioration suggests a disorder such as Alzheimer's disease.
   c. **Associated symptoms** may favor a particular diagnosis; e.g., incontinence and gait apraxia are seen in normal pressure hydrocephalus (NPH).

   d. **Associated psychiatric symptoms,** such as hallucinations, paranoia or personality change, may also implicate a particular diagnosis.
2. **Review of systems** should be completed and include incontinence, gait disturbance, and falls.
3. **A past medical history may reveal risk factors** for stroke (hypertension, obesity, hypercholesterolemia, cigarette smoking, diabetes mellitus, postmenopausal status) or other general medical or neurologic etiologies.
4. **A past psychiatric history may suggest comorbid illness,** such as depression or alcohol abuse, particularly if prior episodes of psychiatric illness are elicited.
5. **Medications are implicated in up to 30% of cases of dementia. Common offenders include anticholinergics, antihypertensives, psychotropics, sedative-hypnotics, and narcotic analgesics.** Any drug is suspect if its first prescription and initiation of symptoms are temporally related.
6. **Family history is a significant risk factor for developing certain dementias, including Alzheimer's disease and frontal dementia.**
7. **A social and occupational history** is useful when assessing premorbid intelligence and education (both of which may confound cognitive screens for dementia) as well as a change in the level of function.

C. Physical Examination

1. A **general medical examination,** with a particular focus on the cardiovascular system, is an essential part of the evaluation of dementia. Endocrine, inflammatory, and infectious etiologies, for example, may also be suggested by physical findings.

2. A **complete neurologic examination,** including function of the cranial nerves, sensory and motor function, deep-tendon reflexes, and cerebellar function, can reveal focal findings which may suggest a vascular dementia or degenerative process (e.g., Parkinson's disease).

3. **Vision and hearing screening** may reveal losses which can masquerade as, or exacerbate, cognitive decline.

D. Psychiatric examination
may reveal evidence of delirium, depression, or psychosis. **On formal mental status testing, such as with the Folstein Mini-Mental State Examination** (MMSE; Table 7-2) **or other supplemental tests** (see Table 7-3), **documentation of particular findings, in addition to the overall score, allows cognitive function to be followed over time.**

E. Laboratory Evaluation

1. **Guidelines established by the American Academy of Neurology for the evaluation of dementia include:** **electrolytes, glucose, blood urea nitrogen (BUN) and creatinine, and liver function tests (which are often included in a comprehensive metabolic panel, or Chem-20); a complete blood count; tests of thyroid function; a vitamin B12 level; and syphilis serology. The likelihood of detecting a reversible cause of dementia with this screen is generally less than 10%. A computed tomography (CT) scan of the brain,** without contrast, can also be useful to rule out a subdural hematoma, hydrocephalus, stroke, or tumor.

2. **Additional investigations are indicated if the initial workup is uninformative, if a particular diagnosis is suspected, or if the presentation is atypical** (see Table 7-4). Such investigations are particularly important in young patients with rapid progression of dementia.

   a. **Neuropsychological testing may be useful,** and is essential in cases where a patient's deficits are mild or difficult to characterize. Briefer **screens, such as the Folstein Mini-Mental State Examination, have poor sensitivity and specificity for dementia, particularly in highly educated or intelligent patients. The MMSE also fails to assess executive function and praxis.**

   b. **Magnetic resonance imaging (MRI)** of the brain is more sensitive for recent stroke and should be consid-

Table 7-2. Folstein Mini-Mental State Examination

Task	Instructions	Scoring
Date: orientation	"Tell me the date"	One point each for year, season, date, day of the week, month
Place: orientation	"Where are you?"	One point each for state, county, town, building, floor/room
Register three objects	Name three objects, ask patient to repeat them	One point for each correctly repeated
Serial sevens	Ask the patient to count backwards from 100 by 7. Stop after five answers. (Or ask patient to spell "WORLD" backwards)	One point for each correct answer or letter
Recall three objects	Ask the patient to recall the registered objects	One point for each correct object
Naming	Point to watch, ask "What is this?" Repeat with a pencil	One point for each correct answer
Repeating a phrase	Ask patient to say, "No ifs, ands, or buts"	One point if successful on first try
Verbal commands	Give the patient a piece of paper, and say, "Take this paper in your right hand, fold it in half, and put it on the floor"	One point for each correct action (out of three total)
Written commands	Show the patient a piece of paper with the words "CLOSE YOUR EYES"	One point if the patient's eyes close
Writing	Ask the patient to write a sentence	One point if the sentence has subject, verb, and makes sense
Drawing	Ask the patient to copy a pair of intersecting pentagons	One point if the figure has ten corners, two intersecting lines
		Total number of points: 30

Table 7-3. Supplemental Mental State Testing for Patients with Dementia

Area	Test
Memory	Recall name and address: "John Brown, 42 Market Street, Chicago"
	Recall three unusual words: "tulip, umbrella, fear"
Language	Naming parts: "lab coat: lapel, sleeve, cuff; watch: band, face, crystal"
	Complex commands: "Before pointing to the door, point to the ceiling"
	Word-list: "In one minute, name all the animals you can think of"
Praxis	"Show me how you would slice a loaf of bread"; "Show me how you brush your teeth"
Visuospatial	"Draw a clock face with numbers, and mark the hands to say 11:10"
Abstraction	"How is an apple like a banana?"; "How is a canal different from a river?"; proverb interpretation

Table 7-4. Supplemental Laboratory Investigations

What	When	Why
Neuropsychological testing	Patient's deficits are mild or difficult to characterize	The sensitivity of the MMSE for dementia is poor, particularly in highly educated or intelligent patients (who can compensate for deficits)
Lumbar puncture (including routine studies and cytology)	Known or suspected cancer, immunosuppression, suspected CNS infection or vasculitis, hydrocephalus by CT, rapid or atypical course	Look for infection, elevated pressure, abnormal proteins
MRI with gadolinium	Any atypical findings on neurologic exam	More sensitive than CT for tumor, stroke
EEG	Suspected toxic-metabolic encephalopathy, partial complex seizures, Creutzfeldt-Jakob disease	Look for diffuse slowing (encephalopathy) vs. focal seizure activity
HIV testing	Risk factors or opportunistic infections	Up to 20% of patients with HIV infection develop dementia, although it is unusual for dementia to be the presenting sign
Heavy metal screening, screening for Wilson's disease or autoimmune disease	Suggested by history, physical exam, laboratory findings	May be reversible

ered when focal findings are detected on the neurologic examination.

c. An **electroencephalogram (EEG)** may be used to identify toxic-metabolic encephalopathy, partial complex seizures, or Creutzfeldt-Jakob disease.

d. A **lumbar puncture** may be informative when cancer, infection of the central nervous system (CNS), hydrocephalus, or vasculitis is suspected.

e. **Testing for human immunodeficiency virus (HIV)** is indicated in patients with appropriate risk factors, as up to 20% of patients with HIV infection develop dementia. However, dementia is uncommon as a *presenting* sign of HIV infection.

f. **Heavy metal screening,** as well as tests for Wilson's disease or autoimmune diseases, should be reserved for patients in which these etiologies are suspected.

V. Alzheimer's Disease (Dementia of the Alzheimer's Type)

A. Diagnosis

A diagnosis of probable Alzheimer's disease (AD) is made when a patient meets the criteria for dementia as above and has **a gradual and progressive course,** once other etiologies have been ruled out. A definite diagnosis of Alzheimer's disease requires histopathologic confirmation and is generally made at postmortem examination.

In the early stages of Alzheimer's disease a patient typically develops subtle **loss of short-term memory**. Subsequently, the individual becomes lost easily and develops **word-finding and naming difficulty**, which results in vague speech, circumlocution, and the use of clichés. At the same time the individual may develop **apraxias** that affect such motor tasks as dressing and eating, and visual-spatial impairments that are apparent when driving or performing similar tasks. Finally, in the late stages, **judgment becomes impaired**, and the patient may develop personality changes, such as apathy or hostility and social withdrawal. Disturbed sleep-wake patterns are also typical at this stage.

Psychiatric symptoms are often prominent in Alzheimer's disease. Depression and anxiety may be presenting complaints; they are seen in up to 40% of cases. **Delusions** are also common, affecting up to 50% of patients; delusions often relate to theft or to other family members. **Hallucinations,** which are most often visual, affect up to 25% of patients with AD. **Agitation** is also a frequent symptom.

B. Risk Factors

Major risk factors for Alzheimer's disease include increasing age and positive family history; other risk factors include a history of head trauma and Down's syndrome. The genetic component of Alzheimer's disease is suggested by the fact that up to 50% of those with a first-degree relative with the disease will themselves be affected by the age of 90 years. **Three chromosomes have been linked to development of early-onset Alzheimer's disease:**

1. **Trisomy 21, or chromosome 21 mutations;** Down's syndrome patients older than age 30 years show Alzheimer's disease pathology in nearly all cases.
2. **Chromosome 14** contains the presenilin 1 gene; mutations here account for most cases of familial early-onset Alzheimer's disease.
3. **Chromosome 1** contains the presenilin 2 gene; mutations here have been associated with Alzheimer's disease in families from the Volga River area in Russia.

Nonetheless, **these mutations account for fewer than 5% of cases of Alzheimer's disease.** Additional **"vulnerability genes" have been identified for Alzheimer's disease; chief among them is the *ApoE-4* allele, which is associated with an increased risk for Alzheimer's disease and with an earlier age of onset.**

C. Histopathology

The typical histopathologic changes in Alzheimer's disease include senile plaques and neurofibrillary tangles. Plaques are extracellular and contain β-amyloid; tangles are intracellular and contain cytoskeletal filaments. Other changes include synaptic degeneration and loss of cortical and subcortical neurons, particularly in the hippocampus, cortex, and nucleus basalis. **Neuron loss occurs first in the entorhinal cortex and the nucleus basalis.**

Neuron loss affects a number of neurotransmitter systems. However, **death of cholinergic neurons in the basal forebrain causes a particularly prominent decrease in levels of cortical acetylcholine.**

The role of imaging in the diagnosis of Alzheimer's disease is not yet clear. On positron-emission tomography (PET) scans, for example, parietal and temporal lobe hypometabolism is typically seen.

D. Course

The average **survival after the onset of symptoms in Alzheimer's disease is 8–10 years.** Predictors of more rapid institutionalization or death include the presence of extrapyramidal signs, the presence of psychotic symptoms, young age at onset, current cognitive dysfunction, and prior duration of illness.

VI. Other Selected Etiologies

A. Vascular dementia (formerly referred to as multi-infarct dementia) accounts for up to 20% of cases of dementia.

1. **Typical features include a stepwise progression of cognitive deficits and associated focal signs and symptoms** (e.g., deficits in sensory or motor function). Clinically, these features are often incorporated into an "ischemic score"; the diagnosis is confirmed by brain imaging.
2. **Risk factors** are those associated with vascular disease, vasculitis, or embolic disease (including atrial fibrillation).
3. A single strategically placed infarct, multiple infarcts, or white matter ischemia may all yield dementia; overall, **stroke yields a nine-fold increased risk of dementia.** The clinical significance of "periventricular white matter changes" or Binswanger's disease, commonly noted on imaging studies, is not yet well established.
4. **Treatment of vascular dementia focuses on secondary prevention by addressing underlying risk factors.** Anticoagulation, with coumadin or aspirin, is often utilized.

B. Dementia with Lewy bodies (DLB) may be more prevalent than previously recognized; postmortem studies reveal the presence of Lewy bodies in up to 25% of dementia cases.

1. Clinically, DLB shares features of both Alzheimer's disease and Parkinson's disease. A patient with

DLB may suffer repeated falls and be unusually sensitive to adverse effects of typical neuroleptics. Common psychiatric symptoms include depression and systematized delusions. **In addition to progressive cognitive decline, the consensus criteria for clinical diagnosis require at least two of the following for a probable diagnosis:**
  a. **Recurrent visual hallucinations,** which are often well formed.
  b. **Parkinsonism.**
  c. **Fluctuating cognition,** with variation in attention and alertness.

2. **Risk factors** for DLB are not yet well understood, but some studies suggest a genetic predisposition may be important. The disease is more prevalent in males by a factor of 2:1; the age at onset varies from 50 to 80 years.

3. **The typical neuropathologic finding in DLB is the Lewy body, a round, eosinophilic intraneuronal inclusion.** Lewy bodies may be found in both cortical and subcortical structures. Of note, Lewy bodies are also detected in many cases of Alzheimer's and Parkinson's disease, as well as in a small number of otherwise well elderly individuals.

4. No specific treatment for DLB has yet emerged, although patients may respond to cholinergic agents (see below).

C. **Frontotemporal dementias** comprise a spectrum of disorders including **Pick's disease.**

1. **Unlike most other dementias which present initially with cognitive change, frontal lobe dementia presents insidiously with behavioral changes. Common psychiatric symptoms include depression, anxiety, and delusions. Language impairments are also seen, including abundant speech and echolalia or repetition. Other typical changes include:**
  a. Decline in personal hygiene
  b. Disinhibition and impaired social awareness
  c. Impulsivity
  d. Inflexibility and rigidity
  e. Repetitive behaviors, particularly involving an obsessive focus on certain foods

2. Typically the age of onset is between 40 and 70 years; a family history of early-onset dementia is often present. In some familial cases linkage has been shown to chromosome 17.

3. Neuropathologic changes typically include intraneuronal inclusions, known as Pick bodies, and loss of cortical neurons, particularly in the frontal and anterior temporal lobes. Structural neuroimaging demonstrates atrophy in these areas; SPECT (single photon emission computed tomography) studies often reveal frontal lobe hypoperfusion.

4. **Treatment** relies on management of behavior.

D. **Normal pressure hydrocephalus typically presents with a "magnetic gait" followed by urinary incontinence and then dementia.** Particular cognitive deficits include impaired concentration and mild memory deficits. On head CT, ventriculomegaly and diffuse cortical atrophy may be noted. Diagnosis relies on clinical improvement following serial lumbar punctures (LPs), known as the Miller Fisher test. If a patient benefits from LPs, ventriculoperitoneal shunting sometimes provides more persistent improvement.

E. **Parkinson's disease is associated with dementia in up to 70% of cases.** However, significant cognitive dysfunction usually occurs later in the disease course. A number of other dementias (including Huntington's disease, progressive supranuclear palsy, and corticobasal degeneration) manifest both neurologic and psychiatric features.

VII. Prevention

Prevention of dementia remains an active area of investigation. Some studies suggest that NSAIDs (nonsteroidal anti-inflammatory drugs), but not acetaminophen or aspirin, and estrogen replacement may reduce the relative risk of developing Alzheimer's disease, or delay its onset.

VIII. Treatment

A. **Reversible etiologies should be addressed first.** Thus, any comorbid medical problems identified in the initial evaluation must be treated, whether or not they contribute directly to the dementia. At the same time, drugs with cognitive side effects should be minimized and eliminated altogether whenever possible; as noted above, medications are implicated in 10–30% of cases of dementia.

B. **Psychosocial or behavioral interventions are essential in treating patients with dementia.**

1. **Educate the patient and the family** in a supportive and caring way, as presentation of an initial diagnosis may be extremely frightening. Seek the family's advice as to how to inform the patient.

2. **Ensure patient safety** by informing both the patient and the family that driving may become impossible.

3. **Address legal issues** (such as wills, health care proxies, and durable power of attorney) **early.**

4. **Suggest assistance with financial management,** such as bill paying.

5. **Continue routine health maintenance** visits every 3–6 months.

6. **When appropriate, raise the possibility of placement,** as nearly 75% of those with dementia will require a long-term care facility. Other options include adult

day care, respite care, home health aides, outreach services, and homemakers.

7. **Address behavioral problems: wandering, agitation, screaming, incontinence, aggression, and psychosis. Most commonly these issues, rather than cognitive decline, precipitate nursing home placement.** Although pharmacotherapy may be beneficial in some cases, behavioral interventions remain a mainstay of treatment.

8. **Care for the caregivers** by providing referral to support groups or other sources of information and coping skills. **Over 50% of caregivers will develop clinically significant depression.**

C. **Pharmacologic treatment should target specific symptoms.** This strategy allows for more accurate assessment of treatment response and course over time. The Folstein Mini-Mental State Examination can be used to approximate cognitive status; similar scales exist for behavioral assessment. **Functional measures include the Activities of Daily Living** (see Table 7-5) **and the Instrumental Activities of Daily Living scales.** However, none of these measures is especially sensitive to change. Clinicians therefore need to attend to particular patient activities, such as hobbies, where treatment effects may be more pronounced.

In treating any geriatric patient, clinicians should in general start medications at low dosages and increase them slowly, paying careful attention to side effects.

1. **Disease-modifying drugs** include free radical inhibitors, such as vitamin E or selegiline, estrogen, and anti-inflammatory drugs, such as NSAIDs.
   a. Vitamin E, selegiline, or both may slow progression of Alzheimer's disease.
   b. Estrogen replacement, in addition to decreasing the relative risk of developing Alzheimer's disease, may slow progression.
   c. NSAIDs, but not acetaminophen or aspirin, have been shown to decrease the relative risk of developing Alzheimer's disease.

2. **Drugs which enhance cognition** in patients with Alzheimer's disease include the cholinesterase inhibitors, tacrine and donepezil. Both have been shown to have modest effects on indices of cognitive function.
   a. **Tacrine** is generally dosed q.i.d. because of its short half-life. Hepatotoxicity may result from its use, and cholinergic effects, such as facial flushing, nausea, vomiting, and diarrhea, may arise.
   b. **Donepezil** is dosed q.d. It has not been associated with hepatotoxicity and it has fewer cholinergic side effects.
   c. **Rivastigmine and eptastigmine** are among the newer cholinesterase inhibitors being tested in ongoing clinical trials.

3. **Drugs which treat psychiatric or behavioral symptoms** are equally important.
   a. For depressive symptoms, SSRIs (selective serotonin reuptake inhibitors) are considered as first-line because of their relative safety.
   b. For hallucinations and psychosis, antipsychotic drugs at low doses may be helpful.
   c. Agitation and anxiety may respond to SSRIs or antipsychotics. **Benzodiazepines may cause disinhibition and can further impair cognition.**

D. **Referral** to a specialist in geriatric psychiatry or neuropsychiatry can be helpful in certain circumstances. **Patients with atypical presentations, with unusual symptoms or rapid progression, as well as those in whom no etiology can be identified, should be referred.** In some cases families may request a referral, particularly when they are interested in participating in a research protocol.

Selected Readings

Cummings JL, Vinters HV, Cole GM, Khachaturian ZS: Alzheimer's disease: etiologies, pathophysiology, cognitive reserve, and treatment opportunities. *Neurology* 1998; 51:S2–S17.

Falk WE, Albert MA: Dementia. In Cassem NH, Stern TA, Rosenbaum JF, et al. (eds): *Massachusetts General Hospital Handbook of General Hospital Psychiatry*, 4th ed. St. Louis: Mosby, 1997:123–147.

Kaye JA: Diagnostic challenges in dementia. *Neurology* 1998; 51: S45–S52.

Papka MP, Rubio A, Schiffer RB: A review of Lewy body disease, an emerging concept of cortical dementia. *J Neuropsychiatry Clin Neurosci* 1998; 10:267–279.

Small GW: Alzheimer's disease and other dementing disorders. In Kaplan HI, Sadock BJ (eds): *Comprehensive Textbook of Psychiatry*, 6th ed. Baltimore: Williams & Wilkins, 1995:2562–2565.

Table 7-5. Activities of Daily Living	
Basic	*Instrumental*
Bathing	Shopping
Dressing	Cooking
Walking	Managing finances
Toileting	Housework
Feeding	Using telephone
Transfers (to/from bed, chair)	Taking medications Traveling outside of home

Chapter 8
Mental Retardation

JOHN N. JULIAN

I. Overview

A. Historical Perspective on Mental Retardation

Although mental retardation and psychiatric illness have had a shared ancestry with a divergent course, they were viewed quite differently in the middle ages. In the 16th century the English Court of Wards and Liveries clearly differentiated "idiots" from "lunatics." Kraepelin in his initial diagnostic scheme listed mental retardation as a distinct form of psychiatric illness. It was not until the late 19th century that mental retardation and psychiatric illness were noted to coexist. The phrase "imbecility with insanity" was noted in the *American Journal of Insanity* in 1888. Since then, mental retardation and psychiatric illness have continued to be investigated but not at the rate at which other areas of psychiatry have developed.

B. Modern Investigations Regarding the Relationship Between Mental Retardation and Psychiatric Illness

1. Several hypotheses have been formulated to explain why individuals with cognitive impairment seem to be at increased risk for psychiatric disorders.
2. With the occurrence of the "Decade of the Brain" and a shift in focus towards neurodevelopmental psychiatry, the relationship between mental retardation and psychiatric illness has generated more interest. Future investigation in this area is likely to shed light on complex issues; e.g., behavioral phenotypes and the relationship between coping abilities and the vulnerability to mental illness.

II. Epidemiology

A. Prevalence

1. **The prevalence of mental retardation is between 1% and 3%** depending on the criteria used, the methods used, and the populations sampled; most investigators believe the prevalence is probably closer to 1%.
2. Mental retardation is a condition with diverse etiologies; **more than 350 causes of mental retardation are known.**
3. However, approximately 40% of cases have no clear etiology.
4. **The three most common causes of mental retardation account for about 30% of identified cases.** They include:

   a. **Down's syndrome** (chromosome 21), which is the most common genetic cause of mental retardation.

   b. **The fragile X syndrome** (X-linked gene *FMR-1*), which is the most common inherited cause of mental retardation.

   c. **The fetal alcohol syndrome** (with triad of growth retardation, developmental delay, and classical facial features), which is the third most common known cause of mental retardation.

B. Comorbid Psychopathology

1. **The mentally retarded population suffers from the full range of psychiatric illness,** and likely is afflicted at a higher rate than the general population.

   a. Some studies estimate that **the prevalence of psychiatric disorders is 4–6 times that of the general population.**

   b. In institutional settings upwards of 10% of the mentally retarded population have some form of psychopathology; percentages are less clear in community samples. One must be cautious of methodological problems when interpreting data regarding this population.

C. Etiology of Psychopathology in the Mentally Retarded

1. Why there appears to be a higher prevalence of psychiatric illness in the mentally retarded population is unclear.

   a. One theory centers on the idea that mental retardation is a manifestation of damage to cortical and subcortical substrate, regardless of whether this damage can be identified with available technology. This damage confers a special vulnerability to psychiatric conditions.

   b. Another theory holds that individuals with mental retardation are chronically exposed to a confusing and stressful world, based on their decreased ability to cope with the demands of a complex society and an inadequate cognitive capacity to resolve emotional conflicts. This constant stress leads to increased psychiatric pathology.

   c. A third theory highlights the lack of psychiatric care in this population. It questions the psychiatric profession's unwillingness to treat psychiatric illness in the mentally retarded due to a prevailing view that behavioral disturbance and psychopathology is somehow more acceptable in individuals with mental retardation.

55

III. Diagnostic Features

A. Definition

1. The definition of mental retardation comes from work done by the American Association on Mental Retardation; it has basically been adopted by DSM-IV.
   a. **"Mental retardation refers to substantial limitations in present functioning. It is characterized by significantly subaverage intellectual functioning, existing concurrently with related limitations ... [in several adaptive areas and] ... manifests before age 18."**
   b. In more objective terms, **mental retardation is defined by having a standardized IQ score at least two standard deviations below the mean and impairment in at least two out of ten areas of adaptive functioning when compared to peers of the same age and culture.** The areas identified include: communication, self-care, home living, social/interpersonal skills, use of community resources, self-direction, functional academic skills, work, leisure, health, and safety. However, it should be kept in mind that these domains were not empirically selected and no single measure of adaptive function exists.

B. Classification of Mental Retardation

1. Mental retardation is classified into four levels of severity based on intellectual impairment as measured by IQ scores. These categories do not reflect functional capabilities; they have a standard error of measurement of approximately 5 points. The levels of severity, their IQ ranges, and their prevalence within the mentally retarded population are as follows:
   a. **Mild** (IQ 55–70): 85%
   b. **Moderate** (IQ 40–55): 10%
   c. **Severe** (IQ 25–40): 3–4%
   d. **Profound** (IQ < 25): 1–2%
2. A substantial proportion of individuals diagnosed with mild mental retardation as children lose this diagnosis in adulthood as their adaptive skills improve and with no psychologist around to test them. Those who retain this label into adulthood tend to be affected more severely.

IV. Evaluation and Differential Diagnosis

A. Evaluation

1. The evaluation for a diagnosis of mental retardation is relatively straightforward; it is based on the previously mentioned diagnostic criteria.
2. History of adaptive functioning from ancillary sources like school and primary caregivers and neuropsychiatric and adaptive behavior testing are the cornerstones of evaluation.
3. **A thorough medical and neurological examination is important to rule out correctable causes (including hearing impairment, vision impairment, and seizures) of observed dysfunction.**
4. These exams are also helpful to identify any physical features that may be associated with specific syndromes, as many syndromes have related psychiatric conditions.
5. There are no laboratory findings that are specifically associated with mental retardation.
6. However, some laboratory findings are associated with a variety of causes of mental retardation (e.g., metabolic disturbances and chromosomal abnormalities). It is helpful to identify these if not done previously, as this information can again lead to diagnosis of syndromes that may have associated psychiatric pathology.

B. Differential Diagnosis

1. The differential diagnosis for mental retardation also includes physical disabilities.
2. In addition, specific learning disorders, communication disorders, and borderline intellectual functioning must be considered.
3. Although pervasive developmental disorders (e.g., autism) are a separate diagnostic category, 75–80% of individuals with a pervasive developmental disorder also have comorbid mental retardation.

V. Treatment Considerations

A. Overview

1. It is unlikely that a psychiatrist will be called upon to treat mental retardation per se, as specialized education and training in adaptive functioning is done in schools and vocational settings. It is more likely that a psychiatrist will be called upon to evaluate and treat a psychiatric or behavioral disorder that interferes with adaptive functioning.
2. The evaluation and differential diagnosis of psychiatric illness in this population is not as straightforward as the diagnosis of mental retardation itself. The full range of psychiatric disorders is found in people with mental retardation, at rates that are probably higher than they are in the general population.
3. **There are also certain behavioral disorders and syndrome-associated disorders that occur in people with mental retardation.**
   a. **Syndrome-associated disorders are specific disorders that have a high probability of being exhibited by people with a given syndrome.**
   b. The terms pathobehavorial syndrome and behavioral phenotype are concepts that have been used to try and conceptualize this phenomenon.
4. Finally, one must bear in mind that definitive diagnosis is both clinically and methodologically a chal-

lenge. This is often due to limited self-reporting by a substantial proportion of the population.

B. Traditional Psychiatric Disorders

What follows is a brief synopsis of traditional psychiatric disorders, behavioral disorders, and syndrome-associated disorders that present in the mentally retarded. In each category, differences in their presentation, if any, and any special treatment considerations will be highlighted.

1. **Affective disorders**
   a. **Depression and bipolar spectrum disorders may present differently in the mentally retarded population, with less subjective reporting and more reliance on change from baseline behavior, than they do in the general population.** Observable mood changes, accompanied by quantifiable neurovegetative symptoms using sleep charts and calorie counts, are helpful. Behavioral difficulties may be primary in those with severe mental retardation.
   b. Treatment can involve both medication and therapy, with the type of therapy chosen based on the individual's strengths. Medication with a high anticholinergic load should be avoided if possible, due to the potential of anticholinergic agents to cause cognitive blunting.

2. **Anxiety disorders**
   a. The full spectrum of anxiety disorders has been reported in the mentally retarded population. **Somatic, more observable aspects of anxiety are often more helpful than is reliance on self-report.** The possibility of trauma must always be considered given the vulnerability of the population. Obsessive-compulsive disorder (OCD) is difficult to distinguish from stereotypy given the critical need for self-reported ego-dystonic feelings.
   b. Treatment consists of behavior therapy and medication. Benzodiazepines may be used, but their potential for disinhibition should be considered.

3. **Schizophrenia**
   a. The co-occurrence of schizophrenia with mental retardation has been noted since the days of Kraepelin and Bleuler. However, diagnostic clarity remains a problem. Observable behaviors related to psychosis must be present in addition to the chronic changes in baseline function associated with major mental illness.
   b. Antipsychotics are the drugs of choice; newer, atypical agents cause fewer extrapyramidal symptoms. While the overuse of neuroleptics has been a problem in the past, it is not clear that extrapyramidal symptoms are worse or more prevalent in the mentally retarded population.

C. Behavioral Disorders

1. **Aggression**
   a. **Aggression is one of the prime reasons for institutionalization and for consultation in the mentally retarded population.** Pain and discomfort, as well as environmental triggers and/or psychopathology, can precipitate aggression.
   b. Behavioral treatment is usually a first-line intervention for aggression, followed by use of medication for any underlying psychiatric disorder or impulse control disorder.

2. **Self-Injurious Behavior**
   a. Self-injurious behavior (SIB) either potentially causes or actually causes physical damage to an individual's body. It usually presents as idiosyncratic, repetitive acts that occur in an identical form.
   b. Behavior therapy is the mainstay of treatment, but medications (e.g., selective serotonin reuptake inhibitors [SSRIs] and neuroleptics with potent D-I blockade) which address compulsive acts have been reported to be successful.

3. **Stereotypy**
   a. **Stereotypies are invariant, pathologic, motor behaviors or action sequences without an obvious reinforcement pattern. They are often seen in circumstances of extreme stimulation or deprivation, and are noted in many institutionalized mentally retarded adults.**
   b. Behavior therapy is the primary treatment; SSRIs have been tried but have yet to be evaluated in a rigorous manner.

4. **Copraxia**
   a. **Copraxia involves rectal digging, feces smearing, and coprophagia.** It is a rare phenomenon that is usually **only found in the profoundly retarded population.**
   b. Behavior therapy is the first line of treatment after medical conditions are ruled out.

5. **Pica**
   a. Pica involves eating inedibles (e.g., dirt, paperclips, and cigarette butts). It usually occurs in severely retarded individuals.
   b. Behavior therapy is the mainstay of treatment. It is unclear that dietary supplements are helpful.

6. **Rumination**
   a. Rumination involves repeated acts of vomiting, chewing, and reingestion of the vomitus. This condition occurs more often in the severely to profoundly retarded population.
   b. Behavior therapy is the treatment of choice; overfeeding should be included in the differential.

D. Syndrome-Associated Disorders

1. **Down's syndrome (trisomy 21)**
   a. Individuals with Down's syndrome have **a classical physical presentation of round face, a flat nasal bridge, and a short stature.**
   b. **Psychiatric comorbidities include Alzheimer's dementia,** which often begins after the age of 40 years, and depression.

2. **Fragile X syndrome (q27, long arm of X chromosome)**

a. Individuals with the fragile X syndrome present with **a triad of long face, prominent ears, and macro-orchidism.**

b. The full range of psychiatric disorders has been reported but by far **the most prominent comorbidity is attention-deficit/hyperactivity disorder (ADHD), which occurs in approximately 80% of affected individuals.**

c. One-third of female carriers may be mentally retarded.

3. **Prader-Willi syndrome (chromosome 15 deletion, 70% of cases)**

a. Individuals with Prader-Willi syndrome exhibit **a short stature, obesity, hypogonadism, and hyperphagia.**

b. Common comorbidities include OCD and depression.

4. **Williams syndrome (chromosome 7 deletion)**

a. Individuals with Williams syndrome present with **elfin-like faces, a starburst iris, as well as supravalvular aortic stenosis and hypertension.**

b. There is also a loquacious communication style, known as cocktail party speech.

c. Comorbidities include ADHD, anxiety, and depression.

VI. Conclusion

There are several important points to consider in the area of mental retardation and psychiatric illness.

A. Mental retardation is a prevalent condition with diverse etiologies and affects approximately 1% of the population.

B. Three of the most common known causes of mental retardation are Down's syndrome, fragile X syndrome, and fetal alcohol syndrome.

C. People with mental retardation are susceptible to the full range of psychiatric illness and likely suffer psychiatric illness at a higher rate than do those in the general population.

D. Certain pathobehavioral syndromes are unique to the mentally retarded population.

E. Individuals with mental retardation are an incredibly underserved population when it comes to psychiatric services, both from a clinical and research perspective.

Suggested Readings

American Psychiatric Association: *Diagnostic and Statistical Manual of Mental Disorders, Fourth Edition.* Washington, DC: American Psychiatric Association, 1994.

Bergman JD, Harris JC: Mental retardation. In Kaplan HI, Sadock BJ (eds): *Comprehensive Textbook of Psychiatry,* 6th ed. Baltimore: Williams and Wilkins, 1995.

Gualtieri CT: *Neuropsychiatry and Behavioral Pharmacology.* New York: Springer-Verlag, 1990.

King BH, State MW, Shah B, Davanzo P, Dykens E: Mental retardation: a review of the past 10 years. Part I. *J Am Acad Child Adolesc Psychiatry* 1997; 36:1656–1663.

Russell AT, Tanguay PE: Mental retardation. In Lewis M (ed.): *Child and Adolescent Psychiatry A Comprehensive Textbook,* 2nd ed. Baltimore: Williams and Wilkins, 1996.

State MW, King BH, Dykens E: Mental retardation: a review of the past 10 years. *J Am Acad Child Adolesc Psychiatry* 1997; 36: 1664–1671.

Volkmar FR (ed): Mental retardation. *Child Adolesc Psychiatr Clin North Am.* Philadelphia: WB Saunders, 1996; 5(4).

Chapter 9

Mental Disorders Due to a General Medical Condition

B.J. Beck

I. Introduction

A. Definition

1. **DSM-IV definition: Mental Disorders Due to a General Medical Condition (DTGMC) are psychiatric symptoms thought to be the direct, physiologic consequence of a nonpsychiatric, medical condition.** The psychiatric symptoms themselves are severe enough to warrant recognition, and treatment, as a problem. This terminology is an attempt to replace the previously used functional versus organic dichotomy, and its unfortunate suggestion that the former has no biologic or physiologic basis, or that the latter is unaffected by psychosocial or environmental influences.

2. **General qualifiers. The mental disorder must:**
   a. **Be the direct pathophysiologic consequence of the medical condition.**
   b. **Not be better accounted for by another, primary mental disorder.**
   c. **Not occur solely during the course of delirium (i.e., a disturbance of consciousness in association with cognitive deficits).**
   d. **Not meet criteria for dementia (i.e., a syndrome with memory impairment and aphasia, apraxia, agnosia, or disturbances of executive function).**
   e. **Not be substance-induced.**

B. Disorders

1. **Mental Disorder DTGMC should be part of the differential diagnosis for any psychiatric syndrome.** Alterations in cognition, behavior, or perception look much the same whether they derive from primary mental disorders, toxins, trauma, tumors, or seizures. For this reason, all but three of the individual disorders are listed in DSM-IV with disorders of similar symptomatology. These disorders are listed below, under the chapter titles in which they are located in DSM-IV:
   a. Delirium, Dementia, Amnestic, and Other Cognitive Disorders
      i. **Delirium DTGMC**
      ii. **Dementia DTGMC**
      iii. **Amnestic Disorder DTGMC**
   b. Schizophrenia and Other Psychotic Disorders
      i. **Psychotic Disorder DTGMC**
   c. Mood Disorders
      i. **Mood Disorder DTGMC**
   d. Anxiety Disorders
      i. **Anxiety Disorder DTGMC**
   e. Sexual Disorders
      i. **Sexual Dysfunction DTGMC**
   f. Sleep Disorders
      i. **Sleep Disorder DTGMC**

2. **Three diagnostic categories do not meet criteria for a psychiatric disorder,** and are listed separately in the chapter, Mental Disorders DTGMC:
   a. **Catatonic Disorder DTGMC**
   b. **Personality Change DTGMC** (coded on Axis I, not Axis II)
   c. **Mental Disorder Not Otherwise Specified (NOS) DTGMC**

II. Psychiatric Differential Diagnosis

A. Primary Mental Disorders

1. **It may be difficult to ascertain whether the mental disorder in question is the direct physiologic consequence of the medical condition, or whether the two merely coexist. Correlation between the onset or severity of the medical and mental conditions is helpful, but inadequate, to establish a causal link.**

   Psychiatric symptoms may be the first symptoms of a medical condition (e.g., depression as the first manifestation of pancreatic carcinoma), or be out of proportion to the severity of the medical condition (e.g., depression or irritability in patients with early or minimal sensorimotor symptoms of multiple sclerosis). Alternatively, the psychiatric symptoms may occur late in the course of the medical condition (e.g., psychosis years after the onset of epilepsy), or may not resolve simultaneously with the medical condition (e.g., depression that continues after hypothyroidism is corrected).

   When treatment of the general medical condition does dissipate the psychiatric symptoms, an etiologic relationship is supported. However, some mental disorders DTGMC are amenable to, and require, treatment in their own right (e.g., interictal depression); this does not imply the diagnosis of primary mental disorder.

2. **Atypical features of primary mental disorder support an etiologic relationship to the medical condition:**
   a. **Age of onset:** e.g., first onset panic attacks in a 65-year-old man
   b. **Course:** e.g., sudden onset of depression
   c. **Associated features:** e.g., cognitive deficits out of proportion to mildly depressed mood

3. **Typical features of the primary mental disorder** suggest that conditions may coexist:

   a. **Recurrent past episodes** (in the absence of the medical condition)
   b. **Positive family history**
4. **The scientific literature supports the causal relationship between some medical conditions and the occurrence of certain psychiatric symptoms.** That is, there is a greater than base-rate occurrence for a mental syndrome in patients with a particular medical condition, compared with an appropriate control group. Or, a mental syndrome may correlate with expected **deficits or symptoms based on the location of brain pathology** or pathophysiology (e.g., disinhibition or decreased executive function with frontal lobe damage). Although such studies may support the causal relationship between medical and mental disorders, the **diagnosis for a given patient must be considered individually.** Less stringent, but helpful, are individual **case studies** which suggest a link between a given medical condition and a mental disorder.

B. Substance-Induced Disorders
Prescription and over-the-counter medications, illicit drugs, or alcohol may be used, misused, or abused during the course of a general medical condition. **A careful history, and possibly the use of urine or blood tests, should alert the clinician to drug use and abuse and be part of every evaluation.** Use, intoxication, or withdrawal can cause mental symptoms which continue for up to a month after discontinuation of a substance. The therapeutic use of some medications causes psychiatric symptoms (e.g., steroids in a patient with systemic lupus erythematosus) that mimic the symptoms of the disease itself (e.g., mood lability).

C. If mental symptoms seem to be substance-induced *and* DTGMC, both conditions should be coded.

D. If one is not sure whether a mental disorder is due to a general medical condition, a primary mental disorder, or is substance-induced, the NOS code should be used.

III. General Medical Conditions

The mnemonic, GENeral MEDical CONDITions (Table 9-1), should help the evaluating clinician recall the broad categories of medical conditions that can cause psychiatric syndromes.

A. Infectious Diseases
Infection of the central nervous system (CNS), and especially the chronic meningitides, are increasingly prevalent as immune suppression is on the rise, either from acquired immunodeficiency syndrome (AIDS) or as a result of immune suppressant therapy for malignancy or organ transplantation.

Table 9-1. Categories of General Medical Conditions

GENeral MEDical CONDITions

Germs (infectious diseases)
Epilepsy
Nutritional deficit

Metabolic encephalopathy
Endocrine disorders
Demyelination

Cerebrovascular disease
Offensive toxins
Neoplasm
Degeneration
Immune disease
Trauma

---

1. **Herpes simplex virus (HSV) has a propensity for the temporal and inferomedial frontal lobes,** and is the most commonly encountered focal encephalopathy. Widely recognized to cause a loss of the sense of smell (anosmia), as well as olfactory or gustatory hallucinations, the limbic distribution of HSV may also result in psychosis, bizarre behavior, or personality change. These personality changes, along with affective lability and decreased cognitive function, may persist. Simple or complex partial seizures may also develop.

2. **Human immunodeficiency virus (HIV) infection is associated with neuropsychiatric symptoms of multiple etiologies, including, but not limited to, direct CNS infection** (e.g., HIV-related metabolic derangements, endocrinopathies, medication side effects, tumors, opportunistic infections). **Accepted terms for the neuropsychiatric syndromes of HIV CNS infection (e.g., HIV-1-associated cognitive/motor complex, AIDS dementia complex, dementia due to HIV disease)** are inadequate descriptors for the range of reported symptoms. The presence, severity, and location of HIV-related CNS pathology does not correlate particularly well with the reported symptoms. Besides the deficits suggested by the above terms (i.e., cognitive deficits: attention, concentration, and visuospatial performance; motor deficits: fine motor control and speed; and dementia: short-term memory loss, word-finding difficulties, and poor executive function), patients may experience depressed mood, apathy, social withdrawal, and a lack of energy, motivation, or spontaneity. Although much less common, mania

and hypomania have also been reported. Psychosis is rarely reported as a new syndrome; when present, it generally occurs in the setting of advanced disease.

3. **Rabies, an acute viral disease of the mammalian CNS, is most often transmitted by exposure to infected saliva through an animal bite.** Rare in the United States, human rabies is more commonly seen following domestic animal bites received during foreign travel. The virus travels centripetally along peripheral nerves to the CNS. The distance the virus travels, along with size of innoculum and degree of host defenses, is thought to be responsible for the extreme variability in incubation period, from 10 days to a year; the mean incubation period is 1–2 months.

   The initial prodrome is similar to that of other viral illnesses, except for the distinct feature of local fasciculations or paresthesias at the inoculation site. Once rabies proceeds to acute encephalitis, brainstem dysfunction, coma, and death usually follow within 4–20 days. The encephalitis is heralded by agitation and motor excitation, followed by periods of confusion, psychosis, and combativeness which may initially be interspersed with lucid periods. Half of infected individuals experience painful, violent spasms of the diaphragm, laryngeal, pharyngeal, and accessory respiratory muscles when attempting to swallow liquids, which leads to classic hydrophobia. There is autonomic dysfunction, upper motor neuron weakness and paralysis, cranial nerve involvement, and often vocal cord paralysis.

4. **Lyme disease is a tick-borne spirochetal infection** most common in parts of Europe and the United States (especially the Northeast, upper Midwest, and Pacific Coastal states). **Because of the confusing array, and unreliable results, of serologic tests, as well as the prolonged, recurrent, and nonspecific nature of the symptoms, the clinician must have a high level of awareness of the neuropsychiatric sequelae of Lyme disease.** Diagnosis may require both Lyme ELISA (enzyme-linked immunosorbent assay) and Lyme Western blot, as well as polymerase chain reaction assay (PCR) or culture.

   A flu-like syndrome and rash (erythema migrans) usually follow the initial tick (*Ixodes scapularis*) bite, with hematogenous spread taking place over days to weeks. Once lodged in the target organs (heart, eyes, joints, muscles, peripheral or central nervous system), the organism (*Borrelia burgdorferi*) may lie dormant for months to years, at which point memory of the initial event has often dimmed. Diagnostic delay is associated with a more chronic course, but **even with early, aggressive, antibiotic**

treatment, symptoms may recur or develop months to years later.

Lyme encephalitis may present with fatigue, mood lability, irritability, confusion, and sleep disturbance. Much less common, encephalomyelitis may mimic multiple sclerosis. **A more chronic encephalopathy may develop with a large range of disturbances in personality, cognition** (short-term memory, memory retrieval, verbal fluency, concentration and attention, orientation, processing speed), **behavior** (disorganization, distractibility, catatonia, mutism, violence), **mood** (depression, mania, lability), **thought processes** (paranoia), and **perception** (hallucinations, depersonalization, hyperacusis, photophobia). Strokes, seizures, and severe dementia are rare sequelae of neurologic Lyme disease.

5. **Neurosyphilis, of the symptomatic, parenchymal, general paretic type, is a form of late (tertiary) syphilis seen in less than 10% of untreated syphilitics, 20 years after primary infection.** Even more rare in the postpenicillin era, **general paresis may be on the rise among individuals with AIDS.** Antibiotics have also changed the classical picture, and patients may have mixed, more subtle, symptoms of late syphilis. With diffuse, but particularly frontal lobe involvement, signs and symptoms of general paresis (Table 9-2) include personality change, irritability, poor judgment and insight, difficulty with calculations and recent memory, apathy, and decreased personal grooming. **If untreated, mood lability, delusions of grandeur, hallucinations, disorientation, and dementia may follow, along with the classical neurological signs of tremor, dysarthria, hyperreflexia, hypotonia, ataxia, and Argyll Robertson pupils (small, irregular, unequal pupils that accommodate, but do not react to light).** Cerebral spinal fluid with elevated protein

---

Table 9-2. Manifestations of General Paresis

PARESIS

Personality

Affect

Reflexes (hyperactive)

Eye (Argyll Robertson pupils)

Sensorium (illusions, delusions, hallucinations)

Intellect (decreased recent memory, orientation, calculation, judgment, and insight)

Speech

SOURCE: Lukehart SA, Holmes KK: Syphilis. In Fauci AS, Braunwald E, Isselbacher KJ, et al. (eds): *Harrison's Principles of Internal Medicine*, 14th ed. New York: McGraw-Hill, 1998:1027.

and lymphocyte count, and positive VDRL, confirms the diagnosis.

6. **Chronic meningitis is a potentially treatable condition that sadly presents with minimal, and subtle, physical signs and symptoms (e.g., low-grade fever, headache) which, especially in the immunocompromised patient, may be overlooked or attributed to an underlying condition (e.g., AIDS).** Likewise, the common psychiatric concomitants (confusion, cognitive dysfunction, memory, and behavioral problems) are nonspecific. **The most common cause of chronic meningitis is *Mycobacterium tuberculosis;*** common fungal agents are cryptococcus and coccidioides.

7. **Chronic and persistent viral or prion diseases of the CNS** are included here more for historic, rather than practical, significance. These tend to be increasingly rare disorders that, once manifest, lead unalterably to death in a matter of months to a few years. The neurologic signs may lag behind the psychiatric symptoms, but are so extreme and rapidly debilitating that they are unlikely to be attributed to primary mental disorders.

   a. **Subacute sclerosing panencephalitis (SSPE) occurs in children and adolescents (usually before age 11 years) following previous measles (rubeola) infection or, rarely, measles vaccination.** SSPE has steadily declined since the advent of widespread measles vaccination. With a predilection for males (3:1, male/female), the first signs are often deterioration in school work, distractibility, behavioral change (opposition and temper tantrums), sleepiness, and hallucinations. **Neurological signs, which appear within a few months, include myoclonic jerks, ataxia, seizures, and further intellectual deterioration.** Patients are generally bed-ridden within 6–9 months, and dead within 1–3 years.

   b. **Creutzfeldt-Jakob Disease (CJD) is a rare, and rapidly progressive, fatal, illness of primarily 50–70-year-olds.** Most cases of this prion disease are sporadic, though **5–15% may be familial.** There is also evidence of person-to-person transmission through corneal transplantation, as well as transmission through cadaveric human growth hormone or cadaveric gonadotropins. The hallmarks of the disease, dementia and myoclonus, may be preceded by intellectual decline (memory difficulties, mood instability, poor judgment), sensorimotor disturbance (dizziness, vertigo, gait problems), and perceptual abnormalities (visual illusions or distortions). Hallucinations, delusions, and confusion may follow. Patients become spastic, mute, and stuporous, and usually die in less than a year. Characteristic electroencephalographic (EEG) changes late in the course, along with cortical and cerebellar atrophy seen on head computed tomography (CT) scan, are suggestive of the diagnosis.

   c. **Kuru, or "trembling with fear," is a fatal disorder of progressive dementia and extrapyramidal signs, which was endemic among a particular tribal group of New Guinea highlanders who ate the brains of their dead.** As this ritual cannibalism declined, so did the incidence of Kuru.

B. **Epilepsy is a common (1% lifetime prevalence), neurologic disorder characterized by episodic, disorganized firing of electrical impulses in the cortex of the brain.** The location of these impulses dictates the seizure phenomena, which may include altered consciousness, as well as motor, cognitive, behavioral, affective, perceptual, and/or memory disturbances. Seizures were often considered to be emotional problems prior to the use of the EEG which demonstrated a correlation between behavioral and objective findings. It is not surprising that psychiatric and neurologic syndromes were confused; the CNS has only certain, nonspecific, modes of response to stimulation, regardless of the source of the input. However, **seizures remain a clinical diagnosis, which may be supported, but not ruled out, by EEG.**

1. **Complex partial seizures,** often of temporal lobe or other limbic origin, are of particular interest to the psychiatrist. It is estimated that 60% of the roughly 2 million epileptics in the United States have nonconvulsive seizures, which are most commonly partial seizures. Of those with partial seizures, 40% do not show the classic, focal findings on EEG. A high level of suspicion must be maintained by the psychiatrist not to uncritically accept the neurologist's dismissal of the diagnosis based on a "normal" EEG.

   a. **Depression occurs in slightly more than half of patients with epilepsy, as compared to 30% of matched (medical and neurologic outpatient) controls.** The incidence is thought to be even higher in patients with partial complex seizures and left hemispheric foci, which suggests that depression may be caused by seizure-induced limbic dysfunction. **The suicide rate in patients with epilepsy is five times that of the general public; in patients with temporal lobe epilepsy, the risk may be 25-fold higher than in the general population.**

   b. **Anxiety** symptoms are also more closely associated with partial seizures than with other types of seizures. **It may be particularly difficult to differentiate partial seizures from panic attacks.** Both may occur "out of the blue," with hyperarousal, intense fear, perceptual distortion, and dissociative symptoms, such as depersonalization or derealization. Both may be responsive to benzodiazepines. Both may appear to begin with hyperventilation, a common symptom of panic which can also lower the seizure threshold in susceptible individuals. However, in panic disorder, the fear of passing out is common, while the actual loss (or alteration) of consciousness is rare; auditory or visual distortions may occur, but usually not olfactory or gustatory hallucinations; automatisms (chewing or lip-smacking movements) are not common; and there is usually no period of confusion following the episode. Panic attacks generally last 10–20 min, with memory of the event intact. It is precisely this memory that leads to the fear of the next attack and promotes the development of agoraphobia. In contrast, **complex partial seizures often start with cognitive (déjà vu, jamais vu, forced thinking), affective (fear, depression, pleasure) or perceptual (illusions, olfactory or gustatory hallucinations) auras, followed by a brief cessation of activity, then a minute or less of automatismic behavior and unresponsiveness, concluding with a brief period of (less than a minute to a half an hour) lack of, or decreased, awareness. There is often incomplete memory of the episode, and agoraphobia is rare.**

c. **Psychosis** is also more prevalent in patients with complex partial seizures. **The risk of psychosis in patients with epilepsy may be as much as 6–12 times that of the general public. Besides the psychotic symptoms experienced as auras or postictal delirium, there are brief episodic, as well as unremitting, chronic psychoses that are thought to result from subictal, temporal lobe dysrhythmias.** The most common symptoms are hallucinations, paranoia, and thought disorders (e.g., circumstantiality, as opposed to the more common schizophrenic symptoms of thought blocking, derailment, and tangentiality). Psychosis often appears after many years of epilepsy, and may be preceded by personality changes. A notable difference in psychotic presentation is that the epileptic's affect is generally intact and warm, as compared to the affective flattening of the schizophrenic.

d. **Personality symptoms** associated with temporal lobe epilepsy are commonly described, but controversial, and not supported by controlled studies using structured, diagnostic tools. Nonetheless, **the interictal traits reported include hyperreligiosity, hypergraphia, hyposexuality, dependence, obsessionality, and a marked humorlessness.** There is better agreement about **a sticky, or viscous, conversational style that is difficult to disengage.**

e. **Violence should be considered a rare ictal event, which is never an organized, purposeful act.** Episodic dyscontrol is a controversial syndrome, described as recurrent outbursts of uncontrollable rage, in response to minor irritations, which may occur more frequently in patients with early onset of temporal or frontal lobe epilepsy. However, such outbursts are also associated with psychosis and multiple psychosocial, educational, intellectual, socioeconomic, and family deficits, as well as a history of abuse. The overwhelming probability is that such attacks are related to (interictal or primary) psychopathology or brain injury (which might also be the cause of seizures), and should not be attributed to seizure activity per se.

2. **The significance of epilepsy in psychiatric practice goes beyond its neuropsychiatric manifestations, and includes the psychosocial ramifications of living with a seizure disorder, the cognitive and affective side effects of common antiepileptic medications, and the seizure threshold-lowering effect of certain neuroleptic and tricyclic antidepressant medications.** Thus the presence of, for instance, mood symptoms, and a seizure disorder does not automatically make the diagnosis of mood disorder due to epilepsy. Yet, interictal mood symptoms deserve to be treated, even when they are most likely caused by the seizure disorder. **Finally, the difficulty or inability of confirming the clinical diagnosis of a seizure disorder, in the setting of psychiatric symptoms resistant to the usual treatments, should prompt a trial of an appropriate antiepileptic medication.**

C. Nutritional Deficits

1. **Niacin (nicotinic acid) deficiency, and deficiency of its precursor, tryptophan, lead to pellagra, which, when untreated, leads to a chronic wasting, diarrheal, neurologic (encephalopathy and peripheral neuropathy) and dermatologic (sun-exposed skin rash, angular stomatitis, and glossitis) syndrome. The early symptoms are nonspecific and may easily be mistaken for depression: insomnia, fatigue, irritability, anxiety, and depressed mood.** Untreated, this progresses to mental slowing, confusion, psychosis, and dementia, which may be accompanied by a spastic spinal syndrome with leg weakness, hyperreflexia, clonus, and extensor plantar responses. Pellagra is rare since the advent of niacin fortification of cereals, but still occurs in alcoholics, refugee populations, and vegetarians in less developed nations. Most symptoms reverse quickly with niacin repletion. Dementia, however, a sign of severe and prolonged deficit, may clear slowly or incompletely.

2. **Thiamine (vitamin B_1) deficiency occurs in two forms: beriberi in areas of poverty or famine, and Wernicke-Korsakoff syndrome in alcoholism.** There are cardiovascular, neuropathic, and cerebral signs and symptoms that generally occur in combination, but can less frequently present as isolated forms. Few alcoholics or malnourished individuals develop clinical deficiency, and other factors (e.g., activity and total calorie intake) affect the presentation. **The syndrome may be precipitated by the administration of glucose to asymptomatic, thiamine-deficient patients. The early symptoms may include decreased concentration, apathy, mild agitation, and depressed mood.** Confusion, amnesia, and

confabulation are late signs of severe, prolonged deficit.

3. **Cobalamin (vitamin B_{12}) deficiency, from lack of absorption (e.g., from absence of intrinsic factor in pernicious anemia or after gastric surgery) or vegetarian diet, leads to megaloblastic macrocytic anemia and neurodegenerative changes in the peripheral and central nervous systems. Neuropsychiatric symptoms, which may precede hematologic findings, include apathy, irritability, depression, and mood lability.** Less common, and indicative of more severe disease, is **megaloblastic madness, a delirium with prominent hallucinations, paranoia, and intellectual decline.** Neurologic signs include peripheral numbness and paresthesias, sphincter dyscontrol, abnormal reflexes, and decreased position and vibratory sensation. Because the axonal demyelination and neurodegenerative changes lead ultimately to cell death, not all neurologic findings clear with treatment.

D. **Metabolic encephalopathy should be considered whenever sudden or abrupt changes in mentation, orientation, behavior, or level of consciousness occur.** Although the waxing and waning presentation of delirium may eventually be evident, early memory impairment, passivity, withdrawal, or anxiety, and agitation, may be wrongly attributed to a primary psychiatric disorder.

1. **Hepatic encephalopathy may result from acute, subacute, or chronic hepatocellular failure, with a range of neuropsychiatric symptoms from mild personality change to coma, many of which may precede the more classical neurologic or physical findings (e.g., asterixis or icterus, respectively).** Earliest signs, apparent only to close family and friends, are mild intellectual difficulties, often covered by intact verbal ability. **Objective mental slowing, mild confusion, decreased concentration, depressed or labile mood, irritability, sleep-wake reversal, and decreased personal grooming are common early signs.** There may be periods of intermittent disorientation, inappropriate behavior, and outbursts of rage before the progressive deterioration in consciousness, speech, cognition, and memory leave the patient somnolent, incoherent, disoriented, confused, and amnestic. The final stage is coma.

2. **Renal insufficiency, acute or chronic, is associated with neuropsychiatric symptoms.** Acute renal failure is most notable for delirium, often with bizarre visual hallucinations. **Chronic renal insufficiency is associated with a wide range of symptoms, from mild difficulties in concentration, problem solving or calculation, to more severe cognitive impairment and lethargy.** While adequate dialysis may improve cognitive function, there are also problems of memory, concentration, and mental slowness associated with dialysis (even though the removal of aluminum has nearly eradicated the incidence of dialysis dementia). Depression also seems more prevalent in renal insufficiency, and in dialysis patients, although associated endocrine dysfunction (e.g., hyperparathyroidism) and disordered neurotransmission are thought to be contributing factors. Finally, uremia is associated with seizures, and complex partial seizures may be an occult cause of altered behavior, affect, perception, cognition, and consciousness.

3. **Hypoglycemic encephalopathy, whether from excess endogenous or exogenous insulin, can present with confusion, disorientation, or hallucinations and bizarre behavior.** Often, but not always, these symptoms are preceded by restlessness or apprehension. **Physical signs and symptoms include nausea, hunger, diaphoresis, and tachycardia.** Untreated, stupor and coma follow. **Repeated hypoglycemic episodes may cause permanent amnesia from hippocampal involvement.**

4. **Diabetic ketoacidosis can also present with nonspecific symptoms of fatigue and lethargy, before the "three Ps" (polyphagia, polydipsia, polyuria), headache, nausea, and vomiting appear.** In a poorly controlled, elderly, diabetic patient, osmotic fluid shifts can cause a slowly resolving delirium that primarily affects cognitive function.

5. **Acute intermittent porphyria (AIP) is a rare, autosomal dominant enzyme deficiency that interferes with heme biosynthesis and causes the accumulation of porphyrins. More common in women than men, it is known for the classical triad of episodic, acute, colicky abdominal pain, motor polyneuropathy, and psychosis, usually with onset in the 20–50 age range.** However, **AIP may present with only psychiatric symptoms:** insomnia, anxiety, mood lability, depression, and psychosis. A small percentage of chronic psychiatric patients have been found to have undiagnosed porphyrias. Neurologic effects, hyponatremia, and other electrolyte imbalances from vomiting and diarrhea, can lead to seizures. **Attacks can be precipitated by drugs, alcohol, low calorie diets, or gonadal steroids (endogenous or exogenous). Porphyrinogenic drugs include most antiepileptic medications, meprobamate, sulfonamide antibiotics, and ergot derivatives.** Phenothiazines, bromides, narcotic analgesics, and glucocorticoids are among the safe medications.

E. **Endocrine disorders** are associated with psychiatric symptoms, most commonly depression and anxiety. In the past, when endocrinopathies were diagnosed later in their course, delirium and dementia were more common.

1. **Thyroid**

   a. **Hypothyroidism, which is at least four times more prevalent in women than in men, has an insidious onset of nonspecific symptoms, such as fatigue, lethargy, weight gain, decreased appetite, depressed mood, cold intolerance, and slowed mental and motor activity.** Later in the course, the physical signs are dry skin, thin and dry hair, constipation, stiffness, a coarse voice, facial puffiness, carpal tunnel symptoms, loss of the outer third of the eyebrow, loss of hearing, and a delayed relaxation phase of deep tendon reflexes. Early symptoms may be attributed to aging, depression, dementia, or Parkinson's disease. Hallucinations and paranoia, the manifestations of the so-called "myxedema madness," are late findings. Roughly 10% of patients have residual psychiatric symptoms after hormone replacement.

   b. **Hyperthyroid patients appear restless, anxious, fidgety, or labile.** Symptoms may overlap with those of anxiety or panic, with palpitations, tachycardia, sweating, irritability, tremulousness, decreased sleep, weakness, and fatigue. Weight loss occurs despite increased appetite. **Elderly patients may manifest apathy, psychomotor retardation and depression, rather than hyperactive symptoms;** proximal muscle wasting and cardiovascular symptoms (failure and atrial arrhythmias) may predominate.

2. **Parathyroid** dysfunction is closely linked to perturbations in calcium, phosphate, and bone metabolism. However, attempts to correlate symptoms with absolute serum calcium levels have been inconclusive.

   a. **Hyperparathyroidism, and the resultant hypercalcemia, may be asymptomatic in as many as half of all patients, or present early on with nonspecific signs of mental slowness, lethargy, apathy, decreased attention and memory, and depressed mood.** Delirium, disorientation, and psychosis are also reported.

   b. In **hypoparathyroidism, a gradual onset of hypocalcemia may cause personality change, or delirium, without the characteristic tetany of a more precipitous drop in serum calcium.**

3. **Adrenal dysfunction**

   a. **Adrenal insufficiency, whether from autoimmune Addison's disease (primary hypocortisolism) or the sudden withdrawal of prolonged glucocorticoid therapy (secondary hypocortisolism), presents with initially mild psychiatric symptoms that may be attributable to depression: apathy, negativism, social withdrawal, poverty of thought, fatigue, depressed mood, irritability, and loss of appetite, interest, and enjoyment.** Other signs and symptoms include nausea, vomiting, weakness, hypotension, and hypoglycemia. Psychosis, delirium, and eventually coma may develop. The treatment is glucocorticoid replacement, although psychiatric symptoms may not fully resolve and may require specific therapy, as well. Care should be taken to choose psychotropic medications that will not exacerbate hypotension. The relative roles of decreased glucocorticoids versus the increased levels of adrenocorticotropic hormone (ACTH) and corticotropin-releasing factor (CRF) versus the lack of normal diurnal and stress modulation in glucocorticoid replacement, in the development and continuation of psychiatric symptoms, are unclear.

   b. **Hypercortisolism may result from chronic hypersecretion of ACTH (ACTH-dependent) from a pituitary adenoma (Cushing's disease) or a nonpituitary neoplasm (Cushing's syndrome); or, less frequently, it may result from the direct, adrenal oversecretion of cortisol from a tumor or hyperplasia (ACTH-independent Cushing's syndrome).** The vast majority of patients will experience psychiatric symptoms, which may precede the (often partial) development of the classical, Cushingoid, stigmata: trunkal obesity, peripheral wasting, hirsutism, moon facies, acne, and striae. **Psychiatric symptoms include anxiety (similar to general anxiety disorder [GAD] or panic disorder) and depression, with crying, extreme irritability, insomnia, decreased interest, energy, concentration, and memory.** Suicidal ideation may be prevalent. Although relatively rare, psychosis may develop. Prolonged administration of exogenous corticosteroids produces a similar syndrome and patients may be extremely responsive, psychiatrically, to small dose adjustments. High dose, exogenous corticosteroids may also precipitate mania. In patients with a history of corticosteroid-induced mania and a need for episodic corticosteroid treatment, the prophylactic use of a mood stabilizer is indicated.

4. **Pituitary dysfunction** can disrupt the normal modulation of multiple systems in the body, and **thus can cause a wide range of psychiatric symptoms.** The postpartum, hemorrhagic destruction of the pituitary (**Sheehan's syndrome**), for example, may cause depression, mental slowness, and mood lability. An overactive pituitary can lead to adrenal hyperplasia and all the symptoms of Cushing's syndrome, described above.

F. **Demyelinating disorders** are associated with neuropsychiatric symptoms as well as motor and sensory changes. These disorders are relatively rare in the general public and may present initially with mild alterations in mood, behavior, cognition, or personality. **When the early physical complaints are intermittent, subjective, and variable, they may be attributed to depression, anxiety, somatization, or even malingering. Multiple sclerosis (MS) is by far the most prevalent of these disorders (50–60 per 100,000), with amyotrophic lateral sclerosis (ALS) a**

distant second (3–5 per 100,000). Others include metachromatic leukodystrophy, adrenoleukodystrophy, gangliosidoses, and SSPE.

1. **Multiple sclerosis (MS), an episodic, inflammatory, multifocal, demyelinating disease of unknown etiology, affects the cerebral hemispheres, optic nerves, brain stem, cerebellum, and spinal cord. MS is more common in cold and temperate climates, with a predilection for women, and an onset between ages 20 and 40 years.**

   Studies suggest that psychiatric symptoms are prevalent throughout the course of MS, do not clear during remission of physical symptoms, and correlate poorly with magnetic resonance imaging (MRI) findings, severity of physical symptoms, or length of illness. In order of prevalence, **95% of MS patients experience some of the following alterations in mood, behavior, or personality: depressed mood, agitation, anxiety, irritability, apathy, euphoria, disinhibition, hallucinations, aberrant motor behavior, or delusions. Depressive symptoms may occur in over 75% of patients, and are associated with an increased rate of suicide.** Although the presence of depression does not vary by gender or age, the risk of suicide in MS is higher in men, the newly diagnosed, and those with onset prior to age 30 years. Despite the common wisdom that MS is associated with euphoria, only about a quarter of patients experience this mildly elevated mood at some point during their course of illness, and persistent euphoria probably occurs in less than 10% of patients. Euphoria should not be considered synonymous with mania, which is rarely seen. Rather, what passes for euphoria in MS is more of an upbeat nature that may seem incongruent with the patient's condition and premorbid personality style.

   Mild to moderate cognitive deficits appear in more than half of MS patients, with more severe decline seen in 20–30%. Memory is most often affected, though severe dementia is not common.

2. **Amyotrophic lateral sclerosis (ALS), the most common degenerative motor neuron disease, is still relatively rare,** with an annual incidence of 1.6 per 100,000 population. It may begin with either upper or lower motor neuron involvement, but eventually both will be affected. It has a relentless course to death within 4 or 5 years, usually from diaphragmatic failure. The sporadic form is more common, although there are familial forms. Dementia may occur in familial ALS, but, even with advanced sporadic disease, cognitive function remains intact. **Uncontrollable laughing and crying (pseudobulbar affect) is the result of degenerative** changes in the cortical bulbar projections to the brainstem.

3. **Lipid storage disorders are a group of rare, inherited (autosomal recessive) enzyme deficiencies** that can present in adulthood with multiple psychiatric and neuromuscular signs and symptoms.

   a. **Metachromatic leukodystrophy** (MLD) is rapidly fatal when it presents in infancy. When it presents in adolescence or adulthood, however, it has an insidious, progressive course with cognitive decline, forgetfulness, deterioration of work or school performance, and personality changes. Mild cerebellar signs follow, with gait disturbances, masked facies, and strange postures. Patients become demented, and finally mute and bedridden.

   b. **Adrenoleukodystrophy** (ALD) also causes adrenal insufficiency (i.e., primary Addison's disease). It may present with aphasia, dementia, asymmetric myelopathic findings (e.g., homonymous hemianopsia, hemiparesis), or the psychiatric symptoms of Addison's disease. A progressive, more symmetric presentation follows, with spastic paraparesis or demyelinating polyneuropathy. Glucocorticoids treat the adrenal insufficiency, but there is no treatment for the overall disorder.

   c. **Gangliosidoses** are a group of lysosomal storage diseases that include the **adult form of Tay-Sach's disease.** Lower motor neuron and spinocerebellar symptoms may present in childhood or adolescence as clumsiness or weakness, with normal intelligence and vision. However, in some patients, psychosis or seizures develop, while the neuromuscular effects are mild.

G. **Cerebrovascular disease** is the third most common cause of death in the United States, behind heart disease and cancer. **The vast majority of strokes are ischemic (85%), and about a third of all strokes are the result of atherosclerotic thrombosis and cerebral embolism.** Essential hypertension is the most common cause of hemorrhagic stroke; spontaneous aneurysmal rupture, or arteriovenous malformation, are much less frequent causes of parenchymal bleeding.

1. **Depression,** either major depression or dysthymia, is the most common post-stroke psychiatric syndrome, which occurs in over half of patients. Roughly two-thirds of these patients experience depressive symptoms in the immediate post-stroke period, while the rest become depressed after about six months. The natural course of untreated, post-stroke depression is about a year, while the course of dysthymia may be more protracted and variable. While the severity of deficits does not correlate with the onset of depression, depression is correlated with poor recovery and with a decreased ability to participate in rehabilitative therapies. Standard

antidepressant therapies have been shown to shorten the course of post-stroke depression, underscoring the importance of timely recognition and initiation of treatment. There is suggestive, but questioned, evidence that stroke location (left hemisphere frontal, prefrontal, or basal ganglia) predisposes to depression; previous stroke, subcortical atrophy, and personal or family history of mood disorder may also increase the risk of post-stroke depression.

2. **Aprosodia,** the inability to affectively modulate speech and gestures (motor aprosodia), or the inability to interpret the emotional components of another's speech or gestures (sensory aprosodia), may follow right (nondominant) hemisphere insults. **The aprosodic patient often appears affectively blunted, or "flat," but this is a disorder of** *expression***, not mood, and it should be carefully differentiated from depression.**

3. **Anxiety,** as an isolated syndrome, is relatively rare in the post-stroke period. However, almost half of patients with post-stroke depression have concomitant anxiety symptoms.

4. **Mania,** although rare, correlates with right-sided lesions of the orbitofrontal, basotemporal, basal ganglia, and thalamic areas. This secondary mania may be more common in those with pre-existing subcortical atrophy, or a personal, or family history of mood disorder.

5. **Affective incontinence** may be seen, with **multiple lacunar infarcts** affecting the descending corticobulbar and frontopontine pathways. This release of cortical inhibition over lower brainstem centers results in uncontrollable outbursts of laughing or crying and loss of more moderate emotional expression, such as smiling. This affective dyscontrol occurs along with dysarthria, dysphagia, and bifacial weakness, which together comprise the syndrome of **"pseudobulbar palsy."**

H. **Toxins,** of various types in miniscule amounts, are gaining notoriety as the putative cause of myriad nonspecific symptoms in certain, sensitive individuals. While there are few data to support the existence of **multiple chemical sensitivity or environmental illness,** there are syndromes from common environmental toxins, such as carbon monoxide or low-level lead exposure, that may be overlooked because of their similarity to common medical or primary mental disorders.

1. **Carbon monoxide** (CO) poisoning, from faulty heating or exhaust systems, may cause a flu-like illness with cough, nausea, and general malaise. More chronic, low-level exposure can cause cognitive deterioration and depression. Severe, but sublethal poisoning can lead to memory dysfunction, visual problems, parkinsonism, confabulation, psychosis, and delirium.

2. **Lead,** a known toxin in young children, also poses a risk to adults who are exposed in a variety of occupational, recreational, and environmental settings. Potentially hazardous activities include home renovation, drinking from leaded crystal, and jogging in areas of heavy traffic. Stained glass, ceramic, and lead figure artisans, as well as artists who use lead-based oil paints, and even art conservators, are at risk. Firearm enthusiasts should also monitor their lead levels. The psychiatric symptoms of low-level lead exposure are nondescript, and easily dismissed as depression: after-work fatigue, sleepiness, depressed mood, and apathy. At higher levels, cognition and memory may be impaired, along with sensorimotor symptoms, restlessness, and gastrointestinal complaints. Organic lead exposure from gasoline, solvents and cleaning fluids can cause psychosis, restlessness, nightmares, and, at very high levels, seizures, and coma.

3. **Mercury exposure from organic mercury,** as from contaminated fish, **results in a primarily neurologic syndrome,** while **exposure to inorganic mercury presents initially with psychiatric symptoms.**

   a. In **organic mercury poisoning,** the prominent neurologic effects include motor-sensory neuropathy, cerebellar ataxia, slurred speech, paresthesias, and visual field defects. The primary psychiatric symptoms, depression, irritability and mild dementia, may be less striking.

   b. With **inorganic mercury poisoning, the** *Mad Hatter* **syndrome,** the initial symptoms are depression, irritability, and psychosis, with less prominent headache, tremor, and weakness. Whereas exposure in the past was occupational or from broken thermometers, present-day sources may be less obvious. Mercury is found in readily purchased botanical preparations and folk medicines. It is also sold in easily broken capsules with instructions to sprinkle it in the home or car, a practice of certain cultural or religious sects.

4. **Drugs: overdose, herbal, nonprescription, prescribed, or recreational.** All should be considered potential toxins when evaluating changes in cognition, behavior, consciousness, or personality. (However, these would be substance-induced mental disorders, and are discussed elsewhere.)

I. **Neoplasm,** unregulated focal or diffuse growth within the cranial confines, can produce any of the symptomatic presentations available to the CNS. As compared to ischemic infarcts, tumors affecting similar brain volume are less symptomatic. The clinical presentation may suggest the type, location, and primary versus metastatic nature of the lesion.

Metastatic brain lesions are more prevalent in adults, than are primary brain tumors. In addition, paraneoplastic syndromes of non-brain tumors also cause psychiatric symptoms.

1. **Brain tumors,** such as **gliomas,** which account for 50–60% of primary brain tumors, **tend to produce diffuse symptoms** (e.g., cognitive decline), as they grow slowly and diffusely throughout the cortex. Multiple metastases or lymphoma can also present this nonfocal pattern. **Meningiomas** (25% of primary brain tumors) grow extrinsically to the brain and **compress a limited area, causing progressive, more focal symptoms. Seizure is the third presentation of intracranial lesions,** which may be the result of abnormal excitation or interference of normal inhibitory mechanisms. Cortical invasion or compression, even from a relatively small meningioma, is more likely than subcortical tumors to cause seizures. Constitutional symptoms (fever, weight loss, fatigue) are more common with metastatic disease.

   Psychiatric symptoms occur in half of patients with brain tumors and, of those, over 80% have tumors in the frontal or limbic areas. Besides depression and personality changes, frontal tumors are associated with bowel and bladder incontinence. Temporal lobe tumors are especially likely to cause seizures, often with ictal or interictal psychosis. Poor memory, or Korsakoff syndrome, aphasia, depression, and personality changes are also seen with temporal lobe tumors. Akinetic mutism, an alert but immobile state, occurs with upper brainstem tumors. Delirium is a sign of rapidly growing, large, or metastatic tumors.

2. **Paraneoplastic syndromes,** most common in small cell carcinoma of the lung, produce neuropsychiatric symptoms that may precede by many months the detection of the causative, non-CNS tumor. Tumors of the breast, stomach, uterus, kidney, testicle, thyroid, and colon may also cause paraneoplastic syndromes. These syndromes may arise from tumor production of hormones, with clinical manifestations of inappropriate antidiuretic hormone secretion (SIADH), hypercortisolism, hypercalcemia, or hyperparathyroidism. Less well understood are the mechanisms responsible for encephalitic paraneoplastic syndromes, which involve nonreversible, often selective, inflammatory and/or neurodegenerative destruction. **Paraneoplastic limbic encephalitis** has an insidious onset over weeks to months, with confusion and agitation. Depressed mood, anxiety, personality change, hallucinations, and catatonia are also reported, and may lead to psychiatric hospitalization. Initial memory loss progresses to dementia. Pathologically, there is neuronal loss in the medial temporal lobe and other limbic areas, along with meningeal and perivascular lymphocytic infiltration.

3. **Pancreatic cancer** is associated with a higher than expected incidence of depression, which may be its initial presentation.

4. **Colloid cysts,** nonmalignant, space-occupying lesions of the third ventricle, exert pressure on diencephalic structures, and may increase intracranial pressure by ventricular obstruction. They have been associated with depression, mood lability, psychosis, personality change, and position-dependent, intermittent headache.

J. Degenerative disorders, especially of the basal ganglia, produce not only motor and sensory dysfunction, but a spectrum of neuropsychiatric symptoms that include depression, psychosis, and dementia. In fact, the severity of the movement symptoms may vary with the level of emotional stress. This association between movement and emotion may be mediated by the largely limbic and cortical inputs to the basal ganglia, and the shared neurotransmitter systems (dopamine, γ-aminobutyric acid [GABA], serotonin, norepinephrine).

1. **Parkinson's disease,** which affects 1% of the population over the age of 65 years, is known for its classical features of bradykinesia, rigidity and tremor, and characteristic disturbances of gait and posture. The major degenerative loss is in the pars compacta of the substantia nigra, although other structures are also involved. Dopamine, and to some extent norepinephrine and possibly other neurotransmitters, are depleted, which may contribute to the depression experienced by over half of patients. Dementia is also more common than in age-matched controls. Psychosis can develop, and is complicated by the dopaminergic and anticholinergic medications used to treat the disease.

2. **Huntington's chorea** is an autosomal dominant disorder of primarily striatal destruction and GABA depletion. Besides atrophy of the caudate and putamen, there is mild frontal and temporal wasting. Most common in the age range of 30–40 years, onset is extremely variable, and juvenile disease has a more rapidly progressive course (average duration of 8, as opposed to 15, years). The prevalence is 10 per 100,000 population. The classic choreiform movement disorder may present with, before, or after, prominent psychiatric symptoms. Early on, memory may be intact, but serious defects in attention, judgment, and executive function are evident. This may be followed by depression, apathy, social withdrawal, and a lack of attention to personal grooming. Irritability and impulsivity

are common. The initial presentation may also mimic obsessive-compulsive disorder or schizophrenia. The depression is responsive to antidepressants and should be treated. The cognitive decline, like the movement disorder, is progressive, and leads to dementia.

3. **Wilson's disease** is an autosomal recessive defect in copper excretion that causes deposition of copper in the liver, brain, cornea, and kidney. This genetic deficiency of ceruloplasmin has a prevalence of 3.3 per 100,000 population. One person in 90 may be a heterozygous carrier. Symptoms are rare before age 6 years and commonly present in the teens. However, some patients remain asymptomatic well into adulthood. About half of patients present with liver manifestations: acute hepatitis, parenchymal liver disease, cirrhosis, or fulminant hepatitis. The vast majority of remaining patients present with neuropsychiatric symptoms, virtually always accompanied by gold or green-brown copper deposits around the cornea, the pathognomonic **Kayser-Fleischer rings.** Copper toxicity in the brain affects the lenticular nuclei and, to a lesser degree, the pons, medulla, thalamus, cerebellum, and cerebral cortex. Neurologic features include tremor, spasticity, rigidity, chorea, dysphagia, and dysarthria. Cognition is generally intact, although the dysarthria may be mistaken for mental retardation. About 10–25% of patients present with psychiatric symptoms, although those who present with neurologic findings also have psychiatric symptoms. Schizophreniform, bipolar, and more typical depressive symptoms may be seen, but bizarre, possibly frontal, behavior is more common. Psychiatric symptoms that respond incompletely to successful, excess copper removal require more specific treatment and psychopharmacotherapy.

K. Immune Diseases

1. **Acquired immunodeficiency syndrome** (AIDS) is caused by HIV infection, and is discussed above (see A.2) and elsewhere in this book.
2. **Systemic lupus erythematosus** (SLE) is an autoimmune, inflammatory disease of unknown etiology that affects women (9:1) more often than men, usually in the third to fifth decades. Tissue damage occurs in multiple systems, which gives the disorder an extremely variable presentation and course. Laboratory tests may be confirmatory, but are not totally specific or reliable. When patients present with depression, sleep disturbance, mood lability, mild cognitive dysfunction, or psychosis, which up to one-half of patients do, the nonspecific nature of their complaints may lead to the erroneous diagnosis of a primary mental disorder, such as major depression or somatization disorder. Correct diagnosis may lead to steroid therapy, which can worsen psychiatric symptoms.

L. **Trauma** to the head is extremely common in the United States, with roughly a million severe traumatic brain injuries per year. Young males are at highest risk. Motor vehicle accidents are responsible for about half of all closed head injuries, with falls, violence, and sports causing most of the rest.

1. **Penetrating head injury,** such as that received from a gunshot wound, is often dramatic; it tends to cause focal symptoms related to the size and location of directly involved brain tissue.
2. **Closed head injury** is far more common, and complicated, causing more diffuse symptoms and prolonged sequelae that do not correlate with the severity of the injury. The neurobehavioral dysfunction, including cognitive, somatic, and emotional symptoms, may clear in 3–6 months, or may persist for years after the injury. The mechanisms of injury in blunt trauma to the head may account for this variable course. Direct impact, acceleration/deceleration, and shearing forces, parenchymal stretching, and microscopic tears cause brain contusion and neuronal damage which may be followed by edema and bleeding. Limbic areas of the brain, the anterior temporal lobes and the inferior surface of the frontal lobes, are the major sites of damage. Cognitive slowing may occur with poor attention, increased distractibility, memory difficulties, perseveration, and poor planning. Personality changes, irritability, impulsivity, depression, anxiety, and mood lability are also common. Among the many somatic symptoms are headache, dizziness, fatigue, and sleep disturbance, which may be attributed to depression. Photophobia, noise sensitivity, tinnitus, and blurred vision also occur. Multiple head injuries, advanced age, drug or alcohol use increase the risk of prolonged impairment. Patients with head injuries are often very sensitive to psychotropic medications, and may require "geriatric" doses.
3. **Postconcussive syndrome** (PCS) is the prolonged duration of cognitive, somatic, and emotional symptoms following "head trauma that caused significant cerebral concussion." DSM-IV has developed research criteria for PCS. A careful history for distant head trauma is necessary to recognize the syndrome.

IV. Evaluation of the Problem

Since Mental Disorder DTGMC should be part of the differential diagnosis for any psychiatric syndrome, the evaluation is the same as for any careful, psychiatric evaluation. A high level of "medical suspicion" is required to gather the necessary information to make the diagnosis.

A. **History:** from records, the patient, other caregivers, and, when possible and appropriate (e.g., when the patient is a poor, or limited historian, or for medical or mental reasons), from family members or others close to the patient.
   1. **Medical**
      a. A careful review of past and present illnesses, treatments, procedures, all medications, exposures, travel, head injury, seizure, habits (caffeine, tobacco), and recreational drug use.
      b. Correlation in time between medical events and psychiatric symptoms.
   2. **Psychiatric:** close attention to onset, course, treatment response, and past episodes, for typical and atypical features of primary mental disorders.
   3. **Family:** the presence of similar symptoms, other psychiatric disorders, medical illnesses that "run" in the family; early, or unexplained deaths.
   4. **Social:** education, occupation, living situation, interpersonal relationships (fights, violence), recreational activities.

B. **Examination of the Patient**
   1. **Laboratory examination** should be focused to support or rule out a suspected diagnosis.
   2. **Imaging** should also be used to confirm a diagnosis, not to discover unsuspected pathology. Sudden onset, focal signs, rapid progression, infectious disease, or trauma are indications for appropriate brain imaging.
   3. A **Mental Status Exam** (MSE) is not specific for general medical conditions, but is comparable to the MSE in similar, primary mental disorders. Certain medical conditions, however, may present patterns of behavior or cognitive deficits that may be found on the MSE.
   4. **Other tests** may be specific to a given medical condition (e.g., a sleep-deprived EEG in suspected complex partial seizures).

V. Treatment Considerations/Strategies

A. **Some general medical conditions are chronic, stable, or unremitting,** and little can be done to change or treat them, or alter their course (e.g., previous stroke or toxic exposures, degenerative or demyelinating diseases). The mental disorder or **psychiatric symptoms should be treated** to the fullest extent possible, regardless of their medical etiology.

B. Whenever possible, **underlying medical conditions should be treated,** controlled, and/or stabilized. For example, infections should be treated with appropriate agents, metabolic perturbations should be normalized, diabetic control and renal function optimized. **Some mental disorders will clear** when the underlying condition is treated, and thus long-term treatment of the mental disorder is unnecessary. Short-term comfort measures, however, may be necessary as the mental symptoms may lag behind the course of the medical condition. An example of this would be the judicious use of benzodiazepines in a patient being treated for hyperthyroidism.

C. **Often the medical condition and the psychiatric symptoms require ongoing treatment.** Maximal seizure control, for instance, may not be perfect, leaving the patient with interictal symptoms, such as depression, that should also be treated. **The psychosocial stresses of chronic or acute medical conditions, as well as other, primary mental or personality disorders, can exacerbate the psychiatric symptoms, interfere with treatment, and generally complicate the clinical picture.**

VI. Conclusions

Neuropsychiatric symptoms may precede, accompany, or follow the onset of a variety of general medical conditions. The psychiatrist must maintain a high level of suspicion, as well as a current knowledge of the broad categories and common features of these more prevalent conditions, to consider Mental Disorder Due to a General Medical Condition in the differential diagnosis of every patient. Few, if any, general laboratory or imaging examinations are necessary, but the judicious use of specific examinations to support or confirm the suspected diagnosis is recommended. Although the underlying condition should be treated, when possible, psychiatric symptoms may also require specific treatment.

Suggested Readings

American Psychiatric Association: *Diagnostic and Statistical Manual of Mental Disorders, Fourth Edition.* Washington, DC: American Psychiatric Association, 1994.

Cassem NH (ed.), Stern TA, Rosenbaum JF, Jellinek MS (co-eds): *Massachusetts General Hospital Handbook of General Hospital Psychiatry,* 4th ed. St. Louis: Mosby, 1997.

Diaz-Olavarrieta C, Cummings JL, Velazquez J, de la Cadena CG: Neuropsychiatric manifestations of multiple sclerosis. *J Neuropsychiatry Clin Neurosci* 1999; 11:51–57.

Fallon BA, Kochevar JM, Gaito A, Nields JA: The under diagnosis of neuropsychiatric Lyme disease in children and adults. *Psychiatr Clin North Am* 1998; 21(3):693–703.

Fauci AS, Braunwald E, Isselbacher KJ, et al. (eds): *Harrison's*

Principles of Internal Medicine, 14th ed. New York: McGraw-Hill, 1998.

Geffken GR, Ward HE, Staab JP, et al.: Psychiatric morbidity in endocrine disorders. *Psychiatr Clin North Am* 1998; 21(2):473–489.

Hartman DE: Missed diagnoses and misdiagnoses of environmental toxicant exposure. *Psychiatr Clin North Am* 1998; 21(3): 659–670.

Jones EA, Weissenborn K: Neurology and the liver. *J Neurol Neurosurg Psychiatry* 1997; 63:279–293.

Kaplan HI, Sadock BJ, Grebb JA (eds): *Kaplan and Sadock's Synopsis of Psychiatry: Behavioral Sciences, Clinical Psychiatry*, 7th ed. Baltimore: Williams and Wilkins, 1994.

Rundell JR, Wise MG (eds): *Textbook of Consultation-Liaison Psychiatry*. Washington, DC: American Psychiatric Press, Inc., 1996.

Skuster DZ, Digre KB, Corbett JJ: Neurologic conditions presenting as psychiatric disorders. *Psychiatr Clin North Am* 1992; 15(2):311–333.

Stern TA, Herman JB, Slavin PL (eds): *The MGH Guide to Psychiatry in Primary Care*. New York: McGraw-Hill, 1998.

Tucker GJ: Seizure disorders presenting with psychiatric symptomatology. *Psychiatr Clin North Am* 1998; 21(3):625–635.

Chapter 10

Alcoholism and Alcohol Abuse

JOHN A. RENNER

I. Introduction

A. Incidence

According to the National Comorbidity Study (1990–1992), the lifetime prevalence for alcohol abuse is 6% in women, and 12% in men; for alcohol dependence it is 8% for women and 20% for men. The 12-month prevalences for alcohol abuse (2% for women and 3% for men) and alcohol dependence (4% in women and 11% in men) are also high.

B. **Alcohol abuse spans the continuum from brief episodes of excessive drinking to chronic patterns** that produce significant problems, yet it never progresses to either psychological or physical dependence (Table 10-1).

C. **Alcohol dependence (alcoholism) is defined as the excessive and recurrent use of alcohol despite medical, psychological, social, or economic problems** (Table 10-1).

D. Diagnostic criteria for alcohol dependence, as classified in DSM-IV, include tolerance and withdrawal symptoms. Although these signs of physical dependence are not required for the diagnosis, they are associated with more severe forms of the disorder. Specifiers can be added to the diagnostic criteria:
   1. With Physiological Dependence: **tolerance or withdrawal.**
   2. Without Physiological Dependence: **no tolerance or withdrawal.**
   3. Early Full Remission: **no criteria for dependence or abuse present for at least 1 month, but less than 12 months of remission.**
   4. Partial Full Remission: **one or more criteria for dependence or abuse present for at least 1 month, but less than 12 months; full criteria not met.**
   5. Sustained Full Remission: **no criteria for dependence or abuse present for 12 months or longer.**
   6. Sustained Partial Remission: **one or more criteria for dependence or abuse present for 12 months or longer, but full criteria not met.**
   7. In a Controlled Environment: **no criteria for dependence or abuse present for at least the past month, but the individual is in an environment in which access to alcohol and controlled substances is restricted.**

E. Comorbid Conditions
   1. **In 1994, the National Comorbidity Survey (NCS) reported that the majority of patients in the United States with serious psychiatric disorders also abuse alcohol or other drugs.** Individuals in this group accounted for more than half of all lifetime psychiatric disorders in the United States; they usually had a history of three or more disorders, one of which was a substance abuse disorder.
      a. **The majority of individuals with an alcohol disorder have at least one other psychiatric disorder.**
      b. Comorbid conditions (in rank order) associated with a substance abuse diagnosis are:
         i. Abuse of a second substance (most common)
         ii. Antisocial personality disorder
         iii. Phobias (and other anxiety disorders)
         iv. Major depressive disorder
         v. Dysthymic disorder (least common)
      c. Most lifetime co-occurring alcohol disorders begin at a later age than at least one other NCS/DSM-III-R disorder.
      d. Anxiety disorders and affective disorders co-occur more frequently with alcohol disorders in women.
      e. Substance disorders, conduct disorder, and antisocial personality disorder co-occur more frequently with alcohol disorders in men.
      f. 25–50% of suicides involve alcohol.
   2. **Alcohol-related problems affect over 10% of drinkers and are the third leading cause of death in the United States. Alcoholism causes 80% of hepatic cirrhosis. Patients injured under the influence of alcohol fill 50% of trauma beds in the United States.**

II. Neurobiology of Alcohol

A. **The positive reinforcement of alcohol appears to be mediated by:**
   1. Activation of γ-aminobutyric acid A receptors (GABA-A) which open chloride channels for a primary central nervous system (CNS) depressant effect.
   2. Release of opioid peptides and dopamine.
   3. Inhibition of glutamate NMDA (N-methyl-D-aspartate) receptors.
   4. Interaction with serotonin systems.

B. **Chronic alcohol use causes:**
   1. Upregulation of excitatory glutamate NMDA receptors

Table 10-1. DSM-IV Diagnostic Criteria

ALCOHOL ABUSE: One or more of the following present at any time during the same 12-month period.

1. Alcohol use results in failure to fulfill **major obligations**.

2. Recurrent use in **physically dangerous situations** (such as drunk driving).

3. Recurrent alcohol-related **legal problems**.

4. Continued use despite recurrent **social or interpersonal problems**.

5. Has never met criteria for Alcohol Dependence.

ALCOHOL DEPENDENCE: Three or more of the following present at any time during the same 12-month period.

1. **Tolerance**.

2. **Withdrawal**.

3. Use in **larger amounts**, or for **longer periods** than intended.

4. Unsuccessful **efforts to cut down** or control use.

5. A great deal of **time spent** obtaining alcohol, using or recovering from alcohol use.

6. **Important activities given up.**

7. **Continued use despite knowledge of problems.**

SOURCE: Adapted from *DSM-IV* Criteria for Substance Abuse and Substance Dependence, American Psychiatric Association, 1994.

2. Downregulation of inhibitory neuronal GABA receptors
3. Increased central norepinephrine activity

C. **The response to the termination of alcohol consumption involves CNS hyperactivity** due to a lack of opposition to an alcohol-induced excitatory state.

III. Alcohol Metabolism

A. **The primary metabolism of alcohol occurs through oxidation in the liver.** Ethanol is metabolized via alcohol dehydrogenase to acetaldehyde, which is converted to acetate via aldehyde dehydrogenase; thereafter, carbon dioxide and water are produced.

B. **Disulfiram (Antabuse)** inhibits the action of aldehyde dehydrogenase and produces toxic blood levels of acetaldehyde.

C. **A healthy liver oxidizes 0.75 oz. of 80-proof alcohol in 1 h; in regular drinkers, the metabolic rate is even faster.**

D. **Elimination of alcohol: 90% is oxidized by the liver; 10% is excreted unchanged by the lungs and kidneys.**

E. **Asians have lower levels of both alcohol dehydrogenase and aldehyde dehydrogenase. Therefore, they metabolize alcohol more slowly and become intoxicated on lower amounts of alcohol than do Caucasians.**

F. **Blood alcohol concentration (BAC) helps determine alcohol intoxication** (Table 10-2). (Note: A 160 lb. man who drinks 5 oz. of whiskey in 1 h develops a BAC of 0.10%.)

A BAC over 150 mg% in a person who does not appear very intoxicated, or over 300 mg% in any awake person, is evidence of physical addiction (tolerance) to alcohol.

G. The decreased gastric oxidation of alcohol by women causes a higher BAC in women than in men.

IV. Physiologic Effects of Alcohol

A. **Cardiovascular Effects**
1. **Increased cardiac output (in alcoholics)**
2. **Elevated blood pressure**
3. **Increased heart rate and cardiac oxygen consumption (in non-alcoholics)**
4. **An increased risk of myocardial infarction**

B. **Increased incidence of cancer:** esophageal, head, neck, liver, stomach, colon, and lung

Table 10-2. Effects of Drinking Alcohol on the BAC and Clinical Findings

BAC	Clinical Findings
0.05%	Exhilaration, loss of inhibitions
0.10%	Slurred speech, staggering gait
0.20%	Euphoria, marked motor impairment
0.30%	Confusion
0.40%	Stupor
0.50%	Coma
0.60%	Respiratory paralysis → death

C. Miscellaneous
1. **Hypoglycemia occurs with acute intoxication.**
2. **Increased blood estradiol levels in women.**
3. **Dysregulation of triglycerides and lipoproteins.**

V. Alcohol-Related Syndromes

A. Acute Alcoholic Hallucinosis (Alcohol Psychotic Disorder, with Hallucinations; 291.3) (see Table 10-3)
1. **This condition occurs after cessation of drinking in an alcohol-dependent person (the onset of symptoms is during withdrawal).**
2. **It can also occur without a drop in BAC (with an onset during intoxication).**
3. **No delirium, tremor, or autonomic hyperactivity develops.**
4. **Hallucinations are usually auditory and paranoid.**
   a. **Symptoms can become chronic.**
   b. **Symptoms are not due to schizophrenia (it has a late onset, and no typical premorbid personality).**

B. Alcohol Withdrawal/Delirium Tremens (DTs) (see Table 10.3)
1. **Minor (early) withdrawal symptoms include:**
   a. Onset 8–9 h after the last drink
   b. Sweating, a flushed face, and insomnia
   c. Hallucinations in 25%
   d. Grand mal seizures (rum fits)
   e. Mild disorientation
2. **Major (late) withdrawal symptoms (DTs) include:**
   a. Onset 48–96 h after the last drink
   b. Tremor, and an increase in psychomotor activity
   c. Vivid hallucinations
   d. Seizures are absent
   e. Profound disorientation
   f. Increased autonomic activity and fever

C. Pathological Intoxication
Idiosyncratic Alcohol Intoxication is classified as Alcohol Use Disorder Not Otherwise Specified (291.9).
1. Intoxication develops after small amounts (4 oz.) of alcohol.
2. Automatic behaviors (usually combative or violent) are manifest.
3. Sleep or amnesia for the event often follows.

D. Alcohol Withdrawal Seizures
1. Involve generalized tonic-clonic seizures.
2. Occur within 24–48 h after the last drink.
3. **Rarely involve more than one seizure, but a second seizure can occur within 3–6 h of the first seizure.**
4. **Hypoglycemia, hyponatremia, and hypomagnesemia in chronic alcoholics are often involved.**
5. **They are easily treated with benzodiazepines.**
6. Status Epilepticus occurs in less than 3% of patients.

E. Fetal Alcohol Syndrome (FAS)
1. **Signs:**
   a. An affected infant may show signs of alcohol withdrawal.
   b. An early stage of liver disease may be evident.
   c. Mental retardation (44% had an IQ of 79 or below) is common.
   d. A retarded weight and height curve may develop.
2. Congenital heart disease and other defects appear: wide-set eyes, short palpebral fissure, short and broad-bridged nose, hypoplastic philtrum, a thinned upper lip, and flattened mid-face.
3. **Incidence: six-fold increase between 1979 and 1993, to 6.7 per 10,000 births** (CDC, 1995).
   a. 17% are stillborn or die shortly after birth.
   b. 20% have birth defects (32% show full "fetal alcohol syndrome").
4. Maternal alcohol use while breastfeeding impairs a child's motor development, but not his/her mental development.
5. Long-term effects of FAS: < 6% able to function in school; most never hold a job. The average IQ in 61 subjects with FAS was 68 (Streissguth, 1991); 72% have major psychiatric disorders (Famy, 1998).

VI. Genetics and the Biologic Correlates of Alcoholism

The Virginia Twin Registry Study supports the findings of other current research that suggests that **genetic factors have a major influence on the development of both alcohol abuse and alcoholic dependence.** The specific biologic mechanisms affected by these genetic factors are less clearly understood. This large population-based

Table 10-3. DTs vs. Acute Alcohol Hallucinosis

Condition	Sensorium	Tremor	Hallucinations	Pupils	Vital signs	Onset	Duration
Delirium tremens	Confused	Yes	Visual	Dilated, slow to react	↑	Gradual	3–10 days
Alcohol hallucinosis	Clear	Rare	Auditory	Normal	±	Rapid	5–30 days

twin study also demonstrated that environmental factors shared by family members had little influence on the development of alcoholism in males (Prescott and Kendler, 1999). The **social use of alcohol, however, is primarily influenced by environmental factors,** such as peer pressure, cultural attitudes, price, and availability.

A. **Summary of Risk Data in the United States**
   Nonfamilial alcoholism accounts for 51% of all alcoholics and is characterized by less severe alcoholism, later onset, better school and work histories, smaller families, higher socioeconomic status, and less psychopathologic or antisocial behavior (Frances, 1980).
   1. **Any drinker** has a 5–10% risk of becoming an alcoholic.
   2. If **one parent** is alcoholic, the risk doubles to 20%.
   3. If **both parents** are alcoholic, the risk is between 20% and 50%.
   4. The risk for fathers, sons, and brothers of alcoholics approaches 50%.
   5. Risk for male and female twins is 28% for fraternal twins and 54% for identical twins.
   6. If the father is severely alcoholic and criminal, the son's risk is 90%.

B. **The Stockholm adoption study** included 862 males and 913 females, adopted and raised by non-relatives; two types of alcoholism were identified (Cloninger et al., 1981):
   1. **Type I, or "Milieu-limited" alcoholism**
      a. Affects both men and women.
      b. Reflects a congenital susceptibility (both parents can have mild, adult-onset alcohol abuse).
      c. Has a severity that is determined by postnatal stress.
      d. Estimates a risk in sons that is twice the normal incidence.
      e. Is associated with a risk in daughters with an alcoholic mother that is three times the normal incidence.
   2. **Type II, or "male-limited" alcoholism**
      a. Is passed only from fathers to sons.
      b. Involves fathers who are both severely alcoholic and criminal.
      c. Sons of affected individuals have nine times the normal incidence.
      d. Has an early onset of alcohol abuse (before age 25 years).
      e. Postnatal environmental has no influence.
      f. Daughters of such fathers have no increased incidence.
   Prospective personality "trait" studies (e.g., involving the Minnesota Multiphasic Personality Inventory [MMPI]) have failed to document a typical pre-alcoholic personality. However, certain constellations of personality traits, and biological findings, may be associated with specific alcoholic subtypes (Cloninger, 1987; Buydens-Branchey et al., 1989). Type II males are three times as likely

to be depressed and four times as likely to have attempted suicide as type I males.

C. **Brain Wave Studies**
   Event-related potential-evoked P300 brain waves studied in 6–13-year-old sons of alcoholic fathers showed a neurophysiological deficit, compared to controls, that was identical to that seen in chronic abstinent alcoholics (Begleiter, 1984).

D. **Abnormal Response Patterns in Males at Risk for Alcoholism**
   1. An enhanced thyrotropin response was seen in sons of familial alcoholics. Daughters showed no abnormalities (Moss, 1986).
   2. Schuckit (1994) demonstrated that a low level of response to alcohol at age 20 years predicts the likely development of alcoholism at age 30.

E. **Neurobiologic Susceptibility to Alcoholism** (Tarter, 1984, 1985)
   1. **Temperamental deviations.** Biologic and psychologic characteristics associated with a vulnerability to alcoholism have been identified in pre-alcoholic males. They manifest cognitive and behavioral deficits and electrophysiologic abnormalities suggestive of dysfunction along the prefrontal-midbrain neuraxis.
   2. **A pre-existing serotonin deficit has been identified in type II alcoholics** (Buydens-Branchey). Low serotonin metabolites in the cerebrospinal fluid (CSF) are associated with depression, impulsivity, and violence (Brown, 1990), early onset alcoholism (Linnoila, 1992), and insomnia.
   3. **A mutation on the D_2 dopamine receptor gene (D_2DR) associated with severe alcoholism, Tourette's syndrome, attention-deficit/hyperactivity disorder (ADHD), autism, and posttraumatic stress disorder (PTSD) has been investigated.** The mutant A-1 allele causes a reduced density of D_2 receptors. Although it does not cause alcoholism, it is a modifier gene that causes a more severe form of alcoholism (Blum, 1990; Comings, 1991; Noble, 1991).

VII. Evaluation of the Patient

A. **General Recommendations**
   Screening for alcohol-related problems should be routine for all mental health patients regardless of setting, and **is mandatory in patients examined for the Boards.** Individuals with alcohol problems are also at high risk for the abuse of other drugs; they should therefore be screened for the abuse of other legal and illegal substances.

B. **Psychiatric and Social Problems Associated with Alcoholism**

1. **Mental disorders commonly comorbid with alcoholism** include other substance abuse, antisocial personality disorder, conduct disorder, mania, and schizophrenia.
2. **Mental disorders sometimes comorbid with alcoholism** include major depressive disorder (especially in females), anxiety disorders, ADHD, and PTSD.
3. An erratic school or employment history.
4. Domestic violence.
5. Marital problems, especially multiple divorces.

C. **Alcoholism Screening Instruments**
   In addition to questions regarding the quantity and frequency of drinking, several instruments are available for detecting less overt problems.
   1. The **CAGE test has four simple questions** (Table 10-4) that can be easily inserted into the psychiatric interview. Two or more positive responses correlate with significant alcohol-related problems. This is a quick and reliable screening tool, even for those patients who try to hide their alcohol abuse; it is a more reliable indicator than elevated liver function tests.
   2. The **Michigan Alcoholism Screening Test (MAST).** This is a 25-question instrument (Table 10-5) that takes longer to administer, but is a more accurate screening tool than the CAGE, especially for women and the elderly.

D. **Interviewing the Patient**
   Suspected substance abuse patients should be approached in a respectful and nonjudgmental manner. A confrontational approach by the clinician does not facilitate the interview process, and has been shown to decrease the rate of successful referral to alcohol treatment. A moralistic approach is never helpful, and is also likely to alienate and to demoralize patients; it may also increase denial and diminish motivation for treatment.

E. **Abnormal Blood Chemistries Commonly Seen in Alcoholics**

No one test is considered diagnostic for alcohol dependence.
1. CDT (carbohydrate-deficit transferrin) is the most sensitive indicator of alcoholism.
2. GGTP (or GGT, γ-glutamyltranspeptidase): a blood level of >30 units/L of this liver enzyme is induced with $4+$ drinks per day for 2 weeks. It returns to normal (<30 units/L) if the patient stops drinking.
3. A MCV (mean corpuscular volume) >95 μm^3 in males and >100 in females.
4. Liver function tests (LFTs): elevated aspartate transaminase (AST) (or serum glutamic-oxaloacetic transaminase [SGOT]), alanine aminotransferase (ALT) (or serum glutamic-pyruvic transaminase [SGPT]), and alkaline phosphatase.
5. cAMP (cyclic adenosine monophosphate) levels in white blood cells (WBC) of alcoholics are three times normal.

VIII. Differential Diagnosis

Many disorders may mimic alcoholism and complicate the diagnostic process.

A. **Medical Problems**
   1. Mild alcohol intoxication is marked by disinhibition; more severe intoxication results in delirium, ataxia, or even coma. The clinician needs to rule out life-threatening conditions (e.g., head injuries) and other neurologic and metabolic problems (e.g., hypoglycemia).
   2. Alcohol use disorders may mimic insomnia and can cause a variety of medical problems, including gastrointestinal bleeding, pancreatitis, cirrhosis, hepatitis, cardiomyopathy, labile hypertension, intracranial hemorrhage, and peripheral neuropathy.

B. **Psychiatric Problems**
   The presence of a nonalcohol-induced psychiatric disorder is suggested by psychiatric symptoms that precede alcohol use, are greater than what would be

---

Table 10-4. The CAGE Questionnaire

"**C**" Have you ever felt you should **C**ut down on your drinking?

"**A**" Have people **A**nnoyed you by criticizing your drinking?

"**G**" Have you ever felt bad or **G**uilty about your drinking?

"**E**" Have you ever had a drink first thing in the morning to steady your nerves or to get rid of a hangover (**E**ye opener)?

SCORING: Item responses on the CAGE are scored 0 or 1, with a higher score indicative of alcohol problems. A score of 2 or more is considered clinically significant.

SOURCE: Published in the American Journal of Psychiatry, 1974, the American Psychiatric Association.

Table 10-5. Michigan Alcoholism Screening Test (MAST)

Clinical utility of instrument	To screen for alcoholism with a variety of populations
Research applicability	Useful in assessing extent of lifetime alcohol-related consequences
Copyright, cost, and source issues	No copyright
	Cost: $5 for copy, no fee for use
	Source:
	Melvin L. Selzer, M.D.
	6967 Paseo Laredo
	La Jolla, CA 92037

Points		YES	NO
( )	0. Do you enjoy a drink now and then?	—	—
(2)	1. Do you feel you are a normal drinker? (By normal we mean you drink less than or as much as most other people.)[a]	—	—
(2)	2. Have you ever awakened the morning after some drinking the night before and found that you could not remember a part of the evening?	—	—
(1)	3. Does your wife, husband, a parent, or another near relative ever worry or complain about your drinking?	—	—
(2)	4. Can you stop drinking without a struggle after one or two drinks?[a]	—	—
(1)	5. Do you ever feel guilty about your drinking?	—	—
(2)	6. Do friends or relatives think you are a normal drinker?[a]	—	—
(2)	7. Are you able to stop drinking when you want to?[a]	—	—
(5)	8. Have you ever attended a meeting of Alcoholics Anonymous (AA)?	—	—
(1)	9. Have you gotten into physical fights when drinking?	—	—
(2)	10. Has your drinking ever created problems between you and your wife, husband, parent, or other relative?	—	—
(2)	11. Has your wife, husband (or other family members) ever gone to anyone for help about your drinking?	—	—
(2)	12. Have you ever lost friends because of your drinking?	—	—
(2)	13. Have you ever gotten into trouble at work or school because of drinking?	—	—
(2)	14. Have you ever lost a job because of drinking?	—	—
(2)	15. Have you ever neglected your obligations, your family, or your work for 2 or more days in a row because you were drinking?	—	—
(1)	16. Do you drink before noon fairly often?	—	—
(2)	17. Have you ever been told you have liver trouble? Cirrhosis?	—	—
(2)	18. After heavy drinking have you ever had delirium tremens (DTs) or severe shaking, or heard voices or seen things that really weren't there?[b]	—	—
(5)	19. Have you ever gone to anyone for help about your drinking?	—	—
(5)	20. Have you ever been in a hospital because of drinking?	—	—
(2)	21. Have you ever been a patient in a psychiatric hospital or on a psychiatric ward of a general hospital where drinking was part of the problem that resulted in hospitalization?	—	—
(2)	22. Have you ever been seen at a psychiatric or mental health clinic or gone to any doctor, social worker, or clergyperson for help with any emotional problem where drinking was part of the problem?	—	—
(2)	23. Have you ever been arrested for drunk driving, driving while intoxicated, or driving under the influence of alcoholic beverages?[c]	—	—
(2)	24. Have you ever been arrested, taken into custody, even for a few hours, because of other drunk behavior? (IF YES, How many times? —)	—	—

^{a}Alcoholic response is negative

^{b}5 points for each Delirium Tremens

^{c}2 points for *each* arrest

SCORING SYSTEM: In general, five points or more would place the subject in an "alcoholic" category. Four points would be suggestive of alcoholism, and three points or less would indicate the subject was not alcoholic.

Programs using the above scoring system find it very sensitive at the five-point level, and it tends to find more people alcoholic than anticipated. However, it is a screening test and should be sensitive at its lower levels.

SOURCE: Selzer ML: The Michigan Alcoholism Screening Test: the quest for a new diagnostic instrument. *Am J Psychiatry* 1971; 127: 1653–1658.

SUPPORTING REFERENCES:
Zung BJ, Charalampous KD: Item analysis of the Michigan Alcoholism Screening Test. *J Stud Alcohol* 1975; 36: 127–132.
Skinner HA: A multivariate evaluation of the MAST. *J Stud Alcohol* 1979; 40: 831–844.
Zung BJ: Factor structure of the Michigan Alcoholism Screening Test in a psychiatric outpatient population. *J Clin Psychol* 1980; 36: 1024–1030.
Skinner HA, Sheu WJ: Reliability of alcohol use indices: the Lifetime Drinking History and the MAST. *J Stud Alcohol* 1982; 43: 1157–1170.
Hedlund JL, Vieweg RW: The Michigan Alcoholism Screening Test (MAST): a comprehensive review. *J Operational Psychiatry* 1984; 15: 55–64.

expected given the amount and duration of the drinking, and last longer than 4 weeks following detoxification. Appropriate diagnostic assessment can not be accomplished while an individual is actively drinking.

1. **Dysthymia and Major Depressive Disorder,** with or without suicidality, can be difficult to distinguish from the depression induced by chronic alcohol consumption. More than 60% of alcoholics are clinically depressed when admitted for detoxification, and many complain of dysthymia during the early months of sobriety. Any alcoholic or intoxicated individual who expresses suicidal ideation should be considered a serious suicide risk, regardless of the presence or absence of Major Depressive Disorder. In most cases, depressive symptoms should clear after 2 weeks of sobriety. If the patient remains depressed beyond 2 weeks, they should be assessed for a comorbid depressive disorder.

2. **Anxiety** is a common symptom during alcohol withdrawal, but it usually clears within a few days. Some alcoholics also complain of generalized anxiety, and/or panic attacks lasting up to 12 months following detoxification. These symptoms are difficult to distinguish from a comorbid anxiety disorder and require a comprehensive psychiatric evaluation after the patient has achieved sobriety.

3. **Schizophrenia** or other psychotic disorders may be confused with the hallucinations associated with delirium tremens or with alcohol hallucinosis.

IX. Treatment Strategies

A. Overview
Effective treatment of drinking problems requires more than management of the medical aspects of detoxification. Psychiatrists must also understand:

1. The distinction between detoxification (the gradual elimination of alcohol from the body) and definitive treatment for alcohol dependence.

2. The stages of the recovery process and the way ambivalence impedes progress toward sobriety.

3. The types of psychiatric problems that complicate the management of these patients.

B. Chronic Disease Model
Although a brief office intervention may be sufficient for people with minor problems, long-term treatment is usually required for individuals who are alcohol dependent. Successful management of such patients can be a long-term process during which treatment interventions must be matched to the particular needs of each patient. Psychiatrists must understand the stages alcoholics usually pass through during the recovery process, the importance of using correct intervention skills, and the need to identify and treat comorbid psychiatric conditions. The Project Match study showed that "matching" patients to a specific type of alcoholism treatment did not improve outcome except in cases of psychiatric severity. Alcoholics Anonymous (AA), cognitive-behavioral therapy (CBT), and motivational enhancement are equally effective for other patients. The critical treatment question is: "Which treatment for which patient at which time?"

C. The Stages of Behavioral Change
The work of Prochaska and DiClemente has provided a paradigm for the process of behavioral change, including change in the addictive disorders. Individuals commonly move through a series of specific stages on the road from abusive drinking to stable sobriety. Successful treatment involves helping the alcoholic move from one stage to the next, through the use of those intervention techniques that are most effective for each stage. Typically, patients cycle through this process several times before achieving stable sobriety. This approach works best when the clinician recognizes the

Table 10-6. The Stages of Behavioral Change

1. **Precontemplation**	Drinker is unaware that alcohol use is a problem, or has no interest in changing drinking pattern.
2. **Contemplation**	Drinker becomes aware of problems, but is still drinking and is usually ambivalent about stopping.
3. **Preparation**	Previous pattern continues, but drinker now makes decision to change. May initiate small changes.
4. **Action**	Behavioral change begins; is typically a trial and error process with several initial relapses.
5. **Maintenance**	New behavior pattern is consolidated; relapse prevention techniques help to maintain change.
6. **Relapse**	Efforts to change are abandoned. Cycle may be repeated until permanent sobriety is established.

SOURCE: Adapted from Prochaska, DiClemente, and Norcross, 1992.

importance of a gradual stepwise progression through the stages of change, rather than demanding instant recovery (Table 10-6).

D. Motivational Interviewing Techniques
Based on the Stages of Change Model, Miller and Rollnick have elaborated a counseling style designed to avoid patient resistance, to resolve ambivalence about drinking, and to induce change. The basic concepts of this approach are:
1. Therapist style is a powerful determinant of patient resistance and change.
2. Confrontation of the problem is a goal, not an intervention style.
3. Argumentation is a poor tool to induce change.
4. When resistance is evoked, patients tend not to change.
5. Motivation can be increased by specific treatment techniques.
6. Motivation emerges from the interaction between patient and therapist.
7. Ambivalence is normal, not pathological.
8. **Helping patients resolve ambivalence is the key to change.**

This interviewing technique suggests the following approaches for use during each stage in the recovery process.

E. Moving Patients from Pre-Contemplation to Contemplation
Many patients may be unaware that their drinking is problematic.
1. Provide **feedback,** and explore the patient's perspective on alcohol and its effects, but don't confront or argue.
   a. Obtain a physical examination and laboratory data (e.g., LFTs, BAC, MCV).
   b. Administer an assessment instrument (CAGE or MAST).
   c. Review the quantity and frequency of a patient's drinking.
2. Summarize your findings and connect drinking to identified problems.
3. **Involve family** in this process whenever possible.
4. If the patient refuses to accept your conclusions, maintain medical follow-up, listen sympathetically to the patient's complaints, and encourage the patient to agree to an "evaluation" of his or her problems.
5. The goal is to help patients connect their problems to their drinking.

F. Moving Patients from Contemplation to Preparation
1. Explore the patient's ambivalence about drinking; start with the positives:
   a. Positive: "What do you like about your drinking?"
   b. Negative: "What problems does the drinking create?"
2. Help the patient internalize this conflict; don't become part of the conflict.
3. Help the patient discuss their anger, humiliation, guilt, and resentment.
4. Search out their wish to control and/or stop their drinking.
5. The goal is to help the patient resolve his or her ambivalence; do not recommend action until the patient has made the decision to stop.

G. Moving Patients from Preparation to Action
1. Clarify the patient's goal: to stop, to control drinking, or to explore problems?
2. Recommend treatment options if the patient wishes to stop drinking.
3. Recommend substance abuse counseling if the patient wishes to "control" use or remains highly ambivalent about his or her drinking.

4. Support the patient's self-efficacy: "You can do it!"
5. **The goal is to develop an action plan; let the patient choose from a menu of treatment options.**

H. Action: Active Quitting Begins

1. Focus on directive behavior-based therapy and other specific prescriptions for gaining and maintaining sobriety (e.g., go to AA, stop socializing with other drinkers, see a counselor).
2. Avoid passive, nondirective, forms of psychotherapy.
3. Anticipate a **trial and error process** to refine treatment needs.
4. Provide ongoing optimism and support.
5. Work with self-help programs
   a. **Alcoholics Anonymous (AA)** is the primary treatment resource for most alcoholics. It relies on group support to guide the alcoholic through a process of spiritual renewal and characterologic change. The emphasis on "one day at a time," reliance on one's "higher power," and spirituality are central to the AA philosophy.
   b. Psychiatrists rely on AA to complement other types of interventions. Its immediate accessibility, the connection to a strong social network of sober individuals, and the provision of free unlimited 24-hours-a-day support make it an invaluable resource.
   c. Schizoid individuals and persons with more severe psychopathology may be uncomfortable in any type of self-help group. Professionally run groups or individual counseling are the preferred options for such patients.
   d. Nonreligious persons may find Rational Recovery or similar self-help programs an effective alternative to traditional AA.
   e. Psychiatrists may need to reassure patients that AA does not discourage psychotherapy or the use of appropriately prescribed medication for the treatment of psychiatric conditions.
   f. Successful referral to self-help programs requires familiarity with the resources available in the local community.
      i. Try to match the program to the patient's age, race, social or professional status, and religious or sexual orientation, if the patient so desires.
      ii. Insist that the patient initially attend four or five different groups, to "shop around."
      iii. Most programs will provide a volunteer to escort a newcomer to his or her first meetings. This will greatly facilitate referral.

I. Maintenance

Relapse Prevention is a specialized form of CBT developed by Marlatt to help maintain sobriety.

1. Alcoholics are taught to identify high-risk situations and predictors of relapse. Feelings, thoughts, and behaviors that trigger craving and relapse are explored and the patient is taught to modify them.

2. Making the distinction between lapses (brief slips) and full relapses helps patients terminate drinking episodes promptly before they experience a complete loss of control. Redefining such events as opportunities for learning reduces guilt and demoralization and enhances the likelihood of successful outcome.
3. These techniques are most helpful after patients have achieved an initial period of sobriety.

X. Medications in the Treatment of Alcoholism

In addition to the drugs used to treat alcohol withdrawal, medications are now available that significantly enhance the long-term management of alcoholism.

A. Detoxification

1. Benzodiazepines are the preferred medications for detoxification because of their excellent side-effect profile.
   a. Long-acting benzodiazepines, such as **chlordiazepoxide** and **diazepam,** are the standards for uncomplicated detoxification. When high enough initial doses (>60 mg diazepam over 24–36 h) are used, these drugs are self-tapering.
   b. The short-acting benzodiazepine, **lorazepam**, is recommended only for patients with significant liver disease, for those who are cognitively impaired, for patients over 65 years, and for any patient with unstable medical problems. This drug needs to be tapered over 4–8 days, but it is metabolized to the glucuronide form and is rapidly excreted by the kidney, giving the clinician more flexibility when managing unstable patients.
2. Symptom-triggered dosing based on withdrawal scales, such as the Clinical Institute Withdrawal Assessment (CIWA-Ar), works best, but requires frequent patient monitoring. This approach provides for adequate control of symptoms, avoids overmedication, and shortens the period of detoxification treatment.

B. Medications for Long-Term Treatment

1. **Naltrexone,** an opiate antagonist, has recently been found to reduce craving and relapse in alcoholics. Given in doses of 50 mg orally per day, it is well tolerated and seems to work best in motivated patients who describe intense craving. It is contraindicated for patients taking opiates or for those patients with acute hepatitis or liver failure. A positive response in terms of reduced craving and/or drinking is usually apparent within 7–10 days. If there is no response at 10 days, the medication should be discontinued.
2. **Disulfiram** inhibits the enzyme aldehyde dehydrogenase, leading to elevated levels of acetaldehyde.

Doses of 250 mg orally per day can produce tachycardia, dyspnea, nausea, and vomiting, if the patient drinks.

a. In controlled trials disulfiram is no better than placebo in producing continuous abstinence, but it does reduce the number of days drinking and the severity of concurrent medical problems.

b. Disulfiram works best in stable, motivated patients who are followed closely by their psychiatrist.

c. Liver function tests (LFTs) need to be monitored periodically for signs of disulfiram-induced hepatitis.

d. Disulfiram inhibits the metabolism of imipramine, desipramine, phenytoin, diazepam, and chlordiazepoxide. The doses of all of these medications need to be lowered when given in combination with disulfiram.

e. Amitriptyline potentiates disulfiram. Lower doses may be used when prescribed with this antidepressant.

f. Disulfiram also inhibits dopamine β-hydroxylase and may exacerbate psychosis in some schizophrenics. Reducing the daily dose to 125 mg, and adding a high-potency dopamine-blocking agent, such as haloperidol, may resolve the problem.

C. Treating Associated Symptoms

Following detoxification, alcoholics may experience various distressing symptoms and may pressure the psychiatrist to provide medication for these complaints. After a careful evaluation to rule out comorbid psychiatric disorders, patients should be reassured that these symptoms **are a normal part of early recovery** and will usually resolve with extended sobriety. Avoiding prescribed medications helps patients learn that they are moving beyond a dependency on exogenous chemicals.

1. **Anxiety.** Relaxation techniques and cognitive-behavioral interventions can be utilized. Avoid the prescription of benzodiazepines because of their abuse potential in this population.

2. **Depression.** The majority of alcoholics entering detoxification programs are clinically depressed. Following detoxification less than 3% of men and 12% of women meet DSM-IV criteria for a depressive disorder. These individuals should be considered for antidepressant therapy. Fluoxetine has been demonstrated to reduce both drinking and depression in severely depressed alcoholics. Paroxetine and nefazodone are also well tolerated by this population, although efficacy data are less clear-cut. For individuals with less severe depressive symptoms, psychotherapy is often helpful in managing guilt and discouragement.

3. **Insomnia.** If appropriate sleep hygiene does not resolve the problem, use of the sedating antidepressant, trazodone (25–100 mg p.o. q.h.s.), may help. It has no significant abuse potential and is effective for long-term use. Sedative hypnotic drugs should be avoided because of their abuse potential.

XI. Managing Dual Diagnosis Patients

Psychiatric diagnoses made during periods of active drinking are highly unreliable. The patient should be observed following a minimum of 2 weeks of sobriety to confirm any diagnosis. Once it is clear that the symptoms are not secondary to the patient's alcoholism, any comorbid psychiatric disorder must be treated. **Failure to adequately diagnose and treat comorbid psychiatric disorders is the most common cause for the failure of alcoholism treatment.**

A. Anxiety Disorders

1. General considerations. If anxiety complaints are associated with alcohol craving or preoccupation, an initial response should be a 2-week trial of naltrexone. If there is no response, or if anxiety symptoms persist despite reduced craving, the patient should be evaluated for an independent anxiety disorder.

2. Specific treatment options for anxiety disorders comorbid with the substance use disorders are outlined in Table 10-7.

3. Use of benzodiazepines. Judicious use of the less abusable benzodiazepines, such as oxazepam or chlordiazepoxide, may be considered for patients with panic disorder or generalized anxiety disorder (GAD) who have failed to respond to the more conservative therapies recommended above. These patients should be monitored carefully for signs of abuse of these medications, and/or relapse to drinking.

a. **Panic Disorder** may precede the development of alcoholism and usually becomes more severe following extended drinking. Behavioral psychotherapy and antidepressants, such as imipramine, paroxetine, and nefazodone, have all proved to be effective treatments.

b. **Posttraumatic Stress Disorder (PTSD)** and comorbid alcohol abuse are very difficult to treat. Such patients should be referred to specialized treatment programs.

B. Major Depressive Disorder

Various tricyclic antidepressants and the selective serotonin reuptake inhibitors have been used with some success in depressed alcoholics, though there are few adequately controlled clinical trials. Nefazodone appears to have particular value in those alcoholics with a combination of anxiety and depressive symptoms. It is well tolerated and rapidly normalizes sleep patterns.

C. Bipolar Disorder

Mood-stabilizing drugs can have dramatic benefits in these cases. Adequate control of manic episodes often eliminates excessive drinking.

Table 10-7. Treatment of Specific Axis I Conditions in the Presence of an Alcohol-Related Disorder

Condition	Primary Treatment	If No Response
Panic Disorder	CBT + nefazodone or SSRI	Alternative SSRI or venlafaxine
Social phobia		
1) Specific type	CBT + beta-blocker	
2) Generalized + depression	CBT + SSRI	
3) Generalized, no depression	Nefazodone or SSRI	
Posttraumatic Stress Disorder (PTSD)	Psychotherapy	Medications as needed
1) Plus depression	Nefazodone or SSRI	Alternative SSRI
2) With related psychosis	New generation antipsychotics	Alternative antipsychotic
3) With severe insomnia	Trazodone	Sedating TCA
Obsessive-Compulsive Disorder (OCD)	SSRI	Clomipramine, if no seizures or suicide ideation
Generalized anxiety disorder (GAD)	Treat any comorbid	
1) 90% are comorbid for panic disorder, PTSD, social phobia, or OCD	anxiety disorders, as above	
2) GAD + depression	Nefazodone or SSRI	
3) GAD, not depressed	CBT/relaxation therapy	Buspirone, up to 60 mg q.d.

1. **Bipolar I:** lithium in the standard dose range is most effective.
2. **Bipolar II:** valproic acid may have some advantage in this group.

D. Schizophrenia

Intensive long-term substance abuse counseling must be provided in conjunction with comprehensive psychiatric management. Schizophrenic patients do poorly in most AA groups, and may be highly ambivalent about sobriety, since they often use alcohol to moderate psychotic symptoms or to reduce the side effects of their antipsychotic medications.

E. Attention-Deficit/Hyperactivity Disorder (ADHD) can be treated with methylphenidate 10–20 mg p.o. t.i.d., though these patients must be followed carefully for signs of stimulant abuse.

XII. Criteria for Referral for Inpatient Detoxification

A. A history of failure in outpatient detoxification, or **multiple relapses**

B. Suicidal ideation or acute psychosis

C. A history of **Delirium Tremens**

D. Comorbid medical problems that require frequent daily monitoring during detoxification

XIII. Criteria for Referral for Specialized Long-Term Alcoholism Treatment

A. A history of **multiple treatment failures.**

B. Serious comorbid psychiatric conditions, especially if they have failed to respond to initial efforts at psychiatric management.

C. Abuse of other drugs (**polysubstance abuse**).

D. Living in very unstable environments, e.g., the homeless.

Selected Readings

American Psychiatric Association: *Diagnostic and Statistical Manual of Mental Disorders, Fourth Edition.* Washington: American Psychiatric Association, 1994.

Begleiter H, Porjesz B, Bihari B, et al.: Event-related brain potentials in boys at risk for alcoholism. *Science* 1984; 255:1493–1496.

Bein, TH, Miller, WR, Tonigan, JS: Brief intervention for alcohol problems: a review. *Addiction* 1993; 88:315–335.

Blum K, Noble EP, Sheridan PJ, et al.: Allelic association of human dopamine D_2 receptor gene in alcoholism. *J Am Med Assoc* 1990; 263:2055–2060.

Brown GL, Linnoila MI: CSF serotonin metabolite (5-HIAA) studies in depression, impulsivity, and violence. *J Clin Psych* 1990; 51(4, suppl):31–41.

Buydens-Branchey L, Branchy M, Noumair D, Lieber C: Age of alcoholism onset, I & II. *Arch Gen Psychiatry* 1989; 46:225–236.

Center for Disease Control and Prevention, reported in *The Boston Globe*, More babies are found to suffer fetal alcohol syndrome,

April 7, 1995.

Ciraulo DA, Renner, JA: Alcoholism. In Ciraulo DA, Shader RI (eds): *Clinical Manual of Chemical Dependence.* Washington DC: American Psychiatric Press, 1991.

Cloninger CR: Neurogenic adaptive mechanisms in alcoholism. *Science* 1987; 236:410–416.

Cloninger CR, Bohman M, Sigvardsson S: Inheritance of alcohol abuse: cross-fostering analysis of adopted men. *Arch Gen Psychiatry* 1981; 38:861–868.

Comings DE, Comings BG, Muhleman D, et al.: The dopamine D_2 receptor locus as a modifying gene in neuropsychiatric disorders. *J Am Med Assoc* 1991; 266:1793–1800.

Famy C, Streissguth AP, Unis AS: Mental illness in adults with fetal alcohol syndrome or fetal alcohol effects. *Am J Psychiatry* 1998; 155:552–554.

Frances RJ, Timm S, Bucky S: Studies of familial and nonfamilial alcoholism. *Arch Gen Psychiatry* 1980; 37:564–566.

Friedman L, Fleming NF, Roberts DH, Hyman SE (eds): *Source Book of Substance Abuse and Addiction.* Baltimore: Williams and Wilkins, 1996.

Kessler RC, McGonagle KA, Zhao S et al.: Lifetime and 12-month prevalence of DSM-III-R psychiatric disorders in the United States. *Arch Gen Psychiatry* 1994; 51:8–19.

Kessler RC, Crum RM, Warner LA, et al.: Lifetime co-occurrence of DSM-III-R alcohol abuse and dependence with other psychiatric disorders in the National Comorbidity Survey. *Arch Gen Psychiatry* 1997; 54:313–321.

Koob GF, Roberts AJ: Brain reward circuits in alcoholism. *CNS Spectrums* 1999; 4:23–33.

Linnoila MI, Virkhunen M: Aggression, suicidality, and serotonin. *J Clin Psych* 1992; 53:46–51.

Mayfield D, McLeod G, Hall P: The CAGE questionnaire: validation of a new alcoholism instrument. *Am J Psychiatry* 1974; 131: 1121–1123.

Miller WR, Rollnick S: *Motivational Interviewing: Preparing People to Change Addictive Behavior.* New York: The Guilford Press, 1991.

Moss HB, Guthrie S, Linnoila M: Enhanced thyrotropin releasing hormone in boys at risk for development of alcoholism: preliminary findings. *Arch Gen Psychiatry* 1986, 43:1137–1142.

Noble EP, Blum K, Ritchie T, et al.: Allelic association of the D_2 dopamine receptor gene with receptor-binding characteristics in alcoholism. *Arch Gen Psychiatry* 1991; 48:648–654.

O'Malley SS, Jaffe AJ, Chang G, et al.: Naltrexone and coping skills therapy for alcohol dependence. A controlled study. *Arch Gen Psychiatry* 1992; 49:881–887.

Osser DN, Renner JA, Bayog R: Algorithms for the pharmacotherapy of anxiety disorders in patients with chemical abuse and dependence. *Psychiatr Ann* 1999; 29:285–301.

Prescott CA, Kendler KS: Genetic and environmental contributions to alcohol abuse and dependence in a population-based sample of male twins. *Am J Psychiatry* 1999; 156:34–40.

Prochaska J, DiClemente C, Norcross J: In search of how people change. Applications to addictive behaviors. *Am Psychol* 1992; 47:1102–1114.

Rollnick N, Heather N, Bell A: Negotiating behavior change in medical settings: the development of brief motivational interviewing. *J Ment Health* 1992; 1:25.

Saitz R, Mayo-Smith MF, Roberts MS, et al.: Individualized treatment for alcohol withdrawal. *J Am Med Assoc* 1994; 272:519–523.

Sandberg GG, Marlatt GA: Relapse prevention. In Ciraulo DA, Shader RI (eds): *Clinical Manual of Chemical Dependence.* Washington DC: American Psychiatric Press, 1991.

Schuckit MA: Low level of response to alcohol as a predictor of future alcoholism. *Am J Psychiatry* 1994; 151:184–189.

Selzer ML: The Michigan Alcoholism Screening Test: the quest for a new diagnostic instrument. *Am J Psychiatry* 1971; 127:1653–1655.

Streissguth AP, Aase JM, Clarren SK, et al.: Fetal alcohol syndrome in adolescents and adults. *J Am Med Assoc* 1991; 265:1961–1967.

Sullivan JT, Syhora K, Schneiderman J, et al.: Assessment of alcohol withdrawal: the revised Clinical Institute Withdrawal Assessment for Alcohol Scale (CIWA-Ar). *Br J Addict* 1989; 84:1353–1357.

Swift RM: Drug therapy for alcohol dependence. *N Engl J Med* 1999; 340:1482–1490.

Tarter RE, Hegedus AM, Goldstein G, et al.: Adolescent sons of alcoholics: neuropsychological personality characteristics. *Alcohol Clin Exp Res* 1984; 8:216–222.

Tarter RE, Alterman AI, Edwards KL: Vulnerability to alcoholism in men: a behavioral-genetic perspective. *J Stud Alcohol* 1985; 46:329–356.

Chapter 11

Substance-Related Disorders: Cocaine and Narcotics

John Matthews

I. Cocaine-Related Disorders

A. **Cocaine abuse involves a pattern of use that is less intense and less frequent than cocaine dependence.** The use is maladaptive and leads to impairment and distress in at least one of the following areas within a 12-month period:
 1. A failure to meet obligations at home, work, or school.
 2. Use of cocaine in situations that are considered physically hazardous.
 3. The development of cocaine-related legal problems.
 4. Continued use of cocaine despite social and interpersonal problems caused or worsened by cocaine use.

B. **Cocaine dependence involves a maladaptive pattern of use that leads to impairment and distress in at least three of the following areas within a 12-month period:**
 1. The development of tolerance defined by either a need for **a significant increase in the amount of cocaine to achieve the desired effect or a significant decrease in the effect of the usual cocaine dose.**
 2. The **development of cocaine withdrawal symptoms** (see below) or the need to ingest cocaine to relieve or to prevent withdrawal symptoms.
 3. The **use of cocaine in larger amounts** and for longer periods than was intended.
 4. The **inability to cut down** or to control the use of cocaine.
 5. The time spent to obtain cocaine and to recover from the effects of cocaine is great.
 6. Social, occupational, or recreational activities are stopped or reduced to maintain cocaine use.
 7. **Cocaine use is maintained despite persistent or recurrent physical or psychological problems** that are caused or exacerbated by its use. Dependence may be episodic or continuous.

C. **Cocaine intoxication involves clinically significant maladaptive behavioral or psychological changes** (e.g., euphoria, interpersonal sensitivity, anxiety, tension, anger, stereotypic behaviors, poor judgment, impaired social and occupational functioning, and hypervigilance) **that developed during or shortly after cocaine use. Two or more of the following symptoms develop during or immediately after the use of cocaine:**
 1. **Tachycardia or bradycardia**
 2. **Pupillary dilation**
 3. **Elevated or lowered blood pressure**
 4. **Diaphoresis or chills**
 5. **Nausea or vomiting**
 6. **Weight loss**
 7. **Agitation or psychomotor retardation**
 8. **Muscle weakness**
 9. **Chest pain**
 10. **Arrhythmias**
 11. **Respiratory depression**
 12. **Confusion**
 13. **Seizures**
 14. **Dyskinesias**
 15. **Dystonia**
 16. **Coma**

D. **Cocaine withdrawal involves dysphoric mood and two of the following physiological symptoms which develop within hours to several days following the cessation of, or a decrease in, cocaine use:**
 1. Fatigue
 2. Vivid and unpleasant dreams
 3. Insomnia or hypersomnia
 4. Increased appetite
 5. Agitation or psychomotor retardation

E. **Other cocaine-induced disorders include:**
 1. Cocaine intoxication delirium
 2. Cocaine-induced psychotic disorder, with delusions
 3. Cocaine-induced psychotic disorder, with hallucinations
 4. Cocaine-induced mood disorder
 5. Cocaine-induced anxiety disorder
 6. Cocaine-induced sexual dysfunction
 7. Cocaine-induced sleep disorder
 8. Cocaine-related disorder not otherwise specified

II. Pharmacology of Cocaine

A. **Cocaine preparations include coca leaves, cocaine hydrochloride, coca paste, free base, and crack** (Gold, 1997).
 1. **Coca leaves.** This form of cocaine is **ingested orally and is the least potent of all of the preparations;** its purity is 0.5–1.0%. The average acute dose is 20–50 mg, the onset of action is 5–10 min, and the dura-

85

tion of the high is 60–90 min. It is used primarily by natives of Central and South America.

2. **Cocaine hydrochloride (oral).** This form of cocaine is a powder; its purity ranges between 20% and 80% and the bioavailability is 20–80%. The average acute dose is 100–200 mg, **the onset of action is 10–20 min, and the duration of the high is about 45–90 min.**

3. **Cocaine hydrochloride (intranasal).** The purity of this form is 20–80% and the bioavailability is about 20–30%. The average acute dose is 30 mg per line, **the onset of action is 2–3 min, and the duration of the high is about 30–45 min.**

4. **Cocaine hydrochloride (intravenous).** Cocaine hydrochloride **powder is dissolved in water to produce an intravenous form.** This is a particularly potent form since it has a bioavailability of 100%. The average acute dose is 25–50 mg, the **onset of action is 30–45 s, and the duration of the high is 10–20 min.** It is on occasion combined with heroin, forming a mixture known as a "speedball."

5. **Cocaine alkaloid (free base).** Cocaine is **separated from its hydrochloride base by heating it with ether, ammonia, or some other solvent.** This is a procedure with risk since the solvent can ignite. The purity is 90–100%. The average acute dose is 250–1000 mg, the **onset of action is 10 s, and the duration of the high is 5–10 min.**

6. **Cocaine alkaloid (crack).** Crack, a cocaine alkaloid, is **extracted from cocaine hydrochloride by mixing it with sodium bicarbonate.** The purity is 50–95%. The average acute dose is 250–1000 mg, the **onset of action is 10 s, and the duration of the high is 5–10 min.**

B. Metabolism
Cocaine is **metabolized to benzoylecgonine,** which can be detected in the urine for up to 36 h.

C. Impact on Neurotransmitters
1. **Cocaine blocks the uptake of dopamine (DA), serotonin (5-HT), and norepinephrine (NE)** from each of their neuron terminals by binding to the presynaptic transporter complexes. The reinforcing properties of cocaine are believed to be mediated by enhancing neurotransmission through the mesolimbic dopamine pathway (dopamine cells in the ventral tegmental area in the brainstem project to the nucleus accumbens). The nucleus accumbens and DA serve as the final common pathway for the rewarding experiences of most recreational drugs of abuse.

2. In animal studies, using microdialysis techniques to measure released DA concentrations in the nucleus accumbens, researchers found a dose-dependent relationship between self-administration of cocaine and DA concentrations.

3. In human studies using positron emission tomography (PET), researchers demonstrated cocaine binding to high-affinity receptor sites on DA transporters in vivo.

D. Physical and Psychological Effects of Cocaine
1. **The acute physical and psychological effects of cocaine include:**
   a. **Vasoconstriction**
   b. An **increased heart rate**
   c. An **increased blood pressure**
   d. **Euphoria; increased energy**
   e. A **heightened alertness** and sensory awareness (confirmed by desynchronization of brain waves on EEG recordings)
   f. Increased **anxiety**
   g. An increased risk of panic attacks (in predisposed individuals)
   h. An increased self-confidence
   i. A **decreased appetite**
   j. An increased **sexual excitement and spontaneous ejaculation**
   k. An increased **risk for psychosis** (including paranoid delusions).

An individual's response to cocaine may be trait-dependent. Individuals who have a low level of arousal may have a positive experience from cocaine use, whereas individuals who have a high level of arousal may have a negative experience.

2. As a result of **chronic use of cocaine,** many individuals **develop symptoms of depression, irritability, agitation, a lack of motivation, insomnia, panic attacks, hypervigilance, paranoia, and hallucinations.** The long-term effects of cocaine may be the result of neurotransmitter depletion.

E. Comorbid Substance Use
Sedating substances, such as alcohol, are frequently used to combat the stimulating effects of cocaine and to prolong the euphoria it produces. Alcohol combines with cocaine to produce cocaethylene which has similar neurochemical, pharmacological, and behavioral properties to cocaine. However, **cocaethylene is believed to have more cardiac toxicity.**

III. Epidemiology of Cocaine-Related Disorders

A. Historical Trends
1. In the 1970s, cocaine was considered by professionals to be a safe and nonaddictive drug. **Cocaine use peaked in 1978 at 25% of the population;** however, cocaine use dropped to a low of 20% of the population in 1989. Reasons provided for the reduction in use include:
   a. Education about the detrimental effects of cocaine

b. Promotion of better health

c. The need to be competitive in today's society; much of the decline in use has been among the middle and upper classes.

2. **A community survey from 1991 demonstrated that 12% of the population had used cocaine at least once during their lifetime,** that 3% had used cocaine within the past year, and that less than 1% had used cocaine within the past month. It is not known how many of those individuals would have met criteria for a substance use disorder.

3. Data from the National Institute of Drug Abuse (1997) demonstrated that **55% of drug-abusing patients, mostly in outpatient treatment programs** (methadone, short-term inpatient, residential, and outpatient), are **dependent on cocaine.**

B. Social Impact
Cocaine use continues to be a serious problem among the disadvantaged, who have easy access to the drug and little hope of becoming a productive part of society. Crack has become very affordable; vials cost as little as $10.00. Cocaine use is more prevalent among African-Americans and is associated with violence and the transmission of acquired immunodeficiency syndrome (AIDS).

IV. Course of Cocaine-Related Disorders

There are two primary patterns of use: episodic and daily use.

A. Episodic use generally occurs during weekends or on one or two occasions during the week. **Binges** are a type of episodic use when large amounts of cocaine are consumed within a few hours or a few days. **Binges end when cocaine supplies are depleted.**

B. Daily use of cocaine generally progresses from small amounts to large amounts due to the development of tolerance to the euphoric effects of cocaine.

C. Progressive Use
The form and route of administration of cocaine also determine the course and progression of use. Intranasal use tends to show a more gradual progression from use to abuse or dependence over months to years, whereas intravenous use and smoking tend to show a rapid progression to eventual dependence over weeks to months.

V. Comorbid Psychiatric and Cocaine-Related Disorders

A. Prevalence
1. **The rate for any psychiatric disorder (excluding other substance abuse) in cocaine abusers seeking treatment is 50%; the lifetime prevalence is 80%.**

Among cocaine abusers the rate for a lifetime diagnosis of major depressive disorder is 50%, for dysthymic disorder it is 25–50%, and for bipolar spectrum disorders it is 25%.

B. Self-Medication
Many cocaine-dependent **patients with comorbid psychiatric disorders use cocaine as self-medication for their psychiatric symptoms:**
1. Depressed patients use to elevate their mood.
2. Bipolar patients use to sustain their highs.
3. Patients with attention deficit disorder use to help their distractibility and their mood.
4. Patients with schizophrenia use to help relieve their negative symptoms.
5. Patients with borderline personality disorder use to help their mood.
6. Patients with antisocial personality disorder use to enhance stimulation and excitement.
7. Patients with narcissistic personality disorder use to further increase feelings of grandiosity.

C. Use of Other Substances
Other substances of abuse, such as alcohol, marijuana, benzodiazepines, and opiates, are associated with cocaine abuse and dependence. Alcohol, marijuana, and benzodiazepines are often used to treat the unpleasant stimulating effects of cocaine, whereas opiates are used to enhance the euphoric effect of cocaine.

D. Comorbid Psychiatric Conditions
Patients with anxiety disorders, especially panic disorder, tend to avoid the use of cocaine since it heightens anxiety and may trigger panic attacks. Panic attacks often continue after stopping the drug in vulnerable individuals.

E. Differential Diagnosis
It can be difficult to distinguish cocaine-induced psychiatric disorders from primary psychiatric disorders. **Cocaine-induced psychiatric symptoms include: depression, panic attacks, anxiety, psychosis, antisocial behaviors, and aggressive behaviors.** In contrast to primary psychiatric disorders, symptoms induced by cocaine resolve within a few hours to a few days.

VI. Medical Complications Associated with Cocaine Use

A. Cardiovascular
Cocaine causes adrenergic stimulation, which may result in **elevation of blood pressure, tachycardia, and arrhythmias. It may also cause vasospasms in coronary arteries.** Adrenergic stimulation, which increases oxygen demand of the heart, in combina-

tion with coronary artery vasospasms, may result in myocardial infarction.

B. Central Nervous System

Cocaine causes vasospasm in cerebral vasculature that results in cerebral vascular accidents acutely as well as multifocal infarcts with prolonged use. Single-photon emission computed tomography (SPECT) has demonstrated significant hypoperfusion in frontal and temporal-parietal areas among chronic users of cocaine. These findings correlate with cognitive impairment (e.g., diminished concentration, attention, and memory as measured by neuropsychological testing). Cocaine can also induce seizures, after either single or repeated use, by a phenomenon called "kindling."

C. Respiratory System

Cocaine-induced respiratory symptoms include **hemoptysis, fever, and productive cough, as well as chest pain due to the build-up of carbon monoxide.** Respiratory disorders secondary to cocaine include asthma, pneumonia, pneumothorax, pneumomediastinum, pneumopericardium, pulmonary edema, and sudden death from cocaine-induced respiratory depression. "Crack lung" is a recently identified condition that is manifest by fever, shortness of breath, chest pain, and pneumonia.

D. Other Systems

Chronic intranasal use of cocaine may cause **nasal septum necrosis** due to its vasoconstricting effects. Cocaine binges may result in **dehydration, malnutrition, and weight loss. Intravenous cocaine use may cause vasculitis, endocarditis, granulomas, hepatitis B and C, human immunodeficiency virus (HIV), pulmonary emboli, and septicemia due to contaminants in the injection solution.**

E. Use in Pregnancy

Cocaine use **increases the risk of fetal hypoxia and placental abruption** due to its vasoconstrictive properties. Cocaine readily crosses the placenta and can have toxic effects on the fetus. Echocardiograms reveal left ventricular hypertrophy in the fetus. Cocaine can cause fetal growth retardation, reduced head circumference, decreased birth weight, congenital anomalies, malformations of the urogenital system, central nervous system (CNS) irritability ("jittery baby"), attentional problems, cerebral vascular accidents, and death. Cerebral vasoconstriction and hypoxia may interfere with brain development. Cocaine is found in breast milk up to 60 h after use. Symptoms observed in babies who ingest cocaine from breast milk include: rapid heart rate, increased blood pressure, apnea, diaphoresis, and mydriasis.

VII. Treatment of Cocaine Use

A. Treatment Settings

The goal is to use the least restrictive environment so that family, social, and occupational responsibilities are minimally disrupted. Most studies demonstrate that patients can be effectively treated in an outpatient setting. However, patients with complicated psychosocial, psychiatric, or medical problems may require a more structured environment. Criteria for inpatient treatment according to Washton (1990) and others include:

1. Lack of motivation to participate in an intensive outpatient program
2. Significant psychological, cognitive, or neurological deficits
3. Serious comorbid psychiatric or medical problems
4. Several failed attempts at outpatient and partial hospital treatments
5. Lack of a support network
6. Use of highly addictive crack, freebase, or intravenous cocaine
7. Significant dependence on alcohol and/or other substances of abuse
8. The risk for aggressive behaviors towards self, others, or property

B. Intoxication

There is no specific antidote for cocaine intoxication. Treatment is generally supportive. Benzodiazepines are helpful to treat aggressive or agitated behavior. Patients with a paranoid psychosis should not be treated initially with antipsychotic medications because of the risk of inducing a seizure. Their psychosis generally resolves within a few hours up to 3–5 days. If the psychosis continues, the diagnosis should be reconsidered and antipsychotic medication started. Although cocaine increases the risk for seizures, prophylactic use of anticonvulsants has not been shown to be beneficial.

C. Withdrawal

There is no specific treatment of the typical withdrawal symptoms from cocaine dependence (see above for typical symptoms of withdrawal). The symptoms begin within a few hours of discontinuing cocaine use and may persist for several days. Dopamine agonists, bromocriptine and amantadine, were initially used to treat cocaine withdrawal symptoms and cravings, but recent studies have failed to support their use.

D. Relapse Prevention

Cognitive-behavioral therapy (CBT) approaches help patients identify the internal (emotions) and external (situations) cues that activate addictive beliefs ("The only way I can have fun is to get high") which trigger cravings and urges to use.

Once cravings and urges are activated, permissive beliefs ("I can stop after one smoke") and rationalizations to use are realized; permissive beliefs lead to strategies ("I'll drive to Bill's to buy crack") to use. The therapist helps the patient to challenge the validity of his or her addictive and permissive beliefs. CBT relapse prevention strategies are particularly effective over a 12-week period with more severe cocaine abusers. Outcome studies at 6–12 months also demonstrate that cognitive-behavioral relapse prevention is significantly more effective than routine clinical management. **A behavioral approach using contingent vouchers has been particularly effective in keeping patients in treatment and maintaining abstinence.** In this approach, patients earn vouchers to purchase predetermined items (books, social events with their family) provided that they maintain clean urines.

E. Self-Help Groups
Cocaine Anonymous (CA) is a 12-step program modeled after Alcoholics Anonymous. A recent study of day hospital cocaine-abusing patients showed that greater participation in self-help groups at 3 months posttreatment predicted less cocaine use at 6 months posttreatment.

F. Pharmacological Treatments
Pharmacological treatment is not indicated for cocaine dependence. Studies of pharmacological treatments that could reduce the subjective effects of cocaine and reduce symptoms of cocaine abstinence have been mixed and inconclusive. Multiple methodological problems (including differences in patient populations, absence of controls, differences in psychosocial interventions, differences in route of cocaine administration, and inconsistent outcome measures) have plagued clinical studies. Dopamine agonists (e.g., amantadine and bromocriptine) and tricyclic antidepressants (e.g., desipramine) initially showed promise in treating cocaine dependence, but more recent studies have failed to confirm earlier findings.

VIII. DSM-IV Opioid-Related Disorders

A. Opioid Abuse
A maladaptive pattern of opioid use leading to clinically significant impairment or distress, as manifested by one or more of the following, occurring within a 12-month period:
1. Recurrent opioid use resulting in a failure to fulfill major role obligations at work, school, or home.
2. Recurrent opioid use in situations in which it is physically hazardous.
3. Recurrent opioid-related legal problems.

4. Continued opioid use despite having persistent or recurrent social or interpersonal problems caused or exacerbated by the effects of the opioid.

B. Opioid Dependence
A maladaptive pattern of opioid use, leading to clinically significant impairment or distress, as manifested by three or more of the following, **occurring at any time in the same 12-month period:**
1. Tolerance, as defined by either of the following:
   a. A need for markedly increased amounts of the opioid to achieve intoxication or desired effect.
   b. Markedly diminished effect with continued use of the same amount of the opioid.
2. Withdrawal, as manifested by either of the following:
   a. The characteristic withdrawal syndrome for opioids.
   b. The same or a closely related opioid is taken to relieve or avoid withdrawal symptoms.
3. The opioid is often taken in larger amounts or over a longer period than was intended.
4. There is a persistent desire or unsuccessful efforts to cut down or control opioid use.
5. A great deal of time is spent in activities necessary to obtain, use, or recover from the effects of the opioid.
6. Important social, occupational, or recreational activities are given up or reduced because of substance use.
7. The opioid use is continued despite knowledge of having a persistent or recurrent physical or psychological problem that is likely to have been caused or exacerbated by the opioid.

C. Opioid Intoxication
Clinically significant maladaptive behavioral or psychological changes (e.g., initial euphoria followed by apathy, dysphoria, psychomotor agitation or retardation, impaired judgment, or impaired social or occupational functioning) **that developed during, or shortly after, opioid use.** Physiological changes include pupillary constriction (or pupillary dilation with severe overdose) and one or more of the following signs developing in the context of opioid use:
1. Drowsiness or coma
2. Slurred speech
3. Impairment in attention or memory

D. Opioid Withdrawal
The development of at least three or more of the following symptoms with either reduction or cessation of opioid use, or administration of an opioid antagonist:
1. Dysphoric mood
2. Nausea or vomiting
3. Muscle aches

4. Lacrimation or rhinorrhea
5. Pupillary dilation
6. Piloerection or sweating
7. Diarrhea
8. Yawning
9. Fever
10. Insomnia

E. Other Opioid-Induced Disorders

According to DSM-IV, the following disorders are diagnosed instead of Opioid Intoxication or Opioid Withdrawal only when the symptoms are in excess of those usually associated with the Opioid Intoxication or Withdrawal syndrome and when the symptoms are sufficiently severe to warrant independent clinical attention:

1. Opioid Intoxication Delirium
2. Opioid-Induced Psychotic Disorder
3. Opioid-Induced Mood Disorder
4. Opioid-Induced Sexual Dysfunction
5. Opioid-Induced Sleep Disorder

IX. Opiate Pharmacology

A. Opiates bind to three types of receptors in the brain, which are referred to as **mu, delta, and kappa. Mu and delta receptors,** when activated, **influence mood, reinforcement, analgesia, respiration, blood pressure, gastrointestinal function, and endocrine functions. Kappa receptors,** when activated, **produce dysphoria and analgesia.** Receptor subtypes (mu1, mu2, kappa 1, and kappa 2) have been identified, but specifics as to what functions they mediate are yet to be determined.

B. Opiate drugs are categorized as to how they are able to bind and activate receptor types:

1. **Agonists readily bind to and activate receptors.**
2. **Antagonists readily bind to but do not activate receptors.**
3. **Partial agonists bind to receptors but only activate them to a limited extent; they may also block receptors from occupation by other agonists or antagonists.**

Morphine, methadone, fentanyl, and sufentanil are primarily pure mu receptor agonists, buprenorphine and pentazocine are partial agonists, and naloxone and naltrexone are pure antagonists. Opiate receptors are located throughout the CNS, parts of the autonomic nervous system, and the gastrointestinal system. The receptors most commonly targeted by prescribed medications are located in the CNS and gastrointestinal system. When CNS receptors are activated, individuals experience tranquillity, reduced apprehension, analgesia, cough suppression, respiratory depression, pupillary constriction, and changes in temperature. When gastrointestinal receptors are activated, individuals experience nausea, constipation, and vomiting.

C. The positive reinforcing effect of opiates is mediated through the ventral tegmental area (VTA) dopamine projections to the nucleus accumbens, and through direct effects of mu and delta agonists on neurons in the nucleus accumbens. Mu and delta agonists inhibit γ-aminobutyric acid-A (GABA-A) interneurons that normally tonically inhibit VTA dopamine cells. The net effect of mu and delta agonists is to increase VTA dopamine cells firing rates, resulting in an increased release of dopamine in the nucleus accumbens. Stimulants, such as cocaine and amphetamine, also increase dopamine release via different receptors. Stimulants combined with opiates significantly increase their euphoric effect without increasing their side effects. As mentioned above, the combination of opiates and cocaine given together intravenously is called a "speedball."

D. Urine Testing

Opioids are measured in blood, urine, saliva, and hair. Heroin is measured as morphine in urine. Most short-acting opioids are detected in the urine 12–36 h after administration. Routine urine screens do not detect meperidine, fentanyl, and oxycodone. Poppy seeds contain small amounts of morphine and codeine, which can result in false positive urine tests for opioid abuse.

X. Epidemiology of Opiate Abuse

A. A United States **community survey from 1991 demonstrated that 6% of the population had used analgesics for nonmedical reasons,** 2.5% used them within the past year, and 0.7% used them within the past month. Most opioid-dependent individuals are not receiving treatment.

B. Heroin abuse and dependence occur three times more frequently in males than in females. The nonmedical use of opioids (excluding heroin) occurs at almost twice the rate in Caucasians than in African-Americans. Some studies suggest that heroin abuse is more frequent among minority groups; however, these data are based on surveys of public treatment facilities, which may exclude a significant number of white middle-class heroin addicts.

XI. Course of Opiate Abuse

A. Studies examining patterns of use in adolescents and young adults have discovered a progression of drug use beginning with cigarettes, alcohol, marijuana, and eventually opioids. **The onset of opioid abuse in general is in the teens and early twenties.**

Once opioid dependence develops, the course is generally longstanding for many years with frequent lapses and relapses. Even after long periods of incarceration, relapse rates are high. According to some experts, the average duration of active opioid addiction is 9 years.

B. **The death rate among opioid addicts is 20 times that in the general population, and the increased rate is due to overdose, infection, AIDS, suicide, homicide, and trauma.**

XII. Etiological Factors Associated with Opiate Use

A. Not everyone who experiments with opioid use develops abuse or dependence. According to the National Comorbidity Survey (1994), **7.5% of individuals who used any opioids for nonmedical purposes and 23% of individuals who used heroin eventually developed opioid dependence.** There are genetic, biological, and psychosocial factors that contribute to opioid dependence.

B. **Genetic and Biological Factors**
   1. Animal studies demonstrate that various strains of rodents exhibit differences with regard to their ability to learn opioid self-administration behavior and to their sensitivity to the effects of opioids.
   2. Family members of opioid addicts exhibit higher rates of addictive disorders and psychiatric disorders.
   3. **Studies of twins have shown that monozygotic twins are more likely than dizygotic twins to be concordant for opioid dependence.**
   4. Environmental stress can sensitize animals to self-administer opioids. Corticotropin-releasing factor (CRF), a peptide important in the brain's response to environmental stress, can stimulate opioid-seeking behavior in opioid-dependent animals, whereas CRF antagonists can reduce stress-related opioid self-administration. There is evidence that corticosteroids can sensitize animals to self-administer opioids and that they also increase the sensitivity of the VTA dopamine neurons to excitatory input. In addition, addicts physically dependent on heroin have high serum levels of glucocorticoids during withdrawal, and there are increases in adrenocorticotropic hormone (ACTH) prior to the onset of withdrawal symptoms. This increase of hypothalamic-pituitary-adrenal axis (HPA axis) activity is thought by some researchers to trigger cravings to use opioids in opioid-dependent individuals via the VTA. Environmental stressors may be influencing drug-seeking behavior through increases in corticosteroids and through increases in VTA activity through excitatory input from prefrontal cortical areas.

C. **Psychosocial Factors**
   1. **The self-medication hypothesis proposed by Khantzian argues that there is a strong relationship between type of dysphoric state and drug preference.** Khantzian emphasizes the "anti-rage" properties of opioids.
   2. In adolescents, risk factors for the development of opioid dependence include: marijuana abuse, symptoms of depression, lack of a close relationship with parents, and leaving school. In general, other risk factors include: availability of opioids, alienation from social institutions, social deviancy, and impulsivity.
   3. Opioid addicts tend to score low on sensation-seeking, and they tend to avoid excessive internal and external stimulation.

XIII. Comorbid Psychiatric and Opiate Use Disorders

A. **Studies show that 80–90% of opioid-addicted individuals carry a lifetime diagnosis of a psychiatric disorder.** Major depressive disorder (25% current and 50% lifetime) and antisocial personality disorder (25–40%) are the two most common comorbid psychiatric disorders in opioid-dependent individuals. There is also an increased risk of posttraumatic stress disorder (PTSD). Children and adolescents with conduct disorder are at greater risk of developing substance abuse problems, especially opioid dependence. Psychiatric treatment of Axis I disorders improves outcome. Those addicts who seek treatment have more depression and anxiety, lower levels of social functioning, and more drug-related legal problems than untreated opioid addicts. Biopsychosocial complications of opioid abuse appear to encourage addicts to seek treatment earlier.

B. **It can be difficult to distinguish the difference between a primary mood disorder from an opioid-induced mood disorder.** Chronic use of opioids may cause symptoms consistent with the diagnosis of major depressive disorder. Depression in opioid addicts could also be related to psychosocial stressor complications from chronic opioid use.

C. **The diagnosis of antisocial personality disorder is questionable in the context of an addiction** unless antisocial behaviors predate the onset of the addiction; addictive disorders tend to promote antisocial behaviors.

D. **Alcohol, benzodiazepines, and cocaine are the most common comorbid substances used by opioid addicts.**

XIV. Medical Complications of Opiate Use

A. Intravenous Opioid Use

1. **Complications from contamination.** The most common injectable opioids are heroin, Dilaudid, and Demerol. Heroin is sold on the streets in "bags" and there is a wide variability of purity and potency. Contamination, both chemical and microbial, of the injectable opioid contributes to multiple medical complications. **Chemical contaminants include talc, starch, and quinine (used as adulterants), and cotton (used as a filter); the primary microbial contaminants include *Staphylococcus aureus*, β-hemolytic streptococci, and anaerobes. Some of the most common medical complications include:**

   a. **Cellulitis**
   b. **Skin abscesses**
   c. **Endocarditis**
   d. **Septic arthritis**
   e. **Hepatitis A, B, C, and D**
   f. **Osteomyelitis**
   g. **Nephropathy**
   h. **Rhabdomyolysis**
   i. **Pulmonary emboli, pulmonary hypertension**
   j. **Pneumonia**
   k. **Meningitis**
   l. **Brain abscess**
   m. **Tuberculosis**
   n. **HIV infection**

2. **Liver disease.** Studies using serological testing show that **two-thirds of intravenous drugs users have been exposed to hepatitis B and C.**

3. **Pulmonary disease. Talc and cotton can cause granulomatous pulmonary reactions.** Heroin is known to cause pulmonary edema but the mechanism is unclear. The common causes of pneumonia include *Haemophilus influenzae* and *Streptococcus pneumoniae*. Tuberculosis (TB) has been on the increase in intravenous drug users over the past few years, thus, TB must be considered in the presence of pulmonary infiltrates. One study showed that, in one population of intravenous drug users, one-quarter had latent TB. The antitussive property of opioids contributes to respiratory infection and pneumonia.

4. **Cardiac disease. Endocarditis occurs in 0.2% of addicts in a 12-month period.** Contaminated needles and opioids cause endothelial damage on heart valves followed by platelet fibrin deposition and bacterial infection. *Staphylococcus aureus* is the most common infectious agent followed by *Streptococcus*. Right-sided endocarditis may result in pulmonary emboli, which are generally not fatal, whereas left-sided endocarditis may result in systemic emboli, which are often fatal.

5. **Renal disease. Intravenous heroin use can lead to focal or diffuse glomerulosclerosis, which may progress to nephrotic syndrome and end-stage renal failure.** Hematuria and proteinuria are found on urinalysis. Frequently occurring skin abscesses and ulcerations may result in renal amyloidosis.

6. **HIV infection. Two-thirds of intravenous drug users in the Northeastern United States, according to one study, are HIV positive.** Twenty-five per cent of individuals with AIDS use intravenous drugs. Infants born HIV-positive may have clinical features similar to fetal alcohol syndrome.

7. **Complications with Pregnancy in the Setting of Opiate Use. Results from several studies indicate that an average of 80% of infants born to mothers addicted to opioids experience a syndrome of opioid withdrawal.** The fetus is exposed to multiple episodes of going in and out of withdrawal as the mother continues to use short-acting opioids, and each episode of withdrawal places the fetus at risk of being aborted. It is now common practice to place pregnant opioid-dependent women on methadone maintenance. The dose of methadone needs to be high enough to block cravings and opioid use and low enough to decrease withdrawal symptoms for the infant at the time of delivery. In general, the goal is to achieve methadone doses of 20 mg/day or less. Pregnant women already stable on methadone, at doses above 20 mg/day, should be tapered slowly at a rate of 1–2 mg per week in order to prevent a miscarriage. The safest time period for tapering methadone is during weeks 14–32 of the pregnancy. The most common withdrawal symptoms in neonates include: hyperactivity, hyperactive reflexes, increased muscle tone, diaphoresis, a high-pitched cry, yawning, insomnia, decreased eating, tremor, and mottling. A few neonates will experience more severe withdrawal symptoms which include: seizures, vomiting, diarrhea, and fever. In general, the mild withdrawal symptoms do not require treatment, but, for severe withdrawal, paregoric (for mu opioid withdrawal) and phenobarbital (for hyperactivity and seizures) are the most frequently used pharmacological treatments. The onset of withdrawal symptoms occurs as early as 12–24 h after birth depending on the half-life of the opioid used. However, since the neonate does not have the enzymes to metabolize and excrete opioids, the presence of withdrawal symptoms may be delayed and last many weeks, compared to adults. Perinatal mortality rates are about 7% for neonatal deaths and 4% for stillbirths.

XV. Treatment of Opiate Use

A. Intoxication

Acute intoxication does not generally require any treatment. With ingestion of large amounts of opioids resulting in respiratory depression and coma, treatment in a hospital setting is required. Life supports, including a ventilator, are essential. **The respiratory depression can be reversed by naloxone 0.4 mg IV;** if there is no response within 2 min, naloxone 0.8 mg IV can be repeated twice, more 5 min apart. Signs of a response to naloxone include: increased respirations, increased blood pressure, and reversal of constricted pupils. Depending on the half-life of the opioid used, naloxone needs to be continued until the effects of the opiate abate. For short-acting opioids like heroin, the crisis resolves in about 4 h; however, for long-acting opioids such as methadone or LAAM (L-α-acetylmethadol), hospitalization may be required up to 48 h.

B. Detoxification

There are four commonly used strategies and two experimental strategies for opioid detoxification: **methadone substitution; clonidine; clonidine-naltrexone ultrarapid detoxification; buprenorphine; lofexidine (experimental); and ultrarapid opioid detoxification under anesthesia/sedation (experimental).**

1. **Methadone substitution.** Methadone has a long half-life, which provides for a smoother withdrawal off opioids. In general, some clinicians believe that it should only be used for detoxification off more addictive substances, such as heroin, morphine, meperidine, or hydromorphone. For less addictive opioids such as codeine, oxycodone, propoxyphene, or pentazocine, simply tapering the dose or using clonidine is the best strategy. The starting dose of methadone can vary between 20 and 40 mg/day. Doses of methadone above 40 mg/day in a patient who is not opioid dependent can be lethal. It may take a few days to determine the stabilizing dose of methadone (based on signs and symptoms of withdrawal) before starting the taper. For inpatients, the stabilizing dose may be decreased at a rate of 5–10% per day; however, for outpatients, the dose should be tapered at a rate of 10% per week until a dose of 20 mg/day and then at a rate of 3% per week for the remainder of the detoxification. Outpatients are more likely to relapse during the detoxification due to the availability of opioids, thus, it is important to provide a more comfortable taper. Patients tend to tolerate the taper to 20 mg/day, but below 20 mg/day they express more sensitivity to withdrawal symptoms and significant fears of being off opioids. For the long-acting opioids (methadone and LAAM) that have been used for long periods of time in a methadone program, a gradual detoxification over a period up to 180 days (in a licensed facility) has been shown to put the patient at less risk for relapse.

2. **Clonidine. Clonidine is an alpha-2-adrenergic agonist which reduces symptoms of opioid withdrawal by inhibiting noradrenergic hyperactivity in the locus coeruleus.** Clonidine suppresses many symptoms of withdrawal, including rapid heart rate, increased blood pressure, sweating, nausea, vomiting, diarrhea, and cramps. Clonidine has no effect on craving, muscle aches, or insomnia, thus adjunctive medications need to be added, such as nonsteroidal anti-inflammatory drugs for muscle aches and possibly benzodiazepines for insomnia. Benzodiazepines need to be used cautiously and for a brief period of time. The most common side effects of clonidine are sedation and hypotension. For short-acting opioids (Kleber, 1999), the starting dose is 0.1–0.3 mg every 4–6 h up to a maximum of 1.0 mg the first day. During days 2–4, clonidine doses are increased based on the need to control withdrawal symptoms, up to a maximum daily dose of 1.3 mg. Beginning day 5, the dose of clonidine is reduced by 0.2 mg/day. For long-acting opioids (methadone, at a dose of 20–40 mg/day) (Kleber, 1999), the starting dose is 0.1 mg t.i.d. on day 1. On days 2–4 the dose of clonidine is increased to a maximum of 0.4 mg t.i.d. This dose is maintained until day 11 at which time the dose of clonidine is reduced by 0.2 mg/day, but not to exceed 0.4 mg/day. During detoxification with clonidine, blood pressure and pulse should be checked before each dose. The dose should be held and the daily dose reduced if the blood pressure is below 90/60 mmHg.

3. **Clonidine patch. The clonidine patch is a transdermal delivery system designed to provide a constant daily dose of clonidine over a 7-day period,** which provides for a smoother withdrawal off opioids. It is available in three strengths that are equivalent to oral clonidine: 0.1 mg, 0.2 mg, and 0.3 mg. For the first 2 days of detoxification, oral clonidine has to be given because it takes 48 h for the transdermal clonidine to reach steady state. On day 1, oral clonidine 0.2 mg t.i.d. or q.i.d. is given along with transdermal clonidine. The patch dose depends on weight: 0.2 mg if 100 lb.; 0.4 mg if 100–200 lb.; or 0.6 mg if the weight is greater than 200 lb. On day 2, the oral dose is reduced by half and discontinued on day 3. The clonidine patch or patches are removed after 7 days and replaced with half the original dose for an additional 7 days if withdrawal symptoms continue. In general, detoxification is complete in

7 days for short-acting opioids and about 10 days for long-acting opioids. The patch or patches are removed if the systolic blood pressure drops to 80 mmHg or the diastolic drops to 50 mmHg.

4. **Clonidine-naltrexone. The addition of naltrexone to clonidine can significantly shorten the time to complete detoxification.** Naltrexone accelerates the withdrawal process and clonidine reduces withdrawal symptoms. Completion rates range between 55% and 95%. During the first day, outpatients need to be monitored for 8 h because of the risk for serious withdrawal due to the naltrexone and the need to monitor blood pressure due to the clonidine. According to a protocol by O'Connor et al. (1995) and Vining et al. (1995), on day 1, the patient is premedicated with clonidine 0.2–0.4 mg and oxazepam 30–60 mg. Two hours later naltrexone, 12.5 mg, is given orally and clonidine 0.1–0.2 mg every 4–6 h (up to 1.2 mg) and oxazepam 30–60 mg are given every 4–6 h for the remainder of the day. On day 2, naltrexone 25 mg orally is given 1 h after the first doses of clonidine 0.1–0.2 mg and oxazepam 30–60 mg. Clonidine 0.1–0.2 mg every 4–6 h (up to 1.2 mg) and oxazepam 30–60 mg every 4–6 h are continued throughout day 2. On day 3, the only change is an increase in naltrexone to 50 mg. After day 3, clonidine and oxazepam are continued for an additional 2–3 days. Medications to treat muscle cramps (nonsteroidal anti-inflammatory drugs) and nausea (prochlorperazine or ondansetron) may also be required. An inpatient protocol using even higher doses of naltrexone can speed up the time to complete detoxification to within 2–3 days.

5. **Lofexidine. Lofexidine is an alpha-2-agonist currently used in England for opioid detoxification.** Its advantages over clonidine include reduced risks for sedation and hypotension. The National Institute on Drug Abuse (NIDA) is now studying lofexidine for possible FDA approval.

6. **Buprenorphine. Buprenorphine is a partial mu agonist analgesic that is very effective for detoxification off opioids.** The only form available to clinicians is parenteral; however, a sublingual form combined with naloxone is being developed. When given intramuscularly, the pharmacological effect has its onset within 15 min and lasts about 6 h. With intravenous use, the onset of action is earlier. The equivalent parenteral dose of buprenorphine compared with 10 mg of morphine is 0.3 mg. Buprenorphine is very safe when taken in overdose due to the "ceiling effect" of being a partial mu agonist; it exhibits very little respiratory depression. There are three strategies used for opioid detoxification with buprenorphine: abrupt discontinuation;

gradual taper; and discontinuation with precipitation of withdrawal with naltrexone. The first step in all three methods is to stabilize patients on buprenorphine for at least 3 days. Studies now available demonstrate that, with abrupt discontinuation, the withdrawal symptoms are minimal and that abrupt discontinuation has higher success rates than gradual withdrawal.

7. **Ultrarapid Opioid Detoxification Under Anesthesia.** The procedure involves the induction of anesthesia with propofol, tracheal intubation, and the precipitation of withdrawal with either intravenous naloxone or naltrexone via intragastric tube. Patients are under anesthesia up to 8 h and they are discharged within 24–48 h. Antiemetics, antidiarrheal medications, clonidine, and benzodiazepines are used to treat breakthrough withdrawal symptoms. There may be serious risks with this approach since deaths have been reported within 24 h of the procedure. There are no controlled or outcome studies to validate its use.

C. Opioid Substitution

1. **Methadone maintenance. Only a facility licensed by a state can dispense methadone maintenance for the treatment of opioid dependence.** The criteria for initiating treatment include: a minimum of a 1-year history of physiological dependence on opioids (episodic or continuous); current signs and symptoms of withdrawal; needle tracks; and positive urines. For previously treated patients, reinstatement into a methadone maintenance program may occur within 2 years of discontinuation of methadone without the presence of current physical dependence and with documentation from a physician that relapse to opioid dependence is imminent. Individuals who are released from a penal institution and who met the criteria for methadone maintenance prior to incarceration may be admitted to a methadone program without the presence of physical dependence. Women who are pregnant are eligible for methadone maintenance if they are physically dependent on opioids or if they were dependent on opioids in the past and are now at imminent risk of relapse. Patients under the age of 18 years must have failed at least two opioid detoxifications in the past and have the consent of a parent, legal guardian, or an adult designated by state authority to enter a methadone maintenance program. Patient characteristics that predict a successful outcome in a methadone program include: brief history of drug abuse; older than 25 years of age; psychological stability; good social support system; good work history; minimal legal problems; and low severity of opioid abuse.

Methadone has a half-life of 24–36 h, thus it can be given orally once daily. The combination of its slow onset of subjective effects and its long half-life results in a reduction in the euphoric peaks and distressing withdrawal symptoms that tend to account for the reinforcing properties of opioid drugs. Methadone is well tolerated, and its main side effects include sedation, constipation, excessive sweating, ankle edema, decreased libido, and mild euphoria. The starting dose of methadone is determined by the intensity of the withdrawal signs and symptoms. For mild withdrawal, the initial dose is about 10 mg/day of methadone, whereas for severe withdrawal the initial dose is 20–40 mg/day. The patient should be monitored for a period of 2 h after the first dose in order to determine the effectiveness of the starting dose in reversing withdrawal signs and symptoms. The maintenance dose is determined by the reduction or the elimination of opioid abuse as determined by negative urine screens, the lack of reinforcing properties such as euphoria, and minimal side effects. Although there is a broad range of effective maintenance doses across patients (10–100 mg/day), recent studies have shown that doses averaging 70–80 mg/day are needed to block opioid cravings and drug use. Methadone blood levels are helpful, and the goal is to achieve trough blood levels of 150–600 ng/mL. The maximum allowable dose according to federal regulations is 120 mg/day. About one-third of methadone maintenance patients do well and about one-third show no benefit. With doses of methadone greater than 60 mg/day, retention rates in methadone programs reach 60% at 6 months and up to a 90% reduction in opioid abuse. Unfortunately, the treatment only reaches 20–25% of opioid addicts. The benefits from methadone maintenance include decreased opioid use, criminal behavior, unemployment, and risk for contracting AIDS.

2. **L-α-Acetylmethadol (LAAM). LAAM is long-acting congener of methadone which has been approved for the use of opioid substitution in methadone programs.** LAAM has the same eligibility criteria as methadone but it is unavailable for pregnant females and individuals under 18 years of age. Its safety in pregnant women has not been determined. Women who are on LAAM must get monthly pregnancy tests.

LAAM has two active metabolites, nor-LAAM and dinor-LAAM, both of which are mu agonists. These two metabolites account for LAAM's slow onset of action, its long half-life of 72–96 h, and its long time to steady state, up to 20 days (time to steady state for methadone is 5–8 days). Because of its long half-life, LAAM is given three days per week: Monday, Wednesday, and Friday. The dose on Friday is 20–40% greater than the other two weekly doses in order to adequately cover the potential for withdrawal over the weekend. The starting dose of LAAM is 20–40 mg, and the usual maintenance dose is 60 mg on Monday and Wednesday and 80 mg on Friday. When starting LAAM, methadone can be given in doses of 5–20 mg/day as a supplement to help the patient during the stabilization period. To switch from methadone to LAAM, the methadone dosage should be multiplied by 1.2, whereas to switch from LAAM to methadone, the LAAM dosage should be multiplied by 0.8. The effectiveness of LAAM compares well with methadone; however, it seems to benefit a different subgroup of opioid addicts.

3. **Buprenorphine. Buprenorphine clinically exhibits characteristics of both methadone and naltrexone. Its mu agonist properties satisfy cravings and prevent opioid withdrawal and its mu antagonist characteristics block the reinforcing effects from abused opioids.** It is these characteristics that have led researchers to test buprenorphine's usefulness for opioid substitution in addicts. It has a half-life of 24–36 h, which allows for once-a-day dosing. It is available to clinicians in an injectable form; however, a sublingual form is available to researchers. The sublingual form has the disadvantage that it has to be held in the mouth for 3 min. Subcutaneous buprenorphine at a dose range of 8–12 mg/day is comparable to methadone 60 mg/day for maintaining abstinence from opioid abuse.

D. Psychosocial Treatment

1. **Psychosocial treatment modalities include: individual, group, and family psychotherapy; therapeutic communities; and self-help groups such as Narcotics Anonymous.** Typical outcome measures are frequency and amount of opioid used, employment status, level of psychosocial functioning, and severity of psychiatric symptoms.

2. **Psychotherapy.** The greater the degree of psychopathology in opioid addicts, the poorer the treatment outcome. However, for opioid addicts with psychiatric disorders, psychotherapy can significantly improve treatment outcome compared to treatment without psychotherapy. Antisocial personality predicts poor response to psychotherapy. Positive predictors of psychotherapy outcome include: establishing a good alliance between therapist and patient; treating psychiatric symptoms such as depression early; assessing and addressing psychosocial problems; and monitoring treatment compliance.

a. **Supportive-expressive therapy** is more effective than drug counseling alone for opioid addicts with a high degree of psychiatric symptoms.

b. **Cognitive-behavioral therapy.** Studies in community-based methadone clinics showed that CBT plus drug counseling, and supportive-expressive therapy plus drug counseling, are each more effective than drug counseling alone at 7 and 12 months in methadone patients with high levels of psychiatric symptoms. All three treatment conditions were equally effective in methadone patients with low levels of psychiatric symptoms.

c. **Behavioral therapy.** Cue extinction and contingency management are two effective behavioral approaches. There is good evidence that cravings can be classically conditioned; thus, through repeated exposures to internal or external cues, cravings are extinguished. With contingency management, the therapist and the patient establish a set of rewards for maintaining abstinence and a set of aversive consequences for opioid use; urine toxicology screens are randomly used to determine treatment compliance. In a recent study of patients in a methadone maintenance program, adding psychosocial services (on-site medical and psychiatric services, family therapy, and employment services) to contingency management and methadone substitution significantly improved outcome. Patients in the methadone substitution alone condition had to be terminated from the study by week 12 due to a high percent of opiate-positive urine samples.

d. **Family therapy.** Family members can be helpful in assisting the treatment team in initiating and monitoring contingency management protocols and helping with compliance issues.

e. **Group therapy.** Relapse prevention groups combined with self-help groups are more effective in reducing opioid use, legal problems, and unemployment than no treatment in detoxified opioid-dependent patients.

f. **Therapeutic communities.** Patients reside in these facilities from 6 to 18 months. The environment is structured and consists of a hierarchy of privileges and responsibilities. The community confronts denial and emphasizes personal responsibility for achieving abstinence. Only highly motivated individuals are successful; 50% drop out by 6 months and only 15–25% graduate.

g. **Narcotics Anonymous (NA).** There are essentially no differences between NA and Alcoholics Anonymous (AA). NA includes patients with an addiction to any illicit drug. The main purpose of NA is to provide a support network, confront denial, and help prevent relapse by addressing thinking and behaviors that often lead to use. Outcome studies are lacking with regard to the efficacy of NA.

Suggested Readings

American Psychiatric Association: Substance-related disorders. In *Diagnostic and Statistical Manual of Mental Disorders*, 4th ed. Washington, DC: American Psychiatric Press, 1994:175–272.

American Psychiatric Association: *Practice Guideline for the Treatment of Patients with Substance Use Disorders: Alcohol, Cocaine, Opioids.* Washington, DC: American Psychiatric Press, 1995.

Franklin JE, Frances RJ: Alcohol and other psychoactive substance use disorders. In Hales RE, Yudofsky SC, Talbott JA (eds): *The American Psychiatric Press Textbook of Psychiatry*, 3rd ed. Washington, DC: American Psychiatric Press, 1999:363–423.

Gold M: Cocaine (and crack): clinical aspects. In Lowinson JH, Ruiz P, Millman RB, Langrod JG (eds): *Substance Abuse: A Comprehensive Textbook*, 3rd ed. Baltimore: Williams and Wilkins, 1997:181–199.

Gold M, Miller NS: Cocaine (and crack): neurobiology. In Lowinson JH, Ruiz P, Millman RB, Langrod JG (eds): *Substance Abuse: A Comprehensive Textbook*, 3rd ed. Baltimore: Williams and Wilkins, 1997:166–181.

Jaffe JH, Knapp CM, Ciraulo DA: Opiates: clinical aspects. In Lowinson JH, Ruiz P, Millman RB, Langrod JG (eds): *Substance Abuse: A Comprehensive Textbook,* 3rd ed. Baltimore: Williams and Wilkins, 1997:158–166.

Jaffe JH, Jaffe AB: Neurobiology of opiates/opioids. In Galanter M, Kleber HD (eds): *Textbook of Substance Abuse Treatment*, 2nd ed. Washington, DC: American Psychiatric Press, 1999:11–19.

Kleber HD: Opioids: detoxification. In Galanter M, Kleber HD (eds): *Textbook of Substance Abuse Treatment*, 2nd ed. Washington, DC: American Psychiatric Press, 1999:251–269.

O'Brien CP, Cornish JW: Opioids: antagonists and partial agonists. In Galanter M, Kleber HD (eds): *Textbook of Substance Abuse Treatment*, 2nd ed. Washington, DC: American Psychiatric Press, 1999:281–294.

O'Connor PG, Waugh ML, Carroll KM, et al.: Primary care-based ambulatory opioid detoxification: the results of a clinical trial. *J Gen Intern Med* 1995; 10:255–260.

Senay EC: Opioids: methadone maintenance. In Galanter M, Kleber HD (eds): *Textbook of Substance Abuse Treatment*, 2nd ed. Washington, DC: American Psychiatric Press, 1999:271–279.

Simon EJ: Opiates: neurobiology. In Lowinson JH, Ruiz P, Millman RB, Langrod JG (eds): *Substance Abuse: A Comprehensive Textbook*, 3rd ed. Baltimore: Williams and Wilkins, 1997:148–158.

Vining E, Kosten TR, Kleber HD: Clinical utility of rapid clonidine-naltrexone detoxification for opioid abuse. *Br J Addiction* 1988; 83:567–575.

Washton AM: Structured outpatient treatment of alcohol vs drug dependence. *Recent Dev Alcohol* 1990; 8:285–304.

Chapter 12
Psychosis And Schizophrenia

DAVID C. HENDERSON AND DONALD C. GOFF

I. Introduction

Psychosis is a gross impairment of reality testing which can result from a variety of psychiatric and medical problems. Psychotic symptoms generally fall into three categories:

A. Hallucinations
Hallucinations are sensory perceptions in the absence of external stimuli. Hallucinations may be in the form of voices, noise, or music (auditory), visions (visual), odors, or taste (olfactory and/or gustatory), and sensations of touch (tactile).

B. Delusions
Delusions are **firmly held false beliefs.** Delusions may be of persecution, of a somatic nature, of grandeur, of jealousy, or of the feeling that someone has been replaced by an impostor (Capgras' syndrome).

C. Thought Disorder
Formal thought disorder **refers to a disruption in the form, or organization of thinking.** A patient may be incoherent and have difficulty communicating their thoughts to others, or have a loosening of associations, overinclusiveness, neologisms, thought blocking, clanging, echolalia, concreteness, or poverty of speech.

II. History of Diagnostic Classification of Schizophrenia

A. Kraepelin
Kraepelin, **in 1896, distinguished "dementia praecox" from "manic depressive psychosis"** and **emphasized a chronic, deteriorating course.** The term "Kraepelinian schizophrenia" has been used by some investigators to refer to a condition in which a patient fails to achieve remission and live independently for a 5-year period.

B. Bleuler
Bleuler, in **1911,** described "schizophrenia" as a splitting of psychic functions. He **described specific fundamental symptoms of schizophrenia as the "Four As": involving autism, ambivalence, loosening of associations, and inappropriate affect.** He emphasized "negative symptoms" and described accessory symptoms which included delusions and hallucinations.

C. Schneider
Schneider, **in the 1970s, described 11 "first-rank symptoms"** of schizophrenia, including hallucinations, delusions, thought withdrawal, thought insertion, imposed feelings, and impulses. He **emphasized the "positive symptoms" of schizophrenia** and believed that the diagnosis of schizophrenia can be made with second-rank symptoms, which include other disorders of perception (not first-rank), sudden delusional ideas, perplexity, emotional impoverishment, and depressive and euphoric mood changes.

III. DSM-IV Diagnosis of Schizophrenia

A. Features
The essential features of schizophrenia include:
   a. **Psychotic symptoms for at least 1 month (less if treated)**
   b. **Functioning below the highest expected level**
   c. **A duration of illness for at least 6 months (including prodromal or residual phases)**

B. Active Phase
The active phase requires either bizarre delusions or hallucinations (where two or more voices converse with each other, or a voice keeps a running commentary of the person's behaviors or thoughts), or two or more of the following symptoms: delusions; hallucinations; disorganized speech; grossly disorganized or catatonic behavior; or negative symptoms.

C. Prodromal or Residual Symptoms
Prodromal and residual phase symptoms include: **social isolation or withdrawal; impairment of functioning; peculiar behavior; impaired personal hygiene; blunted or inappropriate affect; abnormal speech** (e.g., digressive, vague, overly elaborate); **odd beliefs** (e.g., superstitions, extrasensory perception [ESP]); **unusual perceptual experiences; and apathy.**

D. Subtypes of Schizophrenia
1. **Catatonic type:** catalepsy or stupor; negativism or mutism; excessive motor activity; peculiar voluntary movements (posturing, mannerisms, stereopathy, grimacing); echolalia or echopraxia.
2. **Disorganized type: disorganized speech and behavior; flat or inappropriate affect, but not meeting the criteria for catatonic type.**

97

3. **Paranoid type: preoccupation with one or more delusions or frequent auditory hallucinations; the patient does not experience significant disorganization, catatonia, or inappropriate or flat affect.**
4. **Undifferentiated type:** active psychotic symptoms, but not meeting criteria for other types.
5. **Residual type:** the absence of psychosis and not meeting criteria for other types.

IV. Differential Diagnosis of Psychotic Symptoms

A. **Mood Disorders** (if present, they are of brief duration)
   1. Schizoaffective disorder: the mood disorder is prominent and the patient experiences psychotic symptoms when euthymic.
   2. Bipolar disorder: psychosis is present only during manic or depressive episodes.
   3. Psychotic depression: psychosis occurs only during depressive episodes.
B. **Schizophreniform disorder:** involves a prodromal phase, an active phase, and has a residual duration of less than 6 months.

C. **Brief reactive psychosis:** the duration is less than 1 month.
D. **Schizotypal personality disorder:** a condition that fails to meet the criteria for the active phase of schizophrenia.
E. **Delusional disorder:** a persistent condition with nonbizarre delusions.
F. **Organic Etiologies**
   These include (see Table 12-1): substance abuse; use of medications; seizure disorder; delirium; infectious diseases; endocrinopathies; nutritional deficiencies; neoplasms; heavy metal exposures; and neurologic disorders.

V. Evaluation of Psychosis

Most causes of psychosis (Table 12-1) can be ruled out by a good medical history, by a physical and neurological examination, and with screening laboratory examinations (see Table 12-2).

A. **Important diagnostic questions** must be asked to distinguish medical from psychiatric disorders:
   1. Has a reversible, organic cause been ruled out?

Table 12-1. Drugs and Medical/Neurological Conditions Associated with Psychosis

Drugs of abuse	Infectious diseases
Alcohol	Brain abscess
Amphetamines	Hepatic encephalitis
Barbiturates	Infectious mononucleosis
Caffeine	Malaria
Cannabis (THC)	Meningitis
Cocaine	Syphilis
Hallucinogens (LSD, PCP, MDMA)	
Inhalants	**Endocrine disorders**
Opioids	Addison's disease
Sedative-hypnotics	Cushing's syndrome
	Hypo/hyperthyroidism
Neurological disorders	Hypo/hyperparathyroidism
Alzheimer's disease	
Complex partial seizures	**Nutritional deficiencies**
Huntington's disease	Niacin deficiency (pellagra)
Hydrocephalus	Thiamine deficiency (Korsakoff's psychosis, beriberi)
Lupus cerebritis	Vitamin B_{12} (pernicious anemia)
Parkinson's disease	**Other**
Pick's disease	Neoplasms
Wilson's disease	Heavy metal exposures
	Prescription medications

Table 12-2. Evaluation of Psychosis

1. Perform a complete physical and neurological exam
2. Conduct a mental status exam—ordering neuropsychological testing as indicated
3. Obtain a full laboratory screen: electrolytes, BUN, creatinine, calcium, glucose, CBC, thyroid panel, liver enzymes, VDRL, vitamin B_{12}, folate, HIV when indicated
4. Obtain a toxicological screen
5. Order brain imaging (CT or MRI)
6. Obtain an EEG if clinically indicated

2. Are cognitive deficits (e.g., memory impairment) prominent? If so, consideration must be given to delirium or dementia.
3. Is the psychiatric illness episodic or continuous?
4. Have psychotic symptoms been present for at least 4 weeks?
5. Are negative symptoms present?
6. Has evidence of the illness been present for at least 6 months?
7. Are mood episodes prominent?
8. Have there been episodes of major depression or mania?
9. Do psychotic features occur only during affective episodes?

B. Neuropsychological testing is frequently helpful to uncover underlying psychotic symptoms and cognitive impairments.

C. Brain imaging often yields little information in the absence of focal neurologic impairment. However, a brain scan (magnetic resonance imaging [MRI] or computed tomography [CT]) is generally recommended at least once in a patient with an atypical psychosis or with treatment-refractory psychotic symptoms.

D. An **electroencephalogram (EEG)** should be performed if clinically indicated.

VI. Epidemiology of Schizophrenia

A. Prevalence
1. The prevalence of schizophrenia is **1% world-wide.** The prevalence varies by region in the United States.
2. There appears to be a higher incidence of schizophrenia among the urban poor. In part, this may be related to economic drift and to the drift of chronically disabled patients towards urban areas.

3. The incidence of schizophrenia may be decreasing in Great Britain since 1950, but higher among British Afro-Caribbeans.

B. Age of Onset
1. Males manifest the illness earlier (ages 18–25 years) than do females (ages 26–45 years).
2. Twenty percent of cases occur after the age of 40 years; the majority of those are women.

C. Premorbid Deficits
1. Children at risk have lower scholastic test scores.
2. Future schizophrenic children can be identified in home movies by abnormalities of affect and by coordination.
3. Some evidence also suggests that children at risk experience a thought disorder and diffuse developmental abnormalities as early as infancy.

D. Stress and Age of Onset
1. Stress appears to be a significant factor that impacts on the age of onset of schizophrenia. In college, 44% of cases develop in the first semester.
2. Among army draftees, there is an eight-fold higher incidence of first-break psychosis during the first few months as compared with episodes during the second year.
3. Child abuse victims have an earlier age of onset and a poorer course.

E. Gender Differences
The lifetime risk of schizophrenia is approximately equal for males and females, with males experiencing an earlier age of onset and poorer course. The course in females may worsen after menopause. Ninety percent of males and 25% of females develop the illness before the age of 30 years.

F. Season of Birth
1. **There is a modest increase in the prevalence of schizophrenia among those born in the spring and early winter.** In the northern hemisphere, schizophrenic patients are more likely to have been born between January and April.
2. In the southern hemisphere, schizophrenic patients are more likely to have been born between July and September.
3. An increased incidence of schizophrenia exists among individuals exposed to influenza or to other viruses during the late second trimester (6 months).

VII. Patterns of Inheritance

A. No single genetic factor can be identified for schizophrenia. The possibilities for genetic inheritance include several discrete diseases, a multifactorial threshold model, or partial or incomplete penetrance.

B. Monozygotic twins have the highest concordance rate (40–50%) for schizophrenia, and twins raised by adoptive parents have the same rate of developing schizophrenia as do twins raised by their biological parents.

C. Dizygotic twins have an approximately 15% concordance rate for schizophrenia. Biological relatives have an approximately 9% rate of schizophrenia compared to a rate of 2% among adoptive relatives. However, no single genetic pattern has been identified.

D. Most linkage studies, including studies of the gene for the dopamine D_2 receptor **have been negative.** A large number of chromosomes (including chromosomes 5, 11, 18, 19, and X being most commonly reported) have been associated with schizophrenia. Recent evidence also suggests a vulnerability locus in the region 6p24-22 (in 15–30% of pedigrees).

VIII. Biological Abnormalities

A. Enlargement of Cerebral Ventricles
1. Many patients with schizophrenia, at the time of diagnosis, exhibit **bilateral enlargement of the lateral and third ventricles** on neuroimaging studies.
2. The **left ventricles may be slightly larger than the right ventricles;** this change is usually static. Also, the left ventricles are enlarged in affected discordant monozygotic twins.

B. Histopathological Changes
1. **Decreased size of the anteromedial temporal lobe,** along with cytoarchitectural abnormalities of the parahippocampal gyrus, may be found in some patients with schizophrenia.
2. **Reduced neuronal density** has been observed in the **prefrontal cortex, thalamus, and cingulate gyrus.**
3. **Absence of gliosis,** which suggests a developmental abnormality, and evidence of abnormal cell migration in the hippocampus and frontal cortex have also been observed.

C. Hypofrontality
1. In a resting state, **reduced frontal lobe activity,** may correlate with negative symptoms (although results have been inconsistent).
2. Failure to activate the prefrontal cortex with the Wisconsin Card Sort is a highly specific finding in discordant monozygotic twins.
3. These abnormalities are not affected by neuroleptics.

D. Neuropsychological Functioning
1. An individual with schizophrenia generally exhibits **deficits in attention, memory, learning, and an inability to shift sets on neuropsychological testing.**

2. **Cognitive deficits** appear premorbidly and worsen over the course of the illness.
3. **Smooth pursuit eye movements (SPEM) are abnormal in 50–85% of patients** with schizophrenia as well as in 45% of first-degree family members. This finding may represent an alternative expression of an autosomal dominant gene. The SPEM abnormality is nonspecific and occurs in mania (state dependent) and Parkinson's disease.
4. Evoked potentials P50 waveforms decrease after the first of paired stimuli in normal controls, but not in patients with schizophrenia. This may reflect an impairment of gating (filtering) auditory input; up to 50% of first-degree relatives have this defect. Finally, **impaired generation of P300 event-related potentials have been observed** in patients with schizophrenia.

E. Receptors and Neurotransmitters
1. **Dopamine D_2 receptor density may be increased in the striatum and the nucleus accumbens.**
2. **Norepinephrine receptor density may be increased in the nucleus accumbens.**
3. **Glutamate receptors are increased in the frontal cortex and hippocampus.**
4. Altered serotonin activity has also been suspected.

IX. Theories of Etiology

A. Dopamine Hyperactivity
1. **Schizophrenia and acute psychosis are associated with increased mesolimbic dopamine activity** (in the temporal lobes) which may be mediated, in part, by mesocortical hypoactivity (in the prefrontal cortex).
2. Supporting evidence for dopamine hyperactivity includes:
   a. The fact that dopamine agonists, such as amphetamine, produce psychosis.
   b. All conventional antipsychotic agents are dopamine antagonists and the affinity for dopamine D_2 receptors correlates with antipsychotic efficacy.
3. Evidence which complicates the dopamine model includes:
   a. Agents that act at other receptors also produce psychosis (lysergic acid diethylamide [LSD], phencyclidine [PCP]).
   b. The antipsychotic effect may follow a delay of 2–10 weeks after dopamine blockade has occurred.
   c. Evidence of abnormalities in dopamine, its metabolites, or its receptor densities in patients with schizophrenia has been inconsistent.
   d. Negative symptoms are not clearly linked to dopamine.

B. Serotonin Dysfunction
1. LSD, a serotonin (5HT) agonist, and 3,4-methylene dioxymethamphetamine ("ecstasy") (MDMA) toxicity, each produce chronic psychosis.
2. Clozapine, and other atypical antipsychotic agents, are active at the serotonin $5HT_2$ and $5HT_{1c}$ receptors. Unfortunately, evidence of serotonin abnormalities has been inconsistent.

C. Phencyclidine (PCP) Model (Javitt, 1991)
1. PCP and ketamine produce delusions, hallucinations, thought disorder, negative symptoms, and catatonia in normal individuals. These drugs may also produce cognitive deficits and frontal lobe hypometabolism. In those with schizophrenia, ketamine can produce psychotic relapses.
2. Glutamate appears to mediate dopamine activity. The PCP receptor interacts with N-methyl D-aspartate (NMDA)-type glutamate receptor complex by blocking ion channels.

D. Viral Hypothesis
Viral infection during the third trimester is suspected of compromising the development of the medial temporal lobe. This may account for the relationship between the season of birth and the decreasing incidence of schizophrenia in Great Britain.

E. Diathesis and Stress Model (Two-Hit Model)
1. In this model, the first factor (or hit) is an inherited vulnerability to schizophrenia, which may be manifested by neuropsychological deficits (e.g., impaired auditory gating).
2. The second factor is an environmental injury to the hippocampus (e.g., by an obstetrical injury, infection, trauma, or hypoxia).

X. Predictors of Outcome

Negative symptoms, poor premorbid function, insidious onset, and the absence of remissions predict a poor outcome in schizophrenic patients. The outcome most closely correlates with the initial response to medications. The outcome may be worse if pharmacotherapy is significantly delayed.

A. Course of Illness
1. Generally, the outcome is poor. **Approximately 10% recover, and 20% have a good outcome.** With newer atypical antipsychotic agents, more patients are considered to have a good outcome. The outcome is generally better in underdeveloped countries
2. **While the suicide rate for patients with schizophrenia is 10–13%, 18–55% of patients with schizophrenia attempt suicide.** The incidence of suicide and attempts has decreased with the introduction of atypical antipsychotic agent, clozapine.

3. For many patients, negative symptoms worsen over time. **Patients with schizophrenia, paranoid type, experience a later age and a more rapid onset;** they have a better prognosis. **Those with a disorganized type, also called hebephrenia, and the undifferentiated type have an earlier age of onset and a more insidious onset;** they tend to experience a continuous but stable course.
4. **Individuals with schizophrenia have an elevated rate of violence, particularly if they experience paranoia and disorganization.** Homicide rates are best studied in this group and may be increased by a factor of ten compared to the general population. Schizophrenics with the paranoid subtype or with delusions which promote violence are at greatest risk for violence. The presence of auditory command hallucinations is a risk factor in the context of a delusional system.

B. Awareness of Illness
1. **More than half of patients with schizophrenia have impaired insight into their illness.** This may reflect frontal-cortical dysfunction.
2. When evaluating a patient with denial or impaired insight into their illness, a focus on the developmental, education, employment, and social history may provide clues to the nature of the illness.

C. Negative Symptoms
1. **Negative symptoms of schizophrenia often receive less attention than do psychotic symptoms, but they can be just as disabling.**
2. Negative symptoms include anhedonia, asociality (social isolation), affective flattening, alogia (poverty of speech and thought), inattentiveness, and apathy.
3. Response of negative symptoms may occur independently of psychotic symptom response, and follow a different time course.

D. Differential Diagnosis of Negative Symptoms
The evaluation of a patient with negative symptoms should include consideration of other disorders or conditions with similar symptoms. **These disorders include: neuroleptic-induced akinesia; depression; frontal lobe injury; idiopathic or neuroleptic-induced parkinsonism; substance abuse (particularly of stimulants); hypothyroidism; trauma; posttraumatic stress disorder.**

XI. Psychosocial Treatment

A. Acute treatment includes containment, reduction in stimulation, and development of an alliance. Medication side effects should be avoided. Education and support for the patient and their family are vital.

B. Long-term treatment includes individual supportive and problem-solving therapy. The emphasis should be placed on medication compliance, development of social skills, and adjustment to the illness.

C. Family work should be educational and supportive while focusing on an understanding of the illness and development of realistic expectations.

D. Stable housing, improved vocational status, medication compliance, and treatment of positive and negative symptoms are key, while reducing hospitalization rates.

E. Supported employment programs improve employment rates, and reduce positive symptoms, hostility, and affective symptoms, while lowering the rate of hospitalizations.

Suggested Readings

American Psychiatric Association: *Diagnostic and Statistical Manual of Mental Disorders, Fourth Edition.* Washington, DC: American Psychiatric Association, 1994.

Goff DC, Henderson DC: Treatment-resistant schizophrenia and psychotic disorders. In Pollack MH, Otto MW, Rosenbaum JF (eds): *Challenges in Clinical Practice: Pharmacologic and Psychosocial Strategies.* New York: The Guilford Press, 1996:311–328.

Goff DC, Henderson DC, Manschreck TC: Psychotic Patients. In Cassem NH, Stern TA, Rosenbaum JF, Jellinek MS (eds): *Massachusetts General Hospital Handbook of General Hospital Psychiatry*, 4th ed. St. Louis: Mosby, 1997:149–171.

Meltzer HY: Biological studies in schizophrenia. *Schizophr Bull* 1987; 13:77–110.

Chapter 13
Mood Disorders: Depression

John Matthews

I. Overview

A. The Diagnostic and Statistical Manual, Fourth Edition (DSM-IV) denotes three categories of unipolar depressive disorders:

1. **Major Depressive Disorder (MDD),** which is characterized by one or more episodes of persistent depressed mood, or a loss of interest or pleasure, for a minimum of 2 weeks, with four or more of the following symptoms of depression: weight disturbance; appetite disturbance; sleep disturbance; fatigue or loss of energy; feelings of guilt or worthlessness; poor concentration; psychomotor agitation or retardation; suicide attempts or thoughts of death.

2. **Dysthymic Disorder,** which is characterized by a depressed mood, experienced more days than not, over at least a 2-year period, as well as two or more of the following symptoms of depression: poor appetite or hyperphagia; insomnia or hypersomnia; low energy or fatigue; low self-esteem; poor concentration and difficulty making decisions; feelings of hopelessness.

3. **Depressive Disorder Not Otherwise Specified (NOS),** which identifies those individuals who do not meet criteria for MDD or Dysthymic Disorder, or Adjustment Disorder with Depressed Mood, or Adjustment Disorder with Mixed Anxiety and Depressed Mood.

II. Major Depressive Disorder (MDD)

A. DSM-IV Criteria

1. **To diagnose MDD, at least five of the following symptoms must be present during the same 2-week period;** symptoms must result in a deterioration of function. At least one of the symptoms must be either depressed mood or a loss of interest or pleasure. Symptoms due to medical disorders or mood-incongruent delusions or hallucinations are not to be included.

   a. **Depressed mood** most of the day and nearly every day as expressed by either subjective account or observation made by others.

   b. Markedly **diminished interest** or pleasure in all, or almost all, activities most of the day, nearly every day, as expressed by either subjective account or observation made by others.

   c. Significant unintentional **weight loss or weight gain** (e.g., more than 5% of body weight in a month), or a decrease or increase in appetite nearly every day.

   d. **Insomnia or hypersomnia** nearly every day.

   e. **Psychomotor agitation or retardation** nearly every day (observable by others, not merely subjective feelings of restlessness or being slowed down).

   f. **Fatigue or loss of energy** nearly every day.

   g. **Feelings of worthlessness or excessive** or inappropriate **guilt** (which may be delusional) nearly every day (not merely self-reproach or guilt about being sick).

   h. **Diminished ability to think or concentrate,** or indecisiveness, nearly every day (either by subjective account or as observed by others).

   i. **Recurrent thoughts of death** (not just a fear of dying), **recurrent suicidal ideation** without a specific plan, or a **suicide attempt** or a specific plan for committing suicide.

2. The symptoms must cause disruption in social, occupational, or other important areas of functioning.

3. The symptoms are not secondary to a medical condition (e.g., Cushing's disease) or to the physical effects of a substance (e.g., alcohol, recreational drugs, or medications).

4. The symptoms are not secondary to bereavement. After the loss of a loved one, bereavement may be complicated by MDD if the symptoms persist for 2 months or longer, or are characterized by a marked functional impairment, by preoccupation with worthlessness, by suicidal ideations or behavior, or by psychotic symptoms.

5. The symptoms do not occur in the context of schizophrenia, schizophreniform disorder, delusional disorder, or psychotic disorder not otherwise specified.

6. There are several specifiers that may be used to describe MDD: mild severity; moderate severity; severe without psychotic features; severe with psychotic features; in partial remission; in full remission; chronic; with catatonic features; with melancholic features; with atypical features; with postpartum onset; with or without full inter-episode recovery; with seasonal pattern.

B. Specifiers for Major Depressive Disorder

1. **MDD with Psychotic Features.** In this condition, delusions and hallucinations are present in addition to the symptoms of major depression. The psycho-

tic symptoms may be mood-congruent (i.e., the content is consistent with depressive themes, such as guilt, poor self-worth, death, hopelessness, punishment), or mood-incongruent (i.e., where the content is not consistent with typical depressive themes, such as delusions of control, thought broadcasting, thought insertion, persecutory delusions). Both mood-congruent and mood-incongruent psychotic symptoms can be present concurrently. Delusions occur without hallucinations in about one-half to two-thirds of adults, whereas hallucinations occur without delusions in one-fourth or less of adults. Once psychotic symptoms appear, they tend to be present in each subsequent depressive episode.

2. **MDD with Melancholic Features.** During the most severe period of the episode, there is either loss of pleasure in all or almost all activities, or there is lack of reactivity to usually pleasurable stimuli. In addition, three or more of the following must be present: a depressed mood that is experienced as qualitatively different from the feeling experienced after a loss; depression that is worse in the morning; awakening at least 2 h before the usual time; marked psychomotor retardation or agitation; significant anorexia or weight loss; and excessive or inappropriate guilt.

3. **MDD with Atypical Features.** In this condition mood reactivity occurs in response to actual or potential positive events. Two of the following features must be present: significant weight gain or an increase in appetite; hypersomnia; leaden paralysis or a heavy feeling in the arms and legs; and a long-standing pattern of sensitivity to interpersonal rejection that results in social and occupational dysfunction.

4. **MDD with Postpartum Onset.** The onset of episodes in this condition must occur within 4 weeks of delivery.

5. **MDD with Seasonal Pattern.** A temporal relationship exists between the onset of episodes and the season of the year. Episodes of depression generally occur in the fall or winter.

6. **MDD with Catatonic Features.** At least two of the following must be present: motor immobility (including waxy flexibility or stupor); excessive motor activity that is purposeless and not influenced by external stimuli; extreme negativism (manifested by maintenance of a rigid posture or resistance to commands); unusual voluntary movements (manifest by posturing, stereotyped movements, mannerisms, or grimacing); echolalia or echopraxia.

C. Differential Diagnosis

1. **Mood disorder due to a general medical condition with depressive or with major depressive-like episode.** The diagnosis is based on history, physical examination, and laboratory results. A temporal relationship must exist between the onset of depressive symptoms and the development of the abnormal physiological condition.

2. **Substance-induced mood disorder with depressive features.** The diagnosis is based on history, physical examination, and laboratory results. The symptoms of depression must develop during or within a month of substance intoxication or withdrawal; otherwise, the substance use is etiologically related to the depression.

3. **Dysthymic disorder.** This diagnosis differs from major depressive disorder based on its severity, chronicity, and persistence. In dysthymic disorder, the depressed mood needs to be present more days than not for a period of 2 years.

4. **Dementia.** In dementia, there is a premorbid period of cognitive decline; whereas, in depression, the cognitive decline is associated with onset of depression.

5. **Manic episodes with irritable mood or mixed states.** This diagnosis requires the presence of manic symptoms. The presence of symptoms that meet criteria for both a manic episode and a major depressive episode, every day for at least 1 week, would constitute a mixed manic episode.

6. **Attention-Deficit/Hyperactivity Disorder (ADHD).** Distractibility and low frustration tolerance are common to ADHD and to MDD. The disturbance in mood in ADHD is one of irritability rather than sadness or loss of interest.

7. **Adjustment disorder with depressed mood.** This diagnosis is made if the depressive episode occurs in the context of a psychosocial stressor; it is not due to bereavement, and it does not meet criteria for MDD.

D. Epidemiology

1. **The lifetime prevalence for MDD** in community samples for Americans 18 years and older **ranges from 10% to 25% for women and 5% to 12% for men.** The point prevalence for MDD in community samples for adults is 5–9% for women and 2–3% for men.

2. Since World War II, there has been a trend toward both an earlier age of onset of depression and an increased rate of depression.

3. In prepubertal children, the rate of depression for boys is greater than the rate for girls. Between the beginning of puberty and age 50 years, the rate for depression in women is twice the rate for depression

in men. After the age of 50 years, the rates of depression in women and men are equal.

E. Course of MDD

1. **The average age of onset for unipolar depression is 29 years.**

2. **The onset of MDD may be sudden or gradual** and develop over several weeks or months. Early signs may include insomnia, poor appetite, decreased concentration, loss of interest, or any of the other symptoms of depression, but they occur at a subthreshold level. Other prodromal symptoms include anxiety and panic attacks. MDD with a sudden onset often occurs in the context of a severe psychosocial stressor, especially divorce or loss of a loved one. Eighty percent of acute episodes of MDD are associated with a significant stressor in the previous 6-month period.

3. **MDD is a recurrent illness.** The probability of having a recurrence is influenced by the number of previous episodes. **The risk for relapse after one episode is about 50%, whereas the risk of relapse after three episodes is greater than 80%. The average lifetime number of episodes is four.** The inter-episode interval shortens with increasing numbers of episodes from 6 years after two episodes to 2 years after three episodes. The rate of recurrence after a full recovery from an episode of major depression, in patients with recurring illness, ranges from 50% within 2 years and approximately 90% within 6 years.

4. **Full recovery from an episode of MDD occurs in 50% of cases by 6 months.** For individuals evaluated at 1 year postdiagnosis of MDD, 40% will still meet criteria for major depression, 20% will be in partial remission, and 40% will be in complete remission. Twenty percent of individuals evaluated at the end of 2 years, and 12% at the end of 5 years, continue to be significantly depressed.

5. The course of recurrent major depressive episodes is variable. **Factors that contribute to relapse include: a high number of previous episodes; inadequate antidepressant treatment; partial response to treatment; discontinuation of effective treatment; rapid discontinuation of antidepressants; a highly emotional environment; and comorbid medical or non-affective psychiatric disorders.**

6. **Five to 10% of individuals with a single episode of major depression will eventually develop bipolar disorder.** Young individuals with first episodes that are severe or that are associated with psychotic features may develop bipolar disorder. Women with postpartum depression are at greater risk of developing bipolar disorder.

F. Etiology

1. **Family studies**

   a. MDD is common in families. **It is found two to three times more frequently in the first-degree biological relatives of individuals with the disorder than in the general population.** However, more frequent occurrence in families does not prove that the disorder has a genetic etiology.

   b. Family studies of depressed patients demonstrate significantly higher rates of depression in first-degree relatives, who share 50% of the genome, than in second-degree relatives, who share 25% of the genome. These findings suggest a genetic contribution, but they are inconclusive.

2. **Twin studies and adoption studies**

   a. Studies conducted in Europe and in the United States have demonstrated that **the concordance rate for major depression is about 50% in monozygotic twins, compared to 20% in dizygotic twins.** These results argue for a genetic factor in the development of major depressive disorder. However, most of the twins in these studies were raised together, and it has been hypothesized that twins' behavior can influence each other and that identical twins tend to be treated more alike by their environment than fraternal twins or sibs.

   b. Adoption studies attempt to differentiate the influence of genetic and environmental factors on the expression of an illness. A common strategy is to examine differences in rates of the illness among biological relatives versus adoptive relatives. Recent studies of adoptees with MDD have shown that the rates for depression are higher in their biological parents as compared to the rates in their adoptive parents.

   c. Studies of identical twins raised apart have shown a concordance rate of about 70% for unipolar and bipolar disorder, which is similar for identical twins raised together. These results provide further support for a genetic contribution to the development of MDD.

   d. However, in both twin and adoption studies, between 20% and 30% of identical twin pairs are not concordant for depression, thus arguing for an interaction of the environment with a genetic vulnerability in order for major depressive disorder to be expressed. Reviews of recent twin studies have shown that between 20% and 45% of the variance in the risk for depressive disorders is attributed to genetic factors and the remainder to environmental factors.

3. **Biochemical theories**

   a. **Biogenic amine hypothesis**

      i. The biogenic amine hypothesis was the first biochemical theory to explain the biological basis of both depression and mania. The theory evolved out of observations by clinicians that certain medications had either a negative or positive effect on mood. Reserpine, which depletes the brain of norepinephrine, serotonin, and dopamine, had a tendency to make patients feel depressed, whereas iproniazid, which inhibits the metabolism of nor-epinephrine, serotonin, and dopamine, had a tendency to improve the mood of some tuberculosis patients. The hypothesis argued that depression is the result of too little catecholamine or indoleamine neurotransmitter and mania is the result of too much catecholamine or indoleamine transmitter. Further support for the theory emerged with the finding from animal studies that the tricyclic antidepressants (TCAs) block the uptake of nor-epinephrine and serotonin from presynaptic terminals.

ii. Problems with the theory became evident with the observation that the uptake-blocking mechanism takes place within minutes, whereas the therapeutic effect of TCAs takes about 2 weeks. Other explanations for the effectiveness of antidepressants were pursued with the new technological advances in receptor biology. Subsequent animal research demonstrated that TCAs, monoamine oxidase inhibitors (MAOIs), and electroconvulsive therapy (ECT) downregulate beta-adrenergic receptors over a period of time consistent with the time course to achieve a therapeutic effect. The downregulation of beta-adrenergic receptors did not fully explain the biochemical basis of depression since most of the new antidepressants have no effect on these receptors.

iii. Recent studies have demonstrated that norepinephrine and serotonin are important to the therapeutic effect of TCAs and serotonin reuptake inhibitors (SSRIs), respectively. In one study, dietary depletion of L-tryptophan, which decreases the synthesis of serotonin, resulted in a relapse of depression in SSRI-responders. In another study, subjects given α-methylparatyrosine (AMPT), which inhibits the synthesis of norepinephrine, resulted in a relapse of depression in TCA (primarily norepinephrine uptake blockers)-responders.

iv. The SSRIs and atypical antidepressants, except bupropion, increase serotonin neurotransmission nonselectively. However, the two atypical antidepressants, mirtazapine and nefazodone, selectively increase serotonin neurotransmission through the $5HT_{1a}$ receptor subtype by blocking the $5HT_2$ receptor. An increase in $5HT_{1a}$ receptor activity may be important for the therapeutic effect of many of the newer antidepressants.

G. Biological Markers

1. **Sleep dysregulation**

a. Electroencephalographic (EEG) studies in patients with MDD have identified several **architecture abnormalities during sleep, including: shortened rapid eye movement (REM) latency (decreased time from sleep onset to the onset of the first REM cycle); decreased non-REM sleep; increased REM density (increased number of REMs per unit of time during REM sleep); reduced total sleep time; and decreased sleep continuity.** Sleep architecture abnormalities are most commonly associated with the melancholic subtype in unipolar depression.

b. Any single sleep architecture abnormality is not closely associated with MDD. However, **the combination of decreased REM latency, increased REM density, and decreased sleep efficiency discriminates patients with MDD from controls.** These measures, however, are not specific to MDD, thus they are not appropriate for use as a diagnostic test.

2. **Hypothalamic-pituitary-adrenal axis dysregulation**

a. Hypersecretion of cortisol over the 24-h circadian cycle has been repeatedly observed in patients with MDD.

b. **The dexamethasone suppression test (DST) has been used to assess further the finding of hypersecretion of cortisol in depressed patients. The test consists of giving a 1 mg dose of dexamethasone at 11 p.m. and measuring serum cortisol the following day (usually at 8 a.m. and 4 p.m.).** Normally cortisol is suppressed to levels below 5 μg/dL. Decreased or nonsuppression of serum cortisol in response to a 1 mg dexamethasone challenge occurs in about 50% of patients having MDD with melancholia and in about 80% of patients having MDD with psychotic features. Increased activity could occur at any point between the hypothalamus and the adrenal gland. There is evidence of increased release of corticotropin-releasing factor (CRF) from the hypothalamus. CRF is regulated at the level of the hypothalamus, in part, by norepinephrine and serotonin, the same neurotransmitters implicated in the pathophysiology of depression.

c. Consistent with the physiologic abnormalities noted above are the findings that the pituitary and adrenal glands are hypertrophied in patients with MDD.

3. **Hypothalamic-pituitary-thyroid axis dysregulation**

a. Thyroid abnormalities have been associated with mood disorders: about 10% of hospitalized depressed patients have a diagnosis of hypothyroidism; thyroiditis is more common in patients with mood disorders; patients with rapid-cycling bipolar disorder are more likely to exhibit hypothyroidism; and triiodothyronine (T_3) is used to augment antidepressants for treatment-resistant depression.

b. **The thyrotropin-releasing hormone (TRH) stimulation test can be used to challenge the hypothalamic-pituitary axis.** Protirelin, 55 IU, is given intravenously as the standard dose and thyroid-stimulating hormone (TSH) serum levels are measured at 0.5 and 1.5 h after the infusion. An increase in serum TSH less than 5 IU/mL after TRH infusion is considered a blunted response. One-third of euthyroid patients with melancholia have blunted responses. Some studies show the blunted response as a trait marker while others identify it as a state marker. The underlying mechanism for this abnormal response has not been determined.

4. **Brain Imaging**
   a. **Enlarged ventricles are more frequently found in elderly patients with late-onset MDD compared to those patients whose depression had an early onset.** Magnetic resonance imaging studies (MRI) have demonstrated regional abnormalities, including decreased sizes of the caudate and the putamen. These parts of the basal ganglia have connections with the amygdala and the hippocampus that are important in regulating emotions.
   b. Studies utilizing positron emission tomography (PET) have shown decreased metabolic activity in the frontal cortex of unipolar depressed patients. This hypofrontality is reversed with response to antidepressant medications.
   c. Single photon emission computed tomography (SPECT) studies have shown global reductions in cerebral blood flow in unipolar depressed patients compared to controls. However, frontal, prefrontal, cingulate, and temporal regions show greater perfusion deficits.

H. Pharmacological Treatment of MDD

Antidepressants can be classified into several categories: TCAs and tetracyclic antidepressants; monoamine oxidase inhibitors (MAOIs); selective serotonin reuptake inhibitors (SSRIs); and atypical antidepressants (see Tables 13-1 to 13-4).

1. **Efficacy**
   a. Double-blind placebo-controlled studies have demonstrated that **all of the antidepressants are equally effective in treating MDD. Response rates range from 60% to 80% for drugs** and from 30% to 40% for placebo. Remission rates range from 40% to 50% for antidepressants. Response rates are generally defined as a 50% reduction in scores on depression rating scales.
   b. In view of the absence of a difference in response rates or remission rates among the antidepressants, decisions concerning which antidepressant to use are based on side effect profile, history of response, family history of response, potential for drug interactions, risk of aggravating an existing medical condition (e.g., cardiac conduction defect), risk in overdose, depression subtypes (e.g., atypical depression), and cost.
   c. Once an antidepressant has been chosen, the dose must be titrated slowly with most antidepressants in view of the risk of inducing side effects. The SSRIs have a flat dose-response curve that enables the clinician to achieve the therapeutic dose more quickly. With elderly and medically ill patients on multiple medications, the dose should be increased more slowly, and the final maintenance dose may be half or one-third of the usual average dose. An adequate trial for antidepressants is 4–6 weeks at an adequate therapeutic dose. None of the available antidepressants appears to have a more rapid onset of action.

   d. **Blood levels can be obtained for all of the antidepressants, but only three of the TCAs (desipramine, nortriptyline, and imipramine) show a correlation between blood level and therapeutic effect.** Other reasons to obtain blood levels include monitoring compliance, risk for toxicity, and potential drug interactions.

2. **Treatment phases**
   a. Treatment is divided into three phases to assist in treatment decision-making: **the acute phase, the continuation phase, and the maintenance phase. The acute phase has an average duration of about 12 weeks,** which is the time it often takes to achieve full remission once there is evidence of a response to an antidepressant.
   b. **The continuation phase** begins when full remission is achieved. This phase **lasts from 4 to 6 months** and is considered a high-risk period for relapse. It is highly recommended that antidepressant medication be continued throughout this period. When the antidepressant is discontinued, it should be tapered gradually over several weeks or months in order to prevent withdrawal (from SSRIs), anticholinergic rebound (from TCAs), or increased risk for relapse. Psychotherapeutic approaches which focus on reducing stress and maintaining compliance are often helpful in preventing relapse.
   c. **The maintenance phase represents the long-term commitment to prophylactic treatment with an antidepressant.** Research has demonstrated that all classes of antidepressants not only treat the acute symptoms of depression but also prevent recurrence of episodes. Longitudinal studies demonstrate that a history of three or more episodes places patients at greater than 80% risk for recurrence. **There is also evidence that the maintenance dose of an antidepressant should be at the same dose that achieved full remission.** Other factors that contribute to the risk for relapse include: comorbid psychiatric disorders (e.g., panic disorder); comorbid substance abuse; dysthymic disorder; and chronic medical illnesses.

3. **Side effects** (see Tables 13-1 to 13-3)
   a. The side effect profile of antidepressants depends on their unwanted receptor-blocking properties and their effect on increasing certain neurotransmitter transmission.
   b. **Side effects related to receptor-blocking properties are:**
      i. **Muscarinic blockade:** dry mouth, constipation, blurred vision, and difficulty initiating urination
      ii. **Alpha-1-adrenergic blockade:** orthostatic hypotension
      iii. **Histaminic blockade:** weight gain and sedation
   c. **Side effects related to receptor activation are:**
      i. Norepinephrine: rapid heart rate, increased anxiety, insomnia, tremor, and diaphoresis
      ii. Serotonin: insomnia, sexual dysfunction, gastrointestinal disturbances (e.g., nausea, vomiting, diar-

Table 13-1. Tricyclic Antidepressants (TCAs)

Name	Mechanism: Uptake blocker	Alpha-1-adrenergic blockade	Muscarinic blockade	Histamine H1 blockade
Amitriptyline (Elavil)	NE and 5HT	+++	+++	+++
Amoxapine (Asendin)	NE	+++	+	++
Clomipramine (Anafranil)	NE and 5HT	+++	+++	+
Desipramine (Norpramin)	NE	++	+	+
Doxepin (Sinequan)	NE	+++	++	+++
Imipramine (Tofranil)	NE and 5HT	+++	++	++
Nortriptyline (Pamelor)	NE	+++	+	+
Protriptyline (Vivactil)	NE	++	+++	++
Trimipramine (Surmontil)	None	+++	++	+++
Tetracyclic antidepressant				
Maprotiline (Ludiomil)	NE	+++	+	+++

+, weak; ++, moderate; +++, strong.

Table 13-2. Selective Serotonin Reuptake Inhibitors (SSRIs)

Name	Alpha-1-adrenergic blockade	Muscarinic blockade	Histamine H1 blockade
Fluoxetine (Prozac)	+/0	+/0	+/0
Fluvoxamine (Luvox)	++	+/0	+/0
Paroxetine (Paxil)	+/0	+	+/0
Sertraline (Zoloft)	+/0	+/0	+/0

0, none; +, weak; ++, moderate.

Table 13-3. Atypical Antidepressants

Name	Mechanism	Alpha-1-adrenergic blockade	Muscarinic blockade	Histamine H1 blockade
Bupropion (Wellbutrin)	Blocks NE and DA uptake	+/0	+/0	+/0
Mirtazapine (Remeron)	Releases NE and 5HT by blocking D_2 receptors. Blocks $5HT_2$ and $5HT_3$ receptors	+	+	+++
Nefazodone (Serzone)	Blocks $5HT_2$ receptor; Blocks NE and 5HT uptake	+	+/0	+/0
Trazodone (Desyrel)	Blocks $5HT_2$ receptors and blocks 5HT uptake	+++	+/0	+
Venlafaxine (Effexor)	Blocks 5HT and NE uptake	+/0	+/0	+/0

0, none; +, weak; ++, moderate; +++, strong.

Table 13-4. Monoamine Oxidase Inhibitors (MAOIs)

Name	Reversible/Irreversible	Inhibits MAO-A	Inhibits MAO-B
L-Deprenyl (Eldepryl)	Irreversible	$-^a$	$+$
Moclobemide	Reversible	$+$	$-$
Phenelzine (Nardil)	Irreversible	$+$	$+$
Tranylcypromine (Parnate)	Irreversible	$+$	$+$

^{a}L-Deprenyl at doses above 10 mg/day inhibits both MAO-A and MAO-B.

rhea), restlessness (akathisia), headaches, and appetite loss

   iii. Dopamine: psychosis, agitation, and elevated blood pressure

I. Electroconvulsive Therapy (ECT)

1. **The primary indications include: failure of several antidepressant trials; severe depression with psychotic features; high risk of suicide; medical emergency due to severe weight loss; previous good response.**

2. **Contraindications. There are no absolute contraindications to ECT;** however, certain high-risk medical conditions must be reviewed with an appropriate consultant. Some of the high-risk conditions include: hypertension; cardiac arrhythmias; presence of a cardiac pacemaker; myocardial infarction; intracardiac thrombi; anticoagulant therapy; pregnancy; dementia; vascular aneurysms; respiratory disorders (e.g., chronic obstructive pulmonary disease, asthma, emphysema); brain tumor or mass; epilepsy; orthopedic problems; a history or family history of problems with anesthesia.

3. **Efficacy. ECT is more effective than antidepressants in treating MDD,** both with and without psychotic features. Response rates for MDD are between 70% and 90%. The response rate for major depressives with inadequate pre-ECT pharmacotherapy is about 85%, whereas the response rate for major depressives who are medication resistant pre-ECT is 50%.

4. **Procedure. ECT is given 3 times per week with the average number of treatments between 8 and 12.** Unilateral ECT is the preferred procedure since it is less likely to cause confusion and/or memory disturbances. Bilateral ECT is indicated if there is no response to at least 6 unilateral treatments.

5. **Side effects. The primary side effect is memory loss for events close to the time of the treatment (retrograde) and for events 3–6 months after completing ECT (anterograde).** Post-ECT confusion is also common and can take up to 7 days to clear. Factors that contribute to memory loss and confusion include: long seizures; older age; a high-intensity stimulus; bilateral electrode placement;

inadequate oxygenation; large number of treatments; short interval between treatments. Recent advancements that have reduced memory loss and confusion include: brief pulse stimulus; unilateral electrode placement; and hyperventilation with 100% oxygen prior to applying the stimulus.

J. Treatment of Subtypes of MDD

1. **MDD with Psychotic Features.** The standard treatment of psychotic depression includes use of an antidepressant and an antipsychotic medication. The response rate for an antidepressant alone is 40% and for an antipsychotic alone is 20%, whereas the response rate for the combination of an antidepressant and an antipsychotic medication is 70%. Recent studies have suggested that SSRIs are as effective as TCAs in combination with an antipsychotic medication.

2. **MDD with Melancholic Features.** There is controversial evidence that TCAs may be more effective than SSRIs in treating melancholia. However, because of problematic research design, there has been no conclusive evidence for these findings.

3. **MDD with Atypical Features.** The MAOIs and SSRIs have been shown to be more effective in treating atypical depression than TCAs. The response rates for MAOIs and SSRIs are 70%, whereas the response rate for TCAs is 50%. Thus SSRIs and MAOIs are considered first-line treatments for atypical depression.

4. **MDD with Seasonal Features.** Artificial light with an intensity of 2,500 lux placed 1 m from the patient is very effective in treating seasonal affective disorder (SAD). The response rate is as high as 75%, which is similar to antidepressant medications. Light therapy is more effective in treating patients with SAD than patients with nonseasonal MDD. Patients can be exposed to the light at any time of the day; however, some patients require the exposure to occur in the morning. Response to light occurs within a week, and relapse may occur as soon as 3–4 days after discontinuation. Light therapy should begin in the fall and be continued

through the spring. SSRIs, MAOIs, and bupropion have also been shown to be as effective as light therapy for treating SAD.

K. Psychotherapy

1. **Cognitive-behavioral therapy (CBT) and interpersonal psychotherapy (IPT)** have been shown in research studies to be effective in the treatment of mild to moderate depression. Brief forms of psychodynamic psychotherapies and supportive psychotherapy are considered helpful by many clinicians, but their effectiveness has not been demonstrated by using the scientific method.

2. **Cognitive-behavioral therapy (CBT)**

   a. The cognitive-behavioral approach to treating depression focuses on the impact of maladaptive belief systems on patients' views of themselves, their environment, and their future. Patients who are depressed tend to see themselves as defective, their environment as unsupportive and too demanding, and their future as unchanging and hopeless. The primary tasks are to identify distorted beliefs and then to challenge their validity by using a variety of cognitive-behavioral techniques.

   b. **Cognitive therapy has been shown to be as effective as antidepressants in outpatients with mild to moderate acute depression.** However, antidepressants appear to be more effective than CBT in the treatment of acute severe depression in an inpatient population.

   c. In one study, cognitive therapy was as effective as antidepressants in preventing relapse. Another study demonstrated that, for responders to cognitive therapy and responders to antidepressants who had their treatment discontinued, cognitive therapy-treated patients had lower relapse rates compared to antidepressant-treated patients at 2-year follow-up (21% vs. 50%, respectively).

3. **Interpersonal psychotherapy (IPT)**

   a. IPT focuses on interpersonal losses, role disputes and transitions, social isolation, and deficits in social skills as contributing factors for precipitating depression. Techniques such as role-playing are used to develop social skills, and role expectations are clarified in conjoint sessions for role disputes. IPT is focused on the present, and it is conducted by the use of a manual. It is time limited, usually 16 weeks in duration. It makes use of psychoeducation and teaches patients that depression is a medical illness.

   b. **Studies evaluating the efficacy of IPT in the acute treatment of depression have concluded that IPT is more effective than antidepressants in treating mood, suicidal ideations, and lack of interest, whereas antidepressants are more effective for appetite and sleep disturbances.** In comparison to IPT, antidepressants may be more rapid in treatment response.

   c. Studies evaluating the efficacy of IPT in the maintenance treatment of depression have shown that, in a 3-year follow-up study, IPT relapse-free survival rates were 30–40%, whereas supportive care relapse-free survival rates were 10%. Also, patients receiving high-quality IPT had 2-year survival rates similar to antidepressants. The lack of adequate dosing of IPT may account for some of the differences between survival rates for IPT and antidepressants.

L. Combination Psychotherapy and Antidepressant Treatment

1. Due to methodological problems, data from studies combining psychodynamic psychotherapy, cognitive therapy, or IPT with antidepressants have not confirmed any advantage to combined treatment. For the treatment of mild to moderate depression, it is recommended to treat with either an antidepressant or one of the brief forms of psychotherapy. For severe depression, it is recommended to start with an antidepressant.

2. Combined therapy should be used if treatment with one modality is insufficient to produce a complete response, if the depression is chronic, or if the clinical presentation includes multiple symptoms, some of which might be more responsive to one modality over the other. For example, problems with assertiveness would be more amenable to psychotherapy, whereas an appetite disturbance would likely respond best to an antidepressant.

III. Dysthymic Disorder

A. DSM-IV Criteria

1. **Depressed mood** (or potentially an irritable mood in children and adolescents for at least 1 year) **must be present for most of the day, more days than not, for at least 2 years.**

2. When depressed, the patient exhibits at least two of the following symptoms: poor appetite or overeating; insomnia or hypersomnia; low energy or fatigue; low self-esteem; poor concentration or difficulty making decisions; or feelings of hopelessness.

3. During a 2-year period (1 year in children or adolescents) of the disturbance, the person has never been symptom-free for more than 2 months.

4. A lack of evidence for a major depressive episode during the first 2 years of the disturbance.

5. No history of mania, hypomania, or cyclothymia.

6. Symptoms are not caused by a medical condition, drug of abuse, or a medication.

7. The symptoms do not occur exclusively during the course of psychotic disorders.

8. The symptoms cause clinically significant distress or impairment in psychosocial functioning.

B. The lifetime prevalence for Dysthymic Disorder is 6% and the point prevalence is 3%.

C. Course

Dysthymic disorder generally exhibits a slow and insidious onset beginning in childhood, adolescence, or early adulthood. When dysthymic disorder is comorbid with major depressive disorder, the condition is referred to as a "double depression." The presence of dysthymic disorder increases the risk for an episode of major depressive disorder in vulnerable individuals.

IV. Depressive Disorder Not Otherwise Specified

A. DSM-IV Criteria

1. This category includes depressive disorders that do not meet criteria for MDD, Dysthymic Disorder, Adjustment Disorder with Depressed Mood, or Adjustment Disorder with Mixed Anxiety and Depressed Mood.

2. Examples include the following:
   a. **Minor Depressive Disorder,** which is manifest by at least 2 weeks of depressive symptoms but fewer than five of the required symptoms for MDD.
   b. **Recurrent Brief Depressive Disorder,** which is manifest by depressive episodes lasting from 2 days up to 2 weeks, and occurring at least once a month for 1 year.
   c. **Premenstrual Dysphoric Disorder,** which is manifest by markedly depressed mood, marked anxiety, marked affective lability, and a decreased interest in activities during the last week of the luteal phase of the menstrual period. Each of these symptoms resolves within a few days of the onset of menses. The symptoms must be present during most menstrual cycles during the past year, and be totally absent for at least 1 week after the menstrual period, and be severe enough to interfere with work, school, or usual activities.
   d. **Postpsychotic Depressive Disorder,** which is a Major Depressive Episode that occurs during the residual phase of Schizophrenia.
   e. **Depressive Disorder NOS,** which is also used in situations where the clinician has identified a depressive disorder but is unable to determine if it is primary or secondary to a medical condition or to use of a psychoactive substance.

Suggested Readings

American Psychiatric Association: Mood disorders. In *Diagnostic and Statistical Manual of Mental Disorders*, 4th ed. Washington DC: American Psychiatric Press, Inc., 1994:317–391.

American Psychiatric Association: *Practice Guideline for Major Depressive Disorder in Adults.* Washington DC: American Psychiatric Press, Inc., 1993.

Bernstein JG: *Drug Therapy in Psychiatry*, 3rd ed. St. Louis: Mosby, 1995:112–194.

Blackburn I, Bishop S, Glen A, et al.: The efficacy of cognitive therapy in depression: a treatment trial using cognitive therapy and pharmacotherapy, each alone and in combination. *Br J Psychiatry* 1981; 139:181–189.

Dubzovsky SL, Buzan R: Mood disorders. In Hales RE, Yudofsky SC, Talbott JA (eds): *The American Psychiatric Press Textbook of Psychiatry*, 3rd ed. Washington DC: American Psychiatric Press, Inc., 1999:479–565.

Frazer A: Antidepressants. *J Clin Psychiatry* 1997; 58(suppl.6): 9–23.

Klerman G, Weissman M, Rounsaville B, Chevron E: *Interpersonal Psychotherapy of Depression.* New York: Basic Books, 1984.

Parker G, Hadzi-Pavlovic D, Pedic F: Psychotic (delusional) depression: a meta-analysis of physical treatments. *J Affect Dis* 1992; 24:17–24.

Quitkin FM, Harrison W, Stewart JW, et al.: Response to phenelzine and imipramine in placebo nonresponders with atypical depression. *Arch Gen Psychiatry* 1991; 48:319–323.

Rosenbaum JF, Fava M: Approach to the patient with depression. In Stern TA, Herman JB, Slavin PL (eds): *The MGH Guide to Psychiatry in Primary Care.* New York: McGraw-Hill, 1998: 1–14.

Rosenbaum JF, Fava M, Nierenberg AA, Sachs GS: Treatment-resistant mood disorders. In Gabbard GO (ed): *Treatments of Psychiatric Disorders*, 2nd ed. Washington DC: American Psychiatric Press, Inc., 1995:1275–1328.

Rothschild AJ: Management of psychotic, treatment-resistant depression. In Hornig-Rohan M, Amsterdam JD (eds): *The Psychiatric Clinics of North America*, 1996; 19(2):237–252.

Wright J, Thase M, Sensky T: Cognitive and biological therapies: a combined approach. In Wright J, Thaes M, Beck A, Ludgate J (eds): *Cognitive Therapy with Inpatients.* New York: Guilford Press, 1992:193–218.

Chapter 14
Bipolar Disorder
S. Nassir Ghaemi

I. Overview

Mood disorders are among the most common psychiatric conditions. While community studies suggest that around 5–10% of the general population in the United States experience a major depressive episode at least once in a lifetime, **bipolar disorder occurs in about 1–2% of the population.** Milder variations on bipolar disorder, such as hypomania and cyclothymia, may account for another 2–5% of the population. Therefore, roughly 10–20% of the general population develop a mood disorder at some point in life. Bipolar disorder, a treatable condition, is chameleonic in its numerous guises; if left untreated, it is deadly. **Since it shares features with both unipolar depression and schizophrenia, bipolar disorder is frequently misdiagnosed.** Also, it is characterized by numerous phases of illness, which may make it difficult to identify. Although effective treatment can result in almost complete recovery, **the risk of suicide with this condition is high (lifetime estimate 19%).** Bipolar disorder is usually due to a primary mood disturbance, but it can also occur secondary to medical conditions and to substance abuse.

II. Epidemiology

The lifetime prevalence of classical bipolar disorder is approximately 1%. Higher estimates are reported in studies which carefully assess milder symptoms of hypomania and cyclothymia (with a 2–5% lifetime prevalence). Of those identified as bipolar by epidemiologic studies, only one-third have already been diagnosed by a physician, and, of those, **only 27% have ever received treatment.** This rate of undertreatment is worse than for any other psychiatric illness.

A. **Gender**
   The incidence of bipolar disorder is equivalent among males and females, unlike unipolar depression, which is more frequent in women. The rapid-cycling subtype of bipolar disorder is overrepresented among females.

B. **Age**
   According to recent studies, the average age of onset of bipolar disorder is around 19 years (range 15–20 years). The reported age of onset of affective disorders has decreased in the last few decades, which may reflect improvement in diagnosis or be related to other demographic and social factors. **New-onset bipolar disorder is rare after the fifth** decade of life; when it occurs, it is usually secondary to a medical/neurological condition, or to the effects of medications (particularly antidepressants and steroids).

C. **Ethnicity**
   There are no known ethnic characteristics related to bipolar disorder. Some studies suggest that minorities (African-Americans and Hispanics) with bipolar disorder may be more likely to be misdiagnosed with schizophrenia.

D. **Class**
   Bipolar disorder, unlike schizophrenia, is not generally associated with a downward drift of socioeconomic class. Bipolar patients are somewhat more common in middle and upper socioeconomic classes. Also, members of lower socioeconomic classes who have bipolar disorder are often misdiagnosed as having schizophrenia.

E. **Individual Factors**
   Bipolar disorder is associated with a 19% lifetime completed suicide rate. It is associated with extremely high rates of divorce, an occupational history of numerous jobs, often excellent academic achievement followed by a decline in occupational performance, and generally chaotic life histories (both personally and socially). Bipolar disorder is associated with elevated IQ in some studies. Women with bipolar disorder have a life-expectancy that is diminished by 9 years.

F. **Comorbid Conditions**
   Sixty percent of individuals with bipolar disorder are likely to develop substance abuse at some point in their lifetimes. Violence and legal problems are also common.

III. Differential Diagnosis

A. **Differentiation from Other Axis I Disorders**
   Often, the varieties of mood disorders are subsumed under the lay term "depression." Although depressive symptoms are common in all of the varieties of mood syndromes, technically the word "depression" is not a specific diagnosis but a symptom, like "fever." This can lead to confusion among patients and clinicians alike. Hence, it is important to clarify the diagnostic meaning of the

above terms and to diagnose accurately bipolar disorder so that specific treatment can be initiated.

Bipolar disorder needs to be distinguished clearly from unipolar depression. In unipolar depression, no mood swings occur: one is either depressed or average in one's mood, but there is no mood elevation. Bipolar disorder, on the other hand, is an illness where mood swings occur: one either has a depressed or an elevated mood or is euthymic. In other words, it differs from unipolar depression by the fact that **mood elevation occurs. It takes** *only one episode* **of mood elevation for a diagnosis of bipolar disorder to be made, no matter how many times an individual becomes depressed.**

Bipolar disorder is also associated with psychotic features in 50% of individuals at some point in the illness; thus it can be mistaken for schizophrenia. A key difference is that the patient's **affect is flat in schizophrenia,** while there is evidence of elevated mood at some point in bipolar disorder. Lastly, **distractibility is a DSM-IV criterion for bipolar disorder and attention deficit disorder; hence these two conditions can be confused, particularly in children. The key feature that distinguishes bipolar disorder from these other conditions is the manic or hypomanic episode,** particularly when characterized by an elevated or irritable mood, a decreased need for sleep, flight of ideas or increased talkativeness, and increased goal-directed activities. **The presence of a single manic or hypomanic episode trumps all of the above diagnoses:** schizophrenia, unipolar depression, and attention deficit disorder are diagnosed only if bipolar disorder is absent. **Only schizoaffective disorder, bipolar type, remains a possible diagnosis once a manic/hypomanic episode is diagnosed:** when psychosis lasts for 2 weeks outside of a mood episode, schizoaffective disorder, but not bipolar disorder, may be present.

B. **Subtypes of Bipolar Disorder** (see Table 14-1)
In **bipolar disorder, type I,** at least one manic episode is identified, with or without major depression. In **bipolar disorder, type II,** not a single manic episode is identified, but at least one hypomanic episode, and at least one major depressive episode, is identified. In **cyclothymia,** major depressive symptoms do not reach the threshold for diagnosis of a major depressive episode, and mood elevation, while present, does not reach threshold for diagnosis of a manic episode. **The key difference between mania and hypomania is that mania is associated with significant social or occupational dysfunction** (often involving spending sprees, sexual indiscretions, reckless driving, and impulsive travelling), **while hypomania is not.**

Mood elevation involves an irritable or euphoric mood, along with sufficient symptoms of mania. Note it is *not* **just euphoric mood.** While many persons with mania report "high" or "happy" mood, others have only an *irritable* mood. It is a mistake to identify mania when only euphoria is present; one can also have mania without any euphoria. Manic episodes, while classically involving euphoria, can be characterized by an irritable mood. Either type can still be described as pure mania. Depressed mood can coexist with manic symptoms; with other neurovegetative symptoms of depression, this leads to a diagnosis of a mixed episode. Mixed manic episodes are as common as are pure manic episodes.

The diagnosis of a rapid-cycling bipolar disorder identifies an illness with a course of numerous, defined as four or more in a year, mood episodes. According to the kindling hypothesis, rapid-cycling may represent an end-stage and severe phase of bipolar disorder.

IV. Theories on the Etiology and Neurobiology of Bipolar Disorder

A. **The Kindling Hypothesis**
The kindling hypothesis states that bipolar disorder is similar in its clinical course, and possibly in its biological mechanism, to epilepsy. According to this theory, as in epilepsy, **the more episodes that occur early in the illness, the more frequent and severe**

Table 14-1. Subtypes of Bipolar Disorder

- Bipolar disorder type I: mania, with or without depression
- Bipolar disorder type II: hypomania, with major depression
- Cyclothymia: hypomanic symptoms plus subthreshold depressive symptoms for 2 years
- Pure mania: euphoric or irritable mood
- Mixed mania: depressed mood
- Rapid-cycling: four or more mood (of any polarity) episodes in a year

later episodes are likely to be. Thus, earlier episodes will be shorter, less severe, and easier to treat than later episodes. Also, anticonvulsant agents may exert an antikindling effect on neurons in the limbic system, which results in their mood-stabilizing effects.

B. Other Theories

Other theories that have been suggested include:
1. Abnormally fast biological clocks, or **circadian pacemakers,** in the suprachiasmatic nucleus.
2. Elevated **norepinephrine and dopamine** neurotransmitter activity in the limbic system.
3. Abnormal **G-protein** and second messenger functions that mediate mood in key limbic neuronal pathways.

V. The Impact of Genetics and Environment

A. Genetics

Like other major mental illnesses, bipolar disorder has an important genetic component. The genetic basis of bipolar disorder is neither Mendelian nor qualitative, with dominant and recessive gene contributions. Instead, **it is non-Mendelian (i.e., quantitative), with a polygenic influence of numerous genes,** none of which is sufficient to lead to the illness in any significant manner. Studies of twins indicate that this genetic contribution accounts for about 60% of the heritability of the illness; the other 40% is due to environmental effects.

B. Environment

Based on twin studies, the environmental influence is not likely to be familial or shared, but rather due to specific environmental effects ("the slings and arrows of outrageous fortune") that are unique to each individual. Obstetric complications, intrauterine viral infections, neurodevelopmental abnormalities in childhood, use of hallucinogenic ("prokindling") drugs, and psychosocial trauma may be among these specific environmental influences. **It is likely that the most potent environmental influences on the etiology of the illness occur early in life,** before the illness's typical onset in adolescence and early adulthood.

Psychosocial stressors later in adulthood, such as the death of family and friends, the end of romantic relationships, and occupational stress, more likely serve as environmental triggers for specific episodes, acting on the underlying susceptibility to illness established earlier in life. There is some evidence, consistent with the kindling hypothesis, that the influence of psychosocial environmental triggers is less evident later in the course of illness, when episodes occur autonomously and more frequently compared with earlier in the course of bipolar illness, when episodes occur less frequently and are more often triggered by psychosocial stressors.

VI. Course of the Illness

A. Chronicity

Bipolar disorder, unlike unipolar depression, is almost always a recurrent condition. A single manic episode heralds the near certainty of future manic or depressive episodes and the likely need for long-term medication treatment. Unlike major depression, **there is no evidence that any kind of psychotherapy is as effective as medication in the treatment of mania.** However, psychotherapies may be helpful along with medications in the long-run, particularly when they enhance medication compliance and strengthen the therapeutic alliance between clinician and patient.

B. Seasonal Variation

Seasonal features are not uncommon; manic episodes occur more often in the summer, and depressive episodes in the winter or spring. This pattern should not be confused with that of seasonal affective disorder, a diagnosis made only when mood episodes almost always occur solely in certain seasons, and almost invariably fail to occur outside of those seasons for a number of years. Many patients who meet criteria for seasonal affective disorder are diagnosable with bipolar disorder, type II, based on the experience of major depression in the winter followed by hypomania in the spring.

C. Duration of Episodes

Depressive episodes (mean untreated duration of 6–12 months) tend to last longer than manic episodes (with a mean untreated duration of 3–6 months) in bipolar disorder.

VII. Evaluation

A. The Depressed Patient

Individuals with bipolar disorder experience major depressive episodes that are longer in duration than manic episodes are. Also, afflicted individuals are more likely to have insight into depression than they are into mania, and thus are more likely to seek help for their depression. Atypical depressive symptoms (increased sleep, increased appetite, preserved reactivity of mood, leaden heaviness of the limbs, and a personality style characterized by rejection sensitivity) are somewhat more common in bipolar disorder than they are in unipolar depression. Psychotic features (delusions or hallucinations) are also more common in bipolar than in unipolar depression. Further, all patients who meet criteria for major depression need to be screened for the presence of manic symptoms to rule out a mixed episode. Ultimately, the best way to differentiate a currently depressed individual's diagnosis as bipolar or unipolar depression is to determine if manic or hypomanic episodes have occurred in the past.

B. The Manic Patient

To diagnose a manic episode, a patient must experience irritable or euphoric mood, with three (if euphoric) or four (if irritable) of the seven cardinal symptoms of mania, for 1 week. The cardinal symptoms of mania are easily remembered by a mnemonic (**"DIGFAST"**) that reminds one of the excessive activity of mania (see Fig. 14-1).

1. **Distractibility** is the most common manic symptom, but also the most subjective. It involves the inability to maintain one's focus on tasks for any extended duration.
2. **Insomnia** refers to **decreased *need* for sleep.** It differs from the insomnia of depression, which simply involves decreased sleep. An excellent way to differentiate the two is to ask about the patient's energy level. In mania, despite decreased sleep, the energy level is average or high. In depressive insomnia, it is low.
3. **Grandiosity** reflects inflated self-esteem. This can be delusional, or, in milder cases, it involves increased self-confidence out of proportion to one's circumstances.
4. **Flight of ideas,** or racing thoughts, indicates a rapid progression of one's thought processes.
5. **Activities** (i.e., an increase in goal-directed activities), which are functional and often appear useful; they fall into four categories:

Distractibility

Insomnia

Grandiosity

Flight of ideas

Activities

Speech

Thoughtlessness

Mania = Euphoric mood + 3 criteria or Irritable mood + 4 criteria for 1 week (or hospitalized) + significant social/occupational dysfunction

Fig. 14-1.   DIGFAST: a diagnostic mnemonic for mania.

a. **Social:** increased socializing, calling friends, going out more than usual.
b. **Sexual:** increased libido or hypersexuality.
c. **Work:** increased productivity, cleaning the house more than usual.
d. **School:** producing many projects, studying more than usual.

In all cases, usual levels of activity need to be based on a comparison with activity levels during the euthymic state.

6. **Speech** is pressured or the individual is more talkative than usual. Pressured speech may be present in the mental status examination. If not, one can ask the patient to compare their level of talkativeness with their speech during euthymic periods.
7. **Thoughtlessness** (e.g., pleasure-seeking activities which do not display usual judgment, and, unlike increased goal-directed activities, are dysfunctional). Four common varieties are sexual indiscretions, reckless driving, spending sprees, and sudden traveling.

To qualify for a diagnosis of a manic episode, in addition to the above criteria, there must be **significant social or occupational dysfunction** which arises from the above symptoms. If there is no social or occupational dysfunction, then a hypomanic episode is diagnosed. Also, for a diagnosis of a manic episode, the symptoms must last at least 1 week (or lead to hospitalization). If they last less than 1 week, but at least 4 days, then a diagnosis of hypomanic episode is made.

C. Ruling Out Secondary Mood Disorders

The medical causes of secondary mood disorders fall into several large categories; these are discussed below in order of descending importance (see Table 14-2).

1. **Drugs. Substance abuse** is the most common culprit. Cocaine, in particular, causes mania and may "kindle" a new or worsened bipolar illness. Drugs used to treat a variety of medical conditions can cause mania; among these, the most common classes are **antidepressants and steroids.**
2. **Neurological disorders.** These are the most common nonpsychiatric illnesses that cause mood disorders. Probably the most common neurological disorder associated with mania is **multiple sclerosis. Frontal lobe syndromes,** whether due to head trauma, dementia, or stroke, can also simulate manic symptoms, especially impulsivity and hypersexuality. **Temporal lobe epilepsy,** particularly when the focus is in the nondominant hemisphere, is associated with manic symptoms during the ictal period.
3. **Endocrine disorders.** These are less common, and mood disorders usually occur in advanced stages of illness where other more characteristic physical

Table 14-2. Common Secondary Causes of Mania

Substance abuse/intoxication/withdrawal

Alcohol, cocaine, amphetamines, caffeine

Medications

Antidepressants, steroids, L-dopa, amphetamines, barbiturates, adrenocorticotropin (ACTH)

Neurological conditions

Multiple sclerosis, frontal lobe syndromes, temporal lobe epilepsy, stroke, head trauma, subcortical dementias, encephalitis, Huntington's disease, pseudobulbar palsy

Endocrine conditions

Hyperthyroidism, Cushing's syndrome

Other medical illnesses

Infections: herpes simplex encephalitis, HIV encephalitis, syphilis, other viral or parasitic encephalitides

Autoimmune disease: systemic lupus erythematosus

Metabolic states: hypoglycemia, hypoxia

symptoms are present. **Hyperthyroidism** and **Cushing's syndrome** tend to be associated with mania.

4. **Other. Infectious diseases, metabolic states, and immunologic diseases** can produce mood disorders. **Herpes simplex encephalitis,** which affects limbic areas, often simulates manic symptoms. **Human immunodeficiency virus** (HIV) infection is highly associated with mania, possibly as a direct viral effect on neuronal pathways subserving mood. **Systemic lupus erythematosus** is probably the most common autoimmune condition associated with mania. **Hypoglycemia and hypoxia** can each lead to mood instability.

In the treatment of secondary mood disorders, where possible, the offending agent, if a drug, should be removed, or the relevant medical condition treated. In the case of chronic medical conditions, aggressive antidepressant treatment for unipolar symptoms is indicated to minimize the adverse effects of depression.

VIII. Approach to the Bipolar Patient

A. General Strategies

1. **Establish a therapeutic alliance. Noncompliance** with mood stabilizers is a major problem in bipolar disorder. Not only are there the general issues shared with other medications (the hassle factor, numerous side effects), but some bipolar patients appear to prefer to be ill, sometimes due to a wish to experience hypomanic symptoms and frequently due to a marked lack of insight into the nature of their condition.

2. **Don't be fooled by depression or psychosis.** Psychiatrists make two common mistakes that lead to misdiagnosis. The first is to assume that, if patients experience psychotic symptoms, they must have schizophrenia. However, **one cannot make a diagnosis of schizophrenia based solely on the presence of psychotic symptoms.** Instead, the diagnosis of an affective disorder is based on affective symptoms, ignoring the psychotic symptoms; the diagnosis of schizophrenia is only made after having ruled out any affective disorder. Schizophrenia is a diagnosis of exclusion.

The second, and more common, mistake is to assume that when patients experience depressive symptoms, unipolar depression is present. However, **depression is not a diagnosis, it is a symptom.** Like "fever," depressive symptoms need further analysis to determine the underlying diseases. If present, one must ask, what type of depression is this? There are three possibilities: **it is either secondary or primary (i.e., bipolar or unipolar).** Secondary and bipolar depression need to be ruled out before unipolar depression can be diagnosed.

In summary, not all psychosis is schizophrenia, and not all depression is unipolar depression. In both cases, the alternative diagnosis is bipolar disorder (and schizoaffective illness in the case of psychosis).

3. **Don't rely solely on an individual's self-report. As with numerous other psychiatric conditions, one cannot definitively rule out bipolar disorder based on an individual's self-report in a clinical interview,** even after inquiring about all possible manic symptoms.

It appears that *part of the illness* is that the patient does not recognize possessing the illness. This *lack of insight* is more common in bipolar disorder than it is in those with unipolar depression. Thus, it is easier to diagnose unipolar disorder because the patient can help make the diagnosis; in bipolar disorder the patients' denial of their symptoms hinders our attempts at diagnosis. **Thus, it is important to get reliable information from outside sources,** like family and friends. Diagnosis is based on the clinician's judgment, after searching all available sources of clinical information, which include, but are not limited to, the patient's opinion.

4. **Establish safety.** Assess for the possibility of suicide and violence. **Acutely manic patients usually require hospitalization.**

B. **Goals of the Assessment**
   A major goal of an assessment for bipolar disorder is to determine if the patient has had at least one manic or hypomanic episode at any point in their lifetime. This will guide the diagnosis of a bipolar subtype and influence treatment.

C. **Specific Elements of History**
   1. **Obtaining a medical history. Rule out possible secondary medical causes of bipolar disorder.** This requires that one take a careful medical history and obtain blood and urine samples to screen for the illnesses described previously.

   2. **Obtaining a substance abuse history. Rule out secondary substance abuse-related mood disorders.** This requires taking a careful history as well as blood and urine screening samples. Remember that the presence of substance abuse does not establish a secondary mood disorder; 60% of individuals with bipolar disorder experience substance abuse at some point in their lives. Rather, **bipolar disorder would be secondary to substance abuse if episodes of abnormal mood invariably occur during periods of substance abuse and not outside of those periods,** or (in those without a history of abstinence) if consistent substance abuse precedes the onset of a mood disorder.

   3. **Assess manic symptoms. Use the DIGFAST mnemonic. Establish time-frames in which to use the mnemonic.** At least two time-frames are required: current (the past 1–2 weeks), and past. When assessing for past manic symptoms, begin by assessing for mania, requiring that patients recall time-frames of 1 week or longer when they might have experienced elevated or irritable mood, decreased need for sleep, or other manic symptoms. If not volunteered, the stereotypic impulsive behaviors of mania (sexual indiscretions, reckless driving, spending sprees, impulsive traveling) should be assessed. If mania is not identified, then hypomania at any point must be assessed. Special attention should be given to establishing a patient's "normal" baseline in mood and energy (usually "even-keeled" mood of not feeling particularly happy or sad in the absence of specific cause, and "average energy" requiring around 7–9 h of sleep nightly). **Hypomania** represents any deviation above this baseline for 4 days or longer, associated with some manic symptoms but **without significant social or occupational dysfunction.** If significant dysfunction exists, mania should be diagnosed, even in the absence of the stereotypic behaviors described above.

   4. **Assess the family history.** Most patients with bipolar disorder have a family history of psychiatric illness. This may be unipolar depression or schizophrenia, particularly since bipolar disorder has frequently been misdiagnosed as these conditions in the past.

   5. **Assess prior psychiatric treatment.** Frequently, individuals with bipolar disorder have been treated with antidepressants, which can worsen the course of the illness (see below). Periods of antidepressant use are often correlated with diagnostic information regarding manic symptoms. Other hints of a bipolar diagnosis include an initial rapid response to antidepressant agents followed by a loss of response, treatment resistance to multiple antidepressant trials, or response to the addition of a mood stabilizer (like lithium) to antidepressants.

   6. **Assess for the presence of comorbid psychiatric conditions.** Common comorbid conditions include anxiety disorders (e.g., panic disorder and obsessive compulsive disorder [OCD]), posttraumatic stress disorder, cluster B personality disorders (especially borderline personality), past attention deficit disorder, and eating disorders. These comorbid conditions often influence treatment decisions (see below).

   7. **Complete a mental status examination. Focus the examination on affect.** If a patient is currently manic, the **affect is either euphoric, irritable, or labile.** If a patient is currently in a mixed state or is depressed, the affect is usually depressed. Anxiety may or may not be present. Patients may express their mood as "down" or "sad" when depressed, but, when manic, mood may be reported as "fine." In some cases, euphoric mood may be described as "giddy," "high," or "up." Thought content is usually normal, although, in mild cases of mania, paranoid or grandiose ideas of reference may be present. Obsessions may occur with comorbid OCD. In many cases of mania, thought process is characterized by **flight of ideas,** or a sense that

one's thoughts are racing faster than one can speak them. Otherwise thoughts can be normal, circumstantial, or tangential. Looseness of associations tends to occur in patients with psychotic features. **Speech** in mania is often, but not always, characterized by a sense of **pressure**. Patients may be **overtalkative** and unduly prolong conversations. Cognition is generally intact, with normal orientation to person, place, and time, and unimpaired immediate, short-term, and long-term recall. Concentration is often impaired in depression and mania; however, manic patients are often **distractible** and unable to maintain focus without jumping from topic to topic. Suicidal and homicidal ideation should always be assessed.

8. **If current or past manic symptoms are identified, then the following features of the history should be determined:**
   a. Age of onset of first mania or hypomania
   b. Age of onset of first major depression
   c. Number of lifetime manic or hypomanic episodes
   d. Number of lifetime major depressive episodes
   e. Typical cycle of episodes (mania followed by depression followed by well interval, or depression followed by mania followed by well interval, or continuous cycling)
   f. Last and longest periods of euthymia
   g. Age of first psychiatric treatment
   h. Age of first bipolar diagnosis and previous psychiatric diagnoses if present
   i. History of infection or head trauma
   j. Sleep pattern
   k. Menstrual regularity
   l. Intentions for conception, pregnancy, or lactation in females

m. Effect of illness on social and occupational functioning
n. Last period of best occupational functioning

D. Management of the Bipolar Patient
1. **Assess and treat baseline medical and substance abuse conditions.** Medical assessments should be made carefully. **Thyroid function, in particular, should be assessed in an individual with rapid-cycling bipolar disorder, since subclinical hypothyroidism is associated with that condition. Substance abuse** should be assessed and treated aggressively.
2. **Maximize mood-stabilizing treatments. Mood stabilizers are the only treatments that are effective in both the acute and maintenance phases of treatment for bipolar disorder** (whether for manic, or mixed, or depressive episodes). Mood stabilizers can be thought of as possessing some antidepressant properties and some antimanic properties, thus stabilizing patients near euthymia. **Standard mood stabilizers include lithium, valproic acid, and carbamazepine. The newest probable mood stabilizer is lamotrigine.** Since standard mood stabilizers often do not work sufficiently well alone or in combination, other medications with adjunctive mood-stabilizing effects are often added to the standard agents (see Fig. 14-2). Adjunctive mood-stabilizing agents include atypical antipsychotic agents (e.g., clozapine, risperidone, and olanzapine), and other novel anticonvulsants (e.g., gabapentin).
3. **Eliminate and avoid mood-destabilizing agents.** The major concern here are **antidepressant agents.** Antidepressants pose two risks. In the short-term, **they can cause mania;** in this regard, bupropion and paroxetine have a lower risk of switching an individual into acute mania than tricyclic anti-

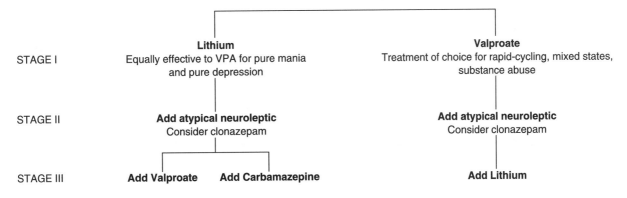

STAGE I	**Lithium** Equally effective to VPA for pure mania and pure depression	**Valproate** Treatment of choice for rapid-cycling, mixed states, substance abuse
STAGE II	**Add atypical neuroleptic** Consider clonazepam	**Add atypical neuroleptic** Consider clonazepam
STAGE III	**Add Valproate** **Add Carbamazepine**	**Add Lithium**

If purely depressed at this stage for > 1 month

Add Antidepressant
Bupropion or Paroxetine preferred
Taper after 1 month of euthymia

Stages II and III can be reversed in order depending on the clinical setting.

Fig. 14-2. An algorithm for the treatment of bipolar disorder.

depressants in acute bipolar depression. In the long-term, **they can lead to rapid-cycling and more manic and depressive episodes** than would have occurred if left untreated. While these agents have a role in the treatment of severe acute bipolar depression (along with mood-stabilizing agents), they can usually then be tapered after the acute phase of treatment is over. When used too aggressively, such as in long-term treatment after resolution of acute depressive symptoms, they often lead to a rapid-cycling course and a long-term worsening of an individual's bipolar illness. As **mood destabilizers** they can counteract the effect of mood stabilizers, such as lithium, and render a patient "treatment-resistant" who might otherwise respond to mood stabilizers (see Table 14-3). Antidepressants are appropriate for acute depression in bipolar disorder, but not necessarily for prophylaxis of future depressive episodes in bipolar disorder.

4. **Educate the patient and establish a therapeutic alliance.** Education is an important component of the long-term treatment of bipolar illness. Many patients have little knowledge or insight into their symptoms. If they improve, they need to understand and come to terms with the need to take medications most of their lives. Often, they must adjust to side effects, or work with their clinicians to adjust medication dosing to minimize the impact of side effects. To enhance compliance, a good therapeutic alliance is of the utmost importance. Psychological factors of the long-term treatment of bipolar disorder may be the missing link between the pharmacological efficacy of medications such as lithium, and their relative lack of effectiveness in naturalistic long-term studies of real-world treatment. Adjunctive individual psychotherapy with a psychotherapist versed in bipolar disorder can be important, as can the use of cognitive-behavioral and interpersonal psychotherapies for the depressive phases of bipolar dis-

order. Self-help and family groups, such as the Alliance for the Mentally Ill (AMI) and the Depressive and Manic Depressive Association (DMDA), are important.

5. **Be cautious about overemphasizing comorbid conditions.** With the exception of substance abuse, the treatment of many comorbid conditions that occur with bipolar disorder can be deferred until the mood symptoms of bipolar illness are effectively under control. This is because many of the treatments (e.g., antidepressants and amphetamines) for comorbid conditions such as panic disorder, OCD, and attention deficit disorder (ADD), can be mood destabilizers and worsen the course of bipolar illness. Also, it is usually self-defeating to emphasize borderline personality traits in the presence of current mood symptoms and unequivocal past mania. Research has shown that, during acute mood episodes, personality traits are excacerbated and personality disorders are evident until after the acute mood episode resolves. Thus, **a definitive diagnosis of personality disorder should often be withheld until a mood episode resolves.** If a personality disorder can be diagnosed during periods of euthymia, then a true comorbid illness can be said to exist and more aggressive treatment for it be justified.

Suggested Readings

Akiskal HS: The prevalent clinical spectrum of bipolar disorders: beyond DSM-IV. *J Clin Psychopharmacol* 1996;16 (Suppl. 1): 4S–14S.

Ghaemi SN, Sachs GS, Chiora AM, et al.: Is bipolar disorder still underdiagnosed? Are antidepressants overutilized? *J Affective Dis* 1999; 52:135–144.

Goodwin FK, Ghaemi SN: Understanding manic-depressive illness. *Arch Gen Psychiatry* 1998; 55:23–25.

Goodwin FK, Jamison KR: *Manic Depressive Illness.* New York: Oxford University Press, 1990.

Harrow M, Goldberg JF, Grossman LS, Meltzer HY: Outcome in manic disorders. *Arch Gen Psychiatry* 1990; 47:665–671.

Kalin N: Management of the depressive component of bipolar disorder. *Depression Anxiety* 1996/1997; 4:190–198.

Keller MB, Lavori PW, Coryell W, et al.: Differential outcome of pure manic, mixed/cycling, and pure depressive episodes in patients with bipolar illness. *J Am Med Assoc* 1986; 255(22):3138–3142.

Pope HG Jr, Lipinski JF: Diagnosis in schizophrenia and manic-depressive illness. *Arch Gen Psychiatry* 1978; 35:811–828.

Sachs GS: Bipolar mood disorder: practical strategies for acute and maintenance phase treatment. *J Clin Psychopharmacol* 1996; 16 (Suppl. 1):32S–47S.

Wehr TA, Goodwin FK: Can antidepressants cause mania and worsen the course of affective illness? *Am J Psychiatry* 1987; 144(11):1403–1411.

Table 14-3. Causes of Treatment Resistance in Bipolar Disorder

- Mood-destabilizing effects of antidepressants
- Medication noncompliance
- Comorbid substance abuse
- Misdiagnosis
- Specificity of response of diagnostic subtype
- Comorbid psychosis
- Comorbid medical conditions

Chapter 15

Anxiety Disorders

D AN V. I OSIFESCU AND M ARK H. P OLLACK

I. Introduction

A. Overview

Anxiety is an expected, normal, and transient response to stress; it may be a necessary cue for adaptation and coping. Pathologic anxiety is distinguished from a normal emotional response by four criteria:

1. **Autonomy:** it has no or minimal recognizable environmental trigger.
2. **Intensity:** it exceeds the patient's capacity to bear discomfort.
3. **Duration:** the symptoms are persistent rather than transient.
4. **Behavior:** anxiety impairs coping, and results in disabling behavioral strategies, such as avoidance or withdrawal.

B. Definition of Anxiety

Anxiety results from an unknown internal stimulus, or is inappropriate or excessive when compared to the existing external stimulus. Anxiety differs from fear, which is a sense of dread and foreboding that occurs in response to an external threatening event.

C. Manifestations of Anxiety

1. **Physical symptoms** are related to autonomic arousal (e.g., tachycardia, tachypnea, diaphoresis, diarrhea, and lightheadedness).
2. **Affective symptoms** that range in severity from mild (e.g., edginess) to severe (experienced as terror, the feeling that one is "going to die" or "lose control").
3. **Behavior** is characterized by avoidance (e.g., noncompliance with medical procedures) or compulsions.
4. **Cognitions** include worry, apprehension, obsessions, and thoughts about emotional or bodily damage.

II. Etiology

A. Neurophysiology

The two prototypic anxiety disorders (panic disorder and generalized anxiety disorder [GAD]) correspond to at least two neurotransmitter systems, which are modulated by other systems as well.

1. **Central noradrenergic systems.** The **locus coeruleus (LC),** a small retropontine nucleus, is the major source of the brain's adrenergic innervation. LC stimulation generates panic attacks; LC blockade (e.g., by tricyclic antidepressants, or alprazolam) decreases panic attacks.
2. The γ-**aminobutyric acid (GABA)** neurons from **the limbic system,** especially the septohippocampal areas, mediate generalized anxiety, worry, and vigilance. The highly concentrated GABA receptors in those structures bind benzodiazepines to reduce this heightened state of vigilance. Neuronal connections exist between the LC and limbic structures.
3. **Serotoninergic systems and neuropeptides** are important modulators of the two systems outlined above. The interconnections of these neuronal systems explain the efficacy of clinical interventions with diverse mechanisms of action (serotoninergic and noradrenergic antidepressants, benzodiazepines and cognitive-behavioral therapy [CBT]) on pathologic anxiety.

B. Cognitive-Behavioral Formulations

Cognitive-behavioral formulations of anxiety focus on the information-processing and behavioral reactions that characterize the anxiety experience. The emphasis is placed on the role of thoughts and beliefs (cognitions) in activating anxiety, as well as on the role of avoidance or other escape responses in the maintenance of both fear and dysfunctional thinking patterns. Faulty cognitions are often characterized by overprediction of the likelihood, or degree of catastrophe, of negative events. Attempts to neutralize anxiety with avoidance or compulsive behavior serve to "lock in" anxiety reactions and contribute to the chronic arousal and anticipatory anxiety that mark anxiety disorders.

C. Developmental (Psychodynamic) Formulations

In Freud's later writing, anxiety was described as a signal of threat to the ego; signals are elicited because current events have similarities (symbolic or actual) to threatening developmental experiences (traumatic anxiety). Object relations theorists emphasize the use of internalized objects to maintain affective stability under stress.

III. Epidemiology

A. Prevalence

1. **Anxiety disorders are among the most prevalent psychiatric disorders in the general population.** Approximately one-quarter of the United States population experiences pathologic anxiety over the course of their lifetime (Table 15-1).

2. **First-degree relatives** of patients with anxiety disorders have a **significantly increased risk** for anxiety disorders compared with those in the general population. For first-degree relatives of patients with panic disorder the risk is increased four- to eight-fold. Limited data from twin studies are also consistent with a genetic contribution.

IV. Course of Anxiety Disorders

A. Physical and Psychosocial Function

1. **Anxiety disorders are associated with marked impairments in physical and psychosocial function, as well as quality of life.** Panic disorder is associated with increased rates of alcohol abuse, marital and vocational problems, and suicide attempts (in individuals with comorbid depression and personality disorders). Panic and phobic anxiety are also associated with increased rates of premature cardiovascular mortality in men. Patients with panic disorder lose workdays twice as often as the general population, with 25% of panic patients becoming chronically unemployed, and up to 30% receiving public assistance or disability. Patients with panic disorder are five to seven times more likely to be high utilizers of medical services compared to non-panic individuals.

2. **Most patients with anxiety disorders improve with treatment.** High rates of relapse after discontinua-

tion of pharmacotherapy support the need for maintenance therapy for many individuals.

V. Differential Diagnosis

Anxiety disorders should be differentiated from medical and psychiatric conditions associated with anxiety. It is also important to recognize when anxiety symptoms mimic the symptoms of medical illness.

A. Organic Causes of Anxiety (medical illnesses that mimic anxiety disorders)

1. In a patient with a known medical illness, the condition, its complications, and its treatment should be suspected as potential causes of anxiety. For example, in a patient with chronic obstructive pulmonary disease (COPD), hypoxia, respiratory distress, and sympathomimetic bronchodilators can all cause anxiety symptoms.

2. **Six factors associated with an organic anxiety syndrome** can help differentiate it from a primary anxiety disorder:
   a. Onset of symptoms after the age of 35 years
   b. Lack of personal or family history of an anxiety disorder
   c. Lack of a childhood history of significant anxiety, phobias, or separation anxiety
   d. Absence of significant life events generating or exacerbating the anxiety symptoms
   e. Lack of avoidance behavior
   f. A poor response to antipanic agents

3. A patient with an organic cause of anxiety may not otherwise meet criteria for panic disorder or generalized anxiety disorder; there is often a significant lack of **psychological** symptoms in the context of severe physical symptoms.

4. **Common medical conditions associated with anxiety include:**
   a. **Endocrine:** hyperadrenalism (pheochromocytoma), hypothyroidism, hyperparathyroidism
   b. **Drug related:**
      i. **Intoxication:** caffeine, cocaine, sympathomimetics, theophylline, corticosteroids, thyroid hormones
      ii. **Withdrawal:** alcohol, narcotics, sedative-hypnotics
   c. **Hypoxia:** all causes of **cerebral anoxia,** including **cardiovascular** (arrhythmias, angina, congestive heart failure [CHF], anemia) and **respiratory** (COPD, pulmonary embolism)
   d. **Metabolic:** acidosis, hyperthermia, electrolyte abnormalities (e.g., hypercalcemia)
   e. **Neurological:** vestibular dysfunction, seizures (especially temporal lobe epilepsy)

B. Anxiety that Complicates Medical Illness

1. **Anxiety in the primary care setting.** Anxiety is particularly common in the general medical setting. The National Ambulatory Medical Care Survey

Table 15-1. Prevalence of anxiety disorders in the United States population

Disorder	Prevalence Lifetime (%)	12 months (%)
Any anxiety disorder	24.9	17.2
Panic disorder	3.5	2.3
Agoraphobia	5.3	2.8
Social phobia	13.3	7.9
Simple phobia	11.3	8.8
Generalized anxiety disorder	5.1	3.1

(1980–1981) revealed that anxiety is the presenting problem for 11% of the patients visiting primary care physicians (PCPs), and is the most common psychiatric problem seen by PCPs. More than 90% of the patients with anxiety present primarily with somatic complaints. Moreover, most patients with anxiety first seek help in primary care settings or emergency rooms. The majority of heavy users of primary care services (including patients with chronic illness) have significantly higher rates of mood and anxiety disorders than do less frequent visitors to PCPs. High rates of anxiety disorders are found in patients presenting with the symptoms of chest pain, dizziness, irritable bowel syndrome, and dyspnea.

2. **Workup of the anxious patient.** The medical workup of the anxious patient should rely primarily on the medical and psychiatric history, the medication and drug history, and on appropriate physical and neurological examination. One should consider the anxiogenic effects of existing medications and medical conditions, as well as the effects of substance use and withdrawal (see above). Targeted physical examination, and laboratory and clinical tests are employed based on clinical assessment, patient characteristics, and the focus of the patient's somatic complaints (e.g., cardiac, pulmonary, gastrointestinal, neurologic).

C. **Psychiatric Disorders, Other than Anxiety Disorders**

Anxiety is also present in psychiatric disorders other than anxiety disorders. In **delusional disorders** there are persecutory fears which may mimic anxiety or phobias. Anxiety symptoms occur in the prodromal phase and during the course of **schizophrenia.** The presence of hallucinations, delusions, or disorganized speech associated with a marked decrease of social functioning for a long period of time differentiates schizophrenia from anxiety disorders.

More than half of all anxious patients also experience significant **depression.** Symptoms such as dysphoria, hopelessness, anhedonia, early morning awakening, psychomotor retardation, and suicidal thoughts are more indicative of depression than anxiety. Anxiety-disordered patients usually do not lose their interest in their activities, but find it hard to negotiate them comfortably. Patients with anxiety should be evaluated for depression, given the high percentage of comorbidity. When anxiety and depression coexist, monotherapy with an antidepressant or the combination of an antidepressant and a benzodiazepine is indicated;

treatment with a benzodiazepine alone is best avoided.

If anxiety develops in reaction to a stressful situation, and within 3 months of a stressor, but lasts less than 6 months after cessation of the stressor, a diagnosis of **adjustment disorder with anxiety** is made. Treatment of this condition is typically aimed at reducing the impact of the known stressor. However, symptomatic relief with an anxiolytic or antidepressant treatment can markedly improve the patient's quality of life and prevent complications.

VI. Primary Psychiatric Disorders

A. **Panic Disorder and Agoraphobia**
1. **Definitions. Panic disorder is a syndrome characterized by recurrent unexpected panic attacks about which there is persistent concern. Panic attacks** are discrete episodes of intense anxiety, which develop abruptly and **peak within 10 min; they are associated with at least four other symptoms of autonomic arousal.** Associated symptoms include:
   a. **Cardiac symptoms:** palpitations, tachycardia, chest pain, or discomfort
   b. **Pulmonary symptoms:** shortness of breath, a feeling of choking
   c. **Gastrointestinal symptoms:** nausea or abdominal distress
   d. **Neurological symptoms:** trembling and shaking, dizziness, lightheadedness, or faintness, paresthesias
   e. **Autonomic arousal:** sweating, chills or hot flashes
   f. **Psychological symptoms:** derealization, depersonalization, a fear of losing control or going crazy, or fear of dying

   Whereas the initial panic attack is usually spontaneous, subsequently, apprehension frequently develops about future attacks (anticipatory anxiety). **Agoraphobia,** a complication of panic disorder, involves anxiety about, or avoidance of, places or situations from which ready escape might be difficult, or from which escape might be embarrassing, or where help may be unavailable in the event of a panic attack. Agoraphobia can significantly restrict a patient's daily activities, to the point where he or she becomes dependent on companions to face situations outside the home; some individuals may become homebound.

2. **Epidemiology. Panic disorder has a lifetime prevalence of 1.5–3.5%;** it is more commonly diagnosed in women (2:1 female/male ratio). This difference may reflect a true gender difference or the fact that men tend to self-medicate with alcohol and are less likely to seek treatment. Many affected individuals recall a significant life event in the year before onset of the disease. The age of onset is typically

between late adolescence and the third decade of life, but many affected individuals experience anxiety dating back from childhood, in the form of inhibited, anxious temperament or childhood anxiety disorders. Panic disorder tends to run in families; however, the relative contribution of genetic and environmental factors is an area of active research interest.

3. **Diagnostic features.** Based on DSM-IV, the diagnosis requires:
   a. Recurrent, unexpected panic attacks.
   b. At least one of the attacks is followed by more than a month of:
      i. Persistent concern about additional attacks
      ii. Worry about the implications of the attack and its consequences
      iii. A significant change in behavior related to the attacks
   c. There is no organic factor (general medical condition, substance use) which generates these symptoms.
   d. Panic attacks are not accounted for by any other mental disorder.
   e. The presence or absence of agoraphobia is specified.

   A large number of patients experience **limited symptom attacks,** where only one or two of the panic symptoms are experienced. Limited symptom panic attacks are also associated with significant morbidity.

4. **Disease course and treatment. Panic disorder is often a chronic disease,** with high rates of relapse after discontinuation of treatment. Untreated panic disorder is often complicated by persistent anxiety and avoidant behavior, social dysfunction, marital problems, alcohol and drug abuse, increased utilization of medical services, and increased mortality (from cardiovascular complications and suicide). Avoidant behavior can lead to a progressive constriction of a patient's social interactions, and restricts the individual from the places where panic attacks have occurred or places where easy escape may be difficult or assistance unavailable. Affected patients may experience chronic distress and demoralization which can trigger depression. While alcohol can temporarily alleviate the anxiety symptoms, patients who abuse it may experience rebound anxiety, tolerance, and withdrawal, which may all exacerbate anxiety.

   The established treatments of panic disorder include use of antidepressants, high-potency benzodiazepines, and cognitive-behavioral therapy (see Chap. 44).

B. **Generalized Anxiety Disorder (GAD)**
   1. **Definition. Patients with GAD suffer from excessive anxiety or worry, that is out of proportion to situational factors;** it occurs more days than not for longer than 6 months. These patients are often considered "worriers" or "nervous" by their families and friends. The anxiety is usually associated with muscle tension, restlessness, insomnia, difficulty concentrating, easy fatigability, and irritability. Affected patients typically experience persistent anxiety rather than discrete panic attacks, as in panic disorder.

   2. **Epidemiology. The prevalence of GAD is about 5% in community samples;** it is more typically diagnosed in women (2:1 female/male ratio). The age of onset is frequently in childhood or adolescence, with some patients having an onset in their twenties. GAD is frequently comorbid with other anxiety disorders (panic disorder, social phobia), depression, and with alcohol and drug abuse. The course of the disease is chronic but fluctuating in severity; it is frequently worsened during periods of stress.

   3. **Diagnostic criteria (DSM-IV)**
      a. Excessive anxiety and worry regarding a number of events or activities, that occurs more days than not for at least 6 months.
      b. The individual finds it difficult to control the worry.
      c. Three out of six symptoms (restlessness, easy fatigability, difficulty concentrating, irritability, muscle tension, insomnia) are present.
      d. The worry is not related to features of other disorders.
      e. The anxiety causes significant distress or impairment in function.
      f. The anxiety is not attributed to an organic cause (e.g., substance use, medical condition).

   4. **Treatment.** The treatment of GAD includes pharmacotherapy (antidepressants, benzodiazepines, buspirone) and cognitive-behavioral therapy (see Chap. 44).

C. **Specific Phobia**
   1. **Definition. Patients with specific phobia have marked and persistent fear of circumscribed situations or objects** (e.g., heights, closed spaces, animals or the sight of blood). Exposure to the phobic stimulus results in intense anxiety and avoidance which interferes with the patient's life.

   2. **Epidemiology. The lifetime prevalence of phobias is about 10% in the general population.** The age of onset varies depending on the subtype. Phobias to animals, natural environments (heights, storms, water), blood, and injections each have an onset in childhood. Situational phobias (e.g., triggered by airplanes, elevators, enclosed places) have a bimodal distribution with one peak in childhood and another peak in the mid-twenties.

   3. **Diagnostic criteria (DSM-IV)**
      a. Persistent, excessive unreasonable fear of an object or situation.

b. Exposure to a feared stimulus invariably provokes anxiety, including panic.

c. Recognition that the fear is excessive or unreasonable.

d. The phobic stimulus is avoided or endured with dread.

e. The fear and the avoidant behavior interfere with the person's normal routine or cause marked distress.

f. In a patient under the age of 18 years, symptoms last longer than 6 months.

g. The symptoms are not better accounted by another disorder (e.g., obsessive-compulsive disorder [OCD], panic disorder).

h. Specific subtypes (e.g., animal, natural environment, blood-injection-injury, situational) should be specified.

4. **Treatment.** Benzodiazepines are useful acutely to decrease phobic anxiety and to facilitate exposure (e.g., to take an airplane flight). However, cognitive-behavioral therapy, involving exposure and desensitization to the feared stimulus, offers more comprehensive and persistent benefits.

D. Social Phobia

1. **Definition. Patients with a social phobia fear being exposed to public scrutiny; they fear that they will behave in a way which will be humiliating or embarrassing.** This perception leads to persistent fear and ultimately to avoidance or endurance with intense distress of the social situation. The anxiety can be limited to circumscribed performance situations, i.e., "performance anxiety" (e.g., speaking, eating, using a public bathroom, writing in public), or can affect more general social interactions. Although discomfort related to public speaking is a relatively frequent occurrence in the general population, a significant degree of distress or the presence of impairment is necessary to warrant the diagnosis of social phobia.

2. **Epidemiology. The prevalence of social phobia varies between 3% and 13% in different studies.** In epidemiological and community studies the prevalence is greater in females than in males; however, the prevalence is greater for males in clinical samples. This may be the result of males experiencing more pressure for social performance and thus becoming aware of existing pathology. The onset of social phobia is usually in adolescence, although most affected individuals have a history of anxiety dating back to childhood.

The symptoms of social phobia may overlap with those of panic disorder, avoidant personality, and shyness. Social phobia is frequently comorbid with depression and with alcohol and drug abuse. The course of the disease is chronic but it fluctuates; it is frequently worsened during periods of stress.

3. **Diagnostic criteria (DSM-IV)**

a. Fear of showing anxiety symptoms or acting in a way that will be embarrassing or humiliating when scrutinized by others.

b. The situation almost invariably provokes anxiety.

c. The patient recognizes that the fear is excessive or unreasonable.

d. The phobic stimulus is avoided or endured with intense anxiety.

e. The fear and the avoidant behavior interfere with the person's normal routine or cause marked distress.

f. In a patient under the age of 18 years, symptoms last longer than 6 months.

g. The symptoms are not better accounted by an organic condition or by another mental disorder (e.g., trembling in Parkinson's disease, stuttering).

h. The subtype ("performance anxiety" vs. generalized) should be specified.

4. **Treatment.** The treatment of social phobia includes pharmacotherapy (antidepressants, such as monoamine oxidase inhibitors [MAOIs] and selective serotonine reuptake inhibitors [SSRIs], benzodiazepines, beta-blockers) and cognitive-behavioral therapy (see Chap. 44).

E. Obsessive-Compulsive Disorder

1. **Definitions. Obsessive-compulsive disorder (OCD) is characterized by recurrent, intrusive, unwanted thoughts (i.e., obsessions, such as fears of contamination), or compulsive behaviors or rituals (e.g., repetitive handwashing).** The obsessions are recurrent, persistent thoughts, impulses or images, characterized by four criteria:

a. They are experienced as intrusive and inappropriate and cause marked anxiety and distress.

b. They are not simply worries about real-life problems.

c. Attempts are made to ignore obsessions or neutralize them with some other thought or action.

d. The person recognizes the obsession as a product of his/her own mind, rather than imposed from the outside as in thought insertion.

The compulsive behaviors take place in response to obsessions or rigid rules. Compulsive behaviors are aimed at reducing distress or preventing a dreaded event; they are clearly excessive or unconnected in a realistic way with the event they are trying to neutralize.

2. **Epidemiology. The lifetime prevalence is 2–3% in the general population.** The mean age of onset is in the mid-twenties; less than 5% of patients develop the disease after the age of 35 years. The disease has a chronic course.

3. **Diagnostic criteria (DSM-IV)**

a. The presence of obsessions or compulsions.

b. The patient is or was able at some point to recognize that the obsessions or compulsions are excessive or unreasonable.

c. The obsessions or compulsions cause marked distress, are time-consuming (more than 1 h/day), or significantly interfere with the person's normal routine.

d. The content of the obsessions or compulsions is not restricted to the features of any concomitant Axis I disorder.

e. The obsessions or compulsions can not be attributed to an organic cause (e.g., substance use, medical condition).

The differential diagnosis includes obsessive-compulsive personality disorder, phobic disorders, depression, schizophrenia, and Tourette's disorder.

4. **Treatment.** The treatment of OCD includes pharmacotherapy (SSRIs and the tricyclic antidepressant clomipramine) and cognitive-behavioral therapy aimed at extinguishing intrusive thoughts and compulsive behavior (see Chap. 44).

F. Posttraumatic Stress Disorder (PTSD)

1. **Definition. Patients with PTSD have experienced an event that involved the threat of death, injury, or severe harm to themselves or others; their response involved intense fear, helplessness, or horror.** Patients frequently re-experience the traumatic event in the form of nightmares, flashbacks, or by marked arousal when exposed to situations reminiscent of the event. PTSD patients avoid situations which remind them of the trauma; they may become emotionally numb, irritable, hypervigilant, or have difficulties with sleep and concentration.

2. **Epidemiology.** The syndrome was initially described long before Vietnam veteran populations; for those who had combat injuries the prevalence of PTSD is about 20%. PTSD can also occur in civilians who suffer life-threatening accidents or assaults; **the prevalence of PTSD is 1% in the general population and 3.5–15% in civilians exposed to trauma.** The syndrome may occur at any age. Symptoms usually begin within the first 3 months after trauma, although they can be delayed for months or years. The course is varied; complete recovery occurs within 3 months in half of those affected. Many others experience symptoms for more than a year after the trauma.

The complications of PTSD include social withdrawal, depression, suicidality, as well as alcohol and drug abuse. Psychosocial risk factors for PTSD include previous personality disorder, early trauma, a chaotic childhood, and previous mental illness. Protective factors include good self-esteem, external control, and social support.

3. **Diagnostic criteria (DSM-IV)**

a. The patient must have experienced, witnessed, or confronted an event that involved actual or threatened death, serious injury or threat to the physical integrity of self or others. The person's response involved intense fear, helplessness, or horror.

b. Persistent re-experience of the trauma in the form of intrusive recollections, nightmares, flashbacks, psychological distress and psychological reactivity occurs on cue exposure.

c. Persistent avoidance of stimuli (thoughts and activities) associated with the trauma; numbing of general responsiveness (detachment or estrangement from others, sense of foreshortened future).

d. Symptoms of increased arousal (sleep disturbance, irritability and anger, difficulty concentrating, hypervigilance, startle response).

e. Symptoms last for more than 1 month.

f. Symptoms cause significant distress and impairment. Subtypes: acute (symptoms for less than 3 months), chronic (symptoms for more than 3 months), and delayed onset (onset more than 6 months after trauma).

The differential diagnosis includes **acute stress disorder,** in which symptoms occur within 4 weeks of the traumatic event and persist for less than 4 weeks.

4. **Treatment.** Pharmacological treatment targets reduction of prominent symptoms (e.g., hypnotics for sleep disturbance, antidepressants for depression). A number of studies have demonstrated the efficacy of the SSRIs for the treatment of the general PTSD syndrome. Exposure-based cognitive-behavioral therapy is very effective for PTSD. Also important is psychotherapy aimed at survivor guilt, anger, and helplessness. Affected patients may benefit from family therapy and from vocational rehabilitation in the context of their significant impairment in social and professional functioning.

VII. Conclusions

Anxiety disorders are a group of psychiatric disorders associated with high morbidity and with significant mortality (through suicide, comorbid substance abuse, and from cardiovascular problems). Given the similarities in presentations between certain medical conditions and anxiety disorders, a comprehensive medical, psychiatric, and substance use history is very important in the diagnostic process. Since most of the anxiety disorders tend to be chronic, many patients may benefit from ongoing pharmacotherapy and/or psychosocial interventions to optimize and maintain benefit.

Suggested Readings

American Psychiatric Association: *Diagnostic and Statistical Manual of Mental Disorders, Fourth Edition.* Washington, DC: American Psychiatric Association, 1994.

Fyer AJ, Manuzza S, Coplan J, et al.: Anxiety disorders. In Kaplan

HI, Sadock BJ (eds): *Comprehensive Textbook of Psychiatry*, 6th ed. Baltimore: Williams and Wilkins, 1995.

Pollack M, Smoller J, Lee D: Approach to the anxious patient. In Stern T, Herman J, Slavin P (eds): *The MGH Guide to Psychiatry in Primary Care*. New York: McGraw-Hill, 1998.

Rosenbaum J, Pollak M, Otto M, Bernstein J: Anxious patients. In Cassem NH, Stern TA, Rosenbaum JF, Jellinek MS (eds): *Massachusetts General Hospital Handbook of General Hospital Psychiatry*, 4th ed. St Louis: Mosby, 1997.

Chapter 16
Trauma and Posttraumatic Stress Disorder

RAFAEL D. ORNSTEIN

I. Overview

A. The puzzling, and disturbing effects of psychological trauma on human functioning have been described for generations, going as far back as Homer's *Iliad*. In more recent times, large numbers of American Civil War veterans complained of generalized weakness, heart palpitations, and chest pain, thought to result from the physical stress of war; it was referred to as **"soldier's heart."** In World War I, psychologically disabled veterans were thought to have suffered from brain damage, or **"shell shock." Kardiner** described a syndrome in World War II veterans that foreshadowed the current diagnosis of posttraumatic stress disorder (PTSD); he labeled it a **"traumatic neurosis of war,"** and made the point that the syndrome was physiological in nature. **Posttraumatic stress was virtually ignored until after the Vietnam War when both veterans groups and the feminist movement spoke out about psychological trauma. Later, Horowitz** helped to formulate the diagnosis that found its way into the DSM-III. Earlier in the century, **Freud** and **Janet** became interested in how psychological trauma led to psychopathology.

B. Since its inception in the DSM-III, **the diagnosis of posttraumatic stress disorder (PTSD) has helped researchers study the connection between psychological trauma and psychiatric morbidity.** Initially, PTSD was described as a normal, expectable response to trauma. It was thought that the severity and chronicity of the syndrome might be related directly to the nature of the trauma. Subsequently, the diagnostic criteria for PTSD included several phenomena: an initial, expectable response to trauma, an initial pathological response, and a more prolonged, pathological state. **The development of PTSD following a trauma is the exception rather than the rule. Current research suggests that individual vulnerabilities play a significant factor in the development of the syndrome.** Some researchers have even proposed that trauma per se may not "cause" PTSD, but rather trigger an endogenous psychiatric illness.

C. **Acute and long-term responses to traumatic events are varied and multidetermined. Nearly every person can be expected to have some disruption in their mental functioning following a significantly traumatic event**—a "normal" stress response. On average, most people are able to adapt following a traumatic event and return to their previous level of function, with or without some chronic symptoms. When the symptoms following a trauma impair functioning, they often appear as syndromes, labeled in the DSM-IV as **Acute Stress Disorder and PTSD. Chronic exposure to trauma, and/or trauma occurring in childhood can produce long-lasting personality disturbances.** When the response to trauma reaches the level of PTSD, there are frequently a host of comorbid psychiatric conditions. Exposure to trauma that does not result in a psychiatric diagnosis may still result in chronic symptoms that may have a significant impact on the individual.

II. Posttraumatic Stress Disorder

The DSM-IV criteria for PTSD define 'trauma' and the three central groups of posttraumatic symptoms: **intrusive/re-experiencing, avoidance/numbing,** and **hyperarousal.** If these symptoms are pervasive, prolonged, and debilitating enough, they reach threshold for a diagnosis. **A typical posttraumatic response may involve alternating symptoms of avoidance and re-experiencing** as the person struggles to come to terms with the trauma and its consequences. **Common difficulties faced in integrating the traumatic experience include: fear of repetition of the trauma, shame over helplessness, loss of a sense of invulnerability, feeling of personal failure, rage at source of trauma and ensuing guilt, and guilt over having survived while others perished.**

A. **The DSM-IV defines "trauma" in a specific way:**
   1. **"Trauma" involves a physical threat to life or bodily integrity;** examples include:
      a. **Exposure to military combat, violent assault, including rape and robbery, domestic violence, automobile accidents, childhood physical and sexual abuse or neglect, natural disasters, and sudden catastrophic medical illness.**
      b. **Witnessing a traumatic event.**
      c. **Being told about a trauma** experienced by a loved one.
   2. **A defining characteristic of a traumatic event, according to the DSM-IV, is that the person's response involves "intense fear, helplessness or hor-**

129

ror." Because of the intensity of the feelings associated with a trauma, **perception of the event may be distorted:** it may be experienced as fragments of sensations; time may be slowed or accelerated. **Feelings may be dissociated from events as they are occurring, and there can be varying degrees of amnesia for all or part of the traumatic event.**

B. **Intrusive, re-experiencing symptoms are a hallmark of PTSD. Traumatic memories** are often quite disruptive; they are vivid, sensory experiences, that can intrude unbidden. **Nightmares** are common, often repetitive, lifelike, and disruptive to sleep; a patient begins to dread sleep and will "fight it," to avoid the frightening nightmares. **Flashbacks, hallucinations,** and other experiences of **reliving the trauma** can occur. **Intense emotional distress** and **physiological reactivity,** such as heart palpitations, shortness of breath, chest tightening, and excessive sweating, occur in response to internal or external reminders of the trauma.

C. **Avoidance** of reminders of the trauma and **psychological numbing** can be the most disabling symptoms following a trauma. Following a trauma, a person may **avoid** anything that may remind one of the trauma, including thoughts or feelings, activities, places or people that are associated with the event. There can be **amnesia** for the trauma itself. Numbing symptoms include an overall sense of **detachment, diminished range of emotions,** and **withdrawal** from important activities.

D. **Hyperarousal** can create interpersonal problems. These symptoms include marked **sleep difficulty, irritability,** and **anger outbursts, difficulty with concentration, hypervigilance,** and an **exaggerated startle response.**

III. Acute Stress Disorder

This disorder describes **an acute response to trauma.** It includes the criteria for PTSD but adds and **emphasizes dissociative symptoms.** An acute stress disorder may follow any trauma, but a typical example includes a soldier responding to battle, becoming acutely disoriented, and being in a "daze." Acute Stress Disorder appears to be a good predictor of subsequent PTSD; the presence or absence of the diagnosis predicted PTSD at 6 months in 83% of cases in one study. The diagnostic criteria are listed below.

A. **Diagnostic Criteria for Acute Stress Disorder**
   1. Exposure to a traumatic event in which both of the following were present:
      a. The person experienced, or witnessed, an event that involved actual or threatened death or serious injury, or threat to the physical integrity of self or others.

b. The person's response involved intense fear, helplessness, or horror.
   2. Either during or after the distressing event, the individual had three or more of the following dissociative symptoms:
      a. A subjective sense of numbing
      b. A reduction of awareness of his or her surroundings (e.g., "being in a daze")
      c. Derealization
      d. Depersonalization
      e. Dissociative amnesia (inability to recall an important aspect of the trauma)
   3. The traumatic event is persistently re-experienced with recurrent images, thoughts, dreams, illusions, flashback episodes, or a sense of reliving the experience.
   4. Marked avoidance of stimuli that arouse recollections of the trauma.
   5. Marked symptoms of anxiety or increased arousal (e.g., difficulty sleeping, irritability, poor concentration, hypervigilance, exaggerated startle response, motor restlessness).
   6. The disturbance causes clinically significant distress or impairment in social, occupational, or other important areas of function
   7. The disturbance lasts from 2 days to 4 weeks and occurs within 4 weeks of the traumatic event.
   8. The disturbance is not due to the direct physiological effects of a substance (e.g., a drug of abuse, a medication) or a general medical condition.

IV. Epidemiology

A. **Prevalence of PTSD in the General Population**
   1. **Results range from 1% to 14%.** The Epidemiological Catchment Area Study showed lifetime PTSD rates of around 1.3% at two sites. More subjects (around 15%) reported subclinical symptoms following a trauma.
   2. A survey of 1,007 young adults in a Detroit HMO showed that 39% had been exposed to a traumatic event; 23.6% of them developed PTSD, leading to a lifetime prevalence of 9.2% (6.0% for males and 11.3% for females).

B. **Prevalence of PTSD Following Specific Traumas**
   1. The rates of PTSD following natural disasters vary. Following the Mt. St. Helens volcanic eruption, a population sample of those exposed showed a lifetime prevalence of PTSD of 3.6%, compared to a rate of 2.6% in controls. Following a dam break and subsequent flood at Buffalo Creek, researchers found a 59% lifetime prevalence of PTSD; 25% still met criteria at 14-year follow-up.
   2. For **war veterans,** rates can vary according to traumatic exposure. Overall, lifetime PTSD rates for

Vietnam veterans are 15%. Those exposed to median levels of combat showed rates of 28% compared to 65% among those exposed to the highest levels of combat. For political prisoners and prisoners of war, rates can range from 30% to more than 70%. For torture victims, rates can be as high as 90%.

3. Among individuals who suffer a **violent assault,** there is a 20% rate of PTSD. Victims of rape have been found to have rates of PTSD near 50% in some studies. Witnessing a person being killed or seriously injured confers a risk of 7%.
4. Following a **traffic accident,** 10–30% still have PTSD 6–18 months following the accident.
5. In a group of individuals who experienced a sudden, unexpected death of a close friend or relative, 14% developed PTSD.
6. The likelihood of developing PTSD is two-fold higher in females than in males. This is due to females' greater vulnerability to assaultive violence.

V. Longitudinal Course of PTSD

A. **PTSD can be a chronic illness.** Of the Vietnam veterans who developed PTSD following the war, 50% of males and 32% of the females suffered from the syndrome in 1988. Among World War II prisoners of war, 50% still manifest PTSD 40 years after their trauma.

B. PTSD is **acute** if symptoms last less than 3 months, **chronic** if symptoms last for more than 3 months, and **delayed** if there is an onset of symptoms at least 6 months after a stressor. PTSD symptoms can be **intermittent** and residual. It is not uncommon for PTSD to be reactivated, years after it has apparently resolved.

C. If the stressor involves interpersonal violence, victims are at greater risk for chronic PTSD.

VI. Risk Factors for Developing PTSD

A. **The nature of the traumatic stressor remains the most important risk factor for developing PTSD.** However, not every person will develop PTSD after exposure to a severe traumatic event. Even "mild trauma" can trigger PTSD in some individuals. The stressors most likely to cause PTSD are (Tomb, 1994):
1. Stressors that are severe, unexpected, prolonged, intentional, and repetitive
2. Stressors that involve threat to physical integrity of self or a loved one
3. Stressors that are isolating, demeaning, or in conflict with one's self-concept

B. **Personal vulnerability is an important risk factor,** especially in less severe trauma. Risk factors include:
1. A psychiatric history, including major depression, anxiety disorders, conduct disorder, neurotic personality, antisocial and narcissistic personality disorders
2. A history of previous trauma, including childhood sexual abuse
3. Low intelligence
4. Limited social supports
5. Childhood separation from parents, or divorce of parents in early childhood
6. Family history of major depression or anxiety disorders, which suggests a genetic component to PTSD

C. **Dissociative symptoms** experienced during or shortly after a traumatic event.

D. The presence of severe symptoms early on appears to predict more severe symptoms later on.

VII. Associated Syndromes and Comorbidity

A. Children exposed to physical or sexual abuse, or adults exposed to prolonged and repeated trauma may develop long-standing problems in psychological and interpersonal function. The younger the person the more vulnerable they may be to long-term difficulties. Although not yet recognized as a distinct diagnosis in the DSM, this syndrome is known in the literature as **Complex PTSD** or **Disorders of Extreme Stress Not Otherwise Specified.** The syndrome describes a range of debilitating symptoms:
1. Difficulty with **affect regulation,** including problems managing anger, self-destructive behavior, impulsive and risk-taking behavior
2. **Dissociative symptoms** and amnesia
3. **Somatization**
4. A range of **characterological difficulties,** including: a damaged sense of self, chronic guilt and shame, a feeling of ineffectiveness, idealization of the perpetrator, difficulty in establishing and maintaining trusting relationships, a tendency to be re-victimized or to victimize others, and a chronic sense of despair and hopelessness

B. Although studies continue to show that PTSD is a distinct syndrome, comorbidity is frequently the rule rather than the exception; typical comorbid conditions include major depression, other anxiety disorders, and substance abuse.

C. Exposure to trauma that does not result in PTSD *can* create long-standing symptoms, including depressed and anxious mood, and damage to the victim's sense of self. However, in the absence of PTSD, exposure to trauma itself does not appear to be a risk factor for specific psychiatric diagnoses.

D. If a person develops PTSD following a trauma, he or she is at far greater risk of developing other psychiatric disorders such as major depression, other anxiety disorders or substance abuse, compared with a person who was exposed to a trauma, but did not develop PTSD.

E. Major depressive disorder is a risk factor for PTSD, and PTSD is a risk factor for major depressive disorder. Often they can develop at the same time.

F. The Epidemiological Area Catchment Study showed 60–80% lifetime comorbidity with PTSD cases compared to 15% in controls.

G. In a study on Vietnam veterans, 50% of veterans with current PTSD met criteria for another DSM-III diagnosis 6 months prior to an assessment compared with 11.5% of veterans without PTSD. Another study showed that lifetime comorbidity in Vietnam veterans with PTSD is near 99%, including substance abuse, depression, anxiety disorders, and antisocial personality disorder.

VIII. Neurobiology of PTSD

The neurobiology of PTSD is a rapidly advancing field of study. Although there is no single model that completely explains the pathophysiology of the disorder, data support the fact that PTSD is a discrete illness with biological correlates.

A. Review of the Neurobiology of the Normal Stress Response
  1. **Norepinephrine** plays a role in orienting to new stimuli, in selective attention, and autonomic arousal. The **locus coeruleus,** located in the pons, contains a large number of the brain's noradrenergic cell bodies that project throughout the brain.
  2. **Cortisol** stimulates metabolic processes that prepare the body for fight or flight. Cortisol also modulates the stress response by counteracting catecholamines and restoring homeostasis; cortisol provides negative feedback for the stress response.
  3. **Endogenous opiates** increase the pain threshold.
  4. Neurotransmitters are linked together in a **web of feedback loops.** For example, during stress, corticotropin releasing factor (CRF) increases the turnover of norepinephrine (NE), and NE increases concentrations of CRF in the locus coeruleus.
  5. **Serotonin** appears to play a role in regulating the stress response.

6. In this theoretical scenario proposed by Rauch et al. (1998), the limbic system and the cerebral cortex process a stressful event. The **thalamus** relays information about threat to the **prefrontal cortex** and **amygdala.** The **amygdala** is a limbic structure that is involved in threat assessment, emotional learning, and fear conditioning; it attaches emotional significance to incoming stimuli and facilitates the flight or fight response. The **amygdala** relays information to the **hippocampus, paralimbic system, sensory processing** systems, and other structures. The **hippocampus,** a limbic structure, is involved in learning and memory, especially verbal information, events, places, and facts; it processes contextual information and provides feedback to the **amygdala** regarding past experience and current context. The **anterior cingulate cortex,** a part of the **paralimbic system,** may set priorities between emotional and cognitive processes and may play a role in regulating the **amygdala.**

B. The Neurobiology of PTSD
  1. It is hypothesized that **abnormalities in the sympathetic branch of the autonomic nervous system** play a role in the symptoms of intrusion and arousal.
    a. Animal models have shown that severe stress can cause dysregulation of the locus coeruleus, causing hypersensitivity to external stimuli.
    b. Combat veterans suffering from PTSD have exaggerated heart rate responses during exposure to combat-related stimuli, as compared with combat veterans without PTSD and veterans with other anxiety disorders.
    c. Some studies have suggested that urinary excretion of norepinephrine is higher in patients with PTSD as compared with controls.
  2. Abnormalities of the **hypothalamic-pituitary-adrenal** (HPA) **axis,** especially in regards to cortisol, are a principle finding in PTSD.
    a. **In PTSD, cortisol levels are chronically decreased,** there is increased glucocorticoid receptor sensitivity, stronger negative feedback, and sensitization of the HPA system. In sharp contrast, in **acute and chronic stress and major depression, cortisol levels are increased,** there is decreased glucocorticoid receptor responsiveness, a decrease in negative feedback, and desensitization of the HPA system (Yehuda, 1998).
    b. Patients with PTSD can show lower cortisol levels up to 50 years following the initial trauma.
    c. Lower cortisol levels immediately following a trauma can be a risk factor for developing PTSD at a later date. Studies have found that, following a rape, low cortisol was associated with prior rape or assault, which in turn was the strongest predictor of subsequent PTSD.
    d. In animal studies, high levels of cortisol are damaging to the hippocampus.

3. The **hippocampus tends to be smaller** in subjects with PTSD. MRI measurement of hippocampal volume in patients with PTSD has been done in a few, very small studies. Findings tentatively suggest that patients with PTSD have slightly smaller hippocampal volumes, correlated with severity of traumatic exposure, cognitive deficits, and PTSD symptoms. The significance of these findings is unclear; lower volumes may represent a premorbid risk factor, a result of exogenous toxins, or the result of elevated cortisol.

4. Functional neuroimaging studies suggest a **typical pattern of brain activation** in the face of traumatic stimuli in patients with PTSD. A very small number of subjects have been studied with functional neuroimaging, while stimulated with traumatic material. The findings very tentatively suggest that PTSD is associated with **exaggerated activation of the amygdala and deactivation of Broca's area.**

5. It has been hypothesized (Rauch et al., 1998), that PTSD may involve a primary hypersensitivity of the amygdala or an inadequate inhibition of the amygdala by the hippocampus or the anterior cingulate. Van der Kolk et al. (1994) have hypothesized that traumatic memories are laid down in the hippocampus under stress, and in this way traumatic memories remain as sensory fragments without an organized narrative.

6. Other biological models for PTSD include stress sensitization, fear conditioning, and learned helplessness.

IX. Evaluation and Treatment Immediately Following a Traumatic Event

Immediately following a traumatic event, survivors rarely come to the attention of psychiatrists. Victims of trauma focus on practical concerns such as re-establishing safety, obtaining information, responding to medical or legal concerns, securing food and shelter, and connection with family and other social supports. Most people adapt to traumatic events without professional help and often decline an offer of such help. There is a great deal of interest in determining whether or not acute psychological intervention can have an impact on the subsequent development of posttraumatic symptoms. A variety of debriefing strategies have been developed and research findings are mixed. Some studies suggest that well-trained clinicians, working in teams, can implement a highly structured debriefing process in a group setting that can diminish the development of PTSD symptoms. Other studies suggest that such interventions can actually worsen outcome, perhaps because of the expression of overwhelming feelings. Current research is evaluating whether such debriefings should be offered to all survivors or only those at high risk. Evaluation and treatment should include and be guided by the following principles.

A. **Help the individual regain a sense of mastery and control.** Communicate a sense of hope and expectation of recovery.

B. **Encourage the use of existing supports** and refer for psychological treatment only those at high risk; the option of follow-up should be made to all.

C. **Pay attention to the practical and immediate concerns** brought about by the traumatic event. Tell the patient any information available about the event.

D. **Assess the patient's mental status** to determine if he or she can manage safely with current available support. Dissociation can be pronounced, and can be an important risk factor for the subsequent development of PTSD.

E. **Gently encourage the patient to review the trauma** and the surrounding events. If possible, identify the aspect of the trauma that was most distressing to the patient. However, the patient's capacity to tolerate the retelling must be considered. It is not necessarily helpful and can be harmful for the patient to become overwhelmed in recounting the trauma. The need for the patient to face the "reality of the trauma" must be balanced with "denial," which may help the patient process the experience in a tolerable fashion. **Appreciate and respect the patient's coping style.**

F. **Assess the patient for risk factors for PTSD.** Those at highest risk may need ongoing treatment.

G. **Victims of rape,** for example, **need specialized follow-up.** They will need a medical workup that evaluates their physical well-being, appropriately documents findings for any legal proceedings, and provides a sense of safety. Referral for specialized psychological services, such as a rape crisis center, can provide support, treatment, and assistance with legal issues.

H. **Assess whether or not the patient is at risk for ongoing trauma,** or is a victim of child or spousal abuse, for example. Children need immediate protection with the help of social service agencies. Victims of domestic violence come from all socioeconomic groups; they will need encouragement to seek help and often are reluctant to acknowledge the extent of their danger. Patients who face persistent threat should be encouraged to write out a safety plan that details concrete steps they will take to avoid future trauma. These steps may include involving local law enforcement authorities. Although the clinician can encourage the patient to take steps to protect him- or herself, it is ultimately the patient who must make that decision.

I. Tolerate the patient's feelings and help put them into context. It can be greatly reassuring for a patient to know that feelings of fear, helplessness, guilt, shame, and anger are expectable responses to a traumatic event. The patient may need to be reassured that he or she is not "going crazy."

J. Educate the patients about the common responses to trauma, which can help them feel more in control of their experiences. Patients should be told that they may experience insomnia, nightmares, intrusive memories, and irritability in the first few months or so after the trauma but that these symptoms should then begin to subside.

K. Educate patients about possible maladaptive responses to trauma. Alcohol abuse is common as patients attempt to manage hyperarousal and intrusive symptoms.

L. Use medication sparingly. There is no long-term benefit from heavily sedating a patient following a trauma. Severe anxiety, agitation, and insomnia may be treated with low-dose benzodiazepines. Supplies should be given for not more than several days and are contraindicated in patients with alcohol or substance abuse.

X. Evaluation of Patients with PTSD

Patients are evaluated for PTSD in a variety of settings; the evaluation may be part of a general psychiatric evaluation in which the PTSD is not yet diagnosed, or part of a course of treatment specific for PTSD. The evaluation needs to be tailored to the needs of the current circumstances. An evaluation should include and be guided by the following principles:

A. The time course of the patient's symptoms has important clinical implications. Symptoms may cause clinically significant impairment in the first month, as acute stress disorder, or in the following 2 months as PTSD. One group of patients will improve and return to an acceptable level of functioning, whereas another group will go on to have chronic PTSD. After 3 months, PTSD is a chronic psychiatric illness.

B. In a general psychiatric evaluation, screen for exposure to traumatic events throughout the lifecycle. **It may be more effective to ask about specific traumas than to ask about trauma in general, but introduce questions in a normalizing and nonjudgmental manner.** For example, a clinician might say, "It is not uncommon for people to have been

touched in ways they didn't want while they were growing up. Did you ever have the experience of being touched in a sexual or harsh way while you were a child?"

C. Be aware of how the interview is affecting the patient. Especially in regards to trauma, straightforward questions may evoke a sudden eruption of powerful and overwhelming feelings. Work with the patient to establish a tolerable level of distress appropriate for the circumstances of the interview. For example, a clinician might say, "I realize that some of these questions may bring up strong feelings, let me know if this is something that might be difficult to talk about." If the patient cannot tolerate talking about the trauma itself, it may be useful for the clinician to shift the focus to the effects of the traumatic event on various aspects of the individual's life.

D. Offer the patient an opportunity to recount the traumatic event. Note the patient's capacity to tell the story. Some patients will find it helpful to talk about the event, some will be so overwhelmed they think or speak of nothing else, others will not be able to speak of the trauma at all.

E. Review the symptoms of PTSD and assess the intensity and the frequency of the patient's symptoms. Patients will frequently report intrusive and hyperarousal symptoms but rarely the avoidance and numbing symptoms that can be so disabling. Ask the patient how they cope with symptoms. Are there ways he or she has learned to come out of a flashback or to manage the irritability of hyperarousal?

F. Evaluate the patient's overall psychological, social, and occupational function. Has the patient been able to resume his or her usual activities? Is there difficulty resuming activities which the patient associates to the trauma? How is the patient relating to family and friends? Is there an increase in social isolation or feelings of alienation? Assess the patient's premorbid functioning; has the trauma changed the patient's self-esteem, their capacity to tolerate loss, their ability to manage dependency, autonomy, and intimacy? Is the patient able to trust and to take risks?

G. Assess how the trauma has affected the individual's "sense of themselves" or self-schema, and how the trauma may impact on any ongoing issues related to the individual's developmental stage. For instance, if a young man is assaulted, this may conflict with his idea of his own masculinity, which may be defined by his physical prowess. In another example, the effects of childhood sexual abuse may become evident as a young woman develops difficulties in a relationship with a man, or is flooded with memories as she cares for a young child.

H. **Formulate a differential diagnosis,** as several psychiatric illnesses share characteristics of PTSD.
   1. **Psychotic disorders** and PTSD can present with hallucinations. Hallucinations in patients with PTSD typically involve a fragment of the traumatic event, or a voice of a perpetrator. At times patients hear their name called out. Patients with PTSD typically do not have delusions or a formal thought disorder.
   2. **Bipolar disorder** and PTSD can both present with irritable and labile mood, anger outbursts, marked sleep disturbance and impulsive, risk-taking behavior. Patients with PTSD do not experience prolonged euphoria or expansive moods.
   3. **Major depressive disorder** and PTSD share a number of symptoms including emotional withdrawal, detachment, social isolation, helplessness, agitation, and sleep disturbance. It is common for PTSD patients to develop secondary depression. Weight loss or gain and generalized feelings of guilt are more typical of a primary depression.
   4. **Other anxiety disorders** and PTSD share a number of characteristics; patients with panic and agoraphobia are also avoidant, panic attacks resemble the autonomic arousal patients with PTSD experience when they have an intrusive memory, and the obsessive thought of a person with obsessive-compulsive disorder (OCD) can resemble the fixation with the trauma seen in PTSD.

I. **Screen the patient for the frequently occurring comorbid conditions** that complicate treatment and recovery.
   1. Alcohol and other substance abuse
   2. Major depressive disorder
   3. Somatoform disorders
   4. Dissociative disorders
   5. Other anxiety disorders

J. **Evaluate the patient's strengths, and note the efforts made to successfully adapt to the trauma.** Patients may present for treatment due to a precipitating factor that disrupts previously successful adaptation to a traumatic event.

K. **Assess the patient's safety.** Is there a risk for ongoing trauma?

XI. Guidelines for the Treatment of PTSD

Patients with PTSD vary in the severity of their illness and the time course of their recovery. Some patients utilize treatment to overcome overwhelming trauma, others appear to make little progress at all. For some patients, the passage of time and life events offer a chance for recovery; for other patients the trauma has made it impossible to move forward in life. The symptoms of PTSD can create a cycle that traps the patient within a world of the trauma. Traumatic memories, vivid, sensory and timeless, threaten to overwhelm the survivor. Efforts are made to cope with such powerful and disorganized memories; the threat from within is that any intense feeling may trigger a traumatic memory, the threat from without is that so many stimuli have become associated with the trauma. The person may withdraw into dissociative states or use alcohol to control intrusive memories and hyperarousal. The person with PTSD feels helpless in coping with the past and helpless in managing the present. The loss of control in the present stimulates traumatic memories and perpetuates the cycle. Psychiatric treatment for PTSD aims to address this cycle and is guided by the following general principles:

A. **Treatment generally involves an integration of several therapeutic approaches**, including **psychodynamic** and **cognitive-behavioral. Medication** often plays an important adjunctive role.

B. **Treatment is phase-oriented.** The initial goal is to **stabilize the patient** and address acute symptoms. The second phase involves **working through the trauma,** and the last phase focuses on **re-establishing social relationships.**

C. **Stabilization can be a prolonged phase**, and in some cases comprises the entire treatment. **Education** about posttraumatic experiences is the cornerstone of therapy. If patients can anticipate expectable posttraumatic responses they can feel less helpless. **Identifying feelings** and putting words to bodily experiences begins to organize a chaotic emotional world. As patients learn to notice how symptoms come and go, they discover that they can exercise more control over their emotional life. **Safety** is facilitated by the connection to the therapist in a treatment that has clear and predictable boundaries. Stabilization involves **addressing any maladaptive behaviors,** such as substance abuse and self-destructive behavior. Ongoing exposure to trauma will undermine improvement, and patients may need to be taught to distinguish safe from unsafe behavior.

D. **Treat comorbid disorders.**

E. Patients can **work through the trauma** in several different ways. Patients can learn to tolerate the traumatic memories and environmental triggers and become desensitized, thereby **diminishing avoidance.** As well, patients can begin to create a narrative of the traumatic event and understand its personal meaning. The reality of the trauma and its impact becomes integrated into the survivor's sense of self.

F. Ultimately, the patient must return to daily life in the community. Facilitating the development of **social relationships** is an important part of recovery from trauma.

G. Treating a patient with PTSD can put the therapist under significant emotional strain. Hearing about the traumatic event and witnessing a patient's distress can be traumatic for the therapist. It can be difficult for the therapist to maintain the necessary balance between seeing the patient as a helpless victim *and* as a survivor capable of taking responsibility.

H. The therapist must balance the need for the patient to review the traumatic event with the danger that the patient will be traumatized by the retelling.

I. Patients with a history of childhood sexual abuse or patients with **complex PTSD** are often challenging to treat. These patients often have significant **difficulties with affect regulation and trust.** It may take years for a patient to develop a relationship with the therapist sufficiently robust to manage the exploration of the trauma. For such a patient, learning **impulse control, affect regulation, boundary management, and basic positive self-regard** are prerequisites for exploration of the trauma itself.

XII. Psychosocial Treatment Modalities for PTSD

A. Psychodynamic approaches are characterized by the following:
1. This approach **emphasizes exploration of the personal meaning of the traumatic event** for the individual patient.
2. **The impact of the trauma on the patient's self-concept is explored;** often feelings of shame, grief, and helplessness emerge. As the treatment progresses, feelings of guilt and anger and fantasies of omnipotent control are frequently encountered.
3. **Unresolved conflicts from earlier in life may be exacerbated** by the trauma and dealt with in the treatment.
4. **The patient's coping styles and defenses are noted.** Patients who are experiencing flooding of affects are helped to organize themselves, and those who are overcontrolled and detached are helped to gain access to feelings. Patients may need to explore their fears of losing control as they begin treatment.
5. **The patient's relationship with the therapist is seen as an integral part of the treatment.** The connection helps contain affects and process transference reactions.

B. Cognitive-behavioral approaches are characterized by the following:
1. The goal of treatment is the **disruption of the link between trauma-related cues and the intense anxiety responses and avoidance that is typical for PTSD.** Patients are taught to distinguish trauma memories and trauma-related emotions from current reality and thereby feel more in control of the world.
2. The technique often stimulates the patient to **experience a traumatic memory in order to modify the response to that memory.**
3. **Patient education** about the nature of the symptoms of PTSD establishes a focus of the treatment.
4. **Patients identify underlying, distorted, "all-or-nothing" beliefs** about the world following the trauma. For example, "I am a helpless person … the world is not a safe place … I am guilty for everything." These distorted thoughts can be addressed and altered.
5. **Patients are taught ways to soothe themselves** with relaxation techniques and guided imagery in order to manage PTSD symptoms
6. **Patients are exposed to traumatic material** and learn to respond in new ways, learning to distinguish real from imagined threat and learning to diminish physiological reactivity.
7. Cognitive-behavioral techniques have been the most studied treatment for PTSD, and they have been found to be helpful for the disorder.

C. Group treatment can be an important component of an overall treatment plan, providing support and information. For some patients, group settings allow for a diffusion of the strong transference reactions that can impede treatment progress.

D. Eye Movement Desensitization and Reprocessing (EMDR)
1. Shapiro (1995) found that negative responses to disturbing memories and thoughts were attenuated with rapid eye movements. She developed a treatment used for PTSD based on the following technique:
   a. An affect-laden image of the trauma is constructed along with a summary statement.
   b. Subjective distress is rated.
   c. An alternate, positive statement is formulated.
   d. Eye movements are initiated by the patient following an object moving across the visual field, while the patient holds in mind the traumatic image.
   e. After 12–24 repetitions, the patient notes his or her subjective distress.
   f. The cycle is repeated 3–15 times until there is significant reduction in distress.

2. The treatment is advocated as an adjunct to other modalities. Proponents suggest that several sessions can significantly reduce PTSD symptoms.

3. The psychiatric community and the scientific literature are bitterly divided over this technique. To date there is no clearly documented method of action. Critics contend that, at best, EMDR is a nonintrusive exposure technique and that its benefits are nonspecific. Advocates contend that, although its method of action is unclear, the benefits are impressive. Although the technique is quite controversial and still considered experimental, its use is growing in clinical practice.

XIII. Pharmacotherapy of PTSD

A. Medication is an important adjunctive treatment for PTSD. Medication should be tailored to the stage of the illness and targeted for specific symptoms. Some level of anxiety may be necessary for the patient to make use of psychological treatment.

B. There are very few controlled studies of medication for PTSD; most recommendations are generally from open trials and documented clinical anecdotes.

C. First-line treatment includes **selective serotonin reuptake inhibitors** (SSRIs) and **anti-adrenergic** agents.

1. **Fluoxetine** has been studied in double-blind, placebo-controlled study, and has been found to be effective for intrusive hyperarousal and numbing symptoms in civilian populations. Other **SSRIs** are also thought to be effective.

2. **Clonidine and propranolol** have been found to be effective for intrusive symptoms, especially flashbacks and nightmares, and for hyperarousal symptoms in open studies.

3. **Nefazodone** has recently been studied and found to be promising in populations of war veterans.

4. **Tricyclic antidepressants** have shown mixed results in controlled studies, but may be more effective in military veterans.

5. **Monoamine oxidase inhibitors** have been shown to be effective in intrusive symptoms, but these medications are rarely used because of dietary restrictions and drug interactions.

D. **Benzodiazepines** can be cautiously and sparingly used for hyperarousal symptoms; dependence and abuse are significant risks. They may also exacerbate dissociative symptoms.

E. **Trazodone** can be useful for insomnia. **Mirtazapine** and **doxepin** can also help with sleep.

F. **Mood stabilizers,** such as valproate, carbamazapine, and lithium, have been studied in small, open studies. They can be used empirically for mood lability and anger outbursts.

G. **Antipsychotic medication** should be reserved for the most disorganized and psychotic patients. However, the use of newer, atypical antipsychotics is being explored as a treatment for PTSD.

Suggested Readings

American Psychiatric Association: *Diagnosis and Statistical Manual of Mental Disorders, Fourth Edition*. Washington, DC: American Psychiatric Association, 1994:424–432.

Breslau N: Epidemiology of trauma and posttraumatic stress disorder. In Yehuda, R (ed.): *Psychological Trauma*. Washington, DC: American Psychiatric Press, 1998.

Foa E, Meadows E: Psychosocial treatments for posttraumatic stress disorder. In Yehuda R (ed.): *Psychological Trauma*. Washington, DC: American Psychiatric Press, 1998.

Freidman M: Current and future drug treatment for posttraumatic stress disorder patients. *Psychiatr Ann* 1998; 28(8):461–467.

Herman JL: Sequelae of prolonged and repeated trauma: evidence for a complex posttraumatic syndrome (DESNOS). In Davidson JRT, Foa EB (eds): *Posttraumatic Stress Disorder: DSM-IV and Beyond*. Washington, DC: American Psychiatric Press, 1993:213–228.

Horowitz MJ: *Stress Response Syndromes*. Northvale, NJ: Jason Aronson; 1986.

Marmar CR, Foy D, Kagan B, et al.: An integrated approach for treating post-traumatic stress. In Oldham JM, Riba MB, Tasman A (eds): *Review of Psychiatry*, Vol. 12. Washington, DC: American Psychiatric Press, 1993:239–273.

Meichenbaum D: *A Clinical Handbook/Practical Therapist Manual for Assessing and Treating Post-Traumatic Stress Disorder*. Waterloo, Ontario: Institute Press, 1994.

Ornstein R: Approach to the patient following a traumatic event. In Stern TA, Herman JB, Slavin PL (eds): *The MGH Guide to Psychiatry in Primary Care*. New York: McGraw-Hill, 1998.

Rauch S, Shin L, Pitman S: Evaluating the effects of psychological trauma using neuroimaging techniques. In Yehuda R (ed.): *Psychological Trauma*. Washington, DC: American Psychiatric Press, 1998.

Shapiro F: *Eye Movement Desensitization and Reprocessing*. New York: Guilford Press, 1995.

Tomb DA, Allen SN: Phenomenology of posttraumatic stress disorder. *Psychiatr Clin North Am* 1994; 17(2):237–250.

Van der Kolk B, McFarlane AC, Weisaeth L, eds: *Traumatic Stress*. New York: Guilford Press, 1996.

Yehuda R: Neuroendocrinology of trauma and posttraumatic stress disorder. In Yehuda R (ed.): *Psychological Trauma*. Washington, DC: American Psychiatric Press, 1998.

Chapter 17

Somatoform Disorders

Cristina Brusco and Edye Geringer

I. Introduction

A. Overview

Somatization can occur either as a symptom, or as a psychiatric syndrome. All somatoform disorders share the feature of the overimportance of physical symptoms and illness in a patient's life, which may lead to the patient feeling misunderstood by health care professionals. This can lead to breakdown in the physician-patient relationship, and to increased attempts to legitimize their quest for care.

1. **Definitions of somatization**
   a. Somatization is characterized by the tendency, in the absence of an organic etiology, to experience and communicate somatic distress in response to psychosocial stress, to attribute this distress to physical illness, and to seek medical help for these symptoms. This can range from normal complaints (e.g., headaches) to the belief that one has an illness (e.g., melanoma).
   b. Somatization also involves a disturbance in the way a person perceives, organizes, attributes and/or expresses physical experiences.
2. **Impact of somatization.** Somatization accounts for a disproportionate number of users of medical care, laboratory tests, procedures, visits, hospital stays, and total health care costs (up to $30 billion per year). However, most individuals report numerous physical symptoms and do not seek medical attention.
3. **Etiologies of somatization.** Various physical, psychological, cultural, interpersonal, and biological theories have been proposed to explain somatization.
   a. The **"wandering womb"** refers to the ancient Egyptian belief that hysteria was caused by the uterus which migrated upwards and displaced other organs to cause discomfort.
   b. Somatization can be used as an **intrapsychic defense,** whereby a patient can ward off unbearable impulses or affects, such as unacceptable bodily sensations, murderous rage, or forbidden sexuality. The pain and suffering are seen as "deserved" and used as atonement for hostile impulses.
   c. Somatization can be a means of **social communication** for some patients, allowing them to tell their doctor and the world that "I am a person deserving of care." A patient may attain the sick role and/or **secondary gain** by virtue of physical complaints.
   d. **"Abnormal illness behavior"** occurs when the provider and the patient have disparate assumptions about the nature of illness. This mismatch can lead to a failure to respond to treatment and to the excessive utilization of health care.
   e. **Learning theory** implicates a patient's ability to recall symptoms from either the patient's own or a role model's past experiences as a means of expressing current distress.
   f. **Cultural stigma of psychiatric illness** can account for why patients express their symptoms physically. For example, it is easier for a Chinese patient to accept "neurasthenia" as a diagnosis than depression.
   g. The presence of lateralized defects on **functional brain imaging studies,** alexithymia, and impaired selective attention on neuropsychological testing may help explain why some psychiatric states can only be expressed with physical symptoms.

B. DSM-IV Somatoform Disorders (see Table 17-1)

1. Somatization Disorder
2. Undifferentiated Somatoform Disorder
3. Conversion Disorder
4. Pain Disorder
5. Hypochondriasis
6. Body Dysmorphic Disorder
7. Somatoform Disorder Not Otherwise Specified

II. Somatization Disorder (Hysteria, Multisymptomatic Hysteria, or Briquet's Disease)

A. Definition

Somatization disorder is a chronic disorder characterized by multiple, clinically significant somatic complaints that results in impairment of function and/or frequent use of medical services.

B. History

Thought of for thousands of years as a disorder of women, **Sydenham, in 1679,** linked the disorder in men and women to psychological stressors, referring to them as "antecedent sorrows." **Briquet, in 1859,** focused on a long course involving multisymptomatic complaints, and labeled the condition "multisymptomatic hysteria." In the 1950s, objective criteria were introduced; **in the 1970s the term "Briquet's disease" was coined.** Modern classification has moved away from etiologic references.

C. DSM-IV Criteria

1. **A history of multiple and recurring physical complaints which begin before the age of 30 years and occur over several years is required. The physical complaints result in medical treatment or cause significant impairment in social, occupational, or other important areas of function.**

2. **To make the diagnosis all four of the following criteria have to be met at some time during the illness:**
   a. **Four pain symptoms,** each in a different area of the body or of a different function, such as headache, back pain, arthralgias, rectal and abdominal pain, dysmenorrhea, dysuria, and dyspareunia.
   b. **Two non-pain-related gastrointestinal symptoms,** such as bloating, nausea, vomiting, diarrhea, and food sensitivity.
   c. **One sexual symptom,** other than pain, such as decreased desire, erectile dysfunction, menorrhagia, or hyperemesis gravidum.
   d. **One pseudoneurological symptom,** including amnesia, fainting, blindness, double vision, aphasia, seizure, ataxia, and paralysis.

3. **The symptoms, after appropriate investigation, are not caused by a known medical condition or substance.** If a medical condition does exist, the complaints or impairments are deemed grossly in excess of expected.

4. **The symptoms are neither intentionally produced nor feigned.**

D. Clinical Features

1. **The patient's history**
   a. The major goal of the patient is apparently to communicate distress through a recitation of symptoms.
   b. The **history is often colorful and dramatic;** there is often little specific information, and it is often inconsistent from visit to visit. It may be presented as an unending laundry list of complaints with great detail.
   c. A patient with this condition may not be able to distinguish between emotional and somatic feelings.
   d. **An afflicted patient is at risk for iatrogenic complications.**
   e. These patients may seek multiple treaters, including alternative health providers, and **doctor-shop** in search of a cure.
   f. **The relationship with treaters is often strained** and ends in mutual frustration and dissatisfaction.

2. **Clinical course**
   a. The onset of symptoms can start in adolescence; the diagnostic criteria are usually met by age 25 years.
   b. The symptoms are chronic and fluctuate; rarely do the symptoms remit completely.
   c. Episodes often last from 6 to 9 months, and may be followed by a 9–12-month period of quiescence.

E. Epidemiology

1. Community surveys reveal that **women have a 0.2–2% lifetime prevalence of somatoform disorders.**

2. **In men the overall prevalence is 0.2%.** Greek and Puerto Rican men account for 5–20% of men with the disorder.

3. Culture may also impact presenting symptoms. For example, burning in the hands and feet is more common in men from Southeast Asia, as compared to North American men. This may alter the review of systems.

F. Psychiatric Comorbidity

1. Axis I: 50% of somatization disorder patients have mood disorders. Anxiety disorders, substance abuse, and posttraumatic stress disorder are also common.

2. Axis II: 72% of patients with somatization disorder have personality disorders, most commonly histrionic, borderline, and antisocial personality disorders.

3. The comorbidity of a history of childhood sexual abuse and neglect and somatoform disorder is high (30–70%).

4. **A family history of somatization disorder is quite common.**
   a. 10–20% of first-degree female relatives of female patients with somatization disorder develop it themselves.
   b. Male relatives of female patients with somatization disorder are more likely to have antisocial personality disorder and problems with substance abuse.
   c. Adoption studies have demonstrated that patients are five times more likely to present with somatoform disorders if either the biologic parents or the adoptive parents have had somatization disorder.

G. Differential Diagnosis

1. Since many medical conditions (e.g., acute intermittent porphyria, multiple sclerosis, systemic lupus erythematosus, endocrine disorders, chronic infections) present with variable and fluctuating courses, it is important to distinguish medical from psychiatric disorders.

2. **Somatization disorder is more likely than an underlying medical condition when there is:**
   a. Multiple organ involvement
   b. An early onset of disease
   c. A chronic course
   d. An absence of any laboratory, radiographic, or physical abnormalities

3. **Other psychiatric disorders can mimic somatization disorder, and include:**
   a. Schizophrenia, when multiple somatic delusions are present
   b. Anxiety disorders, especially during a panic attack
   c. Depressive disorders, during a depressive episode
   d. Another somatoform disorder

H. Treatment

1. The goal of treatment is to **provide care for the patient but not to focus on curing the disease.**

Table 17-1. Comparison of Somatoform Disorders

	Somatization Disorder	Conversion	Pain Disorder	Hypochondriasis	Body Dysmorphic Disorder
Main features	Recurrent, multiple, chronic, somatic complaints not accounted for by medical findings	Symptoms affecting voluntary motor or sensory systems, suggesting neurological disorder, preceded by stress	Pain is the predominant focus of treatment, psychological factors affect onset, severity, exacerbation and maintenance	Fear of, or belief that one has a serious illness despite adequate medical evaluation and reassurance, NOT DELUSIONAL	Imagined ugliness, NOT DELUSIONAL INTENSITY
Age of onset (years)	< 30	10–35	Any age	Early adulthood	Adolescence
Associated features	Repeated workups, multiple physicians, inconsistent history, chaotic lives	"La belle indifference," suggestible, symptoms do not conform to anatomic pathways	Disability, social isolation, search for the cure	Repeated workups, doctor-shopping, childhood illness	Frequent checking, avoidance, feel mocked by others, surgery makes it worse
Comorbid medical illness	+/−	+/−	Common	Infrequent	No
Epidemiology	0.2–2% women, 0.2% men	25% medical outpatients	?	4–9% medical outpatients	?
Gender	Women > men	2:1–10:1, women > men	Equal	Equal	Equal
Course	Chronic	Usually self-limited, 25% recur in 1 year	Variable, often chronic	Chronic, waxes and wanes	Chronic
Secondary gain	+/−	+/−	+	+/−	−
Family history	Somatization disorder, antisocial, substance abuse	Conversion disorder	Depression, alcohol abuse, pain disorder	Illness in family member when a child	
Comorbid psychiatric illness	Major depression, panic, substance abuse, personality disorder	Dissociative disorder, PTSD, depression	Substance abuse, depression, anxiety	Anxiety, depression	Depression, delusional disorder, social phobia, OCD, suicide
Treatment	Regular appointments, maintain vs. cure	Suggest cure, examine stress, no need to confront	Avoid iatrogenesis, multimodal treatment, care not cure	? Selective serotonin reuptake inhibitors	Prevent iatrogenesis, SSRI, ? antipsychotics

2. The best **treatment occurs in the context of a long-term relationship** with an **empathic primary care provider** (PCP). The PCP should be encouraged to:
   a. Allow the patient to **maintain the sick role.**
   b. Schedule **regular follow-up appointments** of a **set length.**
   c. **Set the agenda** of the visit.
   d. **Prevent iatrogenesis** and limit workups to objective findings, and not complaints.
   e. **Do no more and no less for the somatic patient than for any other patient.**
   f. **Set limits** on contacts outside of visit time.
   g. **Introduce psychosocial issues slowly,** using stress or mind-body language.
3. **Psychiatric referral** is useful to treat and manage comorbid psychiatric disorders.
   a. Psychiatric **consultation decreases health care costs** and unnecessary utilization of services.
   b. The goal of psychiatric consultation is to provide a **framework for treatment.** It should not be viewed as the end of the relationship with the PCP.
   c. **Comorbid psychiatric disorders should be treated** and managed.
   d. **Individual or group psychotherapy** can be useful in either a dynamic or cognitive-behavioral model.
4. **Stress-reduction** education can be useful.

III. Undifferentiated Somatoform Disorder (Somatization Syndrome or Subthreshold Somatization Disorder)

A. **Definition**
   This category includes subthreshold somatization disorders, such as chronic fatigue syndrome, ecologic allergies, multiple chemical sensitivities, and fibromyalgia.

B. **DSM-IV Criteria**
   1. **One or more physical complaints** (such as fatigue, loss of appetite, or a gastrointestinal complaint or urinary complaint) **must persist for 6 months or longer.**
   2. Either:
      a. **The symptoms,** after appropriate evaluation, **cannot be fully explained** by a known medical condition or substance; or
      b. **The complaints or impairments are grossly in excess of what would be expected** on the basis of the existing medical condition.
   3. **The symptoms must cause significant distress or impairment** in social, occupational or another important area of functioning.
   4. **The symptoms are neither intentionally produced nor feigned.**

C. **Clinical Features**
   1. The presentation is similar to that of somatization disorder, but it may be more culturally based, as an idiom of distress, or as a manifestation of stigma avoidance.
   2. The course is variable; an eventual diagnosis of a general medical disorder is more common than it is in somatization disorder.

D. **Epidemiology**
   1. This disorder **occurs most commonly in young women of low socioeconomic status.** It is 30 times more frequent than is somatization disorder. Its **lifetime prevalence is 4–11%.**

E. **Differential Diagnosis**
   1. The differential diagnosis includes the same medical disorders that are found along with somatization disorder.
   2. The psychiatric differential diagnosis includes somatization disorder, somatoform disorder not otherwise specified, major depression, anxiety, and malingering.

F. **Treatment**
   The **treatment is similar to that of somatization disorder.** Patients with this disorder may be more responsive to psychiatric referral.

IV. Conversion Disorder (Hysteria, Conversion Reaction, Hysterical Psychoneurosis, Conversion Type)

A. **Definition**
   Conversion disorder involves the presence of symptoms or deficits that affect voluntary motor or sensory function in a fashion that suggests a neurological condition but which is not explained by the medical findings.

B. **History**
   1. Conversion disorders were described as early as **1900 BC** and labeled as hysteria, which led to the description of conversion and somatization disorders as indistinct until the 1850s. **Briquet** developed the first modern concept of conversion disorder as a central nervous disorder. **Reynolds** introduced the idea of conversion as a loss of function secondary to ideas, and **Charcot** elaborated this by linking conversion symptoms and trauma. **Freud** used the concept to analyze the case of Dora. Currently, the importance of unconscious processes in diagnostic criteria has been reduced.

C. **DSM-IV Criteria**
   1. **One or more symptoms or deficits affecting a voluntary motor or sensory function that suggests a neurological or general medical condition are required.**
      a. The sensory symptoms include double vision, blindness, deafness, and loss of touch or pain.

b. The motor loss symptoms include paralysis, aphonia, difficulty swallowing, ataxia, tremor, and urinary retention.

2. **Symptom initiation or exacerbation is preceded by psychological conflict or stress.**

3. **The symptom, after appropriate investigation, cannot be fully explained by a general medical condition,** substance, or culturally sanctioned experience, such as glossalia in religious rituals or hysterical epidemics.

4. **The symptom causes significant distress and is not feigned.**

5. **The symptom is not limited to pain or sexual dysfunction,** and does not occur only in the course of somatization disorder.

6. Conversion disorder should be coded along with the type of deficit involved.

D. Clinical Features

1. **Patients**
   a. The more medically naive the patient, the greater the likelihood of implausible symptoms.
   b. **Patients with this disorder tend to be suggestible.**
   c. Conversion-disordered patients are more likely to have had **prior conversion symptoms** or symptoms of dissociation.
   d. **One-third** of patients with conversion disorder **have concurrent neurological illness.**

2. **Symptoms**
   a. As opposed to the patient with somatization disorder or the patient with hypochondriasis who believes they are gravely ill, the patient with conversion disorder often presents with **"la belle indifference."**
   b. Symptoms are more likely to **occur following extreme stress.**
   c. Rather than following known anatomic pathways, the **symptoms tend to conform to a patient's own ideas** (e.g., a stocking-glove distribution and a midline anesthesia).
   d. Symptoms are **inconsistent with the physical examination.** For example, a "paralyzed" arm doesn't fall on the patient's head, optokinetic nystagmus is maintained in hysterical blindness, and antagonistic muscle function is maintained in paralysis.
   e. The presentation may **resemble the patient's own symptoms** (e.g., epileptics who have pseudoseizures).
   f. The symptoms **rarely cause physical disability.**
   g. The symptoms **tend to recur.**

3. **Course**
   a. Conversion disorder is rarely reported in patients younger than 10 years, or older than 35 years; however, cases have been seen in groups of all ages including 90-year-olds.
   b. Patients with conversion disorder older than 35 years are more likely to have occult neurological disorders.
   c. The syndrome usually remits within 2 weeks after hospitalization, but it has a recurrence rate of 20–25% within the first year.

d. Prior episodes increase the rate of recurrence.
e. 20% of patients with conversion disorder develop somatization disorder within 4 years of their first episode.

E. Etiology

1. A **dynamic hypothesis** suggests that the conversion symptom is a solution to an unconscious conflict. Secondary gain is often an unconscious cause of conversion. For example, a woman whose husband had an affair may become paralyzed rather than walk away from the marriage.

2. **Altered function** of both the dominant and nondominant **hemispheres,** as well as impaired cortical communication, seem to play a role in conversion symptoms.

3. **Hypercritical families** may create "unspeakable dilemmas" predisposing to conversion reactions.

F. Epidemiology

1. Conversion disorder is **the most common somatoform disorder.** Approximately 25–33% of female psychiatric outpatients report an episode of conversion. The annual incidence of conversion disorder in the general population is between 11 and 300 per 100,000. Conversion occurs in 25–30% of hospitalized veterans. Conversion is diagnosed in 5–16% of psychiatric consultations, and in 1–3% of psychiatric outpatients.

2. The **rate of diagnosis is increasing** among rural populations, those with low socioeconomic status, and in developing regions.

3. A **gender bias exists,** with a ratio of 2–10:1, women/men. Left-handed women have a higher incidence.

G. Psychiatric Comorbidity

1. Conversion disorders can be a precursor to depression, somatization, and/or dissociative disorders.

2. Among Axis II-disordered patients (mostly with histrionic, dependent, or antisocial personality disorders), conversion disorder can be an unconscious means to an end.

H. Differential Diagnosis

1. Neurological diseases are diagnosed in one-fifth to one-half of patients with conversion disorder. Early studies reported an even higher incidence.

2. The most common neurological disorders associated with conversion disorder are multiple sclerosis, myasthenia gravis, seizures, and dystonia.

3. Other somatoform disorders may present with conversion symptoms.

I. Treatment

1. **A good prognosis is associated with an acute onset of disease, a clear stressor, a short interval between the onset of symptoms and initiation of treatment, rapid improvement in the hospital, an above-average intel-**

ligence, and a presenting symptom of paralysis, aphonia, or blindness.

2. **A poor prognosis is associated with a presenting symptom of tremor and/or seizure, an increased interval between symptom onset and treatment, and a reduced intelligence level.**

3. The **use of suggestion** and **physical therapy** legitimizes the symptoms.

4. Confrontation of the patient is not helpful, as it results in **"loss of face."**

5. **Indirect examination** of stressors can lead to relief.

6. **Behavioral techniques** should be instituted; referral to family therapy is often indicated.

V. Pain Disorder (Psychogenic Pain Disorder, Somatoform Pain Disorder)

A. Definition

Pain is the predominant focus of this clinical syndrome; it is associated with illness-affirming behavior.

B. History

In recent years there has been a movement away from etiology and towards a descriptive approach to this disorder. DSM-IV includes a subtype of pain associated with a medical disorder that is *not* a mental disorder.

C. DSM-IV Criteria

1. Pain occurs in one or more anatomical sites as the focus of attention.

2. Pain causes significant distress or impairment in social, occupational, or other areas of function. This includes disability, an increased use of health care facilities, an increased use of medications, and family problems.

3. Psychological factors have a role in the onset, severity, exacerbation, and maintenance of the pain.

4. The pain is not intentionally produced.

5. Pain disorder is not due to a mood, anxiety, or psychotic disorder, or to dyspareunia.

6. Subtypes and specifiers

   a. The 307.80 classification is used for a pain disorder that is associated with psychological factors.

   b. The 307.89 classification is a pain disorder associated with both psychological factors and a general medical condition.

   c. The last subtype is a pain disorder associated with a general medical condition (Axis III).

   d. Each subtype specifies an acute or chronic condition.

D. Clinical Features

1. Described as **severe and constant,** the pain may not be consistent with known anatomic pathways.

2. When the pain is consistent with a medical condition, the **severity is disproportionate to clinical findings.**

3. The most frequent sites of pain are the head, the face, the low back, and the pelvis.

4. **Pain is the main life focus** of a patient's energy; they frequently spend their life searching for a cure.

5. This behavior can lead to **disability** and **complications** that include iatrogenic substance abuse (opioid/benzodiazepines), fractured relationships, depression (which occurs in 30–50% of those with chronic pain), anxiety (with acute pain), and insomnia.

6. The **etiology is multifactorial;** primary and secondary gain are often involved.

E. Epidemiology

The **prevalence** of these disorders is **unknown.** Pain disorder consumes a large amount of health resources, with **$10 billion spent in 1980** on disability for chronic pain. The peak incidence occurs in the **third and fourth decade** of life. The **presenting symptoms** for males and females are different: **women** complain of more **headaches, men** complain more of **back pain. A family history** of increased depression, alcohol abuse, and pain disorders is often present. **A significant psychological stressor** is often the precipitating event.

F. Course

1. The **course is variable;** the syndrome can persist for years.

2. **A good prognosis is associated with continued work and the absence of pain as a focus of life.**

3. The differential psychiatric diagnosis includes malingering and factitious disorders.

G. Treatment

1. Emphasize **living with pain** and not removal of pain.

2. Employ a **multimodal treatment** approach, combining physical, family, group, and cognitive-behavioral therapy.

3. **Avoid iatrogenic complications.**

4. **Treat psychiatric illnesses as they arise.**

VI. Hypochondriasis

A. Definition

Hypochondriasis is a syndrome involving an excessive and pervasive preoccupation with fears of having, or the belief that one has, a serious illness that does not respond to reassurance after appropriate medical assessment.

B. History

Although it was described as a modern disease in the 1920s, hypochondrium before the 19th century meant abdomen. Therefore, hypochondriasis referred to disorders below the abdomen.

C. DSM-IV Criteria
1. **Hypochondriasis is a preoccupation with fears of having, or the idea that one has, a serious disease based on one's misinterpretation of bodily symptoms.**
2. **This preoccupation persists despite appropriate medical evaluation and reassurance;** the belief is not of delusional intensity (if so, a diagnosis of delusional disorder, somatic type is made).
3. This **preoccupation causes significant distress or impairment.**
4. **Hypochondriasis lasts at least 6 months** and is not accounted for by another mental disorder.

D. Clinical Features
1. **Symptoms**
   a. The **major presenting symptom** is a **fear of disease** and/or the **belief that one has a serious illness (disease conviction).** The symptoms are presented in excruciating detail as evidence of serious disease. The symptom reports can have a relentless quality.
   b. A patient's preoccupation can involve **any symptom or organ system** (e.g., heart rate, cough, headache). The complaints can be single or involve more than one system. It has been called **"medical student disease,"** when a patient reads about an illness and is convinced that he or she has it.
   c. Hypochondriasis should be evaluated in a patient's **cultural context.**
2. **Doctor-patient relationship.** A patient with this problem frequently **doctor-shops,** which can be a source of frustration for both the doctor and patient. These patients are often **resistant to psychiatric referral.** Workups can become overzealous or inattentive.
3. **Clinical course**
   a. The **onset** is in **early adulthood.**
   b. **A chronic, waxing and waning course is typical.**
   c. During a 5-year follow-up, two-thirds of patients still met criteria for hypochondriasis.
   d. Episodes may be **precipitated by stress,** especially the death of someone close.
4. **Etiology**
   a. **Amplification,** or misattribution hypothesis, refers to a patient that misinterprets a normal somatic sensation as an abnormal symptom.
   b. **Psychodynamic** hypotheses include the notion that hypochondriasis serves as an ego defense against guilt, or as a vehicle for aggressive wishes towards others, or as a result of conflicts transferred to a physical complaint.
   c. **Learning theory** suggests that a patient may find that the sick role, reinforced by social interaction, can fulfill a need to be cared for.

d. Variant theorists believe that **hypochondriasis is a form of another psychiatric disorder** (e.g., obsessive-compulsive disorder [OCD]).

E. Epidemiology
1. **Hypochondriasis occurs in about 3–13%** of the general population in the United States. In Africa it occurs in 1% of the population (based on a survey of 14 countries).
2. It can account for 4–9% of patients in general medical practice.
3. The incidence is equal in males and females.
4. The history often includes a childhood illness, or illness of a significant family member when the patient was a child.

F. Differential Diagnosis
1. An underlying medical condition must be ruled out.
2. Hypochondriasis can occur as a transient response to medical illness.
3. Hypochondriasis can occur as a symptom of or comorbidly with an Axis I disease (e.g., depression, anxiety disorders, specific disease phobia, OCD, somatoform disorders, psychotic disorders, or body dysmorphic disorder).

G. Treatment
1. A **good prognosis** for hypochondriasis **is associated with an acute onset and high levels of general medical comorbidity.** It also includes an absence of a personality disorder, no secondary gain, high socioeconomic status, and less disease conviction.
2. Accompanying psychiatric conditions must be treated.
3. **Regular contact with a caring medical physician** should be maintained with palliation, and not cure, as the goal.
4. Patients may switch to **self-help** regimens.
5. The workups are based only on objective findings.
6. Cognitive-educational **group treatments** which include reattribution, distraction, and attentional tracking have been helpful.
7. Use of **selective serotonin reuptake inhibitors (SSRIs)** may have some benefit in these patients.

VII. Body Dysmorphic Disorder (BDD; Dysmorhophobia)

A. Definition
BDD is a disease of imagined ugliness.

B. History
The disorder was described in European, Japanese, and Russian psychiatric literature over 100 years ago, yet it was not focused on in the United States until the 1960s. Krapelin first described it as a

compulsive neurosis, and Janet described it as an obsession of shame of the body.

C. **DSM-IV Criteria**

BDD is a preoccupation with an imagined defect in appearance, or a markedly excessive preoccupation if a slight anomaly is present. The preoccupation causes significant distress or impairment and is not accounted for by another mental disorder.

D. **Clinical Features**

1. Patients complain often of a **facial deformity** (e.g., asymmetry, size of nose), but it can be of anything.
2. **Patients feel too ashamed to present for treatment,** or to describe their anomaly.
3. Patients may frequently **check and groom** themselves (hair-combing, skin picking, especially in mirrors or in other reflective surfaces).
4. **They may try to compensate for the imagined anomaly** (e.g., wearing a hat if hair loss is imagined, or stuffing their shorts if a small penis is perceived).
5. **Complications** include social isolation (some only go out at night or are house-bound), imagined mockery, functioning below capacity, iatrogenic complications (7–9% of patients who undergo cosmetic surgery meet criteria for BDD), and suicide.

E. **Clinical Course**

The **onset occurs in adolescence;** 30 years is the mean age at the time of diagnosis. It can become **chronic.** The **presentation can be culture-specific:** for example, in Southeastern Asia, there occurs a preoccupation that the penis is shrinking and will disappear into the abdomen and cause death.

F. **Etiology**

Psychodynamic features of the disease are thought to include displacement of a sexual or emotional conflict onto a body part.

G. **Epidemiology**

1. The frequency in males and females is equal. Of patients in a university plastic surgery clinic 2% were diagnosed with this disorder.
2. Depression, delusional disorder, social phobia, and OCD can be comorbid conditions. There is also a relationship between BDD and delusional disorder, somatic type.
3. There is a higher than expected family history of mood disorders and OCD.

H. **Treatment**

1. The **prevention of iatrogenesis** is optimal. After cosmetic surgery, for example, psychiatric pathology can re-emerge.
2. The use of **SSRIs can be helpful.** Relapse is common when the drug is discontinued.

3. **Antipsychotics** should be used for delusional disorder.

VIII. Somatoform Disorder Not Otherwise Specified

A. **Definition**

These disorders are residual categories for disorders for which physical symptoms are the focus of treatment but which do not meet criteria for another somatoform disorder.

B. **Examples**

1. Pseudocyesis, or the belief that one is pregnant. Endocrine changes may be present but are not explained by a general medical condition.
2. Nonpsychotic hypochondriasis lasting less than 6 months.
3. Unexplained physical complaints lasting less than 6 months.

Suggested Readings

Barsky AJ, Borus JF: Somatization and medicalization in the era of managed care. *J Am Med Assoc* 1995; 274:1931–1934.

Barsky AJ, Stem TA, Greenberg D: Functional somatic symptoms and somatoform disorders. In Cassem N, Stern TA, Rosenbaum JF, Jellinek MS (eds): *The MGH Handbook of General Hospital Psychiatry.* St Louis: Mosby, 1997:305–336.

Calabrese LV: Approach to the patient with multiple physical complaints. In Stem TA, Herman JB, Slavin PL (eds): *The MGH Guide to Psychiatry in Primary Care.* New York: McGraw-Hill, 1998:89–98.

Ford CV: *The Somatizing Disorders.* New York: Elsevier, 1983.

Guggenheim FG, Smith GR: Somatoform disorders. In Kaplan HI, Sadock BJ (eds): *Comprehensive Textbook of Psychiatry,* 6th ed. Baltimore: Williams and Wilkins, 1995:1251–1270.

Martin RL, Yutzy SH: Somatoform disorders. In Hales RE, Yudofsky SC, Talbott JA (eds): *The American Psychiatric Press Textbook of Psychiatry,* 2nd ed. Washington, DC: American Psychiatric Press, 1994.

Phillips KA, McElroy SL, Keck PE Jr: Body dysmorphic disorder. 30 cases of imagined ugliness. *Am J Psychiatry* 1993; 150:302–308.

Simon GE, Guerje O: Stability of somatization disorder and somatization symptoms among primary care patients. *Arch Gen Psychiatry* 1999; 56:90–95.

Smith GR: *Somatization Disorder in the Medical Setting.* Washington, DC: American Psychiatric Press, 1991.

Stern TA: Malingering, factitious illness and somatization. In Hyman (ed.): *Manual of Psychiatric Emergencies.* 2nd ed. Boston: Little, Brown, 1988:217–225.

Chapter 18
Factitious Disorders

A D E L E   C .   V I G U E R A   A N D   T H E O D O R E   A .   S T E R N

I. Overview

In factitious disorders, the individual's goal is to produce or feign signs of medical and mental disorder, and to assume the patient role. Factitious disorders are conditions that are, by definition, not real or natural. Although they have a compulsive quality, the behaviors are considered voluntary even if they cannot be controlled. Obvious secondary gain, or such as avoidance from work, monetary gain, or escape from legal authorities, is not a feature of factitious disorders; these are essential features which distinguish these disorders from malingering. Factitious disorders are incapacitating to the patient, who often produces severe trauma or develops untoward adverse effects from repeated surgical or medical interventions. Serial hospitalizations essentially make it impossible for these patients to have meaningful sustained interpersonal or work relationships. **The prognosis in most cases is poor.** Although there are no adequate data about the long-term outcome of these patients, a few of them appear to die prematurely as a result of needless medications, instrumentations, or surgeries without the disorder ever being suspected.

II. Epidemiology

The prevalence of factitious disorders is unknown. Even when the diagnosis of factitious disorder is strongly suspected or confirmed, it is generally not recorded in hospital discharge summaries; determination of the prevalence is therefore difficult.

Although often described as a rare syndrome, **most clinicians have encountered at least one patient with this disorder.** These cases are often memorable because **patients with factitious disorders tend to wreak havoc on the ward and induce strong countertransference feelings of hatred.** Conflicting data exist on whether factitious disorders are more common in males or females. They appear to occur most frequently among people who are health care workers and who have had extensive previous experience with illness, injury, or hospitalization during their early development.

III. Diagnosis

A. Diagnostic Features

There are three cardinal features of factitious disorder: the intentional production of physical or psychological signs or symptoms that are under voluntary control and are not explained by any other underlying physical or mental disorder; the primary motivation for the behavior is to assume the sick role; incentives for the behavior, such as economic gain, and the avoidance of legal responsibility, are absent.

In the DSM-IV, factitious disorders are classified by type: with predominately psychological signs and symptoms; with predominately physical signs and symptoms (also known as Munchausen syndrome); with combined psychological and physical signs and symptoms. DSM-IV also includes the category of factitious disorders not otherwise specified (NOS); the most notable example, factitious disorder by proxy (or Munchausen by proxy), is included in the appendix.

B. Subtypes

1. **Factitious disorder with predominately physical signs and symptoms (also known as Munchausen syndrome)** is a severe form of psychopathology that may account for 10% of individuals with factitious disorders. Studies of fever of unknown origin have determined that 2.2–9.6% were factitious. One study reported a 9% rate of factitious disorders among all patients admitted to the hospital. Patients may present with a diverse array of physical complaints or signs, such as fever, hematoma, hemoptysis, seizures, hypoglycemia, or abdominal pain. These patients characteristically travel from hospital to hospital trying to gain admission with these medical symptoms. **In factitious disorder by proxy (better known as Munchausen syndrome by proxy), someone intentionally produces physical signs or symptoms in another person who is under their care.** The most common scenario involves a mother who purposely deceives medical personnel into believing the child is ill by either giving false information or intentionally inducing illness or injury in the child. The motivation in the disorder is for the caretaker to assume the patient role indirectly.

2. **Factitious disorder with predominately psychological signs and symptoms** is a difficult diagnosis to make; it is often made only after prolonged investigation. The feigned symptoms often include depression,

hallucinations, dissociative and conversion symptoms, and bizarre behavior. Other symptoms, which also appear in the physical type of factitious disorder, include pseudologia fantastica and impostership. Pseudologia fantastica is characterized by extensive and colorful fantasies associated with the presentation of the patient's story. The listener's interest in the story pleases the patient and helps reinforce the symptom. The patient often gives false and conflicting accounts about other areas in their life, such as claiming the death of a parent or child to obtain sympathy. Impostership usually involves assuming the identity of a prestigious person. Men, for example, may claim they are important war heroes who attribute their surgical scars to wounds received in battle.

3. Factitious disorders may present with **combined psychological and physical symptoms.**

IV. Clinical Features

A. **Factitious disorders typically begin in early adult life, although they may appear during childhood or adolescence.**

B. **Personality Disorders**
Many patients with factitious disorders fulfill the diagnostic criteria for borderline personality disorder, especially in terms of their rigid defensive structure and poor identity formation. They may have a masochistic personality in which pain serves as a punishment for imagined or real sins.

C. **Afflicted patients typically have** a normal to above average IQ, absence of a formal thought disorder, strong dependency needs, and confusion over their sexual identity.

D. **A typical admission has several characteristics:**
1. **The patient often arrives in the emergency room late at night or on a weekend.** He or she is familiar with the diagnoses of most disorders that usually require hospital admission or medication. **The patient uses convincing medical jargon and generally presents with an apparent acute illness or pain supported by a plausible and often dramatic case history.**
2. **The patient generally appeals to the qualities of nurturance and omnipotence in the physician** in an attempt to convince him or her to provide treatment.
3. Patients may insist on surgery. In about half the reported cases, the patient demands treatment with specific medications, usually analgesics.
4. **Once in the hospital, the patient's demands for attention increase;** irritation and anger develop when they are not met.
5. **Complaints of misdiagnosis and mistreatment arise and are directed toward staff.**

6. **The deception is often uncovered** by discovering, for example, insulin-filled syringes in a patient's suitcase during his hospitalization for hypoglycemia.
7. **The staff become angry and lose interest in the patient's medical issues.** This results in either swift discharge of the patient or the patient eloping from the hospital.
8. **The patient arrives at a nearby hospital with a similar presentation** shortly after such a discharge.

V. Etiology

A. **Psychodynamic underpinnings of factitious disorders are poorly understood.** The patient may perceive one or both parents as rejecting figures who are unable to form close relationships. Feigning illness is done in an attempt to recreate the desired positive parent-child bond. The disorder may be considered as a form of repetition compulsion. The patient repeats the basic childhood conflict of needing and seeking acceptance and love while expecting that they will not be forthcoming. The physician and staff members are perceived by the patient as representing rejecting parents. Primitive defense mechanisms (including repression, regression, identification with the aggressor, and symbolization) are typically seen in factitious disorders

B. **Many afflicted patients suffered childhood abuse or deprivation that resulted in frequent hospitalization.** The inpatient stay may have been regarded as an escape from a traumatic home life and the patient may have found a series of loving caretakers.

C. **Patients may identify with a close relative who was hospitalized for a particular illness.** They may feign the same illness in order to reunite with that particular relative in a magical way.

D. **These behaviors might represent an unconscious last-ditch effort to ward off further mental disintegration into psychosis.**

VI. Differential Diagnosis

A. **True Physical Disorders**
Factitious disorders must be distinguished from those conditions that are true physical disorders. Failure to diagnose and treat an underlying physical illness could lead to death of the patient.

B. **Somatization Disorders (Briquet's Syndrome)**
Somatization disorders or conversion disorders are distinguished from factitious disorders by the fact that the production of symptoms is not under voluntary control. The symptoms are a result of unconscious conflicts. These patients are typically not savvy about hospital procedures or medical

diagnoses, nor is there any secondary gain from their complaints.

C. Malingering
Unlike patients with factitious disorders, malingerers have an obvious, recognizable secondary gain in producing their signs and symptoms. They generally seek admission to avoid the law, to receive financial compensation, or to avoid work.

VII. Approach to the Patient who Presents with Factitious Disorder

A. General Strategies
1. **Gather information from collateral sources.** The psychiatric examination should emphasize corroboration of a patient's information with any available friend, relative, or other informant. Verification of all the facts presented by the patient concerning prior medical care is essential.
2. **Avoid confrontation.** When verifying facts initially it is necessary to avoid pointed or accusatory questioning that may provoke evasion, defensiveness, or flight from the hospital. It may nearly be impossible to be certain of the diagnosis during the initial encounter.
3. **Be aware of negative countertransference.** Patients with factitious disorders usually evoke feelings of hostility and contempt among staff members. Try to embrace a nonjudgmental approach to the patient. One appropriate intervention is to maintain awareness that, even though the patient's illness is factitious, the patient is still ill.
4. **Be alert to specific elements of the history that typically suggest the presence of a factitious disorder.**
   a. Evidence of addiction or multiple hospital admissions
   b. Numerous forms of identification (e.g., hospital cards, insurance forms)
   c. Itinerant lives
   d. A facility for medical jargon
   e. A paucity of verifiable history
   f. An absence of close interpersonal relationships
   g. A history of having worked in a medically related field
   h. An early history of sadistic or rejecting parents, chronic illness, or an important relationship with a physician
   i. History of personality disorder. Although a wide range of psychiatric diagnoses have been associated with this syndrome, these individuals are usually thought to have personality disorders.
   j. A multiplicity of scars
5. **Recognize typical clinical presentations associated with factitious disorders.**
   a. **The acute abdominal type (laparotomaphilia migrans).** This type is the most common; many of these individuals have been operated on so frequently that abdominal symptoms may, in fact, be a consequence of intestinal obstruction secondary to adhesions.
   b. **The hematologic type.** Profound anemia may have been produced by surreptitious bloodletting and by complications of ingestion and self-administration of anticoagulants.
   c. **Neurologic type (neurologia diabolica),** often presenting with loss of consciousness, paroxysmal headaches, or seizure.
   d. **The dermatologic type (dermatitis autogenica),** frequently the result of self-inflicted wounds or chemical abrasions.
   e. **The febrile type (hyperpyrexia figmentatica).** These individuals often lose their fever when thermometers are placed, monitored, and removed under observation.
   f. **The endocrinologic type,** including those who present for evaluation of hyperinsulinemia, hyperthyroidism, and hypoglycemia.
   g. **The cardiac type,** including those individuals who complain of chest pain or arrhythmia.

VIII. Treatment

A. No specific psychiatric therapy has been effective in treating factitious disorder.

B. Early identification of the disorder is perhaps the most important intervention since determining the diagnosis can help prevent the patient from undergoing multiple, unnecessary, and potentially dangerous interventions.

C. Focus on management, rather than cure. Re-frame the patient's desire for medical attention as a cry for help. However, even the most empathetic therapeutic confrontation may be met with profound denial, resistance, and anger. For this particular patient population, effective psychiatric care cannot be done in the absence of ongoing medical care. Good liaison between the psychiatrist and the medical/surgical staff is strongly advised.

D. Legal intervention is sometimes needed, particularly **in situations of Munchausen by proxy, which generally involves children.** Child welfare services should be notified and arrangements made for ongoing monitoring of the child's health.

Suggested Readings

Asher R: Munchausen's syndrome. *Lancet* 1951; i:339–341.

Barsky AJ, Stern TA, Greenberg DB, Cassem NH: In Cassem NH, Stern TA, Rosenbaum JF, Jellinek MS (eds): *Massachusetts General Hospital Handbook of General Hospital Psychiatry*, 4th ed. St Louis: Mosby, 1997:305–336.

Factitious disorders. In Kaplan HI, Sadock BJ, Grebb JA (eds): *Synopsis of Psychiatry*, 7th ed. Baltimore: Williams & Wilkins, 1994:632–637.

Stern TA: Munchausen's syndrome revisited. *Psychosomatics* 1980; 21:329–336.

Stern TA: Factitious disorders. In Hyman SE, Jenike MA (eds): *Manual of Clinical Problems in Psychiatry*. Boston: Little, Brown, 1990:190–194.

Chapter 19

Dissociative Disorders

S TEVEN C. S CHLOZMAN AND R AFAEL D. O RNSTEIN

I. Introduction

Dissociative Disorders encompass a heterogeneous and sometimes controversial set of disorders. Although the concept of dissociation is more than 100 years old, dissociative phenomena are currently enjoying renewed interest. This increase is in part related to a burgeoning literature addressing the effects of trauma on memory and personality, as well as the apparent epidemic of dissociative disease during the 1980s. There is now a growing consensus that the increase in new cases deserves closer scrutiny and may represent an overdiagnosis of dissociative disorders. Nevertheless, dissociative phenomena have been consistently described throughout the history of psychiatry, and when appropriate should be considered in the differential diagnosis.

Central to the conceptualization of dissociation is the understanding that a person's consciousness may not be fully integrated. Thus, a patient may experience a distinct alteration in personality or experience, in which thoughts, feelings, or actions are not logically integrated with other self-referential experiences. Traumatic experiences are often considered etiologic factors in the development of dissociation. Although the most well known of these disorders is Dissociative Identity Disorder (previously called Multiple Personality Disorder), it is important to note that current nosology also includes Dissociative Amnesia, Dissociative Fugue, Depersonalization Disorder, and Dissociative Disorder Not Otherwise Specified. One must also be careful to consider Factitious or Malingered Dissociative Disorders when individuals present with symptoms of dissociation.

II. History of Dissociative Disorders

A number of historical figures have been instrumental in establishing the current conceptualization of dissociative phenomena.

A. **Franz Anton Mesmer** (1734–1815): **known for his theories of "animal magnetism,"** and today recognized as one of the first clinicians to explore the clinical utility of hypnosis in treating dissociation. (see III, below)

B. **Pierre Janet** (1859–1947): with other clinicians, **he established hypnosis as a clinical intervention for dissociative states.** Most importantly, he was first to connect the etiologic nature of traumatic experiences.

C. **Sigmund Freud:** differed from Janet by suggesting that dissociation results from the ego's vigorous defense against psychological pain. Thus, while Janet felt that the ego collapsed and fragmented under the weight of traumatic experiences, **Freud felt that trauma forced a powerful ego to wall off psychological pain, after which this pain manifests itself only in dissociative states.**

D. **Morton Prince:** published *The Dissociation of a Personality* (1906), in which he describes his patient, Sally Beauchamp, as "The Saint, the Devil, the Woman." His work is **likely the first clinical investigation into the notion of separate dissociative identities.**

III. Etiology of Dissociation

A. **Traumatic experience** is strongly correlated with dissociation. Multiple studies and case series document the relationship of trauma to dissociative states.

B. **Children appear more prone to dissociation than adults, and may develop dissociative traits in response to trauma at a very young age.** Some researchers have theorized that these individuals remain more susceptible to dissociation than similarly traumatized older individuals.

C. Research suggests a potential clinical link between **dissociative states and hypnosis.** For example, patients with dissociative disorders are reportedly more hypnotizable than are control subjects. Moreover, hypnosis may represent a valuable clinical intervention for the treatment of dissociative disorders. Finally, some studies have found that subjects who have had traumatic experiences but who do not manifest a dissociative disorder appear more hypnotizable when compared to nontraumatized individuals.

D. Recently, research has suggested that dissociative states (given the extent to which information about one's self is compartmentalized in those suffering from dissociative disorders) can be explored in terms of **state-dependent learning** (a broad concept meant to suggest that information stored in one "state" may only be retrieved in that specific state).

151

E. Complex partial seizure activity has been suggested as a cause of dissociation. However, a definitive link has not yet been revealed. While some patients with dissociative disorders have concurrent seizure disorders, the seizures themselves do not necessarily cause their dissociative symptoms. **Electroencephalographic (EEG) studies** of patients with dissociative disorders have been contradictory; some studies suggest EEG differences within the same patient during different dissociative states.

F. Neurochemical and pharmacologic agents may be related to dissociative phenomena. Substances such as LSD (lysergic acid diethylamide), phencyclidine, and ketamine appear to provoke dissociative episodes, and some studies suggest a serotonin dysregulation as contributing to dissociative tendencies.

IV. Who Dissociates?

Dissociation can be measured clinically using the Dissociative Experience Scale (DES). This 28-item self-report questionnaire has achieved good reliability and validity. Higher scores represent more dissociative experiences. However, this scale has achieved only face validity, and can be purposefully misrepresented by the subject.

Other standardized assessments include the Structured Clinical Interview for Dissociative Disorders (SCID-D), as well as the Minnesota Multiphasic Personality Inventory (MMPI). Again, one must realize that the SCID-D has also achieved only face validity, and that the MMPI has not been validated for Dissociative Disorders. Nevertheless, using these scales, as well as other means of assessment, several conclusions have been suggested regarding those who experience dissociative states.

A. Gender

Males and females (in both psychiatric and nonpsychiatric samples) have similar DES scores. Thus, no gender differences are apparent in terms of the likelihood to dissociate. Similarly, there are no discernible differences on hypnotizability scores between males and females.

B. Age

There appears to be a negative correlation between age and the tendency to dissociate. Thus, younger individuals are more likely to dissociate. Similar findings have been documented for hypnotizability.

C. Childhood Trauma

Some studies have noted high DES scores in adults who suffered childhood trauma.

D. Different dissociative disorders have epidemiological differences. For example, while the tendency to dissociate is roughly equal in men and women, Dissociative Identity Disorder is more common in women, while Dissociative Fugue might be more common in men (see below).

V. Dissociative Amnesia (Formerly Psychogenic Amnesia)

A. Defined in DSM-IV as **"an inability to recall important personal information, usually of a traumatic nature, that is too extensive to be explained by normal forgetfulness."**

B. Dissociative Amnesia may be global, with total loss of autobiographic information, or it may be episodic, in which patients cannot recall specific episodes of behavior or traumatic experiences. These experiences may include self-mutilation, criminal or sexual behaviors, traumatic events, or even marital or financial crises.

C. Dissociative Amnesia appears to be a common short-term reaction in both men and women to severe stress, such as **civilian disasters.**

D. The **incidence** in both males and females appears roughly equal.

E. Dissociative Amnesia may occur during any age, though its **peak incidence appears in the third and fourth decades.**

F. Three-fourths of cases last **between 24 h and 5 days.**

G. Differential diagnosis includes organic syndromes (secondary to brain injuries, lesions, or seizures) as well as factitious disorders and malingering.

H. Treatment aims at restoring the missing memories, sometimes through psychotherapy and free association, but at times using hypnosis or an Amytal interview.

I. Generally speaking, patients with Dissociative Amnesia recover quickly and completely. However, many patients continue to display a propensity towards amnesia in the setting of trauma.

VI. Dissociative Fugue

A. Dissociative Fugue is characterized in the DSM-IV as **"the sudden unexpected travel away from one's place of daily activities, with inability to recall some or all of one's past."** Often, patients suffering from Dissociative Fugue will **assume entirely new identities** during their fugue episode.

B. Note that Dissociative Fugue is essentially Dissociative Amnesia **plus** travel.

C. Dissociative Fugue appears to be **more common during wartime or after natural disasters.**

D. Dissociative Fugue may be the **rarest of the dissociative disorders.**

E. Patients suffering from Dissociative Fugue may appear normal, though they often become confused and distressed when asked questions about their personal history.

F. Although men appear to be affected as often as women, **the incidence of men suffering from Dissociative Fugue increases during war.**

G. Dissociative Fugue occurs **primarily in adults, usually between the second and fourth decades.**

H. Although fugues may last from a few hours to several years, **most episodes last from a few days to a few months.**

I. **Alternative diagnoses** include brain pathology leading to fugue states, drug-induced fugues secondary to alcoholic or drug-related blackouts, and factitious disorders or malingering. In addition, some cultural syndromes (e.g., Amok and Latah) may mimic fugue states.

J. **Treatment** is similar to that for Dissociative Amnesia; the patient is helped to recall the events preceding the fugue, sometimes through hypnosis or Amytal interview.

K. **Prognosis varies.** When fugue states are of short duration, they tend to resolve spontaneously. Longer-lasting episodes may be intractable.

VII. Dissociative Identity Disorder (Formerly Multiple Personality Disorder)

Among the Dissociative Disorders, Dissociative Identity Disorder (DID) has received the most attention over the last two decades. Thus, **the majority of research focusing on Dissociative Disorders has involved DID, and the diagnosis has endured considerable controversy.** The positive aspects of this controversy involve an ongoing debate about the interplay of society on psychiatric nosology, as well as a careful re-examination of all dissociative phenomena and their relationship to consciousness and pathology.

A. **DID is defined in the DSM-IV as "the presence of two or more distinct identities or personality states (each with its own relatively enduring pattern of perceiving, relating to, and thinking about the environment and the self)."** In addition, the DSM specifies that **"at least two of these identities" must periodically "take control of the person's behavior."** Finally, there must be a demonstrated **"inability to recall important personal information that is too extensive to be explained by ordinary forgetfulness."**

B. An important aspect of DID is the **amnestic quality for alternate personalities** displayed by the primary personality. However, in many instances different personality states have varying levels of awareness of other personalities (often called **"alters"**), and often a **dominant personality state** exists that is cognizant of all of the various personalities. **The term "co-consciousness" has been used to describe the simultaneous experience of multiple entities at one time.** Thus, one personality may be aware of another's feelings regarding an ongoing experience.

C. DID is characterized by **high rates of depression,** and often by affective symptoms that constitute the presenting complaint.

D. From **one-third to one-half of cases of DID experience auditory hallucinations.** Some researchers have suggested that these hallucinations are described as **"inner voices,"** helping to differentiate these symptoms from the external voices heard by those suffering from schizophrenia and other psychotic disorders. Furthermore, in contrast to individuals suffering from schizophrenia, patients with DID are **unusually hypnotizable and do not display evidence of a formal thought disorder.**

E. **The mean number of personality states in DID is approximately 13.** However, case series have shown that the number of alternate identities may vary from one to 50.

F. DID is reported **more commonly in women than in men.**

G. Prevalence estimates range from **rare to 1%.**

H. A number of **somatic symptoms may accompany DID,** including **headaches, gastrointestinal distress, and genitourinary disturbances.** In addition, there is an increased rate of **conversion disorders, pseudo-seizures, and self-mutilation.** Finally, a number of **personality disorders,** including Borderline Personality Disorder, are associated with DID.

I. DID is usually diagnosed in the **third or fourth decade,** though those suffering from DID usually report symptoms during childhood and adolescence. Most case series document a chronic, fluctuating course, characterized by relapse and remission. Making the diagnosis of DID in a particular patient is not without controversy. Some clinicians have proposed that the diagnosis must be persistently pursued if a patient's symptoms even subtly hint at the possibility of dissociation. These clinicians describe patients who are either unaware of, or who wish to hide their disorder, and need to be "educated" about DID. Critics contend that patients with DID are highly suggestible and that clinicians "create" such patients by "suggesting" symptoms. The critics emphasize that the symptoms are reinforced by clinicians showing interest and enthusiasm in the multiplicity of personalities.

J. Extended psychotherapy remains the treatment of choice, although approaches vary widely and remain controversial. Some clinicians describe specialized treatment for DID, including delineating and mapping the alters, inviting each to participate in the treatment, and facilitating communication between the various alters. Through careful exploration of all alternate identities, clinicians attempt to understand past episodes of trauma as experienced by each personality. Hypnosis is sometimes employed to reach dissociated states. Other clinicians focus on the function of the dissociative process in the here-and-now of the patient's life and the ongoing treatment. They help patients become aware of using dissociation to manage feelings and thoughts within themselves and to manage the closeness and distance within relationships. All approaches seek to increase affect tolerance and to integrate the dissociated states within the patient.

K. Psychopharmacologic treatments, such as **antidepressants and anxiolytics,** are often useful in treating the commonly accompanying complaints of depression and anxiety. However, no pharmacological treatment has been found to reduce dissociation per se. Benzodiazepenes reduce anxiety but can also exacerbate dissociation. Although not routinely used for dissociative disorders, neuroleptics are sometimes employed in patients who are grossly disorganized; they should be used in the lowest possible doses and be discontinued if they are unhelpful.

VIII. Depersonalization Disorder

A. According to the DSM-IV, Depersonalization Disorder is characterized by **"persistent or recurrent episodes . . . of detachment or estrangement from one's self."** Often, patients with symptoms of depersonalization will **"feel like an automaton or like he or she is living in a movie."**

B. Reality testing is intact in those who suffer from Depersonalization Disorder. This represents an important distinction from other psychotic disorders.

C. Transient depersonalization is common; such events are not considered pathological. Studies have suggested that as many as 50% of people will at some point endorse transient symptoms.

D. Transient depersonalization occurs equally in both men and women. However, Depersonalization Disorder is much rarer than is transient depersonalization; it occurs roughly twice as often in women.

E. Depersonalization Disorder usually **begins by late adolescence or early adulthood.**

F. Most **episodes last from hours to weeks.**

G. Differential diagnosis includes depression and psychosis, as well as illicit drug ingestion and iatrogenic drug effects. Brain pathology, such as seizures, migraines, or discrete lesions, may lead to depersonalization.

H. Treatment is difficult, and **patients are often refractory to intervention.** Treating accompanying psychiatric conditions, such as depression or anxiety, may help. As with other dissociative disorders, exploration of past traumatic events may prove useful.

IX. Dissociative Disorder Not Otherwise Specified

A. This category is reserved for presentations in which the predominant feature is dissociation without meeting clear criteria for any specific dissociative disorder.

B. Examples include patients who experience **derealization** (the quality of perceiving previously familiar objects in the external world as strange and unfamiliar) but not depersonalization, or patients with ill-defined alternate personalities. In addition, symptoms that result from torture or brainwashing may be classified in this category.

C. Ganser's syndrome (sometimes called **Prison Psychosis**) is classified as a Dissociative Disorder Not Otherwise Specified. It is characterized by the provision of approximate answers, i.e., offering half-correct answers to simple inquiries, such as answering "5" to the question, "What is two plus two?" The correct set of the response is given, but the answer is inaccurate. Ganser's syndrome is often reported in incarcerated populations.

D. Culture-bound syndromes, such as **Amok** in Indonesia or **Latah** in Malaysia, are often characterized by dissociation and sometimes by violence. These syndromes have been included in the DSM-IV as Dissociative Disorder Not Otherwise Specified.

X. Factitious or Malingering Dissociative Disorders

A. Feigned dissociative symptoms may be more common than previously realized. A 1994 case series suggested that as many as 10% of patients with symptoms of DID in fact suffered from

factitious dissociative symptoms. The motivation in this series appeared to be the **assumption of the sick role,** consistent with other presentations of factitious disorders.

B. Case reports detail dissociative symptoms expressed as a form of **malingering.** In these episodes, individuals feign dissociative symptoms for reasons other than assuming the sick role, such as **avoiding criminal or financial responsibilities.**

C. **Individuals attempting to feign dissociative symptoms are often extremely invested in the diagnosis of DID.** They may express their symptoms only when they feel they are being observed or heard, and they may refuse collateral interviews with other individuals in which the clinician attempts to gather additional information. One study suggested that approximately 50% of those with feigned DID admit their simulation of dissociation to a caretaker. Additionally, individuals who simulate these symptoms may have substantially more exposure to popular and scientific explorations of dissociation than do those with genuine dissociative disorders.

XI. Dissociative Trance Disorder

A. This is **not currently a formal classification,** but is listed in the DSM-IV as "Criteria Sets and Axes Provided for Further Study."

B. Dissociative Trance Disorder might include apparent episodes of **demonic possession** or **religious ecstasy.** The feeling of being possessed is reportedly commonly in those who feel guilty about perceived transgressions. Examples might involve an individual who is unfaithful to his spouse and who becomes convinced that demonic possession is responsible for his infidelity.

C. It is important to rule out psychosis, malingering, or factitious disorder when considering this category.

Suggested Readings

Coons PM: The dissociative disorders. Rarely considered and underdiagnosed. *Psychiatr Clin North Am* 1998; 21:637–648.

Nehmiah JC: Dissociative disorders. In Kaplan HI, Sadock BJ (eds): *Comprehensive Textbook of Psychiatry*, 6th ed. Baltimore: Williams and Wilkins, 1995:1281–1293.

Putnum FW: Dissociative phenomena. In Tasman A, Goldfinger SM (eds): *American Psychiatric Press Review of Psychiatry*, Vol. 10. Washington, DC: American Psychiatric Press, 1991:145–160.

Chapter 20
Sexual Disorders and Sexual Dysfunction

LINDA SHAFER

I. Introduction

A. Sexual Problems Occur Frequently and Cause Great Distress
1. 43% of women and 31% of men have experienced some form of sexual dysfunction.
2. 50% of American couples suffer from some type of sexual problem.
3. 24% of Americans will experience a sexual dysfunction at some time in their lives.
4. The primary care physician (PCP) is often the first to see the patient with sexual problems.

B. The *Diagnostic and Statistical Manual of Mental Disorders, Fourth Edition* (DSM-IV) divides sexual disorders into two groups:
1. Sexual dysfunctions: psychophysiologic impairment of sexual desire and/or of the sexual response cycle.
2. Paraphilias: recurrent, intense sexual urges or behaviors that cause marked distress and that involve unusual objects or activities.

II. Evaluation of the Problem: Sexual Dysfunction

A. General Recommendations
1. Sexual dysfunction is best understood by having knowledge of the stages of the normal sexual response, which vary with age and with physical status.
   a. **The four-step model (Masters and Johnson)**
      i. Excitement: arousal.
      ii. Plateau: the phase of maximum arousal prior to orgasm.
      iii. Orgasm: a stage that involves muscular contractions at 0.8 s intervals.
      iv. Resolution: a phase leading to a return to baseline.
      v. Refractory period: in men, a stage which increases with age; in women, there is no refractory period.
   b. **The triphasic model (Kaplan)**
      i. Desire.
      ii. Excitement (arousal): a vascular phenomenon, caused by innervation of the parasympathetic nervous system (2nd, 3rd, and 4th sacral segments of the spinal cord).
      iii. Orgasm: a muscular reaction, caused by innervation of the sympathetic nervous system, whose reflex center is in the lumbar cord.
   c. **Changes in the sexual response associated with aging**
      i. Males are slower to achieve an erection and need more direct stimulation to the penis to achieve an erection.
      ii. Females have decreased levels of estrogen which leads to less vaginal lubrication and to narrowing of the vagina.
   d. **Medications, diseases, injuries, and psychological conditions can affect the sexual response in any of its component phases, and lead to different dysfunctional syndromes** (Table 20-1).
      i. Several types of sexual dysfunction can coexist.
      ii. One sexual dysfunction can be the cause of another.
      iii. A primary sexual dysfunction is one that has been present since the onset of sexual activity.
      iv. A secondary sexual dysfunction is one that occurs after a period of normal functioning.

B. Medical History
1. Although most sexual disorders were thought to have a psychological basis, newer diagnostic testing has identified more conditions having an organic etiology.
2. **Most sexual disorders are multicausal and share a mixed etiology.**
3. Physical disorders, surgical disorders (Table 20-2), use of medications, and drug use or abuse (Table 20-3), can affect sexual functioning directly and/or cause secondary psychological reactions which can cause a sexual problem.
   a. **Sexual dysfunction is a common side effect, which occurs in more than 30% of patients taking a selective serotonin reuptake inhibitor (SSRI).**
      i. Treatment strategies include use of cyproheptadine, bupropion, yohimbine, amantadine, buspirone, sildenafil, ginkgo biloba, and/or a drug holiday.
4. Psychological causes of sexual disorders are complex; they range from superficial issues (e.g., fear of failure) to deep ones (e.g., profound depression).
   a. No direct correlation has been found between specific background factors and certain sexual dysfunctions.
   b. Predisposing, precipitating, and maintaining factors play a role in sexual problems (Table 20-4).

C. Taking a Sexual History
1. Be aware that patients are usually embarrassed to bring up and discuss sexual problems.

Table 20-1. Classification of Sexual Dysfunctions

Impaired Sexual Response Phase	Female	Male
Desire	Hypoactive sexual desire Sexual aversion	Hypoactive sexual desire Sexual aversion
Excitement (arousal, vascular)	Sexual arousal disorder	Erectile disorder
Orgasm (muscular)	Orgasmic disorder	Orgasmic disorder Premature ejaculation
Sexual pain	Dyspareunia Vaginismus	Dyspareunia

Table 20-2. Medical and Surgical Conditions Causing Sexual Dysfunctions

Organic Disorders	Sexual Impairment
Endocrine Hypothyroidism, adrenal dysfunction, hypogonadism, diabetes mellitus	Low libido, impotence, decreased vaginal lubrication, early impotence
Vascular Hypertension, atherosclerosis, stroke, venous insufficiency, sickle cell disorder	Impotence, ejaculation and libido intact
Neurologic Spinal cord damage, diabetic neuropathy, herniated lumbar disc, alcoholic neuropathy, multiple sclerosis, temporal lobe epilepsy	Impotence, impaired orgasm Sexual disorder-early sign, low libido (or high libido)
Local genital disease Male: Priapism, Peyronie's disease, urethritis, prostatitis, hydrocele	Low libido, impotence
Female: Imperforate hymen, vaginitis, pelvic inflammatory disease, endometriosis	Vaginismus, dyspareunia, low libido, decreased arousal
Systemic debilitating disease Renal, pulmonary, or hepatic diseases, advanced malignancies, infections	Low libido, impotence, decreased arousal
Surgical-postoperative states Male: Prostatectomy (radical perineal) abdominal-perineal bowel resection	Impotence, no loss of libido, ejaculatory impairment
Female: Episiotomy, vaginal repair of prolapse, oophorectomy	Dyspareunia, vaginismus, decreased lubrication
Male and female: Amputation (leg), colostomy and ileostomy	Mechanical difficulties in sex, low self-image, fear of odor

Table 20-3. Drugs and Medicines Causing Sexual Dysfunction

Drug	Sexual Side Effect
Cardiovascular	
Methyldopa	Low libido, impotence, anorgasmia
Thiazide diuretics	Low libido, impotence, decreased lubrication
Clonidine	Impotence, anorgasmia
Propranolol	Low libido
Digoxin	Gynecomastia, low libido impotence
Clofibrate	Low libido, impotence
Psychotropics	
Sedatives	
Alcohol	Higher doses cause sexual problems
Barbiturates	Impotence
Anxiolytics	
Diazepam	Low libido, delayed
Alprazolam	ejaculation
Antipsychotics	
Thioridazine	Retarded or retrograde ejaculation
Haloperidol	Low libido, impotence, anorgasmia
Antidepressants	
MAOIs (phenelzine)	Impotence, retarded ejaculation, anorgasmia
Tricyclics (imipramine)	Low libido, impotence, retarded ejaculation
SSRIs (fluoxetine, sertraline)	Low libido, impotence, retarded ejaculation
Atypical (trazodone)	Priapism, retarded or retrograde ejaculation
Lithium	Low libido, impotence
Hormones	
Estrogen	Low libido in men
Progesterone	Low libido, impotence
Gastrointestinal	
Cimetidine	Low libido, impotence
Methantheline bromide	Impotence
Opiates	Orgasmic dysfunction
Anticonvulsants	Low libido, impotence, priapism

2. Remember that physicians, too, are often uncomfortable discussing sexual issues, in part because of fears of offending patients.

3. **Ask routine screening questions as part of the medical history to give the patient a chance to talk about sexual problems;** for example:
   a. Is there anything you would like to change about your sex life?
   b. Have there been any changes in your sex life?
   c. Are you satisfied with your present sex life?

4. **Additional routine questions to ask during the AIDS era include:**
   a. Are you sexually active?
   b. Do you practice safe(r) sex?
      i. Lack of knowledge of safe sex practices can contribute to the spread of AIDS.
      ii. Physicians should be prepared to discuss the benefits of safe sex techniques, including the use of condoms and spermicides that contain nonoxynol-9.
      iii. Failure to ask AIDS screening questions may result in complaints of inadequate treatment or a malpractice suit.

5. **Interview techniques**
   a. Attempt to be sensitive and nonjudgmental.
   b. Move from the more general to more specific topics, in an appropriate context.
      i. Sexual issues can be integrated easily into the medical history during review of the systems, when discussing the initiation or introduction of a new medication, or when the chief complaint involves a gynecological or urological problem.
      ii. Physicians should be aware of covert presentations of sexual problems (e.g., headache, insomnia, and low back or generalized pelvic pain) that have no apparent medical basis.
   c. Vary questions depending on the patient's age, social class/occupation, and the nature of the patient's continuing relationship with you.
   d. Design the taking of the sexual history to fit the patient's needs and your time.
   e. If a sexual problem is uncovered, take a detailed history.
      i. Determine its onset.
      ii. Establish its progression. How often? With all partners? On masturbation? With fantasy?
      iii. Complete an assessment. Avoid use of "why" questions because this tends to make a patient feel defensive. Use "what" questions (e.g., "What do you think caused your problems?").
      iv. Ask about attempts at resolution of the problem. Did they read or seek advice from books, friends, or clergy?
      v. Clarify the patient's expectations and goals. Do they wish to resolve the problem, save their marriage, or use the problem as an excuse for divorce?

Table 20-4. Psychological Causes of Sexual Dysfunction

Predisposing factors
Lack of information/experience
Unrealistic expectations
Negative family attitudes to sex
Sexual trauma: rape, incest

Precipitating factors
Childbirth
Infidelity
Dysfunction in the partner

Maintaining factors
Interpersonal issues
Family stress
Work stress
Financial problems
Depression
Performance anxiety
Gender identity conflicts

D. Examination of the Patient
1. **Physical examination**
   a. A thorough physical examination is indicated on every patient, with special attention paid to endocrine, vascular, neurological, urological, and gynecological systems.
2. **Laboratory examination**
   a. The extent of the laboratory examination depends on the nature of the problem.
   b. The extent of the laboratory examination depends on one's index of suspicion (i.e., is it organic or psychological).
   c. The sexual history and physical examination together help determine the extent of the organic workup, including what special laboratory studies and diagnostic procedures should be performed.
      i. Screening for unrecognized systemic disease should include a complete blood count (CBC), a urinalysis, a creatinine level, a lipid profile, thyroid function studies, and a fasting blood sugar (FBS).
      ii. Relevant endocrine studies for assessment of low libido and erectile dysfunction include levels of testosterone, prolactin, luteinizing hormone (LH), and follicular stimulating hormone (FSH).
      iii. An estrogen level and microscopic examination of a vaginal smear for vaginal dryness should be obtained.
      iv. A sedimentation rate, a cervical culture, and a Pap (Papanicolaou) smear should be obtained for evaluation of dyspareunia.
      v. Diagnostic tests for erectile functioning include nocturnal penile tumescence (NPT) studies, ultrasonography, and angiography.
   d. Referral to a specialist in urology, gynecology, endocrinology, neurology, and/or psychiatry is made on a case by case basis.

III. Psychiatric Differential Diagnosis of Sexual Disorders

A. Depression (Major Depression or Dysthymic Disorder)
1. Consider low libido, or erectile dysfunction.
B. Manic Phase (Bipolar Disorder)
1. Consider increased libido.
C. Generalized Anxiety Disorder, Panic Disorder, Posttraumatic Stress Disorder
1. Consider low libido, erectile dysfunction, lack of vaginal lubrication, or anorgasmia.
D. Obsessive-Compulsive Disorder
1. Consider "anti-fantasies" that focus on the negative aspects of a partner.
2. Consider low libido, erectile dysfunction, lack of vaginal lubrication, or anorgasmia.
E. Schizophrenia
1. Consider low desire, or bizarre sexual desires.
F. Paraphilias
1. Consider deviant sexual arousal.
G. Gender Identity Disorder
1. Consider dissatisfaction with one's own sexual preference or phenotype.
H. Personality Disorder (Passive-Aggressive, Obsessive-Compulsive, Histrionic)
1. Consider low libido, erectile dysfunction, premature ejaculation, or anorgasmia.
I. Marital Dysfunction/Interpersonal Problems
J. Fears of Intimacy/Commitment
1. Consider deep, intrapsychic issues.
2. Consider a range of sexual disorders, including a lack of vaginal lubrication, and erectile dysfunction.

IV. Diagnostic Criteria

A. Sexual disorders not caused by organic factors (medical conditions, medications, or drugs of abuse) or by another (psychological) Axis I disorder, all of which cause marked individual distress and/or interpersonal difficulties.
1. **Desire phase disorders in males and females**
   a. Hypoactive Sexual Desire Disorder (302.71 DSM-IV)

i. Hypoactive sexual desire disorder is a condition with persistently deficient sexual fantasies and an infrequent desire for sexual activity.

ii. Its incidence has increased from 37%, in the early 1970s, to 55% in the early 1980s.

iii. The lifetime prevalence of this condition is 40% in women and 30% in men.

b. **Sexual Aversion Disorder** (302.79 DSM-IV)

i. Sexual aversion disorder is a condition with a persistent and extreme aversion to, and avoidance of, all or almost all genital sexual contact with the sexual partner.

ii. Its exact incidence is unknown, but it is common.

iii. Primary sexual aversion is higher in men, but secondary aversion is higher in women.

iv. The syndrome is associated with phobic avoidance of sexual activity and/or the thought of sexual activity.

v. One-fourth of those with this condition also meet criteria for panic disorder.

vi. Affected individuals engage in intercourse once or twice a year.

vii. Patients tend to respond naturally to sexual relations if they can get past their high anxiety and initial dread.

2. **Arousal phase disorders**

a. **Female Sexual Arousal Disorder** (302.72 DSM-IV)

i. Female sexual arousal disorder is a condition with the persistent inability to attain or maintain the lubrication/swelling response of sexual excitement until completion of the sexual act.

ii. Its lifetime prevalence is 60%.

iii. The condition is linked to problems with sexual desire.

iv. A lack of vaginal lubrication may lead to dyspareunia.

b. **Male Erectile Disorder** (302.72 DSM-IV)

i. Male erectile disorder is a condition involving the inability to attain or maintain a satisfactory erection until completion of sexual activity.

ii. 10–20 million American men suffer from erectile dysfunction.

iii. Between 50% and 85% of cases of erectile dysfunction have an organic basis (see Table 20-5 for risk factors).

iv. Primary (lifelong) erectile dysfunction occurs in 1% of men under the age of 35 years.

v. Secondary (acquired) erectile dysfunction is manifest by the inability to achieve successful intercourse in 25% of attempts; it occurs in 40% of men over the age of 60 years, and increases to 73% in men who are 80 years old.

vi. Erectile dysfunction may be generalized (i.e., it occurs in all circumstances).

vii. Erectile dysfunction may be situational (i.e., it is limited to certain types of stimulation, situations, and partners).

3. **Orgasm phase disorders**

a. **Female Orgasmic Disorder** (302.73 DSM-IV)

Table 20-5. Risk Factors Associated with Erectile Dysfunction
Hypertension
Diabetes mellitus
Smoking
Coronary artery disease
Peripheral vascular disorders
Blood lipid abnormalities
Peyronie's disease
Priapism
Pelvic trauma or surgery
Renal failure and dialysis
Hypogonadism
Alcoholism
Depression
Lack of sexual knowledge
Poor sexual technique
Interpersonal problems

i. Female orgasmic disorder is a condition involving a persistent delay in, or absence of, orgasm, following a normal excitement phase.

ii. Female orgasmic disorder is the most common type of female sexual dysfunction; its lifetime prevalence is 35%.

iii. 5–8% of afflicted individuals are totally anorgasmic.

iv. 30–40% of afflicted individuals are unable to achieve orgasm without clitoral stimulation during intercourse.

v. The ability to reach orgasm increases with sexual experience.

vi. The diagnosis should *not* be made for women who can experience an orgasm with direct clitoral contact, but who find it difficult to reach orgasm during intercourse. This is a normal variant.

vii. Claims that stimulation of the Grafenberg spot, or G spot, in a region in the anterior wall of the vagina will cause orgasm and female ejaculation have never been substantiated.

viii. Consider that the male sexual partner with premature ejaculation is contributing to female orgasmic dysfunction.

b. **Male Orgasmic Disorder** (302.74 DSM-IV)

i. Male orgasmic disorder is a condition with a persistent delay in, or absence of, orgasm following a normal sexual excitement phase.

ii. It is an infrequent disorder with a lifetime prevalence of 2%; it occurs in men who are usually under the age of 35 years and who are sexually inexperienced.

iii. Retarded ejaculation is usually restricted to failure to reach orgasm in the vagina during intercourse.

iv. Orgasm can usually occur with masturbation and/or from a partner's manual or oral stimulation.

v. The condition must be differentiated from **retrograde ejaculation,** where the bladder neck does not close off properly during orgasm, causing semen to spurt backwards into the bladder.

vi. One must rule out retarded ejaculation in a couple presenting with infertility of unknown cause. The male may not have admitted his lack of ejaculation to his partner.

c. **Premature Ejaculation** (302.75 DSM-IV)

i. Premature ejaculation is a condition involving persistent ejaculation with minimal stimulation before or after penetration and before the person wishes it.

ii. The lifetime prevalence of premature ejaculation is 15%.

iii. With the condition, ejaculation usually occurs in less than 2 min or with fewer than ten thrusts.

iv. Premature ejaculation is the most common male sexual disorder, affecting 30% of men.

v. Prolonged periods of no sexual activity make premature ejaculation worse.

vi. If the problem is chronic and untreated, secondary impotence often occurs.

4. **Sexual pain disorders**

a. **Dyspareunia** (302.76 DSM-IV)

i. Dyspareunia involves persistent genital pain before, during, or after sexual intercourse in either the male or the female.

ii. The prevalence of dyspareunia is 15% in females, and 5% in males.

iii. Patients with dyspareunia often seek out medical treatment, but the physical examination is often unremarkable, without genital abnormalities.

iv. If pain is caused solely by vaginismus or a lack of lubrication, the diagnosis of dyspareunia is *not* made.

b. **Vaginismus** (306.51 DSM-IV)

i. Vaginismus is the persistent involuntary spasm of the musculature of the outer third of the vagina that interferes with sexual intercourse.

ii. The frequency of vaginismus is unknown, but probably accounts for less than 10% of female sexual disorders.

iii. The diagnosis of vaginismus is often made on routine gynecologic examination, when contraction of the vaginal outlet occurs as either the examining finger or a speculum is introduced.

iv. There is a high incidence of associated pelvic pathology with vaginismus.

v. Lifelong vaginismus has an abrupt onset, at the first attempt at penetration, and has a chronic course.

vi. Acquired vaginismus may occur suddenly, following a sexual trauma or a medical condition.

5. **Sexual Dysfunction Not Otherwise Specified** (302.70 DSM-IV)

a. Sexual dysfunction not otherwise specified is a condition without subjective erotic feelings despite otherwise normal arousal and orgasm (female analog of premature ejaculation).

b. It is unclear whether the sexual dysfunction is primary, due to a medical condition, or is substance-induced.

V. Treatment Strategies

A. Organically Based Sexual Disorders

1. **Medical-surgical treatments**

a. Treat pre-existing illnesses (e.g., diabetes).

b. Stop, or substitute for, offending medications.

c. Reduce alcohol and/or smoking.

d. Add medications for psychiatric conditions (e.g., depression).

e. Correct hormone deficiencies (e.g., testosterone for hypogonadism, thyroid hormone for hypothyroidism, estrogen/testosterone (Estratest) for postmenopausal females, or bromocriptine for elevated prolactin after neuroimaging of the pituitary).

f. Initiate a trial of fluoxetine, sertraline, paroxetine, or clomipramine for premature ejaculation.

g. Initiate a pharmacologic erection program (PEP) (e.g., alprostadil intracavernosal injections [Cavarject]).

h. Consider transurethral penile suppository of alprostadil (MUSE) for erectile dysfunction.

i. Consider use of an external penile suction device for erectile disorders.

j. Prescribe oral medicine for erectile dysfunction.

i. Consider use of sildenafil (Viagra).

ii. Be prepared to administer apomorphine, which is under FDA review.

iii. Be prepared to administer phentolamine (Vasomax), which is under FDA review.

iv. Prescribe yohimbine (Yocon).

k. Initiate a topical impotence medication, including alprostadil cream (Topiglan), minoxidil solution, or a nitroglycerine ointment, under investigation.

l. Use the above medications (j. and k.) for female sexual dysfunction, which are currently under investigation.

m. Perform surgery for vascular problems (e.g., endarterectomy).

n. Implant a penile prosthetic device.

B. Psychologically Based Sexual Disorders

1. **General principles**

a. If time is limited, schedule another appointment to take a detailed sexual history and to initiate treatment.

b. Conduct discussions about sex in the office, while the patient is fully clothed, *not* in the examining room.

c. Use the pelvic exam to teach the female patient about sexual anatomy.

d. **Use the PLISSIT model** to recall the levels of treatment.

i. **P:** permission. Help reassure the patient regarding sexual activity. Alleviate guilt about activities that a patient feels are "bad" or "dirty." Use statistics to reinforce the range of normal activities.

ii. **LI:** limited information. Provide information about anatomy and physiology. Correct myths and misconceptions.

iii. **SS:** specific suggestions. Apply behavioral techniques used in sex therapy. There are general principles and specific techniques for each of the sexual dyfunctions.

iv. **IT:** intensive therapy. Patients with chronic sexual problems and/or complex psychologic issues may not respond to the above and may benefit from consultation with a mental health professional, skilled in dealing with sexual problems.

2. **Behavior therapy (sex therapy): general principles**
   a. Improve communication between partners verbally and physically.
   b. Encourage experimentation.
   c. Decrease the pressure of performance by changing the goal of sexual activity away from erection or orgasm to feeling good about oneself.
   d. Relieve the pressure of the moment by suggesting there is always another day to try.

3. **Behavior therapy (sex therapy): specific suggestions**
   a. **Hypoactive sexual disorder**
      i. Behavioral treatment for hypoactive sexual disorder may include initiation of sensate focus exercises (non-demand pleasuring techniques) to enhance enjoyment without pressure.
      ii. Use erotic material.
      iii. Consider masturbation training with fantasy to help individuals become aware of conditions necessary for a positive sexual experience.
   b. **Sexual aversion disorder**
      i. Behavioral treatments for sexual aversion disorder are the same as for hypoactive sexual desire.
      ii. When the phobic/panic-type symptoms are displayed, the addition of antipanic medication (antianxiety or antidepressant) may be helpful.
   c. **Female sexual arousal disorder**
      i. Female sexual arousal disorder usually requires referral to a specialist.
      ii. It is helpful to suggest the use of lubrication, such as saliva or KY jelly, for vaginal dryness.
      iii. Postmenopausal women may benefit from topical estrogen cream, given intermittently.
   d. **Male erectile disorder**
      i. Prescribe "sensate focus" exercises.
      ii. Prohibit intercourse, even if erection occurs.
      iii. Prescribe the female superior position (female on top of male) to attempt nondemanding intercourse (heterosexual couple). The female manually stimulates the penis and if erection is obtained she inserts the penis into her vagina and gradual movement is begun.
      iv. Educate the patient about ways to satisfy his partner without penile-vaginal intercourse.

v. Drug therapy (medication, injection, suppository) can be beneficial to restore confidence while exploring psychological issues.

e. **Female orgasmic disorder**
   i. For women who have never had an orgasm suggest self-stimulation, use of fantasy material, and Kegel vaginal exercises (contraction of pubococcygeus muscles).
   ii. For the woman who is anorgastic with her partner, recommend sensate focus exercises (from nongenital stimulation to genital stimulation). Use a back-protected position (male in seated position with female between his legs with back against his chest). Use controlled intercourse in the female superior position.
   iii. If the woman is anorgastic during intercourse, use the "bridge technique," in which male stimulates the female's clitoris manually after insertion of the penis into the vagina.

f. **Male orgasmic disorder (during intercourse)**
   i. When male orgasmic disorder is present, have the female stimulate the male manually until orgasm becomes inevitable.
   ii. Insert the penis into the vagina and begin thrusting.
   iii. Manual stimulation is repeated if ejaculation does not occur.

g. **Premature ejaculation**
   i. When premature ejaculation is present, suggest an increase in the frequency of sex.
   ii. Teach the "squeeze" technique, in which the female manually stimulates the penis. When ejaculation is approaching, as indicated by the male, the female squeezes the penis with her thumb on the frenulum. The pressure is applied until the male no longer feels the urge to ejaculate (15–60 s). Use the female superior position with gradual thrusting and the "squeeze" technique as excitement intensifies.
   iii. "Stop-start" method is an alternative to the "squeeze" technique. The female stimulates the male to the point of ejaculation then stops the stimulation. She resumes the stimulation for several stop-start procedures, until ejaculation is allowed to occur.

h. **Dyspareunia**
   i. Treat any underlying gynecologic problem first.
   ii. Treat insufficient lubrication as described above.
   iii. Treat accompanying vaginismus as described below.

i. **Vaginismus**
   i. When vaginismus is present, the female is encouraged to accept larger and larger objects into her vagina (e.g., her fingers, her partner's fingers, Hegar graduated vaginal dilators, syringe containers of different sizes).
   ii. Recommend the use of the female superior position, allowing the female to gradually insert the erect penis into the vagina.

iii. Use extra lubricant (KY jelly).
iv. Practice Kegel vaginal exercises to develop a sense of control.

VI. Evaluation of the Problem: Paraphilias

A. General Recommendations

1. Definition. Paraphilias are manifest by recurrent, intense sexually arousing fantasies, sexual urges, or behaviors, involving non-human objects, or the suffering or humiliation of oneself or one's partner, children or other nonconsenting persons that occur over a period of at least 6 months (see Table 20-6).
2. The diagnosis should only be made if the individual has acted on the urges or is markedly distressed by them.
3. Some individuals may always need paraphiliac fantasies for erotic arousal.
4. Some individuals have paraphiliac preferences only during periods of stress.
5. Paraphilias almost always occur in males.
6. Paraphilia replaces the older terms "perversion" and "sexual deviation."

Table 20-6. Diagnostic Criteria of Specific Paraphilias

Disorder (DSM-IV Code)	Definition	Features
Exhibitionism (302.4)	Exposure of genitals to unsuspecting strangers in public.	Primary intent is to evoke shock or fear in victims. Offenders are usually male.
Fetishism (302.81)	Sexual arousal using nonliving objects (e.g., female lingerie).	Masturbation occurs while holding the fetish object. The sexual partner may wear the object.
Frotteurism (302.89)	Sexual arousal by touching and rubbing against a nonconsenting person.	The behavior occurs in a crowded public place from which the offender can escape arrest.
Pedophilia (302.2)	Sexual activity with a prepubescent child. The patient must be at least 16 years of age and be 5 years older than the victim.	Pedophilia is the most common paraphilia. Most of the victims are girls. Victims are often relatives. Most pedophiles are heterosexual.
Sexual Masochism (302.83)	Sexual pleasure comes from physical or mental abuse or humiliation.	A dangerous form is hypoxyphilia, where oxygen deprivation enhances arousal, and accidental deaths can occur.
Sexual Sadism (302.84)	Sexual arousal is derived from causing mental or physical suffering to another person.	Sexual sadism is mostly seen in men. It can progress to rape. 50% of those afflicted are alcoholic.
Transvestic Fetishism (302.3)	Cross-dressing in heterosexual males for sexual arousal.	The wife (partner) may be aware of the activity and help in the selection of clothes or insist on treatment.
Voyeurism (302.82)	Sexual arousal by watching an unsuspecting person who is naked, disrobing, or engaging in sexual activity.	Most commonly occurs in men, but it can occur in women. Masturbation commonly occurs. A variant is telephone sex.
Paraphilia Not Otherwise Specified (302.9)	Paraphilias that do not meet criteria for any of the above categories.	Categories include: necrophilia (corpses), zoophilia (animals), urophilia (urine), and coprophilia (feces).

7. Paraphilias may have legal and societal significance, as they may involve nonconsenting partners.

8. A strong association exists between paraphilia and childhood attention deficit hyperactivity disorder (ADHD).

9. A strong association exists between paraphilia and substance abuse (64%), major depression or dysthymia (39%), and phobic disorder (42%).

B. Medical History

1. **Most paraphilias are thought to have a psychological basis.**
   a. Individuals with paraphilias have difficulty forming more socialized sexual relationships.
   b. Paraphilias may involve a conditioned response in which nonsexual objects become sexually arousing when paired with a pleasurable activity (masturbation).

2. **A medical evaluation should be completed to rule out endocrine and neurologic etiologies,** as well as reactions to medications, to drug use, or to drug abuse.

3. **An organic diagnosis underlying a paraphilia should be suspected when:**
   a. The behavior begins in middle age or later.
   b. There is regression from a previously normal sexuality.
   c. There is excessive aggression.
   d. There are reports of auras or seizure-like symptoms prior to or during the sexual behavior.
   e. There is an abnormal body habitus.
   f. There is an abnormal neurologic examination.

C. Sexual History

1. Most people with paraphilias will not spontaneously reveal their behavior and are very secretive about their sexual activities.

2. Many people when questioned will not admit to a paraphilia because of the illegal nature of the behavior and the impact of the behavior on close relationships.

3. Individuals with paraphilias may first come to the attention of others after their arrest by police.

4. A variety of interview techniques exists.
   a. Use screening questions that will not sound judgmental.
      i. When you want to be sexual, do you engage in sexual activity that other people find unusual?
   b. Appreciate the patient's shame and embarrassment when discussing atypical sexual behavior.
   c. Alert the patient of legal reporting requirements if sexual behavior is harmful or illegal (children in need of protection).
   d. If the sexual behavior is not illegal or harmful, assure the patient of confidentiality.
   e. When one form of atypical sexual behavior is found, ask about others in the same individual.

D. Examination of the Patient

1. Perform an appropriate physical examination.

2. Perform an appropriate laboratory examination.
   a. Penile plethysmography is used to assess paraphilias by measuring an individual's sexual arousal in response to visual and auditory stimuli.

VII. Psychiatric Differential Diagnosis of Paraphilias

A. **Mental retardation**

B. **Dementia**

C. **Substance intoxication**

D. **Manic episode (bipolar disorder)**

E. **Schizophrenia**

F. **Obsessive-compulsive disorder**

G. **Gender identity disorder**

H. **Personality disorder**

I. **Sexual dysfunction**

J. **Nonparaphiliac Compulsive Sexual Behaviors**
   1. Compulsive use of erotic videos, magazines, cybersex
   2. Uncontrolled masturbation
   3. Unrestrained use of prostitutes
   4. Numerous brief, superficial sexual affairs

K. **Hypersexuality/sexual addiction**

VIII. Diagnostic Criteria

A. **Disorders may begin in childhood or early adolescence and become better defined during adolescence or adulthood. The disorders are chronic and lifelong, but fantasies and behaviors often diminish with advancing age. The behaviors increase in response to psychosocial stress, other mental disorders, and an increased opportunity to engage in the paraphilia (see Table 20-6).**

IX. Treatment Strategies

A. **General Considerations**
   1. **People with paraphilias rarely seek treatment, unless forced by their arrest or by their discovery by a family member.**
   2. The paraphilia produces intense pleasure and is difficult to give up; it is like an addiction or compulsion.
   3. Paraphiliacs in therapy often try to convince therapists that their behavior has stopped, when actually it continues.
   4. Treatment outcome for paraphilias is poor, and recidivism is high.
   5. Treatment requires active monitoring.

B. **Specific Techniques**
   1. **Psychotherapy:** insight oriented, supportive
      a. Psychotherapy is relatively ineffective for paraphilias.

2. **Behavior therapy**
   a. Aversive therapy is used to reduce the behavior by conditioning.
   b. Desensitization is used to neutralize anxiety of non-paraphiliac sexual situations by gradual exposure.
   c. Social skills training (individual or group) is used to help form better interpersonal relationships.
   d. Orgasmic reconditioning is used to teach the paraphiliac to become aroused by more acceptable mental imagery.
3. **Medications**
   a. Antiandrogen drugs
      i. Intramuscular injections of medroxyprogesterone acetate (MPA) and cyproterone (not FDA-approved) acetate lower testosterone levels by competitive inhibition of androgen receptors and thus decrease aberrant sexual tendencies.
      ii. Intramuscular injections of leuprolide (approved for treatment of prostatic cancer) and triptorelin (although not FDA-approved), synthetic gonadotropin-releasing hormone analogs, decreases testosterone to castrate level (after an initial transient increase) and may completely abolish deviant sexual tendencies.
      iii. Use of oral estrogen (ethinyl estradiol) has a lower success rate.
   b. Antidepressant drugs
      i. Clomipramine and the selective serotonin reuptake inhibitors (SSRIs), including fluoxetine, setraline, and fluvoxamine, may lower aberrant sexual urges by decreasing compulsivity/impulsivity of the act.

Suggested Readings

American Psychiatric Association: *Diagnostic and Statistical Manual of Mental Disorders, Fourth Edition: Primary Care Version*. Washington, DC: American Psychiatric Association, 1995.

Crenshaw TL, Goldberg JP: *Sexual Pharmacology*. New York: W Norton, 1996.

Kafka M, Prentky R: Attention-deficit/hyperactivity disorder in males with paraphilias and paraphilia-related disorders. *J Clin Psychiatry* 1998; 59(7):388–396.

Kaplan HS: *The Sexual Desire Disorders: Dysfunctional Regulation of Sexual Motivation*. New York: Brunner/Mazel, 1995.

Laumann EO, Paik A, Rosen RC: Sexual dysfunction in the United States: prevalence and predictors. *J Am Med Assoc* 1999; 281:537–544.

Leiblum SR, Rosen RC: *Principles and Practice of Sex Therapy, Update for the 1990s*, 2nd ed. New York: Guilford Press, 1989.

Maurice W: *Sexual Medicine in Primary Care*. New York: Mosby, 1999.

Medical Letter 1992; 34(876):73–78.

Medical Letter 1998; 40(1026):51–52.

NIH Consensus Development Panel on Impotence: *J Am Med Assoc* 1993; 270(1):8390.

Rosler A, Witztum E: Treatment of men with paraphilia with a long-acting analogue of gonadotropin-releasing hormone. *N Engl J Med* 1998; 338:416–422.

Shafer L: Sexual disorders. In Hyman S, Jenike M (eds): *Manual of Clinical Problems in Psychiatry*. Boston: Little, Brown, 1990:228–236.

Shafer L: The denial of the risk of aids in heterosexuals coming for treatment of sexual disorders. In Rutan JS (ed.): *Psychotherapy for the 1990s*. New York: Guilford Press, 1992:263–271.

Shafer L: Sexual dysfunction. In Carlson K, Eisenstat S (eds): *Primary Care of Women*. St. Louis: Mosby, 1995:270–274.

Shafer L: Approach to the patient with sexual dysfunction. In Goroll A, May L, Mulley A (eds): *Primary Care Medicine*. Philadelphia: JB Lippincott, 1995:1053–1056.

Shafer L: Approach to the patient with sexual dysfunction. In Stern TA, Herman JB, Slavin PL (eds): *The MGH Guide to Psychiatry in Primary Care*. New York: McGraw-Hill, 1998:271–280.

Shafer L: Approach to the patient with impotence. In Stern TA, Herman JB, Slavin PL (eds): *The MGH Guide to Psychiatry in Primary Care*. New York: McGraw-Hill, 1998:281–287.

Wincze J, Carey M: *Sexual Dysfunction*. New York: Guilford Press, 1991.

Chapter 21
Eating Disorders
ANNE BECKER

I. Overview

Eating disorders are characterized by disordered patterns of eating, accompanied by distress, disparagement, preoccupation, and/or distortion associated with one's eating, weight, or body shape. Both anorexia nervosa and bulimia nervosa are associated with efforts made to lose weight or prevent weight gain, and both bulimia nervosa and binge-eating disorder (BED) are associated with episodic binge pattern eating.

A. **Etiology**
The etiology of eating disorders appears to be multifactorial, with psychological, sociocultural, genetic, and neurochemical contributions.

B. **Course**
Approximately 50% of individuals with anorexia nervosa and bulimia nervosa make a full recovery, whereas 30% partially recover, and 20% follow a chronic course. Individuals with BED appear to have a slightly more favorable outcome. The mortality rate for anorexia nervosa is 0.56% annually, nearly twice as high as the rate for female psychiatric inpatients of similar age.

II. Epidemiology of Eating Disorders

A. **Prevalence**
Anorexia nervosa is the least prevalent eating disorder, affecting approximately 0.28% of young adult females. Bulimia nervosa affects approximately 1.0% of young adult females. BED is the most prevalent eating disorder, affecting approximately 2.6% of young adults (and up to 29% of adults seeking weight treatment). In addition, clinically significant partial syndromes or atypical eating disorders (eating disorders, not otherwise specified), may occur in up to 5–13% of the young adult female population.

B. **Demographics**
Eating disorders typically affect young, adult females with 85–95% of cases of anorexia and bulimia nervosa and approximately 60% of cases of BED occurring among females.

C. **Onset**
Onset of anorexia is typically slightly earlier than the onset of bulimia, but both generally begin during adolescence; however, both disorders can occur at much older ages. Onset of BED tends to be slightly later, generally beginning in late adolescence or the early 20s.

D. **Sociocultural Factors**
Although previously thought to be more common among affluent Caucasian women, eating disorders affect individuals of diverse ethnic and socioeconomic backgrounds. Eating disorders have been reported all over the globe, but they are more prevalent in industrialized and/or westernized societies.

III. Diagnostic Features

Symptoms of eating disorders commonly overlap phenomenologically; these diagnoses are often made consecutively. Up to half of patients with clinically significant disordered eating present with atypical features or with partial syndrome disorders consistent with an eating disorder, not otherwise specified (Fig. 21-1).

A. **Anorexia Nervosa**
Anorexia nervosa is divided into two subtypes: restricting type (in which there is dieting, fasting, or excessive exercise, but no regular bingeing and/or purging), and binge-eating/purging type (in which there is regular bingeing and purging of calories). Anorexia nervosa is characterized by the following diagnostic features:
1. The refusal to maintain a minimally normal weight (often defined as 85% of the expected body weight for height and age).
2. A fear of gaining weight or becoming fat.
3. A disturbance in the way one's weight or body shape is experienced, a self-evaluation which is unduly influenced by weight or body shape, or the denial of the seriousness of low weight.
4. Amenorrhea (in postmenarcheal females).

B. **Bulimia Nervosa**
Bulimia nervosa includes two subtypes: purging type (in which there is regular use of self-induced vomiting or abuse of laxatives, enemas, or diuretics), and nonpurging type (in which the inappropriate compensatory behaviors include excessive exercise or fasting but not the regular use of self-induced vomiting or abuse of laxatives, enemas, or diuretics). Bulimia nervosa is characterized by the following diagnostic features:

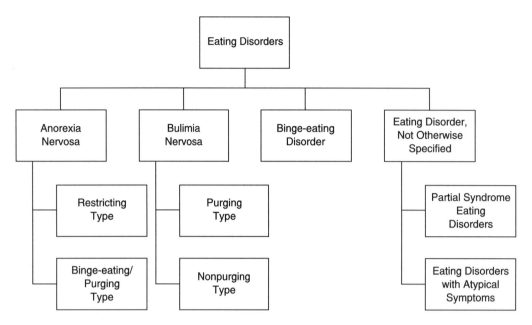

Fig. 21-1. Types and subtypes of eating disorders. (Adapted from Becker AE, Hamburg P, Herzog DB: The role of psychopharmacologic management in the treatment of eating disorders. In Dunner DL, Rosenbaum JF (eds): *Psychiatr Clin North Am: Annu Drug Ther.* Philadelphia: WS Saunders, 1998; 5:18.)

1. Recurrent, episodic binge eating (at least twice weekly for at least 3 months). Binges are characterized by an unusually large amount of food eaten in a discrete period of time and associated with a sense of lack of control.
2. Recurrent, inappropriate compensatory behaviors to prevent weight gain (at least twice weekly for at least 3 months). These compensatory behaviors include self-induced vomiting, laxative, enema, diuretic, stimulant, and diet pill abuse, restrictive pattern eating (e.g., meal-skipping), and exercise.
3. A self-evaluation that is unduly influenced by weight or body shape.
4. Symptoms do not occur exclusively during episodes of anorexia nervosa.

C. **Binge-Eating Disorder**
   Binge-eating disorder is characterized by the following diagnostic features:
1. Recurrent, episodic binge-eating (at least 2 days weekly for at least 6 months) without regular inappropriate compensatory measures to prevent weight gain.
2. The binge-eating episodes are associated with marked distress as well as with at least three of the following:
   a. Eating abnormally rapidly.
   b. Eating until uncomfortably full.
   c. Eating large amounts when not hungry.
   d. Eating alone because of embarrassment.
   e. Feeling disgusted, depressed, or guilty after bingeing.
3. Symptoms do not occur exclusively during the course of anorexia nervosa or bulimia nervosa.

IV. Evaluation and Differential Diagnosis

Because individuals with eating disorders are often reluctant to seek treatment or to disclose their symptoms, their illness may go undetected for years, even in clinical settings. It is also not unusual for some individuals to deny or actively conceal their symptoms, making the diagnostic process a challenge. **Evaluation of the eating-disordered patient should include medical, nutritional, and psychiatric assessments.**

A. **Medical Evaluation**
   Medical evaluation of an eating-disordered patient centers on identification of any complications of undernutrition, obesity, excessive exercise, and/or purging behaviors, and exclusion of any organic causes of appetite or weight change (e.g., thyroid disease) by medical history, physical examination, and laboratory analysis.
1. **Medical history should include a thorough review of systems, a history of weight changes, and an inventory of dietary patterns, purging behaviors, and exercise patterns** (see below). **Current medications should be reviewed** for possible contributions to appetite or weight changes.
   a. **Assessment of individuals with suspected or known anorexia nervosa or bulimia nervosa** should include

questions about: fatigue, postural and nonpostural lightheadedness, palpitations, cognitive changes, peripheral neuropathy, dental caries, abdominal pain, bloating, nausea, constipation, hematemesis, age of menarche, amenorrhea, oligomenorrhea, infertility, intolerance of cold temperature, hair loss, dry skin, and fractures.

  b. **Assessment of individuals with obesity associated with BED** should include questions about potential medical complications of obesity (including hypertension, diabetes mellitus, coronary artery disease, degenerative joint disease, and sleep apnea).

2. **Physical examination should include measurement of height and weight, vital signs, and evaluation of potential complications of weight changes, or inappropriate compensatory behaviors.** An individual with bulimia nervosa will commonly have a normal physical examination.

  a. **Patients with eating disorders should be weighed and measured on initial evaluation;** for anorexia nervosa, weights should be monitored routinely throughout treatment. Clinicians should be sensitive to the discomfort individuals with eating disorders may experience when being weighed, but should avoid estimating weights since individuals with anorexia nervosa commonly wear clothing in such a way so as to disguise their weight.

  b. **Blood pressure, pulse, and temperature should be evaluated periodically** since hypotension, bradycardia, and hypothermia are common among individuals with anorexia nervosa and bulimia nervosa.

  c. **Assessment of individuals with anorexia nervosa should include examination for:** dry skin, yellow skin (due to carotenemia), lanugo, hair loss, acrocyanosis, mitral valve prolapse, arrhythmia, decreased bowel sounds, and peripheral neuropathy.

  d. **Assessment of individuals with bulimia nervosa or binge-eating/purging anorexia should include examination for:** parotid gland enlargement, submandibular adenopathy, dental caries, hand abrasions (Russell's sign), decreased or increased bowel sounds, and rectal prolapse.

3. **Laboratory analysis should routinely include initial and periodic assessment of serum electrolytes for any individual with purging behavior** since hypokalemia and hypomagnesemia are commonly seen in this population. Laboratory examination **for individuals with anorexia nervosa** should also **include a serum glucose** (since hypoglycemia is common in this population) **and a complete blood count** with differential, since leukopenia, neutropenia, anemia, and thrombocytopenia may be seen in association with anorexia nervosa.

  a. Assessment of individuals with electrolyte disturbances, symptomatic arrhythmias, or for whom psychopharmacologic intervention is planned, should

have an electrocardiogram to evaluate whether the QT interval is prolonged or any other abnormalities are present.

  b. Although amenorrhea associated with anorexia nervosa is most often due to decreased gonadotropin releasing hormone pulsatility (leading to hypogonadotropic hypogonadism and low estradiol levels), other causes (e.g., pregnancy) should be excluded.

  c. Since significant osteopenia occurs in half of women with anorexia nervosa, which poses a risk for fractures and kyphosis, women with anorexia nervosa should have a dual-energy X-ray absorptiometry (DEXA) evaluation of lumbar spine bone density to assess severity of bone loss.

B. Nutritional Assessment

Nutritional assessment includes the evaluation of appropriateness of body weight and adequacy of caloric and nutrient intake. Assessment of appropriateness of weight for height can be made by comparing weight and height against the Metropolitan Life Insurance Height-Weight Table or by calculation according to several formulas.

1. **Body mass index (BMI) is calculated by the formula:**

$$BMI = \frac{\textbf{Weight(kg)}}{\textbf{Height(m)}^2}$$

BMI can be used for adult men or women of all heights or weights. A BMI of ≤ 17.5 reflects a weight range consistent with anorexia nervosa. A BMI of 20–25 is considered to be within normal range.

2. **An alternate estimation of an appropriate body weight for height** for adults is made by calculation of the ratio of actual body weight to desirable body weight (percent ideal body weight, or %IBW) as follows:

Women: 100 lb. for the first 5 feet + 5 lb./ inch above 5 feet ± 10%

Men: 106 lb. for the first 5 feet + 6 lb./ inch above 5 feet ± 10%

%IBW of less than 85% is consistent with anorexia nervosa.

C. Psychiatric Evaluation

Psychiatric evaluation of the eating-disordered patient includes establishing the type and severity of the eating disorder and excluding other psychiatric etiologies of appetite or weight changes (e.g., major depression), evaluating comorbid psychiatric illness, and evaluating psychiatric risk.

1. **History of the present illness should evaluate dietary patterns** (i.e., restrictive or binge-pattern eating),

and modalities, frequencies, and durations of any inappropriate compensatory behaviors to lose weight or prevent weight gain as well as the psychosocial context of the illness.

a. Inquire about self-induced vomiting, and whether or not syrup of ipecac is, or has been used, to induce emesis.

b. Inquire about laxative abuse, including frequency of episodes and number of laxatives typically used per episode.

c. Inquire about use of enemas.

d. Inquire about use of diuretics.

e. Inquire about inappropriate use of diet pills, stimulants, or other medications (e.g., methylphenidate or insulin).

f. Inquire about excessive exercise; determine how many hours daily or weekly the individual exercises and whether the individual is likely to exercise when sick or injured.

g. Inquire about fasting, meal-skipping, or restrictive patterns of eating.

h. Inquire about binge-pattern eating. **Clinically, a binge is defined as consuming an unusual amount of food in a discrete period of time while experiencing a lack of control over the eating.**

i. Inquire about psychosocial precipitants to symptoms.

j. Evaluate the need for patient and family education and for family intervention.

2. **Psychiatric history** should include questions about previous treatment as well as history of other psychiatric illness. **Eating disorders are commonly seen in association with mood, anxiety, substance abuse, or personality disorder.**

a. Major depression, dysthymia, and obsessive-compulsive disorder are associated with anorexia nervosa.

b. Major depression, bipolar disorder, substance abuse, anxiety disorders, and personality disorders are commonly seen with bulimia nervosa.

c. Major depression, panic disorder, substance abuse, and personality disorders are associated with BED.

3. **A mental status examination should exclude other possible causes** (such as mood or anxiety symptoms) **of anorexia or hyperphagia,** should evaluate for the presence of comorbid psychiatric illness, and should assess suicidal ideation. Suicidal ideation and behavior are relatively common among individuals with eating disorders.

V. Treatment

Treatment for eating disorders ideally addresses medical, psychological, and nutritional needs, and utilizes a multidisciplinary team approach. Clinicians treating a patient with an eating disorder should communicate regularly about symptoms and therapeutic intervention.

A. **Medical Treatment**

Unless there is a psychiatric emergency, the initial goals of treatment often include medical and nutritional stabilization. Potential complications of low weight (and sometimes overweight) or inappropriate compensatory behaviors are addressed. Regardless of the severity of the disorder, an individual with an eating disorder should be followed routinely by a primary care clinician to monitor weights, vital signs, and, when appropriate, serum electrolytes. Individuals with moderate to severe symptoms will need to be evaluated on a regular basis so that medical interventions can be made when necessary.

1. **Weight restoration is a primary medical goal for the treatment of anorexia nervosa;** a goal weight should be adequate to regain menses and reverse bone demineralization. Individuals with anorexia nervosa are as a rule reluctant to gain weight, so weight restoration generally requires active and collaborative intervention among primary care clinician, mental health specialist, and nutritionist. Patients often respond to behavioral, educational, and psychotherapeutic interventions.

a. Enteral or total parenteral feeding are utilized only in severe cases of anorexia nervosa that fail to respond to the above interventions.

b. Weight gain in severely malnourished individuals must be carefully monitored since complications of refeeding include hypophosphatemia, cardiac arrhythmia, congestive heart failure, and delirium.

2. **Correction of hypokalemia and other electrolyte disturbances is necessary** in this population to prevent cardiac arrhythmias.

3. **Vitamin supplementation** is indicated for individuals with poor nutrition and should include calcium 1000–1500 mg/day, and a multivitamin to provide 400 IU vitamin D daily.

4. **A combination of estrogen and progestin** has *not* been shown to be effective in correcting osteopenia in women with anorexia nervosa **but may be useful for the symptomatic relief of estrogen deficiency symptoms.**

5. Despite menstrual abnormalities and associated infertility seen with anorexia nervosa and bulimia nervosa, pregnancy can occur. Because a variety of obstetric complications are associated with these disorders, **patients should be counseled to avoid conception until the illness has been treated.**

6. Stool softeners or bulk-forming laxatives may be helpful in treating the severe constipation associated with chronic laxative abuse and withdrawal.

7. **Dental care** is indicated for individuals who induce vomiting because of the increased risk of dental caries.

8. **Weight loss treatment is contraindicated for individuals with active bulimia nervosa.** However, it may benefit some individuals with obesity and BED. For those with a history of repeated weight cycling or early-onset BED, it may be optimal to control the binge-pattern eating before embarking upon weight loss treatment.

B. **Nutritional Counseling**

Nutritional counseling is a helpful and often necessary adjunct to medical and psychiatric interventions.

1. **Dietary patterns and weights can be monitored** in this setting and communicated with other members of the team.

2. **Caloric requirements and nutritional deficiencies should be clarified** for patients and clinicians; counseling and suggested meal plans and supplements can be offered to patients who need to gain or lose weight.

3. **Behavioral strategies for establishing healthful patterns of eating can be introduced or reinforced** in this setting (i.e., patients can be assisted with self-monitoring of dietary patterns and identifying and avoiding cues to restrict, binge, or purge).

C. **Mental Health Treatment**

Mental health treatment for eating disorders addresses affective states, emotional conflicts, interpersonal tensions, traumatic losses, and/or maladaptive coping styles that have resulted in disordered patterns of eating and/or excessive preoccupation with body, food, and weight and helps the individual to normalize eating and eliminate inappropriate compensatory behaviors. Psychotherapy with the occasional use of adjunctive pharmacologic therapy is the treatment of choice for these disorders. Because restricting, bingeing, and purging symptoms are often used to modulate unpleasant affective states, many patients will not tolerate their eradication before alternate defenses and coping strategies are in place.

1. **Cognitive-behavioral therapy** (CBT) is the best-studied treatment for bulimia nervosa and for BED. Less is known about its efficacy for anorexia nervosa.

   a. The mean reduction of binge-eating associated with bulimia nervosa with CBT is 73–93% and the mean remission is 51–71%.

   b. The mean reduction of purging symptoms associated with bulimia nervosa with CBT is 77–94% and the mean remission is 36–56%.

2. **Interpersonal psychotherapy** (IPT) has been shown to be equally as effective as CBT for the treatment of bulimia and has been shown effective for the treatment of BED.

3. **Psychodynamic psychotherapy** is less well studied for the treatment of eating disorders, but is a useful approach in many patients. Often, behavioral strategies are employed early in the treatment to assist the patient in controlling the disordered eating or inappropriate compensatory measures.

4. **Family therapy** may be the most effective therapy for the treatment of adolescents with anorexia nervosa and is a useful modality of adjunctive therapy for other eating disorders as well, particularly for adolescents and young adults.

5. **Group psychotherapy** is also a useful adjunctive therapy for anorexia and bulimia nervosa. Group CBT or IPT is effective in the treatment of BED as well.

D. **Pharmacotherapy**

The indications for pharmacotherapy for eating disorders depend largely upon diagnosis, severity, and comorbid psychiatric illness. Since the efficacy of pharmacologic management of disordered eating is limited, **medication management of the eating disorders is optimally offered as an adjunctive treatment to, and not a replacement for, psychotherapy.** Because both individuals with anorexia and bulimia nervosa may be at risk for hypotension, dehydration, hypokalemia, hypomagnesemia, and cardiac arrhythmias among other medical complications, medication therapy may pose additional risks among this population and should be weighed carefully against potential benefits. Medication trials for eating disorders have not been conducted among children or adolescents, so the recommendations below apply only to an adult population.

1. **There is no medication that is generally clinically useful for the primary symptoms of anorexia nervosa.**

   a. There is some evidence that fluoxetine (60 mg/day) may be helpful in stabilizing weight-recovered individuals with anorexia.

   b. Although some medications have been shown to effect some modest weight gain (e.g., cyproheptadine and zinc), these are not routinely used.

   c. Comorbid psychiatric illness or symptoms (e.g., depression or anxiety) may be treated with appropriate pharmacologic therapy but may have limited efficacy in severely underweight patients.

2. **The symptoms associated with bulimia nervosa are moderately responsive to a variety of antidepressant medications in the short term, although remission rates are relatively low. CBT has been shown to be more effective than medication for the treatment of bulimia nervosa, but the addition of medication to psychotherapy is often clinically useful.** The average reduction of bingeing frequency among bulimic

Table 21-1. Summary of Assessment and Management of Eating Disorders

	Assessment	*Management*
General	*Determine onset, course, and patterning of*: • Binge or restrictive pattern eating • Purging or compensatory behaviors • Weight loss, gain, or cycling • Excessive concern and/or distress associated with eating, body, or weight *Exclude* • Alternative medical and psychiatric causes of anorexia, hyperphagia, and weight dysregulation	*Team members should*: • Clarify roles in treatment to patient and to one another • Communicate about symptoms and therapeutic interventions • Identify parameters signaling psychiatric or medical danger or treatment failure and review with the patient
Medical	*Evaluate for complications of purging, excessive exercise, starvation, and/or underweight or overweight with*: • Directed history • Vital signs • Physical exam • Laboratory analyses include: For bulimia nervosa: routinely, serum electrolytes; when indicated, EKG. For anorexia nervosa: routinely, serum electrolytes, glucose, and CBC; when indicated, EKG and DEXA of the lumbar spine. Beta-hCG, FSH, and/or prolactin may be useful in evaluating amenorrhea associated with these disorders	*Routinely monitor*: • Weights and vital signs • Serum electrolytes for patients with purging behaviors *Treat and follow*: • Medical complications initially present or as weight, diet, purging symptoms, or inappropriate compensatory behaviors change *Refer*: • Individuals with self-induced vomiting for dental care
Nutritional	*Evaluate*: • Dietary patterns/caloric and nutrient intakes • Appropriateness of weight (by tables or calculation of %IBW or BMI)	*Introduce and support*: • Nutritional guidelines for weight restoration or control and general health • Behavioral strategies to assist in symptom control
Psychological	*Evaluate*: • Excessive concern with and distress about eating, body shape, or weight • Psychosocial context of symptoms • Comorbid psychiatric illness and suicidality	*Initiate*: • Psychotherapy *Consider*: • Medication (as an adjunctive therapy for bulimia nervosa and BED, and for anorexia nervosa with comorbid psychiatric illness)

individuals on one of the medications shown to be effective is approximately 56% as compared with 11% on placebo; the reduction of frequency of self-induced vomiting is probably similar. Of the agents demonstrated to be effective, no particular medication has been shown to have superior efficacy, so it is recommended that a medication be chosen based on its side effect profile and history of patient response. Consecutive trials of agents may be necessary to treat an individual with a poor response to an initial trial.

a. **Fluoxetine is the best studied among the medications effective against bulimia nervosa and is the only FDA-approved medication for its treatment.** It is generally well tolerated in this population. The recommended dosage is 60 mg/day. Other serotonin-specific reuptake inhibitors have not been studied in controlled trials but are in routine clinical use.

b. **Desipramine and imipramine** (standard antidepressant dosages of up to 300 mg/day, as tolerated) **are effective in reducing the frequency of bingeing and purging in bulimia nervosa.** Amitriptyline has not been found effective in the treatment of bulimia nervosa, and other tricyclic antidepressants have not been studied in controlled trials.

   c. **Isocarboxazid and phenelzine are also effective in reducing bingeing and purging symptoms associated with bulimia nervosa,** but may pose an increased risk for a hypertensive crisis in this population. Spontaneous hypertensive crises have been reported, but the risk may also be increased by dietary indiscretion or dyscontrol and the use of diet pills such as phenylpropanolamine.

   d. **Trazodone and bupropion have been found effective in the treatment of bulimia nervosa** in one study each. Bupropion was associated with an elevated seizure risk, however, and is contraindicated for treatment in individuals with an eating disorder. High dose (200–300 mg/day) naltrexone was also found effective in treatment-resistant bulimic individuals in one study, but is not recommended for routine use since it poses a risk of hepatotoxicity.

   e. **Lithium and carbamazepine have been studied** but not found effective for the treatment of bulimia nervosa, and other mood stabilizers and benzodiazepines have not been studied for its treatment.

3. **Medication management of BED** has not been studied as extensively as for bulimia nervosa.

   a. **Fluvoxamine** (50–300 mg/day in divided doses) **is the only currently available medication that has been found effective in the treatment of BED.**

   b. Desipramine (up to 300 mg/day) has been found effective in the treatment of nonpurging bulimia; however, efficacy among individuals with BED has not been studied.

E. Indications for Inpatient Management

Although eating disorders can often be adequately managed in an outpatient setting, inpatient care or partial hospitalization may be required for some patients.

1. **Indications for inpatient management include:** serious medical risk (e.g., significant hypokalemia or dehydration, ongoing ipecac abuse); very low weight (e.g., $\leq$ 75% expected body weight) or rapid weight loss; growth arrest; psychiatric risk (e.g., risk of self-harm or psychosis); escalating or severe symptoms (e.g., inability to eat, frequent purging throughout the entire day); or failure of outpatient management.

2. It is often helpful to review medical and psychiatric parameters that may signal a need for intensified care with an individual at the onset of treatment.

VI. Conclusions

Eating disorders are common and typically affect young adult women. They are often associated with comorbid psychiatric illness as well as with medical complications. Successful treatment requires collaborative team management with medical, nutrition, and psychiatric intervention (Table 21-1).

Suggested Readings

American Psychiatric Association: Practice guideline for eating disorders. *Am J Psychiatry* 1993; 150:207–228.

American Psychiatric Association: *Diagnostic and Statistical Manual of Mental Disorders, Fourth Edition.* Washington, DC: American Psychiatric Association, 1994:539–550, 729–731.

Becker AE, Hamburg P, Herzog DB: The role of psychopharmacologic management in the treatment of eating disorders. In Dunner DL, Rosenbaum JF (eds): *Psychiatr Clin North Am: Annu Drug Ther.* Philadelphia: WB Saunders, 1998; 5:17–51.

Becker AE, Grinspoon SK, Klibanski A, Herzog DB. Eating disorders. *N Engl J Med* 1999; 340:1092–1098.

Brownell KD, Fairburn CG (eds): *Eating Disorders and Obesity.* New York: Guilford Press, 1995.

Fichter MM, Quadflieg N, Gnutzmann A: Binge eating disorder: treatment outcome over a 6-year course. *J Psychosom Res* 1998; 44:385–405.

Hudson JI, et al.: Fluvoxamine in the treatment of binge-eating disorder: a multicenter placebo-controlled, double-blind trial. *Am J Psychiatry* 1998; 155:1756–1762.

Jimerson DC, Herzog DB, Brotman AW: Pharmacologic approaches in the treatment of eating disorders. *Harvard Rev Psychiatry* 1993; 1:82–93.

Kohn MR, Golden NH, Shenker IR: Cardiac arrest and delirium: presentations of the refeeding syndrome in severely malnourished adolescents with anorexia nervosa. *J Adolesc Health* 1998; 22:239–243.

Paige DM (ed.): *Manual of Clinical Nutrition.* Pleasantville, NJ: Nutrition Publications, 1983; 10:3.

Shisslak CM, Crago M, Estes LS: The spectrum of eating disturbances. *Int J Eating Disord* 1995; 18:209–219.

Sullivan PF: Mortality in anorexia nervosa. *Am J Psychiatry* 1995; 152:1073–1074.

Chapter 22
Sleep Disorders

PATRICK SMALLWOOD AND THEODORE A. STERN

I. Introduction

Sleep, when restorative, becomes so routine as to warrant little more than a passing thought. If altered in even the slightest fashion, however, this once routine process shifts from a benign to a disordered state that can significantly impair any or all facets of daily life. **In this chapter, normal sleep (including sleep stages, cycles, rhythm, and biological mechanisms) is examined. The three major classes of sleep disorders recognized by the *Diagnostic and Statistical Manual, Fourth Edition* (DSM-IV) are then reviewed,** with special emphasis placed on dyssomnias and parasomnias.

II. Normal Sleep

A. History

While the quest to understand sleep is as old as mankind itself, most of what is known about it has occurred in only the last 60 years. During that time, sleep has been redefined as an active state, complete with stages, cycles, and rhythms that are as complex as the waking state. **Loomis (1935) observed that electroencephalographic (EEG) changes were prevalent throughout sleep. Aserinsky and Kleitman (1953) detected various types of eye movements during sleep,** most notably slow rolling eye movements occurring early in sleep and disappearing as sleep progressed, and rapid eye movements associated with irregular breathing and increased heart rate. They named **the sleep phase associated with the slow rolling rhythmic eye movements non-rapid eye movement (NREM) sleep, and the sleep phase associated with the fast erratic eye movements rapid eye movement (REM) sleep. In 1955, Dement and Kleitman discovered that REM sleep was associated with dreaming,** and, 2 years later, that REM and NREM sleep cycled over the course of the night.

B. Polysomnography

Polysomnography, the method used to objectively evaluate sleep, **involves the simultaneous recording of multiple physiological variables in a standardized fashion known as a polysomnogram (PSG). The parameters recorded by the PSG include,** but are not limited to, the following:

1. **Electroencephalogram (EEG):** a recording of the electrical activity of cortical neurons via scalp electrodes that are placed in standardized positions according to the International 10–20 System.
2. **Electrooculogram (EOG):** a recording of eye movements.
3. **Electrocardiogram (ECG):** a recording of heart rhythm.
4. **Electromyogram (EMG):** a recording of the activity of the left and right tibialis anterior muscles and the submental chin muscles.
5. **Respiratory efforts:** a recording of nasal and oral airflow by means of nasal thermistors, and thoracoabdominal movements by means of strain gauges.
6. **Pulse oximetry:** a recording of oxygen saturation in the blood.
7. **Snore monitor:** a recording of snoring by means of a microphone placed on the lateral aspect of the neck. **By employing polysomnography, wakefulness, sleep onset, NREM sleep, and REM sleep can be defined and studied. Table 22-1 summarizes the sleep stages, as well as the EEG, EMG, and EOG findings that define them.**

C. Sleep Cycle and Architecture

NREM and REM do not occur randomly throughout the night, but **alternate in a rhythmic fashion known as the NREM-REM cycle.** In normal healthy individuals, this cycle begins with NREM 1 and progresses to NREM 2, 3, 4, 3, 2, and then REM. **This pattern generally repeats itself at 90–120-min intervals** about three to four times a night. **NREM 3 and 4 are most prominent in the first half of the night** and diminish in the latter half of the night. **REM sleep,** however, is less prominent in the first half of the night and **increases as the night progresses. Sleep latency,** which is usually 10–20 min, is the time from lights out to the first NREM 2. **REM latency** is the time from sleep onset until the first REM, and is usually 90–100 min. **Sleep efficiency** is: [(total sleep time)/(total sleep record time)]×100.

Sleep architecture is the pattern and distribution of sleep stages across an average night and is summarized in Table 22-1.

D. Circadian Rhythm

The circadian rhythm or "biological clock" is **an endogenous rhythm of bodily functions that is**

Table 22-1. Human Sleep Stages and Distribution Across the Night

	EEG Findings	EMG Findings	EOG Findings	Distribution Over the Night
Wake	Alpha waves (8–14 Hz)	Muscle tone and activity present	Variable eye movements	< 5%
NREM 1	Theta waves (4–7 Hz)	Muscle tone and activity present	Slow rolling eye movements	2–5%
NREM 2	Theta waves (4–7 Hz); sleep spindles (12–14 Hz $\geq$ 0.5 sec); K-complexes (triphasic)	Muscle tone and activity present, but slowing	Slow rolling eye movements	45–55%
NREM 3 and 4	Delta waves (0.5–2 Hz) present $\geq$ 50% of the time	Marked decrease in muscle tone and activity	Slow rolling eye movements	13–23%
REM	Relatively low-voltage mixed-frequency waves	Absence of muscle activity	Conjugate rapid eye movements	20–25%

influenced by environmental cues, or *Zeitgebers*. This cycle, unique to each person, **averages 25 h,** but can be as long as 50 h for some. Sleep disorders related to the circadian rhythm emerge when an individual's circadian rhythm clashes with environmental and societal expectations.

E. **Sleep Across the Lifespan**
The amount of time spent in the different stages of sleep varies with age. Infants, for example, spend more than two-thirds of their day sleeping, whereas adults spend less than a third. **The elderly,** on the other hand, **experience a reduction in the intensity, depth, and continuity of sleep,** because of age-related degenerative changes in the sleep mechanisms of the central nervous system (CNS). Specific sleep changes in the elderly include:
1. Increased sleep latency
2. Reduced NREM 3 and 4
3. Decreased REM latency
4. Reduced total REM amount
5. Frequent awakenings
6. Decreased sleep efficiency
Table 22-2 summarizes sleep patterns across the lifespan.

F. **Neuroanatomic Basis for Sleep**
The actual neuroanatomic **basis for the sleep-wake cycle remains elusive.** Most of what is known has been inferred through the observations of early electrolytic lesion studies, which suggest that specific regions of the brain are critical for wakefulness and sleep. By drawing on these results and observing the effects of disease states, Hobson (1974) arrived at the most currently accepted

neuroanatomic model for wakefulness and sleep. Hobson proposed that:
1. Wakefulness is maintained by the ascending reticular activating system (ARAS).
2. Sleep occurred through decreased activity of the ARAS and activation of a hypnagogic sleep system.
3. REM arose through active processes in both the nucleus coeruleus and the gigantocellular tegmental field.
Current research supports this model, as disruption of any of these regions leads to alterations in the sleep-wake cycle, and invariably to sleep disorders.

III. Sleep Disorders

While several classification systems for sleep disorders exist, the DSM-IV classification is perhaps the simplest and easiest to understand. The DSM-IV divides sleep disorders into three major categories: Primary Sleep Disorders, Sleep Disorders Related to Another Mental Disorder, and Other Sleep Disorders. Of the three, Primary Sleep Disorders are the most common, and are therefore emphasized.

A. **Primary Sleep Disorders**
The DSM-IV subdivides the primary sleep disorders into the **dyssomnias** and the **parasomnias.**
1. **Dyssomnias are primary sleep disorders that result in complaints of either sleeping too little (insomnia) or too much (hypersomnia). The DSM-IV subcategorizes dyssomnias into four groups** based in part upon the pathophysiological mechanisms felt to underlie them. The groups include: primary insom-

Table 22-2. Sleep Patterns Across the Lifespan

Age	Time in Bed	Time Asleep	Stage 1	Stages 3 and 4	REM
Birth	17–24 h	16 h	5%	–	50%
12 years	8.5 h	8 h	–	15–20%	20%
25–45 years	7.5 h	7 h	–	–	20%
Old age	8.5 h	6.5 h	15%	0%	20%

nias, primary hypersomnias, breathing-related sleep disorders, and circadian rhythm disorders.

a. **Primary insomnias. Insomnia is the subjective complaint of deficient, inadequate, or unrefreshing sleep. To qualify as a primary insomnia, there must be objective daytime sleepiness and/or subjective feelings of not being rested,** and an absence of psychiatric or medical conditions that better account for it. With **primary insomnia,** the classic form of insomnia, sufferers complain of decreased daytime functioning, and are frequently overaroused and anxious at bedtime. **Sleep-state misperception,** also known as **subjective insomnia** and **nonrestorative sleep,** is a primary insomnia **in which sufferers complain of inadequate and/or poor sleep, but objective findings on the polysomnogram are lacking.** Invariably, patients with sleep-state misperception underestimate total sleep time and efficiency, and overestimate sleep latency. **Idiopathic insomnia is chronic insomnia present from childhood** and is most likely the result of an underlying innate process.

Primary insomnia is perhaps the hardest group of sleep disorders to treat. Once a careful assessment is completed, treatment involves selecting a specific modality based on etiology. Nonpharmacological techniques, such as good sleep hygiene, should be attempted first. If this is unsuccessful, brief intermittent use of sedative-hypnotics may be appropriate. Table 22-3 provides a list of basic sleep hygiene techniques.

b. **Primary hypersomnias. The hallmark of all primary hypersomnias is the complaint of somnolence and excessive daytime sleep.** Like primary insomnias, primary hypersomnias are not the direct result of underlying medical or psychiatric conditions. **The most common type is narcolepsy,** which is **defined by the following tetrad:**

i. **Sleep paralysis** that occurs upon falling asleep or waking up.

ii. **Sleep attacks** with sleep-onset REM periods (SOREMPs). These are usually brief (10–15 min), occur in inappropriate circumstances, and are effectively treated with psychostimulants (dextroamphetamine, methylphenidate, and pemoline).

iii. **Cataplexy** (a condition of transient weakness or paralysis) triggered by strong emotion, often laughter or anger. It frequently lasts only seconds and is **effectively treated with imipramine.**

Table 22-3. Basic Sleep Hygiene

- Limit in-bed time to the amount present before the sleep disturbance
- Lie down only when sleepy, and sleep only as much as necessary to feel refreshed
- Use the bed for sleep only
- Maintain comfortable sleeping conditions and avoid excessive warmth and cold
- Wake up at a regular time each day
- Avoid daytime naps
- Exercise regularly, but early in the day
- Limit sedatives
- Avoid alcohol, tobacco, and caffeine near bedtime
- Eat at regular times daily and avoid large meals near bedtime
- Eat a light snack, if hungry, near bedtime
- Practice evening relaxation routines, such as progressive muscle relaxation, meditation, or taking a very hot, 20-min, body temperature-raising bath near bedtime

iv. **Hypnagogic hallucinations.**

Narcolepsy is rare, with an incidence of 0.07%. The **onset** is usually in **the late teens and early 20s,** and the course is often chronic. The probability of developing narcolepsy is 40 times greater if an immediate family member also suffers from it, suggesting that **genetic factors play a role.** Although sufferers have increased daytime sleepiness with decreased night sleep, total sleep time does not increase over a 24-h period.

c. **Breathing-related sleep disorder. The hallmark of sleep-related breathing disorders is apnea.** Prior to a discussion of sleep apnea syndromes, several terms must be defined. **Apnea is the cessation of nasobuccal airflow for greater than 10 sec. Hypopnea is a 50% reduction of either nasobuccal airflow or thoracoabdominal movements during sleep,** resulting in either a wake pattern on the EEG or at least a 4% decrease in oxygen saturation on the pulse oximeter. The **apnea index** (AI) is the number of clinically significant apneas per hour of sleep; likewise, the **hypopnea index** (HI) is the number of clinically significant hypopneas per hour of sleep. The **respiratory disturbance index** (RDI), perhaps the most sensitive of the indices, **is the sum of the AI and the HI.** An $AI > 5$, or $RDI > 10$ is considered pathologic and warrants treatment.

   i. **Obstructive sleep apnea** (OSA), the quintessential sleep-related breathing disorder, **is the most common organic disorder of excessive daytime sleepiness,** accounting for 40–50% of all patients seen in sleep disorder centers. The estimated **prevalence is 1–2%** of the adult male population in the United States, **increasing to 8.5% of men between the ages of 40 and 65 years.** Women account for 12–35% of OSA patients, with the majority of them being postmenopausal. The most significant risk factors are male sex, age 40–65 years, obesity, smoking, alcohol use, and poor physical health. **The principle defect is occlusion of the upper airway at the level of the pharynx during wake-sleep transitions and sleep proper. First-line therapy includes nasal continuous positive airway pressure (nCPAP) and bilevel positive airway pressure (BiPAP).** Mortality rates for OSA depend on apnea index and treatment modalities. For patients who receive no treatment and have an apnea index > 20, the probability of a cumulative 8-year survival is reported at 0.63 ± 0.17. With the use of nCPAP, regardless of the initial apnea index, the probability of a cumulative 8-year survival rises to 1.0.

   ii. Two other types of sleep apnea are recognized based on etiology and the presence or absence of respiratory effort during apneic events. **Central sleep apnea is a condition of repetitive apneas in which there is cessation of airflow without an attempt to initiate thoracoabdominal respiratory effort.** The etiology of the central sleep apnea, while debated, is felt to lie in abnormal CNS system processes. **Mixed sleep apnea,** as the name implies, is combined repetitive central and obstructive apneas. To qualify as a mixed apnea, an obstructive event follows a central apnea.

d. **Circadian rhythm sleep disorders emerge when societal expectation conflicts with an individual's preferred circadian rhythm.** As a result, the timing of sleep, not its quality and architecture, is adversely affected. The most frequently encountered circadian rhythm disorders are **jet lag syndrome, shift-work sleep disorder, delayed sleep phase disorder ("night owls"), and advanced sleep phase disorder ("larks").** Treatment for these disorders include gradually delaying sleep until achieving the new schedule, light therapy, or melatonin. Virtually all circadian rhythm disorders are self-limited and resolve as the individual adjusts to the new sleep-wake schedule.

e. **Dyssomnias not otherwise specified.**

   i. **Periodic limb movement disorder** (PLM) is a common dyssomnia affecting up to 40% of people over the age of 65 years. **PLM manifests as brief (0.5–5 sec) stereotypic contractions of the lower limbs,** frequently the dorsiflexors of the foot and flexors of the lower legs, **at intervals of 20–60 sec.** Contractions appear during sleep, and although patients are unaware of them, the EEG demonstrates frequent awakenings. **Sleep is often unrefreshing, and hypersomnia is the most common complaint.** While the etiology of PLM is unknown, medications, electrolyte abnormalities, and anemia, exacerbate it. Dopaminergic agents, such as L-dopa, pergolide, and bromocriptine, and benzodiazepines, particularly clonazepam, provide some relief, but definitive treatment is lacking.

   ii. A closely related disorder to PLM is **restless leg syndrome** (RLS). RLS **is a movement disorder characterized by deep sensations of creeping or aching inside the legs and calves when lying or sitting that produce an overwhelming urge to move them.** The disorder is rarely painful, and movement or massage often provides temporary relief. Like PLM, RLS occurs in association with a number of medical problems, especially renal failure, diabetes, iron-deficiency anemia, and peripheral nerve injury. Unlike PLM, it affects sleep initiation more than sleep maintenance. Medications, especially serotonin reuptake inhibitors, can exacerbate the condition. Pharmacological agents such as L-dopa, bromocriptine, and clonazepam can provide symptomatic relief.

   iii. **Recurrent hypersomnia,** also known as **Kleine-Levin syndrome,** is a rare, often self-limiting condition that **primarily affects adolescent males. Symptoms include hypersomnia, hyperphagia, and hypersexuality.** While the exact etiology is unknown, it often follows an acute viral infection.

   iv. **Posttraumatic hypersomnia** is hypersomnia that occurs within 1 year of a head trauma.

   v. **Idiopathic hypersomnia,** as the name implies, is hypersomnia of unknown origin. It is frequently confused with narcolepsy, but can be distinguished from it by the absence of cataplexy and immediate-onset REM sleep. This condition is chronic and often treatment-resistant.

2. **Parasomnias are sleep disorders in which undesirable events arise during specific sleep stages or at the transition between wakefulness and sleep.** Unlike dyssomnias, patients with parasomnias complain mainly about the event itself rather than the quality of sleep. These events are generally bizarre, but not taken seriously by either the patient or physician. **Children are affected more often than adults, and several different parasomnias may occur in the same individual. Typically, individuals are difficult to arouse during an episode, and once awakened, frequently have poor recall for the episode.** The most common parasomnias are **sleepwalking, nightmares, night terrors, and enuresis.**

   a. **Wake-sleep transition disorders. Sleep starts and rhythmic movement disorder** are the most common disorders in this group of parasomnias. Sleep starts, or **hypnogogic jerks,** involve the involuntary contractions of the legs and/or arms at the moment in which the individual enters sleep. This condition is benign, and no treatment, other than reassurance, is warranted. **Rhythmic movement disorder (jactatio capitis nocturna) involves head-banging at sleep onset,** and occurs almost exclusively in children. It is often self-limited and, if treatment is warranted, reduction of stress, benzodiazepines, tricyclic antidepressants (TCAs), and behavioral modification are the treatments of choice.

   b. **Light sleep stage disorders.** This group of parasomnias **arise during NREM 1 and 2, and include sleeptalking and bruxism. Sleeptalking (somniloquism),** as the name implies, **involves vocalizations** ranging from simple words and phrases, to complete conversations. It is frequently spontaneous, but may be elicited by speaking to the sleeper. No treatment is warranted. **Bruxism is repeated tooth grinding during sleep,** and is often the result of underlying stress or dental conditions. Mouth guards are the treatment of choice.

   c. **NREM sleep disorders.** This group of disorders **occur mainly in NREM 3 and 4 (slow wave) sleep.** The most commonly encountered NREM sleep disorders **include sleepwalking, and night terrors.**

      i. Sleepwalking (somnambulism) occurs upon partial emergence from delta sleep. Individuals may walk for some distance and carry out semipurposeful activities. **While most patients are quite adept at avoiding obstacles, serious accidents, such as tripping or falling out of open windows, have been reported.** Sufferers are frequently unresponsive to efforts to wake them, and, once awakened, are amnestic to the event. Common treatments include reassurance, provision of a safe sleep environment, and hypnosis.

      ii. **Night terrors (pavor nocturnus),** like sleepwalking, **occur during partial arousal from delta sleep,** but can begin in NREM stage 2. Patients generally scream, flail about, sit up in bed, and experience autonomic activity, including tachypnea, tachycardia, and mydriasis. These episodes, often 1–10 min in duration, take place early in the night, when NREM duration is at its longest. As with sleepwalking, **patients are often amnestic to the episode.** Treatment options include psychotherapy, stress reduction, and low-dose benzodiazepine (often clonazepam).

   d. **REM sleep disorders.** This group of parasomnias **arises exclusively during REM sleep, and includes nightmare disorder and REM behavior disorder.**

      i. **The hallmark of nightmare disorder is terrifying dreams whose content is often remembered by the patient.** Unlike sleep terror, **nightmare disorder lacks autonomic arousal, frequently occurs late in the night as REM intervals increase, and demonstrates muscle atonia.** Nightmares are associated with increased emotional stress; therefore, the treatment of choice is to decrease the underlying stress.

      ii. **REM behavior disorder** is perhaps the most dramatic of all the sleep disorders. Essentially, **patients appear to be acting out dream content through simple to quite complex movements** that result from the loss of muscle atonia during REM sleep. Although 60% of cases are idiopathic, **up to one-third are due to brainstem pathology and alcoholism.** The disorder is more common in the elderly, and affects males nine times more frequently than females. Low-dose clonazepam can be helpful by decreasing REM sleep density and suppressing REM sleep amount.

   e. **Diffuse sleep disorders.** As the name implies, these disorders appear in any or all sleep stages.

      i. The most common is **nocturnal enuresis, a condition in which involuntary micturition occurs without conscious arousal.** It affects children more than adults, and, while a source of great embarrassment to sufferers, is often self-limited. Treatment involves first ruling out medical causes, such as primary enuresis, and, if none are present, using either behavioral methods, such as bladder training, or low-dose tricyclic antidepressants.

      ii. The final category is **sleep-related seizures,** which is a rare, but important, entity in this group of parasomnias. **Seizures occur mainly during light NREM sleep and usually the first 2 h of sleep.** Because of their similarity to other sleep disorders, nocturnal seizures are often confused for enuresis, night terror, and sleepwalking. The treatment for sleep-related seizures is, as with most forms of seizures, anticonvulsants.

B. Secondary Sleep Disorders

The DSM-IV separates secondary sleep disorders

into those related to mental disorders, medical disorders, and to use of substances.

1. **Sleep Disorders Related to Another Mental Disorder.** This group is further subdivided into insomnia types and hypersomnia types. **As a rule, however, sleep disorders resulting from psychiatric disorders most often present with insomnia rather than hypersomnia as a chief complaint.** Because the mental disorder is the etiology for the sleep disorder, treatment consists of treating the primary psychiatric condition, with occasional symptomatic relief of the sleep complaint. The classic sleep findings associated with each major mental disorder are provided below.

   a. **Psychotic disorders.** The most prevalent findings are difficulty with sleep initiation and maintenance, which are most common in the acute phase of these illnesses. Total sleep time is often decreased, and REM is disrupted early in the episode. Medication side effects must be ruled out, as many of the medications used for treating psychotic disorders can also cause sleep disturbances.

   b. **Mood disorders.** Depression is perhaps the best studied of this group. Classic sleep findings attributed to depressions include early morning awakening, decreased REM latency, long first REM period, increased REM density, nocturnal restlessness, and early morning awakening. However, with atypical depressions, there is often hypersomnia, as well as neurovegetative reversal. With bipolar illness, the percentage of REM sleep increases during the depressed phase and decreases during the manic phase.

   c. **Anxiety disorders are the most common psychiatric cause of insomnia.** Sleep disturbances associated with anxiety include increased presleep worry with difficulty initiating sleep, decreased sleep efficiency, and poor sleep maintenance.

2. **Sleep Disorders Related to a General Medical Condition.** General medical conditions can induce sleep disturbances that mimic virtually any primary sleep disorder. **As a rule, the most frequent sleep complaint is insomnia,** rather than hypersomnia or parasomnia. To make the diagnosis, the history and physical examination must demonstrate a clear connection between the sleep disorder and the underlying medical problem. As with sleep disorders due to mental conditions, **the definitive treatment for this group of sleep disorders is to treat the underlying medical condition.** While the list of medical conditions resulting in sleep disorders is rather lengthy, **the more common ones include seizures, cluster headaches, abnormal swallowing, cardiovascular disease, metabolic disorders, asthma, and gastroesophageal reflux.** A rare condition is **sleep-related hemolysis,** or **paroxysmal nocturnal hemoglobinuria,** which is an acquired hemolytic anemia exacerbated by sleep. Rather than a particular sleep disturbance, however, sufferers complain of rust-colored morning urine.

3. **Substance-Induced Sleep Disorders. Substances, whether prescription medications or recreational drugs, can cause a wide range of sleep abnormalities that are often confused for primary sleep disorders.** To make the diagnosis, the DSM-IV states that the history, physical, or laboratory examination must demonstrate that the substance is related to the sleep complaint, and that the sleep disorder developed during or within a month of intoxication or withdrawal from the substance. Generally, if the substance is a CNS depressant, intoxication causes sedation and withdrawal causes insomnia. Likewise, if the substance is a CNS stimulant, intoxication results in insomnia and withdrawal results in sedation. Because the list of substances is immense, alcohol will be the only substance discussed.

Alcohol is a widely used and abused CNS depressant. In small to moderate amounts, it is sedating, and, while inducing sleep, causes frequent awakenings. In acute intoxication, alcohol decreases REM sleep and increases stages 3 and 4 sleep, while acute withdrawal produces insomnia, increases REM sleep, and decreases stages 3 and 4 sleep. Paradoxically, chronic use frequently results in insomnia, and, if alcohol abuse or dependence is particularly longstanding, insomnia may persist for months or up to a year after detoxification. If the suspected agent of a sleep disorder is alcohol, sleeping preparations are contraindicated, as the combined use of alcohol and sedative can be additive or synergistic, resulting in severe CNS depression, respiratory suppression, and death.

Suggested Readings

Bootzin RR, Lahmeyer H, Lillie JK (eds): *Integrated Approach to Sleep Management: The Healthcare Practitioner's Guide to the Diagnosis and Treatment of Sleep Disorders.* Belle Mead, NJ: Cahners Healthcare Communications, 1994.

Carskadon MA, Roth T: Normal sleep and its variations. In Kryger MH, Roth T, Dement WC (eds): *Principles and Practice of Sleep Medicine,* 2nd ed. Philadelphia: WB Saunders, 1994:3–25.

Culebras A: Update on disorders of sleep and the sleep-wake cycle. *Psychiatr Clin North Am* 1992; 15(2):467–489.

Smallwood P: Obstructive sleep apnea revisited. *Med Psychiatry* 1998; 1:42–52.

Stern TA: Sleep disorders. In: Hyman SE, Jenike MA (eds): *Manual of Clinical Problems in Psychiatry.* Boston: Little, Brown, 1990:140–150.

Williams RL, Karacan I, Moore CA, Hirshkowitz M: Normal sleep and sleep disorders. In Kaplan HI, Sadock BJ, Grebb JA (eds): *Synopsis of Psychiatry,* 7th ed. Baltimore: Williams and Wilkins, 1994:699–716.

Chapter 23
Impulse Control Disorders
K ATHY S ANDERS

I. Introduction

This category of diagnoses in the *Diagnostic and Statistical Manual, Fourth Edition* (DSM-IV) is a "residual." **Diagnoses in this category include kleptomania, pyromania, pathological gambling, trichotillomania, intermittent explosive disorder, and impulse control disorder, not otherwise specified (NOS).**

Each of these conditions involves a drive, or a temptation, to perform some act that is harmful to the person or to others, or the failure to resist an impulse. Other associated features are the experience of increasing tension (of dysphoria or arousal intensity) before committing the act that is followed by a release of tension, a sense of gratification, or a sense of pleasure and relief during and after the act. There may be a sense of guilt, regret, or self-reproach following the behavior.

Controversy surrounds whether these conditions are distinct diagnoses or variants of another Axis I disorder. In some ways they are similar to obsessive-compulsive disorder (OCD), substance dependence, mood disorders, and mental disorders due to a general medical condition. A similar etiology to OCD, eating disorders, mood disorders, paraphilias, and alcohol and substance abuse disorders is postulated because similar treatments work for each of these disorders.

Patients diagnosed with impulse control disorders have an increased risk of being diagnosed with substance abuse disorders, OCD and other anxiety disorders, eating disorders, and mood disorders. Moreover, there is an increased incidence of substance abuse disorders and mood disorders in family members of patients with these impulse control disorders.

Theories place impulse control disorders on a spectrum of affective disorders, as a variant of OCD, or a blend of mood, impulse, and compulsive disorders. While historically these disorders were thought to result from psychodynamic conflicts, recently, since improvement of impulsive symptoms has accompanied use of the serotonergic antidepressants, more biological hypotheses are being explored.

II. Kleptomania

A. Definitions
1. More than 150 years ago, kleptomania was recognized as an **out-of-character behavior of "nonsensical pilfering"** in which worthless items were stolen.

A characteristic increase in tension was relieved only by the act of stealing. Individuals in this category were not known to have a lifestyle of stealing or of premeditated thievery. Since its initial description, few systematic or scientifically rigorous studies have been conducted.

2. **Diagnostic criteria** from DSM-IV include:
   a. A repetitive failure to resist the urge to steal objects that are not needed for personal use or for monetary value.
   b. An increase in tension immediately before committing the theft.
   c. A sense of pleasure, gratification, or relief associated with performing the theft.
   d. The absence of anger or vengeance while stealing; the thefts are not in response to a delusion or hallucination.
   e. Absence of diagnostic criteria for a conduct disorder, a manic episode, or an antisocial personality disorder.

B. Epidemiology
1. **Little is known about the epidemiology of kleptomania.** Few studies have been published on this subject.
2. That said, it is **estimated that the prevalence within the general population is 6 out of 1,000.** Less than 5% of shoplifters meet criteria for kleptomania.
3. Women are more likely than are men to be diagnosed with kleptomania.
4. There is often a lag time of many years (up to several decades) between the onset of the behavior and an individual's presentation for treatment. Women with this disorder on average seek treatment in their 30s, while men seek treatment in their 50s.

C. Evaluation/Examination
1. **This disorder tends to have its onset in later adolescence, followed by a course of chronic, intermittent episodes of stealing** over many years.
2. **Patients generally come to professional attention via court referral or by disclosure during treatment for a related psychiatric disorder.**
3. Ego-dystonic reactions to the behavior and to the unpremeditated nature of the stealing episodes should be examined.
4. **Differential diagnosis** includes:
   a. Criminal acts of shoplifting or stealing
   b. Malingering to avoid prosecution for theft

    c. Antisocial personality disorder

    d. Conduct disorder

    e. Manic episode

    f. Schizophrenia

    g. Dementia

D. Treatment

1. Case series often lack clear definitions and treatment successes are hard to pinpoint.
2. Treatment modalities include:
   a. Insight-oriented psychotherapy
   b. Behavioral therapies that use covert and aversive sensitization
   c. Somatic therapies, including electroconvulsive therapy (ECT) and pharmacotherapy, particularly with serotonergic antidepressants

III. Pyromania

A. Definitions

1. **Pyromania is pathological fire setting without evidence of secondary, monetary, or political gain, intense emotional expression, or fire setting as a criminal act.**
2. **DSM-IV diagnostic criteria** include:
   a. The deliberate act of setting a fire in a purposeful manner on more than one occasion.
   b. Increasing tension and/or affective arousal associated with the act.
   c. Fascination, attraction, and curiosity about fires.
   d. Obvious pleasure, gratification, or relief while setting fires, or when witnessing or participating in the aftermath of the fire setting.
   e. The motivation for fire setting is not due to monetary gain, as an expression of sociopolitical ideology, as a means of concealing criminal activity, as a means of expressing anger or vengeance, as a means of improving one's living circumstances, in response to a delusion or hallucination, or as a result of impaired judgment (e.g., dementia, mental retardation, substance intoxication).
   f. Conduct disorder, a manic episode, or antisocial personality disorder must be ruled out.

B. Epidemiology

1. **True pyromania is rare.**
2. Pyromania is assumed to have a preponderance in males, often with a history of fascination with fires that dates back to childhood or early adolescence.

C. Differential Diagnosis

1. Intentional fire setting for profit, for political interests, or for revenge are exclusions to the diagnosis.
2. Delusions or hallucinations associated with schizophrenia or another psychotic disorder must be ruled out.
3. Fire setting cannot be due to a manic episode with poor impulse control.

4. Dementia or another mental disorder caused by a medical condition may result in behavior due to an impaired ability to acknowledge consequences of an act.
5. Conduct disorder in children and antisocial personality disorder in adults must be considered in the differential.

D. Treatment

There is no definitive treatment modality for fire setting. Typically several modalities, behavioral therapy, pharmacotherapy, family therapy (especially where children are concerned) are used simultaneously.

IV. Pathological Gambling

A. Definitions

1. **Pathologic gambling involves a failure to resist the impulse to gamble in the face of severe disruption in personal, family, or vocational functioning.** This disorder is most similar to addiction disorder; similarities to alcoholism are also noted.
2. **DSM-IV diagnostic criteria:**
   a. **Persistent and recurrent maladaptive gambling behavior as indicated by five (or more) of the following:**
      i. Preoccupation with gambling (e.g., reliving past gambling experiences, planning the next venture, or thinking about ways to get money to continue gambling).
      ii. The need to gamble with increasing amounts of money to achieve the desired excitement.
      iii. Repeated and unsuccessful efforts to control, cut back, or to stop gambling.
      iv. Restlessness or irritability during attempts to cut down or to stop gambling.
      v. Gambling as a means to escape from problems or to relieve dysphoric mood (e.g., feelings of helplessness, guilt, anxiety, or depression).
      vi. Increased gambling activity after losing money ("chasing" one's losses).
      vii. Lying to family members, to one's therapist, or to others, to conceal the extent of involvement with gambling.
      viii. The commission of illegal acts, such as forgery, fraud, theft, or embezzlement to finance gambling.
      ix. Jeopardizing or losing a significant relationship, job, or educational or career opportunity because of gambling.
      x. Reliance on others to provide money to relieve a desperate financial situation caused by gambling.
   b. The gambling behavior is not better accounted for by a manic episode.

B. Epidemiology

1. **The incidence of pathological gambling may be as high as 3% in the general population.**

2. One-third of pathological gamblers are women who make up only 2–4% of Gamblers Anonymous membership.

3. Cultural and sociological factors play a role in the specific manifestation of behavior in the pathological gambler (e.g., cockfights, horse racing, the stock market, ma jong, pai go, and bingo).

C. Evaluation

1. **The differential diagnosis must sort out social gambling and professional gambling from the pathological type.**

2. As with all impulse control disorders NOS, **the clinician must make sure the behavior is not due to a manic episode or an antisocial personality disorder.**

3. Since pathological gamblers exhibit tolerance and withdrawal associated with episodes of gambling, evidence of **irritability, restlessness, poor concentration, and dysphoria can be detected when a gambling episode is delayed or disrupted.**

4. Increasingly bets are made and risks taken as the need for excitement and arousal is chased.

5. Associated alcoholism, workaholic behavior, mood disorders, and antisocial, narcissistic, and borderline personality disorders may be noted.

D. Treatment

1. **Treatment for compulsive gambling is difficult** and the course is characterized by frequent relapses, financial difficulties, and legal problems that work against a commitment to ongoing therapy.

2. No specific treatment modality has been shown to work predictably.

3. Treatment modalities include psychodynamic psychotherapy, behavioral therapy, cognitive therapy, use of psychotropic medications, and electroconvulsive therapy (ECT).

4. The use of Gamblers Anonymous and the associated 12-step programs, Gam-Anon and Gam-a-teen, are important resources in breaking the addiction cycle.

V. Trichotillomania

A. Definitions

1. **The term, trichotillomania, was introduced** to medical literature **by** the French dermatologist, **Francois Hallopeau in 1889** as a compulsive urge to pull out one's own hair.

2. The DSM-IV defines it with the following **diagnostic criteria:**

   a. **Recurrent pulling out of one's hair resulting in significant hair loss.**

   b. **Increased tension immediately before pulling out the hair or when attempting to resist the behavior.**

   c. **The experience of pleasure, gratification, or relief when pulling out the hair.**

d. The disturbance is not better accounted for by another mental disorder and is not due to a general medical condition (e.g., a dermatological condition).

e. The disturbance causes clinically significant distress or impairment in social, occupational, or other important areas of functioning.

B. Epidemiology

1. **Initially considered rare,** there is evidence **that 1–3% of the population have this disorder.**

2. There is **a bimodal presentation.** Some individuals present before 6 years of age; in this group, boys and girls are evenly presented and they are managed with behavioral interventions. This type is time-limited and is treatable. **The second cluster begins in adolescence, and it is made up predominately of girls. This disorder is chronic and poorly treated.**

3. The site of the hair pulling is commonly the scalp (two-thirds of cases) but can include eyelashes, eyebrows, facial hair, and pubic hair.

4. **Comorbidity with other psychiatric diagnoses is common.** Mood disorders, psychotic disorders, eating disorders, anxiety disorders, and substance abuse disorders are prevalent.

5. Trichotillomania can be a symptom of other major mental illnesses including OCD, mental retardation, schizophrenia, depression, and borderline personality disorder. This has raised the controversy whether trichotillomania is a separate diagnostic entity.

C. Evaluation

1. It is important to **differentiate trichotillomania from OCD.** Look for impulsive urges versus goal-associated ideation about the hair pulling.

2. **Factitious disorder** to get medical attention **should be ruled out.**

3. **Alopecia secondary to an organic cause is most difficult to rule out.**

4. Any Axis I mental disorder that has the symptom of trichotillomania due to command hallucinations or delusional beliefs must be considered.

D. Treatment

1. As in most of the impulse control disorders, **many different treatment modalities have been used with variable success.**

2. Psychodynamic psychoanalytic psychotherapy has been successful in anecdotal case reports.

3. **Behavioral treatment has been more successful.** Techniques include:

   a. **Focus on hair pulling as a habit** and substituting other responses.

   b. **Positive reinforcement** for not pulling hair and negative reinforcement of hair pulling, aversive conditioning, relaxation, and competing response training are some of the behavioral techniques.

c. **Hypnotherapy.**

d. **Psychopharmacology** with serotinergic antidepressants, neuroleptics, or lithium.

e. **Personal appearance problems require attention** to both psychotherapeutic and psychopharmacologic interventions for lasting efficacy of treatment.

VI. Intermittent Explosive Disorder

A. Definitions

1. Impulsive and episodic violent behavior that cannot be better defined by a specific organic cause or due to a concomitant psychiatric diagnosis.

2. **The violence associated with this condition is characteristically an aggression out of proportion to the precipitating stressor.**

3. **DSM-IV diagnostic criteria**

   a. **Several discrete episodes of failure to resist aggressive impulses that result in serious assaultive acts or destruction of property.**

   b. The degree of **aggressiveness** expressed during the episodes **is distinctly out of proportion to any precipitating psychosocial stressors.**

   c. The aggressive episodes are not better accounted for by another mental disorder (e.g., antisocial personality disorder, borderline personality disorder, a psychotic disorder, a manic episode, conduct disorder, or attention deficit hyperactivity disorder) and are not due to the direct physiological effects of a substance (e.g., a drug of abuse, a medication) or a general medical condition (e.g., head trauma, Alzheimer's disease).

B. Epidemiology

1. Episodic violence of any type is common in our society. When applying strict diagnostic criteria, **this disorder is considered rare.**

2. **Men make up 80% of the cases.**

3. Intermittent explosive disorder and personality change due to a general medical condition, aggressive type, are the current diagnoses available to label a patient with episodic violent behavior.

C. Evaluation

1. **Most violent behavior can be accounted for by numerous psychiatric and medical conditions.**

2. **The most common diagnosis for violence is personality change due to a general medical condition (e.g., seizures, head trauma, neurological abnormality, dementia, delirium),** aggressive or disinhibited type.

3. Personality disorders of the borderline or antisocial type must be ruled out.

4. Psychosis from schizophrenia or a manic episode may cause this episodic violence.

5. Aggressive outbursts while intoxicated or while withdrawing from a substance of abuse would clearly rule out the diagnosis of intermittent explosive disorder.

D. Treatment

1. **Psychopharmacology is commonly employed** in the chronic management of this disorder. **Anticonvulsants, lithium, beta-blockers, anxiolytics, neuroleptics, antidepressants (both serotonergic and polycyclic agents), and psychostimulants are used** with varying results.

2. **The acute management of aggressive and violent behavior may involve the use of physical restraint and rapid use of a combination of parenteral neuroleptics and benzodiazepines.**

3. Long-term outpatient management of intermittent explosive disorder requires attention to the therapeutic alliance between clinician and patient.

VII. Impulse Control Disorder NOS

A. Definition

1. This category of disorders does not meet diagnostic criteria for any of the previously discussed impulse control disorders or for another mental disorder having the features involving impulse control.

2. Included in this category are diagnoses such as **pathological spending, pathological shopping, repetitive self-mutilation, compulsive sexual behavior, and compulsive face picking.**

B. Epidemiology

1. **Most of the literature on this category focuses on repetitive self-mutilation.**

2. It is **more common in women than in men.** However, it is considered endemic in male prisons.

3. **Two-thirds of self-mutilators have a history of sexual and physical abuse in childhood.**

4. The disorder starts in adolescence and is characterized by severe psychosocial morbidity.

C. Evaluation and Differential

1. The theories about the causes of self-mutilation range from psychodynamic to psychobiologic.

2. Self-mutilation gives a quick sense of relief to stress and is often likened to an addiction.

3. **Differential diagnosis includes:**

   a. A component of borderline, narcissistic, and antisocial personality disorders

   b. Mental retardation, as caused by Lesch-Nyan and deLange syndromes

   c. Hallucinations or delusions from a psychotic disorder

   d. Sexual sadomasochism

   e. OCD

D. Treatment

1. Multimodal treatment is the current recommended treatment.

2. Prognosis is guarded and worsens with comorbidity, with eating disorders, and with substance abuse disorders. Intentional or accidental suicide is common.

3. **Psychopharmacology includes: serotonergic enhancing drugs, and the narcotic antagonist, naltrexone.**
4. Other modalities include psychodynamic psychotherapy, behavioral therapy, and involvement in self-help and 12-step programs.

Suggested Readings

American Psychiatric Association: *Diagnostic and Statistical Manual of Mental Disorders, Fourth Edition* (DSM-IV). Washington, DC: American Psychiatric Press, 1994:609–621.

Beck JC: Legal and ethical duties of the clinician treating a patient who is liable to be impulsively violent. *Behav Sci Law* 1998; 16(3):375–389.

Burt VE: Impulse-Control Disorders not elsewhere classified. In Kaplan HI, Sadock BJ (eds): *Comprehensive Textbook of Psychiatry*, 6th ed. Baltimore: Williams and Wilkins, 1995:1409–1418.

Coccaro EF, Kavoussi RJ, Berman ME, Lish JD: Intermittent Explosive Disorder-revised: development, reliability, and validity of research criteria. *Comp Psychiatry* 1998; 39(6): 368–376.

DeCaria CM, Hollander E, Grossman R, et al.: Diagnosis, neurobiology, and treatment of pathological gambling. *J Clin Psychiatry* 1996; 57 (Suppl. 8):80–84.

McElroy SL, Hudson JI, Pope HG Jr, et al.: The DSM-III-R Impulse Control Disorder not elsewhere classified: clinical characteristics and relationship to other psychiatric disorders. *Am J Psychiatry* 1992; 149(3):318–327.

McElroy SL, Pope HG Jr, Keck PE Jr, et al.: Are impulse-control disorders related to bipolar disorder? *Comp Psychiatry* 1996; 37(4):229–240.

McElroy SL, Soutullo CA, Beckman DA, et al.: DSM-IV Intermittent Explosive Disorder: a report of 27 cases. *J Clin Psychiatry* 1998; 59(4):203–210.

Stein DJ, Hollander E, Liebowitz MR: Neurobiology of impulsivity and the impulse control disorders. *J Neuropsychiatr Clin Neurosci* 1993; 5(1):9–17.

Wise MG, Tierney JG: Impulse control disorders not elsewhere classified. In Hales RE, Yudofsky SG, Talbot JA (eds): *The American Psychiatric Press Textbook of Psychiatry*, 2nd ed. Washington, DC: American Psychiatric Press, 1994:681–699.

Chapter 24

Adjustment Disorders, Grief, and Bereavement

ALICIA POWELL

I. Introduction

Adjustment Disorders are defined as stress-related phenomena in which the sufferer experiences significant dysfunction and symptoms which are relieved when the stressor is removed or a new state of adaptation is reached.

Epidemiologic studies report that **2–5% of outpatients** are given the diagnosis of adjustment disorder, and 11–21% of general hospital patients seen in psychiatric consultation receive the diagnosis.

II. Clinical Features

In contrast to other disorders listed in the *Diagnostic and Statistical Manual, Fourth Edition* (DSM-IV), **no specific set of symptomatic criteria exist** which define an adjustment disorder.

Symptoms may be emotional or behavioral and **must occur within 3 months of the onset of an identifiable stressor. The symptoms must be either in excess of what would be expected from the stressor, or must cause significant impairment in social or occupational functioning.** Somatic concerns may be present.

Adults usually, but not always, present with depressed mood and/or anxiety. Pediatric patients typically present with behavioral symptoms, but they can also have emotional symptoms.

III. Evaluation and Differential Diagnosis

The stress-related problem may not meet criteria for another Axis I disorder, and cannot represent an exacerbation of a previously diagnosed Axis I or Axis II disorder. When presenting a case of adjustment disorder for the Board examiners, it is better to include the appropriate Axis I and/or Axis II disorders as rule-out diagnoses than to exclude them altogether.

The stressor cannot be the loss of a significant person or object; if it is, bereavement (see below) would likely be diagnosed.

The DSM-IV categorizes adjustment disorders based on the predominant symptoms: depressed mood, anxiety, mixed anxiety and depressed mood, disturbance of conduct (seen frequently in pediatric populations), mixed disturbance of conduct and emotions, or not otherwise specified (NOS).

IV. Management of Adjustment Disorders

A. **Treatment of adjustment disorder lies in interventions which reduce the stressor (if possible), strengthen coping mechanisms, and maximize the patient's support system.**

B. **Psychotherapy,** especially supportive individual and/or family therapy, can help the patient express concerns in a safe environment and obtain needed support. For certain common stressors like an illness, support groups can provide a network of information and support.

C. Although not a primary treatment modality, **psychopharmacologic intervention may be indicated to reduce severe symptoms of anxiety or depression.** Treatment should not be withheld just because a patient does not meet strict criteria for a major Axis I disorder. Indeed, some patients diagnosed with adjustment disorder are in the early phase of an Axis I disorder.

V. Introduction to Grief and Bereavement

A. **Grief is a variable but normal response to a significant loss.** The terms **grief, mourning, and bereavement are often used interchangeably. The experience and expression of grief are affected by many factors: cultural norms, personality style, abruptness of loss, significance of the lost person or object to the grieving survivor, extent of preparation for the loss, and the type of death** (natural vs. unnatural).

B. **A complicated grief reaction is one which causes more severe or protracted suffering and loss of functioning** due to inability to grieve appropriately, or the presence of a second psychiatric disorder.

VI. Clinical Features

A. Surveys of bereavement reveal that **most grieving persons are able to cope and recover well from the process,** and few seek psychiatric attention. However, if the survivor does not proceed through a grieving process normally, that person is at risk for development of secondary somatic and emotional problems.

187

B. Grief often appears as a temporary depressive syndrome with sadness, insomnia, diminished appetite, and interests. The survivor may feel guilty about not having done more for the deceased. A passive wish to die may be present, especially as a desire to be with the deceased.

C. The process of grief may be organized into phases:

1. **The initial phase, lasting hours to days, is marked by shock and disbelief.** Early denial is a protective and normal defense against the pain of acute loss.

2. **The next phase may occupy the next several months and ushers in a gradual realization of the loss.** The bereaved person often expresses a variety of emotions, including sadness, anger, hopelessness, emptiness, and helplessness. During this period the survivor may experience many symptoms of major depression, including the feeling that life is no longer worth living. **Active suicidality with plan, intent, or gesture, should be taken as a sign of a complicated grief reaction and managed with appropriate attention to the patient's safety.**

3. **Usually between 6 months and 1 year after the loss, a final phase of grief ensues.** Symptoms of the second phase begin to resolve but may persist, especially if the bond to the deceased was extremely important to the survivor. **The bereaved person fully accepts the reality of the loss during the final phase, and begins to return to a functioning life.** It is normal for the survivor to re-experience symptoms from the first two phases when reminded suddenly of the loss. It is also normal for feelings of anger and anxiety to continue during the final phase. The important measure of the severity of these feelings is the survivor's level of functioning, which usually will be restored during the final phase. If not, the person may be experiencing a complicated grief reaction.

VII. Evaluation and Differential Diagnosis

A. Evaluation should include an assessment of the severity of depression, the presence of psychotic symptoms, alcohol or drug abuse, and suicidal ideation. Additionally, if the survivor witnessed the death, symptoms of posttraumatic stress disorder may appear.

1. **Pay particular attention to those who are bereaved as the result of suicide,** since data suggest that this group of survivors are themselves at increased risk for suicide.

2. **Inquire about the patient's network of social supports.**

B. Symptoms of a second psychiatric condition, if present, **should be investigated** appropriately. The diagnosis of major depression can be difficult in the setting of grief, but if neurovegetative symptoms and signs are severe, or if suicidal ideation is present, the examiner should consider the diagnosis of depression. **Remember that hearing the voice or seeing the face of the deceased may be an accepted symptom of grief in some cultures,** such as Latin cultures.

C. Board examinees should not underestimate the power and importance of simple human compassion for the bereaved. Examiners will expect you to be able to accept and tolerate the patient's feelings. **A listening presence is usually more helpful than directive phrases** like, "Be strong for your children," or false empathy such as, "I know what you're going through." Be sure, however, to **address the patient's grief directly during the interview, and offer a word of sympathy for the patient's loss.**

VIII. Management of Grief and Bereavement

A. Whether or not the grief reaction proceeds normally, **management consists of treatment of dysfunctional symptoms** (like insomnia), or any superimposed disorders, and facilitation of the mourning process. Any intervention should be tailored to the individual, as grief is a personal and variable process.

B. Psychopharmacological treatment is not the primary treatment for grief, but it may promote sleep or relieve anxiety. Unless a secondary depressive or psychotic disorder is present, antidepressants and antipsychotics have no role in the treatment of grief.

C. Mild sedation with benzodiazepines may be indicated for severe anxiety or insomnia. Avoid oversedating the patient, as this only impedes the grieving process. Since rapid relief is desired, avoid agents such as antidepressants or buspirone which can take weeks to work.

D. If major depression, substance abuse, anxiety disorders, or psychosis is present in the grieving person, medical evaluation should be undertaken and the treatment for the disorder initiated.

Suggested Readings

Clayton P, Desmarais L, Winokur G: A study of normal bereavement. *Am J Psychiatry* 1968; 125(64):168–178.

Strain JJ, et al.: Adjustment disorder. In Hales RE, Yudofsky SC, Talbott JA (eds): *The American Psychiatric Press Textbook of Psychiatry*, 2nd ed. Washington DC: American Psychiatric Press, 1994:671–680.

Weisman A: The patient with acute grief. In Stern TA, Herman JB, Slavin PL (eds): *The MGH Guide to Psychiatry in Primary Care.* New York: McGraw-Hill, 1998:177–180.

Chapter 25

Personality Disorders

PATRICK SMALLWOOD

I. Introduction

Defining personality is as frustrating a task as is trying to untie the Gordian knot. To begin this seemingly nebulous task, we offer the following **definition of personality: an enduring pattern of perceiving, relating, and thinking about the environment and oneself that is seen in a wide range of social and personal situations.** Personality is relatively stable and predictable, and, as such, characterizes the individual in ordinary situations. When normal, it is flexible and adaptable. **When disordered, it is implacable, maladaptive, deeply ingrained, and often distressing for both the patient and significant others.** Because of the manipulative quality and ego-syntonic nature of these disorders, personality disorders often lack respectability as valid illnesses; those who make the diagnoses may place partial or full responsibility onto the patient. However, to ignore them as valid illnesses or to choose not to recognize them out of a misguided sense of protecting the patient from a label does a serious injustice and provides inadequate treatment for the whole person.

A. Classification System

Because certain personality disorders share common features, the *Diagnostic and Statistical Manual of Mental Disorders, Fourth Edition* (DSM-IV) has grouped them into three clusters. The **Cluster A personality disorders, which include Paranoid, Schizoid, and Schizotypal, appear to be odd and eccentric ("weird").** The **Cluster B personality disorders, which include Antisocial, Borderline, Histrionic, and Narcissistic, share the common features of being dramatic, emotional, and erratic ("wild").** Finally, the **Cluster C personality disorders, which include Avoidant, Dependent, and Obsessive-Compulsive, have a tendency to be anxious and fearful ("wimpy").** The remaining group, although not a cluster and share no common features, comprises **Personality Disorders Not Otherwise Specified.** In general, **patients frequently exhibit traits of more than one personality disorder,** and, if criteria for more than one disorder are met, then each disorder is diagnosed. Of note, personality disorders are diagnosed on Axis II. For the sake of brevity, only the salient features of each personality disorder will be reviewed in this chapter and the reader is referred to the DSM-IV for specific diagnostic criteria.

B. Epidemiology

Personality disorders are common in the general population, **with an estimated prevalence of 10–18%.** Consequently, these disorders are encountered in a variety of clinical settings. In outpatient populations, for example, the prevalence is estimated at 30–50%, and on inpatient units over 50% have a comorbid personality disorder. **Of patients with Axis I diagnoses, 34%,** most notably anxiety disorders and alcohol abuse, **have comorbid personality disorders.** For patients who demonstrate recurrent suicidal gestures and acts, the prevalence is 48–65%. Of importance, males and females are equally represented.

C. Etiology

Many theories abound as to the etiology of personality disorders. While each provides helpful constructs, none fully explains so complex a process. There is evidence to suggest that genetics play a role. For example, **Cluster A personality disorders are more common in relatives of schizophrenic patients, patients with Cluster B personality disorders have more family members with mood disorders,** and **patients with Cluster C personality disorders appear to have more relatives with anxiety disorders.**

Psychoanalytic theory, however, is by far the best-recognized theory for explaining the etiology of personality and personality disorders. **Freud** believed that personality traits were the product of fixation at a particular stage of psychosexual development. Wilhelm **Reich,** on the other hand, suggested that the personality arose from the particular pattern of defense mechanisms (unconscious mental processes that the ego uses to resolve conflict and thereby reduce anxiety and stress) that the individual consistently used. In nondisordered patients, these defenses are flexible and adaptable. For the disordered patient, they are inflexible and not easily given up, resulting in the impairments that often prompt them to seek treatment. By recognizing the pattern of defense mechanisms that a patient uses, the clinician should be able to determine the personality disorder, and thereby offer appropriate treatment. Table 25-1 lists the more **common defense mechanisms.**

189

Table 25-1. Common Defense Mechanisms

Defense Mechanism	Description
Projection	Unacceptable impulses and feelings are perceived and reacted to as though outside the self
Splitting	Objects are divided into "all good" and "all bad," with rapid shifting from one extreme to another
Regression	An attempt to return to an earlier stage of functioning to avoid tension and conflict at the present level of development
Fantasy	An autistic retreat involving the creation of imaginary lives to avoid conflict and obtain gratification
Dissociation	A temporary and drastic replacement of an unpleasant mood state (or current personal identity) with a more pleasant mood state (or alteration in one's sense of personal identity)
Intellectualization	Excessive use of intellectual processes to avoid expression of affect
Isolation	Separation of a cognitive process from its accompanying affect
Reaction formation	An unacceptable impulse is transformed to the opposite
Repression	A process by which an unwanted idea or feeling is held outside the conscious mind
Acting out	Direct observable action on an unconscious conflict in order to avoid being conscious of either the conflict or the affect that is associated with it
Passive aggression	Aggression toward others is expressed through passivity, masochism, and anger towards self

D. Treatment

Because personality disorders are deeply ingrained and ego-syntonic, they often resist treatment. **The conventional treatment methods for these disorders are psychoanalysis and psychodynamic psychotherapy. The principal goal with these modalities is to assist the patient in identifying and addressing the manner in which personality style is maladaptive, and thereby promote change by transforming what is an ego-syntonic state into an ego-dystonic state.** Recently, pharmacotherapy has been explored. Here, the rationale is to identify those biological dimensions of personality that may respond to medication, such as aggression, impulsivity, anxiety, depression, and psychosis, and treat those symptoms with appropriate medications. Other popular modalities include cognitive-behavioral methods, which attempt to modify specific behaviors, such as impulse control, frustration tolerance, and impaired cognitions, with strategies such as relaxation, role playing, and correction of distorted cognitions by monitoring, correcting, and providing alternative explanations for them.

II. Cluster A Personality Disorders

A. Paranoid Personality Disorder

1. **Core features.** The core feature of paranoid personality disorder is a pervasive, persistent, and inappropriate mistrust of people. **These individuals are reluctant to confide in others; they assume that most people will harm or exploit them in some manner. In new situations, they search for confirmation of these expectations, and view even the smallest slight as significant. They unjustifiably question the loyalty of friends and significant others, and consequently are often socially isolated and avoid intimacy. They pride themselves on being rational and objective, but appear to others as unemotional, affectively restricted, and hypervigilant.** Put simply, these individuals bear grudges, collect injustices, and make mountains out of molehills. Their preferred defense mechanisms include projection, denial, and rationalization. One note of caution: once challenged or stressed in any significant way, these individuals can show profound anger, hostility, referential thinking, or experience brief psychotic states that warrant acute psychiatric treatment.

2. **Differential diagnosis.** The most common differential diagnoses for Paranoid Personality Disorder include Delusional Disorder (paranoid type), Schizophrenia (paranoid type), and Schizoid and

Avoidant Personality Disorders. With Delusional Disorder and Schizophrenia, reality testing is lost, as opposed to Paranoid Personality Disorder, wherein reality testing remains intact. With Schizoid and Avoidant Personality Disorder, the amount and degree of paranoia are significantly less, which distinguishes it from Paranoid Personality Disorder.

3. **Prevalence.** The prevalence of Paranoid Personality Disorder **in the general population is between 0.5% and 2.5%.** There appears to be **an increased incidence in families with Schizophrenia and Delusional Disorder.** By far, the diagnosis is more common in males than females. There is a higher incidence of this disorder in minority groups, immigrants, and the deaf.

4. **Course.** The course of Paranoid Personality Disorder is often **lifelong,** with the best prognosis existing for those individuals with good ego strength and a solid outside support system. A poorer prognosis includes individuals who not only have poor insight and little to no support system, but also those who have comorbid Axis I diagnoses (especially Schizophrenia and substance abuse).

5. **Treatment. Treatment is difficult at best, as these individuals frequently avoid it. If a patient does engage in treatment, psychotherapy is the preferred modality, with the focus being supportive, consistent, and straightforward.** Due to trust issues and need for distance, groups are ineffective for these patients. Long-term pharmacotherapy rarely results in any robust improvement, and is mainly reserved for those times of stress when severe anxiety, hostility, and psychotic decompensation emerge. Under these conditions, short-term use of benzodiazepines and low-dose antipsychotic agents are the treatments of choice.

B. **Schizoid Personality Disorder**
1. **Core features. Individuals with Schizoid Personality Disorder are eccentric loners who are emotionally detached and indifferent to the world around them.** They have little desire for relationships or emotional ties, even with family members. **In social situations, they withdraw, rarely make eye contact, and avoid spontaneous conversation.** Their lack of fashion seems to reflect this pervasive disinterest in the world, as they often don uncoordinated and outdated clothing. With respect to employment, they prefer noncompetitive and isolative jobs with non-human themes, such as mathematics, philosophy, or astronomy. For hobbies, they enjoy solitary pursuits, such as computer games and puzzles. As perhaps a compensation for their lack of involvement in the world, these patients have extraordinary fantasy lives, which also includes their sexual experiences. Despite the apparent oddities, however, they possess clear thinking and intact reality testing. The best caricature of the schizoid personality would be the single, unfashionable, laboratory-oriented, absent-minded professor.

2. **Differential diagnosis.** The differential diagnoses for Schizoid Personality Disorder includes Schizophrenia as well as Paranoid, Obsessive-Compulsive, and Avoidant Personality disorders. Intact reality testing, normal abstracting ability, and the absence of formal thought disorder distinguish Schizoidal Personality Disorder from Schizophrenia. Patients with Paranoid Personality Disorder experience more social involvement than do Schizoid patients. Unlike patients with Schizoid Personality Disorder, patients with Obsessive-Compulsive and Avoidant Personality Disorders, while often socially isolated, view loneliness as ego-dystonic and enjoy a richer interpersonal history.

3. **Prevalence. Schizoid Personality Disorder affects about 7.5% of the population, with males diagnosed twice as often as females.** As with Paranoid Personality Disorder, incidence of psychotic disorders in the relatives of these patients is higher, although this association is less robust. There is also a slightly higher incidence of this disorder in people with solitary and night jobs.

4. **Course.** The onset of Schizoid Personality Disorder is early childhood, and generally remains throughout life. Most individuals function reasonably well and have few problems that require intervention. In a few cases, however, this disorder may progress to schizophrenia or other psychotic states.

5. **Treatment. Psychotherapy is the treatment of choice.** As these patients have the ability to introspect, they may remain in therapy for quite a long time. Supportive therapy is the mainstay, yet some patients may respond to insight-oriented psychotherapy. These patients generally do not desire group therapy, but, after tolerating the interaction with others, may provide a means of improving social skills for some. Pharmacotherapy is often ineffective for the character pathology itself and should be reserved for comorbid Axis I diagnoses.

C. **Schizotypal Personality Disorder**
1. **Core features. The essential features of the schizotypal personality are cognitive, perceptual, and behavioral eccentricities. Patients with this personality disorder frequently embrace beliefs such as telepathy, clairvoyance, and magical thinking to a degree that exceeds cultural and subcultural norms.**

Socially, they are inept and uncomfortable, and therefore prefer to be alone. The style of their clothing may be inappropriate and strange, further reflecting their eccentric nature. Their speech is often vague, digressive, or inappropriately abstract, and they may talk to themselves in public. The content of that speech may also reflect ideas of reference, bodily illusions, and paranoia, but there is usually an absence of formal thought disorders, and reality testing is intact. Under periods of stress, however, these patients may decompensate into brief psychotic states.

2. **Differential diagnosis.** The differential diagnosis for Schizotypal Personality Disorder includes schizophrenia and several personality disorders. Paranoid and Schizoid Personality Disorder shares many of the core features of Schizotypal Personality Disorder, but differs by degree or absence of eccentricity. Borderline Personality Disorder shares some of the unusual speech and perceptual style, but demonstrates stronger affect and connection to others. Patients with Avoidant Personality Disorder, while uncomfortable and inept in social settings, are not eccentric and crave contact with others. Schizophrenia differs from Schizotypal Personality Disorder in that the schizotype possesses good reality testing and lacks psychosis.

3. **Prevalence. Schizotypal personality disorder affects about 3% of the population. There is no known sex ratio, but it is felt to be more prevalent in males.** While there is no known genetic etiology, there appears to be a higher occurrence of this disorder in the biological relatives of schizophrenic patients.

4. **Course. The prognosis for this personality disorder is guarded.** Some patients are able to establish stable relationships, marry, and form families, despite their eccentricities. Others may experience periods of brief reactive psychosis or schizophrenic decompensation, leading some clinicians to believe that schizotypal personality is a premorbid personality state for schizophrenia. About 10% of these patients commit suicide.

5. **Treatment. The treatment for Schizotypal Personality Disorder is mainly psychotherapy.** Because these patients avoid social contact, the first and most difficult task is to establish an alliance. Once accomplished, supportive therapy with social skills training becomes the mainstay for treatment, as these patients are often unable to tolerate exploratory, insight-oriented, or group psychotherapy. **Pharmacotherapy should target comorbid Axis I disorders, with low-dose antipsychotics being used for those periods when these individuals experience brief psychotic decompensation.**

III. Cluster B Personality Disorders

A. **Antisocial Personality Disorder**
   1. **Core features. The key features of Antisocial Personality Disorder are repetitive unlawful acts and socially irresponsible behaviors that began prior to the age of 15 years.** These individuals are so **unconcerned with the feelings and rights of others that they are morally bankrupt and lack a sense of remorse.** Superficially, they are charming and engaging, yet beneath the facade lie individuals who live in a world filled with illegal activity, deceit, promiscuity, substance abuse, and assaultive behavior. Because patients with this disorder are so indifferent to how their actions impact others, antisocial personality disorder is perhaps the most resistant to treatment.

   2. **Differential diagnosis.** The differential diagnosis for antisocial personality disorder includes antisocial behavior, other Cluster B personality disorders, mania, psychosis, substance abuse disorders, mental retardation, and personality changes due to general medical conditions. With antisocial behavior, the actions are similar, but the history lacks a sense of degree and pervasiveness in the activities. Patients with borderline personality disorder may perform illegal acts, yet tend to demonstrate more repetitive suicidal and parasuicidal behaviors, as well as intense affect and self-loathing. Narcissistic personality-disordered patients for the most part adhere to the law as a means to meet their selfish needs. Bipolar mania can be difficult to separate from antisocial personality disorder, as patients with antisocial personalities can also have comorbid bipolar disorders. For the most part, however, patients with bipolar disorder often lack the degree of childhood conduct problems, and the antisocial behavior is usually limited to manic episodes. Once the mania is resolved, bipolar patients frequently display a sense of remorse. Patients with psychotic disorders may also perform criminal acts, but these acts are usually in response to delusions or hallucinations. Substance abuse disorders can be especially difficult to differentiate from antisocial personality disorder, as patients with antisocial personality disorder invariably engage in substance use. However, criminal behaviors associated with substance abuse disorders generally center around using and obtaining the drugs. Patients with mental retardation may perform criminal acts, but they may be unable to appreciate the illegal nature of the actions. Finally, patients with personality changes due to general medical conditions can display antisocial actions, but, for the most part, these

individuals lack a criminal history prior to the pre-cipitating condition.

3. **Prevalence. Antisocial personality disorder affects 3% of men and less than 1% of women.** While encountered more commonly in poor urban areas, up to 75% of the prison population carry the diagnosis. Patients with this disorder have an onset of conduct disorder before the age of 15 years, and frequently suffer comorbid attention deficit hyperactivity disorders, polysubstance disorders, and somatization disorders. While the exact etiology is unknown, it occurs five times more commonly in first-degree relatives of males with the disorder.

4. **Course.** The course for antisocial personality disorder is variable. Some improve during middle age as they come to the realization that society will no longer tolerate their behavior. Others end up in prison, experience the complications of drug dependency, or suffer violent deaths from injury, homicide, or suicide.

5. **Treatment.** As mentioned earlier, **this disorder is difficult, if not impossible, to treat.** Unfortunately, the most effective form of treatment appears to be in confined settings, such as prisons, where external constraints can substitute for their moral deficits. If psychotherapy is attempted, behavioral therapy with a strong emphasis on legal sanctions is the most effective method of treatment. Pharmacotherapy should target comorbid Axis I disorders or dangerous behaviors toward self and others.

B. **Borderline Personality Disorder**

1. **Core features.** Borderline Personality Disorder is perhaps the best studied of all the personality disorders. **The salient features include affect instability with rapidly shifting mood swings, impulsivity, identity disturbance (described as chronic boredom or emptiness), recurrent manipulative suicidal and parasuicidal behaviors (e.g., self-mutilation), and idealization/devaluation ("splitting"). Central to this disorder is an impaired capacity to form stable interpersonal relationships.** Once there is real or perceived separation in those relationships, these patients often react with intense fear and anger. If the fear of abandonment is realized, or if they experience significant stress, the borderline patient may also experience brief reactive psychotic states (also known as "micropsychotic episodes") or dissociative phenomena.

2. **Differential diagnosis.** The differential diagnosis for borderline personality disorder includes other personality disorders, an identity problem, bipolar spectrum disorders, and psychotic disorders.

Borderline patients lack the peculiarity and referential thinking found in schizotypal personality disorder and the extreme suspiciousness seen in paranoid personality disorder. Histrionic, narcissistic, and dependent individuals have stable identities, are capable of forming solid interpersonal relationships, and rarely engage in self-mutilation or chronic suicidal behavior. Identity problem differs from borderline personality disorder in that the former is usually time-limited and linked to a developmental stage (late adolescence or early adulthood). Bipolar spectrum disorders can be difficult to distinguish from borderline personality disorder, as the two may coexist. However, the mood swings displayed by the borderline patient cannot meet criteria for manic or hypomanic episodes. Finally, while the borderline may experience transient psychotic states, patients with major psychotic disorder generally experience a persistent impairment in reality testing.

3. **Prevalence. Borderline personality disorder is the most prevalent personality disorder in all clinical settings (12–15%). It occurs in 2–3% of the population, with a 2:1 female/male ratio.** There is an increased prevalence of mood disorders in families of borderline patients, as well as an increased prevalence of this disorder in mothers of affected children.

4. **Course.** Borderline personality disorder is usually diagnosed before the age of 40 years. While the course can be variable, it rarely changes over time. Some patients improve in middle age and revisit core symptoms only during periods of significant stress.

5. **Treatment.** Depending on the level of personality organization, borderline patients can engage in several modes of psychotherapy, including exploratory, insight-oriented, cognitive-behavioral, and supportive. **The greatest barrier to therapy, however, is the intense countertransference reactions that these patients instill in their treaters, and caution must be taken not to give in to those feelings.** Medications by themselves rarely make dramatic changes in this disorder, but are useful adjuncts to psychotherapy. Target symptoms that respond to medication include impulsivity, emotional lability, intermittent psychosis, and mood symptoms. Vigorous use of pharmacologic agents may be necessary for those periods when these patients pose a significant risk of harm to self or others.

C. **Histrionic Personality Disorder**

1. **Core features. The most notable features of Histrionic Personality Disorder are pervasive over-**

concern with appearance and attention, exaggerated emotional response, poor frustration tolerance that ends in outbursts, and impressionistic speech that lacks detail. They view physical attractiveness as the core of their existence, and, as such, are often provocative in dress, flamboyant in mannerisms, and inappropriately seductive in behavior. While they appear superficially charming, others tend to view them as vain and lacking in genuineness.

2. **Differential diagnosis.** The differential diagnosis for histrionic personality disorder includes other personality disorders, and somatization disorder. Borderline personality disorder differs from histrionic in that the borderline displays more despair and suicidal/parasuicidal behaviors. Likewise, the narcissistic patient is more preoccupied with grandiosity and envy than is the histrionic individual. The dependent personality, while sharing the need for acceptance and reassurance, lacks the degree of emotionality seen in histrionic personality disorder. Somatization disorder can coexist with histrionic personality disorder, but is distinguished by the greater emphasis on physical complaints.

3. **Prevalence. Histrionic personality disorder occurs in 2–3% of the general population. While women receive the diagnosis more often, many clinicians feel that men are underdiagnosed.** This disorder is more common in first-degree relatives of people with this disorder.

4. **Course.** Like most personality disorders, the course is variable. Some experience an attenuation or softening of the core symptoms with age. Others may experience a complicated course, including comorbid somatization, dissociative, sexual, and mood disorders. A few may experience brief reactive psychotic states under stressful situations.

5. **Treatment. Individual psychodynamic psychotherapy, with emphasis on emotional clarification, is the treatment of choice for this disorder.** Long-term pharmacotherapy is reserved for comorbid Axis I disorders. Low-dose benzodiazepines are useful for transient emotional states, and low-dose antipsychotics are often necessary for episodes of dissociation and brief psychotic states.

D. **Narcissistic Personality Disorder**
1. **Core features. The hallmark of Narcissistic Personality Disorder is an overwhelming and pathological self-absorption.** These individuals possess a grandiose sense of self-importance and feel that the people with whom they associate need also to be special and unique. **They are blindly ambitious, often breaking conventional rules and exploiting others to meet their self-serving ends. They lack**

empathy for others, and react with disappointment and rage when another's tragedy compromises their plans. Beneath the facade of self-sufficiency and arrogance lies a fragile individual who is so hypersensitive to issues of self-esteem such that, if they are criticized in even the slightest manner, they react with intense emotion or brief psychotic decompensation.

2. **Differential diagnosis.** What makes the differential diagnosis for narcissistic personality disorder so difficult is that other Cluster B personality disorders often coexist. Nonetheless, a few distinguishing features are helpful. **The borderline patient differs from the narcissist in that the former is more impulsive, has a less cohesive identity, and lives a more chaotic life.** The histrionic patient, unlike the narcissistic patient, is more emotional and deeply involved with others. While the narcissistic and antisocial patient both exploit people, the primary motivation for the narcissistic patient is mainly power rather than material gain.

3. **Prevalence.** The exact prevalence for this disorder is unknown. **The best estimates are that it occurs in less than 1% in the general population and between 2% and 15% in the clinical population. There are no data concerning familial patterns or sex ratio.**

4. **Course. The course of this illness is chronic.** These patients frequently suffer comorbid mood disorders, particularly major depression and dysthymia. Under stress, they may also experience brief reactive psychosis. Aging is the ultimate blow to their self-esteem, as many of the things that they hinge their identity around (e.g., career, health, beauty, and youth) must naturally begin to fade. Consequently, the narcissistic patient is prone to severe mid-life crises.

5. **Course. The treatment of choice for narcissistic personality disorder is individual psychodynamic psychotherapy, including analysis and insight-oriented techniques.** These patients do not tolerate group settings. Pharmacotherapy should target comorbid Axis I disorders, particularly depression. Lithium is helpful for mood swings, and antipsychotic agents are useful for transient psychotic states.

IV. Cluster C Personality Disorders

A. **Avoidant Personality Disorder**
1. **Core features. The core feature of Avoidant Personality Disorder is an excessive discomfort or fear in intimate and social relationships that results in pathological avoidance as a means of self-protection.** For example, to guard against potentially unpleasant situations, these individuals frequently exaggerate the risks of ordinary unplanned tasks

so as not to deviate from a safe daily routine. While genuinely desiring relationships, they are unwilling to enter them due to real or perceived signs of humiliation, rejection, or negative feedback. If, however, they manage to negotiate a relationship, it is only with assurance of uncritical acceptance. Because of this pervasive awkwardness and shyness, they suffer incredibly low self-esteem.

2. **Differential diagnosis.** The differential diagnosis for avoidant personality disorder includes other personality disorders and social phobia. Patients with schizoid personality disorder, unlike patients with avoidant personality disorder, do not desire relationships with others. While dependent personality disorder shares many features with avoidant, the former has greater fear of abandonment, and embraces, rather than avoids, relationships. Social phobia can be very difficult to distinguish from avoidant personality disorder, and many clinicians consider them one and the same. Other clinicians argue, however, that the distinction between the two is that patients with social phobia tend to have specific fears around social performances.

3. **Prevalence. Avoidant personality disorder is common, occurring in about 1–10% of the general population.** Temperament and disfiguring physical illnesses may be predisposing factors. There is no information of sex ratio or familial patterns.

4. **Course.** Patients with avoidant personality disorder are able to function in relationships, marry, and have families, as long as the environment is safe and protective. As with most personality disorders, they are prone to mood disorders, especially depression and dysthymia. Due to the special nature of this disorder, however, they are at especially high risk for anxiety disorders and social phobia.

5. **Treatment.** Treatment for this disorder can be difficult, due to these patients' fear of humiliation and rejection. Once assured of acceptance and safety, they respond to virtually all forms of therapy. Current practice focuses on group settings with strong cognitive-behavioral emphasis. Anxiolytics are helpful in managing situational anxiety, and monoamine oxidase inhibitors (MAOIs) and selective serotonin reuptake inhibitors (SSRIs) are effective for treating comorbid anxiety and depression.

B. Dependent Personality Disorder

1. **Core features. Individuals with Dependent Personality Disorder have a strong desire for others to care for them and an extreme preoccupation with abandonment.** They fear being alone and will go to extreme lengths to preserve any relationship, no matter how physically or emotionally abusive it may be. They are submissive and passive toward others, and fear that any direct expression of anger will end in rejection. Subsequently, they often volunteer for unpleasant tasks, agree with others who may even be wrong, or look to others for assurance about simple daily decisions, to assure being liked or cared for.

2. **Differential diagnosis.** Dependent personality disorder can be difficult to distinguish from other psychiatric conditions, as many disorders have dependency as an underlying feature. The differential diagnosis for dependent personality disorder includes other personality disorders and agoraphobia. Patients with histrionic personality disorder have issues of dependency, but shorter and more numerous relationships. Borderline patients express more affect and anger around real or perceived abandonment, whereas dependent patients become more placating. When faced with rejection or termination of a relationship, avoidant patients withdraw from further contact, unlike dependent patients, who quickly seek out a new relationship to fill the void. Agoraphobia patients, while displaying dependency, tend to demonstrate a higher-level fear around leaving safe environments.

3. **Prevalence. Dependent personality disorder accounts for about 2.5% of all personality disorders,** with females more commonly affected than men. Patients with a history of childhood separation anxiety or chronic illness may be predisposed. There is no known familiar pattern of inheritance.

4. **Course. Many patients with this disorder suffer comorbid dysthymia, major depression, and alcohol abuse.** Because of their dependency and lack of assertiveness, they may also become victims of physical and emotional abuse. Careers are unlikely to advance, due to these patients' need for direction and inability to make decisions without excessive reassurance.

5. **Treatment.** These patients respond well to various forms of individual psychotherapy. Group therapy with emphasis on cognitive techniques, assertive training, and social skills, can be highly useful. Pharmacotherapy should target comorbid Axis I disorders, with benzodiazepines and SSRIs being the most effective medications.

C. Obsessive-Compulsive Personality Disorder

1. **Core features. The major features of Obsessive-Compulsive Personality Disorder are perfectionism and lack of compromise.** These individuals are so preoccupied with rules, efficiency, trivial details, and procedures that the purpose of the activity is often lost or the job is uncompleted. **They maintain**

an inflexible adherence to their own internally strict and unattainable standards, and subsequently dislike delegating tasks for fear that others will not meet those standards. While mindful of the chain of command, they possess a strong need for control and resist the authority and autonomy of others. To their superiors, they appear diligent, as they will tolerate protracted work, even at the cost of pleasure and interpersonal relationships. To their equals or subordinates, they are harsh taskmasters with escalating criteria for job perfection, who are stingy with emotions and compliments.

2. **Differential diagnosis.** The principal differential diagnosis for obsessive-compulsive personality disorder is obsessive-compulsive disorder. While the two are often confused for each other, they differ significantly: patients with obsessive-compulsive disorder have true obsessions and compulsions that they find ego-dystonic, whereas patients with the personality disorder find their behaviors ego-syntonic and rewarded by others. Occasionally, the two disorders coexist, requiring a diagnosis for each.

3. **Prevalence.** This personality disorder is common in the general population, with males receiving the diagnosis more often than females. While the mode of transmission is unknown, it is more common among first-degree relatives of patients with this disorder. There is also an increased concordance in identical twins.

4. **Course.** The course for obsessive-compulsive personality disorder is **variable.** Some patients are able to negotiate intimate long-term relationships, but have few friends, if any, outside those relationships. Others may mellow with age, becoming warm, caring, and generous to those around them. Often, however, depression, somatoform disorders, and alcohol dependence emerge as complications.

5. **Treatment. Unlike other personality disorders, individuals with this disorder often realize the impact of their behavior and seek treatment on their own.** They tend to improve with any number of treatment modalities, but particularly value a nondirective approach. Group therapy may be especially advantageous, as it permits others to point out bothersome behaviors and call for change. While there are few data to support pharmacotherapy, anecdotal evidence suggests that benzodiazepines may be useful in reducing the anxiety associated with their behaviors.

V. Personality Disorder Not Otherwise Specified

The diagnosis of Personality Disorder Not Otherwise Specified is reserved for persistent personality dysfunction that results in significant impairment, but does not reach full criteria for a single personality disorder, or meets criteria for one of the proposed personality disorders in Appendix B of the DSM-IV. These proposed disorders include Passive-Aggressive and Depressive Personality Disorders.

A. **Passive-Aggressive Personality Disorder**
   The major feature of Passive-Aggressive Personality Disorder is passive resistance to authority figures and to any request for adequate performance. This resistance, viewed as covert aggression, reveals itself as obstructionism and procrastination. These patients fail to ask important questions concerning adequate performance expectations, and become sullen or argumentative if those expectations arise. When requested to carry out tasks, they become deliberately inefficient, may make excuses for delays, and frequently complain of being misunderstood or underappreciated. Often, others must pick up their slack.

B. **Depressive Personality Disorder**
   The essential features of Depressive Personality Disorder are pervasive pessimism, anhedonia, and mirthlessness. Patients with this disorder are invariably passive, serious, moralistic, self-denigrating, and suffer low self-esteem. Since many patients with Axis I Dysthymic Disorder share similar presentations, some clinicians believe that this personality disorder and dysthymia are one and the same.

Suggested Readings

American Psychiatric Association: *Diagnostic and Statistical Manual Of Mental Disorders, Fourth Edition.* Washington, DC: American Psychiatric Association, 1994.

Gunderson JG, Phillips KA: Personality disorders. In Kaplan HI, Sadock BJ, Grebb JA (eds): *Synopsis of Psychiatry*, 7th ed. Baltimore: Williams and Wilkins, 1994:731–751.

Phillips KA, Gunderson JG: Personality disorders. In Hales RE, Yudofsky SC, Talbott JA (eds): *The American Psychiatric Press Textbook of Psychiatry* 2nd ed. Washington, DC: American Psychiatric Press, 1994:701–725.

Stone MH: Long-term outcome in personality disorders. *Br J Psychiatry* 1993: 162; 299–313.

Tyrer P, Casey P, Ferguson B: Personality disorder in perspective. *Br J Psychiatry* 1991: 159; 463–471.

Chapter 26

Psychiatric Disorders Associated with the Female Reproductive Cycle

HELEN G. KIM AND ADELE C. VIGUERA

I. Introduction

Reproductive hormone fluctuations mark several important times in the female lifecycle. These particular times around menses, pregnancy, postpartum, and menopause are often associated with mood and anxiety symptoms. **Contrary to popular lore, research has not revealed a consistent association between female reproductive hormones and psychiatric symptoms, but rather supports a more complicated interplay between biological and psychiatric diathesis and psychosocial factors.**

II. Neurobiologic Effects of Estrogen and Progesterone

A. **Estrogen and progesterone affect neurons in the opioid, norepinephrine (NE), serotonin (5HT), dopamine (DA), and γ-aminobutyric acid (GABA) systems.** Estrogen and progesterone receptors have been identified in **multiple areas of the central nervous system (CNS),** including the amygdala, hippocampus, cingulate cortex, locus coeruleus, midbrain raphe nuclei, and central gray matter. Some of the neuromodulatory mechanisms of steroid hormones include: intracellular effects on gene transcription of factors involved in neurotransmission; direct effects on monoamine turnover and metabolism; and direct effects on nerve cell membranes and receptors.

B. **Animal studies have shown that estrogen and other gonadal hormones affect downregulation of central $5HT_2$ receptors.** In addition, estrogen stimulates monoamine oxidase (MAO) degradation, which increases 5HT and other neurotransmitters. **Progesterone, on the other hand, decreases MAO degradation, which decreases these neurotransmitters.** These findings are consistent with the purported antidepressant effects of estrogen and the adverse mood effects of progesterone. However, the exact neuromodulatory mechanism as well as clinical uses of these hormones remain unclear.

III. Depression Through the Female Lifecycle

A. **Epidemiology**
1. **In every age group women have higher prevalence rates of depression than men.** The National Comorbidity Study reported that **the highest depression rates cluster in women during the reproductive years.**
2. The longest naturalistic, prospective study of first-episode major depression revealed no significant gender difference in time to recovery, time to first recurrence, or number of recurrent episodes (Simpson et al., 1997). **The increased female to male prevalence of depression thus may reflect increased risk of a first depressive episode in women of reproductive age.**

B. **Etiology**
1. There has been **no consistent evidence that** premenstrual, pregnancy, postpartum, or perimenopausal associated **psychiatric symptoms are correlated with abnormal levels of steroid hormones or gonadotropin release.**
2. Future research may try to identify subgroups of women who may be vulnerable to changes in the female hormonal milieu and thus may develop mood and anxiety symptoms at these vulnerable periods of hormone flux. In addition, much more work is necessary to delineate the effects of reproductive steroid hormones on CNS neurotransmitter pathways.
3. **History of affective illness also seems to predict potential risk for reproductive cycle-related mood disorders.** This finding has led researchers to wonder whether these disorders represent separate diagnostic entities or exacerbations of underlying mood disorders.
4. Psychosocial and psychodynamic factors also seem to be associated with affective symptoms during different stages of the reproductive cycle.

IV. Premenstrual Syndrome and Premenstrual Dysphoric Disorder

A. **Definitions**
1. **Premenstrual syndrome (PMS)** is a variably defined constellation of emotional and physical symptoms that occur during the luteal phase (i.e., between ovulation and menses) of the menstrual cycle.
2. **Premenstrual dysphoric disorder (PMDD)** is defined by DSM-IV research criteria and includes

the following symptom, timing, and severity parameters:

a. In most menstrual cycles during the past year, five or more of the following symptoms during the last week of the luteal phase with partial remission after the onset of the follicular phase and complete remission in the week postmenses. One of the symptoms must include (i), (ii), (iii), or (iv):
   i. Markedly depressed mood, hopelessness, or self-deprecating thoughts
   ii. Marked anxiety, feeling "keyed up," or "on edge"
   iii. Affective lability
   iv. Marked anger, irritability, or interpersonal conflicts
   v. Decreased interest
   vi. Difficulty concentrating
   vii. Decreased energy
   viii. Changes in appetite, overeating, or specific food cravings
   ix. Sleep disturbance
   x. Feeling out of control/overwhelmed
   xi. Other physical symptoms (e.g., breast tenderness or swelling, joint or muscle pain, "bloating")

b. Symptoms interfere with social or occupational functioning and are not merely an exacerbation of an Axis I diagnosis, such as major depression, panic disorder, or dysthymic disorder.

c. Quality and timing of symptoms must be confirmed by prospective daily ratings during at least two consecutive symptomatic cycles.

B. Epidemiology

1. PMS is extremely prevalent in the general population. Depending on the criteria used, **the estimated prevalence for PMS ranges from 3% to 10%,** though in some reports more than 80% of women experience one or two emotional or physical symptoms premenstrually.

2. **PMDD** affects far fewer women and **has a prevalence rate of approximately 2–5%** of women in the United States.

C. Etiology

1. **Hormone theories**

   a. **There is no consistent evidence that PMS/PMDD is associated with abnormal levels or release of circulating steroid or nonsteroid** (e.g., thyroid hormones, cortisol) **hormones.**

   b. **Certain subgroups of women with pre-existing vulnerability to normal hormone flux may develop mood or anxiety symptoms premenstrually.** In one study, Schmidt (1988) treated women with PMS and controls with leuprolide, a gonadotropin-releasing hormone (GnRH) agonist that suppresses the hypothalamic-pituitary-gonadal (HPG) axis and ceases menstrual cyclicity. Women who had remission of their PMS symptoms were treated with estrogen or progesterone add-back therapy which subsequently induced recurrence of their PMS symptoms. In contrast, controls who were treated with the same regimen of leuprolide and estrogen or progesterone add-back had no PMS symptoms. In this study, women with PMS and controls had differential responses to changes in hormones rather than absolute hormone levels.

   c. In another study by Schmidt and Rubinow (1991), women with prospectively confirmed PMDD were given RU486, an antiprogesterone, which shortened the luteal phase and induced menses. These women had their characteristic PMS symptoms after their RU486-induced menses, while their peripheral endocrine levels were consistent with follicular phase. These results could support one of two conclusions: either PMDD symptoms resulted from hormonal events that occur before the late luteal phase or PMDD represents an autonomous, cyclic disorder linked to the menstrual cycle but capable of being dissociated from the menstrual cycle.

2. The precise role of genetic and environmental factors (e.g., diet and stress) in predisposing women to PMS/PMDD is unknown.

D. Assessment of the Patient with Premenstrual Complaints

1. **Assess the reproductive endocrine status.** To determine the presence of luteal phase symptoms, one needs to determine whether the patient has regular ovulatory cycles. A patient with a history of spontaneous, regular menstrual cyclicity likely has normal menstrual function. To confirm regular ovulatory cycles, a woman can chart her basal body temperature to document a rise in temperature just after ovulation. Alternatively, a patient can measure LH in urine using an over-the-counter kit to detect the LH surge prior to ovulation.

2. **Rule out underlying medical conditions.** Review the medical history for syndromes that could mimic PMDD. For example, endometriosis may cause significant mood symptoms and pelvic discomfort prior to and during menses. In addition, certain conditions, such as migraines, epilepsy, and herpes, may have premenstrual worsening. Careful screening and a physical examination by an internist or gynecologist should be part of the evaluation of dysmenorrhea.

3. **Rule out underlying psychiatric conditions.** Review of the psychiatric history should include a patient's experience during periods of hormone fluctuations, such as during pregnancy and the postpartum period, which may reflect increased vulnerability to PMDD. In addition, different Axis I or II diagnoses can be exacerbated premenstrually rather than constitute PMDD. Excessive alcohol or drug use during the cycle may also affect mood and anxiety states. Axis I diagnoses should be trea-

ted to see if symptoms resolve in the follicular phase but persist in the luteal phase.

4. **Perform prospective daily rating scales.** After ruling out an underlying medical or psychiatric condition, a patient should fill out prospective daily rating scales over two consecutive cycles. Rubinow et al. (1984) reported that less than 50% of women who present with a history of PMDD actually had a premenstrual pattern of symptoms on prospective scales. Documentation of persistent follicular symptoms without luteal worsening rules against PMDD. Careful prospective documentation of symptoms throughout the cycle can help clarify the diagnosis and lead to appropriate workup and treatment.

E. Treatment

1. **Nonpharmacologic treatments**

   a. The role of dietary changes has not been well studied; however, **some women report some symptom improvement in making certain nutritional changes.** Anecdotally, some women have benefited from decreasing salt consumption to decrease fluid retention, or avoiding caffeine to decrease breast tenderness. Consuming carbohydrate-rich, protein-poor evening meals during the late luteal phase may also improve PMS symptoms by increasing synthesis of brain serotonin. The proposed mechanism includes an insulin-mediated reduction of large neutral amino acids which compete with the serotonin precursor tryptophan for receptor-mediated transport across the blood-brain barrier. Some women report benefit from specially formulated, carbohydrate-rich beverages or other changes in diet which include low-fat, complex carbohydrates taken without protein.

   b. **Calcium** (1000 mg/day) **and magnesium** (360 mg/day) **supplements have both been shown to be helpful in reducing PMDD symptoms.** There is more conflicting evidence about the use of different nutritional supplements including vitamins B_6 and E.

   c. There have been no prospective studies of the effects of exercise on PMDD; however, **aerobic exercise often does elevate mood** and certainly has many health benefits. For mood symptoms, women with PMS/PMDD could try regular aerobic exercise, especially through the luteal phase.

   d. **Circadian rhythm manipulations,** such as through sleep deprivation and light therapy, are other anecdotal PMS/PMDD treatments.

   e. Some report benefit from **relaxation techniques, cognitive-behavioral therapy (CBT), and other forms of therapy** in alleviating their premenstrual symptoms.

2. **Hormonal treatments**

   a. **Oral contraceptive pills (OCPs) are sometimes used to treat PMDD** with the hope that constant levels of estrogen and progestin throughout the menstrual cycle will eliminate premenstrual symptoms. OCPs may improve some of the severity of the physical symptoms. However, OCPs often may not affect, or may even worsen, premenstrual depression.

   b. Although once a popular treatment for PMDD, **progesterone** has failed to show consistent superiority over placebo in treating PMDD.

   c. **Gonadotropin-releasing hormone agonists** and synthetic androgens to suppress ovulation may be useful in treating PMDD; however, both have significant side effects which limit long-term treatment.

   d. Without further research, no definitive statements can be made about the utility of hormonal treatments for PMDD.

3. **Psychotropic medications**

   a. Several prospective, double-blind clinical trials have demonstrated that the selective serotonin reuptake inhibitor (SSRI) **fluoxetine**, dosed at 20–60 mg/day throughout the cycle, **is better than placebo in treating PMDD.** Other studies of SSRIs such as sertraline and paroxetine, have also had promising results. In addition, the serotonergic tricyclic antidepressant, clomipramine, dosed at 25–75 mg/day, has been shown to be more effective than placebo. Several ongoing studies of luteal phase dosing of SSRIs are currently underway to confirm anecdotal reports of efficacy.

   b. Although one small crossover study failed to show a significant difference than placebo, another study found that **alprazolam**, dosed at 0.25 mg q.i.d. from day 18 to day 2 of the next menstrual cycle, was **more effective than placebo and oral micronized progesterone.**

   c. **Buspirone,** a $5HT_{1A}$ serotonin receptor partial agonist, at mean doses of 25 mg/day, was shown to be effective in a small, placebo-controlled, double-blind study, though larger controlled trials are needed to confirm this finding.

   d. Other possibly effective antidepressants that have been suggested include nefazodone, other tricyclics (e.g., desipramine, imipramine, and nortriptyline) and the monoamine oxidase inhibitor (MAOI) **phenelzine.**

4. **Treatment of physical symptoms**

   a. For bloating and weight gain, patients should **first try decreasing salt intake and adding calcium and magnesium supplements.** If these recommendations fail, a trial of spironolactone is a reasonable intervention.

   b. For mastalgia, patients can try using support bras and decreasing caffeine intake. When the symptoms persist and do not respond to simple measures, **bromocriptine** has been shown to decrease premenstrual breast tenderness; however, it may cause significant side effects.

   c. For myalgias, arthralgias, or headache, **nonsteroidal anti-inflammatory agents** can be used as needed.

V. Psychiatric Illnesses during Pregnancy

A. **Introduction**
Despite early assumptions about the protective effects of pregnancy on women's psychological health, **few studies have systematically documented the course of psychiatric disorders during pregnancy and the postpartum period. Psychiatrists must help patients weigh the risks of prenatal exposure to psychotropic medications against the risk of unmedicated psychiatric illness.** While there is increasing data to help inform these difficult decisions, there still remain many unanswered questions regarding the risk for relapse in pregnant and postpartum women with and without medications.

B. **Categories of Risk Associated with Pharmacotherapy**
   1. **Risk of teratogenesis.** Teratogenesis is the dysgenesis of fetal organs leading to structural or functional anomalies. Fetal organ formation occurs primarily during the first trimester. The baseline risk of congenital malformations is estimated at 3–4%. Major malformations may be life-threatening and may require major surgery. When in utero drug exposure increases the frequency of congenital malformations above this baseline risk, the drug is labeled a teratogen.
   2. **Risk of perinatal toxicity.** Perinatal syndromes refer to symptoms present in the neonate frequently associated with drug exposure at or near delivery. Different syndromes have been described following in utero exposure to antidepressants, antipsychotics, and benzodiazepines. Potential contributing factors include prolonged drug effects secondary to immature hepatic microsomal activity, or increased free drug levels from decreased plasma protein and protein binding.
   3. **Risk of behavioral teratogenesis**. Behavioral teratogenesis refers to the long-term effects of in utero drug exposure on neurobehavioral development. These long-term effects may have even more important consequences for patients than specific structural anomalies.

C. **Risk of Untreated Maternal Psychiatric Illness**
   1. **Maternal psychiatric symptoms may jeopardize the well-being of both mother and fetus.** For instance, disabling depression and anxiety may lead to decreased self-care, poor appetite, and increased suicidality, which may all undermine a woman's participation in routine prenatal care.
   2. **Untreated depression and anxiety have been associated with poor neonatal outcome and higher rates of obstetric and neonatal complications,** such as lower Apgar scores.
   3. The physiological changes associated with states of depression or anxiety may also pose their own **risks to fetal development.**
   4. **Relapse of psychiatric illness** may increase the risk for recurrent affective illness or increased refractoriness to treatment.

D. **Psychotropic Medications During Pregnancy**
   Patients commonly underestimate the risks of untreated maternal psychiatric illness while overemphasizing potential teratogenicity of their psychotropic medications. In one study, women exposed to nonteratogenic drugs estimated their teratogenic risk to be 25%, which is far above the baseline risk of 3–4% and more in the range of known teratogens, such as thalidomide. **Misperception about risk can lead both physicians and patients to terminate otherwise wanted pregnancies or avoid needed pharmacotherapy.** By informing patients about the nature and magnitude of drug exposure risk as well as the real risks of untreated illness, psychiatrists can help patients reach their own decisions.
   1. **Antidepressants. Tricyclic antidepressants (TCAs) and the SSRI, fluoxetine, are currently considered the safest antidepressants to use during pregnancy.** Prenatal exposure to these agents does not increase the baseline risk of major congenital malformations of 3–4%. There have been case reports of newborns with TCA withdrawal symptoms (e.g., jitteriness, irritability, and seizures), or bowel obstruction or urinary retention presumably due to anticholinergic effects. Overall, the incidence of perinatal toxicity following in utero exposure to TCAs and fluoxetine appears to be low. However, the long-term neurobehavioral effects remain largely unknown.
   Prospective data about reproductive safety for other antidepressants, including sertraline, paroxetine, venlafaxine, nefazodone, fluvoxamine, MAO inhibitors (MAOIs), and stimulants, remain unavailable.
   2. **Mood stabilizers**
      a. **Lithium use during the first trimester has been associated with a 10–20 times greater risk for Ebstein's anomaly.** With the baseline risk for Ebstein's anomaly at 1/20,000, **the risk for Ebstein's anomaly following first trimester lithium exposure is between 1/2,000 (0.05%) and 1/1,000 (0.1%).** Thus, although the relative risk of Ebstein's anomaly is increased, the absolute risk following first trimester lithium exposure is small.
      Prior to discontinuing lithium, one must consider the severity of illness (e.g., chronicity, severity of particular mood episodes, impaired judgment, presence of psychosis). **For women with severe illness, the high risk**

of recurrence of a severe mood episode during pregnancy may overshadow the relatively small risk of Ebstein's anomaly. For such women, maintenance lithium during pregnancy may be the most appropriate course. For women with less compelling histories, slowly tapering off lithium prior to conception and reintroducing lithium later in the second or third trimesters may be the most prudent treatment. Given that the risk of relapse following lithium discontinuation is estimated at 50–60%, decisions to taper off any mood stabilizer should be made with extreme caution. In addition, given that risk for postpartum relapse in bipolar patients is between 50% and 60%, women should strongly consider prophylaxis with mood stabilizers during this high-risk time (either initiated earlier in pregnancy or around delivery).

b. Valproic acid and carbamazepine have a well-established risk of neural tube defects following first trimester exposure of 5% and 1%, respectively. As with other psychotropics, psychiatrists should discuss with women of child-bearing potential the teratogenic risks and the importance of contraception when taking these medications. Valproic acid and carbamazepine treatment during pregnancy should be accompanied by folate to help mitigate the risk of neural tube defects.

The higher teratogenic risk associated with these anticonvulsants compared to lithium suggests that psychiatrists should consider a lithium trial for their women of reproductive age who plan to conceive. Women who have not responded to lithium obviously have more limited choices, and have to consider the stability afforded by particular mood stabilizers, the teratogenic risks of these medications, and the risk of relapse.

3. Neuroleptics. High-potency neuroleptics have not consistently demonstrated increased teratogenicity following first trimester exposure. Low-potency neuroleptics should be avoided in pregnancy given their purported association with increased risk of congenital malformations. Little is known about the reproductive safety of atypical antipsychotics, such as olanzapine, clozapine, and risperidone. Perinatal toxicity has been reported following neuroleptic exposure, including motor restlessness, tremor, difficulty with oral feeding, hypertonicity, dystonia, and extrapyramidal symptoms. In general, high-potency neuroleptics appear to be safer than lower-potency or atypical neuroleptics.

Like many psychotropic medications, antipsychotics are not absolutely contraindicated in pregnancy. Patients and their psychiatrists have to consider whether discontinuing any of these medications poses unacceptable risks for relapse, especially in women with chronic psychotic illness.

4. Benzodiazepines. Early studies of first trimester benzodiazepine use reported a 10-fold increase from baseline risk of oral cleft palate of 0.06%. However, significant controversy exists about the extent of risk associated with benzodiazepine use. Perinatal toxicity associated with benzodiazepine use around the time of delivery has included reports of temperature dysregulation, apnea, depressed Apgar scores, muscular hypotonicity, and failure to feed. However, several studies of low-dose benzodiazepines given to women around the time of delivery was not associated with significant perinatal toxicity. Long-term neurobehavioral data following in utero benzodiazepine exposure is unavailable.

E. Other Nonpharmacological Treatments
   1. Electroconvulsive therapy (ECT). The safety of ECT during pregnancy has been widely reported in the literature. ECT has been used during pregnancy for more than 50 years. For high-risk situations, such as psychotic depression or mania, which require expeditious treatment to protect both mother and fetus, ECT is the treatment of choice. The safe and effective use of ECT during pregnancy requires coordination of care among the patient's psychiatrist, obstetrician, and anesthesiologist.

   2. Psychotherapy. Pregnancy often evokes feelings about one's early life, doubts about one's capacity to mother, and changing family and work roles. Helping women to understand these conflicting feelings can be an important therapeutic intervention both during and after pregnancy. For mild depression and anxiety, many women benefit from supportive, interpersonal, and integrative psychotherapy. For major depression during pregnancy, patients should strongly consider antidepressants and intensive psychotherapy along with other supportive interventions.

VI. Postpartum Psychiatric Illnesses

A. Introduction
   The postpartum period represents a period of increased risk for affective illness in certain subpopulations of women. Despite ongoing controversy regarding the nosology of postpartum psychiatric disorders, studies have consistently demonstrated the deleterious consequences of postpartum psychiatric illness on both mother and child. Recognition and appropriate treatment of these disorders not only alleviate maternal psychiatric symptoms, but also promote healthy mother–infant attachment and infant development.

B. Overview
   Postpartum psychiatric illnesses are conceptualized along a continuum from the more mild, subsyn-

dromal postpartum blues to the more severe psychiatric episodes of postpartum depression or psychosis.

1. **Postpartum blues (PPB) are a self-limited constellation of symptoms which 50–85% of all women experience postpartum. These symptoms usually begin 2–3 days postpartum and consist of depressed mood, crying spells, mood lability, irritability, and anxiety.** These symptoms generally represent a normal part of the postpartum period. However, when symptoms persist beyond 2 weeks or significantly impair functioning, they may represent an evolving major depression.

2. **Postpartum depression (PPD) has been estimated to occur in 10–15% of all postpartum women** depending on **the diagnostic criteria used. These prevalence rates are similar to nonpuerperal cohorts. More than 60% of women have symptom onset within 6 weeks postpartum.** The DSM-IV classifies PPD as major depression that occurs within 4 weeks postpartum. The course of PPD is highly variable and ranges from 3 to 14 months. Clinical features include all the signs and symptoms of major depression. In addition, women with PPD often have prominent anxiety and obsessionality.

3. **Postpartum psychosis (PPP) is a rare condition that occurs in 1–2 of every 1000 postpartum women. PPP begins acutely within the first 48–72 h postpartum and represents a medical emergency.** Clinical features can include delirium, memory impairment, irritability, lability, and psychosis. PPP is a medical emergency requiring immediate hospitalization and treatment in order to protect both mother and infant.

C. Risk Factors

Many etiological theories of postpartum psychiatric illness have centered on the tremendous **hormonal changes** women experience. For instance, levels of estradiol and estriol drop dramatically within the first days postpartum, while other hormones, such as prolactin and cortisol, also change during the course of pregnancy and postpartum. In general, researchers acknowledge the neuromodulatory function of different hormones, but have yet to find consistent associations between different hormones and the emergence of affective symptoms. The multifactorial nature of these illnesses supports a more integrated theory in which hormonal factors play an important causative role only in women with particular vulnerability to psychiatric illness. This predisposition to psychiatric illness may be biologic (evidenced by personal or family history of psychiatric illness), psychological (evidenced by character pathology or limited coping skills), or social/environmental (evidenced by lower occupational/social functioning.)

While no biological, psychological, or social factors have been implicated unequivocally, **there is good evidence to suggest that the following factors are associated with increased risk for postpartum psychiatric illness:**

1. **Psychiatric history of affective illness. Women with a history of postpartum psychosis have a striking 70–90% risk of a recurrent postpartum psychosis.** Women with a history of major depression or bipolar disorder have a 30–50% risk for developing a postpartum mood disorder. Another clear predictor of postpartum depression is depression during pregnancy.

2. **Family history of psychiatric illness**

3. **Limited social support and interpersonal distress,** such as marital conflict and childcare stress

4. **Negative life events** during and after pregnancy

D. Treatment

1. **Postpartum blues.** Women often benefit from education about the normalcy of certain mood symptoms during the postpartum period. They should also be informed of the signs and symptoms of an evolving major depression and the importance of prompt treatment. Most women with the postpartum blues also benefit from reassurance and supportive interventions, such as childcare assistance and referrals to support agencies.

2. **Postpartum depression**

   a. **Supportive interventions.** Grassroots national organizations such as Depression after Delivery (DAD) and Visiting Moms can provide invaluable assistance to women with postpartum depression. Other options for surrogate family support include the services of a doula, a professional caregiver who is trained to help mothers adjust to the responsibilities of motherhood. Some doulas assist in the childbirth, while others provide critical support during the first postpartum weeks by helping with childcare or household tasks.

   b. **Psychotherapy.** Few studies have documented the efficacy of therapy for treating postpartum depression. Pilot studies of interpersonal therapy (IPT) suggest that this time-limited therapy may help treat mild to moderate postpartum major depression. Another small study comparing cognitive-behavioral therapy and fluoxetine found no significant difference in treating postpartum depression. Further research into the efficacy of these nonpharmacologic treatments will help broaden the treatment alternatives for women with postpartum depression.

   c. **Pharmacotherapy**

      i. **Antidepressants.** Despite the high prevalence of postpartum psychiatric illness, there are only a limited number of medication treatment studies. Several studies have demonstrated the efficacy of different antidepressants (e.g., fluoxetine, sertraline, and venlafaxine). In the absence of other studies, the most prudent antidepressant choice depends upon the patient's depressive symptoms and her own history of response to and tolerance of different medications. **Nursing mothers have to consider the relatively unknown risks of nursing on antidepressants.**

Women at increased risk for postpartum depression (e.g., with a history of recurrent major depression or postpartum depression) should consider initiating prophylactic antidepressants either in late pregnancy or early postpartum. Alternatively, women may elect a wait-and-see approach; however, patients, their loved ones, and psychiatrists should be vigilant for early signs of relapse in order to institute prompt treatment.

ii. **Hormonal therapy.** Few studies have looked at the efficacy of estrogen and progesterone treatment for postpartum depression. Despite one limited, open study, progesterone has not consistently proved to be an effective treatment for depressive symptoms. One other study found that estrogen alone or as an adjunct to antidepressants was effective in treating postpartum depression. Both of these studies had significant methodological limitations; however, both highlight the need for further research into hormonal treatments for postpartum depression.

iii. **For severe postpartum depression, inpatient hospitalization and/or ECT may be required** for containment and prompt treatment.

iv. **Lithium.** Women with a history of bipolar disorder, recurrent major depression, postpartum depression, and postpartum psychosis are at heightened risk for a puerperal affective episode. **Prophylactic treatment with lithium initiated either before delivery or within days postpartum may help reduce this risk for relapse.**

E. **Breastfeeding**
All psychotropic medications are secreted in the breast milk at varying concentrations. Physicians should obtain infant serum levels since neonates can have accumulating drug levels, especially infants who are preterm or who have impaired hepatic metabolism. If levels are detectable, women should strongly consider discontinuing nursing. If levels are not detectable, this does not exclude the presence of trace amounts which potentially still may have neurodevelopmental effects on the infant.

1. **Antidepressants.** Despite **anecdotal cases of neonatal toxicity symptoms** (e.g., irritability, colic, and difficulty feeding) reports of adverse consequences **appear limited.** No studies have shown that any one antidepressant has greater safety during breastfeeding. Antidepressant choice should thus be based on patient's past history of response and tolerance of side effects.

2. **Lithium. Lithium can quickly accumulate in the nursing infant and lead to levels exceeding 50% of the maternal level.** Given this risk of lithium toxicity in the nursing infant, breastfeeding while on lithium is not recommended.

VII. Menopause

A. **Introduction**
While some women experience psychiatric, cognitive, or somatic symptoms during the menopausal transition, **no specific psychiatric disorder has been associated with menopause itself.** The relationship between declining estrogen levels and mood symptoms remains controversial. Some studies have demonstrated that certain subgroups of women with histories of mood or anxiety disorders may be more vulnerable to relapse during this phase. As with PMS and postpartum psychiatric disorders, fluctuations in reproductive endocrine functioning rather than absolute hormone levels may drive this increased risk for affective symptoms in some women.

B. **Definitions**
1. **Menopause** is defined as **the cessation of menses for 12 consecutive months.** Women naturally enter menopause with advancing age, usually between 41 and 59 years old. Women can also experience menopause as a result of exogenous hormone treatment or following bilateral oophorectomy.

2. **Perimenopause, the transition from regular menstrual functioning and menopause,** usually lasts between 5 and 10 years. Hormonal changes during this period include declining estrogen levels, which are increasingly unopposed by progesterone due to anovulatory cycles. The perimenopause has been associated with a higher rate of depressive symptoms; however, there is no increased risk of major depression.

3. Following perimenopause, women enter the **postmenopause,** which can account for roughly one-third of a woman's entire lifespan. The reproductive endocrine status of postmenopausal women is characterized by stable low levels of estrogen and progesterone. While the female/male ratio of depression increases after the age of 45 years, the rate of depression in women throughout all ages declines in the postmenopausal period.

C. **Etiology**
1. **Hormonal theories of menopause-associated depression remain controversial.** Support for "estrogen withdrawal" theories include the increased rate of

depression after bilateral oophorectomy compared to women undergoing natural menopause. Some emphasize the potential depressogenic effects of an abrupt decline in estrogen, while others counter that, following surgical menopause, many other complicated hormonal changes also occur, including falling testosterone and progesterone levels.

2. **The "domino theory" of menopause-related affective disorders suggests that certain somatic symptoms,** such as sleep disturbance from nocturnal hot flashes, **may lead to mood disturbance.** This has led some to wonder whether the positive effect on mood some women experience on hormone replacement therapy (HRT) results from a direct effect or from the psychological relief they experience as their menopausal somatic symptoms abate.

3. **Women with a history of major depression appear to be at greatest risk for perimenopausal depression,** which furthers the debate over whether perimenopause-associated depression represents a separate diagnosis or merely an exacerbation of recurrent major depression.

4. **Psychosocial theories** often indict the stress of the life changes that mark the perimenopausal transition. Some of these psychosocial factors include: losing one's reproductive potential, changing family roles, aging, and the onset of physical illnesses. While these factors may be associated with perimenopausal depression, a causal role for psychosocial factors in perimenopausal depression has yet to be established. Furthermore, characterizations of menopause are fraught with culturally bound, pejorative stereotypes (e.g., the "empty nest"), which ignore the positive feelings of personal mastery and maturity some women experience during this life transition.

D. Evaluation
1. **Psychiatric assessment**
   a. **Screen for menopause-associated physical and psychological symptoms,** including whether they reflect minor nuisances or severely impair social and occupational functioning (see Table 26-1).
   b. Determine the symptom onset and course relative to the current hormonal status. While clinical history alone can determine whether a woman is in the perimenopause transition, estradiol and follicle-stimulating hormone (FSH) levels are required to document actual menopause.
   c. Consider mood charts to determine the severity, stability, and pattern of symptoms. Both affective and somatic symptoms, such as hot flashes and vaginal dryness, should be monitored.
   d. Obtain a thorough psychiatric history since **psychiatric history is the best predictor of relapse in the menopausal period.**

Table 26-1. Physical and Psychological Symptoms Associated with Menopause

Vasomotor symptoms
Hot flashes, night sweats, palpitations

Affective symptoms
Depressed mood, anxiety, mood swings

Cognitive symptoms
Poor memory or concentration

Somatic symptoms
Fatigue, headache, joint pain, paresthesias, vaginal dryness, dyspareunia

---

   e. Rule out any Axis I or II diagnosis.
   f. Screen for substance use or illicit drug use which may exacerbate psychiatric symptoms.
2. **Medical assessment**
   a. **Assess reproductive endocrine status.** Hormonal changes in menopause include a decrease in estrogen with subsequent elevations of luteinizing hormone (LH) and FSH. The endocrine profile of menopause is typically defined as an FSH level above 40 IU/L and an estradiol level below 25 pg/mL. Perimenopausal women typically have FSH levels above 25 IU/L and estradiol levels below 40 pg/mL.
   b. **Rule out underlying medical conditions** that can present with anxiety or depression, such as thyroid disease or cardiac arrhythmia.
   c. **Gynecologic history** should include whether a patient has had a chemically or surgically induced menopause versus a natural menopause. Patients who have had bilateral oophorectomy may experience more difficulties with mood and anxiety. Determine whether or not the woman still has her uterus, since estrogen replacement may increase the risk of uterine as well as breast cancer.
   d. **Laboratory tests,** such as thyroid function, FSH, and estradiol levels may be indicated.

E. Treatment Strategies
1. **Pharmacologic strategies**
   a. **Hormone replacement therapy (HRT).** HRT may alleviate mild mood symptoms, along with certain physical symptoms such as vaginal dryness and vasomotor symptoms (e.g., hot flashes, cold sweats). In addition, studies have shown that HRT can reduce the risk of osteoporosis and heart disease. These benefits, however, must be carefully weighed against possible increased risk for breast and uterine cancer in certain subgroups.
      i. **Careful documentation of onset of symptoms and initiation of HRT should be determined.** Some

patients may require dose adjustments or alternative forms of estrogen replacement (e.g., estradiol or conjugated estrogen) before mood improves.

ii. **Mood or anxiety symptoms may result from HRT itself.** Patients may require continuous hormone replacement preparations rather than sequential HRT if they develop cyclical mood or anxiety symptoms. In addition, while progestin added to estrogen replacement decreases the risk of endometrial cancer, it may worsen mood. For these patients a higher estrogen/progestin ratio may attenuate the depressogenic effect of progestin.

iii. If there is no improvement after 2–4 weeks, re-evaluate for a primary Axis I condition and consider the use of standard antidepressant treatment.

b. **Antidepressants.** For menopause-associated major depression, **standard antidepressant treatment should be initiated.** No compelling data support the use of estrogen monotherapy for treatment of major depression.

2. **Psychotherapy strategies.** Cognitive-behavioral, supportive therapy, and psychodynamic therapy alone or in combination with pharmacotherapy may help alleviate mild depressive or anxiety symptoms.

3. **Psychoeducation.** Patients often benefit from reassurance that menopause is not a disease but a natural stage of women's development. Psychiatrists should also educate patients about the hormonal changes and potential vasomotor, cognitive, and psychological symptoms that sometimes accompany menopause. Patient education should also include clear distinctions between these normal symptoms and more disabling conditions, such as major depression and Axis I anxiety disorders.

Psychiatrists should also make clear that HRT alone may treat hot flashes but does not treat major depression.

Selected Readings

Birnbaum C, Cohen L: The psychiatric evaluation and treatment of premenstrual dysphoric disorder. In Pollack MH, Otto MW, Rosenbaum JF (eds): *Challenges in Clinical Practice.* New York: Guilford Press, 1996:408–431.

Cohen LS, Rosenbaum JR: Psychotropic drug use during pregnancy: weighing the risks. *J Clin Psychiatry* 1998; 59 (Suppl. 2):18–28.

Joffe H, Cohen LS: Estrogen, serotonin, and mood disturbance: where is the therapeutic bridge? *Biol Psychiatry* 1998; 44:798–811.

Kessler RC, McGonagle KA, Schwartz M, Blazer DG, Nelson CB: Sex and depression in the National Comorbidity Survey I: lifetime prevalence, chronicity, and recurrence. *J Affect Disord* 1993; 29:85–96.

Nonacs R, Cohen LS: Postpartum mood disorders: diagnosis and treatment guidelines. *J Clin Psychiatry* 1998; 59 (Suppl. 2):34–40.

Roca CA, Schmidt PJ, et al.: Implication of endocrine studies of premenstrual syndrome. *Psychiatr Ann* 1996; 26(9):576–589.

Schmidt PJ, Rubinow DR. Menopause-related affective disorders: a justification for further study. *Am J Psychiatry* 1991; 148: 844–852.

Simpson HB, Nee JC, Endicott J: First-episode major depression. *Arch Gen Psychiatry* 1997; 54:633–639.

Viguera AC, Cohen LS: Approach to the patient entering menopause. In Stern TA, Herman JB, Slavin PL (eds): *The MGH Guide to Psychiatry in Primary Care.* New York: McGraw-Hill, 1998.

Chapter 27

HIV Infection and AIDS

JOHN QUERQUES AND JONATHAN L. WORTH

I. Overview

A. **Human immunodeficiency virus type 1 (HIV-1) is a lentivirus, a type of retrovirus that causes slow, but progressive, immunologic and neurologic disease.** By depleting CD4 T-helper lymphocytes, infection with HIV-1 causes severe immunosuppression that can ultimately lead to fatal opportunistic infections (OIs), neoplasms, and dementing illness, and to a diagnosis of acquired immunodeficiency syndrome (AIDS).

1. Although the majority of AIDS cases in the United States are caused by infection with HIV-1, HIV-2 is responsible for some AIDS cases in West Africa. Therefore, this chapter focuses on HIV-1; for convenience we use the simpler abbreviation, HIV.

B. **HIV infects certain neural cells early in the course of infection,** and, through a variety of direct and indirect means, causes damage throughout the brain, though **subcortical structures and deep white matter are principal targets.**

C. **Provision of care for patients with HIV/AIDS may be complicated** by:

1. The emotional burden of seeing severe, critical illness, often in young patients
2. Countertransference reactions to, and prejudice against, patients from socially marginalized demographic groups
3. Fear of HIV transmission

D. **This chapter addresses key elements of the diagnosis and treatment of psychiatric disorders in HIV-infected and AIDS patients and the neurologic complications of HIV disease.** Because of the rapid pace of research in this area, we caution the reader that some information presented here may be outdated by the time of publication.

II. Epidemiology in the United States

A. The first case of AIDS was reported in 1981, but HIV infection was probably present—but unrecognized—as early as the 1960s.

B. According to the Centers for Disease Control and Prevention (CDC), from 1981 through 1996, 573,800 people in the United States were diagnosed with AIDS, and, as of June 1996, the estimated prevalence was 223,000. **This marked upturn in prevalence reflects improved survival among patients with AIDS due, in part, to combination antiretroviral therapy (ART).**

1. **AIDS is most prevalent among men who have sex with men (MSM), followed by intravenous drug users (IDUs) and people who acquire the disease through heterosexual contact.**

a. The demographics of AIDS is changing. The largest proportionate increase in AIDS prevalence from mid-1995 to mid-1996 occurred in the heterosexual population, largely due to viral transmission from IDUs to their heterosexual partners.

b. **Recently, AIDS has occurred in growing numbers among African-Americans, Latinos, and women.**

2. Despite improvements in treatment and survival rates, in 1995, HIV infection was the leading cause of death among people 25–44 years old.

C. **People at high risk for HIV infection include: older adolescents and young adults, MSM, IDUs and their sexual partners, sexually active heterosexuals living in geographic areas where HIV is prevalent, people with chronic severe mental illness, racial minorities, and children born to the above. Because these same demographic groups are at high risk for psychiatric disorders, patients with HIV/AIDS frequently manifest psychopathology that is unrelated and antecedent to their retroviral illness. The additional burden of HIV/AIDS exacts a heavy toll on an already vulnerable psychosocial state.**

1. People with substance use, bipolar, and severe personality disorders are at increased risk for HIV because of behavioral impulsivity, impaired risk assessment, and the likelihood of swapping sex for drugs of abuse.

2. People at high risk for HIV infection may be more prone to psychiatric illness because, typically, these individuals have poor social supports and are disenfranchised, isolated, and socially marginalized.

D. The CDC first published criteria for AIDS diagnosis in 1987. The revision that followed in 1993 expanded the definition and led to an upturn in the number of AIDS cases. This revised classification system is based on the CD4 count and the presence of complications of HIV. **A CD4 count < 200 or the presence of one of the illnesses listed in Table 27-1 defines AIDS.**

Table 27-1. AIDS-Defining Conditions

Recurrent pneumonia
Recurrent *Salmonella* septicemia
Mycobacterial infection
Pneumocystis carinii pneumonia
Coccidioidomycosis
Candidiasis
Cryptococcosis
Histoplasmosis
Toxoplasmosis of brain
Isosporiasis
Cryptosporidiosis
Cytomegalovirus infection
Herpes simplex virus infection
Progressive multifocal leukoencephalopathy
Kaposi's sarcoma
Lymphoma
Invasive cervical cancer
HIV-related encephalopathy
Wasting syndrome

III. General Approach to the Psychiatric Care of the Patient with HIV/AIDS

A. The differential diagnosis of psychiatric disturbance in a patient with HIV/AIDS is wide. **Affective, behavioral, and cognitive symptoms may be due to primary psychiatric illness, primary effects of HIV in the central nervous system (CNS), secondary effects of systemic HIV disease on the CNS, and side effects of ART and other medications used to treat HIV-related illnesses.** Because two or more of these conditions can coexist and because features of these conditions overlap extensively, diagnosis is often challenging and the etiology of mental status changes may be described as multifactorial (see Table 27-2).

B. **When symptoms are due to HIV CNS infection, systemic HIV disease, or adverse medication effects, response to conventional psychotropic medications is poorer, risk of side effects is greater, and tolerability is reduced,** when compared to the use of these agents in patients with primary psychopathology.

C. **Optimum HIV treatment, targeted at systemic and CNS manifestations, is essential.** Such treatment enhances response to psychotropics and lowers the risk of side effects.

Table 27-2. Differential Diagnosis of Delirium and Mental Status Change in Patients with HIV/AIDS

- Psychiatric disorders
- Psychoactive substance intoxication or withdrawal
- Primary HIV syndromes
  Seroconversion illness
  HIV CNS infection
  HIV dementia
- CNS opportunistic infections
  Fungi
  Cryptococcus neoformans
  Coccidioides immitis
  Candida albicans
  Histoplasma capsulatum
  Aspergillus fumigatus
  Mucormycosis
  Protozoa/parasites
  Toxoplasma gondii
  Amebas
  Viruses
  Creutzfeldt-Jakob papovavirus
  Cytomegalovirus (CMV)
  Adenovirus type 2
  Herpes simplex virus
  Varicella zoster virus
  Bacteria
  Mycobacterium avium-intracellulare
  Mycobacterium tuberculosis
  Listeria monocytogenes
  Gram-negative organisms
  Treponema pallidum
  Nocardia asteroides
- Neoplasms
  Primary CNS non-Hodgkin's lymphoma
  Metastatic Kaposi's sarcoma (rare)
  Burkitt's lymphoma
- Medication side effects (see Table 27-3)
- Endocrinopathies and nutrient deficiencies
  Addison's disease (CMV, *Cryptococcus*, HIV-1, ketoconazole)
  Hypothyroidism
  Hypogonadism
  Vitamin A, B_6, B_{12}, and E deficiencies
- Anemia
- Metabolic abnormalities
- Hypotension
- Complex partial seizures
- Head trauma
- Non-HIV-related illnesses

D. Important data to know include: the severity of the CNS infection, the severity of the systemic HIV disease, the presence of active illness, the medication regimen, the presence of premorbid psychiatric illnesses, and the mode of retroviral infection.

1. **In general, the worse the systemic disease, the more compromised and more vulnerable the CNS is, and the greater the likelihood is that psychiatric symptoms are due to secondary causes** (e.g., medication side effects, OIs).

   a. Stage of systemic HIV disease can be determined by CD4 count, viral load, and history of HIV-related illnesses.

   i. When CD4 counts are < 500, patients are at risk of symptoms.

   ii. When CD4 counts are > 200, the rate of AIDS-defining illnesses increases markedly, and prophylaxis for OIs is instituted.

2. **An answer to the question, "How did you become infected?," asked in a nonjudgmental tone, often reveals who the patient is as a person, how he or she feels about the way he/she was infected, and how he/she has coped with his/her seropositive status. Gathering this information not only helps to forge an alliance with the patient but also directs appropriate management.**

IV. Psychiatric Illness in the Patient with HIV/AIDS

A high index of suspicion should be maintained for "organic" causes of psychiatric symptoms in the patient with HIV/AIDS, especially at advanced stages of illness. In general, mental status changes that are gradual in onset are likely attributable to the primary effects of HIV on the CNS, whereas systemic complications of HIV disease more often cause acute neuropsychiatric disturbances.

This section discusses the diagnostic and therapeutic features of common psychiatric conditions that are distinctive to HIV/AIDS patients. For discussions of these disorders in the general population, the reader is referred to the appropriate chapters in this book.

A. Delirium

One of the most frequent psychiatric complications in hospitalized, HIV-infected patients, **delirium can occur at any stage of HIV infection, but it is more common in patients with advanced disease or with HIV dementia.**

1. **Etiology.** In patients with asymptomatic HIV infection or with a CD4 count > 500, delirium is less likely to be due to HIV infection itself and more likely to be related to abuse of substances (e.g., alcohol, narcotics, steroids, testosterone). In symptomatic patients or in those with a CD4 count < 500 (especially < 100), HIV-related conditions

and medication side effects are likely culprits, though the cause may be multifactorial.

2. **Differential diagnosis.** Table 27-2 lists the conditions that may be responsible for delirium and other mental status changes in patients with HIV/AIDS. Table 27-3 lists the neuropsychiatric side effects of medications commonly used in HIV/AIDS treatment.

3. **Evaluation.** Focused on identification of the underlying cause(s) of delirium, **the history and physical examination are the cornerstones of evaluation of the delirious patient.** Findings dictate the need for laboratory studies, which may include neuroimaging, electroencephalography (EEG), cerebrospinal fluid (CSF) analysis, and blood tests.

4. **Treatment. The hallmark of management is treatment of the underlying cause(s).** Neuroleptics (often given as the equivalent of haloperidol 0.5–5 mg daily) can be used empirically and for symptomatic control of agitation.

   a. High-potency agents are superior to medium- and low-potency neuroleptics, which can worsen delirium because of their anticholinergic effects.

   b. However, **the incidence of extrapyramidal side effects (EPS) from use of high-potency neuroleptics is increased in patients with advanced HIV disease.** Patients with AIDS and, in particular, those with HIV dementia, are at increased risk for neuroleptic malignant syndrome. Alterations in the blood-brain barrier and subcortical injuries seen in HIV dementia may be responsible for the increased frequency of side effects in this population.

   c. With intramuscular administration, thrombocytopenia, coagulopathy, and reduced muscle mass need to be considered.

   d. Short-acting benzodiazepines may be combined with neuroleptics to control agitation but should not be used alone in the treatment of delirium.

B. Major Depression

Although major depression is one of the most frequent major psychiatric complications of HIV infection, whether the occurrence of depression is due to an HIV-specific factor or is attributable to the chronicity of illness is unknown. While CD4 cell depletion per se is not associated with mood disorders, viral effects in the prefrontal cortex-amygdala-pallidum-medial thalamus circuit may contribute to the high rates of depression seen in HIV infection.

1. **Etiology.** Depression can occur at any stage of illness. **In patients with asymptomatic infection or with a CD4 count > 500, depression is likely to be primary.** A recurrence of a premorbid mood disorder or a first depressive episode may be precipitated by

Table 27-3. Neuropsychiatric Side Effects of Medications Commonly Used in Patients with HIV/AIDS

Nucleoside reverse transcriptase inhibitors

Zidovudine (AZT)	Headache, restlessness, agitation, insomnia, mania, depression, irritability, delirium, somnolence, peripheral neuropathy
Didanosine (ddI)	Insomnia, mania, peripheral neuropathy
Zalcitabine (ddC)	Peripheral neuropathy
Stavudine (d4T)	Mania, peripheral neuropathy
Lamivudine (3TC)	Similar to AZT
Abacavir	Headache

Nucleotide reverse transcriptase inhibitor

Adefovir	Asthenia

Non-nucleoside reverse transcriptase inhibitors

Nevirapine	Headache
Delavirdine	Headache
Efavirenz	False positive cannabinoid test, agitation, insomnia, euphoria, depression, somnolence, abnormal dreams, confusion, abnormal thinking, impaired concentration, amnesia, depersonalization, hallucinations

Protease inhibitors

Indinavir	Headache, asthenia, blurred vision, dizziness, insomnia
Ritonavir	Circumoral and peripheral paresthesias, asthenia, altered taste
Saquinavir	Headache
Nelfinavir	Headache, asthenia
Amprenavir	Headache

Other antivirals

Acyclovir	Headache, agitation, insomnia, tearfulness, confusion, hyperesthesia, hyperacusis, depersonalization, hallucinations
Ganciclovir	Agitation, mania, psychosis, irritability, delirium

Antibacterials

Cotrimoxazole	Headache, insomnia, depression, anorexia, apathy
Trimethoprim-sulfamethoxazole	Headache, insomnia, depression, anorexia, apathy, delirium, mutism, neuritis
Isoniazid	Agitation, depression, hallucinations, paranoia, impaired memory
Dapsone	Agitation, insomnia, mania, hallucinations

Antiparasitics

Thiabendazole	Hallucinations, olfactory disturbance
Metronidazole	Agitation, depression, delirium, seizures (with IV administration)
Pentamidine	Hypoglycemia, hypotension, confusion, delirium, hallucinations

Antifungals

Amphotericin B	Headache, agitation, anorexia, delirium, diplopia, lethargy, peripheral neuropathy
Ketoconazole	Headache, dizziness, photosensitivity
Flucytosine	Headache, delirium, cognitive impairment

Others

Steroids	Euphoria, mania, depression, psychosis, confusion
Cytosine arabinoside	Delirium, cerebellar signs

an HIV-related stressor, including unresolved or multiple bereavement. **In patients with symptomatic infection or with a CD4 count < 500, depression is likely to be secondary** to HIV-related complications (see Table 27-2), medication side effects (see Table 27-3), HIV dementia, or substance use.

2. **Differential diagnosis**. The differential diagnosis includes primary depression, new-onset or recurrent; delirium; HIV neurocognitive disturbance; an anergic-apathetic-fatigue state; and secondary causes associated with advanced HIV disease (adrenal dysfunction, euthyroid-sick syndrome, and hypogonadism with low testosterone states).

   a. HIV can cause anergic-apathetic-fatigue states that are due to release of somnogenic lymphokines. They may not be characterized by significant depressive symptoms or by cognitive impairment.

3. **Evaluation.** Evaluation focuses on: identification of psychosocial stressors; medication changes; substance use; and, in advanced cases, underlying conditions that may cause or worsen depression. Laboratory investigations are guided by history and physical findings.

4. **Treatment**

   a. **Pharmacotherapy with tricyclic antidepressants (TCAs) and serotonin reuptake inhibitors (SRIs) is the first line of therapy.** Regardless of agent, start with low doses and increase them slowly. Avoid sedating, anticholinergic, and anti-alpha-adrenergic agents (the latter especially in advanced HIV disease when hypotension is frequent).

   b. TCAs, especially nortriptyline, are particularly useful in patients with diarrhea, dehydration, wasting, and other causes of volume shifts because serum levels can be used to guide dosage.

   c. Bupropion or desipramine may be helpful for depressions with marked fatigue and concentration difficulty, though the use of bupropion is complicated by the heightened seizure risk in HIV-infected patients.

   d. **Psychostimulants may be used as single or adjuvant agents for anergia, apathy, and anorexia.** They may be used as first-line agents when depression is characterized by apathy more than by sadness and when patients have a history of intolerance to other agents.

      i. Because dextroamphetamine can cause severe tremor or persisting movement disorder in patients with advanced disease, some authorities prefer methylphenidate in this population.

   e. **Anticipate treatment intolerance or resistance and the need for polypharmacy in patients with multiple bereavement, unresolved grief, secondary mood disorders, and advanced HIV disease.**

   f. **Psychotherapy** is helpful, especially when psychosocial stressors are evident.

   g. **Electroconvulsive therapy** may also be beneficial.

C. **Suicide**

1. **Many people who are at risk for HIV infection are also at high risk for suicide,** probably because of psychiatric disturbance, substance use, and social disenfranchisement (see II.C). Suicide may be the second leading cause of death among members of high-risk groups who ultimately become infected, second only to AIDS. For many, especially soon after seroconversion, suicidal ideation or a suicide attempt may be an expression of fear and anger about reduced quality of life. In a 1985 study of New York city residents with AIDS, the relative risk of suicide was 66 times greater than in the general population and 36 times greater than among gender- and age-matched controls.

2. Broadly speaking, **reasons for these dramatic suicide rates can be categorized as due to premorbid psychiatric history, psychosocial stressors related to HIV infection, and neuropsychiatric complications of HIV infection.**

   a. **Risk may be most strongly related to concurrent depression.**

   b. Other risk factors include: personality disorders; active substance use; bereavement; pain; coping with a homosexual orientation; HIV-related difficulties at home or at work; fear of and actual disease progression; loss of independence and autonomy; and feeling hopeless, worthless, and burdensome to others.

3. **Evaluation.** Determination of severity of suicidal thought, patient safety, and underlying diagnosis and identification of psychosocial stressors are key elements of the evaluation.

4. **Treatment.** Ensure safety, treat the underlying disorder(s), and provide psychotherapy and psychosocial interventions for stressors.

D. **Difficulty Coping**

Many people who are at risk for HIV infection have substance use disorders, poor self-esteem, and little education. In addition, they are socially isolated, disenfranchised, illiterate, and impoverished. All are risk factors per se for poor coping. Even those with good preparation may have difficulty coping with HIV infection, in part because having critical illness is not an appropriate life-stage situation for many patients. Thus, the people who are least prepared to handle the stresses imposed by HIV/AIDS are those who face these challenges.

1. **The stressors faced by patients with HIV/AIDS are myriad:**

   a. **Diagnosis and treatment of HIV/AIDS:** testing seropositive; serial determination of CD4 count and viral load; initiation of ART; initiation of prophylaxis for OIs; first hospitalization; transfer to hospice care

b. **Experience of symptoms of HIV/AIDS:** wasting; diarrheal illness; treatment-resistant pain and insomnia; vision-impairing disease (e.g., cytomegalovirus retinitis); cognitive and motor dysfunction; side effects of medications (e.g., protease-inhibitor fat redistribution syndrome)

c. **Psychosocial consequences of HIV/AIDS:** disclosure of HIV serostatus; disclosure of sexual orientation (in some cases); loss of health insurance and employment; application for welfare and disability insurance; financial and social impoverishment

2. **Differential diagnosis.** Ineffective coping with these stressors may present as major depression, substance use disorders, acute stress disorder, panic attacks, adjustment disorder, bereavement, or decompensated personality disorders. **If anxious symptoms are prominent, secondary causes** (e.g., hypoxia, hypoglycemia, anemia, medication side effects) **should be considered, especially in patients with symptomatic HIV infection or with a CD4 count < 500. "Anxiety" should also raise suspicion for akathisia and complex partial seizures.**

3. **Evaluation.** Identify the stressors. Use the "marathon model" to identify areas of weakness in the patient's ability to deal with those stressors, and diagnose the psychiatric disorder spawned by the faulty coping mechanism.

   a. **The "marathon model" assesses** the following four areas necessary for effective coping. Deficits in any one may compromise coping.

   i. **Training.** "How did you cope with prior adversity?" Assess how well these strategies will work with HIV infection.

   ii. **Personal team.** Does the patient recognize faces in the crowd along the marathon course? Who specifically comprises the patient's personal support system?

   iii. **Pit stops.** Can the patient take respite from HIV infection (e.g., with drug holidays or a week off without doctors' appointments)?

   iv. **Corporate support.** Does the patient have a primary care physician, HIV specialist, psychiatrist, hospital, health insurance, and employer?

4. **Treatment**

   a. **Nonpharmacologic treatment with supportive and psychoeducational psychotherapy and community- and government-based interventions should focus on establishment of missing components of the "marathon model" and maintenance and strengthening of those elements already present.**

   b. **Pharmacologic treatment** should provide symptomatic control.

   i. Short-term use of **high-potency benzodiazepines** in low doses is helpful for acute anxiety disorders. Long-term use can be problematic because of the potential for abuse and dependence in a population at risk for such disorders. High doses of benzodiazepines risk cognitive and motor side effects, especially in patients with HIV dementia and intracranial lesions.

   ii. **Buspirone** is the treatment of choice in patients with a history of substance abuse or dependence.

   iii. **TCAs** and **SRIs** can be used for chronic anxiety disorders.

E. **Substance Use Disorders**

1. As a powerful stressor, HIV/AIDS complicates both establishment and maintenance of abstinence. **Because substance abuse and dependence occur frequently in patients with HIV/AIDS, regardless of risk group, these disorders (including withdrawal states) should be considered in the differential diagnosis of any Axis I disorder.**

2. **Active abuse or dependence compromises treatment compliance and promotes high-risk behavior.**

3. **Methadone increases zidovudine (AZT) levels,** and **rifampin induces methadone metabolism,** and thus may precipitate acute opiate withdrawal if the methadone dose is not increased.

F. **Psychosis**

One study found that patients with HIV/AIDS and psychosis have a higher mortality rate and tend to have greater global neuropsychiatric impairment when compared to patients without psychosis.

1. **Etiology. In patients with asymptomatic HIV disease or a CD4 count > 500, psychotic symptoms are most likely due to a primary psychosis or to substance use (e.g., steroids, cocaine). In patients with symptomatic disease or a CD4 count < 500, secondary causes should be strongly considered.**

2. **Differential diagnosis.** Secondary causes are identical to those that cause delirium (see Table 27-2). Notable among these are: HIV CNS infection; cytomegalovirus and herpes simplex virus infections; advanced HIV dementia; complex partial seizures; and medication side effects (see Table 27-3).

3. **Evaluation.** Laboratory tests (e.g., neuroimaging, EEG, CSF analysis, blood tests) are ordered as clinically indicated.

4. **Treatment. Management of psychosis proceeds along the same lines as that of delirium** (see IV.A.4). Treatment of the underlying cause is the primary goal; symptoms are controlled with neuroleptics, usually with one-tenth to one-third of the dose required for acute "functional" psychoses.

   a. **Low doses of neuroleptics may be adequate to treat psychosis (and delirium) in HIV-infected patients because of HIV-related damage to subcortical structures, including the basal ganglia. Such injury may also explain the increased sensitivity to EPS in patients with HIV-related psychosis.**

   b. Risperidone is effective and well tolerated.

c. Combination therapy with anticonvulsants and neuroleptics may be helpful.

d. Clozapine should be avoided because of its hematopoietic toxicity.

e. Olanzapine may precipitate or worsen hyperglycemia.

G. Mania

1. **Etiology. In early stages of HIV disease, mania is usually due to premorbid bipolar disorder, substance use, or medication side effects** (see Table 27-3). **In more advanced disease,** these are still possibilities, but **new-onset mania should immediately raise suspicion for secondary causes,** including OIs, toxic/metabolic insults, and CNS space-occupying lesions (see Table 27-2). Mania can also be symptomatic of HIV dementia.

2. **Evaluation.** After determination of medication changes and assessment for substance use, **evaluation focuses on detection of underlying secondary causes.** Cranial magnetic resonance imaging (MRI) and CSF analysis should proceed if the patient has AIDS or a CD4 count < 100.

3. **Treatment. With more advanced disease, there is greater unresponsiveness to, and intolerance of, treatment.**

   a. **Treatment with the Depakote® brand of valproate is highly effective, and is better tolerated than standard combination therapy with lithium and neuroleptics in patients with advanced HIV disease who have abnormalities on neuroimaging studies.**

      i. Aim for symptom control or a low "therapeutic" level.

      ii. Valproate raises AZT levels.

   b. Carbamazepine should be used cautiously, if at all, because of hematopoietic toxicity. It decreases AZT levels.

   c. Clonazepam is helpful, either alone or with valproate.

   d. **Lithium plus neuroleptic is often ineffective and poorly tolerated in patients with advanced HIV disease.** Poor response may be predicted by any brain MRI abnormality, including atrophy.

      i. If lithium is used, be aware of volume shifts secondary to diarrhea and dehydration as these may raise serum lithium levels.

      ii. Lithium toxicity can occur in HIV-infected patients, even when levels are "therapeutic."

      iii. If a neuroleptic is used, guidelines for the use of these agents in patients with HIV/AIDS, as outlined above, should be followed (see IV.A.4).

H. Insomnia

As the CD4 count falls, sleep quality often diminishes, night-time sleep fragments, sleep onset delays, and early morning awakening becomes more frequent.

1. **Differential diagnosis.** Diagnoses include depression, anxiety, fear, pain, systemic HIV disease, HIV CNS infection, and medication side effects (see Table 27-3).

2. **Evaluation.** Assess the severity with visual or numeric analog scales, determine the cause(s), and diagnose comorbid conditions that may worsen the sleep problem. In most cases, a clinical evaluation will suffice without need of polysomnography.

3. **Treatment**

   a. Teach patients the principles of sleep hygiene (see Chap. 22).

   b. Consider using low doses of sedating TCAs, trazodone, nefazodone, or diphenhydramine.

   c. Use of low doses of medium-potency neuroleptics for several days can help with the near-delusional fear at sleep initiation that grips some patients with HIV dementia.

   d. Reserve use of benzodiazepines for short-term treatment of insomnia due to acute pain, exacerbations of chronic pain, adjustment disorders, acute stress disorder, and exacerbations of chronic sleep disorders. When benzodiazepines are used long term for otherwise treatment-refractory cases, different agents should be used alternately (e.g., monthly) to avoid accommodation to any single agent. Avoid agents with long-acting, active metabolites (e.g., diazepam, chlordiazepoxide).

I. Pain

This symptom is frequent in advanced stages of HIV disease.

1. **Pain is most commonly due to a peripheral neuropathy,** which presents as a distal symmetric sensory polyneuropathy with numbness, tingling, and burning in the feet.

   a. It may be due to HIV infection itself or to nucleoside ART (AZT, didanosine, zalcitabine, stavudine). Didanosine is a more frequent culprit than are the others; it sometimes causes an irreversible neuropathy.

2. **Acute demyelinating neuropathy (Guillain-Barré syndrome)** is a self-limited, rapidly evolving symmetrical paralysis with variable sensory signs, beginning in the lower limbs, that sometimes complicates the flu-like illness that accompanies HIV seroconversion.

3. **A chronic progressive or relapsing inflammatory demyelinating polyneuropathy** may complicate the course of advanced HIV disease.

4. **Other causes of pain are herpes zoster, postherpetic neuralgia, myopathy, and headache.**

5. **Evaluation.** Determine the cause(s) and diagnose comorbid conditions that amplify pain (e.g., depression, anxiety, and fear).

6. **Treatment.** Treat the cause(s) and the comorbid conditions and address the bias that may be present among caregivers toward patients with a his-

tory of substance use. The approach is similar to that for any chronic pain syndrome.

a. **Opiates.** Narcotics are recommended only for short-term use for acute pain and for exacerbations of chronic pain.

b. **TCAs.** Low doses of nortriptyline or desipramine can be helpful.

c. **Anticonvulsants.** Low doses of clonazepam can be beneficial, especially for hyperpathia. Carbamazepine should be used cautiously, if at all, because of hematopoietic toxicity. Valproate is generally less effective than is carbamazepine.

d. **Lidocaine.** This agent is useful for herpes zoster and postherpetic neuralgia.

e. As-needed dosing can be difficult for cognitively impaired patients and may result in dangerous overuse.

f. For patients on methadone for opiate dependence, it is preferable to use another analgesic to control pain rather than increase the methadone dose.

g. **Acupuncture.** This technique may be helpful when combined with pharmacotherapy.

V. Neurologic Manifestations of HIV/AIDS

The neurologic manifestations of HIV/AIDS are either primary (i.e., due to HIV itself or to the immunopathological changes precipitated by the retrovirus) **or secondary** (i.e., due to metabolic or toxic derangements, OIs, or neoplasms).

Primary manifestations include HIV dementia, HIV meningitis, vacuolar myelopathy, and neuropathies, the most important of which for the psychiatrist is HIV dementia.

Secondary manifestations include toxoplasmosis, cryptococcal meningitis, cytomegalovirus encephalitis, primary CNS lymphoma, and progressive multifocal leukoencephalopathy.

A. **HIV Dementia**

Known by many other names (e.g., AIDS dementia complex, HIV encephalopathy, HIV-1-associated dementia complex), **HIV dementia presents as a subcortical dementing process caused by HIV CNS infection. Its incidence parallels the progression of systemic disease and depends on the effectiveness of ART within the CNS. Therefore, it is most likely to occur in patients with other AIDS-defining illnesses or a CD4 count < 200.**

1. **Course.** Generally, HIV dementia is slow in onset and of mild to moderate severity, especially when ART is CNS-effective. The longitudinal course varies; some patients experience progressive deterioration, whereas others follow a stable course. Sometimes a long period of relative stability ends in a precipitous decline, but **not all patients with mild dementia progress to the full-blown syndrome.** As with other dementing illnesses, any degree of cognitive impairment renders a patient vulnerable to subsequent neurological insults (e.g., infection, metabolic derangement, sleep deprivation), which, in turn, lead to transient worsening of the cognitive deficits.

2. **Symptoms. HIV dementia is characterized by affective, behavioral, cognitive, and motor symptoms and signs.**

a. **Affective** features include apathy, depressed mood, fatigue, insomnia (see IV.H.3.c), and, in severe cases, depression, mania, or psychosis.

b. **Behavioral** features include a change in social behavior, social withdrawal, anergia, and, in severe cases, agitation (associated with delirium).

c. **Cognitive** features include deficits in attention, concentration, short-term memory, word-finding, visuospatial abilities, and completion of multiple-step activities. Patients may complain that previously automatic activities require effortful concentration. **Aphasia, agnosia, and apraxia occur very late in the course of HIV dementia,** even though the fourth edition of the *Diagnostic and Statistical Manual of Mental Disorders* requires one of these deficits or executive dysfunction for the diagnosis of dementia due to HIV disease.

d. **Motor** features include clumsiness, slowing of movements, and changes in gait and handwriting.

3. **Neurologic examination.** Typical findings include frontal release signs, hyperreflexia, disturbed smooth-pursuit eye movement, and incoordination and weakness (both worse in the lower limbs).

4. **Neuropsychological testing. Psychomotor slowing is the hallmark of HIV dementia,** followed by impaired divided attention and concentration. Therefore, **Part B of the Halstead-Reitan Trail-Making Test is an ideal screening tool for HIV dementia** because it is sensitive to impairments in psychomotor speed and divided attention and it is easy to administer. The Folstein Mini-Mental State Examination, because it mainly tests non-frontal *cortical* areas, is not particularly sensitive for HIV dementia, which affects *subcortical* structures.

5. **Evaluation.** Because HIV dementia is a diagnosis of exclusion, **evaluation focuses on exclusion of other causes of altered mental status** in a patient with HIV/AIDS (see Table 27-2). Laboratory investigations include neuroimaging, CSF analysis, blood tests, and EEG.

a. Cranial **computed tomography** (CT) typically shows cerebral atrophy, ventricular enlargement, and white matter lucencies.

b. Cranial **MRI** reveals cerebral atrophy, ventricular enlargement, and T_2-weighted hyperintense white matter lesions. There is a poor relationship between degree of abnormality on the MRI scan and the severity of dementia.

c. The white matter abnormalities on both CT and MRI occur as multiple punctate lesions or in large confluent areas.

d. Gross anatomical studies find atrophy in subcortical structures and in the frontal, parietal, and temporal cortex; sulcal and ventricular prominences are also seen in brains of patients with AIDS. However, decreased brain weight has not been shown to correspond with the severity of dementia. Similarly, neuropathological changes are seen in brains of HIV-infected patients who do not have dementia.

e. CT and MRI are able to exclude focal lesions, but they are insensitive to the subtle changes detected by functional neuroimaging studies.

f. In early dementia, **functional neuroimaging** studies demonstrate subcortical hypermetabolism, especially in the basal ganglia and thalamus. Later stages are characterized by cortical hypometabolism.

g. **CSF analysis** shows only nonspecific findings and should be ordered only if symptoms are progressive, or severe, or if the CD4 count is < 200.

h. **Blood tests** should be ordered to exclude anemia, electrolyte derangements, endocrinopathies, OIs, syphilis, and vitamin B_{12} deficiency.

i. **EEG** may show mild, nonspecific slowing; it is generally helpful only if a seizure disorder is suspected by virtue of manic symptoms, atypical panic attacks, or formed visual hallucinations.

6. **Treatment.** Treatment is five-pronged:

a. **Optimize ART for primary HIV CNS infection.**

i. **Nucleoside antiretrovirals.** AZT may be the most effective of these agents because it achieves the highest concentration in the CSF. The treatment of choice for HIV dementia, AZT improves cognitive function in the short term and may retard cognitive decline. A full effect may not occur before 2–3 months; moreover, clinical improvement in the long term may be limited by the development of viral resistance to AZT.

ii. **Protease inhibitors.** Because the incidence of HIV dementia parallels the severity of systemic HIV disease, the potent ability of these new agents to decrease viral load may prevent or decrease the symptoms of HIV dementia.

b. **Use neuroprotective agents.** In vitro, these agents block the neurotoxic effects of HIV on neurons. Nimodipine, a calcium-channel antagonist, may help some patients with dementia when used in combination with AZT.

c. **Control symptoms with psychotropic medications** (see appropriate sections above for management of specific psychiatric syndromes).

d. **Provide supportive psychotherapy** to help patients cope with cognitive and functional losses.

e. **Modify patients' activities to capitalize on preserved cognitive strengths.** Maintenance of routine, completion of one task at a time, and reduction of external stimuli are important elements of behavior modification. Neuropsychological test performance can help determine specific modifications.

B. HIV Meningitis

Usually self-limited, but potentially chronic, this aseptic meningitis is a rare complication of the flu-like illness that occurs during seroconversion in one-third of HIV-infected people.

C. HIV Vacuolar Myelopathy

A complication of later stages of HIV/AIDS, this condition presents with bilateral leg weakness, ataxia, loss of vibration and position sense in the lower extremities, as well as bowel and bladder incontinence.

D. HIV Neuropathies (see IV.I)

E. Toxoplasmosis

The most common HIV-related opportunistic neurologic illness, infection with the protozoan, *Toxoplasma gondii*, causes encephalitis and abscesses in immunodeficient hosts, whereas many immunocompetent people are infected but remain asymptomatic.

1. **Symptoms and signs.** These include a rapidly progressive change in mental status, headache, and focal neurologic signs.

2. **Neuroimaging.** CT shows multiple ring-enhancing brain abscesses. T_2-weighted MRI scans demonstrate multiple foci of increased signal that have a predilection for the basal ganglia and are difficult to distinguish from lymphomatous lesions.

3. **Treatment. Pyrimethamine** and **sulfadiazine** lead to clinical and radiologic improvement, but suppressive therapy with pyrimethamine must continue for life because the infection cannot be eradicated.

F. Primary CNS Lymphoma

This neoplastic disease is the second leading cause of neurologic illness in HIV/AIDS patients. It presents as a slowly progressive neurocognitive disorder that can be mistaken for dementia before multifocal signs and elevated intracranial pressure supervene.

1. **Symptoms and signs.** These features depend on the site(s) of the lesion(s).

2. **Neuroimaging.** Lymphoma can be difficult to distinguish from toxoplasmosis.

3. **Treatment.** There is no effective specific therapy, but **radiation** is used to decrease intracranial pressure.

G. Cryptococcal Meningitis

This type of meningitis is caused by the yeast, *Cryptococcus neoformans*.

1. **Symptoms and signs.** Fever, meningismus, cranial nerve abnormalities, and papilledema develop.

2. **Neuroimaging.** CT and unenhanced MRI can be unremarkable, but MRI with gadolinium can show meningeal enhancement.

3. **Treatment. Amphotericin B** and **flucytosine** are effective, but relapse is common; suppressive treatment with amphotericin B or **fluconazole** is required.

H. Cytomegalovirus Encephalitis

A complication of late-stage HIV/AIDS, this condition may be difficult to distinguish from HIV dementia.

1. **Symptoms and signs.** Features include a rapidly progressive delirium, seizures, and fever.

2. **Neuroimaging.** MRI may show periventricular and subependymal abnormal signal.

3. **Treatment. Ganciclovir.**

I. Progressive Multifocal Leukoencephalopathy (PML)

Due to **papovavirus infection,** which is common in the immunocompetent population, PML follows a rapid downhill course in HIV/AIDS patients.

1. **Symptoms and signs.** Multifocal neurologic signs are dependent on lesion location; a progressive delirium is common.

2. **Neuroimaging.** CT shows subcortical nonenhancing lucencies. MRI shows patchy areas of high signal in subcortical white matter.

3. **Treatment.** No specific therapy exists, but temporary improvement may be achieved with **cytosine arabinoside.**

VI. Treatment Considerations

Clinicians must be aware of: the neuropsychiatric side effects of antiretroviral medications and agents used to treat secondary opportunistic infections; the drug interactions between antiretroviral agents and psychotropics; the differences in response to psychiatric medications manifest by patients with HIV/AIDS; and the psychotherapeutic challenges in this population.

A. The antiretroviral armamentarium includes nucleoside reverse transcriptase inhibitors, non-nucleoside reverse transcriptase inhibitors, and, as of 1996, protease inhibitors (PIs).

1. ART is effective in slowing disease progression when the CD4 count is < 500. Combination therapy is more effective than monotherapy.

2. The myriad neuropsychiatric side effects of these medications and others used to treat patients with HIV/AIDS are reviewed in Table 27-3.

B. Many antiretroviral agents are metabolized by the cytochrome P450 system; many are also inducers or inhibitors of this enzymatic pathway.

1. **The three non-nucleoside reverse transcriptase inhibitors are metabolized by, and interact with, the P450 system. Nevirapine and efavirenz induce it; delavirdine inhibits it.**

   a. **Agents whose coadministration with nevirapine requires careful monitoring:** midazolam, oral contraceptives, PIs, and triazolam

   b. **Agents whose coadministration with efavirenz is not recommended:** ergot alkaloids, midazolam, and triazolam

   c. **Agents whose coadministration with delavirdine is not recommended:** alprazolam, amphetamines, carbamazepine, ergot alkaloids, midazolam, phenobarbital, phenytoin, and triazolam

2. **PIs are metabolized by the P450 3A4 isoenzyme and are inhibitors of the P450 system; of these, ritonavir is the most potent.** Ritonavir and nelfinavir may also induce P-450 enzymes.

   a. **Agents that should not be coadministered with PIs:** ergot derivatives, midazolam, triazolam

   b. **Agents that should not be coadministered with ritonavir but can be (in low doses) with other PIs:** alprazolam, bupropion, clorazepate, clozapine, diazepam, estazolam, flurazepam, meperidine, pimozide, propoxyphene, and zolpidem

   c. **Agents whose coadministration with PIs requires low doses and testing of levels:** carbamazepine, clonazepam, hydrocodone, methadone, neuroleptics, oxycodone, psychostimulants, selective SRIs, and TCAs

   d. **Additional agents whose coadministration with ritonavir requires low doses:** maprotiline, nefazodone, trazodone, and venlafaxine

   e. **Agents whose levels may decrease with PIs:** alprazolam (with ritonavir), codeine, ethinyl estradiol (with ritonavir and nelfinavir), hydromorphone, lorazepam, morphine, oxazepam, and temazepam

   f. **Agents that decrease PI levels:** carbamazepine, phenobarbital, phenytoin, rifabutin, and rifampin

   g. When low doses are indicated, a practical approach is to start with half the usual dose.

C. Patients with HIV/AIDS have less lean body mass, metabolize drugs more slowly, and are sensitive to drug side effects. Because of blood-brain barrier compromise, the HIV-infected brain may "see" higher levels of drug than serum levels may predict.

1. Aim for low therapeutic levels.

2. Start with low doses and increase them slowly.

3. Avoid anticholinergic, anti-alpha-adrenergic, and sedating medications.

4. In patients with cognitive impairment, avoid as-needed dosing because patients may accidentally overdose on dangerous medications.

D. Issues that arise in psychotherapy with HIV/AIDS patients include self-blame, self-esteem, death, guilt, health care decisions, and feelings of being punished.

1. Psychotherapists must be aware of their feelings about HIV risk factors (e.g., substance abuse, homosexual sex, sex for trade) and be prepared to ask straightforward, nonjudgmental questions about lifestyles unfamiliar to them.

VII. Legal Considerations

A. The patient's written informed consent is necessary before HIV antibody testing.

1. Statutes vary, but, in some jurisdictions, this permission may be obtained from the patient's attorney-in-fact or the closest relative if the patient is incapacitated.

B. In psychiatric settings, staff are obligated to protect others by monitoring and restricting privileges of HIV-seropositive patients who engage in, or attempt to engage in, high-risk activities while in the hospital.

C. In some jurisdictions, physicians may have a legal requirement to disclose a patient's HIV serostatus against the patient's wishes to protect others without direct identification of the patient. In some jurisdictions, the physician must tell the patient that this information was disclosed. Because statutes vary by geography, clinicians should consult their local medical societies in these cases.

VIII. Conclusions

A. Infection with HIV exerts powerful biological, psychological, and social effects on patients and, directly or indirectly, is responsible for a panoply of affective, behavioral, and cognitive symptoms.

B. The care of these patients, therefore, taps all of a psychiatrist's skills. Not only must the psychiatrist be aware of the differences in the diagnosis and treatment of psychiatric syndromes in HIV-infected patients and the neurologic manifestations of HIV-related illnesses and treatments, he or she must be sensitive to the often fragile and chaotic psychosocial milieu in which many of these patients live.

Suggested Readings

Agenerase (amprenavir) Product Information, April 1999. www. agenerase.com

American Psychiatric Association: *Diagnostic and Statistical Manual of Mental Disorders,* 4th ed. Washington, DC: American Psychiatric Association, 1994:123–163.

Centers for Disease Control and Prevention: 1993 revised classification system for HIV infection and expanded surveillance case definition for AIDS among adolescents and adults. *Morbid Mortal Weekly Rep* 1992; 41 (No. RR-17):1–4, 15.

Centers for Disease Control and Prevention: Update: trends in AIDS incidence, deaths, and prevalence—United States, 1996. *Morbid Mortal Weekly Rep* 1997; 46:165–173.

Drugs for HIV infection. *Med Lett* 1997; 39:111–116.

Flexner C: HIV-protease inhibitors. *N Engl J Med* 1998; 338:1281–1292.

Grant I, Atkinson JH: Psychiatric aspects of acquired immune deficiency syndrome. In Kaplan HI, Sadock BJ (eds): *Comprehensive Textbook of Psychiatry VI*, 6th ed. Baltimore: Williams and Wilkins, 1995:1644–1669.

Greenberg DB, Beckett A: Neuropsychiatric aspects of cancer and AIDS in the intensive care unit. In Irwin RS, Cerra FB, Rippe JM (eds): *Intensive Care Medicine*, 4th ed. Philadelphia: Lippincott-Raven, 1999:2433–2440.

Grinspoon SK, Bilezikian JP: HIV disease and the endocrine system. *N Engl J Med* 1992; 327:1360–1365.

Grunfeld C, Pang M, Doerrler W, et al.: Indices of thyroid function and weight loss in human immunodeficiency virus infection and the acquired immunodeficiency syndrome. *Metabolism* 1993; 42: 1270–1276.

Halman MH, Worth JL, Sanders KM, et al.: Anticonvulsant use in the treatment of manic syndromes in patients with HIV-1 infection. *J Neuropsychiatry Clin Neurosci* 1993; 5:430–434.

Hinkin CH, Van Gorp WG, Satz P: Neuropsychological and neuropsychiatric aspects of HIV infection in adults. In Kaplan HI, Sadock BJ (eds): *Comprehensive Textbook of Psychiatry VI*, 6th ed. Baltimore: Williams and Wilkins, 1995:1669–1680.

Hriso E, Kuhn T, Masdeu JC, et al.: Extrapyramidal symptoms due to dopamine-blocking agents in patients with AIDS encephalopathy. *Am J Psychiatry* 1991; 148:1558–1561.

Marzuk PM, Tierney H, Tardiff K, et al.: Increased risk of suicide in persons with AIDS. *J Am Med Assoc* 1988; 259:1333–1337.

McDonald CK, Kuritzkes DR: Human immunodeficiency virus type 1 protease inhibitors. *Arch Intern Med* 1997; 157:951–959.

Melton ST, Kirkwood CK, Ghaemi SN: Pharmacotherapy of HIV dementia. *Ann Pharmacother* 1997; 31:457–473.

New drugs for HIV infection. *Med Lett* 1996; 38:35–37.

Panel on Clinical Practices for Treatment of HIV Infection: *Guidelines for the Use of Antiretroviral Agents in HIV-Infected Adults and Adolescents.* www.hivatis.org (HIV/AIDS Treatment Information Service), December 1998.

Physicians' Desk Reference, 53rd ed. Montvale, NJ: Medical Economics, 1999:464–469, 484–487, 1204, 1343, 1762–1766, 2675–2680, 2685–2688.

Schaerf FW, Miller RR, Lipsey JR, et al.: ECT for major depression in four patients infected with human immunodeficiency virus. *Am J Psychiatry* 1989; 146:782–784.

Sewell DD, Jeste DV, Atkinson JH, et al.: HIV-associated psychosis: a study of 20 cases. *Am J Psychiatry* 1994; 151:237–242.

Singh AN, Catalan J: Risperidone in HIV-related manic psychosis [letter]. *Lancet* 1994; 344:1029–1030.

Three new drugs for HIV infection. *Med Lett* 1998; 40:114–116.

Worth JL: HIV/AIDS patients. In Cassem NH, Stern TA, Rosenbaum JF, Jellinek MS (eds): *Massachusetts General Hospital Handbook of General Hospital Psychiatry*, 4th ed. St. Louis: Mosby Year Book, 1997:545–569.

Worth JL, Boswell SL: Approach to the patient with HIV infection. In Stern TA, Herman JB, Slavin PL (eds): *The MGH Guide to Psychiatry in Primary Care*. New York: McGraw-Hill, 1998:385–400.

Worth JL, Halman MH: HIV disease/AIDS. In Rundell JR, Wise MG (eds): *The American Psychiatric Press Textbook of Consultation-Liaison Psychiatry*. Washington, DC: American Psychiatric Press, 1996:833–877.

Chapter 28

Catatonia, Neuroleptic Malignant Syndrome, and Serotonin Syndrome

BRAD REDDICK AND THEODORE A. STERN

I. Introduction

The syndromes described in this chapter all allude to the complex interaction of motor, behavioral, and systemic manifestations derived from unclear mechanisms of neurochemical aberration. The clinical similarities among neuroleptic malignant syndrome (NMS), catatonia, and serotonin syndrome have led some to hypothesize a common pathophysiology. Many believe that NMS is but one point along a spectrum of clinical presentations, essentially being an extreme form of catatonia. As our psychopharmacologic armamentarium grows and as drugs potent in their modulation of monoamine action proliferate, the diagnosis and management of these complex disorders becomes even more important.

II. Catatonia

A. Definition

Few disorders are as enigmatic as catatonia. It has been described as a subtype of schizophrenia, but is reported to be more common in affective disorders. Its phenomenology includes a characteristic excitement as well as stupor.

The syndrome of catatonia (derived from the Greek word *katateinein*, to stretch tightly), is made up of an array of motor and behavioral signs and symptoms that often occur in relation to neurochemical insults. The syndrome was characterized as early as 1874 when Karl Kahlbaum first described 21 patients thought to have the disorder, which he proposed was a process of several stages corresponding to symptom severity. Kraeplin included catatonia as a subgroup of his deteriorating psychotic disorders termed "dementia praecox." With the rise in neuroleptic use, catatonia as a subtype of schizophrenia has declined, and a greater proportion of affected patients suffer from affective disorders and general medical conditions.

B. Etiology

The potential etiologies of catatonia are many and are outlined in Table 28-1. The importance of prompt diagnosis is highlighted by the many potential complications associated with catatonia (Table 28-2) and the existence of effective treatments, which may prevent such complications and interrupt progression of the illness.

C. Epidemiology

1. At least one study has looked at the incidence of catatonia upon hospital admission and found its frequency among newly admitted psychiatric inpatients to be approximately 9% (Rosebush et al., 1990).

2. The exact prevalence of catatonia is unknown, although the frequency of catatonic signs arising in affective disorders has remained unchanged since 1922.

3. This is in contrast to the observed decline in prevalence of catatonia associated with schizophrenia from 14% to 8%, which has been attributed to changing patterns in the diagnosis of schizophrenia or to a hypothesized decline of some viral infective disorder which may be involved in the pathogenesis of schizophrenia.

4. Several studies have attempted to outline the association between catatonia and affective disorders. Taylor and Abrams found that 25–50% of patients with catatonic signs and symptoms also meet criteria for affective disorder.

5. Roughly 20% of patients with bipolar illness exhibit one or more catatonic characteristics. Approximately 5–10% of schizophrenic patients will have catatonic features.

D. Diagnosis

1. The *Diagnostic and Statistical Manual, Fourth Edition* (DSM-IV) outlines criteria for catatonia in association with Major Depressive Disorder (MDD), mania, mixed affective state, or schizophrenia, with the presence of at least two of the following:
   a. Motor immobility
   b. Excessive motor activity
   c. Extreme negativism or mutism
   d. Peculiar voluntary movement
   e. Echolalia or echopraxia

2. The syndrome is thought to be the result of a general medical condition when:
   a. The disturbance does not occur during the course of delirium.
   b. The disturbance is not better accounted for by another mental disorder.

219

Table 28-1. Potential Etiologies of the Catatonic Syndrome

Primary psychiatric
Acute psychoses
Conversion disorder
Dissociative disorders
Mood disorders
Obsessive-compulsive disorders
Personality disorders
Schizophrenia

Secondary neuromedical
Cerebrovascular
Arterial aneurysms
Arteriovenous malformations
Arterial and venous thrombosis
Bilateral parietal infarcts
Temporal lobe infarct
Subarachnoid hemorrhage
Subdural hematoma
Third ventricle hemorrhage
Hemorrhagic infarcts
Other central nervous system causes
Akinetic mutism
Pellagra
Alcoholic degeneration and Wernicke's encephalopathy
Cerebellar degeneration
Cerebral anoxia
Cerebromacular degeneration
Closed head trauma
Frontal lobe atrophy
Hydrocephalus
Lesions of thalamus and globus pallidus
Narcolepsy
Parkinsonism
Postencephalitic states
Seizure disorders
Surgical interventions
Tuberous sclerosis

Neoplasm
Angiomas
Frontal lobe tumors
Gliomas
Langerhans' carcinoma
Paraneoplastic encephalopathy
Periventricular diffuse pinealoma

Poisoning
Coal gas
Organic fluorides
Tetraethyl lead poisoning

Infections
Acquired immunodeficiency syndrome
Bacterial meningoencephalitis
Bacterial sepsis
General paresis
Malaria
Mononucleosis
Subacute sclerosing panencephalitis
Tertiary syphilis
Tuberculosis
Typhoid fever
Viral encephalitides (especially herpes)
Viral hepatitis

Metabolic and other medical causes
Acute intermittent porphyria
Addison's disease
Cushing's disease
Diabetic ketoacidosis
Glomerulonephritis
Hepatic dysfunction
Hereditary coproporphyria
Homocystinuria
Hyperparathyroidism
Hyperthyroidism
Idiopathic hyperadrenergic state
Multiple sclerosis
Systemic lupus erythematosus
Thrombotic thrombocytopenic purpura
Uremia

Drug-related
Neuroleptics; typical and atypical (e.g., clozapine, risperidone)
Non-neuroleptics
Alcohol
Anticonvulsants (tricyclics, monoamine oxidase inhibitors, and others)
Anticonvulsants (e.g., carbamazepine)
Aspirin
Disulfiram
Metoclopramide
Dopamine depleters (e.g., tetrabenzine)
Dopamine withdrawal (e.g., levodopa)
Hallucinogens (e.g., mescaline, phencyclidine, and lysergic acid diethylamide)
Lithium carbonate
Morphine
Sedative-hypnotic withdrawal
Steroids
Stimulants (e.g., amphetamines, methylphenidate, and possibly cocaine)

Idiopathic

SOURCE: Adapted from Philbrick KL, Rummans TA: Malignant catatonia. *J Neuropsychiatry Clin Neurosci* 1994; 6:1–13.

Table 28-2. Some Medical Complications Associated with Catatonia

Simple nonmalignant catatonia

Aspiration

Burns

Cachexia

Dehydration and sequelae

Pneumonia

Pulmonary emboli

Thrombophlebitis

Urinary retention and sequelae

Urinary incontinence

Malignant catatonia

Acute renal failure

Adult respiratory distress syndrome

Aphasia and dysarthria

Cardiac arrest

Cheyne-Stokes respirations

Death

Disseminated intravascular coagulation

Electrocardiographic abnormalities

Gait abnormalities

Intestinal pseudo-obstruction

Laryngospasm

Myocardial infarction

Myocardial stunning

Necrotizing enterocolitis

Pneumomediastinum

Pseudomembranous colitis

Respiratory arrest

Respiratory stridor

Rhabdomyolysis and sequelae

Seizures

Sepsis

Severe dysphagia due to muscle spasm

Severe hepatocellular damage

Sudden, profound hypoglycemia

Unresponsiveness to pain

Upper gastrointestinal tract bleeding

c. There is evidence from history, physical examination, or laboratory findings that the disturbance is the direct physiological consequence of a general medical condition.

3. In addition to the criteria outlined in the DSM-IV, it is important to consider subtypes of the syn-drome to facilitate management and treatment. **Catatonic stupor** is characterized by psychomotor withdrawal, whereas **catatonic excitement** is related to psychomotor hyperactivity. Another subtype, **malignant catatonia,** suggested by Philbrick and Rummans, is used when catatonia is complicated by autonomic instability or hyperthermia.

E. **Differential Diagnosis**
With the great number of medical and neuro-logical illnesses which may potentially precipitate catatonia, differentiating among the many possi-ble etiologies can be a formidable task. Table 28-1 outlines **the many potential etiologies of catatonia** that must be considered when the syndrome arises.

F. **Pathophysiology**
The complex array of symptoms and the many potential etiologies make discussion of the mechan-ism by which the syndrome of catatonia develops difficult. **Clinical features (e.g., rigidity) suggest involvement of the basal ganglia and its associated projections.** Given the clinical similarities among neurologic illness involving the frontal lobes, which produce akinetic mutism and idiopathic catatonia, **involvement of dopamine and inhibitory γ-aminobu-tyric acid (GABA) in the prefrontal cortex has been implicated.** Alternatively, subtle **ictal events** invol-ving the prefrontal cortex and the basal ganglia have been postulated, since use of intravenous benzodiazepines (which have antiseizure effects) can treat catatonia.

G. **Evaluation**
1. **A thorough neuromedical workup is essential** so that prompt treatment can be initiated and further medical and psychiatric complications can be pre-vented.
2. **An amobarbital interview may be helpful,** especially in stuporous catatonia; a temporary recovery from catatonic symptoms suggests psychiatric illness.
3. **A physical examination may reveal signs of medical complications. Findings associated with the catato-nia syndrome associated with psychiatric illness** (idiopathic catatonia) include:
   a. Normal optokinetic responses
   b. Normal pupillary responses
   c. Normal ocular nystagmus on cold caloric tests
   d. Extreme negativism
   e. Mutism
   f. Waxy flexibility
   g. (in the case of malignant catatonia and NMS) auto-nomic instability
   h. (in the case of malignant catatonia and NMS) a rise in basal body temperature (hyperthermia as the extreme)

4. **History will often reveal clues to the existence of a premorbid psychotic disorder or underlying medication trial or medical condition,** such as those outlined in Table 28-1. When catatonic mutism precludes obtaining a thorough history, administration of intravenous lorazepam can bring on a temporary lucid interval that may facilitate data collection.

Interviewing the catatonic patient can prove a challenge; it often relies on keen observation of behavior. Many have used rating scales such as **the modified Bush-Francis Catatonia Rating Scale,** which requires two of 14 behavioral signs to make the diagnosis.

5. Studies
   a. **An electroencephalogram (EEG) is needed to detect a potential underlying seizure disorder.** Although a normal EEG may suggest idiopathic catatonia, many psychiatric patients display nonspecific abnormalities on EEG.
   b. **Neuroimaging studies can rule out mass lesions, central nervous system (CNS) ischemic events, and underlying neuromedical illness** that confer vulnerability, although a normal imaging study does not rule out an underlying neuromedical etiology.
   c. **Laboratory tests can illuminate clues to both catatonia and the risk factors for the development of NMS.** Like the physical examination, results of electrolytes, renal function, and the hematocrit may suggest dehydration and raise suspicion for NMS. **An elevated creatine phosphokinase (CPK) typically occurs in both malignant catatonia and NMS;** knowledge of its presence can guide therapy in terms of preventing subsequent renal failure from rhabdomyolysis.

H. **Treatment**
   1. **Pharmacology**
      a. **Discontinuation of any potential offending pharmacologic agent** (e.g., dopamine-blockers such as neuroleptics, Compazine, or metoclopramide), which can cause or worsen catatonia, should be considered.
      b. **Review of the medication record should be accomplished** to determine if dopamine agonists have been withdrawn and consideration given to their resumption.
   2. Since **electroconvulsive therapy** (ECT) continues to be a powerful and important treatment of catatonia, it **should be considered.** Frequently two to three treatments will suffice, although four to six treatments are usually given to prevent relapse.
   3. **Medical/supportive care is essential;** it includes adequate hydration, nutrition, mobilization, and anticoagulation (to prevent thrombophlebitis and pulmonary embolism). Aspiration precautions are also important. Once catatonia is suspected, close observation and frequent vital sign checks are warranted. Throughout the course, a high index of

suspicion should be sustained for the development of medical complications.
   4. **If hyperthermia, autonomic instability, or malignant catatonia emerge, treatment in an intensive care unit may be indicated.**

III. Neuroleptic Malignant Syndrome (NMS)

A. **Definition**
   NMS is a rare complication of neuroleptic therapy that confers high mortality if not treated in a prompt and skillful manner. It is a syndrome defined by its symptoms.

B. **Epidemiology**
   1. **Lack of uniform diagnostic criteria, concurrent use of other medications, and methodological differences used in epidemiology studies have made estimating the frequency of NMS difficult;** its incidence is estimated from 0.07% to 2.2%.
   2. Although there are clinical similarities between NMS and malignant hyperthermia (associated with general anesthesia), **patients with a history of either NMS or malignant hyperthermia do not appear to be at increased risk for developing the other.**
   3. **Mortality rates for patients with NMS have decreased from 20% (prior to 1984) to 11.6%** currently, a decrease thought to be secondary to a greater awareness of the syndrome and its signs and symptoms.

C. **Diagnosis**
   1. **No universally accepted criteria exist for NMS.** However, several attempts have been made to group signs and symptoms into major and minor categories.
   2. **Currently the DSM-IV defines NMS as the development of severe muscle rigidity, and elevated temperature in association with two or more of the following: diaphoresis, dysphagia, tremor, incontinence, changes in level of consciousness, mutism, tachycardia, elevated or labile blood pressure, leukocytosis, and laboratory evidence of muscle injury (elevated CPK).**
   3. Making the diagnosis implies that the symptom complex cannot be better accounted for by a mood disorder with catatonic features, or a general medical or neurological illness.
   4. Attempts to discover risk factors for the development of NMS have been ongoing. Keck and associates examined 18 patients with NMS in a case-controlled fashion. When compared to controls, they identified **several risk factors,** including:
      a. A greater degree of **premorbid psychomotor agitation**

b. **Higher doses of neuroleptics** with greater rates of dose increase

c. A higher number of **intramuscular injections**

d. Concurrent use of **lithium**

D. Differential Diagnosis

1. As the clinical features of NMS resemble those of a host of medical and neurological illnesses, the diagnosis of NMS requires attention to the plethora of potential neuromedical etiologies.

2. Table 28-3 outlines common disorders to consider when the diagnosis of NMS is entertained.

3. Of particular note are those illnesses which present with hemodynamic changes, systemic manifestations, and clouding of the sensorium, which may be confused with NMS.

   a. Although clinically similar to NMS, **malignant hyperthermia** differs from NMS in that it is associated with anesthesia and has a characteristic histologic appearance of skeletal muscle fibers (i.e., they contract on exposure to halothane or caffeine).

   b. **Anticholinergic delirium,** which is manifest by clouding of the sensorium, and an elevated temperature (like NMS), but not by diaphoresis. The diagnosis of anticholinergic delirium can be further clarified by the

---

Table 28-3. Differential Diagnosis of Neuroleptic Malignant Syndrome

Central nervous system disorders

Head trauma

Meningitis

Parkinson's disease

Status epilepticus

Systemic disorders

Hyperthyroidism

Pheochromocytoma

Malignant hyperthermia

Heat stroke

Polymyositis

Sepsis

Psychiatric disorders

Lethal catatonia

Toxic conditions

Anticholinergic syndrome

Serotonin syndrome

Monamine oxidase inhibitor/tricyclic combination

Withdrawal from alcohol or sedative hypnotic drugs

Sudden discontinuation of levodopa

---

administration of physostigmine, which will temporarily ameliorate anticholinergic symptoms.

c. **Serotonin syndrome** is another condition which has similar clinical signs to those of NMS. However, in serotonin syndrome, tremor is a more common peripheral motor finding, fever is present less often, and the laboratory abnormalities seen in NMS are usually absent.

E. Pathophysiology

1. Although poorly understood, **the mechanism thought to be responsible for NMS involves blockade of central dopamine receptors in the basal ganglia, the hypothalamus, and peripherally in postganglionic sympathetic neurons and smooth muscle.**

2. Neuroleptics have been implicated in directly altering basal temperature regulation in the hypothalamus, which may play an added role in the development of fever.

3. Additionally, observations that dantrolene may be beneficial in the treatment of NMS raise the hypothesis that neuroleptics may directly affect skeletal muscle and result in increased cell metabolism and hyperthermia.

4. Some have postulated that the underlying pathophysiology more likely reflects an imbalance in central dopamine and serotonergic and/or adrenergic tone. Case reports of NMS developing from tricyclic antidepressants, selective serotonin reuptake inhibitors (SSRIs), and atypical antipsychotic agents point to the potential involvement of nondopamine monoamines as well.

F. Treatment

1. Given the high morbidity and mortality associated with NMS, **prompt treatment is essential.**

2. Initial management should include transfer to a general hospital where **intensive hemodynamic monitoring and supportive care** can be initiated.

3. Medical and supportive care is crucial once the diagnosis of NMS is made. Suggested supportive measures include provision of **adequate intravenous hydration, active cooling, and close hemodynamic monitoring.**

4. **Electrolyte balance and renal function should be monitored** closely, given the increased risk of renal failure associated with NMS. Dialysis may be necessary.

5. A detailed history and chart review may reveal the use of either neuroleptic or nonneuroleptic dopamine antagonists, or withdrawal of dopamine agonists. Any dopamine antagonists (Table 28-4) should be removed and the agonists resumed.

G. Treatment Hierarchy

1. Discontinue neuroleptics and other dopamine antagonists.

Table 28-4. Dopamine Antagonists

Antipsychotics (neuroleptics)

Phenothiazines

Chlorpromazine (Thorazine)

Triflupromazine (Vesprin)

Mesoridazine (Serentil)

Thioridazine (Mellaril)

Acetophenazine (Tindal)

Fluphenazine (Prolixin, Permitil)

Perphenazine (Trilafon)

Trifluoperazine (Stelazine)

Butyrophenones

Droperidol (Inapsine)

Haloperidol (Haldol)

Thioxanthenes

Chlorprothixene (Taractan)

Thiothixene (Navane)

Dibenzoxepines

Loxapine (Loxitane, Daxoline)

Clozapine (Clozaril)

Indolone

Molindone (Moban)

Diphenylbutylpiperidine

Pimozide (Orap)

Other dopamine antagonists

Antiemetics

Metaclopramide (Reglan)

Promethazine (Phenergan)

Prochlorperazine (Compazine)

Trimethobenzamide (Tigan)

Antihistamines

Hydroxyzine (Atarax, Vistaril)

2. Provide supportive care.
3. **Institute pharmacologic interventions.** These have included **dantrolene,** which may be helpful in reducing muscle rigidity, but it carries a risk of hepatotoxicity. **Bromocriptine** is thought to be effective through its action as a central D_2 agonist, although it may potentially worsen any underlying psychosis. **Other treatments that may be beneficial include: amantadine, levodopa, clonazepam, benztropine, nondepolarizing paralytic agents, and ECT.**

4. **Controversy surrounds the assumption that the development of NMS confers greater risk of developing the syndrome if rechallenged with a neuroleptic.** Most investigators agree that reinstitution of antipsychotic medicines should be delayed for at least 2 weeks after an episode of NMS has resolved, and should include a neuroleptic of lower potency.

IV. Serotonin Syndrome

A. Definition

1. Serotonin plays a major role in multiple psychiatric illnesses. As the number of agents that directly effect central serotonergic tone increases, so has our understanding of the clinical features related to serotonin excess (serotonin syndrome) and the need for heightened clinical awareness in the prevention, recognition, and prompt treatment of the syndrome.
2. Although **its incidence is unknown,** serotonin syndrome is **most commonly the result of the interaction between serotonergic agents and monoamine oxidase inhibitors** (MAOIs), and commonly results in changes in mental status, restlessness, myoclonus, hyperreflexia, diaphoresis, shivering, and tremor.
3. The presumed mechanism involves the brainstem and spinal cord activation of the 1A form of serotonin receptor.
4. **Discontinuation of the serotonergic agents and institution of supportive treatment are the primary treatments,** although the 5HT receptor antagonists may also play a role.
5. Once treatment is initiated, the syndrome usually resolves within 24 h; associated confusion can last for days.

B. Clinical Presentation

1. Serotonin syndrome most commonly occurs in individuals with a history of a psychiatric disorder for which a psychotropic medicine has been prescribed, most commonly some combination of an SSRI, L-tryptophan, an MAOI, an antiparkinson agent, and lithium.
2. **Initially, patients experience peripheral tremor, mild confusion, and incoordination, followed by systemic signs (e.g., hyperreflexia, diaphoresis, shivering, and marked behavioral agitation).**
3. **In severe form patients may develop fever, myoclonus, and diarrhea.**
4. These clinical features can range in duration from 6 h up to 44 h after the initiation of treatment.
5. Table 28-5 outlines the clinical features of serotonin syndrome.

C. Pathophysiology

1. The preponderance of evidence, which relies mostly on animal studies and a few studies in

Table 28-5. The Most Common Clinical Features of the Serotonin Syndrome in Order of Frequency

- Mental status changes
    - Confusion
    - Hypomania
- Restlessness
- Myoclonus
- Hyperreflexia
- Diaphoresis
- Shivering
- Tremor
- Diarrhea
- Incoordination

humans, implicates the role of 5HT in the pathogenesis of serotonin syndrome.

2. The identification of receptor subtypes and subsequent research on the benefits of 5HT antagonism, has implicated $5HT_{1A}$ receptor activation as responsible for serotonin syndrome.

3. Other studies (as in NMS) have implicated both dopamine and serotonergic activation in the syndrome's pathogenesis, arguing that agents with a ratio of greater serotonergic properties to corresponding dopaminergic properties are most likely to precipitate the syndrome.

4. This hypothesis is further supported by peripheral manifestations of serotonergic activation comprising a majority of symptoms observed in the syndrome, along with observations that $5HT_{1A}$ receptors predominate in the caudal brainstem and spinal cord.

5. As these observations are based on animal models of neurotransmission, caution must be used in extrapolating these results to humans.

D. Epidemiology

1. The **incidence of serotonin syndrome is unknown,** and there are no data to suggest that sex or age differences confer any variability in predisposition to developing the syndrome.

2. Given the overlap of symptoms with NMS, serotonin syndrome is often mistaken for NMS and thus may be underreported. Additionally, **the possible existence of varying gradations in symptom severity may also confound full recognition of this syndrome.**

E. Evaluation

1. As with NMS, a detailed history will often reveal concomitant use of at least two psychotropic med-

ications, which confers greater risk for developing the syndrome. As NMS shares many clinical features with serotonin syndrome, prior use of neuroleptics and a history of psychosis are of particular importance.

2. Typically the history is most helpful in establishing a temporal relationship with the initiation of psychotropic agents.

3. **Laboratory testing** is useful to assess a patient's underlying nutritional and hydration status, to screen for elevated CPK raising suspicion of NMS, and to investigate the presence of an underlying medical condition which may raise the risk of developing the syndrome and subsequent complications.

4. Of note, certain monoamine secreting tumors (e.g., carcinoid tumors and oat cell lung malignancies) have been associated with the serotonin syndrome. With these rare malignancies in mind, gastrointestinal and lung roentgenograms may be helpful in the initial investigation.

5. As is the case in catatonia and NMS, an **EEG and neuroimaging** are useful in uncovering an underlying seizure disorder or neurological condition, although normal studies do not rule out the presence of a neuromedical illness.

F. Drug Interactions

1. **As is the case with NMS, drug effects and interactions are the most common precipitant of the syndrome.**

2. Case reports highlight the greater risk of SSRIs, L-tryptophan, and MAOIs in precipitating the syndrome. Specifically, case reports have centered around symptoms arising when SSRIs are combined with either L-tryptophan or an MAOI. Table 28-6 lists **the most common drug interactions associated with serotonin syndrome.**

a. In general, when serotonergic reuptake inhibition is combined with MAO inhibition, the potential for induction of serotonin syndrome is greatly increased. Such a presentation has also been described in combining medications with MAOI properties with either L-tryptophan or lithium.

Table 28-6. The Most Common Drug Interactions Associated with the Serotonin Syndrome in Order of Frequency

- L-Tryptophan and an MAOI (with lithium)
- Fluoxetine and an MAOI
- Fluoxetine and L-tryptophan
- Clomipramine and clorgyline
- Bromocriptine and L-dopa/carbidopa

b. Additionally, the syndrome can be precipitated by overdoses of MAOIs.

c. The potential hazards of using an MAOI and a medicine with any serotonergic properties or reuptake inhibition demand vigilance when prescribing an MAOI.

d. Current treatment practice includes a 2-week washout interval following the discontinuation of an MAOI. In the case of fluoxetine, a minimum of 5-week washout period is required following the discontinuation of fluoxetine and before the initiation of an MAOI.

G. Treatment

1. Given the nonexistence of prospective studies evaluating the treatment of serotonin syndrome, **strategies for treatment are derived primarily from human case reports and data stemming from animal studies.**

2. To date, the literature addressing treatment indicates that **removal of the offending agent will often result in the resolution of symptoms within 24 h.** The first step in treatment is always to discontinue the suspected offending agent.

3. **Supportive measures are essential in both treating and preventing potential medical complications** and often include antipyretics to combat fever, cooling blankets for the development of hyperthermia, clonazepam for myoclonus, anticonvulsants if seizures arise, and antihypertensive agents, such as nifedipine, for severely elevated blood pressure. Rarely does the syndrome progress to respiratory failure, which is usually due to aspiration requiring artificial ventilation.

4. Animal models have suggested that **prophylaxis is possible with pretreatment using $5HT_1$ receptor antagonists.** Agents which confer nonspecific 5HT receptor antagonism and have demonstrated benefit in the treatment or prevention of the symptoms associated with serotonin syndrome include **methysergide** and **cyproheptidine.**

5. Beta-blockers may also be useful in treatment due to their 5HT blocking properties. Specifically, **propranolol** has demonstrated $5HT_{1A}$ receptor antagonism in animal models and, in at least one case report, was successful in blocking the progression of the syndrome after a patient ingested varying amounts of L-tryptophan, isocarboxide, and lithium.

Suggested Readings

American Psychiatric Association: *Diagnostic Statistical Manual, Fourth Edition* (DSM-IV). Washington, DC: American Psychiatric Association, 1994.

Blumer D: Catatonia and the neuroleptics: psychobiologic significance of remote and recent findings. *Comp Psychiatry* 1997; 38:193–201.

Bush G, Fink M, Petrides G, et al.: Catatonia. Treatment with lorazepam and electroconvulsive therapy. *Acta Psychiatr Scand* 1996; 93:137–143.

Fricchione G, Bush G, Fozdar M, et al.: Recognition and treatment of the catatonic syndrome. *J Intensive Care Med* 1997; 12:135–147.

Keck PE, Pope HG, Cohen BM, et al.: Risk factors for neuroleptic malignant syndrome. *Arch Gen Psychiatry* 1989; 46:914–918.

Pope HG Jr, Jonas JM, Hudson JI, et al.: Toxic reactions to the combination of monoamine oxidase inhibitors and tryptophan. *Am J Psychiatry* 1985; 142:491–492.

Prager L, Millham F, Stern TA: Neuroleptic malignant syndrome: a review for intensivists. *J Intensive Care Med* 1994; 9:227–234.

Rosebush PI, Hildebrand AM, Furlong BG, et al.: Catatonic syndrome in a general psychiatric inpatient population: frequency, clinical presentation, and response to lorazepam. *J Clin Psychiatry* 1990; 51:357–362.

Stern TA, Schwartz JH, Shuster JL: Catastrophic illness associated with the combination of clomipramine, phenelzine, and chlorpromazine. *Ann Clin Psychiatry* 1992; 4:81–85.

Stern TA, Herman JB, Slavin PL (eds): *The MGH Guide to Psychiatry in Primary Care.* New York: McGraw-Hill, 1998.

Sternbach H: The serotonin syndrome. *Am J Psychiatry* 1991; 148:705–713.

Chapter 29

Neuroimaging in Psychiatry

DARIN D. DOUGHERTY AND SCOTT L. RAUCH

I. Introduction

In general, neuroimaging is used as an aid in the differential diagnosis of neuropsychiatric conditions; rarely does neuroimaging alone establish the diagnosis. When one is contemplating the use of neuroimaging, a variety of factors must be considered, including the indications, risks, costs, advantages, and limitations. This chapter reviews these factors and provides general guidelines for the use of neuroimaging in neuropsychiatric syndromes.

II. Modalities

A. Structural

1. **Computed tomography (CT)**
   a. Technology
      i. **CT uses X-rays which are differentially attenuated,** depending on the material through which they pass (higher attenuation in dense material, such as bone; lower attenuation in less dense material, such as air and fluid).
      ii. **CT uses serial X-rays acquired in an axial slab-wise (i.e., tomographic) manner.**
   b. **CT with contrast**
      i. Radiopaque iodine-based contrast material introduced intravenously **allows visualization of lesions that compromise the integrity of the blood-brain barrier** (e.g., cerebrovascular accident [CVA], tumor, inflammation).
      ii. **Contrast media** which enhance the visibility of pathology by CT **are either ionic or nonionic.** Nonionic contrast is many times more expensive than ionic contrast. However, **ionic contrast has a greater risk of side effects.**
         - **Idiosyncratic reactions occur in 5% of cases** and include hypotension, nausea, flushing, urticaria, and sometimes frank anaphylaxis. Risk factors include age of less than 1 year or greater than 60 years, and a history of asthma, allergies, cerebrovascular disease, or prior contrast reactions.
         - Chemotoxic reactions can occur in the brain and the kidney. **Chemotoxicity may present as impaired renal function or even renal failure,** with the main risk factor being pre-existing renal insufficiency. In the brain, **chemotoxic reactions manifest as seizures.** Such reactions occur in approximately 1 in every 10,000 cases, but develop in up to 10% of cases in which gross disruption of the blood-brain barrier is present.
   c. **Advantages and limitations**
      i. **CT offers excellent spatial resolution (< 1 mm).**
      ii. **CT is useful for the detection of acute bleeding** (less than 24–72 h old), but is less helpful in subacute bleeding (more than 72 h old) and in severely anemic patients (i.e., with a hemoglobin below 10 g/dL).
      iii. CT is not helpful in visualizing subtle white matter lesions.
      iv. CT uses ionizing radiation and so is strongly contraindicated in pregnancy.

2. **Magnetic resonance imaging (MRI)**
   a. Technology
      i. **MRI exploits the magnetic properties of hydrogen atoms in water molecules to construct a representation of tissue.** Nuclei are excited; as they relax, they give off energy that is used to construct the images. Different components of the relaxation process exist and occur at different rates (called T_1 and T_2) in different tissues. Specific imaging parameters (T_1-weighted vs. T_2-weighted) are selected according to the clinical circumstances.
         - **T_1-weighted images are used for optimal visualization of normal anatomy.**
         - **T_2-weighted images are used to detect areas of pathology.**
      ii. **Diffusion-weighted imaging (DWI)** is a newer MRI technique that detects the tiny random movements of water molecules (diffusion) in tissue. This technique allows a map of the average apparent diffusion coefficient (ADC) to be calculated. Shortly after the onset of an ischemic stroke, the ADC of brain tissue is significantly reduced because of cytotoxic edema. Over several days, the rapid initial drop in ADC is followed by a return to "pseudonormal" values at approximately 1 week and then elevation above normal values subsequently. DWI is **remarkably sensitive in detecting and localizing acute ischemic brain lesions and allows differentiation of acute regions of ischemia from chronic infarcts.**
   b. **MRI with contrast**
      i. **Gadolinium** is used as the contrast medium because of its paramagnetic properties. Like CT contrast, it is introduced intravascularly. The use of **MRI contrast highlights vascular structures and aids in the detection of pathology in areas where blood vessel walls or the blood-brain barrier are**

compromised. Gadolinium causes fewer and less severe side effects than does CT contrast, with one reported death in over 5 million dosings.

c. **Advantages and limitations**

  i. MRI provides **excellent spatial resolution and superior soft-tissue contrast** in comparison to CT (e.g., more useful for the visualization of white matter).

  i. MRI is **superior for surveying the posterior fossa and brainstem.**

  iii. MRI does not use ionizing radiation, and so it is **preferable to CT in pregnancy** although it is still relatively contraindicated.

  iv. MRI is **contraindicated in patients with metallic implants** for the following reasons:

- Metal can cause artifacts in MR images.
- Metal can shift position or absorb heat within the magnetic field, causing burn injuries.
- Mechanical devices such as pacemakers can malfunction within the magnetic field.

3. **CT versus MRI** (Table 29-1)

a. CT is more economical than MRI and is available at more centers.

b. CT is the modality of choice for patients with acute bleeds or acute trauma, **though DWI may soon become the modality of choice for assessing suspected acute brain ischemic events.**

c. **MRI is superior to CT for the differentiation of white from gray matter and the identification of white matter lesions.**

d. **MRI is superior to CT for the detection of posterior fossa and brainstem pathology.**

e. CT is recommended if MRI is contraindicated (i.e., paramagnetic prostheses; inability to tolerate scanner time, noise, or confinement).

f. **MRI is recommended if radiation exposure is contraindicated** (i.e., young children or women of childbearing potential).

B. **Functional**

1. **Positron emission tomography (PET)**

a. Technology

  i. **PET uses positron emission from administered radionuclides to measure cerebral blood flow** (e.g., oxygen-15) **or cerebral glucose metabolism** (e.g., fluorodeoxyglucose [FDG]), **both of which correspond to neuronal activity.**

  ii. With PET one can use inhaled or intravenous radionuclides to look at the brain in the resting state or when activated by specific tasks.

  iii. One can also use radioactive ligands to perform receptor characterization studies.

b. **Advantages and limitations**

  i. PET is **the gold standard of functional neuroimaging modalities.**

  ii. PET **offers excellent spatial resolution (4–8 mm).**

  iii. PET **is very expensive and requires immediate access to the cyclotron,** which produces positron-emitting radionuclides.

2. **Single photon emission computed tomography (SPECT)**

a. **Technology**

  i. **SPECT also uses radionuclides** (e.g., xenon-133, ^{99m}Tc-HMPAO) for functional imaging, but measures single photon emission rather than positron emission.

Table 29-1. Summary Comparisons of CT and MRI

Consideration	CT vs. MRI
Economy	CT $\geq$ MRI
Availability	CT $\geq$ MRI
Speed	CT > MRI
Comfort	CT > MRI
Quality of visualization	
Bleeding	
Acute (< 48–72 h)	CT > MRI
Subacute (> 48–72 h)	MRI > CT
Ischemia	
Acute	DWI > MRI $\approx$ CT
Chronic	DWI $\approx$ MRI > CT
Bone	CT > MRI
Gray matter	MRI > CT
White matter	MRI > CT
Posterior fossa	MRI > CT
Spatial resolution	CT $\geq$ MRI

ii. As with PET, both inhaled and intravenous radio-nuclides are available, as are radioligands for measuring indexes of gross brain activity and performing receptor characterization.

b. **Advantages and disadvantages**

i. SPECT is **more affordable than PET** and does not require a cyclotron for production of radionuclides.

ii. SPECT **provides inferior spatial resolution (≥ 8 mm)** compared with PET.

iii. SPECT **resolution worsens as one attempts to image deeper brain structures.**

3. **PET versus SPECT** (Table 29-2)

a. **PET provides superior spatial resolution, especially for deeper brain structures.**

b. PET offers a broader array of radioligands for use in receptor studies and is the only modality that allows for the measurement of metabolism.

c. SPECT is less expensive than PET and is more widely available.

4. **Functional magnetic resonance imaging** (fMRI) **and magnetic resonance spectroscopy** (MRS)

a. **These modalities remain research tools at this time,** although clinical applications are likely to evolve in the near future.

III. Indications

A. Structural

1. **Computed tomography**

a. There have been numerous studies of the results of CT imaging in psychiatric populations. Across these studies, 12% of patients demonstrated focal abnormalities. **The likelihood of detecting an abnormal finding increased with age, with an abnormal neurologic examination, with an altered mental status, and with a history of head trauma or alcohol abuse.** Weinberger (1984) proposed **criteria for CT imaging in psychiatric settings:**

i. **Confusion or dementia**

ii. **New-onset psychosis**

iii. **Movement disorder**

iv. **Anorexia nervosa**

v. **Prolonged catatonia**

vi. **New-onset major affective disorder or personality change after age 50 years**

2. **Magnetic resonance imaging**

a. When MRI became available in the 1980s, the neuroimaging literature reflected a shift toward the use of MRI in psychiatric populations.

b. Many studies found an increased incidence of white matter lesions in psychiatric populations. However, **studies also revealed that 30% of normals over age 60 years have white matter abnormalities of no apparent clinical significance.**

c. The largest study was done at McLean Hospital over a 5-year period and included all patients who received an MRI during that time (Table 29-3).

d. Finding a structural abnormality on neuroimaging is of questionable value if it does not alter the treatment or outcome.

3. **Pre-ECT therapy neuroimaging**

a. Patients who require electroconvulsive therapy (ECT) often have a more treatment-refractory affective illness and may warrant a more thorough organic workup.

b. Pre-ECT neuroimaging may be helpful in identifying lesions that may lead to an adverse outcome with ECT (aneurysms, tumors, arteriovenous malformations, hydrocephalus, and basal ganglia infarction).

4. **General guidelines for structural neuroimaging**

a. **Criteria**

i. **Patients with acute changes in mental status** (including changes in affect, behavior, or personality) **plus one of three additional criteria:**

- **Age greater than 50 years**
- **Abnormal neurologic exam (especially focal abnormalities)**
- **History of significant head trauma** (i.e., with extended loss of consciousness, neurologic sequelae, or temporarily related to mental status change in question)

ii. New-onset psychosis

iii. New-onset delirium or dementia of unknown cause

iv. Prior to an initial course of ECT

b. Considerations

i. **Adherence to the criteria listed above should yield positive findings in 10–45% of cases. However, only 1–5% will produce findings that lead to specific medical intervention.**

ii. If structural neuroimaging is indicated, one should use MRI unless the problem is an acute trauma, or if an acute bleed is suspected.

5. **Specific pathology**

a. **Hydrocephalus**

i. **In obstructive hydrocephalus, structural neuroimaging studies will reveal enlarged third and lateral**

Table 29-2. Summary Comparisons of PET and SPECT

Consideration	PET vs. SPECT
Economy	
Institutional	SPECT $\gg$ PET
Per scan	SPECT $>$ PET
Availability	SPECT $>$ PET
Spatial resolution	PET $>$ SPECT
Temporal resolution	PET $\geq$ SPECT
Sensitivity	PET $>$ SPECT
Signal/noise ratio	PET $>$ SPECT
Variety of ligands	PET $>$ SPECT

Table 29-3. Brain MRI Results in 6200 Psychiatric Inpatients: Unexpected and Potentially Treatable Findings

MRI Findings	Number of Cases	%
Multiple sclerosis	26	0.4
Hemorrhage	26	0.4
Temporal lobe cyst	22	0.4
Tumor	15	0.2
Vascular malformations	6	0.1
Hydrocephalus	4	0.1
Total	99	1.6

NOTE: Results from 6200 consecutive MR scans performed at McLean Hospital over a 5-year period. Patients receiving MR scans represent approximately 40% of the total number of patients seen during that period.
SOURCE: Adapted from Rauch SL, Renshaw PF: *Harvard Rev Psychiatry* 1995; 2:297–312.

ventricles, small sulci, and possible lucencies at the tips of the ventricles that suggest obstruction of the aqueduct of Sylvius. Asymmetric ventricular enlargement suggests obstruction of the foramen of Monro or a portion of the ventricle.

ii. **In nonobstructive hydrocephalus, structural neuroimaging will reveal enlargement of all four ventricles,** though the fourth ventricle will be less enlarged than the other ventricles.

b. **Cerebral infarct**

i. **Recent infarcts may not be demonstrable with early CT,** though there may be an irregular, low density in the region of the infarct. DWI shows promise in the diagnosis of acute cerebral infarction.

ii. **Older infarcts are generally seen as sharp, semiregular areas of low density,** often abutting the cortical surface or the surface of a ventricle.

c. **Cerebral hemorrhage**

i. **Structural neuroimaging reveals a confluence of a dense area of blood with a surrounding rim of diminished density,** often with mass effect and blood in the subarachnoid space and ventricles.

ii. Note that the scan may be normal in individuals with subarachnoid hemorrhage and lumbar puncture may be required for diagnosis.

d. **Head trauma**

i. **Structural neuroimaging of epidural hematomas is characterized by a lenticular-shaped, biconvex area of low density.**

ii. **Structural neuroimaging of subdural hematomas is characterized by a crescent-shaped area of low density acutely and high density if chronic (aged blood).**

e. **Calcification**

i. If noted in the skull, possible etiologies include osteoma, Paget's disease, metastases, or meningioma.

ii. **Calcification is normally found in the pineal gland, choroid plexus, habenula, and falx.**

iii. **Calcification in other brain regions may indicate aneurysm, tumor** (especially meningioma, oligodendroglioma, or craniopharyngioma in the suprasellar region), **or infection** (especially fungal or parasitic).

f. **Lytic lesions (holes) in the skull**

i. **Single lytic lesions may indicate meningioma, hemangioma, or metastasis.**

ii. **Multiple lytic lesions may be indicative of Paget's disease, myeloma, or metastases.**

g. **White matter abnormalities**

i. **May be indicative of multiple sclerosis, vasculitis, cerebritis, or leukoencephalitis.**

B. Functional

Most applications of functional neuroimaging in psychiatry occur in the field of research. However, a clinical role for functional neuroimaging in dementia and seizures is evolving and showing promise.

1. **Dementia**

a. Characteristic neuroimaging profiles of various forms of dementia are emerging. **Some studies have indicated that functional neuroimaging can offer better than 90% sensitivity and specificity in distinguishing Alzheimer's disease from other kinds of dementia.**

b. However, most forms of dementia are irreversible, and specific diagnoses may not affect the treatment. Furthermore, an adequate clinical examination often is the only thing necessary to reach a diagnosis of dementia.

2. **Seizures**

a. Some seizures, especially complex partial seizures, are not always detected by the electroencephalogram (EEG). EEG measures cortical surface electrical activity but is less efficacious if the seizure focus is deep.

b. **PET and SPECT images demonstrate ictal hyperactivity and interictal hypoactivity. This allows the detection of seizure foci during the predominant interictal period.**

c. To evaluate a possible seizure disorder, functional neuroimaging is performed in conjunction with EEG. **PET also is useful for more precise localization of seizure foci in a patient with a known seizure disorder** if neurosurgical intervention is indicated.

3. **Other**

a. In addition, there is growing potential for the use of functional neuroimaging in the evaluation of movement disorders, stroke, and brain tumors.

IV. Psychiatric Neuroimaging Research

A. What Can We Measure?

1. **Structure**

a. Volumetric parameters (morphometric MRI)

2. **Function**

a. Indices of gross neuronal activity

i. **Cerebral blood flow (CBF)**

- SPECT: HMPAO
- PET: oxygen-15 (water, CO_2, or butanol)
- Functional MRI techniques can be divided into two classes:

"Noncontrast" techniques which make use of endogenous physiological factors to detect changes in cerebral activation. This technique may use T_1-weighted pulse sequences to detect changes in blood flow or T_2-weighted pulse sequences to detect changes in the local concentration of paramagnetic deoxyhemoglobin (often referred to as "blood oxygen-level dependent" imaging, or BOLD).

"Contrast" techniques which utilize intravenous administration of a paramagnetic agent.

ii. **Glucose metabolism**

- PET: FDG

b. **Neurochemistry**

i. Receptor binding capacity: PET and SPECT

ii. Transmitter metabolism: PET

iii. Quantification of chemical concentrations

- Endogenous (e.g., N-acetylaspartate)
- Exogenous (e.g., fluoxetine, lithium)

B. Neuroimaging Research Paradigms

1. **Volumetric studies**

2. **Functional anatomy: PET, SPECT, fMRI**

a. Neutral state

b. Pre/posttreatment

c. Symptom provocation or symptom capture

d. Cognitive-behavioral activation

3. **Receptor characterization: PET, SPECT**

a. Pathophysiology

b. Candidate medications

4. **Moiety concentration quantification: MRS**

a. Endogenous

b. Exogenous

C. Neuroimaging and the Neurobiology of Psychiatric Diseases

1. **Dementias**

a. **Alzheimer's disease**

i. **Accelerated atrophy,** most prominent in temporal structures.

ii. **Hypoactivity in temporoparietal areas** bilaterally.

iii. Functional abnormalities may actually precede symptoms in asymptomatic individuals at genetic risk.

b. **Multi-infarct dementia**

i. **Multiple areas involved,** often both cortical and subcortical lesions with **patchy hypoactivity**

c. **Pick's disease**

i. **Frontotemporal wasting accompanied by frontotemporal hypoactivity**

ii. Often asymmetric or unilateral

d. **Parkinson's disease**

i. **Subtle nigrostriatal degeneration**

ii. **Hypoactivity exhibited in temporoparietal regions bilaterally**

iii. Most similar to Alzheimer's disease

e. **Huntington's disease**

i. **Striatal degeneration** with hypoactivity in striatum

f. **Progressive supranuclear palsy**

i. **Hypoactivity in frontal cortex**

2. **Major depression**

a. **Decreased anterolateral prefrontal cortical activity and increased ventromedial prefrontal cortical activity** regardless of depressive subtype

b. Magnitude of hypoactivity correlated to symptom severity

c. **Hypoactivity resolves with resolution of symptoms**

d. Increased amygdala activity as a trait phenomenon

e. Anterior cingulate metabolism as predictor of treatment response

3. **Schizophrenia**

a. **Global volumetric abnormalities,** as well as decreased volume of left temporal lobe

b. **Decreased anterior to posterior activity ratio** (accentuated with frontal activation task, such as Wisconsin Card Sort)

c. **Increased basal ganglia to cortex activity ratio** (attenuated with neuroleptic treatment)

d. **Decreased frontal activity** correlated with negative symptoms

e. Hallucinations associated with activation in striatum, thalamus, limbic and paralimbic structures, as well as correspondent sensory cortex and language areas

f. Inconsistent findings regarding D_2 receptor density

4. **Anxiety disorders**

a. Inconsistent findings for panic disorder, generalized anxiety disorder, and simple phobia

b. Anxiety states nonspecifically mediated by limbic and anterior paralimbic systems

c. **Obsessive-compulsive disorder** (OCD) studies yield convergent results

    i. **Structural abnormalities involving caudate nucleus and white matter.**

    ii. Increased activity in components of a circuit implicated in the pathophysiology of OCD, including orbitofrontal cortex, caudate nucleus, thalamus, and anterior cingulate cortex.

    iii. Increased frontal and caudate activity normalize with successful treatment regardless of treatment modality (pharmacotherapy or behavioral therapy).

    iv. Elevated anterior cingulate and orbitofrontal activities may predict poor treatment response.

5. **Tourette's syndrome**

a. **Volumetric abnormalities in the striatum,** including replicated finding of rightward shift in lenticulate asymmetry.

b. Functional studies remain somewhat inconsistent, but converge to show hypoactivity within the basal ganglia.

c. Receptor studies implicate increased binding capacity of dopamine transporter sites.

6. **Attention deficit disorder** (ADD) **and attention deficit hyperactivity disorder** (ADHD)

a. **Volumetric abnormalities in the caudate,** with reduced and/or reversed laterality.

b. Functional studies have indicated a failure to normally recruit the anterior cingulate cortex during selective attention tasks.

c. Although stimulant medication has been shown to ameliorate symptoms, no specific or focal change in brain activity profile has been associated with stimulant treatment in ADD.

Suggested Readings

Albers GW: Diffusion-weighted MRI for evaluation of acute stroke. *Neurology* 1998; 51 (Suppl. 3):S47–S49.

Andreasen NC (ed.): *Brain Imaging: Applications in Psychiatry*. Washington, DC: American Psychiatric Press, 1989.

Baxter LR, Schwartz JM, Bergman KS, et al.: Caudate glucose metabolic rate changes with both drug and behavioral therapy for obsessive-compulsive disorder. *Arch Gen Psychiatry* 1992; 49:681–689.

Castellanos FX, Giedd JN, Marsh WL, et al.: Quantitative brain magnetic resonance imaging in attention-deficit hyperactivity disorder. *Arch Gen Psychiatry* 1996; 53:607–616.

Cohen BM, Renshaw PF, Stoll AL, et al.: Decreased brain choline uptake in older adults: an in vivo proton magnetic resonance spectroscopy study. *J Am Med Assoc* 1995; 274:902–907.

Dager SR, Steen RG: Applications of magnetic resonance spectroscopy to the investigation of neuropsychiatric disorders. *Neuropsychopharmacology* 1992; 6:249–266.

Dougherty D, Rauch SL: Neuroimaging and neurobiological models of depression. *Harvard Rev Psychiatry* 1997; 5:138–159.

Dougherty D, Rauch SL, Luther K: Decisions regarding use of neuroimaging techniques. In Stern TA, Herman JB, Slavin PL (eds): *The MGH Guide to Psychiatry in Primary Care*. New York: McGraw-Hill, 1998.

Hollister LE, Shah NN: Structural brain scanning in psychiatric patients: a further look. *J Clin Psychiatry* 1996; 57:241–244.

Holman BL, Johnson KA, Gerada B, et al.: The scintigraphic appearance of Alzheimer's disease: a prospective study using technetium-99m-HMPAO SPECT. *J Nucl Med* 1992; 33:181–185.

Horowitz AL: *MRI Physics for Radiologists: A Visual Approach*. New York: Springer-Verlag; 1992.

Kaufman DM: *Clinical Neurology for Psychiatrists*, 3rd ed. Philadelphia: WB Saunders, 1990.

Malison RT, McDougle CJ, Van Dyck CH, et al.: [^{123}I]B-CIT SPECT imaging of striatal dopamine transporter binding in Tourette's disorder. *Am J Psychiatry* 1995; 152:1359–1361.

Osborn AG: *Diagnostic Neuroradiology*. St. Louis: Mosby Year Book, 1994.

Rauch SL, Renshaw PF: Clinical neuroimaging in psychiatry. *Harvard Rev Psychiatry* 1995; 12:297–312.

Rauch SL, Jenike MA, Alpert NM, et al.: Regional cerebral blood flow measured during symptom provocation in OCD using oxygen 15-labeled carbon dioxide and PET. *Arch Gen Psychiatry* 1994; 51:62–70.

Reiman EM, Caselli RJ, Yun LS, et al.: Preclinical evidence of a genetic risk factor for Alzheimer's disease in apolipoprotein E type 4 homozygotes using PET. *N Engl J Med* 1996; 324:752–758.

Renshaw PF, Rauch SL: Neuroimaging in clinical psychiatry. In Nicholi AM Jr (ed.): *The Harvard Guide to Psychiatry*, 3rd ed. Cambridge, MA: Belknap Press, 1999.

Roland PE: *Brain Activation*. New York: Wiley-Liss, 1993.

Shenton ME, Kikinis R, Jolesz FA, et al.: Abnormalities of the left temporal lobe and thought disorder in schizophrenia: a quantitative magnetic resonance imaging study. *N Engl J Med* 1992; 327:604–612.

Silbersweig DA, Stern E, Frith C, et al.: A functional neuroanatomy of hallucinations in schizophrenia. *Nature* 1995; 378:176–179.

Toga AW, Mazziotta JC (eds): *Brain Mapping: The Methods*. Boston, MA: Academic Press, 1996.

Weinberger DR: Brain disease and psychiatric illness: when should a psychiatrist order a CAT scan? *Am J Psychiatry* 1984; 141:1521–1527.

Chapter 30

Diagnostic Rating Scales and Psychiatric Instruments

D A V I D   M I S C H O U L O N   A N D   M A U R I Z I O   F A V A

I. Introduction

A. Overview

When screening for psychiatric disorders, psychiatrists typically rely on information obtained from the clinical interview, from review of medical records, and from other sources. **However, administration of various standardized diagnostic instruments can be helpful,** and at times necessary. For example, the overwhelming majority of clinical research studies rely heavily on the use of diagnostic instruments. In the clinical setting, a standardized questionnaire often serves as an adjunct to the clinical interview, particularly in cases where the diagnosis is in doubt, or when the efficacy of a treatment is unclear. Psychiatric rating scales attempt to translate clinical observations into objective and (sometimes) quantifiable information. This chapter will review some commonly used instruments, and provide guidelines for the implementation of these instruments.

B. Uses for Diagnostic Psychiatric Instruments
1. To help ensure the accuracy of a diagnosis.
2. To quantify the severity of symptoms.
3. To quantify the effectiveness, or lack thereof, of a given treatment modality.

C. Reliability and Validity
1. **Reliability refers to a scale's ability to convey consistent, reproducible information.** Diagnostic instruments are usually tested for their reliability by having more than one rater administer them, and then comparing the results (i.e., inter-rater reliability). If the instrument is designed to measure phenomena that are consistent over time, test-retest reliability is the measure used.
2. **Validity refers to the scale's ability to measure what it intends to measure.** For a diagnostic instrument to be valid, it must be reliable, although a reliable instrument may not necessarily be valid.

D. Types of Diagnostic Instruments: Self-Rated vs. Clinician-Rated
1. **Clinician-rated instruments.** These are diagnostic instruments which are administered by the clinician. These instruments are advantageous in that they are generally valid and reliable. Most diagnostic instruments are of this kind.

2. **Self-rated instruments.** These are instruments that the patient must complete. Self-rating scales have the advantage that they require less clinician time, which makes them especially useful for screening purposes. However, the reliability of self-rated scales is often difficult to assess, and some patients may be too impaired to complete them. The concordance rate between self-rating and observer scales is not well established.

E. Diagnostic Interviews
Structured clinical interviews were developed because of a perceived unreliability of psychiatric diagnoses. This problem was especially serious with regard to international studies, as psychiatrists from different countries or cultural backgrounds often had a different conceptualization of mental disorders. Several scales were developed, including:
1. The Present State Examination (PSE)
2. The Structured Clinical Interview for Axis I Diagnostic and Statistical Manual of Mental Disorders, Fourth Edition (SCID)
3. The Schedule for Affective Disorders and Schizophrenia (SADS)
4. The Diagnostic Interview Schedule (DIS)
5. The Composite International Diagnostic Interview (CIDI)
6. The Schedules for Clinical Assessment in Neuropsychiatry (SCAN)

The SCID will be reviewed here, as it is the most commonly used diagnostic instrument in psychiatry.

II. The Structured Clinical Interview for DSM-IV (SCID)

A. Overview of the SCID (Note: the DSM-III-R version of SCID is still in use in research settings)
The SCID is essentially a semistructured interview that applies DSM-IV criteria to a patient. It is organized into modules that cover most of the major Axis I disorders (Mood Disorders, Psychotic Disorders, Anxiety Disorders, Substance Use Disorders, Somatoform Disorders, Posttraumatic Stress Disorder, Adjustment Disorders, and Eating Disorders).

B. Administration of the SCID
The SCID is administered by a clinician, sometimes as an exclusive diagnostic tool, often after the

patient has already screened positive for a given disorder (e.g., depression) through a shorter, self-administered questionnaire (such as the Beck Depression Inventory). The SCID begins with a general introductory section on demographics, general medical and psychiatric history, and use of medications. Questions here tend to be more open-ended. It then proceeds by modules to the different Axis I disorders. Questions here are asked exactly as written, and each is based on the individual criteria from DSM-IV. Answers are generally rated on a scale of 1–3 ($1 =$ doubtful, $2 =$ probable, $3 =$ definite), and, based on the number of positive answers, a diagnosis is determined. A SCID-based interview may take up to 2 h to complete, depending on how complicated a patient's history is, and on the patient's ability to provide a good history.

C. **Value of the SCID**

Because the SCID is a time-consuming instrument, **it is used almost exclusively in the research setting.** It is probably the most reliable means of diagnosing psychiatric disorders. In some instances, clinicians may use only a portion of the SCID, such as the mood disorder module.

III. Depression Scales

A. **Hamilton Rating Scale for Depression (HAM-D)**
  1. **Overview of the HAM-D. The HAM-D aims to quantify the degree of depression in patients who already have a diagnosis of major depression.** Questions focus on symptoms experienced only over the past week. It is administered by the clinician, and it generally does not require more than 20 min to complete. The HAM-D is a useful tool for measuring the progress of a patient during the course of treatment, in either the research or the clinical setting.
  2. **Description of the HAM-D.** Several different versions of the HAM-D exist; they differ only in the number of questions included. The longest version includes 31 items; the shortest includes only six items. The longer versions include questions about atypical depression symptoms, psychotic symptoms, psychosomatic symptoms, and symptoms associated with obsessive-compulsive disorder (OCD). The standard form which is generally used in research studies is the 17-item Hamilton D (HAM-D-17).
  3. **Scoring of the HAM-D.** There is a structured version of this instrument in which questions are asked exactly as written, and are rated on a scale of 0–4 or 0–2, depending on the answers given by the patient. Other versions allow more open-ended

questioning. Scores on the HAM-D-17 typically fall into the following ranges:
  a. Not depressed: 0–7
  b. Mildly depressed: 7–15
  c. Moderately depressed: 15–25
  d. Severely depressed: over 25
  4. **The HAM-D as a research tool.** Research studies rely on the Hamilton-D to quantify responses to a given treatment over time. Research studies will often cite a change in Hamilton-D score as a criterion for response. For example, a decrease of 50% or more in the Hamilton-D score is considered to be a positive response to treatment, while a score of 7 or less is considered typical of remission. The HAM-D is the most widely studied instrument for depression, and its reliability and validity are high.

B. **Clinical Global Improvement (CGI) Scale**
  1. **Overview.** The CGI scale is a two-item instrument used as an adjunct in the treatment of psychiatric disorders. It is administered by the clinician after a history has been obtained, and after the HAM-D or other instruments have been completed and reviewed by the clinician. It measures, based on history and scores on other instruments:
  a. CGI-S (severity): the current condition of the patient on a scale of 1–7 (1 being normal, and 7 being among the most severely ill patients).
  b. CGI-I (improvement): the degree of improvement (as perceived by the clinician) since the start of treatment on a scale of 1–7, 1 being very much improved, and 7 being very much worse. Improvement in CGI ratings is also used in research to determine the degree of improvement over time with a given treatment.

C. **Beck Depression Inventory (BDI)**
  1. **Overview of the BDI.** This 21-item questionnaire for assessment of degree of depression is probably the most widely used self-rating scale; it is self-administered by the patient, and can be completed in a few minutes. It is often used as a screening tool for determining the likelihood of a patient meeting criteria for major depression. A clinician may also use it to determine the degree of improvement over time. Questions are different from those found on the Hamilton-D, in that they focus more on cognitive symptoms of depression.
  2. **Scoring of the BDI.** Patients generally must choose between four answers on each item (numbered 0–3 for degree of severity of depression). Scores correlate with severity of depression as follows:
  a. Normal: 0–7
  b. Mild depression: 7–15
  c. Moderate depression: 15–25
  d. Severe depression: over 25

The BDI has been shown to correlate well with the Hamilton-D and CGI, and, because of its sensitivity to change over time, it is often used in drug trials.

D. Zung Self-Rating Depression Scale (SDS)
   1. **Overview of the Zung SDS. This is a 20-item self-administered rating scale.** Items are rated based on frequency rather than intensity.
   2. **Scoring of the SDS.** The raw score is converted into an index score as follows:

$$\text{Index} = \frac{\text{Raw score total}}{\text{Maximum score of 80}} \times 100$$

The SDS index correlates with severity of depression as follows:
a. Normal: below 50
b. Minimal to mild depression: 50–59
c. Moderate to marked depression: 60–69
d. Severe to extreme depression: over 70
The SDS is not thought to be sensitive to change over time, so it is not widely used in clinical trials. However, it is popular for screening purposes, and it has been used on National Depression Screening Day.

IV. Schizophrenia Scales

A. Overview
The complexity of schizophrenia requires that clinicians use several different instruments to assess and study this illness. Scales have been designed to assess positive and negative symptoms, social and vocational adjustment, and medication side effects. Virtually all schizophrenia scales must be administered by a clinician, as many patients would not be able to complete a self-rated form.

B. Description of Scales
   1. **Brief Psychiatric Rating Scale (BPRS).** The BPRS includes 16–24 items, each rated on a scale of 1–7. Items primarily cover symptoms of psychosis, but also address depression, and anxiety symptoms. Ratings are expressed as a sum total of all items. The scale is brief and may be administered in 15–30 min. One limitation of the BPRS is that some definitions of items tend to be vague, and are subject to interpretation. However, the scale has shown high inter-rater reliability.
   2. **Positive and Negative Symptoms Scale (PANSS).** As its name implies, the PANSS, similar to the BPRS, focuses more on the positive and negative symptoms. This scale is frequently used in trials of antipsychotic drugs, largely because of its inclusion of negative symptoms. However, it requires more time to complete than does the BPRS. It has excel-

lent inter-rater reliability and has been validated against other instruments.
   3. **Scale for the Assessment of Positive Symptoms (SAPS).** The strength of the SAPS is its focus on formal thought disorder, which is less emphasized on the previously mentioned scales.
   4. **Scale for the Assessment of Negative Symptoms (SANS).** The SANS was the first scale developed to assess negative symptoms, and it provides the standard against which other scales are compared. It focuses on five groups of symptoms, including alogia, affective flattening, avolition-apathy, anhedonia-asociality, and inattention. Ratings are based on clinical observations of the rater as well as of other staff and family members.

V. Anxiety Scales

A. Anxiety Disorder Interview Scale, Revised (ADIS-R)
The ADIS-R is a semistructured interview used for arriving at DSM-III-R diagnoses of anxiety disorders. It provides information on panic, generalized anxiety, and phobic avoidance, and also measures degree of disability. The scale includes the Hamilton-A and Hamilton-D scales for anxiety and depression, respectively. Its inter-rater reliability is high for most of the anxiety disorders, except generalized anxiety disorder (GAD).

B. Hamilton Rating Scale for Anxiety (HAM-A)
This is the most widely used scale for measurement of anxiety. It is used for patients with diagnosed anxiety disorders. It is similar to the HAM-D, in that it emphasizes somatic symptoms and experiences. It has reasonable validity and reliability.

C. Fear Questionnaire
This is a self-rated instrument used for assessing phobias, including agoraphobia, blood injury phobia, social phobia, and total phobia.

D. Yale-Brown Obsessive-Compulsive Scale (Y-BOCS)
The Y-BOCS is the most widely used scale for assessment of severity of obsessive-compulsive disorder (OCD) symptoms. It includes ten items, and a symptom checklist. Inter-rater reliability is excellent. This scale has been used extensively in medication trials for measuring changes in severity of OCD symptoms.

VI. Mania Scales

A. Manic State Rating Scale (MSRS)
The MSRS is a 26-item scale; it is rated on a 0–5 scale, and is based on the frequency and intensity of symptoms, particularly elation-grandiosity, and paranoid-destructiveness. The MSRS is designed

primarily for use on inpatient units, and has been found to be reliable and valid.

B. Young Mania Rating Scale (Y-MRS)
This scale has 11 items, and is scored following a clinical interview. Four items (irritability, speech, thought content, and aggressive behavior) are given extra weight and scored on a 0–8 scale, while the other items are scored 0–4. The scale has a high inter-rater reliability; scores on the Y-MRS correlate well with length of hospital stay.

VII. Cognitive Impairment Scales

A. Overview
Cognitive scales are useful as an initial screen for organic psychopathology; results of these scales can help the clinician decide whether or not to request formal neuropsychological testing or imaging studies. These scales, however, may be influenced by the patient's intelligence, level of education, and literacy; consequently, clinicians need to be careful not to make erroneous conclusions based on scores of these scales.

B. Description of Scales
1. **Mini-Mental State Examination (MMSE). The MMSE is the most widely used instrument for measuring cognitive impairment.** It is a highly structured instrument, which may be administered by non-clinicians. It includes questions about orientation, memory, attention, naming, as well as ability to follow commands, write a sentence, and copy intersecting polygons. The MMSE may be administered in less than 10 min; it has established reliability and validity.
2. **Blessed Dementia Scale (BDS).** This instrument includes 50 items which assess orientation, recent and remote memory, and the ability to carry out activities of daily living. It is used primarily to diagnose Alzheimer's dementia.

VIII. Personality Disorder Scales

A. Overview
The accurate diagnosis of personality disorders is difficult under most circumstances. Most diagnostic scales have demonstrated poor reliability, largely due to the subjective quality of the criteria, patient unreliability, and the tendency for many patients to meet criteria for more than one disorder at a time. Diagnostic reliability of these scales needs to be improved.

B. Description of Scales
1. **Structured Clinical Interview for DSM-III-R Personality Disorders (SCID-II).** The SCID-II instrument is used for the diagnosis of personality disorders. As with the SCID-I, the SCID-II is organized around different personality disorders; questions are based on the criteria for each personality disorder, and are answered "yes" or "no." This instrument is time-consuming to administer; it is used almost exclusively for research purposes.
2. **Personality Disorder Examination (PDE).** The PDE is a lengthy and semistructured interview consisting of 359 items; it is rated on a 3-point scale (absent, doubtful, or clinically significant). It requires 1–2 h to complete, and provides fairly rich information which places less burden on the assessor's judgment.

IX. Substance Abuse Scales

A. CAGE Questionnaire
This brief instrument is widely used as a screening tool. The name of the scale is an acronym for:
1. Have you ever felt a need to <u>c</u>ut down on drinking?
2. Have people <u>a</u>nnoyed you by criticizing your drinking?
3. Have you ever felt <u>g</u>uilty about drinking?
4. Have you ever had an <u>e</u>ye-opener?

Answering "yes" to two or more of these questions strongly suggests an alcohol-related problem, particularly in a male population.

B. Michigan Alcoholism Screening Test (MAST)
The MAST consists of 25 true-false questions that may be self-rated or administered by the clinician. Briefer versions have been developed, with comparable validity to the original. The Drug Abuse Screening Test (DAST) is similar to the MAST, and may discriminate between alcohol and drug abusers.

C. Addiction Severity Index (ASI)
The ASI assesses severity of problems with drug and alcohol abuse, with medical illness, with the legal system, with the family system, as well as with one's system of support (social and employment). It appears to be a valid instrument that is useful in research as well as in treatment planning. It may be administered in less than an hour.

X. Social Functioning Scales

A. Overview
These scales are often used to assess the outcome of an illness or its overall effect on the patient.

B. Description of Scales
1. **Global Assessment of Functioning Scale (GAF).** The GAF is used on Axis V of the DSM-IV; it is based on collected information on psychological, social, and occupational function. It rates the patient on a scale of 1–100, with a higher score indicating

higher function. Usually there are two ratings made: one for current function, and one for highest function in the past year.

2. **Social Adjustment Scale (SAS).** The SAS assesses social functioning during the past month. Subjects answer questions about work role, household role, parental role, extended family role, sexual roles, social and leisure activities, and overall well-being. This scale covers the widest domain of social function, but may be less useful for severely dysfunctional patients, who may be unable to work and/or who have very limited social contacts.

XI. Drug Side Effect Scales

A. Abnormal Involuntary Movement Scale (AIMS)

The AIMS is widely used to measure late-onset movement disorders, such as tardive dyskinesia. Movements of the head, trunk, and extremities are observed, and rated on a scale of 1–5. It is routinely used in patients receiving antipsychotic medication; typically it is administered every 3–6 months.

B. Systematic Assessment for Treatment Emergent Effects (SAFTEE)

The SAFTEE is used for assessment of side effects in clinical drug trials. It includes a general inquiry form with open-ended questions, and a systematic inquiry form, which asks more specific questions about different systems.

XII. Conclusion

Diagnostic and psychiatric instruments can be useful diagnostic tools, both in psychiatric research as well as in the clinical setting. These tools may be used independently or in conjunction with a thorough clinical interview. They may serve to measure results in a research study, and to help the clinician ascertain the degree of illness and the response to treatment over time.

Suggested Readings

Andreasen NC: Negative symptoms in schizophrenia: definition and reliability. *Arch Gen Psychiatry* 1982; 39:784–788.

Beck AT, Ward CH, Mendelson M, et al.: An inventory for measuring depression. *Arch Gen Psychiatry* 1961; 4:561.

Beigel A, Murphy D, Bunney W: The manic state rating scale: scale construction, reliability, and validity. *Arch Gen Psychiatry* 1971; 25:256.

Blessed G, Tomlinson BE, Roth M: The association between quantitative measures of dementia and of senile change in the cerebral grey matter of elderly subjects. *Br J Psychiatry* 1968; 114:797–811.

Blessed G, Black SE, Butler T, Kay DW: The diagnosis of dementia in the elderly. A comparison of CAMCOG (the cognitive section of CAMDEX), the AGECAT program, DSM-III, the

Mini-Mental State Examination and some short rating scales. *Br J Psychiatry* 1991; 159:193–198.

Di Nardo P, Moras K, Barlow DH, Rapee RM, Brown TA: Reliability of DSM-III-R anxiety disorder categories. Using the Anxiety Disorders Interview Schedule-Revised (ADIS-R). *Arch Gen Psychiatry* 1993; 50:251–256.

Endicott J, Spitzer RL, Fleiss JL, Cohen J: The global assessment scale. A procedure for measuring overall severity of psychiatric disturbance. *Arch Gen Psychiatry* 1976; 33:766–771.

Fenton WS, McGlashan TH: Testing systems for assessment of negative symptoms in schizophrenia. *Arch Gen Psychiatry* 1992; 49:179–184.

Folstein MF, Folstein SE, McHugh PR: "Mini-mental state." A practical method for grading the cognitive state of patients for the clinician. *J Psychiatr Res* 1975; 12:189–198.

Frank E, Prien RF, Jarrett RB, Keller MB, Kupfer DJ, Lavori PW, et al.: Conceptualization and rationale for consensus definitions of terms in major depressive disorder. Remission, recovery, relapse, and recurrence. *Arch Gen Psychiatry* 1991; 48:851–855.

Goodman WK, Price LH, Rasmussen SA, Mazure C, Fleischmann RL, Hill CL, et al.: The Yale-Brown Obsessive Compulsive Scale. I. Development, use, and reliability. *Arch Gen Psychiatry* 1989; 46:1006–1011.

Goodman WK, Price LH, Rasmussen SA, Mazure C, Delgado P, Heninger GR, et al.: The Yale-Brown Obsessive Compulsive Scale. II. Validity. *Arch Gen Psychiatry* 1989; 46:1012–1016.

Gur RE, Mozley PD, Resnick SM, Levick S, Erwin R, Saykin AJ, et al.: Relations among clinical scales in schizophrenia. *Am J Psychiatry* 1991; 148:472–478.

Hamilton M: The assessment of anxiety states by rating. *Br J Med Psychol* 1959; 32:50.

Hamilton M: A rating scale for depression. *J Neurol Neurosurg Psychiatry* 1960; 23:56–62.

Kay SR, Fiszbein A, Opler LA: The Positive and Negative Syndrome Scale (PANSS) for schizophrenia. *Schizophr Bull* 1987; 13:261–276.

Lewis SJ, Harder DW: A comparison of four measures to diagnose DSM-III-R borderline personality disorder in outpatients. *J Nerv Ment Dis* 1991; 179:329–337.

Loranger AW, Sartorius N, Andreoli A, Berger P, Buchheim P, Channabasavanna SM, et al.: The International Personality Disorder Examination. The World Health Organization/ Alcohol, Drug Abuse, and Mental Health Administration international pilot study of personality disorders. *Arch Gen Psychiatry* 1994; 51:215–224.

Marder SR: Psychiatric rating scales. In Kaplan HI, Saddock BJ (eds): *Comprehensive Textbook of Psychiatry*, 6th ed. Baltimore, MD: Williams and Wilkins, 1995:619–635.

Marks IM, Matthews AM: Brief standard self-rating for phobic patients. *Behav Res Ther* 1979; 17:263–267.

Oldham JM, Skodol AE, Kellman HD, Hyler SE, Rosnick L, Davies M: Diagnosis of DSM-III-R personality disorders by two structured interviews: patterns of comorbidity. *Am J Psychiatry* 1992; 149(2):213–220.

Overall JE, Gorham DR: The Brief Psychiatric Rating Scale. *Psychol Rep* 1962; 10:799.

Shear MK, Maser JD: Standardized assessment for panic disorder research. A conference report. *Arch Gen Psychiatry* 1994; 51:346–354.

Spitzer RL, Williams JB, Gibbon M, First MB: The Structured Clinical Interview for DSM-III-R (SCID). I: History, rationale, and description. *Arch Gen Psychiatry* 1992; 49:624–629.

Williams JB: A structured interview guide for the Hamilton Depression Rating Scale. *Arch Gen Psychiatry* 1988; 45:742–747.

Williams JB: Structured interview guides for the Hamilton Rating Scales. *Psychopharmacol Ser* 1990; 9:48–63.

Williams JB, Gibbon M, First MB, Spitzer RL, Davies M, Borus J, et al.: The Structured Clinical Interview for DSM-III-R (SCID). II. Multisite test-retest reliability. *Arch Gen Psychiatry* 1992; 49:630–636.

Young RC, Biggs JT, Ziegler VE, Meyer DA: A rating scale for mania: reliability, validity and sensitivity. *Br J Psychiatry* 1978; 133:429–435.

Zimmerman M: Diagnosing personality disorders. A review of issues and research methods. *Arch Gen Psychiatry* 1994; 51(3):225–245.

Zung WWK: A self-rating depression scale. *Arch Gen Psychiatry* 1965; 12:63.

Chapter 31

Psychological Assessment

MARK A. BLAIS AND SHEILA M. O'KEEFE

I. Introduction

The intent of this chapter is to facilitate a greater understanding of psychological assessment and testing. This will be accomplished by reviewing: the methods used to construct valid psychological instruments; the major categories of psychological tests (including detailed examples of each category); and the application of these instruments in clinical assessment. In addition, issues related to the ordering of psychological testing and tips for understanding the final assessment report will be provided.

II. A Brief History of Modern Psychological Assessment

A. **In the late 1800s the first generation of psychologists, such as Sir Francis Galton** (1822–1911), **focused their efforts on the measurement of sensorimotor functions** (e.g., reaction times), and tried to associate these measurements with life achievement (e.g., educational level, occupation, and social status).

B. **James McKeen Cattell,** an American psychologist, coined the term "Mental Test" in 1890.

C. At about the time that sensorimotor measurement was fading out, **Alfred Binet** (1857–1911) and **Theodore Simon** were commissioned by the French School Board to develop a test to identify students who might benefit from special education programs. **Binet's 1905 and 1908 scales form the basis of our current intelligence tests.** In fact, the development of Binet's 05 scale marked the modern era of psychological testing.

D. The development of instruments to measure personality and psychopathology started around the time of the First World War. To aid in the war effort, **Woodworth developed a self-report test of psychopathology designed to screen army recruits** (called the Personal Data Sheet). Although this effort was unsuccessful, it provided the methodology for the later development of the Minnesota Multiphasic Personality Inventory (MMPI), a self-report test still in use today.

E. **Jung's Word Association Test** (1918) represents the prototype of the projective tests of psychopathology.

F. This was followed by both **Rorschach's Inkblot Test,** which was published in 1921, **and Murray's Thematic Apperception Test (TAT),** published in 1938. The second half of this century has seen intensive efforts focused on the further development of these initial breakthroughs.

III. Psychometrics and the Science of Test Development

A. **Test Development Strategies**
   Three basic test development strategies have guided test construction: rational, empirical, and construct validation methods.
   1. **Rational test construction relies on a theory of personality or psychopathology** (like the cognitive theory of depression) to guide item selection and scale construction. **Scales are developed that reflect a particular theory.**
   2. **Empirically guided test construction uses a large number of items** (called an item pool) **and statistical tests to determine which items differentiate between well-defined groups of subjects** (this is called the empirical keying of items). The items which successfully differentiate one group from another are grouped together to form a scale regardless of their thematic content.
   3. **The construct validation method combines aspects of both the rational and empirical test construction methodologies.** Within this framework, a large pool of items are written to reflect a theoretical construct (e.g., impulsivity), and then these items are tested to determine if they actually differentiate subjects who are either high or low on the construct (impulsive vs. nonimpulsive subjects). Items which successfully differentiate between the groups are retained for the scale. In addition, if theoretically important items do not differentiate between the two groups, this finding may lead to a revision in the theory. **The construct validation methodology is considered the most sophisticated strategy for test development.**

B. **Reliability and Validity**
   To be useful, a psychological test must possess both adequate reliability and validity.
   1. **Reliability represents the repeatability, stability, or consistency of a subject's test score. Reliability is**

usually represented as some form of a correlation coefficient ranging from 0 to 1.0. Research instruments can have reliabilities as low as 0.70, while clinical instruments should have reliabilities in the high 0.80s to low 0.90s. This variation is because research instruments are interpreted as group measures, whereas clinical instruments are interpreted for a single individual. A number of **reliability statistics** are available for evaluating a test:

a. **Internal consistency:** the degree to which the items in a test perform in the same manner.

b. **Test-retest reliability:** the consistency of a test score over time either a few days or a few weeks to a year later.

c. **Inter-rater reliability** for observer-judged rating scales; this is measured by Kappa, and reflects the degree of agreement between raters usually corrected for chance agreement.

Unreliability (the amount of error present in a test score) can be introduced by variability in the subject (subject changes over time), the examiner, or the test itself (given under different instruction).

2. **Validity** is a more difficult concept to understand and to demonstrate, than is reliability. **The validity of a test reflects the degree to which the test actually measures the construct it was designed to measure.** Again, validity measures are usually represented as correlation coefficients ranging from 0 to 1.0. Multiple types of validity data are needed before a test can be considered valid. **Types of validity data include:**

a. **Content validity,** which assesses the degree that an instrument covers the full range of the target construct (e.g., a test of depression which did not include items covering disruptions in sleep and appetite would have limited content validity).

b. **Predictive and concurrent validity,** which demonstrates how well a test either predicts future demonstration of the construct (predictive) or how well it correlates with other current measures of the construct (concurrent validity).

c. **Convergent and divergent validity,** which refers to the ability of a scale to demonstrate significant positive correlations with similar scales, while also having low or negative correlations with scales measuring unrelated traits. Taken together the convergent and divergent correlations indicate the specificity with which the scale measures the intended construct.

It is important to realize that no psychological test is universally valid. Tests are considered valid or not valid for a particular purpose.

C. Definition of a Psychological Test

Ideally, a psychological test is a measurement tool made up of a series of standard stimuli (i.e., questions or visual stimuli). These test stimuli are administered following a standard format under a standard set of instructions. The patient's responses are recorded and scored according to a standardized methodology (insuring that a given response always scored the same way). The patient's test results are interpreted against a normative sample allowing for an accurate evaluation of the patient's performance.

IV. Major Categories of Psychological Tests

A. Intelligence Tests

1. **IQ testing.** Intelligence is a difficult construct to define and to measure. Wechsler wrote that "intelligence, as a hypothetical construct, is the aggregate or global capacity of the individual to act purposefully, to think rationally, and to deal effectively with the environment" (Matarazzo, 1979). This definition helps us see both what the modern tests of intelligence quotients (IQ) try to measure (adaptive functioning) and why intelligence or IQ tests can be important as aids in clinical assessment, particularly in treatment planning. If IQ reflects aspects of effective functioning, then IQ tests measure aspects of adaptive capacity. The **Wechsler series** of IQ tests cover the majority of the human age range. The series starts with the **Wechsler Preschool and Primary Scale of Intelligence** (ages 4–6 years), progresses to the **Wechsler Intelligence Scale for Children-III** (5–16 years), and ends with the **Wechsler Adult Intelligence Scale-III** (16–89 years) (Wechsler, 1991, 1997). All the Wechsler scales provide **three major IQ tests scores: the Full Scale IQ, the Verbal IQ, and the Performance IQ.** All three IQ scores have a mean of 100 and a standard deviation (SD) of 15. This statistical feature means that a 15-point difference between a subject's Verbal IQ and Performance IQ can be considered both statistically significant and clinically meaningful. Table 31-1 presents an overview of IQ categories.

2. **Scoring of the IQ.** It is important to realize that IQ scores represent a patient's ordinal position, their percentile ranking as it were, on the test relative to the normative sample. These scores do not represent a patient's innate intelligence and there is no good evidence that they measure a genetically determined intelligence. They do reflect some degree of the patient's current adaptive functioning. Furthermore, because IQ scores are not totally reliable (all test scores contain some degree of unreliability) they should be reported with confidence intervals indicating the range of scores in which the subject's true IQ would fall.

The Wechsler IQ tests are composed of 10 or 11 subtests which were developed to tap two intellectual domains, **verbal intelligence** (Vocabulary, Similarities, Arithmetic, Digit Span, Information, and Comprehension) and **nonverbal visual spatial intelligence** (Picture Completion, Digit Symbol, Block Design, Matrix Reasoning, and Picture Arrangement). Empirical studies have suggested that the Wechsler subscales can be reorganized to reflect three cognitive domains: verbal ability, visual-spatial ability, and attention and concentration (attention and concentration is tapped by the Arithmetic, Digit Span and by Digit Symbol subtests). Each of the Wechsler subtests is constructed to have a mean score of 10 and standard deviation of 3. Given this statistical feature we know that if two subtests differ by 3 or more scaled score points then the difference is significant. All IQ scores and subtest scaled scores are also adjusted for age.

B. **Tests of Personality, Psychopathology, and Psychological Functioning**
   1. **Objective tests of personality and psychopathology.** Objective psychological tests, **also called self-report tests, are designed to clarify and quantify a patient's personality functioning and psychopathology.** Objective tests use a patient's response to a series of true/false or multiple choice questions to broadly assess psychological functioning. **These tests are called "objective" because their scoring involves little speculation.** Objective tests provide excellent insight into how the patient sees him- or herself and how he wants others to see and react to him.
      a. **The Minnesota Multiphasic Personality Inventory-2 (MMPI-2).** The MMPI-2 (Butcher et al., 1989) is a 567-item true/false, self-report test of psychological functioning. It was designed to provide an objective measure of abnormal behavior, to separate subjects into two groups (normals and abnormals), and then to further subcategorize the abnormal group into specific classes (Greene, 1991). The MMPI-2 contains **ten Clinical Scales** that assess major categories of psycho-

pathology, and **three Validity Scales** designed to assess test-taking attitudes. MMPI-2 validity scales are: **(L) Lie, (F) Infrequency, and (K) correction.** The MMPI-2 Clinical Scales include: **(1) Hs, Hypochondriasis; (2) D, Depression; (3) Hy, Conversion Hysteria; (4) Pd, Psychopathic Deviate; (5) Mf, Masculinity/ Femininity; (6) Pa, Paranoia; (7) Pt, Psychasthenia; (8) Sc, Schizophrenia; (9) Ma, Hypomania; and (0) Si, Social Introversion.** Over 300 "new" or experiential scales have also been developed for the MMPI-2. MMPI raw scores are transformed into T-score and a T-score of 65 or more indicates clinical psychopathology. The MMPI-2 is interpreted by determining the highest two or three scales, called a code type. For example, a 2-4-7 code type indicates the presence of depression (scale 2), anxiety (scale 7) and impulsivity (scale 4) and the likelihood of a personality disorder (Greene, 1991). [Computer scoring and interpretive reports for the MMPI-2 are available through: NCS Assessments, P.O. Box 1416, Minneapolis, MN 55440, (1-800-627-7271).]
      b. **The Millon Clinical Multiaxial Inventory-III (MCMI-III).** The MCMI-III **is a 175-item true/false, self-report questionnaire designed to identify both symptom disorders (Axis I conditions) and personality disorders** (PDs) (Millon, 1994). The MCMI-III is composed of three Modifier Indices (validity scales), ten Basic Personality Scales, three Severe Personality Scales, six Clinical Syndrome Scales, and three Severe Clinical Syndrome Scales. **One of the unique features of the MCMI-III is that it attempts to assess both Axis I and Axis II psychopathology simultaneously.** The Axis II scales resemble, but are not identical to, the DSM-IV Axis II disorders. Computer scoring and interpretive reports are also available from NCS (see above). Given its relatively short length (175 items vs. 567 for the MMPI-2) the MCMI-III can have advantages in the assessment of patients who are agitated, whose stamina is significantly impaired, or who are just suboptimally motivated.
      c. **The Personality Assessment Inventory** (PAI) (Morey, 1991). The PAI is one of the newest objective psycho-

Table 31-1. IQ Categories with their Corresponding IQ Scores and Percentile Distribution

Full-Scale IQ Score Percentile	IQ Categories	Normal Distribution
130 $\geq$	Very superior	2.2
120–129	Superior	6.7
110–119	High average	16.1
90–109	Average	50.0
80–89	Low average	16.1
70–79	Borderline	6.7
69 $\leq$	Mentally retarded	2.2

logical tests available. The PAI was developed using a construct validation framework with equal emphasis placed upon theory-guided item selection and the empirical functioning of the scales. The PAI uses 344 items and a 4-point response format (False, Slightly True, Mainly True, and Very True) to make 22 non-overlapping scales. These 22 scales (four validity scales, 11 clinical scales, five treatment scales, and two interpersonal scales) cover a range of clinically important Axis I and Axis II psychopathology and other variables relevant to interpersonal functioning and treatment planning (e.g., the PAI has scales designed to measure suicidal ideation, resistance to treatment, and aggression). The PAI possesses outstanding psychometric features and is an ideal test for broadly assessing multiple domains of relevant psychological functioning. [The PAI is marketed by Psychological Assessment Resources (PAR) P.O. Box 998, Odessa, FL 33556 (1-880-331-TEST).]

   d. **Validity scales.** Certain response styles or sets can have a negative impact on the accuracy of a patient's self-report. **Validity scales are incorporated into all major objective tests to assess the degree to which a patient's response style may have distorted the findings of the self-report test. The three most typical response styles are: careless or random responding (which may indicate that someone is not reading or understanding the test), attempting to "look good" by denying pathology, and attempting to "look bad" by overreporting pathology (a cry for help or malingering).**

   e. **Objective tests and the DSM-IV.** The computer-generated reports available from objective tests frequently provide suggested DSM diagnoses. At best these diagnoses are informed suggestions and at worse marketing gimmicks. **Psychological tests do not make clinical diagnoses, clinicians do.**

2. **Projective psychological tests.** Projective tests of psychological functioning differ from objective tests in that they **are less structured and require more effort on the part of the patient to make sense of and to respond to the test stimuli.** Even the instructions for the projective tests tend to be less specific than those of objective tests. As a result, **the patient is provided with a great degree of freedom to demonstrate his or her own unique personality characteristics and psychological organizing processes.** While the objective test provides a view of the patient's "conscious" self presentation, **the projective tests provide insights into the patient's typical style of perceiving, organizing and responding to ambiguous external and internal stimuli.** When combined together, data from objective and projective tests can provide a fairly complete picture or description of a patient's range of functioning.

   a. **The Rorschach Inkblot Test.** The inkblot test, developed by Hermann Rorschach, is **a test of whole personality functioning** (Rorschach, 1942/1921). The Rorschach test **consists of ten cards** with inkblots on them (five are black and white, two are black, red and white, and three are various pastels) which are presented to the patient. The test is administered in two phases. First, the patient is presented with the ten inkblots one at a time and asked "what might this be." The responses are recorded verbatim and the examiner tries to get two responses to each of the first two cards. In the second phase, the examiner reviews the patient's responses and inquires **where on the card the response was seen** (known as location in Rorschach language) and **what made it look that way** (known as the determinants) to the patient. For example, if a patient responded to card V with "A flying bat" (inquiry: "Can you show me where you see that?") "Here I used the whole card" ("What made it look like a bat?") "The color, the black made it look like a bat to me," this response would be coded: **Wo FMa.FC'o A P 1.0.**

   In the past, Rorschach "scoring" has been criticized for being too subjective. However, over the last 20 years **John Exner Jr** (Exner, 1986) **and his colleagues have developed a Rorschach system (called the Comprehensive System) which has demonstrated acceptable levels of reliability.** Currently inter-rater Kappa scores of 0.80 or better are required for all Rorschach variables reported in published research studies. For comparison, Kappas in this range are equal to or better than the Kappas reported for structured interview DSM diagnoses. **Rorschach data are particularly useful for quantifying a patient's reality contact and the quality of their thinking.**

   b. **Thematic Apperception Test (TAT).** The TAT **is useful in revealing a patient's dominant motivations, emotions, and core personality conflicts** (Murray, 1938). The TAT **consists of a series of 20 cards depicting people in various interpersonal interactions.** The cards were **intentionally drawn to be ambiguous.** The TAT is administered by presenting eight to ten of these cards, one at a time, with the instructions to **"Make up a story around this picture. Like all good stories it should have a beginning, middle, and an ending. Tell me how the people feel and what they are thinking."** While there is no one accepted standard scoring method for the TAT (making it more of a clinical technique than psychological test proper), when sufficient cards are present, reliable information can be obtained. A few standardized scoring methods have been developed for the TAT. However, these are limited to specific aspects of psychological functioning, such as level of defense operations and degree of psychological maturity. Psychologists typically assess TAT stories for:
   i. Emotional themes
   ii. Level of emotional and cognitive integration
   iii. Interpersonal relational style
   iv. View of the world (is it seen as a helpful or hurtful place). This type of data can be particularly useful

in predicting a patient's response to psychotherapy and to the psychotherapist.

c. **Projective drawings.** Psychologists often employ projective drawings (free-hand drawings of human figures, or of a house, tree, and person) as a supplemental assessment procedure. They represent clinical techniques more than tests, as there are no formal scoring methods. In fact, the interpretation of these drawings often relies heavily upon psychoanalytic theory. Despite their poor psychometric properties, projective drawings can sometimes be very revealing. For example, psychotic subjects may produce human figure drawings that are transparent with internal organs. Still it is important to remember that projective drawings are less reliable and less valid than are other tests reviewed in this chapter.

V. The Assessment Consultation Process and the Report

A. Obtaining the Assessment Consultation

The referral of a patient for an assessment consultation should be like the referral to any professional colleague. Psychological testing cannot be done "blind." The psychologist will want to hear relevant information about the case and will explore with you what question(s) you want answered (this is called the **referral question**) by the consultation. **Based upon this case discussion the psychologist will select an appropriate battery of tests designed to obtain the desired information.** It is helpful if you prepare your patient for the testing by reviewing with him or her why the consultation is desired and that it will likely take a few, perhaps three, hours to complete. You should expect the psychologist to evaluate your patient in a timely manner and to provide you with verbal feedback (a "wet read") within a few days after the testing. The written report should be available within 2 weeks.

B. Using the Test Results

You should review the relevant findings from the consultation with your patient. This helps confirm for the patient the value of the testing and the time they invested in it. If either you or your patient have any questions about the findings you should contact the psychologist for clarification. Ultimately, if necessary, the psychologist should be willing to meet with you or with the patient to explain the test results.

C. Understanding the Assessment Report

The report is the written statement of the psychologist's findings. It should be understandable and it should plainly state and answer the referral question(s). **The report should contain the following information:**

1. **Relevant background information**
2. **A list of the procedures used in the consultation**
3. **A statement about the validity of the test results and the confidence the psychologist has in the findings**
4. **A detailed description of the patient, based upon test data**
5. **Recommendations drawn from the test findings**

The test findings should be presented in a logical manner providing a rich integrated description of the patient (not a description of the individual test results). It should contain some raw data (e.g., IQ scores). This will allow any follow-up testing to be meaningfully compared to the present findings. It should close with a list of recommendations. To a considerable degree the quality of a report (and a consultation) can be judged from the recommendations provided. A good assessment report should contain a number of useful recommendations. You should never read just the summary of a test report; this results in the loss of important information as the whole report is already a summary of a very complex consultation process.

Suggested Readings

Butcher J, Dahlstrom W, Graham J, Tellegen A, Kaemmer B: *MMPI-2: Manual for Administration and Scoring.* Minneapolis: University of Minnesota Press, 1989.

Costa P, Widiger T: *Personality Disorders and the Five Factor Model of Personality.* Washington, DC: American Psychological Association, 1994.

Exner J: *The Rorschach: A Comprehensive System*, Vol. 1, 3rd ed. New York: Wiley, 1993.

Greene R: *The MMPI-2/MMPI: An Interpretive Manual.* Boston, MA: Allyn and Bacon, 1991.

Groth-Marnat G: *Handbook of Psychological Assessment.* New York: Wiley, 1990.

Hathaway SR, McKinley JC: *The Minnesota Multiphasic Personality Inventory*, rev. ed. Minneapolis: University of Minnesota Press, 1943.

Maruish M: *The Use of Psychological Testing for Treatment Planning and Outcome Assessment.* New Jersey: Lawrence Erlbaum Associates, 1994.

Matarazzo J: *Wechsler's Measurement and Appraisal of Adult Intelligence.* New York: Oxford University Press, 1979.

Millon T: *Millon Clinical Multiaxial Inventory-III Manual.* Minneapolis, MN: National Computer Systems, 1994.

Morey L: *The Personality Assessment Inventory: Professional Manual.* Odessa, FL: Psychological Assessment Resources, 1991.

Murray H: *Explorations in Personality.* New York: Oxford University Press, 1938.

Wechsler D: *Manual for the Wechsler Adult Intelligence Scale* rev. ed. New York: Psychological Corporation, 1981.

Wechsler D: *Manual for the Wechsler Adult Intelligence Scale*, 3rd ed. New York: Psychological Corporation, 1997.

Chapter 32

Neuropsychological Assessment

MARK A. BLAIS AND DENNIS K. NORMAN

I. Introduction

Neuropsychology and the field of neuropsychological assessment represent relatively recent developmental lines within applied psychology. In fact, it is only in the last two or three decades that neuropsychology has flourished as a clinical specialty. Prior to the development of clinical neuropsychology, psychologists attempted to differentiate functional from organic impairment based upon a patient's performance on intelligence tests and tests of personality functioning. This crude diagnostic approach sought to identify "signs" of organicity across multiple psychological tests with the goal to be ruling in or out a diagnosis of brain damage (organic impairment). As the scientific understanding of brain-behavior relationships improved, the global concept of "organicity" was increasingly seen as limited, and it became recognized that **organic impairment could be present in a variety of cognitive functions.** This more advanced understanding of brain functioning and damage led psychologists to seek assessment instruments which could evaluate specific cognitive functions and possible sources of cognitive deficits. For example, the evaluation of language functioning alone was broken into such areas as reading and writing, verbal memory, and confrontational naming (to highlight a few relevant functions).

II. History of Neuropsychological Tests

Neuropsychological assessment instruments owe much of their development to the pressures caused by World War II. Due to the increased survival rate of soldiers who suffered head wounds, World War II generated a great deal of interest in studying and measuring the effects of various types of brain damage on behavior and functioning. Out of this interest, **Halstead, in 1947, developed one of the first neuropsychological test batteries. Reitan later refined this series of tests into the battery known today as the Halstead-Reitan Neuropsychological Test Battery.**

III. Modern Neuropsychological Assessment

The modern neuropsychologist is trained to assess brain-behavior relationships using standardized psychological instruments. **The main goal of a neuropsychological evaluation is to relate a patient's test performance to both the status of their central nervous system (CNS) and their real world functional capacity.** In addition to assessing general intelligence, **five major abilities should be evaluated** in a complete neuropsychological assessment: **1) attention and concentration, 2) language (expressive and receptive), 3) memory (immediate and delayed), 4) visual-spatial constructional, and 5) executive functioning and abstract thinking.** This assessment is similar to the mental status examination used in neurology and psychiatry, differing mainly in that it provides a more comprehensive, less subjective, and better quantified assessment of the major cognitive functions. The application of a battery of tests covering these major cognitive areas allows for a broad assessment of the patient's capacities (strengths) and deficits (impairments), and gives some indication as to how these capacities and deficits will impact real world adaptation. More recently, increased attention has been paid to specific functioning related to the diagnosis of developmental and learning disorders in children and adults as our understanding of brain behavior relationships has grown. **A significant number of children receive neuropsychological evaluations to clarify reading, language, and attentional disorders so that proper learning resources can be directed to their learning difficulties. In adult patients, the same evaluations are used to clarify the learning issues necessary for employment or career changes.**

IV. Clinical Application of Neuropsychological Assessment

Neuropsychological assessment is a diagnostic procedure which can greatly add to clinical care. **Common reasons for referring a patient for a neuropsychological assessment include:**

A. Documentation of the functional impairment caused by a neurological disease or injury, such as stroke, seizures, or trauma.

B. Diagnosis of learning disabilities and/or attention deficit disorder.

C. Documentation of the existence of and/or degree of dementia.

D. Differentiation of dementia from depression in the elderly.

E. Assessment of a patient's ability to comprehend and follow treatment instructions.

F. Monitoring of the course of illness through baseline and follow-up testing.

G. Assessment of a patient who has failed multiple psychological or psychopharmacological treatments to better match subsequent treatment plans to the patient's ability level.

V. Approaches to Neuropsychological Assessment: The Standard Battery

A. The Halstead-Reitan (H-R) Battery
The H-R battery is the oldest standardized neuropsychological assessment battery. **The H-R battery is an elaborate and time-intensive set of neuropsychological tests.** It was developed from over 27 tests used by Halstead in the 1940s to measure cerebral functioning and biological intelligence. The Halstead battery was refined by Reitan, and today **the standard H-R battery consists of eight core tests, with supplemental tests being added as indicated.** Analysis of a H-R battery is almost exclusively quantitative. The H-R profile is **interpreted at four levels:**
1. Impairment Index (a composite score reflecting the subject's overall performance)
2. Lateralizing
3. Localizing signs
4. The pattern analysis for inferences of etiology (see Reitan, 1986)

B. The Boston Process Approach
The Boston process approach to neuropsychological assessment is **a newer and more flexible style of neuropsychological assessment.** In the Boston process approach **a small core test battery** (usually containing one of the Wechsler IQ tests) **is given and hypotheses regarding cognitive deficits are developed based on the patient's performance.** Other instruments then are administered to test out and refine these hypotheses about the patient's cognitive deficits. The Boston approach focuses upon both the **quantitative** and **qualitative** aspects of a patient's performance. By qualitative we mean the manner or style of the patient's performance, not just its accuracy. In fact, **review of how a patient failed an item or test can reveal more than the simple knowledge that the item was failed.** In this way the Boston approach reflects an integration of features from behavioral neurology and psychometric assessment.

C. The Luria-Nebraska Battery (L-NB)
The development of the L-NB was an attempt to standardize the innovative work of Luria and his Russian colleagues. Although Luria's work represents a thorough and well-conceptualized approach to neuropsychological assessment, the degree to which the L-NB had been successful in standardizing this approach is not clear. **The L-NB is not widely used in the United States** and a number of prominent US neuropsychologists have criticized the L-NB, suggesting that it is diagnostically unreliable.

VI. The Composite Battery: Using Select Neuropsychological Tests

Many neuropsychologists use a composite battery of tests in their day-to-day clinical work. **A composite battery is usually composed of an IQ test (one of the Wechsler scales) and a number of select tests matched to the population and disorder being studied.** Here we will review some of the specific neuropsychological tests that might be used to compose a battery or to assess specific cognitive functions. [For a description of these tests see Spreen and Strauss (1991).]

A. Attention and Concentration
As attention and concentration are **central to most complex cognitive processes,** it is important to include multiple measures of these functions in a neuropsychological test battery. In fact, some patients who complain of memory disorders will turn out to have impaired attention and concentration rather than memory dysfunction. **Tests of attention and concentration would include: Trail Making Test Parts A and B; Mental Control Subtests of the Wechsler Memory Scale-III; the WAIS-III Digit Span, Digit Symbol, and Arithmetic Subtests.**

B. Receptive and Expressive Language
Because of the importance of documenting deficits in communication skills secondary to brain insults, the evaluation of language functioning is an important part of a neuropsychological assessment. It is important to **assess language from a number of perspectives including: simple word recognition, reading comprehension, verbal fluency, naming ability, and writing. Frequently used measures of language functioning are: the WAIS-III Verbal IQ Subtests; the Boston Naming Test; Verbal Fluency Test; reading (word recognition and reading comprehension); and written expression (a writing sample).** The accurate measurement of reading ability (often using the **North American Adult Reading Tests [NAART]**) improves the estimation of premorbid intelligence and allows the examiner to better gauge the degree of overall cognitive decline.

C. Memory Functioning
The assessment of memory is extremely important in a neuropsychological battery as impaired memory is both a major reason for referral and a strong predictor of worse treatment outcome. **An evaluation of memory should cover both the visual**

and auditory memory systems, measure immediate and delayed recall (usually with a 30-min delay), assess the pattern and rate of new learning, and explore for differences between recognition (memory improvement with a retrieval cue) and free unaided recall.

1. **The Wechsler Memory Scale-III (WMS-III)** (Wechsler, 1987) is one of the principal memory inventories. WSM-III is composed of 11 subtests tapping auditory and visual memory at both immediate and 30-min delayed recall. It also provides indications of auditory and visual learning efficiency (new learning ability). Like the Wechsler IQ scales, this memory test is well standardized. The age-adjusted mean performance for the major memory scores is set at 100 with a standard deviation of 15. The memory subscales all have a mean of 10 and a standard deviation of 3. These statistical properties allow for a fairly detailed evaluation of memory functioning. In fact, the most recent revision of the Wechsler IQ and Memory Scales included joint norming of these tests, which allows for a more meaningful comparison between IQ and memory performance. Given that they share a norming sample it is expected that IQ and memory scores will be basically equal and any statistically significant difference between the two tests can be interpreted as indicating impairment.

2. The **Three Shapes and Three Words Memory Test is a less demanding test of language-based (written) and visual memory.** This brief test also provides measures of learning rate, immediate and delayed recall phases; however, it is not well normed (Weintraub and Mesulam, 1985).

D. **Visual-Spatial Constructional Ability**
   Visual-spatial tests (usually with a motor component—drawing) **help evaluate right hemisphere functions in most (right-handed) adults.** Because these deficits are nonverbal (sometimes called silent), they are often overlooked in briefer nonquantitative cognitive evaluations. **Tests which tap visual-spatial functioning include: the Rey-Ostterreith Complex Figure, Hooper Visual Integration Tests, the Draw a Clock Face Test, and the Performance IQ Subtests of the WAIS-III.**

E. **Executive Functions and Abstract Thinking**
   Executive functioning **refers to a number of higher-order cognitive processes such as judgment, planning, logical reasoning, and the modification of behavior (or thinking) based upon external feedback.** These functions, which are thought to be **associated with the frontal lobes,** are extremely important to effective real world functioning.

1. One of the most frequently used tests of executive functioning is the **Wisconsin Card Sorting Test (WCST),** which requires the patient to match 128 response cards to one of four stimulus cards using three possible dimensions (color, form, and number). While the patient matches these cards the only feedback they are given by the examiner is the response of "right" or "wrong." After ten consecutive correct matches the matching rule shifts to a new dimension (unannounced) and the patient must discover the "new" rule. One of the primary scores from the WCST is the number of perseverative errors committed (a perseverative error is scored when the patient continues to sort to a dimension despite feedback that the strategy is incorrect).

2. Other tests of executive functioning include: **The Category Test, Booklet Format,** the **Stroop Color Word Test,** and the **Similarities and Comprehension subtests of the WAIS-III** (which provide information about abstract reasoning).

F. **Motor and Sensory Functioning**
   Measures of tactile sensitivity and motor strength and speed have long been important in the clinical or bedside neurological examination. Neuropsychologists are also interested in measuring these functions; however, they employ more sensitive instruments and compare a patient's performance to standardized norms. **Typically, neuropsychologists are interested in both the absolute magnitude of the patient's performance (how well did they perform compared to the test's norms) and any noted differences between the two body sides (the left-right discrepancies).**

1. **Tests of motor functioning** include the **Finger Tapping Test** (the average number of taps per 10 sec with each hand) and **Hand Dynamometer** (a test of grip strength).

2. **Sensory ability tests** include **Finger Localization Tests** (naming and localizing fingers on the subject's and examiner's hand) and **Two-Point Discrimination** and **Simultaneous Extinction test** (measures two-point discrimination threshold and the extinction or suppression of sensory information by simultaneous bilateral activation).

G. **General Intelligence**
   Wechsler Adult Intelligence Scale-III (see Chap. 31).

H. **Emotional Function**
   Many psychiatric conditions, particularly anxiety and depression, can produce transient neuropsychological deficits. Therefore, a complete neuropsychological assessment should also include a self-report test of psychopathology, such as the MMPI-2 (see

Chap. 31). Including such a test in the battery allows the neuropsychologist to evaluate the possible contribution of psychopathology to the cognitive profile.

VII. Neuropsychological Tests and Normative Data

One of the main advantages of neuropsychological assessment over a clinical neurological examination is the ability to compare a patient's performance to that of a normative sample. This allows one to determine how well the patient performed relative to an identifiable comparison group. However, **the usefulness of neuropsychological test data can be limited by the quality of the norms employed.** Unfortunately, the quality of norms varies greatly from test to test. Tests like the Wechsler Intelligence and Memory scales have outstanding norms, while other frequently used tests (like the Boston Naming Test) have more limited norms. In working with the elderly it is most helpful to have age- and education-adjusted norms as both of these variables have a substantial mediating effect on the normal (age appropriate) decline of cognitive functioning.

VIII. Brief Neuropsychological Assessment Tools

A number of brief neuropsychological assessment tools are used in clinical practice today. Brief assessment tools are not a substitute for a comprehensive neuropsychological assessment, but they can be useful as screen instruments or when patients can not tolerate a complete test battery. Two such brief tests are the **Dementia Rating Scale (DRS)** and **the Neurobehavioral Cognitive Status Examination** (known as the **COGNISTAT**). **These tests provide a reasonable and brief assessment of the major areas of cognitive functioning (attention, memory, language, reasoning, and construction). Both tests employ a screening methodology** in evaluating these cognitive domains, with the patient first being presented with a moderately difficult item and, if that item is passed, the rest of the items in that domain are skipped (with the examiner moving on to the next domain). However, if the screening item is failed, then a series of items are given to the patient to evaluate more fully the specific cognitive ability.

A. The **DRS is a useful tool for assessing elderly** (65 years and up) **patients who are suspected of having Alzheimer's dementia** (DAT). It takes between 10 and 20 min to administer and it provides six scores. The Total score and the scores from the Memory and Initiation/Perseveration subscales have been shown to be useful in identifying DAT patients. The DRS was designed to a low performance "floor." This means that the test contains many

items tapping low levels of functioning, which allows the test to track patients further as their functioning declines. This quality makes the DRS a useful tool for monitoring DAT patients across the course of their illness.

B. The **COGNISTAT** is conceptually similar to the DRS; however, it **was designed to be used with younger adults** (20–66 years old). This test **provides a rapid and standardized measure of the major areas of cognition.** It is a helpful tool for screening psychiatric patients for cognitive deficits and for assessing patients who are unable or unwilling to complete a comprehensive assessment battery.

IX. Common Neuropsychological Assessment Referral Questions

A. **Depression vs. Dementia**
The differentiation of depression from dementia in the elderly **is the most common neuropsychological referral question** (see Chap. 31 for a discussion of "referral question"). Depression in the elderly is often accompanied by apparent cognitive deficits, making the diagnostic picture somewhat confused with that of early dementia. By evaluating the profile of deficits obtained across a battery of tests a neuropsychologist can help establish the differences between these two illnesses. For example, a depressed patient tends to have problems with attention and concentration and memory (new learning and retrieval), whereas a patient with early dementia has problems with delayed recall memory (encoding) as well as word-finding or naming problems. Each type of patient can display frontal lobe/executive functioning problems. However, the functioning of the depressed patient will often improve with cues or strategy suggestions while this typically does not help the patient with dementia. Although this general pattern will not always be true, it is this type of contrasting performance that allows neuropsychological assessment to aid differential diagnosis.

B. **Independent Living**
Whether or not a patient is capable of living independently is a complex and often emotionally charged question. Neuropsychological test data can provide one piece of the information needed to make a reasonable medical decision in this area. In particular, **neuropsychological test data regarding memory functioning (both new learning rate and delayed recall) and executive functioning (judgment and planning) have been shown to predict failure and success in independent living.** However, any neuropsychological test data should be thoughtfully combined with information from an occupational

therapy (OT) evaluation, assessment of the patient's psychiatric status, and family input (when available) before rendering any judgment about a patient's capacity for independent living.

C. **Attention Deficit Disorder (ADD)**

Neuropsychological assessment has a role in the diagnosis and treatment of adults and children with ADD. However, as in the question of independent living status, it provides just a piece of the data necessary for making this diagnosis. **The evaluation of ADD should include a detailed review of academic performance, including report cards and school records. When possible, living parents should also be interviewed for their recollections of the patient's childhood behavior. The neuropsychological evaluation should focus upon measuring intelligence, academic achievement (expecting to see normal or better IQ with reduced academic achievement), and multiple measures of attention and concentration (with tests of passive, active [shifting] and sustained attention).** While the neuropsychological testing profile might aid in the diagnosis of ADD in adulthood, the diagnosis can usually be done solely based upon historical data. The neuropsychological test data or profile is often more useful in helping the patient, family and treater understand the impact of ADD on the structure and organization of the patient's current cognitive abilities, as well as ruling out comorbid disorders such as learning disabilities, which are very common in ADD.

D. **Neuropsychological Assessment and Treatment Planning**

Neuropsychological assessments can often aid in the treatment planning of patients with moderate to severe psychiatric illness. While this aspect of neuropsychological testing is somewhat under-utilized at present, in the years to come this may prove to be the most beneficial use of these tests. Neuropsychological assessment benefits treatment planning by providing objective data and the test profile regarding the patient's cognitive skills (deficits and strengths). **The availability of such data can help clinicians and family members have more realistic expectations about the patient's functional capacity** (Keefe, 1995). This can be particularly helpful for patients suffering from severe disorders (e.g., schizophrenia). The current literature indicates that neuropsychological deficits are more predictive of long-term outcome in schizophrenic patients than are either positive or negative symptoms.

X. The Neuropsychological Assessment Report

In contrast to the written report from a personality assessment (reviewed in Chap. 31), the written neuropsychological testing report tends to be less integrated. **The test findings are provided and reviewed for each major area of cognitive functioning (intelligence, attention, memory, language, reasoning, and construction). These reports typically contain a substantial amount of raw data** as this is crucial for any meaningful retesting comparison. However, the neuropsychological assessment report should provide a brief summary reviewing and integrating the major findings and also contain useful/meaningful recommendations. As with all professional consultations, the examining psychologist should be willing to meet with you and/or your patient to review the findings and their implications in person.

Suggested Readings

Keefe R: The contribution of neuropsychology to psychiatry. *Am J Psychiatry* 1995; 152:6–14.

Lezak M: *Neuropsychological Assessment*, 3rd ed. New York: Oxford University Press, 1995.

Matarazzo J: *Wechsler's Measurement and Appraisal of Adult Intelligence*. New York: Oxford University Press, 1979.

Milberg W, Hebben N, Kaplan E: The Boston process neuropsychological approach to neuropsychological assessment. In Grant I, Adams K (eds): *Neuropsychological Assessment of Neuropsychiatric Disorders*. New York: Oxford University Press, 1986.

Reitan R: Theoretical and methodological bases of the Halstead-Reitan neuropsychological test battery. In Grant I, Adams K (eds): *Neuropsychological Assessment of Neuropsychiatric Disorders*. New York: Oxford University Press, 1986.

Spreen O, Strauss E: *A Compendium of Neuropsychological Tests*. New York: Oxford University Press, 1991.

Storand TM, VandenBos G: *Neuropsychological Assessment of Dementia and Depression in Older Adults: A Clinician's Guide*. Washington, DC: American Psychological Association, 1994.

Wechsler D: *Manual for the Wechsler Adult Intelligence Scale*, rev. ed. New York: Psychological Corporation, 1981.

Wechsler D: *Wechsler Memory Scale*, rev. ed. New York: Psychological Corporation, 1987.

Weintraub S, Mesulam M-M: Mental state assessments of young and elderly adults in behavioral neurology. In M-M, Mesulam (ed.) *Principles of Behavioral Neurology*. Philadelphia: FA Davis, 1985.

Yozawitz A: Applied neuropsychology in a psychiatric center. In Grant I, Adams K (eds): *Neuropsychological Assessment of Neuropsychiatric Disorders*. New York: Oxford University Press, 1986.

Chapter 33

Laboratory Tests and Diagnostic Procedures

MENEKSE ALPAY AND LAWRENCE PARK

I. Introduction

A. Diagnoses in psychiatry are made by identification of symptom patterns that constitute psychiatric illnesses, as outlined in the *Diagnostic and Statistical Manual, Fourth Edition* (DSM-IV). They are not based on objective, biologically based tests and procedures. These procedures are used to exclude organic etiologies for psychiatric presentations and to monitor illness progression.

B. In the past, numerous attempts have been made to correlate psychiatric illnesses with certain biological correlates, such as the dexamethasone suppression test (DST) in patients with depression. However, despite extensive research on the DST and other biological tests, an accurate and reliable test for major depression has yet to be developed; in fact, a "gold standard" biological test or procedure does not exist for any psychiatric diagnoses.

C. Advances in technology have yielded powerful new methods of examination (e.g., neuroimaging, biochemical and genetic marker analysis). Advances in these techniques may fundamentally change our understanding of psychological states, and change how psychiatry is practiced.

This chapter covers the wide range of tests and procedures currently used for psychiatric assessment.

II. Diagnostic Tests

A. **Overview**
The initial and most important steps in any psychiatric assessment are compilation of a comprehensive history, physical examination, and mental status examination. A carefully conducted initial assessment serves to characterize the nature of psychiatric symptomatology, to suggest an underlying organic etiology, and to direct further tests and studies. A carefully elicited history may reveal evidence of medical conditions, substance-related effects, history of medical or psychiatric illness, family history of medical or psychiatric illness, or psychosocial stressors that could precipitate or aggravate psychiatric symptoms. Physical exam-

ination may reveal further signs and symptoms indicative of an underlying medical condition.

B. **In general, the initial onset of psychiatric symptoms after the age of 40 years suggests an organic etiology**. A history of chronic medical illness, medication use, or alcohol or drug use raises the possibility of recurrence of an illness that presents with neuropsychiatric symptoms. A family history of certain genetic psychiatric illnesses (e.g., bipolar disorder or schizophrenia), or certain heritable medical conditions (e.g., Huntington's disease), is suggestive that these conditions are related to the presentation. The presence of endocrine and metabolic disorders (e.g., thyroid dysfunction, pheochromocytoma) needs to be taken into consideration when making a psychiatric diagnosis.

C. **Physical examination provides information that may aid in either a primary psychiatric diagnosis or an underlying medical diagnosis**. Particularly important elements of the physical exam include vital signs, and the neurological and cardiac examination.

1. Elevated temperature (as well as a decreased temperature in infants and the elderly) indicates possible infectious etiology. If significant temperature abnormalities are present, localizing signs should be assessed to ascertain the location of infection. Significantly elevated temperature, given the appropriate clinical circumstances, could suggest neuroleptic malignant syndrome.

2. Body habitus (including weight and height) may indicate eating disorders.

3. Blood pressure and pulse are important as they serve as markers for cardiovascular function, and for adequate cerebral perfusion.

4. Assessment of level of consciousness can facilitate the diagnosis of a subdural hematoma.

5. Examination of the skin may reveal stigmata of syphilis, liver dysfunction, chronic alcohol use, or intravenous drug administration. New lesions may indicate recent trauma. Previous lesions may be examined to ascertain the severity of past attempts at self-injury.

6. Pupillary examination aids in the diagnosis of substance (particularly opiates) intoxication or withdrawal.

7. Chvostek's sign is an indication of hypocalcemia.
8. A Kayser-Fleisher ring around the pupil is a sign of Wilson's disease.
9. Papilledema, as seen on funduscopic examination, is associated with increased intracranial pressure.
10. In regard to examination of the neck, a positive Kernig or Brudzinski sign may suggest meningitis.
11. Palpation of the thyroid should be conducted to assess for any change in size or consistency, which might suggest thyroid dysfunction.
12. Respiratory and cardiac examinations assess the overall oxygenation of the body (including the brain). Any instability in either system could suggest possible cerebral hypoxia. In addition, respiratory and cardiac examination are important in distinguishing psychiatric symptoms of anxiety and panic from anxiety and panic associated with medical conditions, such as mitral valve prolapse or pheochromocytoma.
13. Examination of the abdomen may yield clues about possible renal, hepatic, gastrointestinal, or urinary tract involvement.
14. Neurological deficits are often associated with psychiatric presentations. Certain physical deficits may represent underlying focal lesions that could also explain psychiatric symptoms (e.g., vascular events, tumors). In addition, certain other neurologic illnesses may have associated neuropsychiatric manifestations (e.g., seizure disorders, Parkinson's disease, Huntington's disease, multiple sclerosis).

D. **The mental status examination is central to the initial evaluation insofar as it characterizes the nature of the patient's mental state. In addition, certain findings may be suggestive of organic dysfunction.**
   1. Decline in level of consciousness or agitation may indicate a state of delirium with an underlying organic etiology.
   2. Decline in memory or cognition may represent dementia.
   3. Impairments of speech, cognition, or behavior may implicate specific areas of brain dysfunction.
   4. Discrete psychiatric symptoms, such as visual hallucinations, delusions, and illusions, are also suggestive of an organic etiology.

III. Types of Studies

A. **Laboratory Tests**
   The most common studies used by psychiatrists are laboratory tests, including analyses of serum chemistries and toxicology (see Tables 33-1 and 33-2). In addition, **endocrine studies** may be particularly important for those with a psychiatric presentation

(see Table 33-3). **Serological studies**, including those for syphilis, human immunodeficiency virus (HIV), hepatitis screen, and rheumatic diseases, may help to detect infectious/immune-mediated etiologies of psychiatric presentations (see Table 33-4). **Hematological studies** may include complete blood count (CBC), erythrocyte sedimentation rate (ESR), bleeding studies, d-dimer, and Coombs test (see Table 33-5). **Analysis of other bodily fluids** (urine, cerebrospinal fluid [CSF]) **and stool** may be indicated as well (see Table 33-6).

B. **Other Techniques**
   1. **Radiologic techniques**
   2. Cardiac function may be assessed through a number of studies, including an **electrocardiogram (EKG), echocardiography, and Holter monitoring.**
   3. Respiratory function may be assessed by **arterial blood gas (ABG), pulse oximetry, and pulmonary function tests.**
   4. **Vascular studies**, such as carotid Doppler ultrasonography, may be used to assess the integrity of the vascular system.
   5. Other studies, such as **electroencephalography (EEG), electrophysiology, and polysomnography,** assess the function of the central (CNS) and peripheral nervous systems.

IV. Routine Screening and Test Choice

A. **In general, the decision to order a test should revolve around the likelihood that a test will be abnormal, as well as the clinical importance of an abnormal (or normal) result.** No clear consensus about routine screening battery for the general psychiatric presentation in medically healthy patients has been reached so far.

   In clinical practice routine screening tests include: CBC, serum chemistries, ESR, vitamin B_{12}, folate, and thyroid stimulating hormone level (TSH). The list of studies of possible relevance to a psychiatric presentation is large. Table 33-7 presents studies to consider for the initial workup of psychiatric presentations.

B. **Beyond the initial routine screening, any further studies should be based on the specific clinical situation.** In those with a history of high-risk behaviors, HIV infection should be assessed. A history of significant weight loss may indicate occult malignancy or infection and may require further workup. In a malnourished patient, nutritional assessment, including the level of vitamins and minerals, should be assessed. Patients with eating disorders may demonstrate a decreased ESR in anorexia, an increased aldolase in bulimia, or a positive phenolphthalein assay in stool or urine in

Table 33-1. Serum Chemistries

Test	Indication	Comments
Alanine aminotransferase (ALT)	Medical workup	↑ Hepatitis, cirrhosis, liver metastasis ↓ Pyridoxine (B_6) deficiency
Albumin	Medical workup	↑ Dehydration ↓ Malnutrition, hepatic failure, burns, multiple myeloma, carcinomas
Aldolase	Ψ: Eating disorders	↑ Ipecac abuse, schizophrenia
Alkaline phosphatase	Medical workup Ψ Psychotropic medication use	↑ Paget's disease, hyperparathyroidism, hepatic disease/metastases, heart failure, phenothiazine use ↓ Pernicious anemia (B_{12} deficiency)
Ammonia	Medical workup	↑ Hepatic encephalopathy/failure, Reye syndrome, GI hemorrhage, severe congestive heart failure (CHF)
Amylase	Ψ: Eating disorders	↑ Bulimia nervosa
Aspartate aminotransferase (SGOT/AST)	Medical workup	↑ CHF, hepatic disease, pancreatitis, eclampsia, cerebral damage, alcohol
Bicarbonate	Ψ: Panic, eating disorders	↑ Bulimia, laxative abuse, psychogenic vomiting ↓ Hyperventilation, panic, anabolic steroid
Bilirubin, total	Medical workup	↑ Hepatic, biliary, pancreatic disease
Bilirubin, direct	Medical workup	↑ Hepatic, biliary, pancreatic disease
Blood urea nitrogen	Medical workup Ψ: Psychotropic medication use	↑ Renal disease, dehydration, lethargy, delirium
Calcium	Medical workup Ψ: Mood disorders, psychosis, eating disorders	↑ Hyperparathyroidism, bone metastasis ↑ Mood disorders, psychosis, eating disorders ↓ Hypoparathyroidism, renal failure ↓ Depression, irritability, delirium, chronic laxative use
Carbon dioxide	Ψ: Panic, eating disorders	↓ Hyperventilation, panic, anabolic steroid abuse
Ceruloplasmin	Medical workup	↓ Wilson's disease
Chloride	Ψ: Eating disorders, panic	↓ Bulimia, psychogenic vomiting ↑ (Mild) hyperventilation, panic
Creatinine phosphokinase (CK, CPK)	Medical workup Ψ: NMS, physical restraint, substance abuse	↑ Neuroleptic malignant syndrome (NMS), IM injection, rhabdomyolysis, restraints, dystonic reactions ↑ Antipsychotic use
Creatinine	Medical workup	↑ Renal disease
Ferritin	Medical workup	↓ Iron deficiency (most sensitive test)
Folate	Ψ: Alcohol, medications	↓ Psychosis, paranoia, fatigue, agitation, dementia, delirium ↓ Alcoholism, phenytoin, oral contraceptive estrogen
γ-Glutamyltranspeptidase (GGT)	Medical workup Ψ: Alcohol	↑ Alcohol, cirrhosis, liver disease
Glucose	Medical workup Ψ: Panic, anxiety, delirium, depression	↑ Delirium ↓ Delirium, agitation, panic, anxiety, depression
Iron-binding capacity	Medical workup	↑ Fe deficiency anemia
Iron, total	Medical workup	↓ Fe deficiency anemia

(continued)

Table 33-1. *(continued)*

Test	Indication	Comments
Lactate dehydrogenase (LDH)	Medical workup	↑ Myocordial infarction, pulmonary infarction, hepatic disease, renal infarction, seizures, cerebral damage, pernicious anemia; associated with RBC destruction
Magnesium	Medical workup Ψ: Alcohol	↓ Alcohol; associated with agitation, delirium, seizures, ↑ Panhypopituitarism
Phosphorus	Medical workup	↑ Renal failure, diabetic acidosis, hypoparathyroidism, hypervitaminosis D ↓ Cirrhosis, hyperparathyroidism, hypokalemia, panic, hyperventilation
Potassium	Medical workup Ψ: Eating disorder	↑ Hyperkalemia acidosis, anxiety in cardiac arrhythmia ↓ Cirrhosis, metabolic alkalosis, laxative abuse, diuretic abuse, bulimia, psychogenic vomiting, anabolic steroid use
Protein, total	Medical workup Ψ: Psychotropic medication use	↑ Multiple myeloma, myxedema, SLE ↓ Cirrhosis, malnutrition, overhydration May affect protein-bound medication levels
Sodium	Medical workup Ψ: Use of lithium	↓ Hypoadrenalism, myxedema, CHF, diarrhea, polydipsia, carbamazepine (CBZ) use, SIADH, anabolic steroids ↓ More sensitive to lithium use
Uric acid	Medical workup	↑ Gout, hematological disorders, renal disorders, endocrine disorders, hypertension, Lesch-Nyhan
Vitamin A	Medical workup	↑ Hypervitaminosis A, depression, delirium
Vitamin B_{12}	Medical workup Ψ: Dementia, mood disorder	↓ Megaloblastic anemia, dementia, psychosis, paranoia, fatigue, agitation, dementia, delirium

SOURCE: Rosse et al. (1995).

↑, increase in lab value; ↓, decrease in lab value; Ψ, psychiatric indication.

SIADH, syndrome of inappropriate antidiuretic hormone.

laxative abuse. Women of childbearing age should be assessed for pregnancy.

C. Psychosis

Initial presentation of psychotic symptoms warrants a full organic workup. Multiple causes of psychosis must be excluded, including CNS lesions, CNS infections, seizure disorders, toxic effects of drugs, alcohol withdrawal, and metabolic or endocrine abnormalities. **Workup should include: comprehensive laboratory testing, lumbar puncture and CSF analysis, syphilis serology, neuroimaging, and EEG.**

D. Depression

Depression is a common psychiatric symptom. While it is often a primary psychiatric symptom, depression may also be associated with a number of medical conditions (e.g., thyroid dysfunction, folate deficiency, Addison's disease, rheumatoid arthritis, systemic lupus erythematosus [SLE], Parkinson's disease, dementia, and the use of certain medications and drugs).

E. Anxiety

Anxiety can be associated with a wide range of organic etiologies as well. Underlying medical conditions that may account for anxiety symptoms include: seizure disorders, postconcussive syndrome, thyroid dysfunction, parathyroid dysfunction, hyperadrenalism, hypoglycemia, pheochromocytoma, drug effects, alcohol or barbiturate withdrawal, cardiac disease (e.g., myocardial infarction [MI], mitral valve prolapse), respiratory compromise (e.g., chronic obstructive pulmonary disease), menopause, and porphyria. **To exclude these organic causes, workup may include: pertinent laboratory testing, serum glucose or glucose tolerance testing, endocrine testing, cardiac workup, respiratory function tests, chest X-ray, urine vanillymandelic acid [VMA], urine porphyrins, and an EEG.**

Table 33-2. Serum Toxicology

Class	Substance	Presentation
Drugs	Alcohol	Intoxication: delirium, psychosis, mood disturbance, anxiety, sexual dysfunction, sleep disturbance Withdrawal: delirium, psychosis, mood disturbance, anxiety, sleep disturbance Persistent use: dementia, amnesia
	Amphetamines	Intoxication: delirium, psychosis, mood disturbance, anxiety, sexual dysfunction, sleep disturbance Withdrawal: mood disturbance, sleep disturbance
	Caffeine	Intoxication: anxiety, panic, sleep disturbance Withdrawal: NA
	Cannabis	Intoxication: delirium, psychosis, anxiety Withdrawal: NA
	Cocaine	Intoxication: delirium, psychosis, mood disturbance, anxiety, sexual dysfunction, sleep disturbance Withdrawal: mood disturbance, anxiety, sleep disturbance
	Hallucinogens	Intoxication: delirium, psychosis, mood disturbance, anxiety
	Inhalants	Intoxication: delirium, psychosis, mood disturbance, anxiety Persistent use: dementia
	Nicotine	Withdrawal: anxiety
	Opioids	Intoxication: delirium, psychosis, mood disturbance, sexual dysfunction, sleep disturbance Withdrawal: sleep disturbance
	Phencyclidine	Intoxication: delirium, psychosis, mood disturbance, anxiety
	Sedative-hypnotics/anxiolytics	Intoxication: delirium, psychosis, mood disturbance, sexual dysfunction, sleep disturbance Withdrawal: delirium, psychosis, mood disturbance, anxiety, sleep disturbance Persistent use: dementia, amnesia
Metals	Lead	Apathy, irritability, anorexia, confusion
	Mercury	Psychosis, fatigue, apathy, decreased memory, emotional lability, "mad hatter-like"
	Manganese	Parkinson-like syndrome, "manganese madness"
	Aluminum	Dementia
	Arsenic	Fatigue, blackouts, hair loss
	Copper	Wilson's disease
Bromides		Psychosis, hallucinations, dementia (especially if serum chloride is elevated)

SOURCE: Rosse et al. (1995).

V. Special Populations

A. The Pediatric Population
In pediatric patients, psychiatric symptoms are relatively uncommon. When psychiatric problems do occur in children, they are often secondary to organic etiologies. For instance, changes in mental status may occur from infection, injury, and exposure to toxins (e.g., heavy metals). CNS infection may be excluded by lumbar puncture and CSF analysis (including culture, fungal, and viral studies). If there is a question of head injury, computed tomography (CT) or magnetic resonance imaging (MRI) may be the definitive study to obtain. Toxic exposures may be assessed through laboratory examination.

B. The Geriatric Population
In geriatric patients, there is an increased likelihood of having concomitant medical conditions. As a result, it is important to recognize that one (or

Table 33-3. Endocrine Studies

Study	Indication	Comments
Thyroid		
TSH (thyroid-stimulating hormone)	Screening for thyroid dysfunction	↑ Hypothyroid ↓ Hyperthyroid
Other thyroid function tests	Thyroid dysfunction	↑ Hyperthyroid ↓ Hypothyroid
Parathyroid	Medical workup Anxiety	↑ Variety of organic mental disorders ↓ Causes hypocalcemia, anxiety
Growth hormone	Schizophrenia, anorexia, depression	↑ Increased response to dopamine (DA) agonist in schizophrenia, anorexia Blunted response to insulin-induced hypoglycemia in depression
Prolactin	Antipsychotic medication use, cocaine, seizures	↑ Antipsychotic use, cocaine withdrawal, generalized seizure Lack of increase suggests pseudoseizure
β-HCG (β-human chorionic gonadotropin)	Pregnancy	↑ Pregnancy
GnRH (gonadotropin-releasing hormone	Psychiatric symptoms	↓ Schizophrenia, anorexia, depression, anxiety
LH (luteinizing hormone)	Panhypopituitarism Depression	↓ Panhypopituitarism, depression
FSH (follicle-stimulating hormone)	Panhypopituitarism, postmenopause, anorexia	↓ Panhypopituitarism ↑ Postmenopausal, anorexia (mild increase)
Estrogen	Menopause, PMS mood disturbance and anxiety	↓ Menopause, depression, PMS Variable changes with anxiety
Testosterone	Steroid/progesterone use, impotence, decreased sexual desire	↑ Anabolic steroid use ↓ Organic causes of impotence, decreased sexual desire, medroxyprogesterone treatment (sexual offenders)
Melatonin	Mood disorders	↓ Seasonal affective disorder
ACTH (adrenocorticotropin hormone)	Medical workup	↑ Steroid use, seizures, psychosis, Cushing's, stress response
Cortisol	Medical workup Mood disorders	↑ Cushing's disease, anxiety, depression
CCK (cholecystokinin)	Eating disorders	Blunted postprandial response in bulimia (may normalize after antidepressant treatment)
Erythrocyte uroporphyrinogen-1-synthetase	Medical workup Psychosis	↑ Acute porphyria, psychosis

SOURCE: Rosse et al. (1995).
PMS, premenstrual syndrome.

more) organic causes may underlie psychiatric symptoms in the elderly. Similar to younger patients, there is no consensus as to which studies to obtain. Kolman (1984) reported five tests of **relatively high usefulness in the elderly: midstream urine (urinalysis, culture, and sensitivities), chest X-ray, serum vitamin B$_{12}$, EKG, and blood urea nitrogen (BUN).** Medical conditions that may contribute to psychiatric symptoms in the elderly include: urinary tract infection, anemia, thyroid disease, and dementia.

Anemia affects greater than 30% of all elderly patients, and can lead to symptoms of weakness, fatigue, depression, lack of motivation, agitation,

Table 33-4. Serology

Test	Agent/Indication	Psychiatric Indication	Comment
RPR, VDRL, FTA-ABS	Syphilis	Dementia, variable	Tertiary syphilis neurological involvement
ELISA, Western blot	HIV	Dementia, psychosis, personality disorder, mood disturbance, variable synptoms	CNS involvement
Hepatitis screen	Hep A antigen (Ag)	Anorexia, depression	Less severe, better prognosis than Hep B
	Hep B surface Ag	Depression	Active Hep B infection
	Hep B core Ag		Active Hep B infection
	Hep B surface antibody (Ab)		Previous infection/vaccination, immunity
Monospot	Epstein-Barr virus (EBV)	Mood disturbance, anxiety	Infectious mononucleosis (may present with depression, fatigue, personality change)
CMV	CMV	Mood disturbance, anxiety, confusion	
Lyme titer	Borrelia burgdorferi	Mental status changes	Erythema chronica migrans, meningitis, arthritis, cardiac problems
ANA	Antinuclear antibody	Delirium, psychosis, mood disturbance	Systemic lupus erythematosus (SLE), drug-induced lupus
LA	Lupus anticoagulant	Phenothiazine use	Elevated with phenothiazine use, especially chlorpromazine
LE cell preparation	Lupus erythematosus	Depression, psychosis, delirium, dementia	Associated with systemic LE

SOURCE: Rosse et al. (1995).
CMV, cytomegalovirus.

or confusion. While a CBC will document hemoglobin and hematocrit, other studies aid in the diagnosis of the anemia.

Thyroid disease is also common (especially in the elderly, and may be atypical in presentation). Checking serum thyroid-stimulating hormone (TSH) now constitutes thyroid screening. If the TSH is abnormal, additional thyroid function tests (TFTs) are then performed.

The National Institutes of Health Consensus Development Conference recommended a careful history and physical examination as the "best diagnostic test" for dementia since different dementing illnesses have different characteristic presentations. In addition, they recommended **CBC, serum chemistries, TFTs, and possibly a screening test for syphilis, a vitamin B_{12} level, and folate studies. If clinically indicated, further testing could include CT, EEG, MRI, and LP.** Other writers have suggested that chest X-ray, carotid studies, HIV testing, immunologic screens, LP, screening for toxins/medications may also be useful.

C. Patients with Substance Abuse
Substance use (intoxication, overdose, and withdrawal) is a major cause of mental status changes. Commonly, serum and urine are tested for substances (see Table 33-8). Alcohol is also routinely checked through breath analysis (breathalyzer). Other methods (e.g., hair or saliva analysis) have also been developed but are not routinely used in clinical practice. Chronic alcohol use may damage the liver and result in increases in liver transaminases. In addition, liver damage is reflected by decreased serum proteins and by an elevated partial thromboplastin time (PTT). A

Table 33-5. Hematology

Test		Indication	Comment
CBC	Hemoglobin, hematocrit	Anemia	Associated depression, psychosis
	White blood cell count	Medical workup, infection, psychotropic use	Leukocytosis associated with lithium, NMS Leukopenia, agranulocytosis associated with phenothiazine, carbamazepine, clozapine use
	Platelets	Medical workup, psychotropic use	↓ Certain psychotropic medications (CBZ, clozapine, phenothiazine)
	Mean corpuscular volume	Alcohol history	↑ Alcohol, vitamin B_{12} or folate deficiency
	Reticulocyte count	Medical workup, carbamazepine use	↓ Megaloblastic, iron deficiency anemia, anemia of chronic disease Monitor when using carbamazepine
ESR	Erythrocyte sedimentation rate	Medical workup	↑ Non-specific infection, inflammation, autoimmune, malignant process
PT	Prothrombin time	Medical workup	↓ Cirrhosis
Coombs test		Medical workup	Hemolytic anemia associated with psychotropic medication use (chlorpromazine, phenytoin, levodopa, methyldopa)

SOURCE: Rosse et al. (1995).

macrocytic anemia may develop as a result of a decreased folate level. In advanced alcohol dependence, a global decrease in mass of the cortex and cerebellum often results and may be noted on head-imaging studies. Clinical correlation may include Wernicke's encephalopathy and Korsakoff's amnestic syndrome. Regarding alcohol withdrawal, serum levels of alcohol do not correspond to severity or timing of withdrawal symptoms.

VI. Neuroimaging

Neuroimaging in psychiatry is used to narrow the differential diagnosis and to determine the prognosis of patients with neuropsychiatric disorders. It is a noninvasive and powerful tool, helpful to assess brain structures and function. Contemporary neuroimaging modalities include structural and functional neuroimaging.

A. **Structural Neuroimaging**
   1. **Computed axial tomography (CT or CAT scan) with or without contrast.** CT scanning uses X-ray beams to determine the attenuation when passing through different densities of the organ systems. The beams from different angles penetrate different organs. Detectors are arranged in a ring-like fashion (the patient in the center) to generate images. During the process, the patient is advanced through the

gantry of the scan after each slice is completed. When the films are completed, areas of high attenuation (e.g., bone) appear white, those of low attenuation (e.g., gas) appear black, and those of intermediate attenuation (e.g., soft tissue) appear in shades of gray.

When contrast material is used, it travels intravascularly and leaks out in areas where the blood-brain barrier (BBB) is compromised. Contrast enhancement occurs in the CNS with tumors, bleeding, infection, inflammation, metastasis, and abscesses.

   2. **Magnetic resonance imaging (MRI) with or without contrast.** MRI uses the magnetic properties of the water molecules of the body. In the magnetic field of the MRI scanner, hydrogen atoms in water molecules align themselves as dipoles with or against the magnetic field. When radiofrequency is applied, some of the dipoles will absorb the energy and align against the magnetic field (high-energy dipoles). When the radiofrequency is turned off, they will return to the lower energy state where they are aligned with the magnetic field. This emission of energy (dipoles from high-energy alignment against the magnetic field to low-energy alignment with the magnetic field) is detected by a coil, and an MRI scanner measures the signal. Images are

Table 33-6. Urine, Stool, CSF Studies

Test	Indication	Comment
Urine	Urinalysis	Urinary tract infection, renal disease, diabetes, alcohol use, acute starvation, urinary tract bleeding, tumor
	Culture and sensitivities	Urinary tract infection
	Chemistries (osmolarity, Na, K, Cl, HCO_3, creatinine)	Renal disease, prelithium workup
	Porphyrins, coproporphyrin, uroporphyrin	Porphyria
	Catecholamines, vanillylmandelic acid (VMA)	Pheochromocytoma
	Myoglobin	
	Copper	Wilson's disease
CSF	Opening pressure	↑ Infection, CNS mass, abscess, hematoma
	Appearance	Cloudy: infection Xanthochromic: CNS hemorrhage
	Glucose	↓ CNS infection
	Protein	↑ CNS infection
	Cells	+WBC: CNS infection +RBC: traumatic tap, CNS hemorrhage
	Culture and sensitivities	CNS infection
Stool	Culture and sensitivities	GI infection
	Ova and parasites	GI parasitic infestation
	Leukocytes	GI infection
	Clostridium difficile toxin	*Clostridium difficile* infection
	Heme	GI bleed
	Phenophthalein	Laxative use/abuse

SOURCE: Rosse et al. (1995).

constructed by applying magnetic field gradients during the radiofrequency irradiation.

MRI images are obtained using different acquisition parameters referred to as T_1 weight and T_2 weight. T_1-weighted images represent neuroanatomy clearly, whereas T_2-weighted images highlight areas of pathology. On T_2-weighed images regions with extravasated blood appear dark, due to the paramagnetic effects of iron; areas with tumor, plaques, and edema appear light due to increased water content. As in CT, contrast material can be used to highlight areas of compromised BBB.

MRI is contraindicated in patients with paramagnetic prostheses or an inability to tolerate scanner time or confinement.

3. **When is structural neuroimaging indicated?** Decisions about when to obtain structural imaging need to be made on a case-by-case basis after a thorough evaluation of the patient. The following

conditions represent populations in whom neuroimaging decreases the possibility of missing a brain lesion associated with a treatable general medical condition:

a. New-onset psychosis
b. New-onset delirium
c. New-onset dementia
d. Onset of any psychiatric problem in patients > 50 years old
e. Abnormal neurologic examination
f. History of head trauma
g. Initial workup for electroconvulsive therapy

4. **Which one is indicated: CT versus MRI?**
   a. A CT scan is preferred in:
      i. Acute hemorrhage and acute trauma.
      ii. Identification of calcification
      iii. If MRI is contraindicated
   b. MRI is preferred when:
      i. Higher soft-tissue resolution is required

Table 33-7. Studies to Consider for Psychiatric Presentations

First-line tests to consider	Serum/breath alcohol
CBC	Serum toxicology
Serum chemistry panel	Heavy metal screen
Thyroid function tests	Serum medication levels
Syphilis serology (RPR, VDRL)	ESR
HIV	ANA
Vitamin B_{12} and folate	LP/CSF analysis
UA	Serum/urine copper
Urine toxicology	Serum ceruloplasmin
Urine uroporphyrins/porphobilinogen	Monospot (EBV)
Erythrocyte uroporphyrinogen-1-synthetase	Blood cultures
Serum ceruloplasmin	Skin test—tuberculosis, brucellosis
CXR	Pregnancy test
EKG	Urine uroporphyrins
	Urine/serum osmolality
Second-line tests to consider, if indicated	Polysomnography
CT—head	Nocturnal penile tumescence
MRI—brain	Evoked potentials
Skull X-rays	Stool tests for occult blood
EEG	ABG

SOURCE: Morihisa et al. (1994).

Table 33-8. Detection of Drugs in Urine

Class of Agent	Agent	Serum	Urine	Hair
Barbiturate		Variable	3 days to 3 weeks	—
Alcohol		1–2 days	1 day	—
Stimulant	Amphetamine	Variable	1–2 days	~ 90 days
	Cocaine (benzolecgonine)	Brief	2–3 days	~ 90 days
Opiate	Propoxyphene	8–34 h (half-life)	1–2 days	~ 90 days
	Codeine, morphine, heroin	Variable	1–2 days	~ 90 days
	Methadone	15–29 h (half-life)	2–3 days	~ 90 days
Anxiolytic	Benzodiazepine	Variable	2–3 days	—
Cannabinoids	Delta-9-THC	—	~ 30 days	~ 90 days
Phencyclidine		—	8 days	~ 90 days

SOURCE: Gastfriend and O'Connell (1998).

ii. Posterior fossa pathology is suspected

iii. Radiation exposure is contraindicated (e.g., children, young women)

B. Functional Neuroimaging

Functional neuroimaging modalities (positron emission tomography [PET] and single photon emission computed tomography [SPECT]) demon-

strate neuronal activity, cellular metabolism, and neuroreceptor profiles with the use of radioactive substances (tracers), which are given intravenously or by inhalation. The tracer arrives in the CNS and is distributed according to regional blood flow, glucose metabolism, and receptor metabolism. It emits a signal that is detected by the scanner, and blood flow or glucose or receptor metabolism are recorded by tomographic imaging.

1. **PET scan.** PET scan requires an on-site cyclotron to prepare the positron emitter tracers, which have a short half-life. Its resolution is greater and more uniform when compared to SPECT, but it is much more expensive. It uses fluorodeoxyglucose (FDG) to assess glucose metabolism, oxygen-15 to assess brain blood flow, and specific radioligands to assess receptors for specific neurotransmitters.

2. **SPECT scan.** SPECT scan uses single photon-emitting nucleotides rather than positron-emitting nucleotides. Major tracers used are xenon-133, ^{99m}Tc-MPAO to determine blood flow and, as in PET scanning, specific radioligands to assess receptors for specific neurotransmitters.

   Functional MRI (fMRI) and magnetic resonance spectroscopy (MRS) are new imaging modalities that offer a great promise as tools for research and clinical applications in the future.

3. **When functional imaging is helpful:**
   a. **Seizures.** PET scanning is done contemporarily with EEG to determine the location of a seizure focus, especially in patients with complex partial seizures. During an ictus the seizure focus is hyperactive; inter-ictally the focus will be hypometabolic. This EEG-PET combination is useful in localizing foci in the preoperative assessment of neurosurgical intervention in patients with refractory seizure disorders.

   b. **Dementia.** Several profiles for dementias exist. Functional imaging studies of patients with Alzheimer's disease demonstrate decreased activity in bilateral parietal and temporoparietal cortices ("ear muff" sign). Parkinson's disease-related dementia mimics Alzheimer's disease. In vascular dementia, there are multiple areas of asymmetric cortical and subcortical hypoactivity. In Pick's disease, frontotemporal cortex hypoactivity is seen. In Huntington's disease caudate hypoactivity is present.

   c. **Major depression.** In patients with major depression, there is a decrease in anterolateral prefrontal cortex activity, more on the left than on the right. The magnitude of decrease of this defect correlates with symptom severity. Functional neuroimaging is used in the differential diagnosis of major depression, and other mood disorders, as well as dementia.

   d. **Schizophrenia.** In patients with schizophrenia, there is a decrease in the ratio of anterior to posterior metabolism. Decreased frontal activity correlates with negative symptoms. Hallucinations are associated with activation of Broca's area, the striatum, and the anterior cingulate cortex.

   e. **Obsessive-compulsive disorder.** There is increased activity in the orbitofrontal cortex-caudate nucleus-thalamus-anterior cingulate cortex circuitry.

   Increased frontal and caudate activity normalizes with successful treatment.

   f. **Posttraumatic stress disorder.** Hippocampal volume is decreased in patients with PTSD compared to healthy controls. Additionally, there is inadequate activation of the anterior cingulate and medial frontal cortex. There is an exaggerated activation of the amygdala in response to threat and exaggerated deactivation in Broca's area.

VII. Electrophysiology

A. Electroencephalogram (EEG)

1. **Waveforms.** The EEG records low-voltage electrical activity of the brain. In organic brain disease, there are changes in this electrical activity, and the EEG is helpful in the diagnosis and differential diagnosis of these disorders. The frequency of the electrical activity is measured in hertz (Hz), a measure of cycles per second. These frequencies are named with Greek letters.
   a. Delta: 0–4 Hz
   b. Theta: 4–8 Hz
   c. Alpha: 8–12 Hz
   d. Beta: > 12 Hz

   Amplitude refers to voltage of the EEG. The normal range is 10–100 μV on a scalp EEG. Usually low-voltage fast activity indicates severe CNS pathology other than sleep. High-voltage slow activity is seen in delirium.

2. **Most common EEG patterns**
   a. **Normal:** posterior alpha rhythm, often low-voltage beta anteriorly, often low-voltage theta in frontotemporal or temporal region.
   b. **Sleep**
      i. **Stage 1:** drowsiness, disappearance of alpha rhythm, onset of frontal, central, and temporal beta
      ii. **Stage 2:** vertex sharp waves (high-voltage single or complex theta or delta waves), predominant runs of sinusoidal 12–14 Hz activity called **sleep-spindles**
      iii. **Stage 3–4:** delta (1–3 Hz) activity.
      iv. **Rapid eye movement (REM):** Low-voltage fast with ocular movement artifacts
   c. **Seizure**
      i. **Generalized seizures:** bilateral, symmetric, synchronous, paroxysmal spike, and sharp waves followed by slow waves
      ii. **Absence: 3-Hz spike-wave complexes** accompanying blinking
      iii. **Complex partial seizures:** spikes, polyspikes, and waves over temporal region
      iv. **Pseudoseizures:** normal EEG
   d. **Delirium:** generalized theta and delta activity (generalized slowing); hepatic, uremic encephalopathies both show **triphasic** waves.

e. **Dementia:** Alzheimer's disease and vascular dementia show alpha slowing of the background (from 10–12 Hz to 8 Hz); with advanced disease the EEG becomes disorganized. Subacute sclerosing panencephalitis (SSPE) and Creutzfeldt-Jakob disease both show **periodic complexes accompanying myoclonic jerks.**

f. **Locked-in syndrome:** normal EEG

g. **Persistent vegetative state:** slow and disorganized EEG

h. **Death:** electrocerebral silence

i. **Medications:** benzodiazepines and barbiturates cause beta activity; neuroleptics and antidepressants may cause nonspecific changes.

j. **Focal lesion:** focal slowing, usually delta, referred to as polymorphic delta activity

k. **Increased intracranial pressure:** frontal, intermittent, rhythmic delta activity (FIRDA)

The EEG should always be interpreted in concert with the clinical presentation. Final determination rests on the overall clinical picture. Activation with hyperventilation, photic stimulation, sleep, and sleep deprivation are helpful in activating seizure foci.

B. Evoked Potentials (EPs)

Any neural activity, internal or external, can cause small changes in the EEG. In EP recordings, stimuli are repeated many times and EEG changes are averaged and recorded to see deviations from the norm. In this way, the integrity of sensory and cognitive pathways can be assessed. For example, in multiple sclerosis (MS), when the myelin sheath is damaged, conduction will be slowed and EPs will be delayed.

The main categories of EPs are:

1. **Brainstem EPs (auditory stimuli)**
2. **Somatosensory EPs (brief electrical stimuli)**
3. **Visual EPs (checkboard stimuli: alternating black and white squares)**
4. **Auditory EPs (click)**

a. During the assessment of auditory EPs a click is applied and the early component recorded is P50. In healthy subjects, when a conditioned paired click is applied, the P50 to the second click is reduced. In patients with schizophrenia, it is not. This is interpreted as a dysfunction of sensory gating in patients with schizophrenia.

b. Another important EP for psychiatrists is the EP P300. The P300 is related to information processing. It is seen in tasks requiring a behavioral response to a target stimulus. Several patient populations (e.g., demented individuals, patients with schizophrenia) show low amplitude and increased latency in P300.

C. Procedures/Challenges

Diagnostic procedures are not regularly used in the clinical setting. Two types of procedures exist: endocrine stimulation procedures, and sedative/hypnotic interviews.

1. **Endocrine stimulation procedures.** The concept behind endocrine stimulation procedures assumes that some relationship exists between endocrine dysfunction and certain types of mental illness.

a. **Dexamethasone suppression test (DST).** The assumption behind the DST is that dysfunction of the hypothalamic-pituitary-adrenal axis underlies major depression, particularly melancholic depression. To test this, an exogenous corticosteroid, dexamethasone 1 mg at bedtime, is administered. Then cortisol levels are drawn at various times throughout the next day (usually at 08:00, 16:00, and 23:00 h). The normal effect is suppression of cortisol and other adrenocorticosteroid release. An abnormal effect is absence of suppression of cortisol release. Nonsuppression is defined as a cortisol > 5 $\mu g/dL$. Nonsuppression is thought to result because of dysfunction of the feedback loop, in which dexamethasone blocks the release of corticotropin-releasing factor from the hypothalamus.

Although extensively tested, the sensitivity of the DST in detecting major depression is about 40–70% (with better correlation with severe psychotic affective disorders). Its specificity ranges from 70% to 90%. False positives may occur in a variety of medical conditions, including significant weight loss, alcohol use, and other drug use (e.g., barbiturates, anticonvulsants). Overall, the DST demonstrates only limited success in identifying major depression.

b. **Thyrotropin-releasing hormone (TRH) stimulation test.** TRH normally stimulates the release of TSH from the pituitary. **It has been reported that a blunted response of TSH release is associated with major depression.** Sensitivity is low, with a blunted TSH response occurring in only 25% of depressed patients. In addition, **the blunted response is also seen with alcoholism, bulimia, borderline personality disorder, panic disorder, and hyperthyroidism.**

c. **Panic provocation tests.** In panic provocation tests, it is theorized that relative states of **hypercarbia result in anxiety or panic.** Numerous agents have been shown to induce panic attacks in people with a history of panic attack. These agents include: CO_2, intravenously (IV) administered lactate, intraveous caffeine, isoproterenol, β-carboline, and flumazenil administration. Intravenous lactate infusion has been demonstrated to be 72% sensitive in detecting persons with panic disorder. Panic provocation tests are not typically used for clinical diagnostic purposes.

2. **Sedative/hypnotic interviews.** The sedative/hypnotic interview (e.g., the Amytal interview) continues to have a role in clinical diagnosis. This technique has been used to aid in differentiation between primary physical versus primary mental dysfunc-

tion. **The theory behind this technique is that administration of amobarbital (Amytal) or any sedative/hypnotic agent decreases the conscious guardedness and facilitates free communication.** While this procedure typically employs intravenous amobarbital infusion, any sedative/hypnotic agent is effective if sufficient sedation is achieved.

VIII. Monitoring Psychotropic Medications

A. Antidepressants

There are no established guidelines for monitoring levels of antidepressants. In the treatment of the medically ill, physicians should consider side effects of the antidepressants as well as the effects of the illness on the metabolism of psychotropics. In patients with liver disease, the antidepressant dosage needs to be carefully adjusted, and liver function tests (LFTs) need to be monitored for the possibility of increased LFTs by the psychotropic. Use of tricyclic antidepressants (TCAs) in the cardiac patient needs to be monitored closely (levels of TCAs and electrocardiogram [EKG] should be checked at baseline and during ongoing care) due to the effects of TCAs on cardiac conduction (PR, QRS, and QT_c prolongation), which may lead to lethal arrhythmias. **It is recommended that blood levels of TCAs be monitored in patients with:**

1. **Noncompliance**
2. **Poor response while taking a therapeutic dose for a reasonable time**
3. **Older age and medical illness**
4. **Serious depression (e.g., suicidal ideation)**

B. Mood Stabilizers

a. **Lithium.** Lithium is commonly used in patients with mood disorders, and affects many organ systems including kidneys, thyroid, heart, and CNS. It is recommended that serum electrolytes, BUN, creatinine, thyroid function tests, and EKG be checked routinely. Additionally, in patients with kidney problems, a 24-h urine test for creatinine and protein clearance is recommended. Steady states of lithium are reached in 3 days ($t_{1/2} = 12$ h), or can be as long as 8 days in patients with kidney problems due to prolonged $t_{1/2}$.

b. **Carbamazepine.** Carbamazepine affects mainly hepatic, hemopoietic, and cardiac conduction systems. A fatal side effect is agranulocytosis. Therefore, it is important to check a complete blood count before the initiation of treatment, every 2 weeks for the first 2 months, and once every 3 months thereafter. Platelet count, reticulocyte count, serum electrolytes, EKG, and liver function tests (aspartate aminotransferase [AST], alanine aminotransferase [ALT], lactate dehydrogenase [LDH], alkaline phosphatase) need to be checked, before and 1 year after the initiation of treatment. In patients of childbearing age, a pregnancy test needs to be done before initiation due to the teratogenic side effects of carbamazepine.

Discontinuation is recommended when the white blood cell count is $< 3,000/mm^3$, hemoglobin is < 11 mg/dL, the platelet count is $< 100,000/mm^3$, and the reticulocyte is $< 0.3\%$.

c. **Valproic acid.** Valproic acid mainly affects the liver, but it can also affect the hemopoietic system and the pancreas.

For details about mood stabilizers see Table 33-9.

C. Antipsychotics

Clozapine is the only antipsychotic that requires close laboratory monitoring due to the possibility of

Table 33-9. Mood Stabilizers

Agent	Half-life (h)	Dose Range (mg/day)	Protein Binding	Blood Levels
Lithium	24	300–2400	Low	0.5–1.2 mEq/L (weekly $\times 1$ month, monthly $\times 3$ months, then every 3 months)
Valproic acid	16	200–2000	Very high	50–150 μg/mL (weekly $\times 2$ weeks, then every 3 months)
Lamotrigine	12	100–700	Medium	–
Gabapentin	6	900–1800	None	–
Carbamazepine	8–30 (variable due to autoinduction)	200–1200	High	6–12 μg/mL (weekly $\times 2$ weeks, then every 3 months)

agranulocytosis in 1% of patients taking this medication. Baseline and weekly CBCs are mandatory when prescribing this medication. If the white blood cell count (WBC) drops significantly ($< 3,000$), even though it may be in the normal range, or in case of mild leukopenia (WBC $= 3,000-3,500$), the patient needs to be monitored closely and CBCs should be checked twice weekly. In the case of leukopenia (WBC $= 2,000-3,000$) or granulocytopenia (granulocytes $= 1,000-1,500$), the medication needs to be stopped, CBCs need to be checked daily, and the patient needs to be hospitalized. Clozapine therapy may be continued after normalization of the blood count. **If agranulocytosis develops (WBC $< 2,000$, or granulocytes $< 1,000$), clozapine is discontinued for life.** Under this condition, the patient needs to be hospitalized and placed under a hematologist's care. Use of other bone-marrow suppressants needs to be avoided; a biopsy may be necessary.

Additionally, an EEG may be helpful if the dosage of the clozapine needs to be raised beyond 600 mg because of an increased incidence of seizures. Clozapine can be reintroduced carefully in patients who experience clozapine-induced seizures.

In patients with cardiac disease, who are taking antipsychotics (e.g., thioridazine), the EKG needs to be checked due to the risk of serious cardiac conduction disturbances.

Table 33-10. Genetic Markers

Genetic Finding	Disorder	Comments
Chromosome 4, short arm	Huntington's disease	Autosomal dominant, 100% penetrance
Chromosome 21	Alzheimer's dementia	Near gene for amyloid precursor protein
X chromosome	Fragile X	Association with infantile autism, pervasive developmental delay
X chromosome	Fragile X carriers	Possible association with schizophrenic spectrum, chronic mood disorders
A1 allele of D_2 receptor	Alcohol, Tourette's, ADHD, autism, PTSD	Mutation of allele may act as modifying gene

Table 33-11. Biological Markers

Biological Marker		Comments
Homovanillic acid (HVA) (plasma)	DA metabolite	Decrease with antipsychotic treatment predicts good treatment response
3-Methoxy-4-hydroxyphenylglycol (MHPG) (24-h urine)	NE activity	Lower levels in bipolar than unipolar depressed Low levels may predict imipramine response High levels associated with learned helplessness Low CSF levels may be associated with increased risk of suicidal behavior
5-Hydroxyindoleacetic acid (5-HIAA) (CSF)	5HT metabolite	Low levels associated with suicidal behavior, aggression, impulsivity, disturbed childhood behavior, violent suicide attempts, depression, seizures, alcohol use High levels associated with anxiety, obsession, inhibited behavior
Tryptophan (serum)	Amino acid	Low levels reported in depression Low tryptophan diet precipitated some depression
Serine (serum)	Amino acid	High levels associated with some psychotics (serine hydroxymethyltransferase activity low)

IX. Genetic Testing and Biological Markers

Recently, research has focused on attempts to identify genetic markers that might underlie psychiatric illnesses. Although no firm relationships have been identified, some possible associations have been identified (see Table 33-10). A related area of research is attempting to identify biological markers of psychiatric illnesses. No firm relationships have been identified, but the list of potential markers is growing (see Table 33-11).

Suggested Readings

Anfinson TJ, Kathol RG: Screening laboratory evaluation in psychiatric patients: a review. *Gen Hosp Psychiatry* 1992; 14:248–257.

Dolan JG, Mushlin AI: Routine laboratory testing for medical disorders in psychiatric inpatients. *Arch Intern Med* 1985; 145:2085–2088.

Falk W: Approach to the patient with memory problems or dementia. In Stern TA, Herman JB, Slavin PL (eds): *The MGH Guide to Psychiatry in Primary Care*. New York: McGraw-Hill, 1998:207–220.

Fenton GW: The electroencephalogram in psychiatry: clinical and research applications. *Psychiatr Dev* 1984; 2:53–57.

Gastfriend DR, O'Connell JJ: Approach to the cocaine or opiate-abusing patient. In Stern TA, Herman JB, Slavin PL (eds): *The MGH Guide to Psychiatry in Primary Care*. New York: McGraw-Hill, 1998:455–460.

Kolman PBR: The value of laboratory investigations of elderly psychiatric patients. *J Clin Psychiatry* 1984; 45:112–116.

Morihisa JM, Rosse RB, Cross CD: Laboratory and other diagnostic tests in psychiatry. In *APA Textbook of Psychiatry*. Washington, DC: American Psychiatric Association, 1994: 277–310.

Rosse RB, Deutsch LH, Deutsch SI: Medical assessment and laboratory testing in psychiatry. In Kaplan HI, Sadock BJ (eds): *Comprehensive Textbook of Psychiatry VI*. Williams and Wilkins: Baltimore, 1995:601–618.

SECTION III

Neurologic Disorders

Chapter 34

Functional Neuroanatomy

Stephan Heckers

I. Overview

There are about 10^{11} neurons in the central nervous system (CNS), and each neuron establishes about 10^3–10^4 connections to other neurons. How are these neurons arranged to process information? This question may serve as a guide to understand, in a systematic fashion, the basic principles of human neuroanatomy.

II. Information Processing in the Brain

The processing of sensory information involves three steps: the collection of sensory information through perceptual modules, the creation of a representation, and the production of a response.

Sensory organs provide information about physical attributes of incoming information. **Details of physical attributes** (e.g., temperature, sound frequency, or color) **are conveyed through multiple segregated channels within each perceptual module.** The anatomical systems involved in reception are the sensory organs, the thalamus, and primary sensory cortex. **Integration of the highly segregated sensory information occurs at several levels.** The first integration occurs in **unimodal association areas** where physical attributes of one sensory domain are linked together.

A second level of integration is reached in multimodal association areas, which link physical attributes of different sensory qualities together, and **a third level of integration is provided by the interpretation and evaluation of experience.** It is at this third level of integration that the brain creates a representation of experience that has the spatiotemporal resolution and full complexity of the outside world. The representation of experience is evaluated and interpreted, which involves conscious and nonconscious processes. Evaluation and interpretation involve comparison of new information with previously stored information. This allows the brain to classify information (e.g., as new or old, or as threatening or not threatening).

Based on the result of the evaluation and interpretation, the brain can then create a response through a variety of channels (e.g., language, affect, and motor behavior).

III. Anatomical Systems

A. Anatomical Areas

Four major anatomical systems are involved in the
processing of information: the thalamus, the cortex, the medial temporal lobe, and the basal ganglia (Figure 34-1). The function of these four systems is modulated by several groups of neurons that are characterized by their use of a specific neurotransmitter. Most of psychopharmacology is aimed at strengthening or inhibiting these modulatory systems.

1. **The thalamus is the gateway to cortical processing of all incoming sensory information:** somatosensory (S), auditory (A), and visual (V).
2. **Primary sensory cortex (i.e., S1, A1, V1) receives sensory information from the appropriate sensory modules** (sensory organ + thalamus). **The association cortex integrates information from primary cortices, from subcortical structures, and from brain areas affiliated with memory, to create the representation of experience.**
3. **The medial temporal lobe serves** two major functions in the brain: **to integrate multimodal sensory information** for storage into and retrieval from memory, **and to attach limbic valence to sensory information** (e.g., pleasant or unpleasant, fight or flight).
4. **The basal ganglia are primarily involved in the integration of input from cortical motor areas.** They modulate the activity of thalamocortical projections, thereby creating a cortico-striato-thalamic loop.

B. Neurotransmitter Systems

Four groups of densely packed neurons provide diffuse projections to all areas of the brain to modulate their functions:

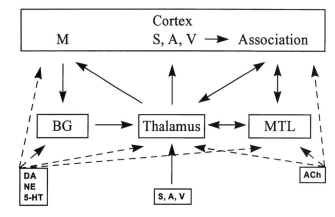

Fig. 34-1. Basic circuitry of information processing.

269

1. **Cholinergic neurons in the basal forebrain (BF) and brainstem**
2. **Dopaminergic neurons in the substantia nigra (SN) and ventral tegmental area (VTA)**
3. **Noradrenergic neurons in the locus coeruleus (LC)**
4. **Serotonergic neurons in the raphe nuclei (R)**

We will now review in some detail the four major anatomical systems (the cortex, the thalamus, the basal ganglia, and the medial temporal lobe) and their modulation by the neurotransmitter-specific projection systems.

IV. Cortex

The association cortex is a six-layered cortex, the so-called isocortex. **Layers 2 and 4 of the human isocortex are defined by a high density of small interneurons** (i.e., neurons that do not send long-ranging projections to other cortical or subcortical areas). **In contrast, layers 3 and 5 are defined by a high density of pyramidal cells, which collect input through their dendrites and project to other cortical or subcortical areas. Interneurons are GABAergic cells** (GABA is γ-aminobutyric acid) **and exert an inhibitory influence on their targets** (via $GABA_A$ receptors), whereas **pyramidal cells are glutamatergic and have an excitatory influence.** Normal cortical function depends on an intricate balance of GABAergic inhibition and glutamatergic excitation. Seizures, for example, are caused by a decrease of GABAergic tone and an increased firing of pyramidal cells. Sedation, on the other hand, can be caused by an increased GABAergic tone.

Cortical neurons are targets for many ascending fibers arising from the underlying white matter. Some of these inputs originate from other cortical areas or from the thalamus. Others arise from neurotransmitter-specific projection systems, such as the dopaminergic neurons of the ventral tegmental area (VTA) and the serotonergic neurons of the raphe nuclei. These two systems, the dopamine (DA) and the 5-hydroxytryptamine (serotonin, 5HT) systems, modulate the function of cortical areas by specific effects on cortical neurons. **The effect of DA on cortical neurons is conveyed by three DA receptors, the D_1, D_4, and D_5 receptors. The D_1 and D_5 receptors are expressed primarily on pyramidal cells, whereas the D_4 receptor is primarily expressed on GABAergic interneurons.** The other important neurotransmitter-specific projection system in the cortex is the serotonergic system. One serotonergic receptor, **the $5HT_{2A}$ receptor, is of particular relevance for the pathophysiology of psychosis.** Hallucinogens (e.g., lysergic acid diethylamide [LSD]) act as agonists at the $5HT_{2A}$ receptor, and several antipsychotic compounds, especially the atypical neuroleptics, block the activity of this receptor. Modulation of cortical function, via the D_1, D_4, D_5, and $5HT_{2A}$ receptors, leads to fine tuning of information processing, for example by increasing the signal-to-noise ratio during corticocortical and thalamocortical neurotransmission. This modulation is one of the important mechanisms for the action of neuroleptic drugs.

V. Thalamus

The thalamus serves several important functions in information processing in the human brain.

The relay nuclei (ventral posterior lateral [VPL], medial geniculate nucleus [MGN], and lateral geniculate nucleus [LGN]) convey sensory information from the sensory organs to the appropriate areas of the primary sensory cortex (S1, A1, and V1) (Figure 34-2).

The association nuclei, especially the mediodorsal nucleus, establish reciprocal connections with the association cortex.

The motor nuclei (i.e., ventral nuclei) relay input from the basal ganglia to the motor and premotor cortex.

VI. Basal Ganglia

The basal ganglia include the ventral striatum, the dorsal striatum (caudate and putamen), and the globus pallidus (Figure 34-3).

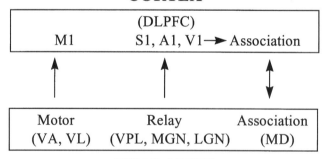

Fig. 34-2. Thalamo-cortical connections.

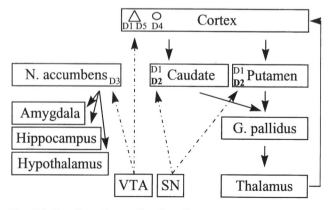

Fig. 34-3. Basal ganglia circuitry.

The dorsal striatum (caudate, putamen) receives input from motor cortex and projects to the globus pallidus. The globus pallidus relays the neostriatal input to the thalamus. The thalamus, in turn, projects back to the cortical areas that gave rise to the corticostriatal projections, thereby closing the cortico-striato-pallido-thalamo-cortical loop. This loop is involved in the generation and control of motor behavior.

In contrast, the ventral striatum (the nucleus accumbens) is connected with the amygdala, hippocampus, and hypothalamus and is therefore considered part of the limbic system. Reward and expectancy behavior and their derailment during drug addiction involve the recruitment of the nucleus accumbens.

All basal ganglia structures are modulated by neurotransmitter-specific projection systems, in particular by dopaminergic neurons. Dopaminergic neurons of the SN project to the neostriatum (nigrostriatal fibers), and dopaminergic neurons of the VTA project to the nucleus accumbens (mesolimbic fibers) and cortex (mesocortical fibers). The two major DA receptors in the dorsal striatum are the D_1 and D_2 receptors. The nucleus accumbens expresses primarily the D_3 receptor.

VII. Medial Temporal Lobe

The medial temporal lobe contains the amygdala, the hippocampal region, and superficial cortical areas that cover the hippocampal region and form the parahippocampal gyrus (PHG) (Figure 34-4).

The hippocampal region can be subdivided into three subregions: the dentate gyrus, the cornu ammonis sectors, and the subiculum. The neurons of the human hippocampal region are arranged in one cellular layer, the pyramidal cell layer. Most pyramidal cell layer neurons are glutamatergic whereas the small contingent of nonpyramidal cells is GABAergic. The serial circuitry of the glutamatergic neurons provides the structural basis for long-term potentiation, a physiological phenomenon crucial for formation of memory. The glutamatergic receptor crucial for the creation of long-term potentiation is the NMDA (N-methyl-D-aspartate) receptor.

The PHG receives many projections from multimodal cortical association areas and relays them to the hippocampal region. Intrinsic connections within the hippocampal region allow further processing before the information is

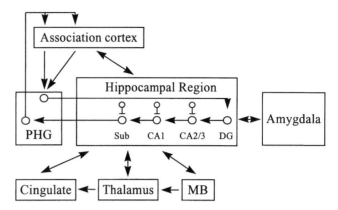

Fig. 34-4. Medial temporal lobe circuitry.

referred back to the association cortex. Some authors have argued that the reciprocal connections between the hippocampal formation and one association area, the prefrontal cortex (either directly or via the PHG), are particularly prominent.

The hippocampus is closely connected with the limbic system (e.g., via the Papez circuit). It has been proposed that the hippocampal formation is recruited via these connections to regulate emotion or to modulate information processing by attaching limbic valence to sensory stimuli.

Interactions between the frontal lobes and the medial temporal lobe are particularly important for declarative memory (i.e., the acquisition and retrieval of information about facts and events). An intricate balance of hippocampus and frontal lobes ensures that the constructive process of memory encoding and retrieval creates accurate representations of experience. Interactions between the hippocampus and the frontal cortex are crucial for the formation of memory, for conscious awareness, and for self-awareness.

Suggested Readings

Fogel BS, Schiffer RB: *Neuropsychiatry*. Baltimore: Williams and Wilkins, 1996.

Kandel ER, Schwartz J, Jessel T: *Principles of Neural Science*, 4th ed. New York: Elsevier, 1996.

Mesulam M-M: *Principles of Behavioral Neurology*. Philadelphia: FA Davis, 1985.

Chapter 35
The Neurologic Examination

ANTHONY P. WEISS AND MARTIN A. SAMUELS

I. Introduction

A. The Importance of the Neurologic Examination in Psychiatric Practice

The neurologic examination, as taught in its unabridged form, can intimidate both medical students and seasoned clinicians alike. Filled with eponymic signs and a multitude of complex maneuvers, the standard neurologic examination is often a source of confusion. Perhaps for this reason, the neurologic exam is all too often omitted by the busy clinician. It has, unfortunately, become commonplace to see the entire examination summarized as "grossly intact."

Including a thorough neurologic examination as part of a patient evaluation is especially relevant to the practice of psychiatry for several reasons:

1. **Psychiatric symptoms (affective, behavioral, or cognitive) may result directly from underlying neurologic disease** (e.g., a stroke causing mood lability). Associated sensory-motor findings on examination may uncover the underlying illness.

2. **Psychiatric symptoms may be highly comorbid in certain neurologic diseases** (e.g., the high rate of depression in Parkinson's disease, and of psychosis in Huntington's disease). In some cases, the psychiatric symptoms may predate other features of the illness, and a thorough examination by the psychiatrist may lead to early recognition and treatment.

3. **The neurologic exam is crucial for distinguishing "real" neurologic deficits from simulated deficits associated with conversion disorders or malingering.** The psychiatrist will often be called upon to clarify this diagnostic dilemma.

4. **Many psychotropic medications affect the motor systems of the brain, and lead to neurologic side effects** (e.g., dystonias, and other movement disorders). Recognition of these adverse effects is critical in the overall management of the psychiatric patient.

This chapter presents a straightforward approach to the neurologic examination, and provides the busy psychiatrist with the clinical tools necessary to handle the situations described above. This chapter assumes at least a rudimentary knowledge of neuroanatomy (see Chap. 34). While a few pertinent clinical situations will be described, the reader is referred to other chapters for discussion of specific neurologic illnesses.

B. Overview of the Complete Neurologic Examination
The neurologic examination does not need to be comprehensive in every patient. Belief to the contrary has contributed to the notion that this examination is too time-consuming and cumbersome for the busy physician. The complete neurologic exam, like any new skill, needs to be taught and practiced in its entirety. While it may be intimidating to the trainee, it is the only way to learn all of the skills that may be called upon in clinical practice. Like a football team that learns an entire play-book only to use a small portion of it in any one game, the physician needs to be facile with all of the exam tools available to be able to use specific techniques when indicated. Examination of the snout reflex may be unnecessary (and perhaps off-putting) to the 20-year-old with a numb hand, but may be an important part of a dementia evaluation.

II. Mental Status

A. Overview of the Mental Status Examination
As with the general neurologic examination, the mental status examination can appear formidable when considered in its entirety. Indeed, formal neuropsychological testing can take several hours or even days to complete. This should not dissuade the clinician from assessing a few basic components of the patient's mental state.

Given the incredible complexity of human cognitive function, it should not come as a surprise that the full mental status exam has several components (Table 35-1). In this section we will highlight a "bare bones" approach to the mental status; the reader is referred to Chapter 2 for further detail.

B. The "Psychiatric" Mental Status
The mental status examination has historically been separated into "psychiatric" and "neurologic" components. While this division is clearly arbitrary, the distinction is used here for convenience. The main components of the psychiatric mental status evaluation include (Table 35-1):

273

Table 35-1. The Complete Mental Status Examination

I. "Psychiatric"
   A. Observational assessment
      1. Dress
      2. Demeanor
      3. Attitude toward examiner
      4. Speech (rate, volume, and prosody)
      5. Motor behavior
   B. Mood/affect
   C. Thought process
   D. Thought content
      1. Obsessions
      2. Delusions
   E. Perceptual disturbances
      1. Hallucinations
      2. Illusions

II. "Neurologic"
   A. Level of consciousness
   B. Memory (verbal and nonverbal)
      1. Registration
      2. Recall
      3. Remote
   C. Language
      1. Expression (spontaneous)
      2. Comprehension
      3. Repetition
      4. Naming
      5. Reading/writing
   D. Visual-spatial/constructional
   E. Calculation
   F. Abstraction
   G. Praxis
   H. Right-left orientation
   I. Face and object recognition

1. **Observational assessment. This includes general observations of the patient's appearance, attitude toward the examiner, and overall demeanor. It also includes a description of the patient's speech and motor behavior.** These observations usually provide important clues into the patient's internal state. For example, a disheveled, unshaven man with minimal eye contact, sparse, hypophonic speech, and a general slowness of movement, might be expected to have a depressive disorder.

2. **Mood and affect.** These terms are analogous to the symptom and sign of emotional disturbance. **Mood represents how the patient feels, while affect is how the patient displays that mood to the world.** Incongruence of mood and affect, while not specific, is an important finding since it may be related to an underlying "organic" deficit.

3. **Thought process.** The expression of thought should be a goal-directed process, in which thoughts are connected and presented in a logical manner. **Abnormality of thought process lies on a continuum from subtle parenthetical comments to a complete lack of connection between ideas.** Such an abnormality will often leave the examiner confused or even wondering what question was originally asked.

4. **Thought content.** Our inner world of beliefs, convictions, and moment-to-moment ideas is hidden from even the savviest psychiatrist. **Thought content can therefore be assessed only by direct inquiry ("What are you thinking about?"), an analysis of speech, or inference from behavior.** While the line between normal and abnormal thought is sometimes blurry, most clinically relevant abnormalities (e.g., delusions) are clear.

C. **The "Neurologic" Mental Status**

This section of the mental status focuses on specific cognitive functions, and, as noted above, can involve hours or days of detailed testing (Table 35-1). **For routine purposes, the following four components comprise an adequate exam.** Unlike other features of the neurologic exam, **it is important that these components be done in order, since basic functions must be intact in order to perform more complex tasks.**

1. **Level of consciousness.** Consciousness lies on a continuum from full alertness to coma. While the two extremes are generally obvious, the middle ground of attentional deficit can be subtle. Since inattention is a hallmark of delirium (acute confusional state), a common and emergent medical condition, **attention should be tested in all patients.** Sustained attention is also a critical component for all other cognitive functioning. Some common tests of attention include:
   a. **Serial 7s.** Ask the patient to subtract 7 from 100, and then continue to serially subtract 7 from the remainder. This test is limited by its reliance on calculation, which may be more a function of education than attention.
   b. **Digit span.** Have the patient repeat a randomly presented list of digits. A normal capacity is between five and seven. Alternatively, have the patient spell a five-letter word (e.g., WORLD) backwards.

2. **Language.** Language is the means by which we present our thoughts to each other. Like other cog-

nitive functions, language can be extraordinarily complex, with entire texts of aphasiology dedicated to its study. **In general, three simple questions allow the examiner to draw valid conclusions about language in the individual patient:**

a. **Is the language *fluent* or *nonfluent*?** Independent of the actual words, does the speech sound like a language? Loss of the normal inflection and spacing of normal speech leads to nonfluent language production.

b. **Is *comprehension* normal or abnormal?** Does the patient seem to understand what you are saying? A request to complete a one- to three-step command (though complex commands may test more than just receptive language function) best assesses this. Asking simple "yes/no" questions (e.g., "Were you born in Mexico?" or "Are we in the kitchen?") is another common method.

c. **Is *repetition* normal or abnormal?** Have the patient repeat a phrase such as "no ifs ands or buts." This particular phrase is quite sensitive, given the difficulty of repeating conjunctions.

3. **Memory.** Memory function is generally divided into three components:

a. **Immediate recall.** This is the ability to hold information long enough to use it (remembering a phone number given by the operator long enough to dial it). Immediate recall is heavily dependent on attention and is tested by both digit span and phrase repetition (see above). Asking the patient to repeat three named items (piano, monkey, and blue) is another commonly used method.

b. **Short-term memory.** Short-term memory involves the ability to store information for later use. Asking the patient to reproduce the three previously named items after a span of 2–5 min is a common test.

c. **Long-term memory.** Long-term memory involves the recall of past events. This is nearly impossible to test accurately at the bedside, since the examiner is rarely privy to details of remote events from the patient's life. Asking about well-known national events or people (e.g., "How did JFK die?") is dependent on the age and educational background of the patient. Accurate assessment often requires a standardized battery of questions available in full neuropsychological testing.

4. **Visual-spatial Skills**

a. **Writing.** Have the patient write his name, address, and a sentence about the weather. Look for grammatical errors, as well as errors in spacing and overall presentation.

b. **Clock.** Have the patient fill in a circle with numbers in the form of a clock. Then ask her to set the hands at 10 minutes to 2. Abnormalities can occur in planning (poor spacing of numbers) or in positioning of the hands, which may belie a frontal lobe lesion. Complete absence of detail on one side of the clock (usually left) may represent a hemineglect syndrome associated with a (right) parietal lobe lesion.

III. Cranial Nerves

A. Olfactory Nerve (CrN I)

Testing of the first cranial nerve is almost uniformly neglected, with the entire cranial nerve examination often described as "II-XII WNL." This notation not only indicates little regard for the first cranial nerve, but also communicates little about the individual features of the exam. It should therefore be abandoned.

The first cranial nerve runs along the orbital surface of the frontal lobe, an area that is otherwise clinically silent. Lesions in this area (e.g., frontal lobe meningioma) may produce unilateral anosmia, occasionally as a unitary symptom. Routine testing of smell is therefore quite important.

Carrying a small vial of coffee is a simple and convenient method for testing smell. Each nostril should be tested separately.

B. Optic Nerve (CrN II)

The optic nerve and its posterior radiations run the entire length of the brain and produce different patterns of symptoms and signs depending on where they are compromised. **A thorough visual examination can therefore be quite informative, and involves five components:**

1. **Funduscopic examination.** The optic nerve is the only nerve that can be visualized directly. The physician should take advantage of this fact in assessing its integrity. A good funduscopic exam will also reveal much about the systemic vascular system and is a critical guide to the presence of increased intracranial pressure.

2. **Visual acuity.** Testing of visual acuity (i.e., the actual strength of vision) is frequently ignored in the adult patient. This is unfortunate since poor vision can profoundly impair a patient's functioning and is often reversible with corrective lenses or surgery. Acuity should be assessed in each eye separately while wearing current corrective lenses.

3. **Pupillary measurement.** Pupillary size represents the delicate balance between sympathetic and parasympathetic input to the ciliary muscles of the eye. The presence of abnormally large or small pupils reflects an imbalance, and may be an important sign of disease. Similarly, an inequality in pupillary size (anisocoria) can be an important hallmark of severe intracranial pathology. Each pupil should be measured in millimeters, with measurements clearly documented for further reference.

4. **Pupillary reaction.** The direct and consensual pupillary reaction to light, and the near reaction (accommodation), should be tested routinely. This

will assess any damage in either the afferent or efferent pathways that comprise the pupillary response. A penlight and close observation are all that is necessary.

5. **Confrontational visual fields.** As noted above, the visual system runs from the retina to the occipital cortex, involving a substantial area of the central nervous system (CNS). Lesions anywhere along this pathway will lead to visual field cuts. Importantly, the patient is almost never aware of this abnormality of vision; careful testing is therefore required to elucidate it. Sit directly in front of the patient, and have him look in your eyes. Test each eye separately by bringing an object (pin or wiggling finger) into each visual quadrant. For the patient who is unable to cooperate in this fashion, simply having him count fingers displayed in each quadrant is another option.

C. **Eye Movement (CrNs III, IV, and VI)**

These three cranial nerves are considered together given their relation to innervation of the extra-ocular musculature involved in eye movement. **There are two main categories of eye movement:**

1. **Saccades.** These are rapid eye movements that allow for brisk transition between items in the visual field. Saccades are tested by having the patient look to the ceiling, floor, left, and right sequentially. Asking the patient to look quickly at your finger and then the opposite thumb is another method.

2. **Pursuits.** These are slow voluntary eye movements that allow for smooth tracking of a moving target. They are tested by having the patient follow your finger through a full range of motion (up, down, left, and right).

   In assessment of eye movements, the examiner should take note of the resting position of the eye (is there a gaze preference?), the fullness of movement (are there any limitations in eye movement?), and the presence of any nystagmus (involuntary oscillation of the eyes). Any abnormality should be noted descriptively.

D. **Trigeminal Nerve (CrN V)**

The trigeminal nerve provides sensory innervation to the face (including the afferent limb of the corneal reflex), and motor innervation to the muscles of mastication. It is evaluated as follows:

1. **Facial sensation.** As with sensory testing in general (see V, below), testing sensory integrity of the face can be a frustrating exercise if the examiner insists on precision. Unless the patient has a specific sensory complaint (e.g., numb chin or facial pain), thorough testing of all sensory modalities is probably unnecessary. Testing light touch (by stroking the face with your fingers) or temperature sensitivity (using a cold metal tuning fork) is usually adequate. Asking the patient to "quantify" the degree of difference ("If this side is a dollar, how much is this side?") is generally not a fruitful exercise. Simply asking, "Does this feel normal on both sides?" saves time and will generally detect any abnormalities worth further investigation.

2. **Corneal reflex.** The corneal reflex involves the direct and consensual blink response to corneal irritation. While it can be helpful in localization of brainstem dysfunction (usually in the comatose patient), it is unfortunately both nonspecific and insensitive. It is therefore not done routinely. The reader is referred to other sources for more detailed information.

3. **Muscles of mastication.** The motor branches of the trigeminal nerve innervate the muscles that open and close the jaw. Denervation abnormalities lead to noticeable jaw malalignment. Palpation of the major muscles (masseter) and brief observation of jaw motion are sufficient in the patient without localized complaints.

E. **Facial Nerve (CrN VII)**

The facial nerve provides motor innervation to the muscles of facial expression. To assess its function, observe the overall appearance of the face, realizing that subtle facial asymmetries are common. Next, ask the patient to wrinkle her forehead, shut her eyes tightly, and smile (or show her teeth). Weakness in these muscle groups should be apparent.

The distinction between *central* and *peripheral* facial nerve palsies can be a source of great confusion (and frequent debates during morning rounds!). Central facial nerve palsy refers to a disruption of the upper motor neuron (cortico-bulbar) fibers that innervate the facial nuclei, while peripheral facial nerve palsy is a disruption of the facial nerve itself. Since there is bilateral corticobulbar innervation only to the portion of the facial nerve that subserves the forehead, a unilateral upper motor neuron (UMN) lesion will spare the forehead. A lesion of the facial nerve itself (Bell's palsy) will cause complete hemifacial weakness. This differentiation is critical since a peripheral lesion is often benign, while the central lesion may represent important intracranial pathology.

F. **The Acoustic/Vestibular Nerve (CrN VIII)**

Lesions of this nerve are an important cause of dizziness. Examination of the dizzy patient, including an assessment of the 8th cranial nerve, is covered in full detail elsewhere.

G. **Glossopharyngeal and Vagus Nerves (CrNs IX and X)**

These two nerves innervate the palate, pharynx, and larynx and are critical for speech and swallowing. Lesions of CrNs IX and X are usually clinically obvious, since they produce dysarthric or hoarse speech and drooling (due to an inability to swallow secretions). The usual method of testing these nerves, the gag reflex, is highly variable and often unhelpful. Inspection of the oral cavity is probably sufficient in the asymptomatic patient.

H. **Spinal Accessory Nerve (CrN XI)**

This nerve provides motor innervation to two muscles: the trapezius and the sternocleidomastoid. A strong shoulder shrug and head turn provide evidence of intact innervation of each muscle, respectively.

I. **Hypoglossal Nerve (CrN XII)**

The hypoglossal nerve provides motor innervation to the tongue. Denervation is usually not subtle and will often cause an audible lisp. Have the patient protrude his tongue and look for deviation to one side. Dyskinesias related to the use of neuroleptic medication (e.g., tardive dyskinesia) may be apparent. Small spontaneous movements of the protruded tongue can be a normal finding.

IV. The Motor Examination

A. **Motor Tone**

Motor tone refers to the resistance of a limb to passive movement through its normal range of motion. To examine for tone, have the patient fully relax her arms and/or legs to allow you to determine the degree of stiffness during passive motion. An increased level of tone, noted by rigidity or spasticity, is an important finding that may belie a UMN or extrapyramidal lesion (parkinsonism). Rigidity as a feature of Parkinson's disease is further discussed elsewhere in this book.

B. **Muscle Bulk**

Muscle atrophy is an important sign of lower motor neuron disease. Assessment of muscle bulk can be extraordinarily difficult, even for the seasoned clinician, due to natural variations in body habitus and the role of weightlifting or exercise (i.e., "bulking up"). Muscles that are unaffected by weightlifting or exercise (e.g., the facial muscles or the intrinsic muscles of the hand) may therefore provide the best estimate of overall muscle bulk.

C. **Motor Power (Strength)**

It is impractical (and unnecessary) to test each of the several hundred muscles in the human body. Should the patient have a focal motor complaint, knowledge of major muscle groups in the proximal and distal limbs becomes important. Muscle strength is graded from 0 (no motion) to 5 (normal strength).

Observation of gait is an excellent screening test for the patient without focal weakness. If the patient is able to rise briskly and independently from a seated position and walk independently, gross motor deficits can be confidently ruled out. The ability to walk on heels and toes further assures distal lower-extremity strength. Gait must be tested in all patients, particularly in the elderly, for whom falls are a life-threatening event.

D. **Abnormal Movements**

Abnormal involuntary movements should be noted and described. They are discussed in detail in the chapter on movement disorders (see Chap. 42).

V. The Sensory Examination

A. **Primary Sensory Modalities**

Sensation allows tactile exploration of our environment. Even the most thorough examiner could not test every square inch of the body for intact sensation, nor would this be necessary. Knowledge of the full sensory exam is important for the patient with a focal sensory complaint, and the reader is referred to other texts for detailed information on this peripheral nerve exam. The main sensory modalities include:

1. **Pain:** tested by pinprick (using disposable sterile pins).
2. **Temperature:** tested by touching the skin with a cold metal object (tuning fork).
3. **Light touch:** tested by simply brushing the patient's skin with your hand or a moving wisp of cotton.
4. **Vibration sense:** tested by applying a "buzzing" tuning fork to the distal lower extremities.
5. **Proprioception:** best tested by the Romberg maneuver (can be assessed during gait observation). Ask the patient to stand with his feet as close together as possible, while still maintaining stability. Ask him to close his eyes while assuring him that you will not let him fall. The patient with poor proprioception will begin to sway and lose balance after closing his eyes.

B. **Cortical Sensory Modalities**

The primary sensory modalities discussed above provide input to the brain about the external environment. The sensory cortex integrates these "building blocks" to form complex sensory experiences. Since higher-level sensory processing requires reliable primary input, testing these cortical sensory modalities is unnecessary in the patient with primary sensory deficits. **Two types of advanced sensory processing are recognized:**

1. **Stereognosis:** the ability to reach into your pocket and distinguish a quarter from a dime is an example of stereognosis. Simply, it is the ability to recognize objects using touch. It is tested by simply placing common objects in the patient's hand and asking her to name them with her eyes closed.

2. **Graphesthesia:** the ability to recognize numbers or letters "written" on the skin, most often using the palm. As with stereognosis, primary sensory modalities must be intact for this test to have meaning.

VI. Coordination Testing

A. Gait Testing

Coordination reflects the ability to orchestrate and control movement, and is crucial in the translation of movement into productive activity. While the cerebellum probably plays the lead role in motor coordination, several other structures (basal ganglia, red nucleus) are also clearly involved.

Walking is an extraordinarily complex motor skill that requires significant coordination of trunk and limbs. Its actual complexity makes it an ideal screening test for coordination ability. The human has a particularly narrow base when standing upright; with any degree of incoordination (ataxia), the patient will need to widen the base to remain upright. Balance becomes even more difficult when other sensory information is removed, forming the basis for the Romberg maneuver.

The sensitivity of screening is increased by having the patient walk heel to toe (as on a tightrope). The ability to do this smoothly and quickly rules out any major impairment in coordination.

B. Diadochokinesia

This term reflects the paired nature of agonist and antagonist muscle activity in coordinated limb movement. Abnormalities of this function are given the lengthy label dysdiadochokinesia, and are detected by several simple maneuvers:

1. **Finger to nose.** Have the patient alternate between touching your finger and touching her nose. Look for inaccuracy of movement (dysmetria) and presence of tremor (intention tremor).

2. **Heel to shin.** Have the patient run the heel of one foot down the shin of the opposite leg (from knee to ankle) as accurately as possible.

3. **Rapid alternating movements.** Include rapid pronation/supination of the forearm (e.g., screwing in a lightbulb), finger tapping, or toe tapping. Having

the patient tap out a rhythm is an excellent way to assess coordination ability. With cerebellar damage, the rhythm will be poorly timed, with emphases in the wrong places.

VII. Reflex Testing

A. Proprioceptive Reflexes

These reflexes, also known as deep tendon reflexes (DTRs), are based on the simple reflex arcs that are activated by stretching (or tapping). **Since they are influenced by the descending corticospinal tracts, DTRs can provide important information on the integrity of this pathway at several levels.** The reader is likely familiar with the methods used to elicit the five major DTRs: biceps, triceps, brachioradialis, quadriceps (knee), and Achilles (ankle). The grading of each reflex is on a 4-point scale, with $2 (2+)$ designated as normal.

B. Nociceptive Reflexes

These reflexes are based on reflex arcs located in the skin (rather than muscle tendons) and are therefore elicited by scratching or stroking. These include the abdominal reflexes, cremasteric reflex, and anal wink, none of which is extensively used clinically.

The major nociceptive reflex of clinical value is the plantar reflex. Stroking the sole of the foot should elicit plantar flexion of the toes. Babinski's sign, marked by an extensor response (i.e., dorsiflexion) of the toes, often with fanning of the toes and flexion of the ankle, is seen in pyramidal tract disease. It has become one of the most famous eponymic signs in all of medicine.

C. Primitive Reflexes (Release Reflexes)

These reflexes are present at birth but disappear in early infancy. Their reappearance later in life is abnormal and is often reflective of frontal lobe disease. Amongst others, they include:

1. **Grasp reflex.** Stroking the patient's palm will lead to an automatic clutching of your finger between his thumb and index finger.

2. **Snout reflex.** Gentle tapping over the patient's upper lip will cause a puckering of the lips. This may also elicit a **suck response,** or a turning of the head toward the stroking stimulus (**root reflex**).

VIII. Conclusion

The brain is an organ that is unmatched in its eloquence. Unlike the anginal grip of cardiac disease or the choking dyspnea of respiratory dysfunction, illness of the brain can send many different messages. Deciphering these messages, using the neurologic examination, can be complex, and at times bewildering. This should not discourage the practicing psychiatrist from using the examination described in this chapter as a routine part of every patient evaluation.

Suggested Readings

DeGowin RL: *DeGowin and DeGowin's Diagnostic Examination*, 6th ed. New York: McGraw-Hill, 1994.

Glick TH: *Neurologic Skills*. Boston: Blackwell Scientific, 1993.

Haerer AF: *DeJong's The Neurologic Exam*, 5th ed. Philadelphia: Lippincott-Williams and Wilkins, 1992.

Lishman WA: *Organic Psychiatry*, 3rd ed. Oxford: Blackwell Science, 1998.

Samuels MA: *Videotextbook of Neurology for the Practicing Physician*, Vol. 2: *The Neurologic Exam*. Boston: Butterworth-Heinemann, 1996.

Samuels MA: *The Manual of Neurologic Therapeutics*. Philadelphia: Lippincott-Williams and Wilkins, 1999.

Samuels MA, Feske S: *Office Practice of Neurology*. Philadelphia: WB Saunders, 1996.

Chapter 36

Neuropsychiatric Dysfunction

Stephan Heckers

I. Introduction

Psychiatrists are often challenged to bridge the disciplines of medicine, neurology, and psychiatry when faced with a patient who has behavioral abnormalities. **The neuropsychiatric evaluation combines medical, neurologic, and psychiatric skills, and includes documentation of the history, examination of the patient, and often the ordering of additional tests.**

II. General Evaluation

A. **Specific Features of the Neuropsychiatric Evaluation**
   1. **History**
      a. **An acute onset of behavioral change should always lead to a thorough search for traumatic events, including physical** (e.g., traumatic brain injury), **chemical** (e.g., hypoxia during stroke), **or psychological** (e.g., stress during a disaster) **insults. Often overlooked are neuropsychiatric sequelae of a medical condition that present some time after the initial symptoms have disappeared** (e.g., depression and anxiety after stroke).
      b. **The age of onset** of several neuropsychiatric disorders (e.g., autism, schizophrenia, mania, or dementia) is relatively well defined. When considering a diagnosis that is rare (e.g., late-onset schizophrenia or early-onset dementia) other more prevalent conditions should be ruled out.
      c. **The course and temporal pattern** (e.g., stable, progressively deteriorating, episodic, ictal) of the expression of symptoms can provide clues for the diagnosis of specific disorders, such as seizures or dementia.
   2. **Baseline mental functioning** of the patient. It is crucial to assess the degree of deficits, such as memory loss, language difficulties, or impaired judgment, and determine how this differs from the premorbid level of functioning.
   3. **Findings of the physical and mental status exam. It is helpful to organize the pattern of behavioral abnormalities along the lines of cortical and subcortical structures.** If the patient demonstrates deficits in one behavioral domain, related functions should be examined (see Table 36-1).

B. **Medical History**
   The history of present illness should document any recent surgical procedures or medical problems. For example, delirium is often seen postoperatively, after myocardial infarction, or with infections (especially when fever is present). Depression is frequently seen after stroke or can accompany a malignancy. **Particularly challenging are paraneoplastic syndromes,** such as limbic encephalitis, when neuropsychiatric deficits predate the onset of other signs of the underlying malignancy. **Any previous neurologic event or recurrent psychiatric illness,** such as psychotic disorder, anxiety, mood disorder, or drug abuse, **should be documented. Any current drug use** (including prescription, over-the-counter, and illicit drugs) **should be documented.**

C. **Examination**
   1. **Physical examination.** Abnormal **vital signs,** especially fever and tachycardia, should prompt a thorough search for systemic or central nervous system (CNS) abnormalities that could explain the neuropsychiatric dysfunction. If **signs of meningeal irritation** (neck stiffness, Kernig or Brudzinski signs) are present, a computed tomography (CT) scan of the head and lumbar puncture should be performed.
   2. **Neurological examination.** The **examination of the cranial nerves** should include **a funduscopic exam** and the testing of extraocular movements, sensory **and motor function of the face, and the gag reflex.** Tests of smell are important in patients with a history of traumatic brain injury, if an orbitofrontal process (stroke, tumor) is suspected, or in patients reporting olfactory or gustatory hallucinations. **Abnormal muscle tone** and abnormal movements of face and limbs may be seen in patients with extrapyramidal movement disorders or in patients treated with psychotropic medication. Examination of reflexes typically includes deep tendon reflexes, Babinski reflex, and primitive reflexes (snout, grasp, glabellar, and palmomental as frontal release signs). **Coordination** can be tested easily with the finger-nose-finger test or heel-shin-heel test.
   3. **Laboratory tests** to rule out many medical conditions that can lead to neuropsychiatric dysfunction should include **electrolytes, calcium, glucose, kidney, liver and thyroid function tests, a complete blood count, levels of vitamins B_{12} and folate, lues serology (such as the rapid plasma reagin [RPR]),**

281

Table 36-1. Mapping of Behavioral Abnormalities

Behavior	Region				
	Frontal	Parietal	Temporal	Striatum	Thalamus
Language	• Motor aphasia [L] • Confabulation	• Dyslexia [L] • Dysgraphia [L]	• Sensory aphasia [L]	• Dysarthria • L caudate nucleus: fluent aphasia	• Confabulation • Anterolateral thalamus: logorrheic aphasia
Affect	• Apathy • Inappropriate, disinhibited • Motor aprosodia [R]	• Sensory aprosodia [R]			
Memory	• Impaired working memory		• Impaired encoding/ recall of information		• Impaired encoding/ recall of information
Others	• Impaired attention • Poor planning, insight • Reduplicative paramnesia	• Impaired attention [R] • Dyscalculia [L]	• Prosopagnosia [L + R]		• Impaired attention
Motor	• Paresis • Abulia • Echopraxia • Perseveration • Frontal release signs	• Dyspraxia [R]		• Extrapyramidal movement disorder	

[L] and [R] indicate left (dominant) and right (nondominant) hemisphere, respectively; in some right hemisphere dominant, left-handed subjects, the hemispheric asymmetry is reversed.

GLOSSARY

Abulia	Lack of will or motivation
Agnosia	Lack of sensory ability to recognize objects
Aphasia	Impairment of language function due to brain damage
Aprosodia	Lack of pitch, rhythm, and modulation in speech
Dysarthria	Disturbance of articulation
Dyscalculia	Difficulty in computing
Dysgraphia	Difficulty in writing
Dyslexia	Difficulty in reading
Dyspraxia	Difficulty in executing purposeful movements
Echopraxia	Involuntary imitation of movements made by another person
Prosopagnosia	Difficulty in recognizing faces
Reduplicative paramnesia	Delusion that a person is replaced by an imposter (Capgras syndrome)

and a test for antibodies against the human immunodeficiency virus (HIV). Screening for drugs (illicit, therapeutic, and over-the-counter) in serum, and for cocaine and marihuana (i.e., tetrahydrocannabinol [THC]) in urine, requires permission of the patient except in an emergency.

III. Evaluation of Behavioral Domains

A. **Level of Consciousness**
The alert patient responds promptly and appropriately to sensory stimulation. **Fluctuation of the level of consciousness between alertness, drowsiness, and stupor is a hallmark of acute confusional states (delirium).** Hyperalertness can be seen in drug-induced states or severe anxiety.

B. **Appearance and Psychomotor Activity**
The patient's posture, hygiene, and clothing may provide valuable information about the patient's affect, thinking, and reality testing. **The patient's attitude** towards the physician and how he engages in the interview may provide information about his personality structure.

Abnormal motor behavior can be due to cortical, basal ganglia, cerebellar, or lower motor neuron disease. **Repetitive movements** may represent tremor, dyskinesia, or tics. **Psychomotor retardation** is often seen in depression but can also be due to hypokinetic movement disorders (e.g., Parkinson's disease), degenerative diseases (e.g., Alzheimer's disease), stroke, or catatonia. **Waxy flexibility** (i.e., the patient remains in a position modeled by the examiner) is sometimes seen in a catatonic state. **Increased psychomotor activity,** to the degree of agitation, is seen in anxious or psychotic patients, as a side effect of psychotropic medication (akathisia) mainly due to neuroleptics and selective serotonin reuptake inhibitors, or in the hyperactive form of delirium.

C. **Speech**
The flow, volume, and rate of speech should be noted.

Pressured speech often accompanies a manic state, whereas **a decreased rate of speech** may be due to depressed mood, and unexpected pauses may represent the psychotic symptom of thought blocking.

If speech is not coherent or goal-directed, more formal language testing (see below) and detailed examination of the thought process are warranted.

Prosody, the affective modulation of speech, is often impaired in patients with right hemisphere lesions, with parietal lesions affecting more the perception (sensory aprosodia) and frontal lesions more the production (motor aprosodia) of affectively modulated speech. However, aprosodia is also seen in depression or hypokinetic movement disorders.

Abnormalities of the larynx, tongue, or mouth can lead to **dysarthria,** a pure motor dysfunction which should be differentiated from aphasia.

D. **Affect**
The outward display of emotion, affect, should be differentiated from the internally felt emotion, mood. Affect is normally appropriate to the situation and congruent with mood and thinking.

Inappropriate and incongruent affect is seen in patients with schizophrenia, mania, or after frontal lobe damage. Pseudobulbar palsy can result in markedly inappropriate and incongruent affect, so-called pathological laughter or pathological crying. The range of affect and appropriate modulation can be restricted to a consistently dysthymic or anhedonic level, as in depression, or to a consistently elevated level, as seen in mania or frontal lobe damage.

E. **Thought**
Thinking is assessed appropriately by listening to the patient talking freely. The thought process should be coherent, logically organized, and goal-directed.

Loosely organized and **incoherent speech (flight of ideas and loose associations)** and an excessive use of words in response to a question, ending in the appropriate answer **(circumstantiality)** or not answering at all **(tangentiality)** are typically seen in mania. Also consider **aphasia** in a patient with incoherent speech (see below).

Poverty of thought with lack of associations is seen in depression, some forms of schizophrenia, after frontal lobe damage, and in basal ganglia disorders such as Parkinson's disease. **The thought content is the material of the patient's conversation.** Excessively recurring themes might indicate a preoccupation or a delusion. It is important to question the patient about the character of his thoughts and rule out clearly psychotic symptoms, such as thought insertion or withdrawal, and ideas of reference (e.g., the television is sending messages specifically to the patient).

F. **Perception**
The correct reception and interpretation of sensory input can be altered due to abnormalities of the peripheral sensory organs, their projections to unimodal cortical areas, or higher-order cortical areas and subcortical structures. Sensory deficits can occur at any of these three levels.

Illusions typically occur with abnormalities of the sensory organs, in drug-induced states, or in acute confusional states.

Hallucinations are often seen in psychotic disorders, but can also be found in patients with seizure, stroke, or tumor, and secondary to drug intoxication or withdrawal.

G. **Cognition**

1. **Orientation. The patient should be oriented to person, place, and time. Orientation to person is almost always preserved,** even in acute confusional states.

   Nonaphasic patients disoriented to person should be evaluated for a dissociative disorder or malingering.

   Orientation to place (by asking for the name of the city, building, floor, and type of room) or time (by asking for year, month, day, time of day) are often impaired in dementia, delirium, or an amnestic disorder. Orientation changes rapidly in acute confusional states and answers should be recorded to compare the degree of impairment.

2. **Attention. The attentional matrix provides the background for all other cognitive faculties and includes vigilance, perseverance, concentration, and resistance to interference. The reticular activating system, the thalamus, and the association cortical areas, primarily those of the frontal lobes, all contribute to the attentional matrix.** Serial recitation tasks (such as the **serial 7s**) or the **digit span** test (repeating a string of numbers forward or backwards, 6 ± 1 correct numbers in one string is normal) **are very helpful, easy to use tests to assess attention.**

   Patients with frontal lobe damage, delirium, or metabolic encephalopathy often score very poorly on such tests. However, anxious and depressed patients might also do poorly. Poor attention is seen in patients with dementia, or in children, adolescents, and adults with attention deficit disorder.

   One form of impaired attention, **unilateral neglect, is seen after lesions of the parietal cortex, the cingulate cortex, the frontal eye field, the thalamus, or the striatum.** Simple bedside tests (e.g., asking the patient to either bisect lines of varying lengths drawn on a piece of paper or cancel all letters of one type on a piece of paper covered with many different letters) are often better than testing for sensory extinction on one side after bilateral sensory stimulation.

3. **Language.** The disruption of language function interferes significantly with everyday functioning of the patient. **The assessment should include testing of repetition, comprehension, naming, reading, and writing.**

   a. Repetition can be tested with sentences such as **"No ifs, ands, or buts."** Repetition is impaired in all four major aphasic disorders involving perisylvian structures (**Broca's area** in motor aphasia, **Wernicke's area** in sensory aphasia, both areas in global aphasia, and the **arcuate fasciculus** connecting the two areas in conduction aphasia) (Table 36-2). Paraphasic errors while repeating should be recorded. Correct repetition does not mean comprehension of the language.

   b. **Comprehension can be tested by asking the patient to perform one-, two-, or three-step tasks.** Alternatively, especially when the patient is apraxic, simple yes/no questions or commands to point to body parts may be used. If a temporoparietal lesion involves Wernicke's area or its vicinity (as in lesions resulting in the sensory transcortical aphasia), comprehension will be impaired.

   c. **Naming is usually assessed by confrontation naming of objects or body parts.** Alternatively, words from a given category (e.g., animals) can be requested; normal subjects should be able to name about 12 in 1 min. Word-finding difficulties (**dysnomia**) are also seen in metabolic encephalopathy, as a side effect of psychotropic medication, and in exhaustion, anxiety, and depression. It is then important to rule out other language deficits.

   d. **Reading should be tested** by asking the patient to read individual words, sentences, or paragraphs. **Alexia** is the inability to comprehend written material. Alexia is associated with agraphia if the lesion is located in the left inferior parietal lobule.

Table 36-2. Differential Diagnosis of the Main Types of Aphasia

Type of Aphasia	Repetition	Comprehension	Speech
Global	Impaired	Impaired	Nonfluent
Wernicke	Impaired	Impaired	Fluent
Broca	Impaired	Intact	Nonfluent
Conduction	Impaired	Intact	Fluent
Transcortical			
Motor	Intact	Intact	Nonfluent
Sensory	Intact	Impaired	Fluent

e. **Writing tests** should include dictation of sentences rather than just phrases (e.g., "I'm fine"). Purely mechanical agraphia due to motor dysfunction should be excluded. Aphasia is typically associated with agraphia, but agraphia not always with aphasia.

4. **Memory. Short-term memory** may be tested by asking the patient to encode a list of three or four words and then testing the immediate and delayed recall after 5 min. Remote memory can be tested by asking for past events or famous people.

Impaired memory is seen in psychiatric disorders and as a result of a neurologic insult. In psychogenic amnesia personal events cannot be recalled, but nonpersonal information of the same time period is often spared. Psychotic disorders and depression often lead to impaired encoding of memory.

It is always important to distinguish between amnesia, an isolated memory deficit, and more global neuropsychiatric dysfunction, such as dementia or delirium, that affect more cognitive domains than just memory. Hippocampal damage due to hypoxia and hypoglycemia or damage to thalamus, mamillary bodies, and periventricular structures due to thiamine deficiency (i.e., Wernicke-Korsakoff syndrome) are well-known causes of amnestic syndromes.

5. **Visuospatial skill. Drawing intersecting geometric figures or drawing a clock (with hands indicating, for example, "10 to 2") are simple tests of visuospatial skills.** Demented or confused patients or those with lesions of the association cortex in the parietal, temporal, and frontal lobes typically show significant impairment. However, damage of the visual pathways from the retina to primary visual cortex can also result in impairment. **Damage to the parietal lobe of the nondominant hemisphere is especially prone to produce visuospatial deficits.** Such patients might also show dyspraxia (i.e., a difficulty in executing purposeful movements, such as brushing teeth, combing hair, or dressing).

H. **Abstracting Abilities**
Testing for abstract similarities (What do a plane and a car have in common?), interpretation of proverbs, or assessing practical judgment (How many slices are in a loaf of bread?) **is a helpful probe for abstracting abilities, affiliated with the dorsolateral frontal cortex.** Patients with frontal lobe damage also tend to perseverate, often adhere concretely to the material presented, and have difficulties shifting attention. However, frontal lobe deficits might not be apparent during formal testing in the office but more so by assessing the patient's level of functioning at home. Bilateral frontal lobe damage may lead to **abulia,** the lack of motivation to speak, move, or act. Other syndromes associated with frontal lobe damage are **reduplicative paramnesia (Capgras syndrome;** i.e., the delusion that a person is replaced by an imposter), and echopraxia (the involuntary imitation of movements made by another person).

I. **Insight/Judgment**
Neurologic insults leading to **unilateral neglect or anosognosia** typically cause impaired awareness and insight. Moreover, psychiatric conditions, such as mood disorders, schizophrenia, dementia, and amnestic disorders, also produce poor insight. **To assess the quality of the patient's insight, ask the patient how much the observed deficits affect him or others around him.**

IV. Summary

Patients with neuropsychiatric dysfunction present a complex diagnostic and management challenge. At times, the diagnosis can easily and quickly be made with an abnormal blood test or a very specific clinical finding. **With a good foundation in the general principles of neuropsychiatry the physician can streamline and optimize the evaluation and consultation process.**

Suggested Readings

Crum RM, Anthony JC, Bassett SS, Folstein MF: Population-based norms for the Mini-Mental State Examination by age and education level. *J Am Med Assoc* 1993; 269:2386–2391.

Damasio AR: Aphasia. *N Engl J Med* 1992; 326:531–539.

Fogel BS, Schiffer RB: *Neuropsychiatry*. Baltimore: Williams and Wilkins, 1996.

Folstein MF, Folstein SE, McHugh PR: "Mini-Mental State": a practical method of grading the cognitive state of patients for the clinician. *J Psychiatr Res* 1975; 12:189–198.

Hier DB, Gorelick PB, Shindler AG: *Topics in Behavioral Neurology and Neuropsychology*. Boston: Butterworths, 1987.

Mesulam M-M: *Principles of Behavioral Neurology*. Philadelphia: FA Davis, 1985.

Chapter 37

Clinical Neurophysiology and Electroencephalography

SHAHRAM KHOSHBIN

I. Overview

A. The Electroencephalogram

1. **Characteristics of recordings**
   a. **The electroencephalogram (EEG) records low-voltage electrical activity produced by the brain.** Recordings are often characteristic of certain ages and states of consciousness; in addition, it is possible to recognize generalized malfunction of the brain, as well as localized or paroxysmal abnormalities. **Ordinarily, the EEG is recorded from the scalp with small surface electrodes.** Although the precise origin of the electrical activity is unknown, most investigators believe that most of the activity represents dendritic synaptic potentials in the cortical pyramidal cells.
   b. **Electrical activity is recorded from a variety of standard sites on the scalp, according to the international electrode placement system.** The nasopharyngeal lead may also be employed; this is a long electrode that is passed through the nose and which rests on the back of the throat near the medial aspect of the temporal lobe.
   c. **Recording electrical activity requires the measurement of the voltage between two electrodes.** It is impossible to record from all pairs of electrodes at the same time. The typical EEG machine has eight or 16 channels. Thus, a series of electrode pairs are evaluated.
   d. **Two different styles of recording exist. In the referential (or monopolar) method,** a series of different electrodes are referred to the same reference electrode, which is presumed to be relatively electrically inactive. Commonly used reference points are the ears, the vertex, or a noncephalic reference. In another method, **the bipolar method,** electrodes placed in a line are recorded serially as successive pairs. (The first recording would be from the first and second electrodes, the second recording would be from the second and third electrodes, and so on.) Creation of different montages gives various views of the electrical activity at different parts of the brain.
   e. **The electrical activity from any electrode pair can be described in terms of amplitude and frequency.** Amplitude ranges from 5 V to 200 V. Frequency of EEG activity ranges from 0 Hz to about 20 Hz. **The frequencies are described by Greek letters: delta (0–4 Hz), theta (4–8 Hz), alpha (8–12 Hz), and beta (more than 12 Hz).**
2. **Recordings during sleep**
   a. **In the normal awake adult (with eyes closed), alpha rhythm seen in the posterior part of the head predominates.** The amplitude of the alpha waves falls off ante-

riorly and it is often replaced by low-voltage beta activity. Often, some low-voltage theta activity can be seen in frontocentral or temporal regions. **The alpha rhythm, which is prominent posteriorly, disappears (or is blocked) when the eyes open.**
   b. **When a normal adult becomes drowsy, the alpha rhythm gradually disappears, frontocentral beta activity may become more prominent, and frontocentral-temporal theta activity becomes predominant.**
   c. **Drowsiness is stage I sleep.** As sleep becomes deeper, high-voltage single or complex theta or delta waves, called vertex sharp waves, appear centrally.
   d. **Stage II sleep is characterized by increased numbers of vertex sharp waves, and centrally predominant runs of sinusoidal 12–14 Hz activity, called sleep spindles, occur.**
   e. Deeper sleep, characterized by progressively more and higher-voltage theta and delta activity, is not usually seen in routine EEG recordings.
   f. In routine EEG studies, some **"activations" (3 min of hyperventilation and a flashing strobe light at different frequencies) are employed to try to bring out abnormalities** not apparent in the record without the activations. Drugs can be used in certain circumstances to activate epileptic activity. Convulsants (such as pentylenetetrazol) could be used for this purpose.
3. **EEG abnormalities**
   a. **Abnormalities of the EEG are either focal (only one area of the brain), or generalized (whole brain).** Additionally, abnormalities are **either continuous or intermittent. An abnormality which appears and disappears suddenly is called paroxysmal.**
   b. **Increased "slow activity"** (i.e., theta and delta activity in a waking record) **is nearly always abnormal.**
   c. Focal delta activity is usually irregular in configuration and is termed polymorphic delta activity (PDA). PDA is usually indicative of a focal lesion of brain. Another type of delta activity is called **FIRDA (frontal intermittent rhythmic delta activity);** this is indicative of increased intracranial pressure in young people and is a less specific sign of some brain abnormality in the elderly. Generalized theta and delta activity is a sign of an encephalopathy. As a general rule, the EEG is a sensitive test for abnormalities, but it is not specific.
   d. Increased beta activity is often a sign that the patient is taking some kind of sedative.
4. **Seizure disorders**
   a. **The EEG has been particularly useful in the analysis of patients with seizure disorders. Paroxysmal abnormal-**

ities are common between overt seizures (interictally) as well as during seizures (ictally). Paroxysmal abnormalities include the spike and the sharp wave.

b. A **spike** is a single wave which stands out from the background activity and has a duration of less than 80 msec. A **sharp wave** is similar with a duration of more than 80 msec. A spike or sharp wave is often followed by a slow wave and spikes and slow waves can alternate at frequencies from 2 Hz to 5 Hz.

c. **Epileptic paroxysmal abnormalities can be generalized or focal.** The classic generalized abnormality is the 3 Hz spike and wave pattern which underlies the petit mal absence attack. A typical focal abnormality is a focal single spike followed by a slow wave. This abnormality can be seen in focal epilepsy or in grand mal epilepsy if the abnormal electric activity spreads rapidly to the entire brain.

d. **Activations, such as hyperventilation, photic stimulation, sleep, sleep deprivation, and use of drugs, are useful in bringing out epileptic activity.** On any one record, it is possible to miss epileptic activity that is infrequent; for this reason multiple recordings are useful.

e. The relationship of any of these abnormalities to the particular patient is complex. For example, **paroxysmal activity on an EEG may or may not mean that the patient's problem is related to epilepsy;** the final determination typically rests on the overall clinical picture and on the results of a therapeutic trial. One should resist the temptation to consider the EEG independently. In particular, a normal EEG does not exclude epilepsy, since (to cite an extreme case) the EEG may be normal during a focal seizure which is observed clinically. Reading EEGs is tricky; it takes experience since there are a wide variety of normal variant wave forms and artifacts that must be recognized.

II. Evoked Potentials

A. Overview

1. **A sensory stimulus in any modality (visual, auditory, or somatosensory) will produce a change in the EEG.** The change is usually small in magnitude compared to the background EEG; **the exact configuration of the change depends on the nature of the stimulus and the site of recording on the scalp.**

2. **The evoked potential is the change in the EEG which is dependent on and time-locked to the stimulus; to see it, the stimulus must be repeated many times and the EEG averaged.**

3. **Evoked potentials can be used to test the integrity of a pathway in the central nervous system (CNS). The most common use of evoked potentials at present is to test the speed of conduction in a particular pathway.** Multiple sclerosis is a disease of central myelin; if myelin is damaged, conduction is slowed and the evoked potentials will be delayed. Although many multiple sclerosis plaques are clinically silent they show themselves with this electrical test. Hence, evoked potentials are quite useful in making the diagnosis of multiple sclerosis.

B. Visual Evoked Potentials

1. Visual evoked potentials (VEPs) were the first to become popular. They **are ordinarily obtained with a checkerboard stimulus that alternates black and white squares repetitively. Each eye is stimulated individually and then responses are measured from the occipital area of the scalp.** The major wave measured is a large positive wave at a latency of about 100 msec. In multiple sclerosis or optic neuritis, the wave is delayed. Delayed or absent VEPs can be seen in many other conditions, including ocular conditions (e.g., glaucoma), compressive lesions of the optic nerve (e.g., pituitary lesions), and pathological conditions of the optic radiations or the occipital cortex.

C. Auditory Evoked Potentials

1. **Auditory stimulation produces complex waveforms.** Stimulation with brief clicks produces six small waves in the first 10 msec. Quite surprisingly, **the sources of this electrical activity are in serial ascending structures in the brainstem.** It becomes possible to study the integrity of the brainstem with these waves, and the test has also been used to assess "brainstem death" in cases suspected of "brain death." The waves are also delayed in multiple sclerosis.

D. Somatosensory Evoked Potentials

1. Somatosensory evoked potentials (SEPs) **are the averaged electrical responses in the CNS to somatosensory stimulation.** Like sensory action potentials (SAPs) in the peripheral nervous system, **most components of SEPs represent activity carried in the large sensory fibers of the dorsal column** (medial lemniscus primary sensorimotor cortex pathway). SEPs can be used to test the integrity of the pathway and to test the speed of conduction in the pathway.

2. SEPs from the upper extremity are commonly produced by stimulation of the median nerve at the wrist. The cerebral SEP to this type of stimulation was the first EP to be discovered (by Dawson in 1947). The cerebral SEP to median nerve stimulation is best recorded from a site approximately 2 cm posterior to the contralateral central electrode. SEPs from the lower extremity are produced by stimulation of the posterior tibial nerve at the ankle or the peroneal nerve at the fibular head.

3. **It is possible to localize a lesion in the somatosensory pathway by using short latency SEPs from subcorti-**

cal structures. Several systems of electrode placement can be used, but the one which seems to produce potentials of greatest amplitude is where the active electrode is placed over the cervical spine and referred to an "inactive" site. By stimulating leg nerves, it is possible to obtain EPs at all levels of the neuraxis, including over the spinal cord.

III. Nerve Conduction

A. Sensory Nerve Conduction

1. **The cell bodies of sensory neurons are located in the dorsal root ganglia.** Each neuron has a central process entering the spinal cord through the dorsal horn and a peripheral process connecting to a sensory receptor in the skin or deep tissues of the limb. **The receptors transduce somatosensory stimuli into electrical potentials, which eventually give rise to action potentials in the axons which are transmitted along the peripheral process to the central process.** There are a variety of sensory neurons, each with a characteristic spectrum of axonal diameters. Some neurons are myelinated while some are unmyelinated; in routine studies the unmyelinated fibers cannot be measured. **Many sensory axons with differing function and size run together with motor axons.**

2. **The goals of sensory nerve conduction studies are:**
   a. To assess the number of functioning axons.
   b. To assess the state of the myelin of these axons.

3. Nerve conduction studies
   a. **In the usual sensory nerve conduction study, all of the axons in a sensory nerve are activated with a pulse of electric current.** Action potentials travel along the nerve and the electric field produced by these action potentials is recorded at a site distant from the site of stimulation. **Each axon makes a contribution to the magnitude of the electrical field and thus the amplitude of the recorded sensory action potential is a measure of the number of functioning axons.**
   b. **Utilizing the distance between the site of stimulation and the site of recording and the time between stimulation and the arrival of the action potentials at the recording site, it is possible to calculate a conduction velocity which reflects the quality of myelin of the axons.**
   c. **In axonal degeneration neuropathies, the primary feature is reduced sensory action potential amplitudes.** The conduction velocity may be slightly slowed, but only to the extent that the normally largest axons are gone and the measured conduction velocity reflects the velocity of the largest remaining axons. In demyelinating neuropathies, the primary feature is slowing of conduction. In radiculopathies, sensory action potential amplitudes and conduction velocities are fully normal. This is because the lesion is virtually always proximal to the dorsal root ganglion and the cell body and its peripheral process remain normal. Sensory action potential similarly remains normal with lesions of the CNS.

B. Motor Nerve Conduction

1. **There are significant differences between sensory and motor nerve conduction which depend in large part on the differences of the anatomy in the two situations.** Motor neurons have cell bodies in the anterior horn of the spinal cord and send their axons to innervate muscle fibers. **Motor axons are always intertwined with sensory axons; there are no nerves that are pure motor nerves. Hence, the electrically stimulated compound action potential of any nerve with motor fibers in it is really a mixed nerve action potential.** Consequently, it is not possible to deduce the number of functioning motor axons by looking at the amplitude of a nerve action potential.

2. It is possible to study motor nerve axons separately from sensory axons by electrically stimulating a nerve and by recording from the muscle fibers innervated by the motor axons in that nerve. Since each motor axon typically innervates hundreds of muscle fibers, the compound muscle action potential is very much larger than the nerve action potential.

3. The number of axons can be diminished and the action potential normal if the process of collateral re-innervation by the remaining axons has been complete. The number of axons can be normal and the action potential diminished if there is a neuromuscular junction deficit or if there is loss of muscle fibers. As a neuropathy progresses and collateral re-innervation fails to keep pace, then the muscle action potential will decline.

4. **The time interval between delivery of the electrical stimulus and the onset of the muscle action potential may be difficult to interpret.** This time period is composed of the time it takes for the motor nerve action potential to travel down the terminal branches of the axon, the time for the release of acetylcholine into the neuromuscular junction, the time for the acetylcholine to produce an endplate potential, the time for generation of a muscle action potential, and, depending on the position of the recording electrodes, the time for the muscle action potential to propagate to the recording electrodes. Calculation of a conduction velocity for these neurons is not as straightforward as it is for the sensory nerve. The time period itself, if obtained under standard conditions, can be a useful measure of the conduction time in the terminal part of the axon; it is called the distal motor latency.

5. The conduction velocity of motor axons can be determined for parts of the axon proximal to the distal portion. If the nerve is stimulated supramaximally in two places, then virtually identical muscle action potentials will result; the major difference will be the different latencies from the time of stimulation. The difference in the latencies is due to the difference in the distances from the sites of stimulation to the muscle. Dividing the difference in the distances by the difference in the times produces a conduction velocity for the segment of nerve between the two sites of stimulation. Similar to the measurement of the sensory action potential, measurements of the muscle action potential are ordinarily made to the time of onset; hence, the calculated conduction velocity refers to the fastest (and largest) axons in the nerve.

6. **In axonal degeneration neuropathies, motor nerve conduction studies are not significantly abnormal until the process is moderately advanced.** Total reliance on motor nerve conduction would result in failure to detect many significant neuropathies. Typically, there will be a slight slowing of conduction velocity and prolongation of the distal motor latency since the largest axons are lost. There may be loss of action potential amplitude when the process is advanced. In demyelinating neuropathies, there will be slowing of conduction velocity and prolongation of distal motor latency.

7. **A focal lesion of a nerve will lead to slowing of conduction and to a decrement of amplitude across the segment, including the area of the lesion, but studies of the nerve distal to the lesion will be fully normal.** Studies of nerve segments proximal to the lesion will show normal conduction velocity with an unchanging and reduced action potential amplitude. Quite dramatic nerve conduction findings are seen with a focal, total lesion. The nerve is fully normal below the lesion but electrical stimulation proximal to the lesion produces no response (similar to the patient's attempts to activate the muscle).

8. **In radiculopathy, motor nerve conduction studies will ordinarily be normal.** There may be slight slowing of conduction velocity in direct relation to the amount of loss of large fibers. In CNS disease, there will ordinarily be no change in motor nerve conduction unless there is involvement of anterior horn cells.

C. Late Responses
1. **Studying the most proximal segments of nerves is difficult, because they are deep and not easily accessible as they leave the spinal column.**

However, it is useful to study the proximal segments of nerves since processes, such as radiculopathies from disc protrusion and certain neuropathies (e.g., Guillain-Barré), affect this segment predominantly. **The so-called late responses (the E-reflex and the F-response) provide a relatively easy technique for study of the proximal segments of nerves. These responses are produced in certain circumstances after an electrical stimulus to a peripheral nerve, and are late with respect to the muscle response (the M-response) produced by the orthodromic volley of action potentials traveling to the muscle directly from the electrical stimulus.**

2. **The H-reflex is a monosynaptic reflex response similar in its pathway to that of the tendon jerk.** The electrical stimulus activates the I-a afferents (coming from the muscle spindles) and action potentials travel orthodromically to the spinal cord. In the cord, the I-a afferents make excitatory monosynaptic connections to the alpha motor neurons; a volley of action potentials is set up in the motor nerve which runs orthodromically the entire length of the nerve from the cell bodies to the muscle. Hence, action potentials travel through the proximal segment of the nerve twice during the production of the H-reflex (once in the sensory portion of the nerve and once in the motor portion). **Obtaining an H-reflex depends on the ability to stimulate the I-a afferents.** If a motor axon is electrically stimulated, then an action potential will travel along the axon antidromically toward the spinal cord as well as orthodromically toward the muscle. The antidromic action potential will collide either in the proximal motor axon or in cell body with the developing H-reflex in that axon and nullify it. In routine clinical practice, it is possible to get this differential stimulation and to produce E-reflexes only in the posterior tibial division of the sciatic nerve while recording from the triceps surae.

3. **The F-response or F-wave has an advantage over the H-reflex in that it can be found in most muscles. It is a manifestation of recurrent firing of an anterior horn cell after it has been invaded by an antidromic action potential.** After a motor nerve is stimulated, an action potential runs antidromically as well as orthodromically; a small percentage of anterior horn cells that have been invaded antidromically will produce an orthodromic action potential that is responsible for the F-response. Thus, to produce an F-response, action potentials must travel twice through the proximal segment of the motor nerve.

IV. Electromyography

A. The Physiology Underlying EMG

1. Understanding the concept of the motor unit is central to the understanding of the physiology of electromyography (EMG). **A motor unit is composed of all the muscle fibers innervated by a single anterior horn cell. In most proximal limb muscles there are hundreds of fibers in each motor unit. In the normal situation, the muscle fibers from the same unit are not clumped together, but are intermingled with fibers from other motor units. When a motor axon fires, each muscle fiber in its motor unit is activated in a constant time relationship to the other fibers in the unit.**

2. **EMG activity is ordinarily recorded with a needle placed into the muscle.** Because the muscle fibers of a single motor unit are not packed closely together, **the EMG needle records from only about ten fibers from each motor unit. The amplitude, duration, and configuration of the electrical activity recorded from a motor unit varies as the needle changes its orientation to the muscle fibers.** Despite its variability it is possible to specify a normal range for the amplitude, duration, and configuration of motor unit action potentials (MUAPs) for each muscle and each age.

3. **When an EMG needle is placed in a normal muscle at rest, there is no electrical activity. With weak effort, first one and then several motor units are activated.** At this low level of activation, it is possible to see the individual MUAPs and evaluate their parameters. With maximal effort so many units are brought into action that individual MUAPs cannot be discerned; all that can be seen is a dense electrical pattern, called an interference pattern, which can be characterized by its density and peak-to-peak amplitude. The normal density would be either "full," if there are no gaps, or "highly mixed," if there are a few, short gaps. Some people are not willing or able to exert a maximal effort and the pattern will be less dense as a result. Hence, the degree of effort has to be taken into account when assessing the interference pattern.

B. Findings on the EMG

1. **Acute partial injury (e.g., a partial laceration of a nerve).** Motor axons that are injured undergo Wallerian degeneration over the course of about 5 days, leaving muscle fibers previously innervated by those axons in a denervated state. **Within approximately 10–14 days, denervated muscle fiber action potentials are recorded by the EMG needle as fibrillations and positive sharp waves.** There is nothing different about fibrillations and positive sharp waves other than a slight difference in the particulars of the recording; both are simply small, diphasic potentials beginning with a positive phase. The motor units that can be activated will be normal; it will not be possible to activate voluntarily the denervated muscle fibers. Descriptive terminology for these patterns is "high mixed," "mixed," "low mixed," and "single unit," in order of decreasing density.

2. **Chronic partial injury. After weeks to months there will be collateral sprouting from surviving motor axons to innervate denervated muscle fibers.** Spontaneous activity will cease. Motor units will now contain more muscle fibers than normal; hence, MUAPs will be long in duration, high in amplitude, and more complex in shape or polyphasic. The interference pattern may improve in density, but probably will remain less than full although the amplitude will increase.

3. **Complete injury. In this circumstance no voluntarily initiated motor nerve action potentials can reach the muscle due to a focal demyelinating injury. Muscle fibers will not be denervated so they will not fibrillate.** EMG examination will reveal no spontaneous activity, no MUAPs, and no interference pattern. This is no different from the first few days of a total injury; after these first days the denervated muscle fibers begin to fibrillate.

4. **Myopathy. The simple model of myopathy is characterized by dropout of individual muscle fibers from their motor units. In active myopathies, especially polymyositis, there may be some segmental muscle necrosis.** This process divides a muscle fiber into an innervated segment and an uninnervated segment. The uninnervated segment might fibrillate and, hence, result in active myopathies, some fibrillation, and positive sharp waves; most commonly spontaneous activity is lacking.

Suggested Readings

Aminoff MJ: *Electrodiagnosis in Clinical Neurology*. New York: Churchill Livingstone, 1980.

Asselman P, Chadwick DW, Marsden CD: Visual evoked responses in the diagnosis and management of patients suspected of multiple sclerosis. *Brain* 1975; 98:261–282.

Goodgold J: *Anatomical Correlates of Clinical Electromyography*. Baltimore: Williams and Wilkins, 1974.

Halliday AM, McDonald WI, Mushin J: Delayed visual evoked response in optic neuritis. *Lancet* 1972; i:982–985.

Johnson EW (ed.): *Practical Electromyography*. Baltimore: Williams and Wilkins, 1980.

Jones SJ: Short latency potentials recorded from neck and scalp following median nerve stimulation in man. *Electroencephalogr Clin Neurophysiol* 1977; 43:853–863.

Khoshbin S, Hallet, M: Somatosensory evoked potentials in the diagnosis of MS: Comparison with other evoked potentials and blink reflex. *Neurology* 1978; 28:388.

Khoshbin S, Hallet M: Pattern reversal visual evoked potentials in patients with multiple sclerosis. In Smith JL (ed.): *Neuro Ophthalmology-Focus.* 1980:229–235.

Khoshbin S, Hallet M: Multimodality evoked potentials and blink reflex in multiple sclerosis. *Neurology* 1981; 31:138–144.

Kiloh LG, McComas AJ, Osselton JW: *Clinical Electroencephalography*, 3rd ed. London: Butterworths, 1972.

Klass DW, Daly DD: *Current Practice of Clinical Electroencephalography.* New York: Raven Press, 1979.

Kosi KA, Tucker RP, Marshall RE: *Fundamentals of Electroencephalography*, 2nd ed. Hagerstrom, MD: Harper and Row, 1978.

Picton TW, Hink RF: Evoked potentials, How? What? and Why? *Am J EEG Technol* 1974; 14:9–44.

Robinson J, Rudge P: Abnormalities of auditory evoked potentials in patients with multiple sclerosis. *Brain* 1977; 100:19–40.

Shahrokhi F, Chiappa K, Young R: Pattern shift visual evoked responses. *Arch Neurol* 1978; 35:65–71.

Shibasaki H, Yamashita Y, Tsuji S: Somatosensory evoked potentials: diagnostic criteria and abnormalities in cerebral lesions. *J Neurol Sci* 1977; 34:427–439.

Starr A: Sensory evoked potentials in clinical disorders of the nervous system. *Annu Rev Neurosci* 1978; 1:103–137.

Starr A, Joseph A: Auditory brain responses in neurologic disease. *Arch Neurol* 1979; 29:827–834.

Stockard J, Stockard J, Sharbrough FW: Detection and localization of occult lesions with brainstem auditory responses. *Mayo Clin Proc* 1977; 52:761–769.

Chapter 38
Seizure Disorders (Epilepsy)

SHAHRAM KHOSHBIN

I. Overview

Psychiatrists often play an important role in the diagnosis, initiation of therapy, and long-term management of seizure disorders. Frequently, one must rely on behavioral manifestations to make the diagnosis, yet epileptic behavior is often difficult to distinguish from nonepileptic behavior. **A seizure is defined as an episodic and paroxysmal change in behavior, usually associated with an alteration in or loss of consciousness.** It can be precipitated by a variety of systemic pathophysiological processes (e.g., fever), or by metabolic derangements (e.g., hypoglycemia), or by toxic reactions. **Epilepsy is characterized by recurrent paroxysmal abnormalities in brain function associated with abnormal electrical discharges from neuronal aggregates.** Epileptic seizures are usually brief and self-limited.

Both in terms of its physical and psychological effects, and its associated social stigma, epilepsy can be disabling (e.g., seizures may prevent an epileptic patient from driving a car, or piloting an aircraft), and also presents special problems during pregnancy. Management is often challenging, because an individual patient may require different types of treatment at different times, and because inappropriate therapy may actually *worsen* the patient's condition.

II. Models for Classifying Epilepsy

A. Focal Models

In the mid-19th century, **John Hughlings Jackson,** the father of the British school of neurology, proposed **the focal model of epilepsy.** Jackson hypothesized that, when a lesion developed in a particular part of the brain, function of that area would be affected during a seizure. In 1860, Jackson described the case of Dr Z (the pseudonym of a British physician who often corresponded with Jackson). Dr Z had written that he had spells during which he smelled a noxious odor. On the basis of this description, Jackson suggested that these spells were epileptic seizures, a revolutionary idea, since Jackson's contemporaries viewed epilepsy as a disorder that caused a person to fall on the ground, jerk uncontrollably, and foam at the mouth. Jackson also guessed that Dr Z must have had a lesion in the uncinate region of the temporal lobe, a portion of the brain associated with the sense of smell. His hypothesis was later confirmed on autopsy.

B. The Centrencephalic Model

In the 1950s, the prominent **Canadian neurosurgeon, Wilder Penfield,** proposed **the centrencephalic model of epilepsy.** Working with the **American electroencephalographer, Jasper,** Penfield found that **some of his epileptic patients had seizures in which the electroencephalographic (EEG) manifestations were bilateral and symmetrical.** He postulated that these seizures originated in the central area of the brainstem, a region Penfield named the centrencephalon.

C. The International Classification of Epilepsy

These two models (focal and centrencephalic) provide the basis for the current international classification of epilepsy adopted by epileptologists in 1971 and modified twice in the interim. According to this classification (Table 38-1), **epileptic seizures are considered as either partial (consistent with the focal model) or generalized (consistent with the centrencephalic model).** In persons with partial seizures, neuroimaging techniques, such as magnetic resonance imaging (MRI), have made it relatively easy to detect brain lesions (e.g., tumors, stroke, vascular malformations), and even ventricular asymmetries or very small lesions that previously could be detected only on biopsy. **In contrast, findings on neuroimaging in patients with generalized seizures are usually unremarkable. In most cases of generalized seizures, the etiology is either metabolic or unknown.**

D. Seizure Symptoms

1. **Changes in consciousness provide important clues to the nature of the seizure. Patients invariably lose consciousness during generalized seizures, or when a partial seizure spreads to the centrencephalon and becomes secondarily generalized. The important difference, however, is that in partial seizures the loss of consciousness is preceded by a sensation known as an "aura"** (from the Greek word for "cold breeze"). In AD 175, the Greek physician Galen first used the term aura to describe the case of a young boy who mentioned that prior to his seizure he felt a "breeze blowing upon him," referring to what we now know to be a partial

Table 38-1. Classification of Epileptic Seizures

Generalized seizures (convulsive or nonconvulsive)
- Tonic-clonic seizures (grand mal)
- Absence seizures (petit mal)
- Minor motor seizures (myoclonic and atonic)

Partial seizures (focal, local)
- Simple partial (without impairment of consciousness)
  Focal motor seizures (Jacksonian)
  Somatosensory and special sensory
  Autonomic
  Psychic
- Complex partial (with impairment of consciousness)
  Motor symptoms (automatisms)
  Sensory symptoms
  Affective symptoms
  Psychic (cognitive) symptoms

seizure that becomes secondarily generalized. Patients with temporal lobe epilepsy (complex partial seizures) often describe the feeling that something is rising over the chest towards their throat. An aura may take one of several forms, from sensations of dizziness to attacks of fear and depression. As in the case of Dr Z, the type of aura may offer a clue to the location of the lesion.

2. In order to classify seizure disorders, the physician should carefully question the patient about his or her state of consciousness at the time of the seizure. **If the patient remains conscious during the episode, the seizure is classified as "partial;" if the patient loses consciousness with no warning, the seizure is "generalized," or "secondarily generalized" if an aura precedes the loss of consciousness.**

3. Once the seizure has been classified, appropriate additional tests can be selected. For strictly generalized seizures, the physician should evaluate the patient for metabolic disorders, including hyponatremia, hypokalemia, hypocalcemia, and hypoglycemia, as well as withdrawal from alcohol or other drugs. In the adult population, de novo generalized seizures nearly always have a metabolic origin. **Since some apparently generalized seizures are actually secondarily generalized, all adult patients should be evaluated for brain lesions.**

4. The incidence of partial seizures is very high in adults. In such cases the physician should rely on computed tomography (CT) or MRI to detect the associated scar, tumor, or other lesion.

5. Although it was once believed that patients should not be examined immediately after a seizure because the findings would be meaningless, in fact the opposite is true. **Patients should always be examined after a seizure to detect any evidence of asymmetry** (e.g., weakness or twitching that is more pronounced in one arm than in the other). Such evidence would indicate a focal rather than a generalized seizure.

6. **Since patients often have preconceived notions about the type of epilepsy they have, the physician should always ask for a detailed description of the seizures rather than accepting the patient's reported "diagnosis" or accepting it at face value.** Patients often mistakenly assume that "petit mal" simply means a relatively minor seizure and that "grand mal" means a major seizure. However, the distinction between the different types of epilepsy is considerably more complex. Nearly half of all adult patients will claim they have petit mal epilepsy, but this condition usually occurs in children between the ages of 2 and 9 years and is almost never seen in adult patients.

III. Generalized Seizures

Although there are seven distinct types of generalized seizures, the events are usually classified into three major groups: major motor seizures, absence seizures, and minor motor seizures.

A. Grand Mal (Tonic-Clonic or Major Motor) Seizures

1. **Grand mal seizures are the most common type of generalized seizure;** they also occur when a partial seizure becomes secondarily generalized.

2. **In a purely generalized grand mal seizure the first event is loss of consciousness; the patient will be unaware of what has happened.**

3. **The second event is the tonic stage, characterized by contraction of the skeletal muscles, extension of the axial musculature, upward deviation of the eyes, and paralysis of the respiratory muscles** due to thoracoabdominal contractions. This stage is brief, ranging from only about 3 sec to a maximum of 30 sec, although it may seem longer because of its dramatic appearance.

4. **The most striking feature is extension of the upper and lower extremities into a semi-opisthotonic posture.** Sudden spasm of the respiratory muscles results in forced exhalation that may sound like scream, the so-called epileptic cry. **Although contraction of the respiratory muscles causes the patient to stop breathing, it is not a cause for concern, since the tonic stage lasts only a few seconds.**

5. As the muscles of mastication go into spasm the patient may bite down hard. Contrary to popular belief, the patient will not swallow his or her tongue, so objects such as a spoon or tongue

depressor should not be inserted forcefully into the patient's mouth. In the young patient, this action could also dislodge a loose tooth, which could later be aspirated. Once the tonic phase is over, insertion of a short, plastic airway will prevent injury.

6. **Eye movements that occur during the tonic stage can provide clues as to the nature of the seizure. In a generalized seizure, the eyes deviate directly upwards, whereas in focal seizures, particularly those involving the frontal lobe, the eyes deviate to either the right or the left.** Even inexperienced observers tend to notice whether the patient's eyes moved straight up or to one side.

7. The best approach to the tonic stage is to observe the patient and to take any necessary measures to prevent inadvertent injury.

8. **Once the tonic stage ends, the patient enters the clonic stage, which is characterized by rhythmic jerking movements.** Clonic movements have a high amplitude and low frequency, unlike myoclonic movements, which are very brief, or tremors, which have a low amplitude and high frequency. **In a generalized seizure, clonic movements are symmetrical, with the arms and legs moving in unison.** Clonic arm movements generally have greater amplitude than clonic leg movements, and the trunk is usually not involved. You may recall that, on drawings of the homunculus which is used to represent parts of the body and the corresponding areas of the brain that govern them, the face and hands are large but the body is very small. **(This relative lack of trunk movement is an important point to recognize because it may help distinguish a grand mal seizure from a pseudoseizure.** When patients experiencing pseudoseizures are attempting to move, they will often move their trunk.)

9. The clonic stage generally lasts between 3 and 7 min, after which time the patient is usually conscious but confused. **If after 7 min the patient either does not wake up or has another seizure, the diagnosis is status epilepticus.**

10. Grand mal seizures are also characterized by symptoms (some of which may alarm the inexperienced physician) involving the autonomic nervous system. **Hippus, in which the pupils alternately contract and dilate in a rhythmic pattern, is common, but occasionally the pupils may either contract or dilate.** It is often useful to examine the pupils during a seizure, even in patients on a respirator, since hippus can be a sign of seizures. Other common autonomic signs include changes in facial color to either pallid or flushed, excessive salivation to the point of drooling, increased heart rate and blood pressure, increasing intravesicular pressure, and

---

Table 38-2. Management of Status Epilepticus

Immediate
- Insert short oral airway/suction
- Establish continuous ECG and monitor blood pressure every 2–3 min
- Sample venous blood for glucose, electrolytes, BUN, and levels of anticonvulsant drug
- Measure arterial pO_2, pCO_2, and pH

Within 5 min
- Administer normal saline and thiamine IV
- Administer 50 ml 50% normal glucose
- Administer a benzodiazepine IV
  EITHER diazepam (2 mg/min, max 10 mg), for short action
  OR lorazepam (2 mg/min, max 8 mg), for longer action
- Start phenytoin IV in normal saline, no faster than 50 mg/min, to a total dose of 15–20 mg/kg
- Watch for hypotension!

Within 30 min (if seizures have not stopped)
- Intubate
- Add
  EITHER phenobarbital IV, no faster than 100 mg/min, for a total dose of 10–20 mg/kg
  OR benzodiazepine-diazepam (50 mg in 500 ml D5W at 40 ml/h)
  OR midazolam (0.1–0.4 mg/kg/h)
  OR paraldehyde (0.1–0.2 ml/kg rectally)
  OR lidocaine (50–100 mg IV push)

Within 1 h (if seizure persists)
- General anesthesia with halothane and neuromuscular blockade

---

relaxation of the urinary and anal sphincters (resulting in incontinence or defecation).

11. **Once patients regain consciousness after a grand mal seizure, they enter the postictal period in which they typically fall asleep for about 2 h and wake up with headache.**

12. Physicians rarely see their epileptic patients in the throes of a grand mal seizure because the 3–7-min event is usually over by the time they arrive. Because the event ends naturally within a few minutes, it may not be necessary to administer medication unless the patient has repeated seizures.

B. Absence Seizures

1. **The second group of generalized seizures, which includes petit mal, are referred to as absence seizures. Absence seizures occur mainly during childhood and are rare after puberty. They are characterized by the arrest or suspension of consciousness for 5–10 sec.** Although a mother might say that her son appears healthy, and may not notice the typically brief seizures, his teacher will report that the boy stares absently for short intervals throughout the day. **Without treatment, petit mal seizures occur about 70–100 times a day,** and such frequent blackouts can seriously impair a child's school performance.

2. **If petit mal epilepsy is suspected, the physician can usually confirm the diagnosis by asking the child to hyperventilate, since this maneuver will precipitate an attack.**

3. **Once you have seen a petit mal attack, you will never forget it. The child will seem to be looking straight through you.** Other signs include **rhythmic blinking** (at a rate of 3 blinks/sec), and **rudimentary motor behaviors called automatisms,** which also occur in adult temporal lobe epilepsy. Petit mal epilepsy is the easiest seizure disorder to diagnose because of its pathognomonic EEG (a spike-and-wave pattern that occurs at a frequency of 3 cycles/sec), especially when the child hyperventilates.

C. Minor Motor Seizures

The most common types of minor motor seizures are myoclonic and akinetic seizures. Although these seizures usually occur in childhood, adults may sometimes experience them.

1. **Myoclonic seizures are characterized by sudden, brief muscular contractions that may occur singly or repetitively.** One type of myoclonic epilepsy of childhood is **West syndrome or infantile spasms,** which typically appear at about 6 months of age and consist of sudden abduction of the upper extremity and flexion of the hip and knees. This disorder has a poor prognosis in terms of both intellectual development and long-term survival. Myoclonic seizures may also occur in adolescents with gray matter disease and in adults with viral infections, such as encephalitis. Unfortunately, these seizures will probably become more common in the years ahead as a result of the increasing prevalence of infections due to the human immunodeficiency virus (HIV); they may also occur in association with dialysis dementia.

2. Unlike myoclonic seizures, **akinetic seizures are characterized by a loss of muscle tone.** The appearance depends on the muscles affected. "Head bobbing" occurs if the neck loses muscle tone, "bending seizures" occur if the upper extremities are affected, and "drop attacks" occur if the lower extremities are involved. However, it is much more common for children to faint than to have akinetic seizures. Although not diagnostic, the EEG is often helpful in identifying akinetic seizures. **A typical pattern consists of slow spikes and waves (or polyspikes and waves), even during the periods between seizures.** In contrast, patients with syncope have a normal EEG.

IV. Partial Seizures

As described above, partial seizures follow Jackson's focal model of epilepsy and are associated with brain lesions. **These disorders are usually classified as either simple or complex, depending on whether or not consciousness is affected.**

A. Simple Partial Seizures

1. **In a simple partial seizure, consciousness is maintained.** Since much of the motor cortex is devoted to controlling the face and hands, focal motor seizures most commonly affect these parts of the body. **Motor movements may spread along the body, usually starting in the hands and then affecting other areas, such as the face and the upper half of the body. This is known as the "Jacksonian march."** (There is almost never movement of the hip or trunk.) Motor seizures may also occur when the lesion (particularly a tumor) affects the frontal lobe. Turning of the head and eyes away from the side of the focus is an adversive seizure. In what is sometimes called a **fencing seizure,** the arm also flexes ipsilateral to the focus and extends contralateral to the focus. These signs indicate frontal lobe lesions affecting areas 6 and 8.

2. **Sylvian seizures are benign motor seizures that involve the tongue and may lead to aspiration.** They are seen in adolescents, usually at night, and generally disappear once the child reaches adulthood. Although the seizure itself is benign, the potential for fatal aspiration makes it essential to diagnose and treat this condition appropriately. Fortunately, sylvian seizures are easily controlled with phenytoin.

3. **Simple partial seizures also include a large subgroup of sensory seizures that can sometimes be difficult to diagnose. The vertiginous seizure, originating in the temporal lobe, is probably the most common type of sensory seizure;** unfortunately, dizziness has a broad differential diagnosis. Somatosensory seizures are usually described as a tingling feeling (paresthesia), or by a sensation of heat or water

running over the affected area; this sensation may spread rapidly from one body part to another. Rarely, a patient will report pain or a burning sensation as well as various auras. When a somatosensory seizure causes tingling of the hands and face the physician may attribute this finding to a transient ischemic attack (TIA) involving the middle cerebral artery. **Unlike TIAs, which may start abruptly but end gradually, somatosensory seizures both begin and end abruptly.** Although the differential diagnosis of tingling of the hands and face should also include migraines, which begin gradually and spread slowly to other parts of the body, these differ from somatosensory seizures, in which spread is rapid.

4. **Auditory seizures are produced by discharges in the anterior transverse temporal gyrus (Heschl's convolution) and the superior temporal convolution. The patient reports tinnitus typically in the form of hissing, buzzing, or roaring sounds. Visual seizures, produced by discharges from the occipital focus, take the form of flickering lights or flashing colors (usually red or white), and are distinct from the "zigzag" pattern of light sometimes reported by patients experiencing migraine. It is worth noting that nearly all epileptic patients have migrainous headaches and many migraine sufferers have abnormal EEGs.** Despite the overlap between these two conditions, the visual features just described can help one distinguish migraine from simple partial seizures due to epilepsy.

B. **Complex Partial Seizures**

These are the most common type of seizures seen in adult medicine. They are characterized by an alteration of consciousness as well as by other complex manifestations; they are also the most difficult to diagnose and to treat. **Patients *may* experience any or all of four symptom types: psychomotor, psychosensory, cognitive, and affective.**

1. **Psychomotor symptoms or "automatisms" may take the form of simple vegetative movements, or complex actions, such as disrobing. The most common automatisms are oral and buccal movements (e.g., lip smacking, licking, or chewing), and the picking behavior sometimes seen in patients with dementia.** In some cases, these individuals may pick at their skin to the point of maceration. Walking is one of the most interesting automatisms that may occur during a complex partial seizure. The physician should not attempt to prevent such behavior during a seizure because the patient may become violent if restrained. When questioned about their behavior, patients often say they have the urge to leave their present location, and some may drive off or go to the bus station or airport out of a desire to travel. **Psychomotor symptomatology also includes staring behavior similar to that seen in petit mal epilepsy. However, unlike petit mal seizures, which last only about 6 sec, staring episodes in complex partial seizures typically last about 1–3 min (i.e., long enough to be recognized).**

2. **Psychosensory symptoms include visual, auditory, and other sensory symptoms. Although psychosensory symptoms are most often due to a lesion in the temporal lobe, they may also be caused by a parietal lobe lesion. Patients generally describe their psychosensory symptoms as being similar to some other sensation or experience.** For example, the patient may describe the sensation of insects crawling under the skin—a common paresthesia called formication (from *formica*, the Latin word for "ant"). This may at least partially explain the scratching or picking automatisms seen in some patients. The visual phenomenon is not merely flashes of lights, but true hallucinations, such as the detonation of a bomb or "fireworks." **Olfactory or uncinate fits are also common and usually take the form of a noxious smell** (e.g., burning rubber) or a metallic taste. It is important to question patients about olfactory or gustatory symptoms, because they generally do not mention these sensations unless asked directly.

3. **Cognitive symptoms may be simple or take the form of hallucinatory experiences similar to those reported by patients with psychosis. Unlike psychotic hallucinations, which may take various forms in the individual patient, the hallucinations that occur as part of a complex partial seizure are stereotypical and repetitive.** Patients commonly envision scenes involving water.

   a. **Visual distortions.** The perception that objects are getting bigger (macropsia) or smaller (micropsia) may also be reported. The British mathematician and author Lewis Carroll had temporal lobe epilepsy. In a sense, Carroll's *Alice in Wonderland* may be considered a long description of visual phenomena such as those experienced in temporal lobe epilepsy—things shrinking and growing, passing through mirrors, and so forth.

   b. **Other cognitive symptoms include the feeling of familiarity known as *déjà vu* (French for "already seen") and, more commonly, the feeling of unfamiliarity referred to as *jamais vu* (French for "never seen").** Children generally find it easy to describe jamais vu, whereas adults find the sensation confusing and disturbing.

4. **Affective symptoms, or ictal emotions, are another characteristic of complex partial seizures.** In some cases patients with affective symptoms do not rea-

lize they are having a seizure. **Since fear and anxiety are the most common affective symptoms reported in temporal lobe epilepsy, it is always important to rule out this possibility during the differential diagnosis of panic disorders.** The diagnosis of complex partial seizures is further complicated by the fact that depression is such a common affective symptom in the general population. However, unlike other types of depression, depression related to seizures begins and ends abruptly. Pleasant ictal feelings may also occur, but they are very rare. Some females may experience orgasms; the only corresponding feeling in the male genitalia is an uncomfortable penile sensation.

   a. Although rage reactions and aggression are sometimes reported in temporal lobe epilepsy, these behaviors are extremely rare.

   b. Aggressive behavior generally occurs late in a seizure and is usually undirected. For instance, a patient might punch into the air, but he is unlikely to attack his mother-in-law.

V. Evaluation of Seizure Disorders

A. Obtaining a Description of the Seizure
As described above, the physician should begin by obtaining a detailed description of the patient's seizures. Although the physical examination is almost always normal, a few signs may provide clues to the diagnosis. Since patients with epilepsy often have a history of brain lesions at an early age, the physician should **look for evidence of hematrophy.** For example, if a patient is asked to place his hands palm to palm, you may find that one hand is smaller than the other. In partial complex seizures, the physical expression of an emotional response may be asymmetrical (e.g., a smile is almost always one-sided). **In about 80% of patients with asymmetrical emotional responses or reflexes, the responsible brain lesion is in the hemisphere opposite the weaker side of the body.**

B. Obtain an EEG
Although the EEG is a valuable tool for diagnosing seizure disorders in pediatric patients, it has only limited value in adults. Nevertheless, **physicians should obtain an EEG if they suspect a seizure disorder. It is often possible to increase the yield of an EEG by asking the patient what events or stimuli seem to trigger a seizure and then trying to reproduce these in a controlled setting.** For instance, if a patient says he has seizures after a sleepless night, you might ask him to remain awake one night and then come in for an EEG the following day. In other patients, you might be able to induce abnormal brain activity by asking them to hyperventilate or by exposing them to a flashing light. To detect EEG abnormalities one must be careful to place the electrodes in the proper positions. Most temporal lobe lesions are on the mesial aspect of the lobe, so the physician should ask the EEG technician to place nasopharyngeal electrodes or surface electrodes on the zygoma or to use special sphenoidal electrodes.

For patients with focal seizures, MRI is better than CT, in which bone artifact can obscure the temporal lobe. If a patient has a lesion on the temporal lobe, a coronal MRI section will usually reveal that the entire lobe is smaller, the ventricle is dilated, or the hippocampus is smaller. MRI scans may also reveal gliosis, which cannot be detected on CT scans. CT should be used only if MRI is not available or if there is no time to arrange for an MRI evaluation.

VI. Behavioral Changes in Epilepsy

A. Interictal Personality Changes
Geschwind described the following five interesting types of personality changes associated with partial complex epilepsy: hypergraphia, hyperreligiosity, hyposexuality, aggressivity, and viscosity. The Russian author Fyodor Dostoyevsky is perhaps the best-known example of an epileptic with hypergraphia, which is the tendency to write prolifically.

Some patients with epilepsy are **deeply interested in religion,** although not necessarily one of the world's major religions.

In some adult patients the onset of seizures coincides with a **sudden loss of interest in sex.** Since patients rarely volunteer this information, the physician should make a point of asking whether they have noticed any change in their sexual desire. Some patients with temporal lobe epilepsy also report a change in their sexual preference.

Aggressivity, the fourth type of personality change associated with epilepsy, **is distinct from the automatic aggressive behavior occasionally seen during seizures.** Again, patients often do not volunteer information about this type of personality change. If patients are asked about their temper, they may become defensive or evasive. Upon further questioning, you might learn that they engage in aggressive behavior, such as breaking dishes or throwing objects out of a window.

Finally, some epileptic patients develop a personality trait Geschwind called viscosity, meaning that the patients tend to be "sticky." For example, some patients with temporal lobe epilepsy may call you every night, and, once they start talking, they won't stop.

These five characteristic personality disturbances provide evidence that brain lesions can cause long-term changes in behavior.

VII. Therapy of Seizure Disorders

A. Historical Notes

1. Perhaps the first description of an authentic treatment for epilepsy appeared in the Book of Mark in the New Testament. Mark described how Jesus advised a man with falling sickness (epilepsy) to pray for 3 days. For Jesus (who was still Jewish at the time), prayer also implied fasting. When the man prayed and fasted for 3 days, he naturally developed ketosis, which stopped his seizures. Physicians now recognize that **a "ketogenic diet"** (i.e., **a diet high in saturated fats,** such as butter and cream) is one of the most effective ways to halt myoclonic and akinetic seizures. Thus, Jesus might be considered the world's first epileptologist.

2. Despite this promising beginning nearly 2,000 years ago, the treatment of seizure disorders remained in the "Dark Ages" until relatively recently. The dramatic seizures and interictal behavioral changes, which are seen particularly in patients with complex partial seizures, may account for the fear and superstitions that have impeded the scientific study of epilepsy.

3. **Initially, bromides were used by Sir Charles Lockock to treat catamenial disorders, including epilepsy. In the early 20th century, physicians first recognized the anticonvulsant effects of phenobarbital,** and, later, of other barbiturates. Today, phenobarbital is reserved for those epileptic patients who cannot take drugs orally, other than phenytoin and the benzodiazepines. Phenobarbital is the only antiepileptic agent that may be given intravenously. Only one other barbiturate, primidone, is still used because it is effective in treating complex partial seizures.

B. Phenytoin

1. **Oral and intravenous phenytoin has been the mainstay of epilepsy treatment since it was first used in the 1930s by two Boston physicians, Houston Merritt and Hillary Putnam. Although the usual oral dosage for adults is 100 mg three times a day, the dose prescribed should actually be based on serum levels, which should be in the range of 10–20 μg/mL,** which is easy to achieve in the oral form. If phenytoin is given intravenously, it must be delivered in a normal saline solution; if a 5% dextrose solution is used, the drug will precipitate out and be ineffective. One can determine when the drug has reached therapeutic levels by measuring the serum concentration or looking for nystagmus. If the concentration reaches toxic levels, ataxia will develop.

2. **The main side effect of phenytoin is drowsiness,** which may be a major concern to many patients. To ensure compliance, the physician should warn patients about this potential effect and assure them that it is only temporary. Phenytoin is generally not prescribed during adolescence since it may induce hirsutism, acne, and gingival hyperplasia.

3. **Some patients may develop important medical complications, including megaloblastic anemia and osteopenia.** In general, the anemia will develop quickly and should be treated with vitamin B_{12} and folate. Osteopenia may develop over a long period of time in female patients and may lead to pathologic fractures. Some patients are allergic to phenytoin and develop erythema multiforme and Stevens-Johnson syndrome up to 2 months after the start of therapy. It is important to inform patients about the manifestations of Stevens-Johnson syndrome and emphasize that they should seek immediate medical attention at the first sign of this potentially fatal condition.

C. Carbamazepine

The anticonvulsant carbamazepine is the drug of choice for temporal lobe epilepsy. The typical dosage for adults is 200 mg three times a day, with **serum levels in the range of 4–12 μg/mL. The major side effects of this agent are bone marrow suppression and hepatic toxicity.** Like the related drug imipramine, carbamazepine also acts as an antidepressant.

D. Valproate

Although valproate is considered the drug of choice for generalized seizures in children, it is now widely used in adult epilepsy. The usual adult dosage is 250 mg three times a day, with **serum levels in the range of 50–100 μg/mL.** The most significant side effects of valproate are alopecia and hepatotoxicity.

E. Other Anticonvulsants

For more detailed information on newer anticonvulsants (e.g., lamotrigine, gabapentin, topiramate, tigabine, and vigabatrin) see Chap. 49 (Anticonvulsants).

Suggested Readings

Bear DM, Fedio P: Quantitative analysis of interictal behavior in temporal lobe epilepsy. *Arch Neurol* 1977; 34:454–467.

Blumer D: Temporal lobe epilepsy and its psychiatric significance. In Benson D, Blumer D (eds): *Psychiatric Aspects of*

Neurological Disease. New York: Grune and Stratton, 1975.

Delgado-Escuela AV, et al.: Current concepts in neurology. Management of status epilepticus. *N Engl J Med* 1982; 306:1337.

Furkenstein H, Khoshbin S: Seizure disorders. In Branch WT (ed.): *Office Practice of Internal Medicine*. Philadelphia: WB Saunders, 1987.

Gastaut H: Clinical and electroencephalographical classification of epileptic seizures. *Epilepsia* 1969; 10 (Suppl.):1–28.

Geschwind N: Behavioral change in temporal lobe epilepsy. *Arch Neurol* 1977; 34:453.

Hughes JR, Olson SF: An investigation of eight different types of temporal lobe discharges. *Epilepsia* 1981; 22:421–435.

Khoshbin S: Van Gogh's malady and other cases of Geschwind's syndrome. *Neurology* 1986; 36 (Suppl.):213–214.

Khoshbin S: Clinical neurophysiology of aggressive behavior. *Clin Electroencephalogr* 1989; 1:74–75.

Khoshbin S, Dawson DM: Epilepsy. An update. In Tyler HR, Dawson DM (eds): *Current Neurology*, Vol. 2. Boston: Houghton-Mifflin, 1979:219–229.

Khoshbin S, Levin L, Milrod L, Carlson L, Hallett M: Cortical evoked potential mapping in complex partial seizures. *Neurology* 1984; 34 (Suppl.):219.

Mayeux R, et al.: Interictal memory and language impairment in temporal lobe epilepsy. *Neurology* 1980; 30:120–125.

Penfield W, Jasper M: *Epilepsy and Functional Anatomy of the Human Brain*. Boston: Little, Brown, 1954.

Slater E, Beard AW: Schizophrenia-like psychoses of epilepsy. *Br J Psychiatry* 1963; 209:95–150.

Stevens JR: Interictal clinical manifestations of complex partial seizures. *Adv Neurol* 1975; 11:85–107.

Waxman SG, Geschwind N: Hypergraphia in temporal lobe epilepsy. *Neurology* 1974; 24:629–634.

Woodbury DM, et al. (eds): *Antiepileptic Drugs*, 2nd ed. New York: Raven Press, 1982.

Chapter 39
Headache

EDWARD R. NORRIS AND MARTIN A. SAMUELS

I. Introduction

Headache is one of the most frequent complaints heard in medical practice, and is the most common reason for referral to a neurologist. Headache is so common that almost everyone has had at least one headache, and 90% of Americans have at least occasional headaches. The majority of these are migraine, tension, or cluster headaches. **While most headache sufferers treat themselves, patients who do see a doctor are always in pain and are often worried about a serious underlying disease, often brain tumor, aneurysm, or stroke.**

II. Evaluation of the Patient with a Headache

A. **Medical History**
   Taking a good headache history is the most important step in the diagnosis of the patient. Typically, with the information derived from the history and the physical examination, a diagnosis can be made reliably.
   1. The optimal history begins with the asking of open-ended questions in a supportive environment.
   2. The history must identify:
      a. The severity and character of the headache
      b. The onset and duration of the headache
      c. Precipitating and ameliorating factors
      d. The effect of medications
      e. Other associated symptoms
   3. Acute or steadily progressive headaches are often signs of life-threatening diseases of the brain, including temporal arteritis, intracranial mass lesions, pseudotumor cerebri, meningitis, and subarachnoid hemorrhage.
B. **Examination**
   The examination of a headache patient must include a neurological examination, a funduscopic examination, and a physical examination of the head.
   1. The neurological examination is aimed at excluding lateralized or focal findings, especially on visual field confrontation, and testing of strength and gait.
   2. A funduscopic examination searches for papilledema.
   3. A physical examination of the head includes observing, palpating for tenderness or masses, and listening over the temples and eyes for bruits.

C. **Ancillary Tests**
   It is unusual for any test to demonstrate an abnormality not suggested by the history and the physical examination. A test is indicated when the history suggests a specific diagnosis (e.g., epilepsy or tumor), **the headaches develop a new quality or become intractable, the history is atypical** (e.g., trigeminal neuralgia in a young patient that may suggest multiple sclerosis), **or when the neurological examination is abnormal.**
   1. Imaging with a noncontrast, computed tomography (CT) scan of the head has no risk and will pick up all important causes of headache; magnetic resonance imaging (MRI) of the head is more sensitive and expensive.
   2. A lumbar puncture is indicated when elevation of intracranial pressure or infection is suspected.
   3. An elevated erythrocyte sedimentation rate (e.g., 70–80 mm/h) suggests giant cell arteritis in an elderly person with new-onset headache.
   4. An electroencephalogram (EEG), evoked responses, and an angiogram are rarely indicated in the evaluation of headache.

III. Headache Syndromes

A. **Migraine**
   Migraine headaches are a type of vascular headache. The term vascular headache is somewhat of a misnomer because the name implies that the cause is entirely related to blood vessels, **whereas most evidence indicates that the cause is an abnormality in neurotransmitters** (e.g., substance P), which deal with pain perceptions, with inconsistent secondary vascular phenomena. **The term vascular is meant to emphasize the pulsating nature of the pain.** The frequency and severity of vascular headaches occur on a spectrum from infrequent brief pains to daily severe migraine headaches.
   1. Migraine headaches are common and **prevalence in females is estimated at 20%. The ratio of females to males is 3:2. There is a family history in 90% of patients.**
   2. **Individual migraine symptoms are usually stereotypic** and recurrent for every patient. Migraine headaches present with a **unilateral pulsating headache,** often in the frontotemporal region. **Photophobia**

301

and phonophobia are common features, indicative of sensory hypersensitivity. Autonomic dysfunction and disability often accompany the migraine and can cause nausea, vomiting, and slow gastric emptying. Personality changes can also occur.

3. Migraine patients usually have a life history that varies with age. The history starts early with infants who have colic, and the young child often has episodic abdominal pain. The headaches begin in puberty and wax and wane throughout life, often with long headache-free intervals. Vascular headaches often improve in middle age. **The headache can last from seconds to days, but usually lasts from 4 to 24 h.**

4. Patients are usually the best informants on what precipitates their headaches. Many foods, such as **aged cheese, red wine, chocolate, and peanuts,** can precipitate migraines. **Skipping meals, too little or too much sleep,** and other **psychological stresses can aggravate vascular headaches.** Birth control pills can make headache better or worse, and pregnancy often ameliorates the vascular headache.

5. Common migraines (migraine without aura) are more frequent. However, **migraine headaches can be preceded by an aura** (migraine with aura). Auras can be moving visual lights, but can include visual field cuts (**scotoma**) and flashing zigzag lines (**scintillations**). The aura usually lasts 20 min. **The aura can consist of any particular transient alteration in any neurological function.**

6. There are a range of treatments available for the migraine patient. Reduction of aggravating factors (e.g., caffeine intake, alcohol [especially red wine], chocolate, and peanuts) can reduce headache frequency.

   Abortive treatment is effective for patients who have infrequent headaches. It is important to treat early at the onset of headache or aura. The most common reason for poor efficacy of treatment is the time delay until the patient takes the medication. **The two most effective treatments are subcutaneous sumatriptan or rectal indomethacin.** Oral medications are not well absorbed due to poor gastric emptying. However, metoclopremide (Reglan) can be used to empty the stomach; then oral sumatriptan or indomethacin can be administered.

   Prophylactic treatment is necessary for patients with frequent headaches. Lipophilic beta-blockers are the most effective (e.g., propranolol, atenolol, or nadolol). Ciproheptadine (Periactin), a weak serotonergic blocking drug, is effective in many cases. Anticholinergic tricyclics (e.g., amitriptyline) are used effectively.

Status migrainosis is diagnosed when a migraine lasts longer than 72 h. Steroids in a rapid taper can abort longer migraine headaches. When this is ineffective, intravenous barbiturates are used to induce coma.

B. Cluster Headaches

1. Unlike migraine headaches, **cluster headaches do not have a family history. The prevalence is estimated at less than 0.4%. The ratio of males to females is 5:1.**

2. The aptly named **cluster headache occurs in clusters of one to eight times daily for several weeks.** The headache **pain is often sharp and retro-orbital. Autonomic dysfunction is present,** with injected conjunctiva, nasal blockage, profuse sweating, facial flushing, ptosis, or miosis.

3. The onset is usually in middle-aged men and may have a cyclical pattern that occurs in the spring. **The cluster headache pain peaks in 5–10 min and can last up to 3 h.**

4. Persons with cluster headaches are sensitive to alcohol. Cluster headaches often occur several hours after going to sleep and are not relieved by sleep. Tobacco smoking can also precipitate headache.

5. **Treatments to abort headaches include 100% oxygen by mask for 15 min, or vasoconstrictive medications and sumatriptan.** Prophylactic treatment includes use of calcium channel blockers (e.g., verapamil), or lithium carbonate (aimed at achieving blood levels of 0.6–1.0 mmol/L).

C. Tension-Type Headaches

1. **Tension headaches are a misnomer because no associated muscle tension can be demonstrated.** A family history is common and the prevalence is higher in women than in men.

2. **The pain is band-like around the head.** It can be generalized or located in the frontal, occipital, or cervical areas. It is not associated with photophobia or phonophobia.

3. The onset is usually brief and the pain is worse during the day.

4. **Tension-type headaches can be precipitated by stress.** They are **often relieved by alcohol.** Exercise, jogging, neck massage, hot bath, or other stress-relieving activity can often ameliorate symptoms.

5. Many **nonmedical treatments,** including biofeedback, relaxation techniques, physical therapy, and stress reduction, are effective. Patients should avoid expensive or potentially harmful strategies. Benzodiazepines and narcotics, although effective, should be avoided.

D. Headaches Due to Substances and/or Their Withdrawal
1. **Iatrogenic headaches are caused by medicines.** The addition or withdrawal of a medication or substance can precipitate them. People who have migraine or other headaches and who use medications to treat their original headache encounter these headaches. The diagnosis is confirmed after exclusion of other causes.
2. These headaches are not usually associated with nausea, a throbbing sensation, or hypersensitivity. They can mirror the symptoms of tension headaches.
3. **The onset occurs after the discontinuation or addition of a substance.** This type of headache can last many weeks without treatment.
4. These headaches are precipitated by the addition of nitroglycerin or isosorbide. The withdrawal of external substances, including caffeine, can cause headache. The withdrawal of any substance used to treat headaches, including aspirin, acetaminophen, nonsteroidal anti-inflammatory drugs (NSAIDs), and narcotics, can precipitate headaches.
5. **Discontinuation of the causative substance or reintroduction of the substance that was withdrawn effectively stops the headache.** A brief course and taper of steroids (e.g., prednisone 30 mg/day, 20 mg/day, 10 mg/day) can help break the cycle.

IV. Secondary Headaches

These headaches often do not follow a characteristic pattern of the preceding headaches. Structural causes should be suspected with an abnormal neurological examination or when the headache is acute or progressive.

A. Trigeminal Neuralgia (Tic Douloureux)
1. **This type of headache is common in patients over the age of 60 years. The usual cause is compression of the trigeminal nerve root by a cerebral blood vessel** at its origin from the brainstem. Occurrence in young people may suggest multiple sclerosis with a plaque involving the trigeminal nerve root.
2. **Trigeminal neuralgia is manifested by brief (20–30 sec) jabs of sharp pain that extend along the three divisions of the 5th cranial nerve.** The pain usually subsides at night.
3. Unlike other headaches, **stimulation of affected areas by touch, eating, or drinking cold liquids results in a sharp pain.**
4. Injection of an anesthetic in the nerve root can stop the pain. Use of carbamazepine is often helpful. In refractory cases, surgical placement of a barrier between the vessel and the trigeminal nerve may be necessary.

B. Temporal Arteritis (Giant Cell Arteritis)
1. **Patients with temporal arteritis are usually older than 55 years.** Although the etiology is unknown, **histology reveals inflammation of giant cells of arteries.** The erythrocyte sedimentation rate (ESR) is usually greater than 40 mm/h.
2. The pain is typically a dull, continuous headache in the temples; in advanced stages, the temporal arteries appear inflamed.
3. Chewing can precipitate the pain (**jaw claudication**).
4. Treatment with high-dose steroids is standard; untreated arteries can occlude, causing blindness or stroke.

C. Intracranial Mass Lesions
1. **Headaches from mass lesions are caused by an increase in intracranial pressure.**
2. **The pain is often bilateral, dull, and mild.** Papilledema is often absent. Subtle personality and cognitive changes are usually present. **Lateralized neurological signs often occur** within weeks of the onset of symptoms.
3. An increase in intracranial pressure by bending or coughing can worsen headaches.
4. Treatment is the removal of the mass-causing lesion.

D. Pseudotumor Cerebri (Benign Intracranial Hypertension)
1. **These headaches usually occur in young obese women,** sometimes with menstrual abnormalities. **They have idiopathic cerebral edema.**
2. The headache is a dull, generalized pain. Papilledema is usually present. Unlike the mass-lesion headache, there is no alteration in personality or cognitive function.
3. **Treatment includes serial lumbar punctures to relieve symptoms.** Diuretics are helpful, as is a steroid taper. Dieting can also reduce headache severity. Surgical placement of a shunt may be used in refractory cases.

E. Headaches Secondary to Infections
1. **Acute meningitis is usually caused by *Meningococcus* or *Pneumococcus*;** it often occurs in small epidemics in confined areas. **Acute meningitis is associated with a rapid onset of a severe headache with photophobia, fever, nuchal rigidity, and malaise.**
2. **Chronic meningitis occurs most frequently in people with compromised immune systems,** especially people with acquired immunodeficiency syndrome (AIDS), those on steroids, or the elderly. Chronic meningitis is associated with a continuous dull headache, with symptoms of systemic illness and cognitive decline.

3. **Herpes simplex encephalitis has a predilection for the inferior surface of the frontal and temporal lobes. It causes fever, somnolence, delirium, and complex partial seizures with amnesia.**

4. **Diagnosis is facilitated by lumbar puncture and a head scan. Treatment with appropriate antibiotics is the cure.**

F. **Subarachnoid Hemorrhage**

1. **The cause of subarachnoid hemorrhage is rupture of a cerebral artery, usually from the circle of Willis.** This is usually caused by a poor joining of vessels of the circle of Willis during development.

2. Hypertensive crises by ingestion of tyramine by patients on monoamine oxidase inhibitor (MAOI) antidepressants can also cause subarachnoid hemorrhage.

3. **A severe headache with nuchal rigidity is the most common symptom. A sentinel bleed or leak with milder headache can occur during exercise, with straining, or during sexual intercourse.**

4. **Diagnosis is made by lumbar puncture or a head scan.**

5. **Treatment is the repair of the leaking or ruptured blood vessel.** Intravanous phentolamine (Regitine), an alpha-adrenergic blocking agent, should be used in patients with MAOI-related hypertensive headaches.

G. **Posttraumatic Headache**

1. **Up to half of all people with concussions can have headaches for 2 months after the incident.** Acceleration and deceleration forces of the injury can cause shear injury to neurons. Litigation is often the pathogenesis of the headache.

2. **Posttraumatic headaches usually occur within 14 days of head injury and resemble migraine or tension headaches.** Nausea, vomiting, dizziness, vertigo, and mood symptoms can occur.

3. Treatment is the same as for tension and migraine headaches. Benzodiazepines and narcotics should be avoided.

H. **Low Cerebrospinal Fluid (CSF) Pressure Headaches**

1. Postlumbar puncture headaches are the most common of this type, but headaches can occur following trauma, an operation, or with idiopathic CSF leaks.

2. **Pain is bilateral, and nausea, blurred vision, photophobia, and postural syncope are often present.** They usually last several days and rarely persist for weeks.

3. **The pain is worse within 15 min of the patient sitting or standing, and worsened by cough, strain, or head movement. It is relieved within 30 min of lying flat.**

4. **Remaining flat in bed and taking analgesics are the most effective treatments.** Injection of sterile autologous blood (blood patch) in the epidural space can seal the leak.

V. Conclusions

1. **Headache is common; 90% of Americans have at least occasional headache.** Patients who are seen for evaluation of headache are always in pain and worried about a serious underlying disease.

2. Evaluation of headache involves taking a careful history with identification of the severity and character of the pain, the onset and duration of the pain, the precipitating and ameliorating factors, the effect of medications, and other associated symptoms.

3. **Examination of the patient must include a neurological examination** focused on excluding lateralized or focal findings, **a funduscopic examination, and a physical examination of the head.**

4. **Migraine, cluster, and tension-type headaches account for the majority of headache syndromes.**

5. Patients with headaches that do not follow a characteristic pattern or have an abnormal neurological examination require a thorough workup for organic etiologies.

Suggested Readings

Baldassano C: Approach to the patient with headache. In Stern TA, Herman JB, Slavin PS (eds): *The MGH Guide to Psychiatry in Primary Care.* New York: McGraw-Hill, 1998:61–65.

Kaufman DM: *Clinical Neurology for Psychiatrists*, 4th ed. Philadelphia: WB Saunders, 1995:197–220.

Samuels MA: *Video Textbook of Neurology for the Practicing Physician.* Butterworth-Heinemann, Boston, 1997.

Singer EJ: Neuropsychiatric Aspects of headache. In Kaplan HI, Sadock BJ (eds): *Comprehensive Textbook of Psychiatry VI*, 6th ed. Baltimore: William and Wilkins, 1995:251–257.

Chapter 40

Pain

MENEKSE ALPAY AND NED H. CASSEM

I. Introduction

Pain is a common, yet complex and challenging symptom. It is defined by the International Association for the Study of Pain as "an unpleasant sensory and emotional experience arising from the actual or potential tissue damage or described in terms of such damage." Nociception is the neural mechanism of detection of noxious stimuli; it is not synonymous with pain. An individual's affective state, previous conditioning, and endogenous system of analgesia all affect the experience of pain. Frequently, a multidisciplinary approach is effective in pain control and restoration of function. To manage pain in a timely and effective manner, a variety of terms and mechanisms need to be understood.

II. Pathophysiology of Pain

A. Nociception
Differentiation of somatic pain (involves activation of nociceptors in peripheral tissues) and visceral pain (involves activation of nociceptors in bodily organs) can be problematic. Somatic pain is usually well localized, is attributable to certain anatomical structures or areas, **and is characteristically described as stabbing, aching, or throbbing. Visceral pain is typically poorly localized,** not necessarily attributable to the involved organ (e.g., referred pain), **and is characteristically described as dull and crampy.**

B. Peripheral Conduction of Nociception
Pain originating from the skin is often used as the model for nociception. Nociceptors in the skin transduce mechanical, thermal, and chemical stimuli into action potentials. **When tissue is injured, nociceptors are stimulated by the liberation of prostaglandins, arachidonic acid, histamine, and bradykinin.** Aspirin, acetaminophen, steroids, and nonsteroidal anti-inflammatory drugs (NSAIDs) act at this stage of the pain pathway.

Subsequently, axons transmit the pain to cell bodies in the dorsal root ganglia in the spinal cord. **Three different types of axons are involved in transmission of painful stimuli from skin to the dorsal horn. They are classified by their diameters; their velocity increases as the diameter and thickness of the myelin sheath increase** (see Fig. 40-1).

1. **A-β fibers** are the largest and most heavily myelinated fibers that transmit light touch.
2. **A-Δ fibers** and **C fibers** are the primary nociceptive afferents.
   a. A-Δ fibers are 2–5 μm in diameter and are thinly myelinated. They conduct immediate, rapid, sharp, and brief pain (first pain) with a velocity of 20 m/sec.
   b. C fibers are 0.2–1.5 μm in diameter and are unmyelinated. They conduct prolonged, burning, and unpleasant pain (second pain) at a speed of 0.5 m/sec.

C. Central Conduction of Nociception
1. **The dorsal horn of the spinal cord**
   a. **A-Δ and C fibers enter the dorsal root and ascend or descend one to three segments before synapsing with neurons in the lateral spinothalamic tract** (laminae I, II, and V of the substantia gelatinosa in the gray matter).
   b. **The major pain neurotransmitter, substance P, an 11-amino-acid polypeptide, is released from the fibers at many of these synapses.** Capsaicin, which is extracted from red-hot pepper, inhibits nociception by inhibiting substance P.
   c. Inhibition of nociception in the dorsal horn is functionally quite important. Stimulation of the A-Δ fibers excites some neurons but also inhibits others. This inhibition of nociception by A-Δ fiber stimulation may explain the salutary effects of acupuncture and transcutaneous electrical nerve stimulation (TENS).

D. Spinothalamic Tract
The lateral spinothalamic tract crosses the midline after synapsing with A-Δ and C fibers, and ascends towards the thalamus. At the level of the brainstem more than half of this tract synapses in the reticular activating system (in an area called the spinoreticular tract), in the limbic system, and in other brainstem regions. The close relationship of pain, affect, and sleep may be explained by these synapses. Another site of projections is the periaqueductal gray (PAG) (see Fig. 40-1), which plays an important role in the brain's endogenous analgesia system.

The lateral spinothalamic tract has two parts:
1. **The neospinothalamic tract, which serves to localize pain,** is phylogenetically recent and **ends in the ventroposterolateral (VPL) and ventroposteromedial (VPM) nuclei of the thalamus.** These nuclei project to the primary somatic sensory cortex in the parietal lobe.

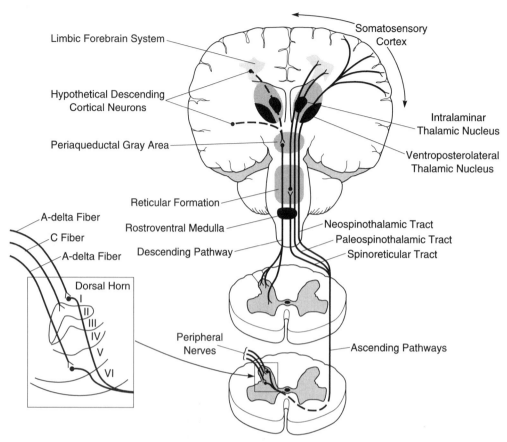

Fig. 40-1.   Schematic diagram of neurologic pathways for pain perception. (Source: Hyman SH, Cassem NH, *Pain*, 1989.)

2. **The paleospinothalamic tract** is a phylogenetically older pain system; it **projects to the intralaminar nucleus of the thalamus,** which has widespread cortical projections. These projections, which are involved in the affective nature of pain, serve to alert to, rather than to localize, pain.

E. **Cortex**
   After synapsing in the thalamic nuclei, pain fibers project to the somatosensory cortex, located posterior to the sylvian fissure in the parietal lobe (Brodmann areas 1, 2, and 3).

III. Endogenous Analgesic System

A. **Overview**
   There are at least 18 endogenous peptides with opiate-like activity in the central nervous system (CNS). They are the products of three precursor proteins:
   1. **Pro-opiomelanocortin** is the precursor of β-endorphin and adrenocorticotropic hormone.
   2. **Proenkephalin** is the precursor of met-enkephalin and leu-enkephalin.
   3. **Prodynorphin** is the precursor of dynorphin and related peptides.

B. **Central Opiate Receptors**
   1. **Mu receptors are involved in the regulation of analgesia, respiratory depression, constipation, and miosis.** They are the receptors (located in the PAG, rostraventral medulla, medial thalamus, and dorsal horn of the spinal cord) mainly responsible for supraspinal analgesia.
   2. **Kappa receptors are involved in spinal analgesia, sedation, and miosis.** They are located in the dorsal horn (spinal analgesia), deep cortical areas, and other locations; pentazocine preferentially acts on these receptors.
   3. **Delta receptors,** like kappa receptors, **mediate spinal analgesia, hypotension, and miosis.** Enkephalins have a higher affinity for these receptors than do opiates. They are located in the limbic system, the dorsal horn, and in other locations unrelated to pain. **Delta receptors also mediate psychotomimetic effects** (i.e., psychosis) in the CNS. Their effects are not reversed by naloxone, an opiate antagonist.

IV. Descending Analgesic Pain Pathway

The descending analgesic pain pathway starts in the PAG (rich in endogenous opiates), projects to the rostroventral

medulla, and from there descends through the dorsolateral funiculus of the spinal cord to the dorsal horn. The neurons in the rostroventral medulla use serotonin to activate endogenous analgesics (enkephalins) in the dorsal horn. This effect inhibits nociception at the level of the dorsal horn since neurons containing enkephalins synapse with spinothalamic neurons.

Additionally, there are noradrenergic neurons that project from the locus coeruleus (the main noradrenergic center in the CNS) to the dorsal horn, thereby inhibiting the response of dorsal horn neurons to nociceptive stimuli. The effect of tricyclic antidepressants (TCAs) is thought to be an increase in serotonin and norepinephrine that inhibits nociception at the level of the dorsal horn.

V. Categories of Pain

A. **Acute pain is usually related to an identifiable injury or to a disease;** it is self-limited, and resolves over hours to days or in a time frame that is associated with healing. Acute pain is usually associated with objective autonomic features (e.g., tachycardia, hypertension, diaphoresis, mydriasis, or pallor).

B. **Chronic pain is pain that persists beyond the normal time of healing or lasts longer than 6 months.** This type of pain does not have a well-defined neurologic mechanism. Characteristic features include vague descriptions of pain, including its timing and localization, accompanied by forceful assertions of its existence. Unlike acute pain, chronic pain typically lacks signs of heightened sympathetic activity, which may be due to chronic adaptation of the autonomic nervous system. Depression, anxiety, and premorbid personality problems are common to these patients. Usually the major problem is a lack of motivation and incentives to get better. It is usually helpful to:
   1. **Determine the presence of a dermatomal pattern.**
   2. **Determine the presence of neuropathic pain.**
   3. **Assess pain behavior.**

C. **Continuous pain in the terminally ill** originates from well-defined tissue damage due to the terminal illness (e.g., cancer). It is a variant of nociceptive pain. Stress, sleep deprivation, depression, and premormid personality may exacerbate this pain.

D. **Neuropathic pain is caused by an injured or dysfunctional central or peripheral nervous system; it is manifest by spontaneous, sharp, shooting, or burning pain that is usually distributed along dermatomes** (see Fig. 40-2). Neuropathic pain is often referred to as deafferentation syndrome, reflex sympathetic dystrophy, diabetic neuropathy, central pain syndrome, trigeminal neuralgia, or postherpetic neuralgia.

Terms commonly used to describe neuropathic pain:
1. **Hyperalgesia** is an increased response to stimuli that are normally painful.
2. **Hyperesthesia** is an exaggerated pain response to noxious stimuli (pressor or heat).
3. **Allodynia** is pain with a stimulus that is not normally painful (e.g., light touch or cool air).
4. **Hyperpathia** is pain from a painful stimulus with a delay and a persistence that is distributed beyond the area of stimulation.

E. **Reflex sympathetic dystrophy (RSD) is a syndrome of sympathetically maintained pain, or a complex regional pain syndrome in an extremity that is mediated by sympathetic overactivity;** it does not involve a major nerve or involve sensory, autonomic, motor, or trophic changes. The syndrome is usually caused by injury; however, the cause is unknown in approximately 10% of cases. It may be the result of microtrauma or macrotrauma (e.g., a sprain, a fracture, or a contusion); iatrogenic causes include amputation, lesion resection, myelography, and intramuscular injections. RSD may be disease-related (e.g., due to myocardial infarction, shoulder-hand syndrome, herpes zoster, cerebrovascular accidents, diabetic neuropathy, a disc herniation, degenerative disc disease, neuraxial tumors or metastases, multiple sclerosis, or poliomyelitis).
   1. **A sensory component includes spontaneous pain** and evoked pain in the affected extremity.
   2. **Autonomic changes** occur (marbled, hyperemic to cyanotic skin color, edema), as well as changes in blood flow and asymmetrical skin temperatures and perspiration in the affected limbs.
   3. **Motor changes** involve decreased strength and range of motion, tremor, hypotonia, atrophy, and dystonias (which are rare).
   4. **Trophic changes** are seen in approximately 30% of cases and rarely occur within the first 10 days of initial symptoms. These changes include disturbed nail growth, increased hair growth, palmar/plantar fibrosis, thin glossy skin, hyperkeratosis, and distal osteoporosis.

The clinical course (which may last up to 6 months) starts with an acute phase involving pain, edema, and warm skin. Subsequently, dystrophic changes dominate the picture with cold skin and trophic changes (3–6 months after the onset of the untreated acute phase). Irreversible atrophic changes (atrophy and contractures) eventually occur.

There may be symptom improvement with inhibition of sympathetic output; sympathetic blockade may be both diagnostic and therapeutic.

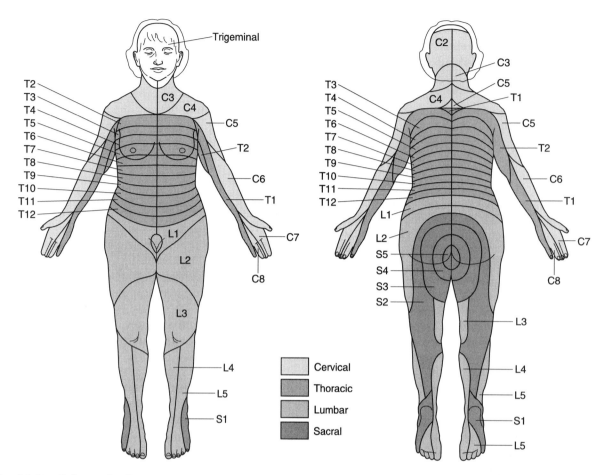

Fig. 40-2.　Schematic diagram of segmental neuronal innervation by dermatomes. (Source: Hyman SH, Cassem NH, *Pain*, 1989.)

F. Idiopathic pain, previously referred to as "psychogenic pain," is poorly understood. The presence of pain does not imply or exclude a psychological component. Typically, there is no evidence of an associated organic etiology or an anatomical pattern of symptoms, which are often grossly out of proportion to identifiable organic pathology.

Jurisigenic pain results from perceived physical or emotional damage related to medical, personal, work, or product injury. Patients with this pain syndrome usually must maintain the sick role for as long as possible to maximize financial return. It is important to recognize the existence of a conflict and to educate patients and attorneys; maintenance of a helping and neutral posture is critical.

G. Phantom pain refers to severe and excruciating pain after amputation, presenting a major obstacle in the treatment of the amputee. It is usually localized to the distal amputated limb and tends to vanish 2–3 years after the amputation. The pathophysiology of this pain is poorly understood. The chaotic innervation of the amputation site, changes in the spinal cord after the amputation, and supraspinal

mechanisms (e.g., attention and stress) may contribute to this pain syndrome.

VI. Psychopathology and Pain

A wide variety of psychotropics (antidepressants, anticonvulsants, benzodiazepines, neuroleptics, stimulants, alpha-2 agonists) can treat pain syndromes.

A. Mood disorders are commonly comorbid with pain:
　1. Depressive disorders have been found in 30–87% of pain patients.
　　a. Major depression develops in 8–50% of pain patients.
　　b. Dysthymia is seen in more than three-fourths of patients with chronic pain.
　2. Anxiety disorders (including panic disorder, generalized anxiety disorder, and posttraumatic stress disorder) are found in more than half of patients with chronic pain.

B. Somatoform disorders, including body dysmorphic disorder, conversion disorder, hypochondriasis, somatization disorder, and pain disorder, are detected in patients with chronic pain. In somatoform pain disorder, pain is a major part of clinical presentation and it causes significant impairment in function.

C. Other psychiatric states may also be comorbid with pain:

1. **Factitious disorders** involve the intentional production or feigning of physical or psychological symptoms (unconscious motivation, conscious production).

2. **Malingering** involves the intentional production or feigning of physical or psychological symptoms motivated by clear external incentives (conscious motivation, conscious production).

3. **Psychoactive substance use disorders:** dependence and abuse may develop as a result of chronic pain.

4. **Personality disorders**

5. **Adjustment disorder**

VII. Analgesic Therapies

A. Overview

1. **The initiation of analgesic therapy involves a multifactorial decision process.**

a. At times analgesia may be delayed until psychopathology can be identified and managed.

b. Efficiency of analgesia needs to be monitored. Function needs to be assessed to guide treatment.

2. **Pharmacological approaches**

a. Pharmacological approaches (including opiates and non-opiates) vary depending on whether pain is acute or chronic (see Tables 40-1 and 40-2 for the various agents and dosing details).

3. **Nonpharmacological approaches include:**

a. Invasive techniques (e.g., nerve blocks, implantable devices, neurosurgery)

b. Noninvasive approaches (e.g., physical therapy, acupuncture, massage, biofeedback, cognitive-behavioral therapy, relaxation techniques, hypnosis)

B. Acute Pain

1. **Acute pain is usually treated medically via treatment of the underlying disorder.**

2. **Management follows the analgesic ladder of the World Health Organization (WHO)** (see Fig. 40-3).

3. **Severe acute pain typically requires use of strong opiates** (e.g., hydromorphone, levorphanol, or

Table 40-1. Nonsteroidal Anti-Inflammatory Drugs

Drug	Dose (mg)	Dosage Interval (h)	Daily Dose (mg)	Peak Effect (h)	Half-Life (h)
Diclofenac	25–75	6–8	200	2	1–2
Etodolac acid	200–400	6–8	1200	1–2	7
Fenoprofen	200	4–6	3200	1–2	2–3
Flurbiprofen	50–100	6–8	300	1.5–3.0	3–4
Ibuprofen	200–400	6–8	3200	1–2	2
Indomethacin	25–75	6–8	200	0.5–1.0	2–3
Ketoprofen	25–75	6–8	300	1–2	1.5–2.0
Ketorolac[a]					
Oral	10	6–8	40	0.5–1.0	6
Parenteral	60 load, then 30	6–8	120		
Meclofenamic acid	500 load, then 275	6–8	400		
Mefenamic acid	500 load, then 250	6	1250	2–4	3–4
Nabumetone	1000–2000	12–24	2000	3–5	22–30
Naproxen	500 load, then 250	6–8	1250	2–4	12–15
Naproxen sodium	550 load, then 275	6–8	1375	1–2	13
Oxaprozin	60–1200	Every day	1800	2	3–3.5
Phenylbutazone	100	6–8	400	2	50–100
Piroxicam	40 load, then 20	24	20	2–4	36–45
Sulindac	150–200	12	400	1–2	7–18
Tolmetin	200–400	8	1800	4–6	2

SOURCE: Borsook et al., 1995.

[a] Use no longer than 5 days.

Table 40-2. Pharmacological Treatment of Acute Pain with Opiates

Drug	Approximate Equianalgesic Oral Dose	Approximate Equianalgesic Parenteral Dose	Recommended Starting Dose (adults more than 50 kg body weight)	
			Oral	Parenteral
Opiate agonist				
Morphine	30 mg q. 3–4 h	10 mg q. 3–4 h	30 mg q. 3–4 h	10 mg q. 3–4 h
Codeine	130 mg q. 3–4 h	75 mg q. 3–4 h	60 mg q. 3–4 h	60 mg q. 2 h
Hydromorphone (Dilaudid)	7.5 mg q. 3–4 h	1.5 mg q. 3–4 h	6 mg q. 3–4 h	1.5 mg q. 3–4 h
Levorphanol (Levo-Dromoran)	4 mg q. 6–8 h	2 mg q. 6–8 h	4 mg q. 6–8 h	2 mg q. 6–8 h
Meperidine (Demerol)	300 mg q. 2–3 h	100 mg q. 3 h	Not recommended	100 mg q. 3 h
Methadone (Dolophine, others)	20 mg q. 6–8 h	10 mg q. 6–8 h	20 mg q. 6–8 h	10 mg q. 6–8 h
Oxycodone (Roxicodone, also in Percocet, Percodan, Tylox, others)	30 mg q. 3–4 h	Not available	10 mg q. 3–4 h	Not available
Oxymorphone (Numorphan)	Not available	1 mg q. 3–4 h	Not available	1 mg q. 3–4 h
Opiate agonist-antagonist and partial agonist				
Buprenorphine (Buprenex)	Not available	0.3–0.4 mg q. 6–8 h	Not available	0.4 mg q. 6–8 h
Butorphanol (Stadol)	Not available	2 mg q. 3–4 h	Not available	2 mg q. 3–4 h
Nalbuphine (Nubain)	Not available	10 mg q. 3–4 h	Not available	10 mg q. 3–4 h
Pentazocine (Talwin, others)	150 mg q. 3–4 h	60 mg q. 3–4 h	50 mg q. 4–6 h	Not recommended

NOTE: Published tables vary in the suggested doses that are equianalgesic to morphine. Clinical response is the criterion that must be applied for each patient; titration to clinical response is necessary. Because there is not complete cross-tolerance among these drugs, it is usually necessary to use a lower than equianalgesic dose when changing drugs and to retitrate to response.

CAUTION: Recommended doses do not apply to patients with renal or hepatic insufficiency or other conditions affecting drug metabolism and kinetics.

CAUTION: Doses listed for patients with body weight >50 kg cannot be used as initial starting doses in children and patients <50 kg. Consult the *Clinical Practice Guideline for Acute Pain Management: Operative or Medical Procedures and Trauma* (section on management of pain in neonates) for recommendations. For morphine, hydromorphone, and oxymorphone, rectal administration is an alternate route for patients unable to take oral medications, but equianalgesic doses may differ from oral and parenteral doses because of pharmacokinetic differences.

CAUTION: Codeine doses >65 mg often are not appropriate due to diminishing incremental analgesia with increasing doses but continually increasing constipation and other side effects.

CAUTION: Doses of aspirin and acetaminophen in combination with opiate/nonsteroidal anti-inflammatory drug preparations must also be adjusted to the patient's body weight.

SOURCE: Adapted from Borsook et al., 1995.

morphine). These may be delivered by patient-controlled analgesia (PCA) or by the epidural route, either with or without local anesthetics (see Table 40-1 for prescription guidelines).

C. Chronic Pain

Chronic pain is usually treated with a multidisciplinary approach, since long-standing pain has far-reaching effects on many physical and psychological systems.

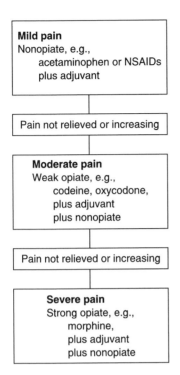

Fig. 40-3.   The analgesic ladder. (Source: Borsook et al., 1995.)

1. **Neuropathic pain is typically treated with anticonvulsants** (carbamazepine, phenytoin, gabapentin, clonazepam) **or antiarrhythmics** (lidocaine, mexiletine, TCAs). Response may also be seen with other analgesics (e.g., opiates or NSAIDs). Nerve blockade and nerve transection rarely offer persistent relief.
2. **Chronic regional pain syndrome (e.g., RSD) involves initial treatment with conservative therapy (i.e., mild analgesics and physical therapy).** Sympathetic interruption may be both diagnostic and therapeutic. Direct sympatholysis usually involves lumbar sympathetic or stellate ganglion block, or a systemic drug challenge with sympatholytic agents (phentolamine, phenoxybenzamine).
3. **Idiopathic pain or pain that fails conventional therapy**
   a. This type of pain requires a multidisciplinary approach, including anesthesia, psychiatry, behavioral medicine, surgery/neurosurgery, physiatry, physical therapy, occupational therapy, nursing, pharmacy, social work, and case management.
   b. Invasive interventions are of unclear value.
   c. Some severe cases in which function is impaired may warrant use of opiates.

D. The Use of Opiates
This is the gold standard for severe or unremitting pain.

1. **The basic principles of opiate use follow the guidelines put forth in the WHO analgesic ladder.** Physicians should explain to patients that opiates are not curative, may be addictive, and have no prophylactic value. When used chronically, function rather than pain should be followed (see Table 40-2 for agents and doses).
2. **Efficacy: opiates are equally efficacious when used in equianalgesic dosages;** however, for unknown reasons one individual may respond better to one agent than to another.
3. **Synergy: analgesia may be potentiated by other drugs** (e.g., NSAIDS, antihistamines, clonidine, neuroleptics, TCAs).
4. **Administration:** an as-needed (p.r.n.) dosing may reinforce the pain cycle, whereas long-acting agents may be preferable for long-term use.
5. **Routes of administration:** oral, PR (per rectum), SL (sublingual), IM (intramuscular), IV (intravenous), PCA, epidural, spinal.
6. **Adverse effects** are common and often limit the use of a drug. Such effects are usually idiosyncratic; it is unclear why some patients are more sensitive than others. Predictors of which patients will experience which side effects and which narcotics will produce them are lacking. Thus, one should expect side effects and take preventive actions. Tolerance to the adverse effects (except constipation) of opiates, occurs.
   a. **Common adverse effects from opiates include:**
      i. **Constipation** is the most common side effect of opiates; it persists over time, requires use of a daily stimulating cathartic, and may respond to oral dosages of naloxone.
      ii. **Respiratory depression** is a potentially serious complication. Tolerance occurs early in chronic therapy, and significant respiratory depression can be managed with naloxone.
      iii. **Severe nausea and vomiting** caused by opiates is rare; it is usually mild.
      iv. **Pruritus** probably occurs through a central mechanism, is rare with oral agents but is very common with spinal and epidural opiates. If tolerance to pruritus does occur it can be treated with naloxone, antihistamines (except when caused by spinal opiates), and by propofol (10 mg IV every 10 min given in two to three doses).
7. **Tolerance** to analgesia may require dose escalation. Changing agents may allow dosing at lower than equianalgesic dose, as cross-tolerance between opiates may be incomplete. Tolerance impairs the ability to assess the appropriate opiate dosage.
8. **Use of opiates for chronic nonmalignant pain is highly controversial,** but there is growing acceptance in well-selected cases. Such management has been avoided owing to high abuse potential,

Table 40-3. DEA Guidelines for the Prescription of Controlled Substances

1. A prescription for a controlled substance is lawful only if issued for a legitimate medical purpose by an individual practitioner acting in the usual course of professional practice. Prescriptions under the law may not be issued for narcotic drugs for the purpose of detoxification or maintenance of narcotics addicts.

2. All prescriptions for controlled substances must bear the following information:
   a. Name of patient
   b. Home address of patient
   c. Name of practitioner
   d. Address of practitioner
   e. Registration number of practitioner
   f. Name of the drug, strength, and quantity of the medicine to be dispensed
   g. Directions for use

3. All prescriptions must be dated with the day when issued to the patient and must be signed manually on that day by the practitioner.

4. It is illegal under both federal and state law to issue a prescription for other than a legitimate bona fide medical need or to date a prescription other than the date when it is issued to the patient and signed by the practitioner.

5. Schedule II controlled substances require written prescriptions prior to dispensing. They may not be refilled. A schedule II drug may be dispensed in an emergency by a pharmacist upon oral prescription of a practitioner if the quantity is limited to the emergency period, if the prescription is reduced immediately to writing by the pharmacist and contains all the information required of written prescriptions except the signature of the prescriber, if the pharmacist knows the prescriber, or makes a reasonable effort to verify the order's validity, and if the prescriber issues to the pharmacist a written prescription within 48 h of the oral order. If the pharmacist does not receive a written prescription from the prescriber within 72 h, he or she must by law notify the DEA regional office.

6. A controlled substance prescription must be for no more than 30 days of medicine.

SOURCE: Borsook et al., 1995.

tolerance, dependence, and other adverse effects. However, opiates may be a reasonable option for patients with chronic nonmalignant pain who have failed other reasonable conventional non-opiate interventions.

   a. **Guidelines for using opiates in chronic nonmalignant pain include:**
      i. Individualized therapy with opioids.
      ii. Use of a single opiate agent, if possible.

      - Use of long-acting preparations.
      - Mixing a single short-acting agent and a single long-acting agent.
      - For daily usage, use around-the-clock dosing rather than p.r.n. dosing.

      iii. Document the efficacy of opiate analgesia.

      - Function is of greater interest than analgesia.

      iv. Use opiate contracts and provide informed consent.
      v. Discuss side effects and risks of addiction, dependence, tolerance, cognitive impairment, fetal dependency in pregnancy, rules of usage and pre-

scribing, and consequences of breaking the contract.
      vi. Designate a single prescriber for all opiates.
      vii. Designate a single pharmacy for distribution of all opiates.
      viii. Maintain a symptom diary.
      ix. Do not provide over-the-phone prescriptions.
      x. Maintain close follow-up.
      xi. Maintain a high level of suspicion of toxicity and addictive tendencies.

      - Watch for evidence of drug hoarding, acquisition of opiates by multiple physicians, uncontrolled dose escalations, or other aberrant behaviors.

      xii. Follow usage guidelines.
      xiii. Consult with an addictions specialist.
      xiv. Periodically review the case with a multidisciplinary team.
      xv. Be aware of relative contraindications (e.g., a history of substance abuse, a severe character disorder, an inability to follow rules). For those with a substance abuse history, the relative nature of these contraindications must yield to compassionate use of narcotics.

E. Analgesic Adjuvants

1. Use of adjuvants, such as NSAIDs, antihistamines, clonidine, corticosteroids, neuroleptics, psychostimulants, and tricyclics can be effective.

2. Partial analgesic effects may be achieved with tricyclics, clonidine, baclofen, muscle relaxants, corticosteroids, antiarrhythmics, and anticonvulsants.

3. Antidepressants: TCAs but not selective serotonin reuptake inhibitors (SSRIs) are well established as having independent analgesic properties.

   a. Efficacy of specific TCAs
      i. TCAs supported as analgesics by controlled studies include amitriptyline (Elavil), nortriptyline (Pamelor), desipramine (Norpramin), imipramine (Tofranil), and maprotiline (Ludiomil).
      ii. TCAs supported as analgesics by anecdotal reports include doxepin, trazodone, and clomipramine.

   b. TCA analgesia strategy. Complete analgesia is rare and side effects are common with the use of TCAs, so usually one must accept mild side effects in exchange for analgesia. TCAs are particularly compelling when pain is accompanied by comorbid depression or by insomnia. Reasonable goals of therapy include decreasing pain intensity by 10–50%, or by decreasing pain from unbearable to bearable levels.

   c. Analgesic TCA dosages may be lower than antidepressant dosages, but some patients require higher dosages.
      i. Start at a dose of 10–25 mg; very low doses should be used for those aged >65 years.
      ii. Slowly increase the dosage to minimize side effects and avoid overshooting the minimal analgesic dose.
      iii. Intolerable side effects may be alleviated by changing to desipramine or nortriptyline.
      iv. Relief may be exhibited in 1–7 days to several weeks (but maximal analgesia may require 2–4 weeks).
      v. TCA-induced analgesic effects persist over time.

F. Nonpharmacological Approaches

1. **Invasive**
   a. **Nerve blocks and implantable devices:** trigger point injections, epidural injections, selective nerve root injections, stellate ganglion and lumbar sympathetic nerve blockade can be employed.
   b. **Neurosurgery**
      i. **Augmentative**
         - An intrathecal pump, which typically delivers an opiate, but may involve baclofen (for spasticity) or a local anesthetic (less common).
         - A spinal cord stimulator (dorsal column stimulator) is a catheter device placed in the epidural space that electrically stimulates the spinal cord. It is used in neuropathic pain and in sympathetically maintained pain states.
      ii. **Ablative therapy**
         - Radiofrequency lesions are used in peripheral pain (e.g., trigeminal and glossopharyngeal neuralgia).
         - Treatment for spinal cord lesions include ganglionectomy (with ablation of the dorsal ganglia), dorsal rhizotomy (with sensory loss in lesioned distribution), and with midline myelotomy (for bilateral pain).
         - Central techniques include mesencephalotomy (for lesions of midbrain spinothalamic and secondary trigeminal tracts—for unilateral head and neck pain), thalamotomy (which is sometimes used with bilateral analgesia), and **cingulotomy (for diffuse chronic pain associated with affective disorders).**

2. **Noninvasive techniques** include physical therapy, TENS, acupuncture (relatively noninvasive), massage, cognitive or behavioral therapy, and distraction (e.g., hypnosis or biofeedback).

G. The Multidisciplinary Approach

1. Goals of the multidisciplinary approach include improving coping, planning a focus on function rather than on analgesia, and decreasing addictive behaviors, including detoxification. This approach offers alternatives to drugs, injections, or surgery for pain control, and improves overall physical and psychological well-being. It strives to decrease behaviors that negatively impact on pain and function, to improve social supports, to decrease social isolation, and to decrease dependence on the health care system.

2. Multidisciplinary team meetings include practitioners from medicine, neurology, pediatrics, physiatry, psychiatry, surgery, anesthesia, neurosurgery, and physical therapy.

3. **Alternative therapies** are of unknown efficacy. Examples include acupuncture, yoga, tai chi, massage, and herbal remedies.

Suggested Readings

Acute Pain Management Guideline Panel: *Acute Pain Management: Operative or Medical Procedures and Trauma. Clinical Practice Guideline.* AHCPR Publ. No. 92-0032. Rockville, MD: Agency for Health Care Policy and Research, Public Health Service, US Department of Health and Human Services, 1992.

Bonica JJ (ed.): *The Management of Pain*, 2nd ed. Philadelphia: Lea and Febiger, 1990.

Borsook D, Lebel AA, McPeek B: *MGH Handbook of Pain Management.* Boston: Little, Brown, 1995.

Breitbart W: Psychiatric management of cancer pain. *Cancer* 1989; 63:2336–2342.

Fields HL: *Pain*. New York: McGraw-Hill, 1987.

Foley KM: The practical use of narcotic analgesics. *Med Clin North Am* 1983; 66:1091–1104.

Hyman SH, Cassem NH: Pain. In Rubenstein E, Fedeman DD (eds): *Scientific American Medicine: Current Topics in Medicine*, Subsection II. New York: Scientific American, 1989:1–7.

NIH Consensus Development Conference: The integrated approach to the management of pain. *J Pain Symptom Manage* 1987; 2:35–41.

Portnoy RY: Chronic opioid therapy in nonmalignant pain. *J Pain Symptom Manage* 1990; 5:S46–S62.

Sternbach R: *Pain Patients: Traits and Treatments*. New York: Academic Press, 1974.

Wall PD, Melzack R (eds): *Textbook of Pain*, 3rd ed. New York: Churchill-Livingstone, 1995.

Chapter 41
Stroke
Schahram Akbarian and Martin A. Samuels

I. Introduction

Stroke is the third leading cause of mortality and morbidity in North America. At present, there are ongoing, important changes in the way stroke is diagnosed and treated; many large medical centers have stroke services available, with multidisciplinary teams offering systemic and/or local invasive treatment in intensive care settings "around the clock." Analogous to the treatment of cardiac patients in coronary care units, the prognosis for a patient suffering an acute stroke nowadays depends to a great deal upon rapid referral to a stroke service. Therefore, practitioners should be able to diagnose an acute stroke and to identify those patients at imminent or high risk for stroke.

The psychiatrist should be familiar with three important topics associated with the neurological disorder, "stroke": the definition and classification of stroke; stroke syndromes and symptoms, including those that could be confused with manifestations of psychiatric disease; and psychiatric disorders as possible sequelae of stroke.

II. The Definition and Classification of Stroke

A. Definition

Stroke is defined as the "sudden or rapid onset of a neurological deficit in a vascular territory that lasts longer than 24 h and that is due to an underlying cerebrovascular disease." A transient ischemic attack (TIA) is defined as the "sudden or rapid onset of a neurological deficit in a vascular territory that lasts less than 24 h and that is due to an underlying cerebrovascular disease."

Presently, most physicians work with these two definitions; previously, a variety of terms (e.g., reversible ischemic neurologic deficit [RIND], a condition that resolved within 1 week) were used.

Pathological changes provide the basis for a widely used classification schema that includes four major types: hemorrhagic (intracerebral hemorrhagic stroke, and subarachnoidal hemorrhagic stroke), and ischemic (thrombotic stroke, and embolic stroke).

B. Cerebrovascular Diseases that Cause Ischemic Stroke

1. **Diseases and conditions**

   a. **Atherosclerosis accounts for 50% of all ischemic strokes. It is typically a "large vessel disease" that involves the arteries of the circle of Willis.**

   b. **Lipohyalinosis accounts for 20% of all ischemic strokes.** Usually the result of hypertension, **it is a "small vessel disease" that causes lacunar strokes.**

   c. **Cerebral embolism accounts for 20% of all ischemic strokes.** Most emboli are derived from a cardiac source. **Emboli that originate from arterial sources (primarily from the aortic arch) are usually smaller in size and thus are less detrimental than are cardiac emboli.** Emboli from a venous source may enter the left side of the heart through a patent foramen ovale.

   d. **Miscellaneous causes account for the remaining 10% of ischemic strokes.** Stroke in a younger patient is often due to a dissection of the carotid or vertebral arteries. Another cause is a hypercoagulable state, which may be a result of a variety of conditions (e.g., pregnancy, pseudopregnancy due to oral contraceptives, sickle cell crisis, antiphospholipid antibody syndrome, or selected cases of migraine that may be related to indolamine-induced alterations in platelet adhesion).

2. **Management**

   a. Until recently, management of ischemic strokes in the acute phase was confined to monitoring the neurological deficit and the careful use of heparin. Neuroimaging methods were comparatively limited in the acute phase (since an ischemic infarct of the brain may not be evident on noncontrast computed tomography (CT) within the first 36–48 h) and were used primarily for ruling out hemorrhagic stroke.

   b. **Modern imaging techniques, such as "diffusion-weighted MRI" are able to localize accurately an evolving ischemic brain infarction, without use of intravenous contrast and within 30 min of the vascular occlusion.** Ongoing clinical trials are attempting to assess systemic treatment options (e.g., tissue-plasminogen activator [TPA]) and local invasive treatment strategies (the latter performed in collaboration with a neuroradiologist or neurosurgeon).

C. Cerebrovascular Diseases that Cause Hemorrhagic Stroke

1. **Diseases and conditions**

   a. **Berry (saccular) aneurysms are due to an inherited weakness of the arterial walls. Berry aneurysms usually bleed into the subarachnoid space.** Aneurysms are **typically located at bifurcations of the arteries of the circle of Willis. The mortality associated with a ruptured**

315

aneurysm is 30%. A moderate or severe headache, that is characteristically "maximum at onset," is associated with a bleeding aneurysm; a transient loss of consciousness is possible. Focal neurological findings are less typical for a ruptured aneurysm. Occasionally, an unruptured aneurysm that expands in size may present with focal findings, such as cranial nerve abnormalities. Intracerebral hemorrhages are usually evident on a noncontrast CT, but the rate of false negatives is 5%. A nondiagnostic CT could be due to the small volume of a hemorrhage, or due to a gravity-induced translocation of the blood into the subarachnoid spaces of the spinal cord. If the index of suspicion remains high despite a normal CT, a lumbar puncture should be performed. Xanthochromic cerebrospinal fluid (CSF), due to lysis of red blood cells, is characteristic of subarachnoid hemorrhages.

Incidentally detected aneurysms that are less than 5 mm in diameter are usually monitored at regular intervals using magnetic resonance or CT angiography.

b. **Charcot-Bouchard small vessel aneurysms are caused by degenerative changes in the walls of small arteries, as a consequence of chronic hypertension.** These small vessel aneurysms are an important cause of intracerebral hemorrhage; **they present with a combination of headache and focal neurological findings. Of the bleeds associated with these aneurysms, 50% occur in the putamen, 20% occur in the thalamus, 10% occur in the cerebellum, 10% occur in the pons, and 10% occur elsewhere** (e.g., lobar hemorrhage). Bleeding into the subcortical structures of the forebrain can present in the early phase with dramatic clinical symptoms; however, it carries a better long-term prognosis than does pontine bleeding. Hemorrhages in the cerebellum demand immediate neurosurgical consultation for possible evacuation of an expanding mass lesion. If not dealt with expeditiously, life-threatening complications, primarily due to compression of the brainstem, may ensue.

Lobar hemorrhages, related to amyloid angiopathy, are becoming more prevalent as the population ages, and fewer hypertensive intracerebral hemorrhages have occurred in the population treated for long-term hypertension.

c. **Arteriovenous malformations (AVMs) result from developmental abnormalities;** constituent vessels proliferate with the passage of time. They are **one-tenth as common as berry (saccular) aneurysms.** Bleeding is partly intracerebral and partly subarachnoid; **in 50% of patients with AVMs, bleeding is the first manifestation of the AVM. In 30% of cases, a seizure is the first manifestation, and in 20%, the first manifestation is a focal neurological finding.**

Other vascular malformations (e.g., capillary telangiectasias and cavernous hemangiomas) may also bleed, leading to some combination of subarachnoid and intracerebral hemorrhage. Episodes of hypertension, such that occur with cocaine use, may lead to rupture of an otherwise silent vascular malformation. To emphasize this point, 50% of cocaine users who develop a cerebral hemorrhage will be found to harbor a vascular malformation. This very high proportion is probably due to the unmasking of a vascular malformation with episodes of hypertension induced by the cocaine.

d. **Subdural and epidural hematomas** are not technically strokes and they do not represent forms of cerebrovascular disease. Acute subdural and epidural hematomas **are usually the result of severe head trauma;** they can progress rapidly over a period of hours or progress over the course of days. **Chronic subdural hematomas (SDH), on the other hand, are not always caused by significant head trauma;** symptoms tend to progress gradually over days to weeks. SDH may result from tears of bridging veins in the subdural space, or from rebleeding of vascular malformations. **Headache is the most frequently encountered clinical symptom with SDH.** With increasing intracranial pressure, other symptoms (including confusion and fluctuations in the level of consciousness, inattention and memory loss, apathy, drowsiness, and coma) develop. Focal findings may be present.

III. Stroke Syndromes

A. **Stroke Syndromes** (listed by vascular territory)
  1. **Strokes of the anterior circulation**
    a. **Carotid artery occlusions.** Clinical manifestations associated with occlusion of the internal carotid artery vary, and depend on the acuity of the occlusion and the efficacy of collaterals. **While clinically silent in up to 50% of cases, occlusion of the internal carotid artery may potentially cause massive infarction of the anterior two-thirds of the cerebral hemisphere.** Occlusion of the internal carotid artery can present with some or all of the clinical symptoms that occur after occlusion of its three major branches (the ophthalmic, the middle cerebral, and the anterior cerebral arteries).
      i. **Amaurosis fugax.** The ophthalmic artery branches off from the distal portion of the internal carotid artery and provides the major blood supply to the optic nerve and to the retina. Although permanent blindness due to occlusion of this artery is rare, **transient monocular blindness may occur in up to 20% of patients that suffer a stroke from carotid artery occlusion.** Therefore, amaurosis fugax is a very important clinical warning sign.

      High-grade (70–99%) stenosis of the carotid arteries, the most common single vessel to be diseased, ultimately leads to occlusion. The risks (approximately 3% mortality and morbidity in good centers) of carotid endarterectomy need to be weighted carefully along with other factors (e.g., age, medical illness).
    b. **Middle cerebral artery (MCA) occlusions**
      i. **MCA occlusions may lead to infarction of the inferior and lateral frontal lobes and affect gaze, motor**

functions, and the somatomotor cortex (with resultant paresis/paralysis of the contralateral arm, face, and leg, and of conjugate gaze to the contralateral side, with deviation of the eyes to the ipsilateral side). Bilateral frontal lobe infarction can result in a gait disturbance and a syndrome manifest by disinhibition and by disturbances in motivation and problem solving.

ii. **Lesions of Broca's area result in a nonfluent aphasia,** in which understanding remains intact, but the ability to speak is compromised (manifest by dysarthric, telegraphic speech, and by poor repetition).

iii. **Lesions of the posterior perisylvian cortex result in central (Wernicke's) aphasia, with fluent, but jargon-filled speech, poor comprehension of language, and poor repetition.** Paraphasias, alexia, and agraphia are also present.

iv. **Lesions of the parietal and temporal white matter can result in an homonymous hemianopia** (reflecting a lesion of the optic radiations from the lateral geniculate to the primary visual cortex).

v. **Lesions of the lateral parietal lobe result in impaired somatosensory sensations in the contralateral arm, face, and leg.** Contralateral apraxias and hemineglect syndromes may develop.

vi. **Lesions of the supramarginal and angular gyrus may result in a loss of optokinetic nystagmus.** Most cases of conduction aphasia (associated with intact comprehension of speech and writing, fluent speech output, paraphasias, and its most obvious clinical hallmark, severe impairment of repetition) are due to a lesion of the supramarginal gyrus of the dominant hemisphere, or of the arcuate fascicle, which interconnects the frontal and temporal cortex, including Broca's and Wernicke's areas.

vii. **Lesions of the posterior limb of the internal capsule result in a pure motor hemiplegia.**

c. **Anterior cerebral artery occlusions**

i. The anterior cerebral artery supplies the medial parts of the cerebral hemisphere. Infarction may lead to sensorimotor deficits in the contralateral foot and leg, and the appearance of contralateral grasp and suck reflexes. Bilateral occlusion may result in urinary incontinence, paraplegia, and abulia.

2. **Strokes of the posterior circulation**

a. **Posterior cerebral artery occlusions**

i. **Lesions of the occipital lobe may result in an homonymous hemianopia.** Bilateral lesions cause cortical blindness, with the patient being unaware of their deficits (anosognosia).

ii. **Lesions of the inferomedial temporal lobe often result in memory deficits.**

iii. **Lesions of the posteroventral thalamus result in sensory disturbances on the contralateral side, with an intention tremor.**

iv. **Lesions of the rostral midbrain can result in paralysis/paresis of vertical eye movements.**

b. **Vertebral artery occlusions**

i. The vertebral artery is the major artery for the medulla and the posterior inferior parts of the cerebellar hemispheres. **Occlusion of this artery typically causes the lateral medullary syndrome (Wallenberg's syndrome), which involves contralateral impairment of pain and temperature sensation on the body (via the ipsilateral spinothalamic tract), ipsilateral impairment of pain and temperature of the face (via the ipsilateral spinal tract and the nucleus of the trigeminal), an ipsilateral Horner's syndrome with miosis, ptosis, and decreased sweating (via the ipsilateral descending sympathetic tract), dysphagia and hoarseness (via the ipsilateral vagus and ambiguous nuclei), vertigo and nystagmus (via the vestibular nuclei), and ipsilateral ataxia (via the inferior cerebellar peduncle).** This syndrome results from an occlusion of the vertebral artery in 80% of cases and is due to an occlusion of the posterior inferior cerebellar artery, a major branch of the vertebral artery, in 20% of cases.

ii. **Isolated infarction of the inferior part of the cerebellum with the sudden onset of vertigo, nausea, vomiting, ataxia, and nystagmus, should not be mistaken for an acute attack of labyrinthitis.** In this setting, a localized posterior headache is highly suspicious for cerebellar infarction. Severe vertigo and an inability to walk also suggest cerebellar infarction, particularly when nystagmus is absent.

c. **Basilar artery occlusion**

i. The basilar artery supplies the midbrain, the pons, and the cerebellar hemispheres. **Basilar artery occlusion involves the corticospinal and corticobulbar tracts, the cerebellar peduncles, the medial and lateral lemnisci, the various nuclei of the pons, and cranial nerves III, IV, V, VI, VII, and VIII.** A complete basilar occlusion results either in a comatose patient (due to lesions of the reticular activating system), or a conscious but paralyzed ("locked-in syndrome") patient. Vertical eye movements and blinking are usually spared.

ii. **Occlusion of branches of the basilar artery causes variable syndromes, with alterations of consciousness, and disturbances of gaze and of the somatomotor system.** Early warning signs of basilar vascular disease include vertigo, blurred vision, diplopia, dysarthria, as well as somatosensory and somatomotor disturbances.

iii. Small penetrating vessels of the basilar arteries supply parts of the pons. **Pontine lesions are often accompanied by disturbances in conjugate eye movements.** The gaze paresis that occurs with these occlusions is on the side of the lesion. ("The eyes look away from a brainstem lesion and towards a hemispheric lesion.") Other symptoms of pontine lesions include ataxia, diplopia, paralysis, nystagmus, deafness or tinnitus, sensory disturbances, and internuclear ophthalmoplegia (i.e., difficulties in adducting the eye past the midline on the side of lesion, due to lesions of the median longitudinal fasciculus).

IV. Neuropsychiatric Symptoms of Stroke that Could Be Confused with Manifestations of Primary Psychiatric Disease

Certain stroke syndromes may produce neuropsychiatric symptoms that could be mistaken for symptoms of primary psychiatric disease, especially in the acute setting (e.g., the emergency department). The following list is not intended to be complete, and it remains good clinical practice to carefully rule out organic factors (including focal brain lesions) in a patient with a suspected primary psychiatric disease.

A. Akinetic mutism is characterized by poverty of speech, apathy, abulia, and immobility. It may occur after bilateral lesions of the medial frontal lobes and the cingulate areas (frequently caused by occlusion of the anterior communicating artery). Akinetic mutism may resemble psychotic withdrawal, but it lacks negativism or catatonic waxy flexibility.

B. Frontal lobe syndromes, including impairments of problem-solving ability, repetition, and inhibition, as well as an altered sense of spontaneity and personality changes may occur after strokes of the anterior part of the cerebral hemisphere. Depending on the predominant symptoms, frontal lobe syndromes could be mistaken for several psychiatric disorders, including personality disorders and depression.

C. Delirium, with a clouded sensorium and agitation, has been observed after bilateral infarctions of the thalamus and the midbrain, and may reflect damage to the ascending reticular activating system. Confusion, with dream-like states, has on occasion been observed in the acute phase of strokes involving the right temporal lobe.

D. Auditory hallucinations of an elementary nature (e.g., hearing music or sounds as opposed to voices), without concomitant confusion or disorientation, has been described after pontine lesions ("pontine auditory hallucinosis") and after lesions of the temporal lobe. Simple visual hallucinations are often symptomatic of lesions in the occipital cortex, whereas more complex formed visual illusions and hallucinations typically occur with temporal lobe dysfunction. Midbrain lesions may cause vivid dream-like hallucinations (termed peduncular hallucinosis).

E. Aphasic syndromes, including motor (Broca's) aphasia and central (Wernicke's) aphasia, are among the most frequently misdiagnosed stroke syndromes. Central aphasias, where a patient may echo the words of the examiner with faulty pronunciation or repeat them in a slavish manner, may be misinterpreted as "mannerism" or "echolalia." Formal verbal paraphasias ("mouse" for "house") and semantic verbal paraphasias ("hotel" for "hospital") are characteristic of central aphasias, but may be misinterpreted as signs of a "formal thought disorder" associated with a psychotic process. Broca's aphasia, on the other hand, with its paucity of spontaneous speech and monosyllabic answer pattern, may be mistaken for the "negative symptoms" of schizophrenia or as a manifestation of psychotic withdrawal. Many patients with Broca's syndrome have some awareness of their disability and may be frustrated, overwhelmed, anxious, or agitated, which, again, may be misinterpreted as a manifestation of a psychiatric illness.

V. Psychiatric Disorders as Sequelae of Stroke

A. Post-Stroke Depression

1. **Major depression, with its characteristic neurovegetative, cognitive, and emotional disturbances, may occur in more than 20% of stroke victims.** Early neuroimaging studies suggested that infarction of the left anterior hemisphere, in particular of the left rostral prefrontal cortex and the left rostral caudate, carry the highest risk for post-stroke depression. Posterior lesions of the right hemisphere, involving the occipital and/or parietotemporo-occipital cortex, may also be accompanied by higher rates of post-stroke depression. Some more recent studies have not found an association between post-stroke depression and location of the lesion.

2. **Three-fourths of patients with post-stroke depression develop a mood disorder within the first 6 months following stroke.** In contrast to "endogenous" major depressive disorder, post-stroke depression appears to have no gender bias. Full-blown major depression secondary to a stroke has an average duration, if left untreated, of 12 months.

3. **Treatment of post-stroke depression is similar to that of other types of depression.** Nortriptyline, citalopram, and other specific serotonin reuptake inhibitors (SSRIs), as well as stimulants and elec-

troconvulsive therapy, have been used with success in the treatment of post-stroke depression. Stimulants have the advantage of inducing an antidepressant response within days of initiation of treatment. This could be a critical factor for mental well-being, early rehabilitation, and avoidance of serious medical sequelae associated with prolonged immobility.

In the DSM-IV, post-stroke depression is listed under Mood Disorder with Depressive Features due to a General Medical Condition.

B. **Aprosodia may resemble the major depression in stroke patients. Prosody is the variation in pitch, rhythm, and the stress of pronunciation that bestows certain semantic and emotional meaning to speech.** Prosody, in the context of vocabulary and grammar, is part of propositional speech. Prosody in the context of emotional content and nonlinguistic aspects of communication is part of emotional speech.

Prosody appears to be primarily a right hemisphere function. Lesions of the right frontal lobe are often accompanied by motor aprosodia, recognized by difficulties in the spontaneous use of emotional inflection in language or by difficulties in emotional gesturing. Sensory aprosodia is defined by difficulties in the comprehension of the gestures and emotional inflections in language due to lesions of the right parietal lobe. Sensory aprosodia may lead to difficulties in the patient's social interactions and relationships. Motor aprosodia, especially if unrecognized, can confound a mental status examination and be mistaken as the "constricted affect" or "psychomotor retardation" of depression. Alternatively, a patient with a motor aprosodia and a concomitant mood disorder might be unable to express his/her inner emotional state; as a consequence, the mood disorder might avoid detection by the clinician. Similar to aphasias, aprosodias should be manifest during the acute stroke phase. Often, it may be impossible to decide if a patient has an aprosodia or if he/she is suffering from post-stroke depression, or both. Given the comparatively low side-effect profile of the newer generation antidepressants, a trial with an antidepressant medication should be initiated even if the diagnostic alternatives (aprosodia or poststroke depression) haven't been clarified.

C. **A catastrophic reaction with restlessness, hyperemotionality, sudden outbursts of tears, irritability, cursing, displays of strong emotions towards the examiner and the examination are part of a syndrome associated with localized brain lesions, predominantly with left hemispheric lesions and with Broca's aphasia.** Initially described in patients suffering from brain injuries in war, the catastrophic reaction may occur after a wide range of brain diseases. Psychological factors in response to the sudden experience of disability and insufficiency may play an important role. Some believe that the catastrophic reaction is a special subtype of post-stroke depression. Of note, the DSM-IV does not list a "catastrophic reaction" as a separate entity. Potential DSM-IV diagnoses for these patients includes Mood Disorder due to General Medical Condition, Acute Stress Disorder, and Adjustment Reaction.

D. **Post-stroke secondary mania or hypomania are rare syndromes and occur in less than 1% of all stroke patients.** Infarctions of the right frontal lobes and other parts of the right hemisphere, including basal ganglia, thalamus, and medial temporal lobe, predominate. The first onset of mania in an elderly patient should be considered as organic until proven otherwise (or, in DSM-IV "language," as Mood Disorder with Manic Features due to a General Medical Condition).

E. **An indifference reaction may result from right hemisphere lesions manifest as a lack of interest in family and friends, or with signs of disinhibition (e.g., telling foolish jokes) and minimization of physical difficulties.** Left spatial hemineglect syndromes may also be accompanied by an indifference reaction. Frontal lobe infarctions may lead to indifference, disinhibition, and literal sophomoric humor (Witzelsucht). DSM-IV does not list the indifference reaction as a diagnostic entity.

F. **Multi-infarct or vascular dementia can occur after multiple localized infarctions affecting the cortical gray matter. Binswanger's subcortical encephalopathy is associated with multiple ("small vessel") lesions affecting subcortical white matter in the border zone between the penetrating cortical and basal ganglionic arteries.**

G. **A pseudobulbar state may result from bilateral infarctions (or other lesions) in the corticobulbar tracts with hyperreflexia, spasticity, dysphagia, and pathologic laughing or crying.** This incontinence of emotion may be considered hyperreflexia of emotional responses, and reflects an underlying mood but with an exaggerated affect. It can be successfully treated with antispasticity agents (e.g., baclofen), or an antidepressant (e.g., a polycyclic drug or an SSRI).

Suggested Readings

Adams RD, Victor M, Ropper AH: *Principles of Neurology*, 4th ed. New York: McGraw-Hill, 1998.

Fricchione G, Weilburg JB, Murray GB: Neurology and neurosurgery. In Rundell JR, Wise MG (eds): *Textbook of Consultation-Liaison Psychiatry*. Washington, DC: American Psychiatric Press, 1996:697–719.

Robinson RG, Forrester AW: Neuropsychiatric aspects of cerebrovascular disease. *The American Psychiatric Textbook of Neuropsychiatry*. Washington, DC: American Psychiatric Press, 1987:191–208.

Samuels MA: *Stroke. Video Textbook of Neurology for the Practicing Physician*. Boston: Butterworth-Heinemann, 1997.

Chapter 42

Movement Disorders

SCHAHRAM AKBARIAN AND MARTIN A. SAMUELS

I. Introduction

Movement disorders, like few other areas of neurology, are of considerable importance for clinical psychiatry. Alterations of movement and posture frequently accompany major psychiatric diseases, including major depression, psychosis, and conversion disorder. On the other hand, a variety of neurodegenerative disorders affect motor systems as well as the neuronal circuits serving cognitive and emotional function. In addition, abnormalities of movement are frequent side-effects of psychotropics. Furthermore, catatonia and neuroleptic malignant syndrome, two potentially life-threatening conditions, are accompanied by disturbances in motor function.

II. Classification of Movement Disorders

John Hughlings Jackson (1835–1911) subdivided movement disturbances into two categories: those with too little movement and those with too much movement.

A. Signs Defined by Too Little Movement

1. **Paralysis** is the complete, and **paresis** the incomplete, loss of motor function in a body part due to neurologic dysfunction. Causes of these signs include lesions of the upper motor neurons (including the giant Betz pyramidal cells in layer V of the primary motor cortex) and/or lesions of the lower motor neurons (in the spinal cord and brainstem). **Paresis and paralysis are the clinical hallmarks of motor neuron disease** (e.g., amyotrophic lateral sclerosis [ALS], also known as Lou-Gehrig's disease), and of poliomyelitis. **Lesions of peripheral nerves and spinal nerve roots that disrupt the flow of action potentials along the axons of anterior horn cells also result in paralysis.**

2. **Rigidity is defined as "too much tone" in a muscle or group of muscles;** it causes impaired motor function with too little movement. Several types of rigidity exist:

   a. **Spasticity is a stiffness that is defined classically by the clasp-knife phenomenon.** With spasticity, muscles do not contract until they are stretched a bit; later when stretched, the augmentation in muscle tone quickly ceases. Spasticity is indicative of upper motor neuron lesions. Baclofen, a γ-aminobutyric acid B ($GABA_B$) receptor agonist that crosses the blood-brain barrier, is the main pharmacologic treatment for spasticity.

Sectioning the posterior spinal roots abolishes spasticity by disrupting the afferent input of muscle spindles into the spinal circuitry.

   b. **Lead pipe stiffness** is thought of as a functional defect in extrapyramidal corticostriatal circuits. It is observed in the setting of relative dopamine deficiency, as seen with Parkinson's disease, neuroleptic malignant syndrome, or acute withdrawal from dopaminergic, antiparkinsonian medications (including L-dopa and bromocriptine).

   c. **Paratonia ("Gegenhalten")** includes the examiner as part of the definition: **"The harder the examiner tries (to move the affected limb) the more resistance is found"** despite all efforts of the patient to relax. Lesions of the prefrontal cortex or the presence of hydrocephalus may present with paratonia. Patients who try to feign paresis on occasion produce paratonia-like signs during physical examination.

   d. The **cogwheel phenomenon** refers to the rhythmically jerky resistance of a passively stretched hypertonic muscle, a finding often observed in Parkinson's disease.

3. **Akinesia (the tendency not to move)** and **bradykinesia (the presence of abnormally slow movements)** may be manifestations of lesions in the basal ganglia or disruption of nigrostriatal pathways; causes include idiopathic, toxic or postencephalitic parkinsonism, pharmacologic blockade of striatal dopamine (D_2) receptors, and head trauma as observed in boxers (i.e., dementia pugilistica).

B. Signs Defined by Too Much Movement

1. **Tremor is an involuntary oscillatory movement.** In contrast to myoclonus, tremor does not occur during sleep.

   a. **Rest tremors.** Two tremors are maximal in the position of repose:

      i. **Parkinson's tremor,** which improves upon action and is typically asymmetric. Parkinsonian tremor often involves several muscle groups and produces oscillations at more than one point (as in the case of the "pill-rolling tremor" of the upper extremities).

      ii. **Rubral tremor** is due to lesions in the cerebellar outflow tract; this type of tremor often results from demyelinating disease or from head trauma. The tremor is alternating and rhythmic when the patient is in repose and becomes ataxic on goal-directed action.

b. **Action tremors.** Several types of action tremor exist. They include:

   i. Goal-directed action tremors due to cerebellar defects, and postural action tremors, which are antigravity posture tremors of a fast and distal nature. As an enhanced physiological tremor, it is typically caused by effects of catecholamines, as observed in anxiety states or after caffeine intake.

   ii. **Familial essential tremors** are also action tremors; they are often treated with primidone or propanolol.

c. **Physiological, postural, and familial tremors** in the hands have a frequency of approximately 8–15 Hz. **Parkinsonian pill-rolling tremor,** in contrast, is approximately 4 Hz in repose and may be accompanied by a finer 7–8 Hz tremor on action.

2. **Myoclonus consists of very quick movements** that are often interrupted by, or follow, a brief loss of tone in affected muscles (e.g., asterixis). Myoclonus and asterixis, commonly seen together, are observed in the setting of renal or hepatic failure, drug intoxication or degenerative disease, including Alzheimer's disease and Creutzfeldt-Jakob disease. Clonazepam is frequently the drug of choice for the treatment of myoclonus.

3. **Fibrillation is defined as muscle fiber contraction in the absence of neuronal signals;** it indicates denervation and is a pathological sign. **Since it cannot be observed with the naked eye it must be demonstrated using electromyography.**

4. **Fasciculations are caused by spontaneous activation of motor units.** In most cases fasciculations are considered physiological. These "muscle twitches" may follow prolonged muscle activity, caffeine intake, or be due to anxiety. However, anterior horn cell disease may be accompanied by fasciculations. A variety of drugs cause fasciculations and myoclonic jerks. Meperidine (Demerol), due to accumulation of its long-lasting, central nervous system (CNS) excitatory metabolite, normeperidine, is a relatively frequent cause of drug-induced fasciculations and myoclonic jerks. Trains of fasciculations produce muscle cramps, which can be treated with a sodium channel blocker (e.g., quinine).

5. **Chorea is defined by continuous, randomly distributed, jerky and abrupt movements that resemble an incomplete gesture.** Chorea may occur after any type of damage (e.g., caused by strokes, encephalitis, cerebral palsy, and chronic neurodegenerative disorders) to the basal ganglia.

   a. **Sydenham's chorea,** which is usually self-limited, is a delayed manifestation of rheumatic fever.

   b. **Senile chorea** may have multiple causes.

   c. With the exception of **Huntington's chorea,** most other choreas appear to occur more frequently in females than in males.

   d. **Estrogen receptors** may play a role in the pathophysiology of some types of chorea, such as **chorea gravidarum** and chorea associated with birth control pills.

   e. Dopamine (D_2) receptor blockers, such as haloperidol, may ameliorate chorea.

6. **Dystonia is characterized by slow, tonic, and sustained muscle contractions,** often of the face and jaw, the tongue and the neck, and of the whole body in the extreme case. Dystonia may also be described as having twisting or repetitive movements.

   a. **Acute dystonia** is an extrapyramidal side effect from a variety of drugs, including, but not limited to, the dopamine (D_2) receptor blockers, such as neuroleptics.

   b. **Meige's syndrome (orofacial dystonia)** is recognized by tonic, symmetric and nonrhythmic contractions of orofacial muscles, interspersed with clonic contractions of the same muscles. It may be idiopathic, or an acute or late-onset side effect of a variety of drugs, including neuroleptics and L-dopa.

   c. **Blepharospasm** resembles Meige's syndrome but affects only the orbicularis oculi muscles.

   d. **Torticollis (cervical dystonia)** is limited to the neck muscles. Another example of these focal dystonias is **writer's cramp,** which is the most frequent type of so-called "occupation cramps." Upon attempting to write, hand muscles undergo tonic and slow contractions, and painful spasms. After abandoning the attempt to write, the symptoms disappear. All of these focal dystonias are considered to be true neurological diseases; contrary to an earlier theory, psychodynamic factors appear to play no significant role in most cases. Local injections of botulinus toxin can result in a dramatic improvement of dystonic symptoms; currently these injections are the treatment of choice. Benzodiazepines may also be helpful in some cases.

   e. **Dystonia musculorum deformans** leads to dystonic contractions across the entire body. Usually the disease begins in childhood, initially affecting only one body part. Both hereditary and symptomatic forms have been described.

7. **Athetosis is a slow, recurrent but continuous movement of an extremity or body part between two extreme positions,** such as pronation and supination. It is symptomatic of striatal lesions, particularly of the putamen.

8. **Hemiballism is characterized by irregular, sudden movements of the proximal muscles of the extremities,** giving the impression that the patient is throwing their arms and legs wildly in all directions. An

acute lesion (typically a stroke) of the subthalamic nucleus is the usual underlying cause.

9. **Akathisia is a type of restlessness with the inability to sit still.** Besides the observable (objective) manifestations of restlessness, akathisia also causes a subjective inner feeling associated with the compulsion to move.

10. **Restless legs syndrome is characterized by an unpleasant sensation in the lower extremities, accompanied by an urge to move the legs.** Restless legs syndrome appears only at rest. It may be a manifestation of a variety of medical diseases, including anemia, diabetes, and hypovitaminosis. It is good clinical practice to initiate a comprehensive medical workup, including tests for iron-deficiency anemia, in patients with restless legs syndrome. A variety of drugs, including neuroleptics, lithium, and mianserin may cause restless legs syndrome. Hereditary factors and pregnancy are other causes. Drugs used to treat restless legs syndrome include clonazepam, carbamazepine, L-dopa, and bromocriptine.

11. **Tics are brief, repetitive, and stereotyped muscle contractions lasting only tenths of a second.** Tics most frequently affect facial muscles (giving rise to blinking, sniffing, facial grimacing, or tongue darting). They are accompanied by subjective symptoms which consist of an urge to perform the tic and an internal discomfort that increases if the tic is suppressed by conscious will power. Tics frequently begin in childhood; the incidence peaks between 5 and 10 years of age. Three out of four children with tics are boys. The syndrome is closely related genetically and phenomenologically to obsessive-compulsive disorder.

III. Movement Disorders Frequently Accompanied by Psychiatric Symptoms

A. **Disorders with Prominent Parkinsonism**

1. **Parkinson's disease.** Parkinson's disease affects 0.3% of the general population and 3% of people over the age of 65 years. Elderly patients with Parkinson's disease suffer from dementia seven times more frequently than do elderly controls; 30% of the elderly with dementia and Parkinson's disease also suffer from Alzheimer's disease, and another 10% from Lewy body disease, which is the second most common cause of neurodegenerative dementia. In 55% of patients with dementia and parkinsonism, no additional neuropathological changes other than those of Parkinson's disease are found. The disease is recognized by the classical triad of tremor, rigidity, and akinesia.

"Bradyphrenia," which is defined as slowing of cognitive processing, is analogous to the bradykinesia of the motor systems. Dopaminergic anti-parkinsonian drugs may improve bradyphrenia. The underlying pathology is a progressive degeneration of dopaminergic neurons in the pars compacta of the substantia nigra. Neuronal degeneration is also found in selected catecholaminergic, cholinergic, and serotonergic nuclei in the brainstem and in selected neuronal populations of the hypothalamus and the cerebral cortex. L-Dopa and other dopaminergic agents that are the mainstay of treatment cause a variety of neuropsychiatric side effects, including hallucinations, mania, hypersexuality, paranoia, vivid dreams, nightmares, and other sleep disturbances. **Major depression occurs in 15–25% of patients with Parkinson's disease.**

The treatment of depression in patients with Parkinson's disease does not differ from that of depression in patients without Parkinson's disease. However, it has to be kept in mind that antidepressant drugs such as the tricyclics (TCAs) and selective serotonin reuptake inhibitors (SSRIs) may cause akathisia and other extrapyramidal symptoms, including dystonia, dyskinesia, and classical drug-induced parkinsonism. Therefore, these drugs may aggravate the motor disturbances in some patients. In selected patients, the monoamine oxidase B inhibitor, selegiline, may be useful for the treatment of depression and may protect dopaminergic neurons from oxygen radical-induced toxicity; this matter is still the subject of investigation. Electroconvulsive therapy (ECT), which is thought to increase the dopaminergic tonus of the striatum, is very effective for the treatment of depression and the motor symptoms of Parkinson's disease.

Antipsychotic agents that block dopamine (D_2) receptors should be avoided in patients with Parkinson's disease because they carry the risk of prolonged, severe exacerbations of akinesia and rigidity. If antipsychotics are indicated in a patient with Parkinson's disease, clozapine (Clozaril), a very weak D_2 but strong D_4 and serotonin ($5HT_2$) receptor blocker, is the drug of choice. Clozapine has a significant antipsychotic effect in patients with Parkinson's disease at doses (25–50 mg/day) that are much lower than those needed for the treatment of schizophrenia. Low-dose clozapine may even improve parkinsonian tremor, probably due to the drug's anticholinergic effects. Low-dose clozapine does not worsen other motor symptoms of Parkinson's disease. Selective $5-HT_2$ (serotonin) receptor blockers, such as quietapine (Seroquel), may also be used as antipsychotics in Parkinson's patients.

2. **Dementia with Lewy bodies is,** after Alzheimer's disease, **the second most common cause of dementia.** The disorder is characterized by parkinsonism, with rigidity usually being more prominent than either bradykinesia or tremor. Dementia is often present in the early stages of the disease. Spontaneous hallucinations and fluctuating levels of cognition are also characteristic. These patients, in a fashion similar to patients with Parkinson's disease, have a pronounced sensitivity to neuroleptic-induced extrapyramidal side effects (EPS).

3. **Progressive supranuclear palsy involves degeneration of nigrostriatal neurons and of oculomotor centers. Cognitive and behavioral changes may occur.**

4. **Multiple system atrophy involves striatonigral degeneration, sporadic olivopontocerebellar atrophy, and the Shy-Drager syndrome.** Parkinsonism, early signs of dysautonomia (e.g., orthostatic hypotension), cerebellar dysfunction, and pyramidal tract signs may be present.

B. **Disorders Associated with Degeneration and/or Dysfunction of Basal Ganglia Circuitry**

1. **Huntington's chorea** is a manifestation of Huntington's disease (HD), **an autosomal dominant inherited disorder that affects 7–10/100,000 of the general population. It is recognized by the triad of choreiform movements, dementia, and a family history of the disease.** Early in the course of the disease, the purposeless movements may be misinterpreted as habit spasms or tics. Dementia is usually present in the later stages of the disease, which is in general fatal 10–20 years after its onset. In 60–75% of HD patients, psychiatric symptoms, such as anxiety, depression, or psychosis, may be among the earliest presenting symptoms of the disease, either with or without concomitant neurological symptoms. Treatment of the psychiatric disturbances is symptomatic, using standard antipsychotics and antidepressant drugs. Neuropathological changes in HD are most marked in the striatum, due to a loss of the GABAergic medium spiny neurons; other anatomical areas, such as the internal layers of the cerebral cortex, are also significantly affected. Positron emission tomography (PET) studies demonstrated that striatal hypometabolism precedes the onset of the clinical symptoms and striatal degeneration. The **HD gene (termed "huntingtin")** has been cloned; an extension of a CAG triplet (encoding the amino acid glutamine) that gives rise to a polyglutamine tract 11–34 amino acids long in normal individuals is abnormally expanded to 36–125 triplets in HD patients. While symptoms of HD usually first appear around the fourth decade, patients with very long **CAG triplet extension** tend to develop the disease as early as in the first decade of life. There is, at present, no cure for HD. Moreover, the relative ease of genetic testing for the disease can cause problems for the first-degree relatives (who have a 50% chance to carry the mutant gene) of an HD patient. Trinucleotide repeat expansion is the underlying molecular defect in a variety of neurogenetic disorders, including (but not limited to) HD, certain spinocerebellar ataxias, spinal and bulbar muscular atrophy, myotonic dystrophy, dentatorubral-pallidoluysian atrophy, and fragile X syndrome.

2. **Wilson's disease is an autosomal recessive disorder of copper metabolism, causing copper depositions in a variety of tissues.** Symptoms are related to dysfunction of liver and brain; they include dystonia, cerebellar ataxia, an intention tremor, and a plethora of psychiatric symptoms, ranging from poor school performance and behavioral disturbances to severe mood disturbances, psychosis, and intellectual deterioration. Although Wilson's disease is rare (prevalence $25/10^7$) it can be diagnosed early (by the detection of a low serum coeruloplasmin, by an abnormal elevation of 24-h urinary copper, and by copper deposition in liver tissue). Early treatment with dietary copper restriction and D-penicillamine may reverse symptoms. Patients with neurological and psychiatric symptoms may have brownish copper depositions (the Kayser-Fleischer rings) at the corneoscleral junction. If not visible by the naked eye, slit-lamp examination should be performed in suspected cases.

3. **Fahr's disease is due to abnormal calcifications of vessels and neuronal tissue in the basal ganglia.** Rigidity and choreoathetosis may be present. A rare familial form, inherited as an autosomal recessive trait, has been described.

    Hypoparathyroidism, and on occasion, hyperthyroidism, may lead to calcification of basal ganglia and cerebellum.

4. **Tourette's disorder** shares with other tic disorders a male/female ratio of 3:1 and an onset in childhood. The prevalence for the disease is 0.05–0.09%. **Tourette's disorder is characterized both by motor and vocal tics and, in 10% of cases by coprolalia and echolalia.** Tourette's disorder may be accompanied by obsessions and compulsions. Hyperactivity, impulsivity, and learning disabilities are also frequent in patients with Tourette's disorder. To make a diagnosis of Tourette's disorder the DSM-IV requires the presence of multiple motor and at least one vocal tic for a period of at least 1 year, with the age of onset before 18 years. The

disease is characterized by a waxing and waning course, but without progressive deterioration. Spontaneous remissions lasting as long as two decades have been described. Complete remission occurs in 10% of Tourette's patients, while 25–65% of patients with simple tic disorder experience complete remission.

Tics are thought of as manifestations of excess dopaminergic activity, presumably within the circuits of the basal ganglia. Tics are ameliorated by dopamine (D_2) receptor blockers and by other molecules that decrease dopaminergic signal transduction. Haloperidol and pimozide are frequently used in the psychopharmacologic management of tic disorders. Doses are, in general, lower than those used for the treatment of psychosis. In some patients, tics are exacerbated by stimulants that increase dopaminergic tonus; in other patients, however, stimulants are therapeutically effective.

IV. Extrapyramidal Side Effects of Psychotropic Drugs

A. **Psychotropics cause a wide variety of extrapyramidal side effects (EPS), including acute dystonia, parkinsonism, akathisia, tardive dyskinesia, and tardive dystonia.** Dopamine antagonists, such as neuroleptics and antiemetics (e.g., metoclopramide [Reglan], prochlorperazine [Compazine]), and acute withdrawal from dopamine agonists (e.g., L-dopa, bromocriptine) are likely to cause EPS. TCAs and SSRIs are also known to cause EPS. Akathisia is the most frequently encountered antidepressant-induced EPS, but classical drug-induced parkinsonism and acute dystonias were also reported.

B. **Acute dystonia is experienced by 10% of neuroleptic-treated patients within the first hours and days of treatment;** 90% of all acute dystonias occur within the first 3 days of treatment. Acute dystonias usually last only for hours and disappear completely within 24–48 h after discontinuation of the offending agent. Young males are at highest risk for acute dystonia. Acute dystonias respond quickly to anticholinergic drugs, such as benadryl or cogentin. Benzodiazepines may also be helpful. Amantadine, an antiviral drug affecting dopamine release, has also been useful in the treatment of drug-induced EPS. However, direct dopamine agonists (e.g., bromocriptine) or indirect agonists (e.g., L-dopa) are not preferred because they may aggravate psychotic symptoms and worsen agitation. Anticholinergics, benzodiazepines or amantadine may be started concurrently with neuroleptics, in order to prevent acute dystonia. Anticholinergics should be used with great caution in patients at risk for delirium (e.g., the elderly patients who are already taking anticholinergic TCAs), sinus tachycardia, glaucoma, ileus, urinary retention, or prostatic hypertrophy.

C. **Drug-induced parkinsonism** occurs in most cases within 5–30 days after starting an antipsychotic. Symptoms include shuffling gait, propulsion, rigidity, cogwheeling, bradykinesia, and tremor. The "rabbit syndrome" is a perioral tremor that responds, as do other symptoms of drug-induced parkinsonism, to anticholinergic drugs. Rabbit syndrome should not be confused with tardive dyskinesia of the facial muscles.

D. **Akathisia** is caused by a variety of drugs, including neuroleptics, TCAs, lithium, SSRIs, and methysergide. Lipophilic beta-blockers, such as propranolol, may ameliorate akathisia, especially when given in the higher dose range. In contrast to drug-induced acute dystonia, anticholinergic drugs often lack a beneficial effect. Benzodiazepines may be helpful in some patients. Ritanserin, a serotonin ($5HT_2$) receptor antagonist, and the irreversible monoamine oxidase B inhibitor, selegiline, may also be useful for treating akathisia in selected patients.

E. **Tardive dyskinesia** (TD), including its variant, tardive dystonia, **is a potentially irreversible late-onset extrapyramidal hyperkinetic movement disorder often caused by long-term administration of dopamine-blocking agents.** It is also observed in some never-medicated schizophrenics and in the general geriatric population. TD frequently affects the mouth and tongue (lip smacking, sucking, or facial grimacing), or causes choreoathethoid movements of the limbs. Symptoms of TD worsen with emotional arousal and decrease when there are voluntary movements of the affected muscle groups. **TD is observed in 10–20% of patients treated with an antipsychotic for more than 1 year.** After the first year, the risk appears to be about 5% per patient per year. However, there is no clear relationship between TD and life-time antipsychotic dose. Three months of cumulative exposure to dopamine receptor blocking agents is considered the minimal exposure necessary for the development of TD. Increased sensitivity to dopamine receptors may play a role in the pathophysiology of TD. Patient groups at highest risk for TD appear to be mood-disordered patients, elderly women, children, and African-Americans. Clozapine, an antipsychotic with a unique receptor profile (including strong D_4 receptor and $5HT_2$

receptor blockage, but very weak D_2 receptor blockage) has only rarely been associated with TD. Other atypical antipsychotics with less affinity for the D_2 receptor (e.g., olanzapine, quietapine, and risperidol) may also have a lower risk for TD, compared with typical antipsychotics.

TD appears not to take a progressive, deteriorating course; it develops rapidly, then stabilizes and often improves to some degree, even if the offending drug is continued. The differential diagnosis of TD includes all conditions (including strokes, mass lesions, and chronic neurodegenerative disease) accompanied by defective basal ganglia circuitry.

The management of TD includes a dose reduction of the dopamine receptor blocker, although this may cause a transient worsening of symptoms ("withdrawal dystonia"). Switching to the atypical antipsychotic, clozapine, has proven useful for some patients. Clozapine is the antipsychotic least likely to cause EPS and TD, and it appears to have a beneficial effect on already existing TD. Increasing the dose of the dopamine receptor blocker may be an additional option, in the event that dose reduction or switching to clozapine is not an option. Vitamin E and calcium channel blockers may be useful, but this matter is still subject to investigation. In the majority of patients, anticholinergics are not useful. Every patient who takes a dopamine antagonist for more than 3 months should be monitored for EPS and TD; documentation of movement disorders should include use of scales such as the Abnormal Involuntary Movement Scale (AIMS).

V. Catatonia and Neuroleptic Malignant Syndrome

Catatonia and neuroleptic malignant syndrome (NMS) are two potentially life-threatening conditions. Disturbances of motor functions are among the cardinal clinical signs of these conditions, and therefore they are mentioned briefly in this chapter.

A. **Catatonia is a syndrome defined by motor immobility (including waxy flexibility) and/or excessive motor activity, extreme negativism (with maintenance of a rigid posture against attempts to be moved), peculiarities of voluntary movement with bizarre posturing, a variety of stereotyped movements, mannerisms, and grimacing.** Malignant catatonia includes, in addition to these motor symptoms, signs of autonomic instability (with fluctuating vital signs), high temperature, and delirium. Untreated cases have a high mortality rate (> 50%), hence the terms "lethal catatonia"

and "pernicious catatonia" found in the older literature. The catatonic syndrome may be a manifestation of a wide range of neurological and psychiatric disorders (including, but not limited to, acute mood disorders and psychosis, nonconvulsive status epilepticus, poisoning, strokes, systemic infections, inflammation of the CNS, as well as metabolic and endocrine derangements). An imbalance involving dopaminergic; and GABAergic signal transduction in the striatum is thought to be involved in the pathophysiology of catatonia.

The current treatment of choice involves use of intravenous benzodiazepines, preferably those without metabolites or a long half-life. Intravenous lorazepam, in doses of 2 mg, may result in dramatic improvement, but its effects may not be long-lasting, necessitating repeated administration. Electroconvulsive therapy (ECT) is also an effective treatment. Supportive measures, if necessary in an intensive care setting, are also important in management of catatonia. Antiparkinsonian agents, such as bromocriptine, and the muscle relaxant, dantrolene, may be helpful in selected cases. Neuroleptics should be used with extreme caution and are probably best avoided altogether in cases of catatonia associated with autonomic signs, hyperthermia, and delirium.

B. **Neuroleptic malignant syndrome (NMS) is associated with use of neuroleptics, including all atypical antipsychotics (even clozapine) and other dopamine antagonists, including metoclopropamide (Reglan) and prochlorperazine (Compazine).** NMS has also been described in Parkinson's patients who have had dopaminergic drugs, such as L-dopa, stopped. NMS is defined by fever, autonomic dysfunction, muscular rigidity, and mental status changes. The mortality rate of full-blown NMS is approximately 10%. NMS is clinically indistinguishable from catatonia. Laboratory abnormalities, such as an elevation in creatine phosphokinase (CPK), leukocytosis, and a reduced serum iron level may occur in both conditions. The muscle rigidity in NMS is often described as a "lead pipe rigidity," while the rigidity in catatonia may be more variable. However, these differences are hardly helpful at the bedside. **Estimates about the frequency of NMS range from 0.05% to 2% among the population of patients treated with neuroleptics.** This variability in the literature is not surprising, given the fact that these critically ill "NMS" patients have coexisting conditions that make accurate diagnosis of NMS difficult. In addition, the clinical symptoms of NMS show considerable variability on a case-to-case basis, and clinicians may have different standards and thresholds for the diagnosis of NMS. In some Parkinson's patients, for example, acute withdrawal from L-dopa, bromocriptine, and other dopaminergic agents may result "only" in hyperthermia and an exacerbation of parkinsonian symptoms, while full-blown NMS with severe autonomic instability is less frequently encountered.

The risk for NMS in males is roughly twice as high as it is in females. It has been suggested that high-potency neuroleptics and rapid-dose escalation may pose a special risk for NMS. It should be kept in mind that a catatonic syndrome has been associated with a wide variety of different drugs (e.g., disulfiram, alcohol, TCAs and MAOIs, hallucinogens, lithium, anticonvulsants, and steroids), some even being functionally antagonistic (for example, both neuroleptics and stimulants, such as amphetamines, methylphenidate, and cocaine have been associated with drug-related catatonia).

Treatment of NMS includes supportive measures in an intensive care setting. Benzodiazepines, ECT, bromocriptine, amantadine, dantrolene, and anticholinergics have been successful in individual cases. In patients with a history of NMS it may be advantageous to switch to clozapine or a low-potency neuroleptic.

VI. Alterations of Movement in Conversion Disorder

Alterations of movement are among the most frequent manifestations of conversion disorder. A diagnosis of conversion disorder should be made only after a thorough neurological and medical examination. Caution must be exercised, because many patients may have both a neurological illness and conversion symptoms. In addition, some medical or neurological conditions may take years to become apparent.

If paralysis is due to a conversion disorder, tendon reflexes must be retained and severe muscular atrophy must be absent. In "hysterical hemiparesis," the typical circumduction of the paretic leg is missing; instead the patient tends to drag the limb like a useless adjunct. Patients who have a disturbance of gait, but who move their legs while lying in bed, often have a conversion disorder. However, there are important exceptions: with lesions of the rostral vermis of the cerebellum, with normal pressure hydrocephalus, and with lesions

of the frontal lobes isolated disturbances of gait may be present.

At the bedside, two tests may provide useful information in the assessment of conversion disorder where paralysis of the lower extremities is present:

1. **Babinski's trunk-thigh test.** The examiner asks the recumbent patient to sit up while keeping his arms crossed in front of his chest. In the patient with organic hemiplegia, there is an involuntary flexion of the paretic lower limb; in paraplegia, both limbs are flexed as the trunk is flexed. In the case of "hysterical hemiplegia," only the normal leg will be flexed; in the case of "hysterical paraplegia," neither leg is flexed.

2. **Hoover's sign.** The examiner places both hands under the heels of the recumbent patient, who is asked to press the heels down forcefully. The examiner then removes his hands from under the nonparalyzed leg, places it on top of the nonparalyzed foot, and asks the patient to raise that leg. In true hemiplegia, no added pressure will be felt by the hand that remained beneath the heel of the paralyzed leg. If conversion symptoms are present, the heel of the "paralyzed" leg will press down the palm.

Tremor as a conversion symptom is difficult to distinguish from neurological tremors. A tremor that is gross in nature, that moves to another body part if the originally affected limb is restrained by the examiner, and that disappears with distraction, may be a "hysterical tremor."

Suggested Readings

Adams RD, Victor M, Ropper AH: *Principles of Neurology*, 6th ed. New York: McGraw-Hill, 1997.

Fricchione G, Bush G, Fozdar M, Francis A, Fink M: Recognition and treatment of the catatonic syndrome. *J Intensive Care Med* 1997; 12:135–147.

Kaplan HI, Sadock BJ: *Comprehensive Textbook of Psychiatry*, 6th ed. Baltimore: Williams and Wilkins, 1995.

Lang AE, Lozano A: Parkinson's disease. *N Engl J Med* 1998; 339: 1044–1053.

Prager LK, Millham FH, Stern TA: Neuroleptic malignant syndrome: a review for intensivists. *J Intensive Care Med* 1994; 9: 227–234.

Samuels MA: *Movement Disorders. Video Textbook for the Practicing Physician.* Boston: Butterworth-Heinemann, 1997.

Samuels MA, Feske S: *Office Practice of Neurology.* Philadelphia: WB Saunders, 1997.

SECTION IV

Treatment Approaches

Chapter 43

Basic Psychopharmacology

STEPHAN HECKERS

I. Overview

Modulation of neuronal activity via neurotransmitters is a fundamental mechanism of brain function. The premier therapeutic avenue of psychiatry is, arguably, the facilitation or inhibition of neurotransmitter systems in the brain, either through the administration of drugs or through psychotherapy. The release of neurotransmitters, their mechanisms of action, and their effect on target neurons are complex and still poorly understood. **However, despite the diversity of neurotransmitters and receptors in the human brain, they have one common goal: to modulate neuronal activity. This is achieved by changing either the electrical or the chemical properties of the cell.** A balance of intracellular and extracellular ions maintains the electrical properties of a neuron. At rest, this balance is called the resting membrane potential. Decreasing the resting potential leads to excitation, increasing it leads to inhibition. The expression of specific genes, the production of proteins, and the creation of a distinct metabolism characterize the chemical properties of a neuron. Regulation of gene expression and protein function determines the biochemical status quo of the cell.

II. Basic Principles

A. Anatomy of the Neuron

Neurons have three compartments: dendrites, cell body (perikaryon), and axon. The cell body integrates the different inputs provided by the dendrites. This integration can occur through modulation of the membrane potential or at the level of the nucleus (regulation of gene expression). **The axon is the output station of the neuron.** The axon can be short (local circuit neuron) or long (projection neuron). If a deviation from the resting membrane potential is above a certain threshold, an action potential is created and travels downstream rapidly. **The nerve terminal is the widened terminal part of the axon. It provides a small area of close contact with dendrites of neighboring cells: a synapse** (see Fig. 43-1).

B. The Synapse

1. **The presynaptic neuron, which releases the neurotransmitter into the synapse, can express two proteins that affect synaptic communication:**
   a. **Membrane-bound receptors bind the intrinsic neurotransmitter (autoreceptor) or transmitters of neighboring neurons (heteroreceptor) and affect the cell via intracellular messengers.** One response, for example, is the modulation of neurotransmitter release.
   b. **Membrane-bound reuptake transporters pump the released neurotransmitter back into the cell.**
2. **The neuron receiving the input (postsynaptic cell) can be modulated via two different types of receptors:**
   a. **Fast-acting, class I (ionotropic) receptors.** The neurotransmitter binds to the receptor protein and within milliseconds leads to a change in the permeability of the associated ion channel, allowing the influx of ions such as Ca^{2+}, Na^+, K^+, or Cl^-.
   b. **Slow-acting, class II (G-protein-coupled) receptors.** The neurotransmitter binds to the receptor protein and thereby changes the protein conformation. This change is relayed to an associated G-protein, so called because it binds guanidine triphosphate (GTP) in order to be activated. G-proteins regulate two major classes of effector molecules: ion channels and second messenger-generating enzymes.

C. Intracellular Information Processing

1. **The activity of receptors and ion channels influences gene and protein expression in neurons. Gene expression is regulated by transcription factors that bind to specific sequences of the DNA in the nucleus.** Therefore, membrane-bound receptors or ion channels in distal parts of the neuron must be able to activate intraneuronal signal transduction pathways that can span long distances and translocate to the nucleus. Since proteins assemble the neuron and determine neuronal properties, gene expression regulates neuronal function and may cause malfunction. Many psychopharmacological agents with delayed therapeutic effects are thought to produce their therapeutic benefits through modulation of gene expression.
2. **Release of neurotransmitters from the presynaptic neuron into the synapse activates receptors on the postsynaptic neuron.** Upon activation of ionotropic receptors, ions such as Ca^{2+} enter the cell and act as second messengers. **Activation of G-protein-coupled receptors facilitates the opening of neighboring ion channels, or the synthesis of second messengers,** such as cyclic AMP (cAMP). **Second messengers (Ca^{2+}, cAMP) regulate the activity of protein kinases** (proteins that transfer phosphate

331

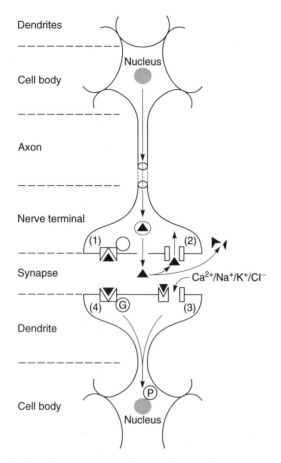

Fig. 43-1. A neurotransmitter released into the synapse may affect the presynaptic neuron (top) via membrane-bound receptors (1) and reuptake transporters (2) and the postsynaptic neuron (bottom) via ion-channel-coupled receptors (3) and G-protein-coupled receptors (4).

groups to a substrate protein) **and phosphatases** (proteins that remove phosphate groups from a substrate protein). In all cases investigated to date, the activation of neurotransmitter receptors changes the state of phosphorylation of neuronal proteins.

3. Since neurotransmitters and receptors influence gene and protein expression in the brain, small but persistent abnormalities in neurotransmission can have far-reaching consequences. An understanding of signal transduction pathways and of transcription factors will be instrumental in providing us with new therapeutic avenues in psychopharmacology.

D. Neuronal Circuitry

How are neurons arranged to process information? **There are about 10^{11} neurons in the central nervous system (CNS) and each neuron establishes about 10^3– 10^4 connections to other neurons.** Here we focus on

four major anatomical systems: the cortex, the thalamus, the basal ganglia, and the medial temporal lobe. The function of these four systems is modulated by several groups of neurons that are characterized by their use of a specific neurotransmitter. **Most of psychopharmacology is aimed at strengthening or inhibiting these modulatory systems.**

1. **The thalamus is the gateway to cortical processing of all incoming sensory information.** Primary sensory cortices receive information from the appropriate input modules (sensory organ + thalamus).

2. **The association cortex integrates information from primary cortices, from subcortical structures, and from brain areas affiliated with memory.**

3. **The medial temporal lobe** (i.e., hippocampus, amygdala) **serves** two major functions in the brain: **to integrate multimodal sensory information** for storage into and retrieval from memory, **and to attach limbic valence to sensory information** (e.g., pleasant or unpleasant, fight or flight).

4. **The basal ganglia are primarily involved in the integration of input from cortical areas.** The basal ganglia modulate cortical activity via a cortico-striato-pallido-thalamo-cortical loop. The most prominent projections to the striatum arise from the motor cortex.

5. **Four groups of densely packed neurons provide diffuse projections to all areas of the brain** to modulate their functions: **cholinergic neurons** in the basal forebrain and brainstem, **dopaminergic neurons** in the substantia nigra and ventral tegmental area, **noradrenergic neurons** in the locus coeruleus, and **serotonergic neurons** in the raphe nuclei. Although there are many more neurotransmitter systems in the brain, in clinical psychopharmacology **we have to be primarily concerned with six systems: the glutamatergic, GABAergic, cholinergic, serotonergic, noradrenergic, and dopaminergic systems.** These six systems can be divided into two groups based on their anatomical characteristics.

   a. **The first group includes the glutamatergic and GABAergic systems.** Their neurons are by far **the two most prevalent and most widely distributed types in the human brain.** The widespread distribution of these two neurotransmitter systems has functional implications: the modulation of glutamatergic and GABAergic neurotransmission affects many neural systems.

   b. **The second group of neurotransmitter systems comprises the cholinergic, serotonergic, noradrenergic, and dopaminergic neurons.** These four systems project to their target areas typically by long-ranging projection fibers. Since these neurotransmitter-specific projection systems reach selected neural systems, **their modulation leads to more circumscribed effects.**

III. Six Neurotransmitter Systems

A. **Glutamatergic Neurotransmission**
Glutamate (Glu) is the most abundant amino acid in the CNS.

1. **Anatomy. Prominent glutamatergic pathways are the corticocortical projections, the connections between thalamus and cortex, and the projections from cortex to striatum (extrapyramidal pathway) and to brainstem/spinal cord (pyramidal pathway).** The hippocampus and the cerebellum also contain many glutamatergic neurons.

2. **Synthesis. Glutamate is synthesized in the nerve terminals from two sources: from glucose via the Krebs cycle and from glutamine by the enzyme glutaminase.** The production of glutamate in releasable pools (i.e., the neurotransmitter portion of the intracellular glutamate) is regulated by the enzyme glutaminase. **Glutamate is stored in vesicles and released by a Ca^{2+}-dependent mechanism.**

3. **Synapse. Glutamate acts at three different types of ionotropic receptors and at a family of G-protein-coupled (metabotropic) receptors.**
   a. **Binding of glutamate to the ionotropic receptor opens an ion channel** allowing the influx of Na^+ and Ca^{2+} into the cell.
   b. NMDA (N-methyl-D-aspartate) receptors bind glutamate and NMDA. The NMDA receptor is highly regulated at several sites.
   c. AMPA (aminomethylphenylacetic acid) receptors bind glutamate, AMPA, and quisqualic acid, while kainate receptors bind glutamate and kainic acid.
   d. The metabotropic glutamate receptor family includes at least seven different types of G-protein-coupled receptors (mGluR$_{1-7}$). They are linked to different second messenger systems and lead to the increase of intracellular Ca^{2+} or the decrease of cAMP.
   e. Glutamate is removed from the synapse by high-affinity reuptake; two transporter proteins are expressed in glial cells and one in neurons.

4. **Function. Glutamate affects many brain functions.** Some examples include:
   a. Glutamatergic neurons and NMDA receptors in the hippocampus are important in the creation of **long-term potentiation (LTP), a crucial component in the formation of memory.**
   b. **Cortical neurons use glutamate as the major excitatory neurotransmitter.** Excess stimulation of glutamatergic receptors, as seen in seizures or stroke, can lead to unregulated Ca^{2+} influx and neuronal damage.

B. **GABAergic Neurotransmission**
γ-Aminobutyric acid (GABA) is an amino acid with high concentrations in the brain and the spinal cord. It acts as the major inhibitory neurotransmitter in the CNS.

1. **Anatomy. GABAergic neurons can be divided into two groups: short-ranging neurons (interneurons, local circuit neurons)** in the cortex, thalamus, striatum, cerebellum, and spinal cord; **medium/long-ranging neurons** with the following projections:
   a. Caudate/putamen→globus pallidus→thalamus, substantia nigra
   b. Septum→hippocampus
   c. Substantia nigra→thalamus, superior colliculus

2. **Synthesis. GABA is synthesized via decarboxylation of glutamate by the enzyme glutamic acid decarboxylase (GAD).**

3. **Synapse. GABA acts at two types of receptors:**
   a. **The GABA$_A$ receptor is a receptor-channel complex comprising five subunits. Activation leads to the opening of the channel, allowing Cl^- to enter the cell, resulting in decreased excitability.** Five distinct classes of subunits (six variants of α, four variants of β, three variants of γ, one δ, and two variants of ρ) are known. The receptor can be modulated by various compounds that bind to several different sites.
      i. Benzodiazepines bind to the α subunit and open the channel if a γ subunit is present and if GABA is bound to the GABA site on the β subunit.
      ii. Barbiturates and ethanol bind near the Cl^- channel and increase channel open time even without GABA present.
   b. **The GABA$_B$ receptor is a G-protein-coupled receptor with similarity to the metabotropic glutamate receptor.** The GABA$_B$ receptor is linked to G_i (decreasing cAMP and opening of K^+ channels) and G_o (closing Ca^{2+} channels). The net effect is prolonged inhibition of the cell.
      i. GABA is removed from the synapse by a sodium-dependent GABA uptake transporter.

4. **Function. GABA is the major inhibitory neurotransmitter in the CNS.** Examples of normal and perturbed function include:
   a. **Cortical and thalamic GABAergic neurons are crucial for the inhibition of excitatory neurons.** Benzodiazepines or barbiturates are efficacious in the treatment and prevention of seizures.
   b. **Modulation of GABA$_B$ receptors is beneficial in the treatment of anxiety disorders, insomnia, and agitation,** most likely due to a general inhibition of neuronal activity.
   c. **Benzodiazepines and ethanol use the same mechanism to influence GABA$_A$ receptors.** This property is the basis for ethanol detoxification utilizing benzodiazepines.

C. **Cholinergic Neurotransmission**
Acetylcholine (ACh) has been known as a neurotransmitter since the mid-1920s. In the peripheral nervous system, ACh is found as the neurotransmitter in the autonomic ganglia, the parasympathetic postganglionic synapse, and the neuromuscular endplate.

1. **Anatomy. Cholinergic neurons in the CNS are either wide-ranging projection neurons or short-ranging interneurons:**
   a. Cholinergic projection neurons in the basal forebrain (septum, diagonal band, nucleus basalis of Meynert) project to the entire cortex, the hippocampus, and the amygdala.
   b. Cholinergic projection neurons located in the brainstem project predominantly to the thalamus.
   c. Cholinergic interneurons in the striatum modulate the activity of GABAergic striatal neurons.

2. **Synthesis. ACh is synthesized by the enzyme choline acetyltransferase (ChAT) from the precursors acetyl-coenzyme A (acetyl-CoA) and choline.** High-affinity and low-affinity transporters pump choline, the rate-limiting factor in the synthesis of ACh, into the cell.

3. **Synapse. ACh acts at two different types of cholinergic receptors:**
   a. **Muscarinic receptors bind ACh as well as other agonists** (muscarine, pilocarpine, bethanechol) **and antagonists** (atropine, scopolamine). There are at least five different types of **muscarinic receptors (M_1–M_5). All have slow response times.** They are coupled to G-proteins and a variety of second messenger systems. When activated, the final effect can be to open or close channels for K^+, Ca^{2+}, or Cl^-.
   b. **Nicotinic receptors are less abundant** than the muscarinic type in the CNS. **They bind ACh as well as agonists** (e.g., nicotine) or antagonists (e.g., d-tubocurarine). The fast-acting ionotropic nicotinic receptor allows influx of $Na^+ > K^+ > Ca^{2+}$ into the cell.
   c. **ACh is removed from the synapse through hydrolysis into acetyl-CoA and choline by the enzyme acetylcholinesterase (AChE).** Removing ACh from the synapse can be blocked irreversibly by organophosphorous compounds and in a reversible fashion by drugs such as physostigmine.

4. **Function. ACh modulates attention, novelty seeking, and memory via the basal forebrain projections to the cortex and limbic structures.**
   a. Alzheimer's disease (AD) and anticholinergic delirium are examples for a deficit state. Blocking the metabolism of ACh by AChE strengthens cognitive functioning in AD patients.
   b. Brainstem cholinergic neurons are essential for the regulation of sleep-wake cycles via projections to the thalamus.
   c. **Cholinergic interneurons modulate striatal neurons by opposing the effects of dopamine.** Increased cholinergic tone in Parkinson's disease and decreased cholinergic tone in patients treated with neuroleptics are examples for an imbalance of these two systems in the striatum.

D. Serotonergic Neurotransmission

Serotonin, or 5-hydroxytryptamine (5HT), is a monoamine widely distributed in many cells of the body, with about 1–2% of its entire body content present in the CNS.

1. **Anatomy. Serotonergic neurons are restricted to midline structures of the brainstem.** Most serotonergic cells overlap with the distribution of the raphe nuclei in the brainstem. A rostral group (B6–8 neurons) projects to the thalamus, hypothalamus, amygdala, striatum, and cortex. The remaining two groups (B1–5 neurons) project to other brainstem neurons, the cerebellum, and the spinal cord.

2. **Synthesis. Serotonin is synthesized by the enzyme amino acid decarboxylase (AAD) from 5-hydroxytryptophan** (itself derived from tryptophan via tryptophan hydroxylase). **The rate-limiting step of the pathway is the production of 5-hydroxytryptophan by tryptophan hydroxylase.**

3. **Synapse. Serotonin acts at two different types of receptors.** With the exception of the $5HT_3$ receptor, all serotonin receptors are **G-protein-coupled receptors.**
   a. **The $5HT_1$ receptors ($5HT_{1A-F}$) are coupled to G_i and lead to a decrease of cAMP.** The $5HT_{1A}$ receptor is also directly coupled to a K^+ channel, leading to increased opening of the channel. The $5HT_1$ receptors are the predominant serotonergic autoreceptors.
   b. **$5HT_2$ receptors ($5HT_{2A-C}$) are coupled to phospholipase C and lead to a variety of intracellular effects** (mainly depolarization). Three receptors ($5HT_{4,6,7}$) are coupled to G_s and activate adenylate cyclase. The function of the $5HT_{5A}$ and $5HT_{5B}$ receptors is poorly understood.
   c. **The $5HT_3$ receptor is the only monoamine receptor coupled to an ion channel, probably a Ca^{2+} channel.** It is found in the cortex, hippocampus, and area postrema. It is typically localized presynaptically and regulates neurotransmitter release. **Well-known antagonists are ondansetron and granisetron.**
   d. **Serotonin is removed from the synapse by a high-affinity serotonin uptake site** that is capable of transporting serotonin in either direction, depending on the concentration. **The serotonin transporter is blocked by the selective serotonin reuptake inhibitors (SSRIs), as well as by tricyclic antidepressants.**

4. **Function. Serotonin is linked to many brain functions due to the widespread serotonergic projections and the heterogeneity of the serotonergic receptors.** Examples include:
   a. **Modulation of serotonergic receptors** and the reuptake site **is beneficial** (among others) **in the treatment of anxiety, depression, obsessive-compulsive disorder, and schizophrenia.**
   b. **Blockade of $5HT_3$ receptors** in the area postrema **decreases nausea and emesis.**
   c. **Hallucinogens** (e.g., lysergic acid diethylamide [**LSD**]) **modulate serotonergic neurons** via serotonergic autoreceptors.

E. Noradrenergic Neurotransmission

Norepinephrine (NE), a catecholamine, was first identified as a neurotransmitter in 1946. In the peripheral nervous system it is found as the neurotransmitter in the sympathetic postganglionic synapse.

1. **Anatomy. About half of all noradrenergic neurons** (i.e., 12,000 on each side of the brainstem) **are located in the locus coeruleus (LC). They provide** the extensive noradrenergic innervation of cortex, hippocampus, thalamus, cerebellum, and spinal cord. The remaining neurons are distributed in the tegmental region. They innervate predominantly the hypothalamus, basal forebrain and spinal cord.

2. **Synthesis. NE is synthesized by the enzyme dopamine-β-hydroxylase (DβH) from the precursor dopamine** (itself derived from tyrosine via dihydroxyphenylalanine [dopa]). **The pathway's rate-limiting step is the production of dopa by tyrosine hydroxylase,** which can be activated through phosphorylation.

3. **Synapse. NE is released into the synapse from vesicles; amphetamine facilitates this release.** NE acts in the CNS at two different types of noradrenergic receptors (alpha and beta):

   a. **Adrenergic alpha-receptors can be subdivided into alpha-1-receptors** (coupled to phospholipase and located postsynaptically; prazosin is a typical antagonist) **and alpha-2-receptors** (coupled to G_i and located primarily presynaptically; clonidine and guanfacine are potent agonists, and yohimbine an antagonist).

   b. **Adrenergic beta-receptors in the CNS are predominantly of the beta-1-subtype.** Beta-1-receptors are coupled to G_s and lead to an increase of cAMP. cAMP triggers a variety of events mediated by protein kinases, including phosphorylation of the beta-receptor itself, and regulation of gene expression via phosphorylation of transcription factors.

   c. **NE is removed from the synapse by two mechanisms:**
      i **Catechol-O-methyltransferase (COMT)** degrades intrasynaptic NE.
      ii. **The norepinephrine transporter (NET), a Na^+/Cl^--dependent neurotransmitter transporter, is the primary way of removing NE from the synapse.** The NET is blocked selectively by desipramine and nortriptyline. Once internalized, NE can be degraded by the intracellular enzyme monoamine oxidase (MAO).

4. **Function. Noradrenergic projections modulate sleep cycles, appetite, mood, and cognition by targeting the thalamus, limbic structures, and cortex.** These functions are targets of antidepressant drugs.

   a. The locus coeruleus (LC) receives afferents from the sensory systems that monitor the internal and external environments. The widespread LC efferents lead to an inhibition of spontaneous discharge in the target neurons. Therefore, the LC is thought to be crucial for fine tuning the attentional matrix of the cortex. Anxiety disorders may be due to perturbations of this system.

   b. The neurons of the LC express a variety of autoreceptors: LC firing can be decreased by clonidine and increased by yohimbine; morphine decreases LC firing and withdrawal leads to increased firing (this is the rationale for clonidine use in the treatment of opiate withdrawal).

F. Dopaminergic Neurotransmission.

Dopamine (DA) was initially considered as merely an intermediate monoamine in the synthesis of norepinephrine and epinephrine. However, in the late 1950s DA was discovered to be a neurotransmitter in its own right.

1. **Anatomy. Dopaminergic neurons can be divided into three major groups based on the length of their efferent fibers:**

   a. **Ultrashort systems** in the retina and olfactory bulb
   b. **Intermediate-length systems** originating in the hypothalamus and projecting, among others, to the pituitary gland
   c. **Wide-ranging systems** originating from two areas:
      i. Substantia nigra (SN) neurons ($=A9$), projecting primarily to caudate and putamen
      ii. Ventral tegmental area (VTA) neurons ($=A10$) projecting to: limbic areas (nucleus accumbens, amygdala)—mesolimbic projections; and cortex (frontal, cingulate, entorhinal)—mesocortical projections

2. **Synthesis. DA is synthesized by the enzyme L-aromatic amino acid decarboxylase from dopa** (which is produced from tyrosine via tyrosine hydroxylase [TH]). The turnover rate of dopa is extremely high and DA levels can be elevated if extra dopa is supplied to the brain.

3. **Synapse. DA is released into the synapse from vesicles; this process is facilitated by amphetamine and methylphenidate.**

   a. **DA acts at two different classes of DA receptors in the CNS: the D_1 receptor family and the D_2 receptor family.** The D_1 receptor family includes the D_1 and D_5 receptors. Both are coupled to G_s and lead to an increase of cAMP. The D_2 receptor family includes the D_2, D_3, and D_4 receptors. All are coupled to G_i and lead to a decrease of cAMP. There is a predilection of the different DA receptors for expression in specific brain areas:
      i. D_1: striatum, cortex, SN, olfactory tubercle
      ii. D_2: striatum, SN, pituitary gland, retina, olfactory tubercle
      iii. D_3: nucleus accumbens
      iv. D_4: GABAergic neurons in cortex, thalamus, hippocampus, SN
      v. D_5: hippocampus, hypothalamus

b. **Presynaptic dopaminergic receptors are typically of the D_2 type and are found on most portions of the dopaminergic neuron (as autoreceptors). They regulate DA synthesis and release, as well as the firing rate of DA neurons.** Autoreceptors are 5–10 times more sensitive to DA agonists than postsynaptic receptors.

c. **DA is removed from the synapse by two mechanisms. First, COMT degrades intrasynaptic DA. Second, the dopamine transporter (DAT),** a Na^+/Cl^--dependent neurotransmitter transporter, transports DA in either direction, depending on the concentration gradient. The DAT is blocked selectively by drugs such as cocaine, amphetamine, bupropion, benztropine, and nomifensine.

4. **Function. DA affects several brain functions, primarily by modulation of other neurotransmitter systems:**

   a. **Dopaminergic neurons of the SN project to the striatum and modulate the function of striatal GABAergic neurons.** Parkinson's disease and extrapyramidal side effects due to treatment with neuroleptics are examples of decreased dopaminergic function.

   b. **Dopaminergic projections of the VTA to limbic structures,** such as the nucleus accumbens, **are known to be involved in reward behavior** and in the development of addiction to drugs, such as ethanol, cocaine, nicotine, and opiates.

   c. Dopaminergic projections from the VTA to the cortex play a role in the fine tuning of cortical neurons (i.e., better signal-to-noise ratio). Dopaminergic projections from the hypothalamus to the pituitary gland tonically inhibit the production and release of prolactin via D_2 receptors; blockade of these receptors leads to hyperprolactinemia.

IV. Conclusion

Psychopharmacology uses molecules to modulate human brain function. Three basic principles of neurotransmission may help to understand the current practice of clinical psychopharmacology. **First, the anatomic organization of neurotransmitter systems determines their behavioral affiliation. Second, neurotransmitter receptors modulate the electrical properties (via ion channels) or the chemical properties (via second messenger systems) of neurons. Third, the intracellular integration of receptor-mediated responses leads to immediate and/or delayed effects on neuronal function.**

Suggested Readings

Cooper JR, Bloom FE, Roth RH: *The Biochemical Basis of Neuropharmacology,* 7th ed. New York: Oxford University Press, 1996.

Hyman SE, Nestler EJ: *The Molecular Foundations of Psychiatry.* Washington, DC: American Psychiatric Press, 1993.

Kandel ER, Schwartz J, Jessel T: *Principles of Neural Science,* 4th ed. New York: Elsevier, 1996.

Nieuwenhuys R: *Chemoarchitecture of the Brain.* Berlin: Springer-Verlag, 1985.

Siegel GJ, Agranoff BW, Albers RW, Molinoff PB: *Basic Neurochemistry,* 5th ed. New York: Raven Press, 1994.

Chapter 44
Treatment of Anxiety Disorders

DAN V. IOSIFESCU AND MARK H. POLLACK

I. Introduction

Anxiety disorders tend to be chronic and to fluctuate. They are associated with considerable morbidity and impairment, yet **they respond well to pharmacological and cognitive-behavioral treatments.**

II. Panic Disorder

Panic disorder is characterized by fear of recurrent unexpected panic attacks, and by a persistent concern related to the autonomic arousal which accompanies such attacks. Traditionally, **treatment of panic disorder has focused on blocking panic attacks, diminishing anticipatory or generalized anxiety, and reversing phobic avoidance.** At the same time, comorbid conditions, among which depression and alcohol abuse are particularly relevant, need to be treated.

A. Pharmacotherapy

The pharmacotherapy of panic disorder aims to prevent panic attacks and to treat comorbid conditions, such as depression. The goal of treatment is to reduce the patient's distress and impairment to the point of remission, or to the point where the patient is capable of participating in other forms of therapy (e.g., cognitive-behavioral therapy [CBT]). (See Table 44-1 for recommended dosages of the most commonly prescribed medications.)

1. **Antidepressants.** The first medications shown to be effective in panic disorder were tricyclic antidepressants (TCAs); monoamine oxidase inhibitors (MAOIs), then selective serotonin reuptake inhibitors (SSRIs) demonstrate efficacy.

   a. **Selective serotonin reuptake inhibitors (SSRIs)** are now the "first-line" treatment of panic disorder, which likely involves dysregulation of the central serotoninergic system. In 1996, paroxetine (Paxil) was the first antidepressant labeled for treatment of panic disorder. Since then other SSRIs (sertraline [Zoloft], fluoxetine [Prozac], fluvoxamine [Luvox]) have demonstrated antipanic efficacy, both in double-blind and open trials. However, direct comparison among different SSRIs in the treatment of panic disorder are lacking.

      i. **Advantages of SSRIs** include a favorable side-effect profile, a broad spectrum of efficacy for comorbid disorders, a low potential for abuse, safety in overdose, and single daily dosing.

      ii. **Disadvantages of SSRIs** include restlessness, "jitteriness," increased anxiety on initial dosing, and a delayed onset of action (3–6 weeks).

   Given the fact that SSRIs have the potential to cause initial restlessness, insomnia, and increased anxiety, and that panic patients are sensitive to somatic sensations, the starting doses should be low (e.g., paroxetine 10 mg/day, sertraline 25 mg/day, fluvoxamine 50 mg/day, fluoxetine 10 mg/day). SSRI doses can then be titrated up, based on clinical response. The average effective doses of SSRIs are in the typical antidepressant range, and somtimes higher (e.g., paroxetine 20–40 mg/day, sertraline 50–150 mg/day, fluvoxamine 150–200 mg/day, fluoxetine 20–40 mg/day, and citalopram [Celexa] 20–40 mg/day).

   b. **Tricyclic antidepressants (TCAs).** Imipramine (Tofranil) was the first pharmacological agent shown to be efficacious in panic disorder. Clomipramine is now considered to have superior antipanic properties when compared with other TCAs (possibly related to its selectivity for serotoninergic uptake).

      i. **Advantages of TCAs** include their lower cost (when compared to SSRIs), the fact that they are well studied, the fact that they are efficacious in SSRI nonresponders, and that they can be administered once a day.

      ii. **Disadvantages of TCAs** include a wide-ranging adverse effects profile (with anticholinergic effects, orthostatic hypotension, effects on the cardiac conduction system, weight gain, restlessness, "jitteriness"), heightened anxiety on initial dosing, a delayed onset of action (3–6 weeks), cardiotoxicity in overdose, and a total cost of care that may be higher than that associated with SSRIs.

   The adverse effect profile of TCAs accounts for a high drop-out rate (30–70%) in published studies. Treatment should be initiated with lower doses (e.g., 10 mg/day for imipramine) to minimize the "activation syndrome" (restlessness, "jitteriness," palpitations, increased anxiety) noted upon initiation of treatment. Typical antidepressant doses (e.g., 100–300 mg/day for imipramine) may ultimately be used to control the symptoms of panic disorder. Blood levels of TCAs, especially for imipramine, nortriptyline (Pamelor), and desipramine (Norpramin), can be checked after achievement of a steady state (about 5

Table 44-1. Recommended Dosage of Most Commonly Prescribed Antianxiety Medications

Drug	Daily Dose Range (mg)	Initial Dose (mg)	Dosing Schedule
SSRIs			
Paroxetine (Paxil)	10–50	10	q.d.
Sertraline (Zoloft)	25–200	25	q.d.
Fluvoxamine (Luvox)	50–300	50	q.d.
Fluoxetine (Prozac)	10–80	10	q.d.
Citalopram (Celexa)	20–60	10–20	q.d.
TCAs			
Imipramine (Tofranil)	100–300	10–25	q.d.
Clomipramine (Anafranil)	100–250	12.5–25	q.d.
Amitriptyline (Elavil)	100–300	10–25	q.d.
MAOIs			
Phenelzine (Nardil)	60–90	15	b.i.d.
Tranylcypromine (Parnate)	30–60	10–60	b.i.d.
Atypical antidepressants			
Venlafaxine (Effexor-XR)	75–300	37.5	q.d.
Nefazodone (Serzone)	300–600	50	b.i.d.
Benzodiazepines			
Alprazolam (Xanax)	2–10	0.25–0.5	q.i.d.
Clonazepam (Klonopin)	1–5	0.25	b.i.d.
Diazepam (Valium)	5–40	2.5	b.i.d.
Lorazepam (Ativan)	3–16	1.0	t.i.d.-q.i.d.
Azapirones			
Buspirone (Buspar)	15–60	5	b.i.d.-t.i.d.
Beta-blockers			
Propranolol (Inderal)	10–60	10–20	b.i.d.
Anticonvulsants			
Valproate (Depakote)	500–2000	250	b.i.d.
Gabapentin (Neurontin)	300–5400	300	b.i.d.-t.i.d.

days after a dose change), and may be useful in cases of poor response.

c. **Monoamine oxidase inhibitors (MAOIs),** such as phenelzine (Nardil) and tranylcypromine (Parnate), are potent antipanic agents.

   i. **Advantages of MAOIs** include their efficacy in treatment-resistant patients.

   ii. **Disadvantages of MAOIs** include their adverse effects profile (anticholinergic effects, orthostatic hypotension, weight gain, and sexual dysfunction), the need for dietary restrictions (to prevent hypertensive crisis), drug interactions, and their toxicity in overdose.

Due to the danger associated with consumption of tyramine-containing foods while taking a MAOI, with drug interactions, and with toxicity in overdose, MAOIs are usually reserved for panic-disordered patients who remain symptomatic after treatment with safer and better tolerated agents. Optimal doses for phenelzine range between 60 and 90 mg/day, while doses of tranylcypromine generally range between 30 and 60 mg/day.

d. **Other antidepressants.** Venlafaxine (Effexor-XR) is generally efficacious in individuals with panic disorder at doses between 75 and 300 mg/day; its starting dose is 37.5 mg/day. Nefazodone, a $5HT_2$ antagonist, is efficacious and tolerable at doses between 300 and 600 mg/day.

2. **Benzodiazepines**

a. **Initiation of treatment.** Benzodiazepines are frequently used in the treatment of panic disorder, due to their efficacy, their rapid onset, and their favorable side effect profile. Common side effects noted at the beginning of treatment include sedation and ataxia, which can be minimized by initiating treatment with low doses and gradually titrating the dose upward. Treatment with benzodiazepines is associated with lower drop-out rates compared with use of TCAs.

   i. **Advantages** include being highly efficacious, rapidly acting, and having a favorable side effect profile.

   ii. **Disadvantages** include the propensity to develop a withdrawal syndrome, a potential for abuse, initial sedation and ataxia, increased sedation in the elderly, interactions with alcohol, and short-term memory impairment.

b. **Pharmacokinetics.** High-potency benzodiazepines (e.g., alprazolam and clonazepam) are equally as effective as TCAs and often better tolerated in the treatment of panic disorder. Treatment with alprazolam should be started with 0.25–0.5 mg b.i.d.-t.i.d., and then gradually increased to maintenance doses (0.5–3 mg q.i.d.). However, alprazolam's short half-life may generate interdose rebound anxiety and withdrawal symptoms. The need to treat interdose anxiety with extra medication may foster a cognitive dependence on the medication. Therefore, a longer-acting high-potency benzodiazepine, such as clonazepam, may be preferred. Clonazepam is also effective in treating panic-disordered patients and its antipanic benefits are sustained over time without escalation of dose. Usually an initial bedtime dose of 0.25–0.5 mg is gradually titrated up to 1–3 mg/day, which may be divided b.i.d. Lower-potency benzodiazepines may also be effective for panic disorder at equivalent doses (e.g., 40 mg/day diazepam).

c. **Discontinuation syndromes. Discontinuation of treatment with benzodiazepines should be done gradually,** sometimes over as long as several months. The taper should be slower near its end. Rapid taper of benzodiazepines or abrupt discontinuation is frequently followed by a withdrawal syndrome, associated with rebound anxiety, weakness, and insomnia. The withdrawal syndrome, which has been described after treatments as short as 4–8 weeks, can be sufficiently severe to cause seizures, confusion, and psychotic symptoms, and is more intense with shorter-acting agents. One strategy to minimize withdrawal is to convert shorter-acting agents to longer-acting benzodiazepines (e.g., clonazepam) prior to initiating the taper. The potential for withdrawal generally decreases after discontinuation of benzodiazepines. Symptoms that persist more than 2 weeks after discontinuation may be more likely interpreted as a return of the original anxiety disorder.

d. **Abuse and dependence.** Clinicians should consider the **potential for abuse and dependence** when prescribing benzodiazepines, especially in patients with a history of alcohol and substance abuse. A history of substance abuse does not represent an absolute contraindication to benzodiazepine treatment, but warrants particular caution on the part of the clinician.

e. **Use in the elderly. Benzodiazepines should be used cautiously in elderly patients,** who, due to decreased pharmacokinetics, may be more sensitive to sedation, ataxia, risk of falls, memory impairment. The elderly may also experience paradoxical agitation on benzodiazepines more often than younger patients.

3. **Other agents.** Buspirone (Buspar) has antianxiety properties but does not appear to be effective in panic disorder. Beta-blockers are not useful as primary treatment of panic, but they may reduce some somatic symptoms of autonomic arousal and may be used as adjuvants to other agents. Some anticonvulsants (valproate [Depakote], gabapentin [Neurontin]) have been used efficaciously in typical, atypical, and treatment-resistant panic disorder.

B. **Cognitive-Behavioral Therapy**

CBT models of panic disorder focus on the information-processing and behavioral reactions that characterize the experience of panic attacks. The initial panic episodes typically emerge at a time of intense stress, which activates the firing of the fight-or-flight alarm system. In vulnerable individuals, the somatic sensations experienced during the initial panic episodes become cognitively associated with intense stress and danger. Subsequently, catastrophic misinterpretations of the meaning of somatic sensations (e.g., "I'm going to have a heart attack") may trigger similar alarm reactions, even in the absence of danger. The misinterpretations trigger intense anxiety, which further intensifies somatic sensations in a positive feedback loop, resulting in a dramatic increase of anxiety into full panic. Later in the course of panic disorder, the alarm reactions (panic attacks) may become the focus of fear themselves.

The CBT of panic disorder aims to eliminate catastrophic misinterpretations and the conditioned fear of somatic sensations, as well as to eliminate avoidance behavior. Most CBT for panic disorder, typically lasting 12–15 sessions, includes four components:

1. **Informational interventions** (i.e., explanations about the nature of the disorder) aim to demystify the somatic sensations experienced during panic

attacks and to instruct patients about self-perpetuating patterns that maintain the disorder.

2. **Cognitive restructuring** aims to de-catastrophize beliefs about the meaning and the consequences of somatic symptoms. The catastrophic misinterpretations often distort the meaning of somatic sensations (e.g., "I'm going to have a heart attack"), or overestimate the probability or the degree of severity of feared outcomes (e.g., "I'm going to lose control"). The patients are asked to record their thoughts in panic diaries and to later analyze these thoughts as hypotheses, evaluating the evidence for or against them. The goal is to help patients reduce catastrophic interpretations and bring their thoughts in accordance with actual consequences.

3. **Exposure interventions** attempt to extinguish the conditioned response (fear) to certain somatic sensations or external situations in which panic may occur (i.e., agoraphobia). **Interoceptive exposure** is designed to induce somatic sensations usually associated with panic (e.g., running up the stairs to induce tachycardia). **In vivo exposure** targets patients suffering with agoraphobic avoidance, by exposing them to the avoided situations. The exposure methods are utilized in a gradual manner.

4. **Anxiety management skills** (e.g., slow breathing techniques, muscle relaxation training) provide patients with skills for prevention of anxious responses to initial anxiety sensations. CBT is efficacious as an initial treatment for panic disorder, or as an adjuvant to pharmacological treatment. CBT can be used also for patients who failed to respond to pharmacotherapy or who wish to discontinue it. The integration of pharmacotherapy and CBT often produces the optimal outcome.

III. Generalized Anxiety Disorder

Generalized anxiety disorder (GAD) is characterized by unrealistic or excessive worry about life circumstances and is accompanied by chronic symptoms of autonomic arousal.

A. **Pharmacotherapy**

Most pharmacological agents used in panic disorder are also effective in GAD. However, there are some differences:

1. **Benzodiazepines** have been the mainstay of treatment for GAD and are utilized for the majority of patients with GAD. There is no proof that any benzodiazepine is more effective than others in the treatment of GAD. The characteristics of treatment with benzodiazepines discussed for panic disorder also apply for GAD.

2. **Buspirone,** a $5HT_{1A}$ partial agonist, has been shown to be effective in the treatment of GAD. Its efficacy has been comparable to benzodiazepines in some studies. The starting dose is usually 5 mg b.i.d., which is then gradually increased to the average therapeutic dose of 10–30 mg b.i.d. (20–60 mg/day).

3. The **antidepressant agents (SSRIs, TCAs, MAOIs)** are also effective treatment for GAD. Considerations in the use of antidepressants for GAD are similar to those for panic, although less well studied.

4. **Beta-blockers (propranolol, atenolol)** are useful as adjuvants to other agents; they may reduce some somatic symptoms of autonomic arousal. When effective, beta-blockers may begin to work within the first week of treatment.

B. **Cognitive-Behavioral Therapy**

Many of the same CBT interventions discussed for panic disorder also apply in GAD.

1. **Informational interventions** identify maladaptive cognitions and the worry process as a primary cause of anxiety.

2. **Cognitive restructuring.** Patients are asked to record their maladaptive cognitions as they occur in high-anxiety situations. Later, they analyze these thoughts logically, as hypotheses, evaluating the evidence for and against them. As patients get better at evaluating the content of their thoughts, specific "worry times" may be assigned to help them gain control over the constant tendency to worry.

3. **Exposure interventions.** Imaginary exposure to core worries is used to help patients decrease their worries about specific concerns.

4. **Anxiety management skills.** Relaxation training (e.g., slow breathing techniques, muscle relaxation training) is used to decrease the arousal that accompanies worry and provides patients with coping tools to use in high-anxiety situations.

IV. Social Phobia

Patients with social phobia are primarily concerned about humiliation, embarrassment, or a negative evaluation by others.

A. **Pharmacotherapy**

An increasing number of pharmacological studies have addressed social phobia. **Medications with demonstrated efficacy in social phobia include MAOIs, benzodiazepines, SSRIs, beta-blockers, and gabapentin.**

1. **MAOIs.** In double-blind studies, phenelzine has proven effective in social phobia. Doses used are

similar to those used for depression and for panic disorder.

2. **High-potency benzodiazepines,** especially alprazolam (Xanax) and clonazepam (Klonopin), are effective in social phobia.

3. **Beta-blockers** have been used with mixed results in the treatment of social phobia. Doses (10–40 mg) of propranolol have been shown to benefit patients with performance anxiety, but beta-blockers are not effective for the generalized subtype of social phobia.

4. **SSRIs.** All SSRIs as well as nefazodone and venlafaxine XR have been reported efficacious in the treatment of social phobia at typical antidepressant doses. Recently, paroxetine became the first agent to receive FDA approval for this indication. Of note, TCAs are not generally effective for the treatment of social phobia.

5. **Gabapentin (neurontin)** (dose range, 300–3600 mg/day) recently demonstrated efficacy in the treatment of social phobia.

B. **Cognitive-Behavioral Therapy**
Fear of critical evaluation by others in social interactions is the key cognitive aspect of social phobia. This fear motivates avoidance of social situations and ultimately prevents the acquisition of social confidence and skills. The CBT for social phobia includes:

1. **Informational interventions,** which are designed to clarify to the patient the anxiogenic nature of their thoughts and the role of avoidance in heightening socially phobic patterns.

2. **Cognitive restructuring,** which is designed to modify the maladaptive cognitions that detract from competent social performance. Typical cognitive distortions include negative expectations of social performance ("I will not know what to say"), distorted evaluations of the self ("Everyone can do it but me"), and distorted anticipation of the reaction of others ("They will think I'm stupid"). Patients are taught to self-monitor their cognitive distortions and to analyze them logically, as hypotheses, evaluating the evidence for and against them.

3. **Exposure interventions,** which aim to provide patients with the ability to practice in social situations and to evaluate their cognitions in that context. Patients rehearse feared interactions in group and homework assignments.

4. **Social skills training** includes instructions and programmed practice in a role-playing format.

V. Specific Phobia

Patients with specific phobia are fearful of circumscribed situations or objects. Those fears lead to significant distress and disability.

A. **Exposure-based interventions,** a form of CBT, **are the mainstay of the treatment for specific phobia.** Adding medications to these interventions appears to bring no additional benefit. Benzodiazepine treatment may be used to help an individual cope with a feared event that is rarely encountered (e.g., dentist visit).

B. **The treatment consists of systematic desensitization and participant modeling.** The systematic desensitization consists of relaxation training combined with gradual exposure (frequently imaginary) to the feared stimulus. In participant modeling, the therapist enacts a behavior and then encourages the patient to repeat that behavior.

VI. Obsessive-Compulsive Disorder

Obsessive-compulsive disorder (OCD) is characterized by recurrent, intrusive, unwanted thoughts (i.e., obsessions, such as fears of contamination) and compulsive behaviors or rituals which attempt to reduce the anxiety caused by obsessive thoughts.

A. **Pharmacotherapy**

1. **Antidepressants. Agents that inhibit serotonin reuptake are the pharmacological treatments of choice for OCD.** Clomipramine, a TCA with potent serotonin reuptake inhibition, has been studied for more than 20 years and has been proven efficacious in the treatment of OCD. The effective doses tend to be high, up to 250 mg/day.

   More recently, several SSRIs (e.g., fluvoxamine, fluoxetine, sertraline, paroxetine, and citalopram) have been shown to provide safe and effective treatment for OCD. SSRIs are generally effective in OCD at higher doses compared with antidepressant doses: fluvoxamine (up to 300 mg/day), fluoxetine (up to 80 mg/day), sertraline (up to 200 mg/day), and paroxetine (up to 60 mg/day).

   Few OCD patients achieve a symptom-free state in response to therapy with serotonergic agents; partial relief from obsessional thinking is the more usual outcome. Most patients who respond to SSRI therapy obtain partial relief from obsessional thinking; their subjective experience of anxiety and their use of compulsive behaviors to decrease anxiety are often reduced but not eliminated.

   Response to SSRI therapy may require 8–10 weeks of therapy. Failure to respond to SSRI therapy may reflect inadequate dosing or inadequate duration of treatment. If a patient does not respond to an SSRI at adequate high doses, another SSRI may frequently be tried with success.

2. **Buspirone,** a $5HT_{1A}$ partial agonist, has been helpful in treatment-refractory OCD, as an adjuvant to SSRIs. The medication is started at a dose of 5 mg b.i.d., then gradually increased to the average therapeutic dose of 10–30 mg b.i.d. (20–60 mg/day).

3. **Benzodiazepines** (e.g., clonazepam) have been used successfully to treat comorbid anxiety in the OCD patient. However, benzodiazepines are not effective when used alone in the treatment of OCD. Some benzodiazepines (e.g., diazepam, alprazolam) are reported to have increased plasma levels when used in combination with SSRIs such as fluvoxamine.

4. Other agents (e.g., trazodone and lithium) have been used as adjuvants to potentiate the effect of SSRIs. Their efficacy in OCD is still controversial.

B. **Cognitive-Behavioral Therapy**
   The goal of CBT for OCD patients is to interrupt the chronic cycles of intrusive concerns and the compulsive rituals used by patients to ameliorate their obsessions. CBT is very effective in OCD, especially in combination with pharmacological treatment. The CBT methods utilized in OCD involve exposure and cognitive interventions.

1. **Exposure and response prevention.** The exposure consists of gradually confronting the patient with situations which are likely to trigger obsessive thoughts and compulsive rituals. For example, patients who fear contamination might be given a "dirty" hand towel and encouraged to hold the "contaminated" towel for an hour or longer. The response prevention used at the time of exposure requires patients to resist performing their compulsive rituals, such as hand washing, for a progressively longer period of time. The repeated exposure without performing the compulsive rituals gradually decreases anxiety.

2. **Cognitive interventions** provide patients with additional skills for breaking the link between intrusive thoughts and compulsive responses.

VII. Posttraumatic Stress Disorder

Patients with posttraumatic stress disorder (PTSD) have experienced an event that involved the threat of death, injury, or severe harm to themselves or others. The severe trauma disrupts the patient's sense of safety to the extent that PTSD patients avoid situations which remind them of the trauma; they may become emotionally numb, irritable, hypervigilant, or have difficulties with sleep and concentration. PTSD patients frequently re-experience the traumatic event in the form of nightmares, flashbacks, or by marked arousal when exposed to situations reminiscent of the event.

A. **Pharmacotherapy**
   The role of pharmacotherapy in PTSD has traditionally been related to symptomatic relief and to facilitate the onset of trauma-focused psychotherapy. As a general rule, pharmacologic agents have been shown to have more effect on the positive symptoms of PTSD (e.g., increased arousal, flashbacks) and limited effects on the negative symptoms (e.g., avoidance and withdrawal). However, recently the SSRIs have demonstrated efficacy for reducing the core symptoms of PTSD.

1. **Antidepressants.** TCAs (e.g., amitriptyline and imipramine) have been shown to be effective in reducing PTSD symptoms in double-blind studies. SSRIs (e.g., fluoxetine, sertraline, paroxetine), bupropion, and MAOIs (e.g., phenelzine) have all been reported to have some efficacy in PTSD. Sertraline recently became the first pharmacological agent to receive FDA aproval for PSTD. The drugs are used in doses similar to those listed in Table 44-1; the doses for bupropion are 225–450 mg/day.

2. **Buspirone** has been reported to reduce the anxiety and increased arousal in PTSD patients at doses of 30–60 mg/day.

3. **Mood stabilizers** have been reported in some studies to be efficacious in PTSD, often at lower doses than are used in bipolar disorder (e.g., lithium 300 mg b.i.d., carbamazepine 100 mg b.i.d., valproate 250 mg b.i.d., gabapentin 300–3600 mg/day). Explanations related to a reduction of the kindling effect have been used to explain the positive effects of those medications in PTSD.

4. **Beta-blockers** (e.g., propranolol, nadolol, atenolol) may be useful in some patients with PTSD in order to decrease persistent symptoms of autonomic hyperarousal. Also beneficial in these patients is **clonidine,** at doses of 0.2–0.6 mg/day.

5. **Benzodiazepines** can reduce anxiety in PTSD, but may have negative therapeutic effects including disinhibition and irritability.

6. **Neuroleptics** may reduce psychoses and impulsiveness in PTSD patients.

B. **Individual Psychotherapy**
   Crisis intervention in the immediate aftermath of a trauma is effective in reducing the development of chronic PTSD. The interaction is focused on establishing support and restoring a sense of security for the patient, and providing an understanding and acceptance of the traumatic events.

For the chronic PTSD patient, exposure-based therapies, such as CBT, appear to be the most successful.

C. Cognitive-Behavioral Therapy
CBT interventions aim to disrupt the link between trauma-related cues and the severe anxiety responses and hypervigilance which characterize PTSD.
1. **Informational interventions** aim to help patients understand their symptoms. Discussion of dissociation and flashbacks may normalize and decrease the fear triggered by these symptoms.
2. **Cognitive restructuring** aims to help patients identify distortions in their thoughts which may have been generated by trauma (e.g., "The world is an unsafe place" or "I am helpless").
3. **Exposure interventions** aim to help patients control their emotional reactions associated to trauma. PTSD patients experience a diffuse association with trauma of objects and situations which are only remotely linked to it. With repeated exposure, patients learn to differentiate between the diffuse, exaggerated fears generated by trauma and the actual safety of current situations. The intensity of exposure therapy can vary. Implosive therapy, a more intense form of exposure therapy, is effective but depends on the ability of the patient to tolerate intense levels of arousal. Systematic desensitization implies a more gradual exposure and can be beneficial in overcoming the phobic avoidance related to trauma.
4. **Relaxation training** may be used as in other anxiety disorders to provide patients with skills for preventing anxious responses to initial stages of exposure treatment.

D. Group Therapy
There appear to be advantages for some patients in group therapy for PTSD, compared with individual therapy. Patients involved in group therapy experience the understanding and support provided by fellow victims; also, groups can sometimes generate and process more intense affects than individual therapy. Some researchers also report a greater effect of group therapy on avoidance and the numbing symptoms present in PTSD, but no conclusive comparisons have been made yet.

VIII. Conclusions

Anxiety disorders benefit from specific and effective treatments, both psychopharmacologic and psychotherapeutic. For many patients, a combination of treatment modalities is the most effective treatment solution, although this issue requires further study. Most treatments have been studied for short periods, generally up to 6 months. However, a large number of patients (20–50%) experience a recurrence of their initial anxiety when the treatment is interrupted. For a large number of patients maintenance pharmacological treatment is recommended.

Suggested Readings

Fyer AJ, Manuzza S, Coplan J, et al.: Anxiety disorders. In Kaplan HI, Sadock BJ (eds): *Comprehensive Textbook of Psychiatry*, 6th ed. Baltimore: Williams and Wilkins, 1995.

Hyman SE, Arana GW, Rosenbaum JF: *Handbook of Psychiatric Drug Therapy*, 3rd ed. Boston: Little, Brown, 1995.

Otto MW, Reilly-Harrington NA, Harrington JA: Cognitive-behavioral strategies for specific disorders. In Stern TA, Herman JB, Slavin PL (eds): *The MGH Guide to Psychiatry in Primary Care*. New York: McGraw-Hill, 1998.

Pollack M, Smoller J, Lee D: Approach to the anxious patient. In Stern TA, Herman JB, Slavin PL (eds): *The MGH Guide to Psychiatry in Primary Care*. New York: McGraw-Hill, 1998.

Taylor CB: Treatment of anxiety disorders. In Schatzberg AF, Nemeroff CB (eds): *The American Psychiatric Press Textbook of Psychopharmacology*, 2nd ed. Washington, DC: American Psychiatric Press, 1998.

Chapter 45

Antipsychotic Drugs

DAVID C. HENDERSON AND DONALD C. GOFF

I. Introduction

Selection of antipsychotic agents has generally been guided by side effect profiles as conventional neuroleptics are all of comparable efficacy. Recently, with newer atypical antipsychotic agents, treatment approaches to psychotic patients have changed. In both the Written and Oral Psychiatry Boards, knowledge of different antipsychotic agents (including their generic names), mechanisms, dosing schedules, side effects, drug interactions, and reasons for choosing one over another are vitally important. This chapter will review the above areas as well as approaches to the treatment-resistant patient.

When choosing an antipsychotic agent it is important to focus on specific target symptoms, which should be monitored closely to determine efficacy for a particular agent. These target symptoms include:
1. Psychosis (hallucinations, delusions, disorganization)
2. Negative symptoms (apathy, flat affect, social withdrawal, poverty of speech)
3. Agitation (hyperkinesis, tension, distractibility)
4. Cognitive impairment (attention, memory, judgment, insight)

II. Antipsychotic Agents

A. **Conventional Antipsychotic Agents**
Conventional (typical) antipsychotics or "neuroleptics" **are agents with dopamine D_2 antagonism** and **may produce extrapyramidal symptoms (EPS).** Conventional agents also may **elevate prolactin levels.** Finally, all conventional agents are equally effective, but differ in their potency and side effects. **Potency,** often described as chlorpromazine equivalency, **often determines side effect profiles.** Table 45-1 lists common conventional agents, their dosing schedule, their potency, and their class (e.g., phenothiazine). The class of an agent is a common question on the written boards examination.

B. **Atypical Antipsychotic Agents**
Atypical antipsychotics (**"second generation" antipsychotics or serotonin-dopamine antagonists) are agents with dopamine D_2 and serotonin $5HT_2$ antagonism. They offer reduced or absent EPS with little or no elevation of prolactin.** They are also generally **more effective for negative symptoms** compared to conventional agents. Of note, clozapine is the only agent clearly more effective for psychotic symptoms. Finally, risperidone is more appropriately classified as a "partial atypical" as it may produce EPS at higher doses and can elevate prolactin.

III. Basic Pharmacology of Antipsychotic Agents

A. **Dopamine D_2 Blockade**
Conventional agents acutely block 75–90% of D_2 receptors, while clozapine blocks only 40–60% of D_2 receptors. Blockade of presynaptic D_2 autoreceptors leads to an increase in electrical activity and to release of dopamine acutely.

B. **Delayed Effects**
The delayed effects of conventional agents are due to an increase in the density of postsynaptic D_2 receptors (supersensitivity) and to depolarization blockade in A9 (substantia nigra) and A10 (ventral tegmental) dopamine neurons.

C. **A9 and A10 Blockade**
Atypical agents produce depolarization blockade only in A10 neurons. All agents increase c-fos in the nucleus accumbens, while conventional agents also increase c-fos in the striatum. **The A9 nigrostriatal (midbrain to neostriatum) pathway appears to be responsible for EPS. The A10 mesolimbic (midbrain to limbic structures) is possibly associated with psychosis,** while the A10 mesocortical (midbrain to frontal and temporal cerebral cortex pathway) may be responsible for negative symptoms.

D. **Side Effects with Conventional Agents**
1. **Dystonia, akathisia, and parkinsonism** are more commonly associated with high-potency conventional agents than with low-potency agents.
2. Low-potency agents tend to produce **sedation, hypotension, weight gain** (although molindone may produce weight loss), and **anticholinergic symptoms** (dry mouth, urinary retention, constipation, and blurred vision).
3. **Hyperprolactinemia** (associated with amenorrhea, galactorrhea, and sexual dysfunction), **tardive dyskinesia, and neuroleptic malignant syndrome** may occur with all D_2 antagonists, unrelated to their neuroleptic potency.

345

4. Other potential side effects include: impaired heat regulation (i.e., **poikilothermia** with hyper- or hypothermia); **pigmentary retinopathy** (thioridazine >800 mg/day); and **electrocardiographic (EKG) changes** (especially with pimozide, chlorpromazine, and thioridazine).

IV. Extrapyramidal Side Effects

A. Dystonia

1. Dystonia is **an involuntary muscle contraction that may involve the tongue, neck, back, and eyes.** It is extremely uncomfortable and can jeopardize future compliance with antipsychotics. It may be life-threatening when laryngeal spasms occur. **Generally, it occurs within the first 4 days of neuroleptic treatment or following an increase in the neuroleptic dose.**

2. **Risk factors** include **youth** (age less than 40 years) and the **use of high-potency neuroleptics.** All patients under the age of 30 years started on high-potency neuroleptics should receive prophylaxis with benztropine 1–2 mg b.i.d. for 10 days, followed by a taper. Often, benztropine is

initiated for prophylaxis and continued needlessly for weeks, months, or years.

3. **Treatments for acute dystonia include benztropine 1–2 mg IM or PO, diphenhydramine 25–50 mg IM or PO, or diazepam 5 mg, slow IV push.** After the initial dystonic reaction has resolved, a standing dose of benztropine or another anticholinergic agent is recommended. Dystonias are less common with atypical agents; they do not occur with clozapine. "Tardive dystonia" is a variant of tardive dyskinesia that appears to respond well to atypical agents, particularly clozapine.

B. Akathisia

1. Akathisia is **the sensation of motor restlessness which is most prominent in the lower extremities.** It is most commonly associated with high-potency agents and it is dose-related. Akathisia is often mistaken for agitation, which may lead to a dose increase of an antipsychotic agent and worsening akathisia.

2. **Possible treatments include:** switching to an atypical agent; **lowering the neuroleptic dose;** adding a **beta-blocker** (e.g., propranolol 20 mg q.i.d.), an

Table 45-1. Conventional and Atypical Antipsychotic Agents

Agent	Starting Dose	Dose Range (mg/day)	Class
Atypical			
Clozapine (Clozaril)	12.5 mg	25–900	Dibenzapine
Olanzapine (Zyprexa)	2.5–10 mg	5–20	Thienobenzodiazepine
Quetiapine (Seroquel)	25–50 mg/day	25–750	Dibenzothiazepine
Risperidone (Risperdal)	1–2 mg/day	0.5–16	Benzisoxazole
High-potency conventional			
Haloperidol (Haldol)	0.5–6 mg/day	2–100	Butyrophenone
Trifluoperazine (Stelazine)	2–10 mg/day	5–60	Phenothiazine (C)
Pimozide (Orap)	1–2	1–10	Butyrophenone
Fluphenazine (Prolixin)	2.5–10	5–60	Phenothiazine (C)
Thiothixene (Navane)	2–10 mg/day	5–60	Thioxanthenes
Mid-potency conventional			
Perphenazine (Trilafon)	8–24 mg/day	8–64	Phenothiazine (C)
Loxapine (Loxitane)	10–50 mg/day	30–250	Dibenzapine
Molindone (Moban)	50–75 mg/day	10–225	Indole
Low-potency conventional			
Chlorpromazine (Thorazine)	100–200 mg/day	100–2000	Phenothiazine (A)
Thioridazine (Mellaril)	50–300 mg/day	100–600	Phenothiazine (B)
Mesoridazine (Serentil)	50–150 mg/day	100–400	Phenothiazine (B)

A, aliphatic phenothiazine; B, piperidine phenothiazine; C, piperazine phenothiazine.

anticholinergic agent (e.g., benztropine 1 mg b.i.d.), or a **benzodiazepine** (e.g., lorazepam 0.5 mg t.i.d.).

C. Parkinsonian Symptoms

1. Antipsychotic-induced parkinsonism can be mistaken for negative symptoms or depression. Clinically, it may appear as idiopathic Parkinson's disease, with **rigidity, tremor, and bradykinesia.** It tends to be associated with use of high-potency agents and it is dose-related.

2. **Possible treatments include lowering the neuroleptic dose, switching to an atypical agent, or adding an anticholinergic agent** (benztropine 1–2 mg b.i.d.; in the elderly start with 0.25 mg) or amantadine (100–200 mg b.i.d.).

3. The elderly are most sensitive to the anticholinergic agents; therefore, long-term use of these agents should be avoided.

D. Tardive Dyskinesia

1. Tardive dyskinesia is **a late-developing involuntary choreiform movement disorder,** most commonly of the mouth, tongue, or upper extremities. Tardive dystonia is a syndrome of chronic dystonic posturing.

2. Studies suggest that **the risk for developing tardive dyskinesia is approximately 4–5% per year of exposure.**

3. **Risk factors** for tardive dyskinesia include **old age, neuroleptic exposure of more than 6 months, a history of parkinsonian side effects, diabetes, affective disorders, and use of high doses of conventional agents.**

4. **Tardive dyskinesia does not appear to be associated with clozapine, olanzapine, or quetiapine,** while risperidone may also be associated with a reduced risk of tardive dyskinesia.

5. **A "withdrawal dyskinesia" may occur when a neuroleptic dose is decreased or when a switch is made to an atypical agent.** This type of dyskinesia usually resolves within 6 weeks. Anticholinergic agents may produce a reversible worsening of tardive dyskinesia. Also, tardive dyskinesia usually does not worsen with continued neuroleptic exposure.

6. **Neuroleptics should not be used if there is no clear benefit.** One should also use the lowest effective dose.

7. **The Abnormal Involuntary Movement Scale (AIMS) should be performed twice yearly** to monitor for tardive dyskinesia. Patients should also be warned and educated when taking neuroleptics for more than 6 months.

8. **Treatment for tardive dyskinesia includes discontinuation or lowering of the neuroleptic dose, addi-**

tion of vitamin E (α-tocopherol) 800–1,200 IU/day (if the duration is less than 5 years), **or switching to an atypical antipsychotic agent.**

9. Clozapine is associated with an increased rate of remission (especially with tardive dystonia). Other atypical agents are promising but their efficacy in suppressing tardive dyskinesia has not yet been established.

E. Neuroleptic Malignant Syndrome

1. Neuroleptic malignant syndrome (NMS) is **a rare, potentially lethal complication of neuroleptic treatment, characterized by hyperthermia, autonomic instability, diaphoresis, confusion, elevated creatine phosphokinase (CPK), and fluctuating levels of consciousness, and rigidity.**

2. The symptoms may evolve over time; they usually start with mental status changes and culminate with fever and elevated CPK. **NMS represents a medical emergency** and treatment should begin, in the hospital, immediately.

3. **Treatment includes discontinuation of the neuroleptic, hydration, and temperature control, and possibly bromocriptine or dantrolene** (although it is unclear if these agents improve recovery).

4. **Two weeks should elapse before restarting an antipsychotic agent.** Cases of NMS with clozapine have been reported, but the incidence appears to be lower than with conventional agents.

V. Antipsychotic Dosing

A. Dosing Schedules

In general, one should use a moderate, fixed dose (e.g., haloperidol 5–15 mg/day, risperidone 3–6 mg/day, olanzapine 10–15 mg/day) of an antipsychotic agent for an adequate period (approximately 4–6 weeks) (see Table 45-1). Benzodiazepines can also be administered for agitation (e.g., lorazepam 1–2 mg q.i.d.).

B. Blood Levels

Blood levels should not substitute for titration of doses based on clinical response. While some have considered there to be a "therapeutic window" (5–15 ng/mL) for haloperidol, the data are inconsistent (see Table 45-2). Blood levels may be useful in cases of nonresponse, noncompliance, or when drug interactions occur.

C. Metabolism

Some patients are poor metabolizers (due to low levels of P450 2D6) and may develop toxic levels even at low doses. Drug interactions range from useful, to benign, to dangerous. For example, the addition of fluoxetine may elevate haloperidol blood levels (see Table 45-3).

Table 45-2. Potential Therapeutic Blood Levels for Antipsychotic Agents

Agent	Therapeutic Range (ng/mL)
Haloperidol	5–15
Chlorpromazine	30–100
Fluphenazine	0.2–2.0
Perphenazine	0.8–2.4
Clozapine	>350
Thioridazine	1–1.5
Loxapine	30–100
Thiothixene	2–15

VI. Patients with First-Break Psychosis

A. Response
First-break patients respond better than do chronically psychotic patients, in that 74% achieve a complete remission and 12% achieve a partial response. In general, patients with first-break psychosis respond to lower doses of antipsychotic agents.

B. Early Treatment
Early treatment is **associated with a better outcome.** When treating first-break patients, it is important to avoid side effects and to provide prophylaxis for dystonia, if conventional neuroleptics are used.

C. Alliance
Development of an alliance and education of the patient and family about the illness and its treatments is vital.

VII. Maintenance Treatment

A. Relapse
Relapse rates in schizophrenia range from 41% in the first year to 15% in the second year following hospital discharge. Low and conventional doses are of approximately equal efficacy against relapse in the first year, while conventional doses may be superior during the second year for the prevention of relapse. Lower doses produce significantly fewer EPS and dysphoria.

B. Depot Neuroleptics
Depot neuroleptics can be used in patients where compliance is an issue. **Fluphenazine decanoate** has a half-life of 6–9 days; its recommended injection interval is 14 days. A low dose would be 5–6.25 mg every 2 weeks, while a conventional dose would be 25 mg every 2 weeks.

Haloperidol decanoate has a half-life of 21 days; it can be given at 4-week intervals.

C. Conversion to Depot Neuroleptics
Conversion to a depot neuroleptic requires approxi-

Table 45-3. Drug Interactions with Antipsychotic Agents (Most Metabolized by Cytochrome P450 2D6)

Alcohol	Additive sedation, incoordination, haloperidol increases alcohol levels
Antacids	Impair absorption of chlorpromazine
Anticonvulsants (except valproate)	Lower antipsychotic blood levels
Tobacco	Lowers antipsychotic blood levels
Erythromycin	Increases clozapine levels
Fluvoxamine	Increases clozapine levels
SSRIs	Increase neuroleptic levels and worsen EPS
Tricyclic antidepressants	Levels increased by some neuroleptics, increase antipsychotic blood levels
Anticholinergics	Additive anticholinergic effects
Antiarrhythmics (class I)	Additive conduction impairment
Antihypertensives	
Methyldopa	Hypotension and confusion
Guanethidine	Reverses the antihypertensive effect
Propranolol	Increases antipsychotic blood level
Lithium	May increase chlorpromazine levels
Disulfiram	Lowers chlorpromazine levels

mately four dosing intervals to achieve a steady-state blood level. In general, one should start with a loading dose and supplement with oral agents. **Tolerability with an oral preparation should be established before initiating the decanoate preparation.** The loading dose of haloperidol decanoate is approximately 20 times the oral dose that had been given, in divided doses, during the first week. The decanoate dose is then decreased by 25% for each of the next two injections. The maintenance dose (given every 4 weeks) is approximately ten times the oral dose.

VIII. Atypical Antipsychotic Agents

A. Clozapine

1. Clozapine (Clozaril), an atypical agent, rarely causes EPS and does not elevate serum prolactin levels. Its major benefit is that it is **more effective than conventional agents for treatment-resistant patients. A weak D_2 antagonist, with relatively greater D_1 and D_4 antagonism, clozapine does not cause D_2 receptor supersensitivity or depolarization blockade in A9 neurons.** However, it releases dopamine in the frontal cortex.

   Clozapine has significant interactions with other neurotransmitter systems; it is an alpha-adrenergic antagonist, a histaminergic (H_1) antagonist, a serotonin ($5HT_2$) antagonist, and is highly anticholinergic. Clozapine is effective in 30% of treatment-resistant patients within 6 weeks in controlled trials and in 60% at 6 months in uncontrolled trials.

2. **Clozapine appears to prevent relapse, to stabilize mood, to improve negative symptoms, to improve polydipsia and hyponatremia, to reduce hostility and aggression, and it may reduce the risk of suicide in patients with schizophrenia. Clozapine may also reduce cigarette smoking and substance abuse in individuals with schizophrenia.**

3. **Clozapine produces many troublesome side effects,** including sedation, tachycardia, hypersalivation, dizziness, constipation, nausea, headache, hypotension, fever, dose-related seizures, weight gain, diabetes, and agranulocytosis (in approximately 1% of patients).

4. **Agranulocytosis** (granulocytes $< 500/mm^3$) occurs in 1.6% of patients after 1 year. The clozapine monitoring system involving weekly complete blood counts has reduced the incidence in the United States. Risk factors may include being an Ashkenazi Jew (with blood markers of HLA B38, DR4, DQw3) or Finnish. Usually, other cell lines (platelets, red blood cells) are preserved. The maximum risk appears to be between 4 and 18 weeks, when 77% of cases occur. Patients usually recover

within 14 days if clozapine is stopped. There appears to be no cross-sensitivity with other drugs. However, carbamazepine, captopril, sulfonamides, and propylthiouracil (PTU) should be avoided in clozapine-treated patients. **Patients who develop agranulocytosis should not be rechallenged with clozapine.**

5. Clozapine is usually started at 12.5–25 mg at bedtime. The dose is then increased by 25 mg/day as tolerated over the first week. It is best to overlap with the previous antipsychotic agent (and to watch for additive side effects) and to taper it when the clozapine dose reaches 100 mg/day. In general, clozapine should be stopped at 600 mg/day or when side effects emerge. The usual therapeutic dose is 300–600 mg/day and the maximum dose is 900 mg/day. Clozapine is metabolized by the cytochrome P450 1A2 and 3A4 system. Agents which affect these enzymes may alter clozapine metabolism (see Table 45-3).

B. Risperidone

1. **Risperidone (Risperdal) is an atypical antipsychotic with significant $5HT_2$ and D_2 antagonism.** Risperidone antagonizes D_4, noradrenergic, and histaminergic receptors. Risperidone offers a lower incidence of EPS, which increases as doses increase above 6 mg/day. Unlike other atypical antipsychotic agents, risperidone causes a sustained increase in prolactin levels in some patients. Risperidone appears to be more **effective for negative symptoms** (partly the result of fewer EPS) compared to conventional agents. It also may be more effective for psychotic symptoms in some treatment-resistant patients.

2. Side effects of risperidone include dizziness, hypotension (particularly after the first few doses), headache, nausea, vomiting, anxiety, rhinitis, coughing, hyperprolactinemia, weight gain, and QT interval prolongation (usually clinically insignificant).

3. The mean optimal dose of risperidone is 4–6 mg/day. The usual starting dose is 1–2 mg/day. Treatment-naïve patients may require only 2–4 mg/day. Elderly patients should be started at very low doses (0.5 mg/day), with a dose range of 0.5–2.0 mg/day. Risperidone is metabolized by cytochrome P450 2D6 isoenzymes and it has a half-life of 24 h (therefore, it can be given once daily).

C. Olanzapine

1. **Olanzapine (Zyprexa) is an atypical antipsychotic agent with a high $5HT_2/D_2$ ratio that most closely resembles clozapine.** Olanzapine possesses anticholinergic activity in vitro (with minimal effects in

vivo), as well as histaminergic and alpha-adrenergic antagonism. Olanzapine exhibits antipsychotic efficacy comparable to haloperidol, yet it is more effective for negative symptoms. Olanzapine also appears to have a substantial antidepressant and antimanic effect when compared to placebo.

2. **Side effects of olanzapine** include **somnolence, dizziness** (without hypotension), **constipation, dry mouth, elevation of SGPT** (serum glutamic-pyruvic transaminase) (but without evidence of hepatotoxicity), and **weight gain.**

3. Starting doses of olanzapine are usually 5–10 mg, and the optimal dose is 10–20 mg/day for adults. Elderly patients should be started at lower doses (2.5 mg/day), but may be increased to 2.5–5 mg/day. Olanzapine is metabolized by cytochrome P450 1A2 and 3A4 isoenzymes; it has a half-life of approximately 20 h (therefore, it can be given once daily).

D. Quetiapine

1. **Quetiapine (Seroquel) is an atypical antipsychotic agent with a high $D_2/5HT_2$ ratio** (it may be effective with $< 60\%$ D_2 blockade) and a very low incidence of EPS. Quetiapine is without significant anticholinergic effects; however, it exhibits alpha-adrenergic antagonism. It has a comparable antipsychotic efficacy to chlorpromazine and is more effective for negative symptoms.

2. Side effects include postural hypotension, somnolence, elevation of liver function tests (LFTs) (reversible), **headache, weight gain, decreased serum T_3 and T_4 levels,** and cataracts (in beagles; the risk in humans has not been established, so eye examinations are recommended every 6 months).

3. The starting dose, in nonelderly patients, is 25 mg twice daily, after which doses are titrated upwards. Clinically effective doses range from 250 to 750 mg/day. Doses should be titrated with care to reduce the risk of postural hypotension, particularly in the elderly. Quetiapine is metabolized by the cytochrome P450 2D6 isoenzyme system; it has a half-life of approximately 6 h (and requires multiple dosing).

IX. Treatment Resistance

A. Alternative Diagnoses

Patients with a poor response to treatment must have their diagnosis reassessed. Alternative diagnoses include **substance (alcohol, PCP, stimulants) abuse, neurological disorders** (e.g., partial complex seizures), **psychotic depression, drug toxicity/delirium** (e.g., steroid psychosis, anticholinergic delirium), **dissociative disorders, hysteria, and posttraumatic stress disorder.**

B. Dose Adjustment

Adjustment of the neuroleptic dose and assessment of compliance are often required. A time-limited trial at a higher dose is often indicated, if tolerated. Alternatively, if one is taking moderate to high doses, a dose reduction may provide symptom relief. The use of adjuvants when symptoms persist may help. Possible adjuvants include:

1. **Risperidone (or olanzapine),** added to clozapine for clozapine partial responders, may improve both positive and negative symptoms. Use of this strategy often enables the dose of clozapine to be reduced, which minimizes side effects.

2. **Lithium** (with blood levels of 0.8–1.2 mEq/L for 3–5 weeks), which is necessary to determine efficacy, particularly if affective symptoms are present. Cotreatment may improve positive and negative symptoms. Drug interactions with antihypertensive agents, and nonsteroidal anti-inflammatory drugs (NSAIDs) may develop.

3. **Electroconvulsive therapy** (ECT), which is helpful for catatonia and for affective symptoms, is most effective early in the course of illness. Its long-term efficacy is unclear.

4. **Antidepressants.** Tricyclic antidepressants (TCAs) may delay a positive response in acute psychosis; selective serotonin reuptake inhibitors (SSRIs) may improve depressive and negative symptoms and increase neuroleptic blood levels.

5. **Buspirone** is helpful with agitation and anxiety (15–45 mg/day).

6. **Anticonvulsants** may decrease tension, suspiciousness, manic symptoms, and electroencephalographic (EEG) abnormalities. Carbamazepine increases P450 activity, and thus may lower neuroleptic blood levels.

7. **Benzodiazepines** can decrease agitation, psychotic symptoms, and social withdrawal. Disinhibition and abuse need to be monitored.

8. **Beta-blockers,** often at high doses, may decrease agitation, violence, and impulsivity.

9. **Anticholinergics,** which may be used for dystonia and EPS; however, they may worsen tardive dyskinesia.

X. Conclusion

If treatment failure occurs, despite adequate doses of conventional agents, a switch to an atypical agent is warranted. Atypical agents differ in their patterns of efficacy; each agent is worthy of consideration. **Clozapine remains the most effective agent for treatment-resistant patients.**

Suggested Readings

Breier A, Wolkowitz OM, Doran AR, Roy A, et al.: Neuroleptic responsivity of negative and positive symptoms in schizophrenia. *Am J Psychiatry* 1987; 144:1549–1555.

Christison G, Kirch D, Wyatt R: When symptoms persist: choosing among alternative somatic treatments for schizophrenia. *Schizophr Bull* 1991; 17:217–245.

Gelenberg AJ, Bassuk EL (eds): *The Practitioner's Guide to Psychoactive Drugs*, 4th ed. New York: Plenum, 1997.

Goff DC, Henderson DC: Treatment-resistant schizophrenia and psychotic disorders. In Pollack MH, Otto MW, Rosenbaum JF (eds): *Challenges in Clinical Practice: Pharmacologic and Psychosocial Strategies*. New York: The Guilford Press, 1996:311–328.

Goff DC, Henderson DC, Manschreck TC: Psychotic patients. In Cassem NH, Stern TA, Rosenbaum JF, Jellinek MS (eds): *Massachusetts General Hospital Handbook of General Hospital Psychiatry*, 4th ed. St. Louis: Mosby, 1997:149–171.

Kane JM: Antipsychotic drug side effects: their relationship to dose. *J Clin Psychiatry* 1985; 46:16–21.

Meltzer HY: Biological studies in schizophrenia. *Schizophr Bull* 1987; 13:77–110.

Chapter 46

Antidepressants and Somatic Therapies

JOSHUA ISRAEL AND MAURIZIO FAVA

I. Overview

Antidepressants represent an effective treatment for major depression. More than 50% of depressed patients will fully recover when an adequate dose of any antidepressant is used for an adequate amount of time (at least 6 weeks); 10–15% will show some improvement, and 20–35% will not improve substantially.

After a first episode of major depression a patient should receive at least 6 months of treatment with an antidepressant at the dosage to which they responded; any tapering of the antidepressant should be done slowly to minimize risk of relapse.

The antidepressant medications are commonly grouped into several classes:

1. Selective serotonin reuptake inhibitors (SSRIs)
2. Cyclic antidepressants, most often the tricyclic antidepressants (TCAs)
3. Monoamine oxidase inhibitors (MAOIs)
4. The growing category of "others" or "atypical antidepressants"

II. Classes of Antidepressant Medications

A. Selective Serotonin Reuptake Inhibitors

1. **Mechanism of action. Serotonergic blockade at neuronal synaptic clefts occurs within hours of initiation of SSRI treatment.** However, the typical time to response in depression for all antidepressant medications, including the SSRIs, is 3–6 weeks; therefore, serotonin reuptake inhibition on its own cannot account for antidepressant efficacy. One postulated mechanism of action of the SSRIs involves **desensitization of serotonergic feedback receptors** in conjunction **with blockade of serotonergic neuronal reuptake;** this allows for a build-up of serotonin in the synaptic cleft with continued neuronal firing. Beta-adrenergic receptor downregulation has also been postulated, and further evidence may show that **changes in intracellular second messenger systems and gene regulation** are responsible for the therapeutic actions of these medications.

2. **Side effects.** All currently available SSRIs are equally efficacious; they differ primarily in their side effects and their half-lives. Some side effects are more common with some SSRIs than with others; however, one patient may find a particular SSRI sedating, while another might find the same SSRI activating.

   The most common side effects of all the SSRIs are: nausea (which tends to be worst during early treatment), reduced appetite, weight loss, excessive sweating, headache, insomnia, jitteriness, sedation, dizziness, and sexual dysfunction (including decreased libido, impotence, and anorgasmia). Other side effects include rash, dry mouth, prolonged bleeding time, and weight gain (during long-term treatment).

   For reasons of tolerability and their benign side effect profile, the SSRIs have become the first-line treatment for depressive disorder illnesses, ranging from dysthymia to severe major depression.

3. **Half-life. Half-lives vary greatly among the SSRIs.** Although a drug's half-life does not affect its treatment efficacy or its onset of action, it is significant in terms of its side effects, its interactions with other agents, and its discontinuation-emergent symptoms. Medications with shorter half-lives may be useful when abrupt discontinuation is desired due to intolerable side effects or to medication interactions. However, medications with shorter half-lives are more likely to cause the discontinuation-emergent symptoms (e.g., tachycardia, anxiety, irritability, worsening of mood, dizziness, jitteriness, and nausea). An SSRI with a longer half-life is more likely to "self-taper," and may be beneficial for a patient who is apt to miss occasional dosages.

4. **Dosing.** Although dose-response curves have not been definitively established for the SSRIs, some patients who do not respond at a lower dose may benefit by having their dosage increased. SSRIs are hepatically metabolized and renally excreted; therefore, lower dosages may be required in hepatically compromised patients, and this is also true to a lesser degree in patients with renal failure.

5. **Drug interactions.** SSRIs should not be co-administered with MAOIs, because of the possibility of causing serotonin syndrome, characterized by myoclonus, tremor, hypertension, diarrhea, and confusion (see II.C below for more detail).

   Cytochrome P450 isoenzymes, including the isoenzymes 1A2, 2C, 2D6, 3A3/4, are located on microsomal membranes throughout the body.

353

Their mechanism of metabolism is best known in the liver and bowel wall, where they oxidatively metabolize medications as well as prostaglandins, fatty acids, and steroids. Alteration in function of these isoenzymes may cause clinically significant pharmacokinetic drug-drug interactions, via changes in drug levels. Some of the SSRIs inhibit the 2D6 and/or 3A4 isoenzymes.

B. Tricyclic Antidepressants

Cyclic antidepressants have been in use for nearly 50 years. All are equally efficacious and are as effective as SSRIs. However, they have a more problematic side effect profile and may be lethal in overdose. The term "tricyclic" signifies a shared chemical structure with two joined benzene rings.

1. **TCA categories**
   a. **Tertiary amine TCAs**
      i. Amitriptyline (Elavil)
      ii. Clomipramine (Anafranil)
      iii. Doxepin (Sinequan)
      iv. Imipramine (Tofranil)
      v. Trimipramine (Surmontil)
   b. **Secondary amine TCAs**
      i. Desipramine (Norpramin)
      ii. Nortriptyline (Pamelor)
      iii. Amoxapine (Asendin)
      iv. Protriptyline (Vivactil)
   c. **Tetracyclic antidepressants**
      i. Maprotiline (Ludiomil) **is a tetracyclic compound composed of four benzene rings.**

2. **Categorization of side effects**
   a. **Anticholinergic effects. Anticholinergic side effects result from the affinity of TCAs for muscarinic cholinergic receptors. Anticholinergic symptoms include dry mouth, blurred vision, constipation, urinary hesitancy, and tachycardia.** Bethanachol (Urecholine), a cholinergic smooth muscle stimulant, may relieve such peripheral anticholinergic signs and symptoms, including ejaculatory difficulties, which can occur with TCAs together with other sexual dysfunction symptoms. Secondary amine TCAs tend to cause fewer anticholinergic effects than tertiary amine TCAs.
   b. **Antihistaminergic effects.** Antihistaminergic side effects result from **histaminergic H_1 receptor blockade. Common side effects include** sedation, carbohydrate craving, and weight gain. Secondary amine TCAs tend to cause less sedation than tertiary amine TCAs.
   c. **Alpha-1-adrenergic receptor blockade.** Orthostatic hypotension results from alpha-1-adrenergic receptor antagonism.
   d. **Serotonin $5HT_2$ receptor blockade.** Sedation may be related to this pharmacological action.
   e. **Cardiac effects.** Cardiac toxicity may occur in susceptible individuals and following TCA overdose; the TCAs should be avoided in patients with bifascicular heart block, left bundle branch block, or a prolonged

QT interval, because they **may slow conduction through the AV (atrioventricular) node.** TCAs are **classified as class I antiarrhythmics** and must be used with great caution with other drugs from this class, including quinidine, procainamide, and disopyramide. TCAs may block the antihypertensive effects of clonidine, methyldopa, guanabenz, guanethadine, reserpine, and guanadrel, and can potentiate the effect of prazosine. TCAs can cause severe orthostatic hypotension in patients with congestive heart failure due to alpha-1 receptor blockade.

TCAs have a low threshold for toxicity; **overdose of even a 1-week supply may be lethal.** Due to the lethality after overdose, it may be safer to treat acutely suicidal depressed patients with non-TCA antidepressants or to prescribe limited quantities of TCAs.

3. **Toxicity. Manifestations of anticholinergic toxicity** may include dilated pupils, blurred vision, dry skin, hyperpyrexia, ileus, urinary retention, confusion, delirium, and seizures. Additionally, arrhythmias, hypotension and coma may develop. Although TCAs are highly plasma-bound and are not removed by hemodialysis, they are metabolized by hepatic microsomal enzymes. Patients who have overdosed on TCAs may require alkalinization of their serum, as well as pressors or ventilatory support to maintain survival.

TCAs should be avoided in patients with narrow angle glaucoma or prostatic hypertrophy, as symptoms related to these conditions may worsen because of anticholinergic effects. TCAs are also contraindicated with MAOIs (see below).

4. **Blood levels.** In general, **TCAs have a linear relationship between increasing levels and effectiveness; some researchers have suggested that with nortriptyline there may be a "U"-shaped curve,** with decreasing efficacy at blood levels above therapeutic range, **although the evidence for such view is unconvincing due to methodological issues present in such studies.** Blood levels can guide treatment with amitriptyline, imipramine, nortriptyline, or desipramine.

C. Monoamine Oxidase Inhibitors

Monoamine oxidase (MAO) is found on the outer membrane of cellular mitochondria, where it catabolizes intracellular monoamines, including the monoamines of the central nervous system (CNS): dopamine, norepinephrine, serotonin, and tyramine. In the gastrointestinal tract and the liver, MAO catabolizes dietary monoamines, such as dopamine, tyramine, tryptamine, and phenylethylamine. The MAO inhibitors (MAOIs) are active on both MAO-A and MAO-B. The MAOIs **phenelzine** (Nardil) and **tranylcypromine** (Parnate) increase synaptic monoamine concentrations. **Both**

phenelzine and tranylcypromine are relatively irreversible blockers of MAO activity (A and B).

MAOIs have a proven efficacy for unipolar major depression. In "atypical" depression (characterized by mood reactivity plus hypersomnia, hyperphagia, extreme fatigue when depressed, and/or rejection sensitivity), **MAOIs are more effective than are the TCAs.** The MAOIs are primarily hepatically metabolized.

1. **Side effects.** The most common side effects include postural hypotension, insomnia, agitation, sedation, impotence, delayed ejaculation, or anorgasmia. Others include: weight change, dry mouth, constipation, urinary hesitancy. Peripheral neuropathies occur and may be avoided by concomitant therapy with vitamin B_6.

2. **Toxic interactions.** When patients on MAOIs ingest dietary amines, rather than being catabolized in the intestines and the liver they are taken up in sympathetic nerve terminals and may cause the release of endogenous catecholamines with a resulting **adrenergic crisis. This is characterized by hypertension, hyperpyrexia, and other adrenergic symptoms** (e.g., tachycardia, tremulousness and cardiac arrhythmias). The amine most commonly associated with these symptoms is tyramine, but others (e.g., phenylethylalamine and dopamine) may be involved.

3. **Dietary interactions. Dietary amines can be avoided by adherence to dietary restrictions and avoiding tyramine-containing foods.** The diet must be strictly followed, but need not be as restrictive as was once thought. **Patients must be instructed to avoid:** all matured or aged cheese, fermented or dried meats (e.g., pepperoni and salami), fava and broad bean *pods* (not the beans themselves), tap beers, marmite yeast extract, sauerkraut, soy sauce and other soy products (e.g., tofu and tempe). All meats and cheese must be fresh and must have been stored and refrigerated or frozen properly. Up to *two* glasses of beer may be consumed safely; this restriction includes non-alcoholic beers.

   Since endogenous MAO activity does not return to baseline immediately upon MAOI discontinuation, 2 weeks should transpire before discontinuing the MAOI diet after MAOI discontinuation, or before beginning a contraindicated medication.

4. **Drug-drug interactions.** Avoidance of toxic drug-drug interactions with MAOIs is critical. **Medications with affinity for serotonergic receptors** (serotonergic TCAs [e.g., clomipramine], SSRIs, venlafaxine, nefazodone and buspirone [Buspar]) **may result in the serotonin syndrome,** with myoclonic jerks, tremor, hypertension, diarrhea, confusion, tachycardia, fever, ocular oscillations; in its severe form it may include hyperthermia, coma, convulsions, and death. MAOIs must be used with caution in patients with diabetes (due to possible potentiation of oral hypoglycemics and worsened hypoglycemia). Low-dose MAOIs may increase *sensitivity* to insulin, and high-dose MAOIs may increase insulin *resistance*.

   Sympathomimetics, both prescribed and over-the-counter, and relatively potent norepinephrine reuptake inhibitors, such as TCAs, may precipitate hypertensive crises. Sympathomimetics are most commonly found in nasal decongestants (e.g., pseudoephedrine, ephedrine, and oxymetazoline [Afrin nasal spray]), and also include amphetamines and cocaine. The cough-suppressant dextromethorphan can have similar toxic effects. **The hypertensive crisis is characterized by headache, stroke, pulmonary edema, and cardiac arrhythmias.** Co-administration of meperidine (Demerol) is contraindicated since it is known to cause a syndrome of fever, vascular instability, delirium, neuromuscular irritability, and death.

   The antiparkinsonian agent selegeline (Eldepryl) is a MAO-B inhibitor which becomes a MAO-A inhibitor as well at higher doses. It is not primarily used for psychiatric disorders. SSRIs and TCAs should not be given to patients on this medication due to the risk of developing a serotonin syndrome, though co-administration of bupropion is not contraindicated, at least at lower doses.

   Prior to beginning an MAOI after discontinuation of a contraindicated antidepressant, the necessary drug-free time varies depending on the half-life of the previous antidepressant. At least five half-lives of the contraindicated medication are required, with 2 weeks required after paroxetine and 5 weeks required after use of fluoxetine.

5. **Medical interactions.** MAOIs are contraindicated in patients with pheochromocytoma, congestive heart failure, and hepatic disease.

D. **Other Agents (Atypical Antidepressants)**
1. **Bupropion (Wellbutrin). Bupropion increases dopamine and norepinephrine turnover in the CNS.** It is hepatically metabolized. Common side effects include agitation, insomnia, weight loss, dry mouth, headache, constipation, and tremor. It has been noted to **cause seizures, at a rate of 4/1,000 in its immediate release form. Its sustained release (SR) form is associated with a seizure risk comparable to that of the SSRIs. However, the risk of seizure markedly increases at doses > 450 mg/day in divided doses** and may be more likely to induce seizures in **patients with bulimia nervosa. It**

is generally safe in overdose, though fatalities have been reported. **Bupropion is one of the safest, if not the safest, antidepressant in patients with cardiac disease.** It rarely induces sexual dysfunction, is less likely to induce it than the SSRIs, and can even be **beneficial as an adjunct in SSRI-induced sexual dysfunction.** Its use is contraindicated with the MAOIs.

2. **Mirtazapine** (Remeron). **Mirtazapine is an antagonist at inhibitory alpha-2-adrenergic auto- and heteroreceptors,** leading to increased release of both serotonin and norepinephrine at the synaptic level. It is also **a relatively potent histaminergic H_1 receptor antagonist and a serotonin 5-HT$_2$ and 5-HT$_3$ receptor antagonist.** Common side effects include somnolence, weight gain, dizziness, dry mouth, constipation, and orthostatic hypotension.

3. **Trazodone** (Desyrel). **Trazodone inhibits serotonin uptake, blocks serotonin 5HT$_2$ receptors** and may act as a serotonin agonist through an active metabolite. It is also an antagonist of **alpha-1-adrenergic receptors.** Metabolism is hepatic. Trazodone is less lethal in overdose than the TCAs, though slightly more lethal than the SSRIs. **The most common side effects are sedation, orthostatic hypotension, and headache.** Priapism is a rare but serious side effect that requires immediate medical attention. Trazodone may induce arrhythmias in those with pre-existing heart disease and may increase levels of digoxin and phenytoin (Dilantin). Trazodone is **most commonly used** as an adjunctive medication **for insomnia** due to its sedating properties.

4. **Nefazodone** (Serzone). Nefazodone is **chemically related to trazodone,** with serotonin blockade but with less alpha-1 blockade and fewer side effects. It is less likely to cause sexual dysfunction than SSRIs, and is less anticholinergic and histaminergic than the TCAs. Metabolism is hepatic. Common side effects include somnolence, dizziness, dry mouth, nausea, constipation, headache and amblyopia, and blurred vision. **Nefazodone is a potent inhibitor of cytochrome P450 3A4 isoenzymes,** and by interacting with cisapride (Propulsid), terfenadine (Seldane) or astemizole (Hismanal) may lead to QT prolongation and torsades de pointes. It is contraindicated with MAOIs.

5. **Venlafaxine** (Effexor). Venlafaxine inhibits both serotonin and norepinephrine uptake, though it is slightly more selective for SRI. Its side effects are similar to those of the SSRIs: nausea, insomnia, sedation, and dizziness; 5–7% of patients experience an increase in baseline diastolic blood pressure. Venlafaxine use is contraindicated with MAOIs.

6. **Psychostimulants.** Although the psychostimulants **dextroamphetamine** (Dexedrine), **methylphenidate** (Ritalin), and **pemoline** (Cylert) have not shown clear benefit in the long-term treatment of depression, they are frequently beneficial in apathetic geriatric patients, and as adjunctive medication in the treatment of refractory depression. Side effects include insomnia, tremors, appetite change, palpitations, blurred vision, dry mouth, constipation, and dizziness. Arrhythmias and tachycardia have also been reported. Pemoline has been associated with hepatic toxicity.

7. **Alprazolam** (Xanax). Alprazolam is a triazoloenzodiazapine used primarily for panic disorder, generalized anxiety disorder, and for sedative-hypnotic purposes. It is hepatically metabolized, and it reduces norepinephrine turnover. Its half-life is 12–15 h, yet it must be given on a t.i.d or q.i.d. basis. Common side effects include drowsiness, ataxia, and headache. Physical and psychological dependence can occur with protracted treatment, and seizures are possible with abrupt discontinuation. Studies have found it to have an antidepressant effect superior to placebo, but this may represent an epiphenomenon of its anxiolytic efficacy.

8. **Antipsychotic agents.** There is no evidence supporting the use of antipsychotic agents alone in nonpsychotic, unipolar depression, though these agents are often beneficial in major depression with psychotic features and mixed episodes of Bipolar Disorder.

III. Special Populations

A. The Elderly
Depression in the elderly should be treated as thoroughly as it would in any patient. Since renal clearance and hepatic metabolism are frequently reduced in the elderly, lower dosages are often called for. Although TCAs are more likely to cause orthostatic hypotension than the SSRIs, they do not appear to cause a greater risk of falls.

B. Pregnancy
No clear link has been established between antidepressant treatment in pregnant women and birth defects, though the risks have not been definitively disproved either. As with all medications, it is prudent to avoid fetal exposure to psychotropics as much as possible. However, the high morbidity and mortality of depression often make this unwise. **Data regarding the TCAs, particularly imipramine, do not indicate a clear increased risk of fetal malformation; fluoxetine, the best studied of the SSRIs, also shows no clear risk of**

Table 46-1. Currently Available SSRIs

Available SSRIs	Half-life (h)
Fluvoxamine (Luvox)	17
Paroxetine (Paxil)	21
Sertraline (Zoloft)	26 (its active metabolite has a 40-h half-life)
Citalopram (Celexa)	36
Fluoxetine (Prozac)	84 (together with its active metabolites, in vivo half-life is 7 days)

fetal malformation. **Electroconvulsive therapy (ECT) is safe to perform during pregnancy.**

C. **Patients with Bipolar Disorder**
The risk of bipolar patients cycling into mania is 30–50% when they are treated with antidepressant medications while not on a mood-stabilizing agent. Antidepressants may even initiate and maintain rapid cycling. The risk is improved, but not eliminated, by mood-stabilizing agents. Bupropion may have the lowest rate of "switch" into mania of the antidepressants.

D. **Patients with Major Depression with Psychotic Features**
Major depression with psychotic features is treated with full dosages of antidepressants. Treatment usually requires the addition of an antipsychotic as well, although atypical antipsychotic agents, which may be associated with intrinsic antidepressant effects, may be used alone in this condition.

E. **Patients with Dysthymia**
Dysthymia is a chronic, mild form of depression which is associated with a high risk of superimposed major depressive episodes (double depression). There is evidence that all antidepressant classes may be useful in the treatment of this condition, although full recovery from double depression may be less likely to occur than in major depression alone.

F. **Patients with Treatment Refractory Depression**
Medical conditions, such as hypothyroidism, anemia, occult malignancy, or confounding substance abuse, must be ruled out. Often depression is labeled "refractory" before adequate medication trials have been conducted. If a patient does not respond to antidepressant treatment of adequate duration and dose, it is reasonable to increase the dosage until benefits are seen or until side effects become problematic. Duration of medication use is equally important, with at least 6 weeks of a

medication trial necessary before treatment failure can be declared. A patient who has not responded to a medication in one class may still respond to a different medication of the same class, to switch to an antidepressant of another class, or to the addition of an antidepressant which acts on different receptors, such as the addition of bupropion, mirtazapine, or a psychostimulant to an SSRI. Other options include the addition of triidothyronine (T_3), lithium augmentation, buspirone, or ECT.

IV. Other Indications for Antidepressants

A. **Chronic Pain**
TCAs are useful in many pain conditions. These include diabetic neuropathy, fibromyalgia, chronic fatigue, postherpetic neuralgia, trigeminal neuralgia, migraine, and tension headache prophylaxis. Frequently TCAs have been useful for these conditions at blood levels lower than those required to achieve antidepressant response.

B. **Potentiation of Pain Medications**
Both the TCAs and psychostimulants potentiate narcotic analgesia.

C. **Bulimia**
High doses of SSRIs are effective in reducing bingeing/purging behaviors. MAOIs and TCAs may also be helpful, but the dietary restrictions associated with MAOI treatment may not be feasible among patients with eating-related impulsivity.

D. **Obsessive-Compulsive Disorder**
Obsessive-compulsive disorder (OCD) responds to medications with serotonergic effects, specifically SSRIs and clomipramine. Obsessions respond better than do compulsions. Typically, these medications are used in dosages higher than those needed for antidepressant response and need to be used for longer periods of time. Trichotillomania and body dysmorphic disorder may similarly respond to SSRIs.

E. **Panic Disorder**
SSRIs have become the first-line treatment for panic disorder. Dosing should begin at low doses, due to the jitteriness and anxiety frequently experienced at the beginning of treatment. MAOIs and TCAs are also effective, though their side effects, particularly at higher dosages, are less tolerable. It is not clear whether the atypical antidepressants are as effective as the other classes of antidepressants in this condition. Anticipatory anxiety and phobic avoidance may respond less

well to antidepressant treatment and may benefit from the addition of cognitive-behavioral therapy.

F. Posttraumatic Stress Disorder

Higher dosages of SSRIs and MAOIs do not remove but may reduce symptomatology of post-traumatic stress disorder (PTSD), although SSRIs are clearly superior to placebo.

G. Smoking Cessation

Bupropion has been shown to be effective in smoking cessation when used as part of an overall treatment program.

Suggested Readings

Alpert JE: Drug-drug interactions: the interface between psychotropics and other agents. In Stern TA, Herman JB, Slavin PL (eds): *The MGH Guide to Primary Care in Psychiatry*. New York: McGraw-Hill, 1998:519–534.

Cohen L, Altshuler LL: Pharmacologic management of psychiatric illness during pregnancy and the postpartum period. *Psychiatr Clin North Am* 1997; 4:21–58.

Fava M, Rosenbaum JF: Pharmacotherapy and somatic therapies. In Beckham EE, Leber WR (eds): *Handbook of Depression*. New York: Guilford Publications, 1995:280–301.

Fava M, Rosenbaum JF: Approach to the patient with depression. In Stern TA, Herman JB, Slavin PL (eds): *The MGH Guide to Primary Care in Psychiatry*. New York: McGraw-Hill, 1998:1–14.

Gardner DM, Shulman KI, Walker SE, Tailor SAN: The making of a user-friendly MAOI diet. *J Clin Psychiatry* 1993; 57:99–104.

Hyman S, Arana GW, Rosenbaum JF: *Handbook of Psychiatric Drug Therapy*, 3rd ed. Boston, MA: Little, Brown, 1995.

Preskorn S: *Clinical Pharmacology of Selective Serotonin Reuptake Inhibitors*. Caddo, OK: Professional Communications, 1996.

Sackheim HA, Prudic J, Devanand DP, et al.: Effect of stimulus intensity and placement on the efficacy and cognitive side effects of electroconvulsive therapy. *N Engl J Med* 1993; 328(12):839–846.

Stern TA, Herman JB, Slavin PL (eds): *The MGH Guide to Primary Care in Psychiatry*. New York: McGraw-Hill, 1998.

Chapter 47

Electroconvulsive Therapy

ANTHONY P. WEISS AND CHARLES A. WELCH

I. The Importance of Education about Electroconvulsive Therapy

A. **The Expanded Role of ECT as a Psychiatric Treatment**
Despite the development of several new antidepressant medications with more favorable safety and tolerability profiles, **the past decade has seen a resurgence in the use of electroconvulsive therapy (ECT) in the treatment of affective illness. The reasons for this increase in the use of ECT include:**
1. **Its excellent safety profile.**
2. **Its superior efficacy,** particularly in the 15–20% of depressed patients for whom adequate drug treatment is unattainable due to treatment resistance, inability to tolerate medication side effects, or an inability to take an oral medication.
3. **Its economic benefits** due to shorter hospital stays.
4. **The decreased societal stigmatization of ECT.**

B. **Importance of Knowledge about ECT for the Practicing Psychiatrist**
Since ECT remains an important part of the psychiatrist's armamentarium against severe affective illness, thorough knowledge of the indications, risks, techniques, and benefits of ECT remains an integral part of a complete psychiatric curriculum. **While only a small minority of psychiatrists are involved in the actual administration of ECT, knowledge of ECT is essential** for the practicing psychiatrist in order to:
1. Know when to make appropriate referrals for convulsive therapy.
2. Educate the patient about the risks and benefits of this treatment.
3. Participate in the post-ECT management of the patient.

II. Historical Overview

A. **Early Theories**
The notion that convulsions might have a beneficial effect on mental illness dates back to Hippocrates, who documented the cure of insane patients following malaria-induced seizures. The first deliberate use of convulsions as a therapeutic agent did not occur until the 1500s, when the Swiss physician **Paracelsus** induced seizures with oral camphor to treat mania and psychosis.

B. **Meduna's Theory of "Biological Antagonism"**
The use of chemically induced seizures did not gain widespread acceptance until 1934, when a Hungarian physician, Ladislaus von Meduna, reported the beneficial effects of seizures induced by intramuscular injections of camphor in oil on a catatonic patient. Meduna, apparently unaware of previous work in this area, based his work on the idea that there was an inherent "biological antagonism" between schizophrenia and epilepsy. While the theory was later disproved, camphor-induced seizures were nevertheless somewhat successful.

C. **Electrically Induced Seizures**
In 1937, the Italian team of Ugo Cerletti and Lucio Bini became the first clinicians to apply electricity to the head to induce a therapeutic seizure. Like Meduna's patient, their first patient had catatonia, which quickly responded to the use of this new technique. More reliable and generally safer than the use of chemically induced seizures, ECT rapidly gained widespread acceptance throughout Europe and the United States.

D. **Improvements in Anesthesiology**
While subtle alterations in the delivery of electricity have been made since its first application (from constant-voltage sine wave stimulation to constant-current brief-pulse stimulation), the major change has come in the realm of anesthesia. Early attempts at ECT were riddled with problems, most notably bone fractures (due to the violent muscular contractions associated with the seizure), and patient discomfort (physical and mental) during the procedure. **Two major breakthroughs have largely alleviated these difficulties:**
1. **The use of curare as a muscle relaxant by the psychiatrist AE Bennett in 1940** allowed complete paralysis of the patient during the seizure, eliminating physical injury.
2. **The development of short-acting intravenous barbiturates in the 1950s allowed for both rapid induction of sedation and for amnesia surrounding the procedure.**

III. Proposed Mechanisms of Action

A. **Overview**
Despite decades of experience with ECT, **the specific mechanism of the antidepressant effect of**

ECT remains unknown. As noted by Sackeim (1994), more than 100 theories have been proposed to explain the therapeutic action of ECT. The most commonly cited ideas are briefly mentioned here.

B. Psychodynamic Theories
Early psychodynamic theories ascribed the beneficial effect of ECT to its fulfillment of the need for punishment in the self-loathing, depressed patient. The fact that ECT retained its effectiveness despite the use of anesthetic agents which eliminated the pain associated with ECT argues against this theory.

C. The Placebo Effect
Many writers have remarked on the dramatic and ritualized nature of ECT, believing that its beneficial effects were due to wishful thinking on the part of the staff and the patient. Several studies have demonstrated that ECT works better than "sham" ECT, largely eliminating the possibility that the beneficial effects are due solely to the placebo effect.

D. ECT as a "Memory Eraser"
Some authors have linked the beneficial effects of ECT to its ability to disturb recent memory, thereby "erasing" the recall of recent traumas that led to the depressive episode. Studies that confirmed that the efficacy of ECT was not correlated with the resultant degree of cognitive impairment debunked this theory.

E. The Seizure as Curative Agent
Since ECT is ineffective when the seizure is either pharmacologically blocked or is subthreshold, it is clear that having a generalized seizure is crucial to the antidepressant effect of ECT. Given the lack of efficacy when a unilateral stimulus is only marginally suprathreshold, it appears that just having a seizure alone may not be adequate.

F. ECT as the Agent of Neurochemical Changes
ECT is associated with a myriad of biochemical changes in the brain. These changes involve the same neuroamines that are implicated in the therapeutic effect of antidepressant medication (i.e., serotonin and norepinephrine). Alteration in the concentration of these neuroamines, and upregulation of their receptors, may be at the heart of ECT's efficacy.

G. Therapeutic Effects of the Rise in Seizure Threshold
Alternatively, some believe that the chemical changes responsible for *terminating* the generalized seizure may play the largest role in ECT's effect. These chemical changes lead to a gradual rise in the seizure threshold over a course of ECT, a change that is correlated with ECT efficacy.

IV. Indications for ECT

A. Well-Established Indications for ECT
Although the exact mechanism by which ECT leads to improvement remains unclear, several neuropsychiatric illnesses are well-established indications for ECT:
1. **Major depression**
2. **Mania**
3. **Schizophrenia** (generally acute exacerbations rather than chronic illness)
4. **Catatonia** (of either organic or affective etiology)

B. Other Indications for ECT
Other illnesses for which ECT may be beneficial (but where less evidence exists) include:
1. **Parkinson's disease**
2. **Intractable epilepsy, status epilepticus, and intra-ictal psychosis**
3. **Neuroleptic malignant syndrome** (in conjunction with dantrolene, bromocriptine, and intensive medical support)

C. First-Line Indications for ECT
While ECT is generally used only after medication failure, it may be regarded as a first-line therapy among patients with major depression who are:
1. **Severely malnourished or dehydrated**
2. **Medically ill and where the use of appropriate antidepressant medication is precluded (e.g., ventricular arrhythmia), or who are unable to take oral antidepressant medication**
3. **Delusionally depressed**
4. **Previous ECT responders**
5. **Requesting ECT**

V. Contraindications to the Use of ECT

A. Absolute Contraindications
There are no absolute contraindications to the use of ECT. In fact, with careful anesthesiologic management, ECT has been safely applied to patients with a variety of conditions once thought to prohibit the use of ECT.

B. Relative Contraindications
Several situations do pose relative contraindications, to ECT. In these cases, the risks and benefits of ECT must be carefully weighed. By reviewing the expected physiologic effects of ECT, two areas of concern become clear:
1. **Cardiovascular conditions.** Autonomic hyperactivity associated with ECT leads to significant cardiovascular effects. Initially, parasympathetic discharge predominates; it may cause bradycardia, premature ventricular contractions, or several seconds of asystole. Other signs of increased vagal tone (e.g., hypotension and salivation) may also

occur. Sympathetic stimulation, an effect prolonged by circulating catecholamines, occurs later. This leads to hypertension and tachycardia. Clearly, standard ECT can place a significant strain on the cardiovascular system, and mimic the response to an exercise tolerance test. **Patients with coronary artery disease, hypertension, vascular aneurysms, and cardiac arrhythmia merit special observation and attention.**

2. **Cerebrovascular effects.** Changes in cerebrovascular dynamics can be equally dramatic, with a fourfold increase in cerebral blood flow. As a result, large rises in intracranial pressure can be seen. **Patients with space-occupying intracerebral lesions, cerebral aneurysms, or recent strokes warrant close attention.**

3. **Other conditions.** Other patients who require close anesthetic monitoring include **those who are pregnant and those who are deemed to be of high anesthetic risk** due to underlying medical or surgical conditions.

VI. Evidence for the Efficacy of ECT

A. **Overview**
Despite being developed for the treatment of schizophrenia, ECT has been studied predominantly in the treatment of affective disorders. While ECT remains useful and effective for a wide variety of neuropsychiatric illnesses (see IV), **the most rigorous clinical evidence exists for its use in treating major depression.**

B. **Acute Treatment**
ECT has been shown to be more effective than either placebo or simulated ("sham") ECT for the treatment of major depression. More importantly, ECT has compared favorably to several active antidepressant treatments, including tricyclic antidepressants (TCAs) and monoamine oxidase inhibitors (MAOIs). While some studies have shown no difference in the efficacy between medication and ECT, others have shown an advantage for ECT (see Janicak et al., 1997). The overall response rate for ECT is approximately 75–90%.

C. **Maintenance Treatment**
Given the nature of major depression as a relapsing and remitting illness, treatment of the acute episode is often followed by a recurrence of depression. This may be even more of a concern after successful treatment with ECT. For this reason, the use of ECT as a maintenance treatment has been explored. At the present time, there is little prospective, randomized data to support this practice. **Existing reports, albeit largely retrospec-**tive and uncontrolled, strongly indicate the efficacy of ECT in preventing depressive relapse.**

VII. Practical Management of the ECT Patient

A. **Pretreatment Evaluation**
A thorough pre-ECT evaluation is essential to the safety and efficacy of ECT. This is routinely conducted in association with an anesthesiologist and includes a complete medical and psychiatric history, full physical examination, complete blood count, determination of electrolytes, an electrocardiogram, and a chest X-ray. Other tests, depending on the patient's underlying medical condition and current medications, may be indicated. The goal is to stabilize the patient's medical condition prior to ECT.

B. **Informed Consent**
As with any procedure, full informed consent must be obtained from the competent patient (or from a designated surrogate in the case of an incompetent patient) prior to the initiation of ECT. More than just a medicolegal formality, the process of informed consent is an opportunity for the psychiatrist to fully explain the risks and benefits of the procedure, and for the patient to ask questions. Both aspects of this process help to allay patient anxiety, to improve the patient-doctor rapport, and to increase satisfaction with the treatment. Videotapes and information sheets augment, but they do not supplant, the process of informed consent.

C. **Patient Care**
ECT is generally administered in the early morning hours. As with any procedure that requires general anesthesia, **a patient should be kept NPO for 6–8 h prior to ECT.**

D. **Use of Concurrent Medications**
Typically, psychotropic medications are discontinued during a course of ECT to avoid interactions with ECT. Medications often used in conjunction with ECT include:

1. **Antidepressants.** TCAs and MAOIs are discontinued routinely, largely to minimize possible cardiovascular complications. The use of newer generation selective serotonin reuptake inhibitors (SSRIs) is probably safe during ECT.

2. **Lithium.** Lithium has been known to cause delirium when co-administered with ECT; therefore, it is usually withheld during the course of ECT.

3. **Anticonvulsants.** Anticonvulsants are not contraindicated in a patient undergoing ECT, although they will raise the electrical stimulus necessary to induce a therapeutic seizure. For those patients

with a pre-existing seizure disorder, it is probably safest to continue anticonvulsants and simply use a higher-intensity stimulus.

4. **Benzodiazepines. Benzodiazepines raise the seizure threshold, and may increase the degree of postictal confusion, particularly in the elderly patient.** Therefore, benzodiazepines are usually withheld during ECT. Pre-ECT anxiety or insomnia are often managed by prescribing a small dose of a neuroleptic or a nonbenzodiazepine hypnotic, such as diphenhydramine.

E. Use of Anesthesia during ECT

The anesthetic goals for ECT are three-fold:

1. **Rapid induction with amnesia.** Over the past 20 years, **methohexital has become the agent of choice for induction of anesthesia for ECT.** As a result of its rapid onset and a short duration of action, its use is ideal for ECT. Moreover, methohexital has little impact on the seizure threshold. The usual intravenous dose of methohexital is between 0.5 and 1.0 mg/kg.

2. **Prevention of injury from tonic-clonic seizure activity.** While curare was the first muscle relaxant used in the modification of ECT, **succinylcholine is the most commonly used agent today.** Its popularity is based on its rapid onset, its lack of effect on seizure threshold, and its relatively low cost. In situations where succinylcholine is contraindicated (e.g., pseudocholinesterase deficiency), other agents have been used with good results.

3. **Attenuation of the sympathetic response to ECT. In patients with pre-existing cardiovascular pathology, for whom tachycardia or hypertension may be life-threatening, pretreatment with beta-blockers may be indicated.** Labetolol (10–20 mg IV) or esmolol (100–200 mg IV) prior to induction of anesthesia have both been used to attenuate the sympathetic response to ECT.

F. Seizure Induction

1. **Electrode placement. Two standard electrode placements are currently employed for the delivery of electricity to the brain. In unilateral placement (the d'Elia placement), both electrodes are placed over the same hemisphere, typically the non-dominant right hemisphere. In bilateral placement, the electrodes are positioned symmetrically over the fronto-temporal areas.**

2. **Stimulus intensity. Newer ECT devices deliver a constant-current, brief-pulse stimulus of electricity.** This technical advance has helped minimize the degree of cognitive dysfunction associated with ECT. The ability to elicit a seizure is necessary, but not always sufficient, for an antidepressant effect. Particularly with unilateral ECT, supplying a stimulus at least 50% above the seizure threshold appears to be most efficacious. This observation is complicated by the natural elevation in seizure threshold noted over the course of ECT.

3. **Seizure properties. For ECT to be effective, the induced seizure must generalize. The optimal duration of the generalized seizure is thought to be greater than 25 sec.** Since the use of muscle relaxants started, the psychiatrist can no longer simply observe the convulsing patient to assess the quality and duration of seizure activity. In some cases, electroencephalographic (EEG) monitoring is used to determine the nature of the induced seizure. In other cases, an inflated blood pressure cuff is placed on a single extremity during the administration of succinylcholine. In this fashion, the isolated limb remains unaffected by the muscle relaxant and can be observed to convulse during the seizure.

VIII. Complications of ECT

A. Mortality

The current mortality rate of ECT is estimated at 0.01–0.03% per patient (i.e., 1–3 per 10,000). The majority of ECT-associated deaths are due to cardiovascular complications.

B. Cardiovascular Complications

The cardiovascular complications of ECT were discussed previously (see V).

C. Cognitive Complications

The cognitive side effects of ECT have been both overdramatized by detractors and under-researched by clinicians. Careful explanation of the major types of cognitive disturbance can help alleviate a patient's concern about this feared complication.

1. **Posttreatment confusion. A brief (15–30 min) period of confusion immediately following treatment is seen in up to 10% of patients.** This is generally time-limited; it may be related to the seizure, to the effects of general anesthesia, or both factors.

2. **Delirium. Confusion associated with slowing of the EEG is common;** such confusion often delays treatment or leads to its discontinuation. The cause of post-ECT confusion is unclear, but it appears more commonly in the elderly, in patients with pre-existing dementia or neurological impairment, and in those treated with bilaterally applied ECT. With cessation of ECT, delirium typically clears within days to weeks.

3. **Memory loss. ECT is associated with both antero-grade and retrograde amnesia.** As with ECT-related delirium, memory impairment is more severe in association with bilateral ECT.

a. **Anterograde amnesia.** During the course of ECT, the ability to learn new information is impaired, leading to anterograde-type amnesia. This difficulty persists briefly after ECT, and returns to baseline 2–6 months post-ECT.

b. **Retrograde amnesia.** Loss of memory for events prior to ECT may also occur. In general, this is more severe for events closest to the time of treatment (i.e., for events leading up to hospitalization) than it is for remote events. Usually, recall is impaired for events during the previous 6 months, though memory disturbance for events occurring up to 2 years prior to ECT is not infrequently reported. For many patients, retrograde amnesia is the most significant side effect of ECT.

IX. Conclusion

ECT is the oldest biological treatment still used by psychiatrists. Although other treatments with better side effect profiles have been developed, ECT retains an important role in the treatment of affective illness.

Suggested Readings

Dubovsky SL: Electroconvulsive therapy. In Kaplan HI, Sadock BJ (eds): *Comprehensive Textbook of Psychiatry*, 6th ed. Baltimore: Williams and Wilkins, 1995.

Janicak PG, Davis JM, Gibbons RD, Ericksen S, Chang S, Gallagher P: Efficacy of ECT: a meta-analysis. *Am J Psychiatry* 1985; 142:297–302.

Janicak PG, Davis JM, Preskom SH, Ayd FJ: *Principles and Practice of Psychopharmacotherapy*, 2nd ed. Baltimore: Williams and Wilkins, 1997.

Miller AL, Faber RA, Hatch JP, Alexander HE: Factors affecting amnesia, seizure duration and efficacy in ECT. *Am J Psychiatry* 1985; 142:692–696.

Sackeim HA: Central issues regarding the mechanisms of action of electroconvulsive therapy: directions for future research. *Psychopharm Bull* 1994; 30:281–308.

Sackeim HA, Devanand DP, Prudic J: Stimulus intensity, seizure threshold, and seizure duration: impact on the efficacy and safety of electroconvulsive therapy. *Psychiatr Clin North Am* 1991; 14:803–843.

Welch CA: Electroconvulsive therapy in the general hospital. In Cassem NH, Stern TA, Rosenbaum JF, Jellinek MS (eds): *The Massachusetts General Hospital Handbook of General Hospital Psychiatry*, 4th ed. St. Louis: Mosby, 1997.

Chapter 48

Lithium

S. Nassir Ghaemi

I. Overview

Lithium was the first medication to be found effective in the treatment of manic-depressive illness. It remains one of only two FDA-approved agents for mania (the other being divalproex). It is most effective in pure mania, and in classical bipolar disorder (i.e., with euphoria and grandiosity). Lithium is less effective in mixed episodes, rapid-cycling disorders, or in patients with comorbid substance abuse. Evidence exists for its prophylaxis of bipolar disorder, although naturalistic outcome studies suggest lower real-world effectiveness. Use of lithium clearly decreases the risk of death by suicide and decreases the overall mortality associated with bipolar disorder. **Unfortunately, lithium has a narrow therapeutic index, is associated with potentially life-threatening toxicity, and has numerous nonlethal side effects.** Thus, noncompliance with lithium is a major clinical problem.

II. History

In the 1940s, lithium was first reported by John Cade, an Australian physician, to be effective in mania. Double-blind studies in the 1960s led to FDA approval in 1970. Lithium was the only standard treatment for bipolar disorder until the anticonvulsant carbamazepine was found to be effective for mania in the 1980s, after which time the efficacy of valproic acid efficacy was noted in the early 1990s. **Divalproex, a formulation of valproic acid, is now the only other FDA-approved agent for use in mania.**

III. Indications

Lithium is FDA-approved for the treatment of **acute mania** and for the **maintenance prophylaxis of bipolar disorder.** Controlled data also exist for its use in **acute depression occurring in bipolar disorder,** and as an **augmentation of antidepressants for unipolar depression.** Lithium is also probably effective in the treatment of **schizoaffective disorder, bipolar type.** It has not been shown to be effective, alone or as an adjunct to other agents, in the treatment of schizophrenia, obsessive-compulsive disorder, anxiety disorders, posttraumatic stress disorder, or personality disorders.

IV. Pharmacology

Lithium is a naturally occurring cation. The standard lithium formulation is lithium carbonate. Other lithium formulations are lithium citrate, which may be better tolerated than the carbonate compound in the setting of severe nausea, and Eskalith CR, a controlled release type of lithium. Eskalith leads to lower serum peaks of lithium and may be associated with fewer cognitive side effects, such as poor concentration or sedation; however, it may be associated with more renal side effects.

The usual dosage of lithium is around 900–1200 mg/day (range 600–1500 mg/day). It often is given two or three times daily, but it can be given in a one-time dose since its mean half-life is about 24 h. It is dosed to a serum therapeutic range of 0.6–1.2 mEq/L, somewhat lower in the elderly (0.4–0.8 mEq/L). A standard level for acute and maintenance treatment is 0.8 mEq/L (0.4 mEq/L in the elderly). **Lithium is not metabolized in the liver; it is excreted unchanged by the kidney.** Thus, its only drug interactions involve other medications that affect its renal excretion (see Table 48-1).

V. Mechanisms of Action

For many years, the mechanism of action of lithium was unknown. **Lithium has mildly proserotonergic effects,** but it does not significantly affect other major neurotransmitters (e.g., dopamine or norepinephrine). **Recent data strongly indicate that lithium's main effects do not occur at the synapse with neurotransmitters, but postsynaptically, at the level of G-proteins and other second messengers (e.g., phosphatidylinositol phosphate, PIP).** It is these cellular effects that probably mediate lithium's clinical utility. **Specifically, lithium inhibits the alpha unit of G-proteins, especially those connected to beta-adrenergic receptors via cyclic adenosine monophosphate (cAMP).** By blocking the G-protein transmission of messages from these noradrenergic receptors, lithium may interfere with the neuronal activity that occurs with mania. **Similar effects on G-proteins linked to other neurotransmitters may produce lithium's antidepressant effects.** Further, lithium may inhibit PIP function when PIP is excessively active, but lithium has no effect when PIP is normally active. Thus, by its complex second messenger functions, lithium may essentially be re-establishing intracellular homeostases that underlie larger neural cir-

Table 48-1. Lithium Drug Interactions: Drugs that Increase Lithium Levels

- NSAIDs (nonsteroidal antiinflammatory drugs)
- Thiazide diuretics
- ACE (angiotensin-converting enzyme) inhibitors
- Calcium channel blockers

Table 48-2. Rank Order of Reasons for Noncompliance with Lithium

- Side effects
- Indefinite intake/chronicity of illness
- Felt less creative
- Felt well, saw no need to take lithium
- Felt less productive
- Missed highs
- Less interesting to spouse
- Disliked idea of moods being controlled by medication
- Hassle to remember
- Felt depressed, thought mood would improve off medication

NOTE: Noncompliance was based on self-report by patients that they did not comply with lithium (from Jamison et al., 1979).

cuits subserving mood, accounting for its mood-stabilizing effects.

VI. Side Effects and Toxicity

Lithium has four groups of side effects: nuisance, medically serious, toxic, and teratogenic.

A. **Nuisance side effects** occur at therapeutic levels and lower, are often related to noncompliance, and are experienced as troublesome. These **include sedation, cognitive difficulties (e.g., poor concentration and memory), a sense of decreased creativity, dry mouth, hand tremor, increased appetite, weight gain, increased fluid intake (polydipsia), increased urination (polyuria), nausea, diarrhea, psoriasis, and acne.** Polydipsia and polyuria persist in about 25% of patients during maintenance treatment with lithium. When severe, this increased urination may represent nephrogenic diabetes insipidus, a condition due to lithium's inhibition of the kidney's sensitivity to the pituitary's antidiuretic hormone (ADH, or vasopressin). Some of these side effects are treatable: sedation and cognitive effects may improve with the controlled release formulation; dry mouth can be minimized by use of sugar-free candy; increased appetite and weight gain can be responsive to carbohydrate restriction (since lithium has a mild insulin-like effect) and exercise; nausea and diarrhea may respond to the citrate formulation; hand tremor may improve with the use of propranolol; and polydipsia and polyuria can improve with the use of thiazide diuretics (e.g., the hydrochlorothiazide/triamterene combination). **Since thiazide diuretics increase lithium levels, lithium doses should be decreased by about 50% when co-administered and lithium levels followed.** It should be noted that, because of lithium's mild insulin-like effect, the insulin regimen of diabetic patients receiving lithium may also need to be altered. Frequently, despite these measures, individuals are unable to tolerate lithium solely due to these nuisance side effects,

which are the main source of lithium noncompliance (Table 48-2).

B. **Medically serious side effects** (excluding toxicity) fall into three categories: **thyroid abnormalities, chronic renal insufficiency, and cardiac effects.**

1. **Lithium's thyroid effects can occur early in treatment,** but often appear after years of use as well. Lithium has a direct reversible antithyroid effect, and thus it can lead to hypothyroidism (usually in about 5% of patients). It inhibits the thyroid gland's sensitivity to thyroid-stimulating hormone (TSH). High TSH levels on laboratory tests indicate a need to either discontinue lithium or supplement it with thyroid hormone replacement. Either T_4 or T_3 formulations can be used, alone or in combination; the most common practice is to use T_4 (L-thyroxine), since it is metabolized in the body to T_3 naturally.

2. **Lithium's kidney effect is more long-term,** usually seen after 10–20 years of chronic therapy. Unlike the acute direct inhibition of renal concentrating ability (including diabetes insipidus), this long-term effect of lithium is often irreversible and may involve renal glomerular function, resulting in a mild azotemia (mildly elevated creatinine levels) in most cases. Lithium appears to reduce the glomerular filtration rate slightly. In rare instances, it can lead to severe chronic renal insufficiency and nephrotic syndrome, with glomerular pathologies of varying types. In the setting of new azotemia, the clinician needs to consider switching from lithium to another agent, although sometimes

lithium can safely be continued, as long as future kidney function tests do not worsen beyond mild abnormalities.

3. **Lithium's cardiac effects** mainly consist of some decrease in cardiac conduction efficiency, which can result in **sick sinus syndrome.** Lithium can produce **blockade of the sinoatrial node,** premature ventricular beats, and atrioventricular blockade. If lithium use is essential in a patient with these effects, a cardiac pacemaker may be necessary. Otherwise, the use of a different mood stabilizer may be indicated.

4. It is noteworthy that lithium **mildly increases free calcium levels,** possibly by stimulating direct release of parathyroid hormone from the pituitary gland, but this effect has little clinical significance, and hypercalcemia is not a serious problem

5. Lithium can also produce a **mild leukocytosis,** although this also is without clinical sequelae.

C. Toxicity
Lithium toxicity occurs in nonelderly adults, usually beginning at a level of 1.2 mEq/L (Table 48-3), with minimal side effects of tremor, nausea, diarrhea, and ataxia. Levels of 1.5–2.0 mEq/L are associated with a higher **risk of seizures.** Above 2.0 mEq/L, acute renal failure can occur and dialysis may be warranted. Above 2.5 mEq/L, coma and death can occur and dialysis is indicated. In the elderly, these signs of toxicity can occur at half the levels. **A special warning is appropriate for the elderly depressed patient who experiences diminished appetite: decreased fluid intake will raise lithium levels to toxic ranges quickly.** If renal failure is produced, lithium levels rise exponentially, greatly increasing the risk of death. Thus, dialysis is essential in such cases.

D. Teratogenicity
Early reports based on retrospective data found that lithium was associated with increased levels of congenital cardiac malformations in children of mothers treated during pregnancy. Specifically, **Ebstein's anomaly, a malformation of the tricuspid valve, was associated with lithium use in the first trimester of pregnancy.** Recent prospective studies report lower risks than in the past. However, cardiac malformations, specifically Ebstein's anomaly, are still generally thought to be a risk with lithium use during pregnancy. **These risks are probably lower than the risks of neural tube defects associated with the use of anticonvulsant mood stabilizers (e.g., divalproex and carbamazepine) in pregnancy.** Thus, in the severely ill manic patient who requires treatment, lithium use, with or without high-potency conventional antipsychotics, may at times be necessary, ideally after the first trimester of pregnancy. However, if possible, lithium use is still generally avoided during pregnancy.

VII. Clinical Effectiveness

A. Acute Mania
Lithium is quite effective in pure mania (i.e., euphoric mood), as are anticonvulsants (e.g., valproate or carbamazepine). Lithium is less effective than the anticonvulsants in mixed (depressive, dysphoric) mania.

Table 48-3. Lithium Toxicity: Blood Levels for Nonelderly Adults (divide levels in half for the elderly)

Lithium level (mEq/L)	Side effects
Below 1.2	**Generally nontoxic:** sedation, nausea, diarrhea, cognitive effects, polyuria, polydipsia, weight gain, psoriasis, tremor
1.2–1.5	**Borderline toxicity:** moderate nausea and diarrhea, more polyuria/polydipsia, increasing tremor, mild ataxia, more severe cognitive difficulties, fine hand tremor
1.5–2.0	**Mild to moderate toxicity:** coarse hand tremor, dizziness, vomiting, severe diarrhea, ataxia, confusion
2.0–2.5	**Moderate to severe toxicity:** delirium, abnormal EEG, abnormal renal function, cardiac arrhythmias, risk of coma
Above 2.5 (dialysis indicated)	**Severe toxicity:** acute renal failure, seizures, death

SOURCE: Adapted from Maxmen (1991).

B. Prophylaxis

Lithium has been shown in double-blind studies to be **effective in the prevention of manic and depressive episodes.** Anticonvulsants have not yet been proven in double-blind controlled studies to have this preventive effect, although clinical experience suggests that they do.

C. Acute Depression

Most studies suggest that **lithium is about as effective as tricyclic antidepressants in the treatment of bipolar depression. Lithium is safer in the treatment of bipolar depression than standard antidepressants, since those agents have a serious risk of causing mania, unlike lithium.** Lithium is also effective as an add-on treatment for unipolar depression, when given with standard antidepressants, for treatment-resistant cases.

D. Rapid-Cycling

Lithium is probably not as effective as anticonvulsants in the treatment of rapid-cycling bipolar disorder (manifest by four or more mood episodes of any kind in a year).

E. Comorbid Substance Abuse

Comorbid substance abuse is **a predictor of poor response to lithium.**

F. Reduction in Mortality from Suicide

Randomized prospective studies have established that **lithium exerts a preventive effect on suicide,** whereas carbamazepine failed to demonstrate that effect. Lithium reduces mortality in bipolar disorder by reducing the suicide risk.

G. Clinical Factors Impacting Response

Chronic use of antidepressants, which often have mood-destabilizing effects, can interfere with lithium response in bipolar disorder. Psychotic features may predict suboptimal response to lithium. Undetected or subclinical hypothyroidism may lead to rapid-cycling, and a resulting poor response to lithium.

For instance, some evidence indicates that subtle thyroid dysfunction (such as normal TSH but low or low-normal free T_4 levels) may be associated with impaired response to mood stabilizers like lithium. Thus, in summary, lithium response may be enhanced by minimizing antidepressant use, targeting nonpsychotic patients, and optimizing thyroid function.

Suggested Readings

Bowden C, Brugger A, Swann A, et al.: Efficacy of divalproex vs lithium and placebo in the treatment of mania. *J Am Med Assoc* 1994; 271:918–924.

El-Mallakh, RS: *Lithium: Actions and Mechanisms.* Washington, DC: American Psychiatric Press, 1996.

Gelenberg AJ, Kane JM, Keller MB, et al.: Comparison of standard and low serum levels of lithium for maintenance treatment of bipolar depression. *N Engl J Med* 1989; 321(22):1489–1493.

Goodwin FK, Jamison KR: *Manic Depressive Illness.* New York: Oxford University Press, 1990.

Goodwin FK, Murphy DL, Dunner DL, et al.: Lithium response in unipolar versus bipolar depression. *Am J Psychiatry* 1972; 129(1):44–47.

Harrow M, Goldberg JF, Grossman LS, et al.: Outcome in manic disorders. *Arch Gen Psychiatry* 1990; 47:665–671.

Hetmar O, Brun C, Ladefoged J, et al.: Long-term effects of lithium on the kidney: functional-morphological correlations. *J Psychiatr Res* 1989; 23(3/4):285–297.

Jamison K, Gerner R, Goodwin F: Patient and physician attitudes toward lithium: relationship to compliance. *Arch Gen Psychiatry* 1979; 36:866–869.

Manji HK, Hsiao JK, Risby ED, et al.: The mechanisms of action of lithium I: Effects on serotoninergic and noradrenergic systems in normal subjects. *Arch Gen Psychiatry* 1991; 48:505–512.

Manji HK, Potter WZ, Lenox RH: Signal transduction pathways: molecular targets for lithium's actions. *Arch Gen Psychiatry* 1995; 52:531–543.

Maxmen JS: *Psychotropic Drugs: Fast Facts.* New York: Norton, 1991.

Sachs GS, Lafer B, Truman CJ, et al.: Lithium monotherapy: miracle, myth and misunderstanding. *Psychiatr Ann* 1994; 24:299–306.

Schou M: Lithium treatment of manic-depressive illness. *J Am Med Assoc* 1988; 259(12):1834–1836.

Chapter 49
Anticonvulsants
Adam Savitz and Gary Sachs

I. Introduction

Over the last 10 years anticonvulsants have increasingly been used to treat psychiatric illness. Initially this was confined mostly to the use of carbamazepine and valproate for the treatment of bipolar disorder. More recently, with the approval of newer anticonvulsants, the use of these drugs for treatment of other disorders has expanded. This chapter will focus on both the properties and uses of different anticonvulsants. Because of the preponderance of controlled, blinded trials using carbamazepine and valproate, these agents will be extensively discussed; gabapentin and lamotrigine will also be covered because of their extensive clinical use. Of note is that, **of the drugs in this class, valproate is the only drug approved by the Food and Drug Administration (FDA) for a psychiatric illness (acute mania). All of the newer anticonvulsants are FDA-approved as adjunctive medications and not as stand-alone anticonvulsants.**

We will discuss each medication and compare it to the ideal anticonvulsant. The ideal anticonvulsant would have highly consistent oral bioavailability, a low protein binding, a long half-life to allow once or twice a day dosing, linear kinetics, no active metabolites, renal elimination, no hepatic enzyme induction or inhibition, and no drug interactions. The older anticonvulsants have only a few of these properties, which makes their use difficult in the polypharmacy common in severe mental illness. Even though their efficacy in mental illness has not been demonstrated in controlled trials, the newer anticonvulsants are popular because of their ease of use.

II. Carbamazepine

A. Overview
Carbamazepine (Tegretol) is an iminostilbene anticonvulsant that is structurally similar to tricyclic antidepressants. **It is used to treat partial seizures, with and without complex symptomatology, as well as generalized, tonic-clonic seizures. Carbamazepine acts by inhibiting voltage-dependent sodium channels** (thereby decreasing the repetitive firing of neurons) **and presynaptic sodium channels** (preventing the depolarization of the axon terminal and the release of neurotransmitters).

B. Pharmacology
Carbamazepine is absorbed erratically and unpredictably; peak blood levels are achieved within 4–8

h. **Approximately 65–80% of the drug is protein-bound.** It is **metabolized by the liver,** resulting in an active metabolite with levels of up to 20% of the parent compound. **The initial elimination half-life is 18–55 h;** this decreases to 5–20 h after hepatic enzymes are induced. **Carbamazepine induces its own metabolism,** which results in the need to increase the dose after 2–3 weeks to maintain the same blood level. This enzyme induction also leads to the lower levels of many other drugs, including antipsychotics, antidepressants, benzodiazepines, oral contraceptives, other anticonvulsants, and warfarin. Co-administration of phenytoin, phenobarbital, and primidone can cause decreased levels of carbamazepine, while some selective serotonin reuptake inhibitors (SSRIs), cimetidine, erythromycin, and isoniazid lead to higher carbamazepine levels. Blood levels can be monitored to assure adequate dosing and to prevent toxicity; carbamazepine has a low therapeutic index. **When used to treat patients with epilepsy, carbamazepine's therapeutic level is 4–12 μg/mL;** although the evidence regarding treatment of bipolar disorder is less clear, the accepted carbamazepine blood level is 8–12 μg/ml. Carbamazepine is typically started at 200 mg at night and gradually increased until therapeutic levels are reached or side effects are encountered. Carbamazepine is usually given in divided dosages two to three times a day.

C. Toxicity
Carbamazepine can cause agranulocytosis and liver failure. However, these adverse effects are very rare and are thought to be prevented by routine monitoring. **Aplastic anemia and agranulocytosis occur at a rate of less than 1 in approximately 20,000 people treated. Rarer still is non-dose-related idiosyncratic hepatitis,** which can be fatal; when it occurs, it develops during the first month of treatment. To prevent lethal outcomes, routine blood monitoring of the complete blood count (CBC) and liver function tests (LFTs) before starting treatment and approximately every 2 weeks for the first 2 months of treatment; thereafter, laboratory tests can be checked approximately every 3 months. **Most clinicians believe that carbamazepine should be stopped if the white blood**

cell count (WBC) drops below 3,000/μL, if the neutrophil count falls below 1,500/μL, or if the LFTs increase by three-fold. Common side effects include neurological (dizziness, ataxia, clumsiness, sedation, and dysarthria), gastrointestinal (nausea and gastrointestinal upset), rash (including very rarely exfoliation), hyponatremia, and cardiovascular (it slows intraventricular conduction, especially in overdose) problems. Side effects are usually managed by slow titration and maintenance of the dose within the therapeutic range. Carbamazepine should be used with caution in pregnancy because it can lead to spinal malformations and possibly to liver damage.

D. Uses

Multiple studies have shown that **carbamazepine is effective for the treatment of acute mania.** Several placebo-controlled trials have demonstrated that carbamazepine works as quickly as neuroleptics in mania and may be better tolerated. Response rates are typically in the range of 55–70%. The efficacy of carbamazepine for the prophylaxis of mood swings in bipolar disorder is less clear; however, numerous studies have shown maintenance rates similar to that of lithium. Furthermore, lithium and carbamazepine have often been used in combination for the treatment of refractory bipolar illness. Some evidence exists to show that **carbamazepine may be better than lithium for treatment of rapid-cycling bipolar and mixed episodes.** The evidence for carbamazepine's efficacy in depression (bipolar or unipolar) is less convincing because only a few patients (20–50%) respond to monotherapy. Carbamazepine has also been used for the treatment of mood liability in patients with schizophrenia and schizoaffective disorder. Even with its efficacy established, carbamazepine has fallen out of favor because of its drug interactions (enzyme induction) and low tolerability.

However, **carbamazepine may be the drug of choice for the treatment of psychiatric symptoms associated with complex partial seizures (temporal lobe epilepsy).** It is better for treatment of the symptoms associated with ictal events than it is for the treatment of residual interictal psychotic or mood symptoms. It remains unclear if the suppression of ictal events with carbamazepine reduces or prevents the development of the interictal syndrome.

Carbamazepine is also effective for treatment of pain syndromes; it was originally used to treat paroxysmal pain syndromes such as trigeminal neuralgia (for which it is more effective than phenytoin); currently, it is used for the treatment of diabetic neuropathy, postherpetic neuralgia, phantom limb pain, and multiple sclerosis. **Carbamazepine has also been used in the treatment of behavioral outbursts and violent behavior;** this therapeutic effect seems to be most potent in cases associated with seizures or mania. In addition, multiple uncontrolled reports have documented carbamazepine's efficacy in the treatment of behavioral outbursts in patients with head injuries, other organic syndromes, and mental retardation. Carbamazepine has also been **studied in the treatment of withdrawal symptoms,** especially those due to high-potency benzodiazepines. One study showed that carbamazepine was as effective as oxazepam for severe alcohol withdrawal and that it produced fewer symptoms of psychological distress. Carbamazepine may treat symptoms of protracted withdrawal.

III. Valproate

A. Overview

Valproate (valproic acid [Depakene] and divalproex sodium [Depakote]) is **an anticonvulsant used for generalized seizures (both petit mal and grand mal) and to a lesser extent for partial seizures. Its mode of action is to increase brain levels of γ-aminobutyric acid (GABA),** the principle inhibitory neurotransmitter. **It is FDA-approved for use in seizure disorders, acute mania, and migraine headache.**

B. Pharmacology

Valproate is **rapidly absorbed after oral ingestion;** peak plasma levels are achieved 1–2 h after taking valproate on an empty stomach, and longer (3–8 h) with food in the stomach or when the divalproex formulation is employed. **It is metabolized by the liver and has no active metabolites. Valproate is highly protein-bound,** a property that can lead to interactions with other protein-bound medications (e.g., Coumadin, digitalis, other anticonvulsants). It has a short biological half-life (8 h); for epilepsy, the typical dosing pattern is three times a day. **When used as an anticonvulsant, blood levels should typically be 50–100 μg/mL,** though they may be higher; blood levels for treatment of mania are not well established. Co-administration of enzyme inducers (e.g., carbamazepine and phenytoin) can lead to lower serum levels of valproate. Co-administration of valproate leads to higher serum levels and to increased toxicity of lamotrigine. Although valproate is often started at low doses (250 mg/day) and gradually increased, valproate can be started with a loading dose of 20 mg/kg/day for the acute treatment of mania.

C. Toxicity

The most worrisome effects of valproate are on the liver. A sizeable proportion (15–30%) of patients will develop a mild and transient rise in transaminases, which usually occurs only in the first 3 months; patients generally remain asymptomatic. Cases of fatal hepatotoxicity have been reported with the use of valproate in children under the age of 10 years, usually when valproate is used along with another anticonvulsant for a neurological problem. Very rare major toxicities include hemorrhagic pancreatitis and aplastic anemia.

Common side effects of valproate are mostly gastrointestinal, such as nausea, vomiting, heartburn and diarrhea (which occur less often with the divalproex formulation or when valproate is taken with food), and sedation which usually improves over time. Other side effects include dizziness, ataxia, tremor, and thrombocytopenia (which rarely leads to a bleeding problem).

Long-term problems that can affect compliance are alopecia and significant weight gain (especially when used in combination with lithium). Routine monitoring with LFTs and CBCs should be done, especially during initiation of therapy.

Valproate should be avoided in pregnancy since there is a high incidence (about 4%) of neural tube defects and neonatal liver disease. Valproate may also lead to polycystic ovarian disease and to menstrual irregularities, especially for women who start the drug in their teenage years.

D. Uses

Valproate has been shown in double-blind, controlled studies to **be effective in the treatment of acute mania** at response rates similar to that seen with lithium and carbamazepine. **Valproate may be more effective than lithium in the treatment of mixed bipolar states and rapid-cycling bipolar disorder.** A few controlled studies have shown that valproate is as effective as lithium in the maintenance treatment of bipolar disorder and may be more effective in the prevention of bipolar depression. Little evidence exists for valproate's effectiveness as an antidepressant.

Although not extensively studied, valproate is an adjuvant treatment for schizophrenia and schizoaffective disorder to control mood swings and aggression. **In patients treated with more than 500 mg of clozapine, valproate is often added to prevent seizures.**

Valproate is also useful in the treatment of some pain syndromes. In controlled studies, prophylaxis with valproate was effective in 65% of migraine sufferers. Valproate may also be effective in the treatment of trigeminal and postherpetic neuralgias. Two open trials have shown valproate to be efficacious for panic disorder. Case reports and a small study have shown that valproate may also be used in the treatment of benzodiazepine withdrawal. In cases of alcohol withdrawal, valproate improved symptoms more rapidly and decreased the need for benzodiazepines. Like carbamazepine, **valproate is effective in preventing complex partial seizures** and reducing the psychiatric symptoms associated with them. In addition, case reports indicate that valproate may reduce behavioral outbursts in patients, especially those with head injuries or other organic brain syndromes.

IV. Clonazepam

A. Overview

Clonazepam (Klonopin) is a high-potency benzodiazepine that is FDA-approved for the treatment of childhood epilepsy, absence seizures (petit mal), infantile spasms, myoclonic epilepsy, and complex partial seizures. Its use in epilepsy requires high doses which lead to significant side effects. **Clonazepam acts as an agonist at the benzodiazepine-binding site of the $GABA_A$ receptor.**

B. Pharmacology

Compared to other benzodiazepines, clonazepam has an **intermediate rate of onset,** achieving peak levels within 1–3 h. Its **biological half-life varies from 15 to 50 h.** Clonazepam has no significant active metabolites; it is metabolized by the liver and its levels can be increased by 3A3 inhibitors (e.g., selective serotonin reuptake inhibitors [SSRIs], cimetidine, and erythromycin). Clonazepam levels can be lowered by enzyme inducers (including carbamazepine, phenytoin, and barbiturates). Clonazepam can interact with other central nervous system (CNS) depressants to cause confusion and stupor.

C. Toxicity

The most common side effects of clonazepam are **sedation and ataxia,** which occur more frequently when high doses are used. In addition, some patients become behaviorally disinhibited with use of benzodiazepines. Like other high-potency benzodiazepines, clonazepam has the potential to create physiological tolerance and dependency, and severe withdrawal symptoms if it is discontinued suddenly. Though not well studied in pregnancy, there is some suspicion that it may be associated with cleft palates and lips.

D. Uses

Several studies have shown that clonazepam **is effective as an adjunctive agent in acutely manic patients.** Its use is associated with a reduced need for neuroleptics in manic individuals. It is unclear if clonazepam can function alone as a mood stabilizer to prevent mania or depression. A recent study in unipolar depressed patients demonstrated that addition of clonazepam to an SSRI may lead to remission of depressive symptoms sooner, as well as preventing some side-effects of SSRIs.

Clonazepam is **very effective in the treatment of panic and other anxiety disorders** (see Chap. 44). Unlike other benzodiazepines, clonazepam seems particularly effective in treating certain neuralgias and peripheral neuropathic pain syndromes; its use is complicated by its addictive potential and by its propensity to induce sedation. It is sometimes used to facilitate withdrawal from shorter-acting high-potency benzodiazepines. Clonazepam is also used to treat neuroleptic-induced akathisia, restless leg syndrome, and some forms of agitation.

V. Lamotrigine

A. Overview
Lamotrigine (Lamictal) is a relatively new drug approved **as adjunctive treatment for refractory partial seizures. Its mechanism of action is thought to be the inhibition of glutamate (an excitatory neurotransmitter) release and the inhibition of voltage-gated sodium channels.**

B. Pharmacology
Lamotrigine is rapidly (1–3 h) and completely (nearly 100%) absorbed orally. It is moderately protein-bound (50–60%) and is unaffected by use of other anticonvulsants. **Its biological half-life is 25 h,** though it is shorter (15 h) when used with enzyme-inducing drugs. Valproate inhibits the metabolism of lamotrigine and can cause toxicity and side effects when co-administered. Lamotrigine does not affect the metabolism of other medications. It is conjugated by the liver and may cause some autoinduction at higher doses. To prevent side effects, the initial daily dose is typically 25 mg/day and increased by 25–50 mg/day every 1–2 weeks, or until a maintenance dose of 75–250 mg/day is achieved. The titration needs to be slower when used with valproate and faster when used in conjunction with an enzyme inducer. Lamotrigine can be given once or twice a day (especially with the co-administration of an enzyme inducer).

C. Toxicity
The most serious side effect of lamotrigine is rash, which may lead to Stevens-Johnson syndrome. Rash occurs in up to 40% of patients in some studies, especially when initial doses are high. A slower titration seems to reduce the incidence of rashes. Severe rashes usually appear during the first 8 weeks of treatment and require hospitalization in 3 out of 1,000 adults and in 1 out of every 100 children. Common dose-related side effects include headaches, blurred vision, ataxia, dizziness, nausea, and fatigue. Its safety in pregnancy is unknown.

D. Uses
Multiple case reports and open trials point to **lamotrigine's effectiveness in treating bipolar disorder.** These effects were initially investigated because use of lamotrigine seemed to improve energy and alertness in epilepsy patients and may have improved some cases of depression. A recent placebo-controlled blinded trial showed that lamotrigine 200 mg/day was effective in treating half of the patients with bipolar (type I) depression. Lamotrigine may also be beneficial in the maintenance treatment of bipolar disorder, especially those with rapid-cycling. In addition, lamotrigine has been investigated in the treatment of **various pain disorders;** it seems to be effective in treating neuralgia, central pain, and neuropathic pain syndromes. In some cases, lamotrigine worked when carbamazepine and valproate failed.

VI. Gabapentin

A. Overview
Gabapentin (Neurontin) is a novel anticonvulsant indicated for **the adjunctive treatment of partial and generalized seizures.** It was synthesized as a GABA analog but does not modulate $GABA_A$ receptor activity. Most likely, **it interacts with the GABA transporter and increases levels of GABA.** Pregabalin is an investigational drug that is structurally similar to gabapentin and may be longer lasting and more potent.

B. Pharmacology
Gabapentin's unique properties have made it a very popular drug. The drug **is well absorbed orally** (approximately 60%). However, its absorption is nonlinear because it is primarily absorbed by intestinal amino acid transporters which are saturable at higher dosages. Gabapentin is not metabolized by humans; **it is excreted unchanged by the kidneys. It does not bind to plasma proteins. Gabapentin's serum half-life is 6–7 h,** though its CNS half-life appears to be longer. The serum level of gabapentin is increased in renal failure and is effectively cleared by hemodialysis. Its use is associated with few drug interactions. Cimetidine may decrease renal clearance, and aluminum/magnesium antacids may decrease absorption. Typically, dosing begins at 300 mg/day and is

increased, as tolerated, to 900–3,000 mg/day in two to three times a day divided dosages. Some patients cannot tolerate an initial dose of 300 mg and need to be started at 100 mg/day.

C. Toxicity

Significant side effects are not common with gabapentin. The most common adverse effects are somnolence, ataxia, dizziness, dry mouth, and fatigue. Often these are minimal with a slow titration of dose. Systematic data have not been accumulated on gabapentin's use in pregnancy.

D. Uses

Because of gabapentin's low side effect profile and lack of drug-drug interactions, it has been used for a wide variety of psychiatric disorders; at the present time **there are no placebo-controlled, blinded trials of its efficacy in mental illness.** Initially, epilepsy patients treated with gabapentin showed an improved mood and quality of life. Open and retrospective trials of gabapentin in bipolar disorder have shown it to be beneficial as both adjunctive therapy and monotherapy. It seems that it may be particularly beneficial in decreasing the frequency of cycling, irritability, and anxiety. As a sole treatment of mania, it has not been effective in a large number of patients. In addition, case reports indicate that gabapentin can cause mood elevation and mania.

Gabapentin has been used extensively in the treatment of anxiety disorders. It has the advantage of having a high degree of safety and a lack of abusability. Although case reports and open trials of the efficacy of gabapentin exist, double-blind studies are in progress to evaluate its effects on panic disorder. One controlled study of gabapentin in social phobia showed that after 14 weeks there was a moderate response of 39% in the gabapentin group, compared to 19% in the placebo group.

Gabapentin has become the first-line anticonvulsant for many pain specialists. Placebo-controlled, blinded trials have shown its efficacy in treating neuropathies (diabetic and mixed) and neuralgias. Case studies of the open use of gabapentin in the treatment of sedative-hypnotic withdrawal have appeared. A controlled study showed that gabapentin is effective in reducing symptoms in Parkinson's disease.

VII. Other New Anticonvulsants

A. Topiramate

Topiramate is a drug approved for the **adjunctive treatment of partial epilepsy in adults. It inhibits the rapid firing of sodium channels, enhances GABA effect at $GABA_A$ receptors, and antagonizes kainate at AMPA (aminomethylphenylacetic acid) receptors.** It is well absorbed orally and has a half-life of 20 h. **It has low protein-binding; 80% is excreted by the kidney unchanged, and 20% is metabolized by hepatic oxidation.** In the presence of enzyme-inducing drugs, more topiramate is metabolized by the liver, and its half-life is decreased. Though it does not induce the metabolism of other drugs, it seems to decrease the effectiveness of oral contraceptives. The main adverse effects are somnolence, dizziness, ataxia, weight loss, kidney stones, and cognitive difficulties. Cognitive difficulties affecting speech and language are insidious in onset and affect up to 25% of patients. The typical starting dose is 25–50 mg/day, increasing slowly to 200–400 mg/day. Open studies of treatment-resistant mood disorders and mania have shown that topiramate may be effective in some patients, though the prevalence of adverse events is high.

B. Tigabine

Tigabine is a new adjunctive anticonvulsant whose **mechanism involves the blockade of the reuptake of GABA and elevation of extracellular levels of GABA. It is well absorbed orally with peak levels achieved in 1 h. It is highly protein-bound (95%) and extensively metabolized by the liver.** It has **a half-life of 8 h,** which is reduced by enzyme inducers. There are no known drug-drug interactions. The most common side effects are dizziness, somnolence, tremor, poor concentration, and confusion. One report of three patients with bipolar spectrum disorders noted improvement on low dosages.

C. Vigabatrin

Vigabatrin is an **investigational anticonvulsant available in Europe.** It works by **increasing GABA levels through the inhibition of GABA transaminase.** Like gabapentin, **vigabatrin is renally excreted, it has a half-life of 5–8 h, and it is not protein-bound.** Side effects are common, and include weight gain, sedation, fatigue, behavioral disturbances, depression, and psychosis. Though it was withdrawn from trials in the United States because of toxicity, recent studies have shown that it may be a very effective drug for addiction; it has been studied in animal models of cocaine and nicotine addiction.

Suggested Readings

Hyman SE, Arana GW, Rosenbaum JF: *Handbook of Psychiatric Drug Therapy*, 3rd ed. Boston: Little Brown, 1995:124–144.

Morris HH: Pharmacokinetics of new anticonvulsants in psychiatry. *Cleveland Clinic J Med* 1998; 65:S8–15.

Perucca E: The new generation of antiepileptic drugs: advantages and disadvantages. *Brit J Clin Pharm* 1996; 42:531–543.

Sussman N: Background and rationale for use of anticonvulsants in psychiatry. *Cleveland Clinic J Med* 1998; 65:S1–7.

Chapter 50

Stimulants, Beta-Adrenergic Blocking Agents, and Alpha-Adrenergic Blocking Agents

JEFFERSON B. PRINCE

I. Stimulants

A. Indications

Stimulant medication is currently FDA-approved for use in **attention deficit hyperactivity disorder (ADHD) and narcolepsy.** However, stimulants may also have efficacy **as adjunctive agents in the treatment of depression and apathy,** and they **can potentiate the effects of narcotic analgesics.** Stimulants most commonly used are **methylphenidate (Ritalin), dextroamphetamine (Dexedrine), a mixture of amphetamine salts (Adderall), and pemoline (Cylert)** (see Table 50-1).

B. General Properties

1. **Actions.** Stimulants have been shown to **increase intrasynaptic concentrations of dopamine (DA) and norepinephrine (NE)** by occupying and blocking the DA transporter protein. In addition, **stimulants cause the release of DA and NE from presynaptic neurons into the interneuronal space.**

2. **Pharmacodynamics and pharmacokinetics. After oral administration, stimulants are rapidly absorbed** and preferentially taken up into the central nervous system (CNS). Food has little impact on their absorption. **Stimulants bind poorly to plasma proteins** and are rapidly metabolized by both hepatic and extracellular routes. Acidification of the urine may enhance excretion.

   a. **Methylphenidate. Oral administration of immediate-release methylphenidate results in a variable peak plasma concentration within 1–2 h, with a half-life of 2–3 h.** Behavioral effects of methylphenidate peak 1–2 h after administration, and tend to dissipate within 3–5 h. **Plasma levels of the sustained-release preparation of methylphenidate peak in 1–4 h, with a half-life of 2–6 h.** Peak behavioral effects of this preparation occur 2 h after ingestion, and last up to 8 h. While generic methylphenidate has a similar pharmacokinetic profile to Ritalin, it is more rapidly absorbed and peaks sooner.

   b. **Dextroamphetamine achieves peak plasma levels 2–3 h after oral administration, and has a half-life of 4–6 h.** Behavioral effects of dextroamphetamine peak 1–2 h after administration, and last 4–5 h. For dextroamphetamine spansules, these values are somewhat longer.

   c. **Adderall** is a racemic mixture of d- and l-amphetamine. The two isomers have different pharmacodynamic properties, and some children with ADHD may have a preferential response to one isomer over the other. Recent data in children with ADHD suggest that, **when compared to immediate-release Ritalin, peak behavioral effects of Adderall occur later and are more sustained.**

   d. **Pemoline.** Pemoline is a CNS stimulant that is structurally different from both methylphenidate and amphetamine, and which seems to enhance central dopaminergic transmission. **Pemoline reaches peak plasma levels 1–4 h after ingestion, and has a half-life of 7–8 h in children and 11–13 h in adults.**

   Tolerance to the effects of stimulants on ADHD symptoms does not appear to develop.

C. Using Stimulants

1. **Attention deficit hyperactivity disorder**

   a. **Short-acting stimulants are generally used for ADHD** and are typically initiated at low doses (2.5–5 mg/day for children and adolescents, 5–10 mg/day in adults), given in the morning with food. Every few days the dose may be increased (usually in increments of 2.5–5 mg/day in children and adolescents, 5–10 mg/day in adults), generally given in divided doses. Suggested daily dose ranges are 0.3–1.5 mg/kg/day for dextroamphetamine and for Adderall, and 0.5–2.0 mg/kg/day for Ritalin. Frequently, immediate-release dextroamphetamine and Ritalin are combined with their longer-acting preparations, although the efficacy of this practice has not been well demonstrated. Adderall may be effective when administered as a single daily, morning, dose; however, it often requires two daily doses.

   b. Several **longer-acting formulations** of methylphenidate are under development. Pemoline is a longer-acting agent that is usually dosed once daily in adults and twice daily in children, in the range of 1–3 mg/kg/day. Pemoline is typically started at 18.75 mg, and gradually increased in increments of 18.75 mg every several days until the desired clinical effect is achieved or side effects preclude further increases. Unfortunately, serum stimulant levels do not appear helpful in determining an effective dose.

   c. Numerous short-term (less than 12 weeks) clinical trials show that **approximately 70% of patients with ADHD respond to stimulant treatment;** a positive

Table 50-1. Stimulants

Brand Name	Generic Name	Daily Dose (mg/kg)	Dosing Schedule	Preparations Available
Ritalin	Methylphenidate	0.3–2.0	q.d.-q.i.d.	5, 10, 20 mg regular-release tablets 20 mg sustained-release tablets
Dexedrine	Dextroamphetamine	0.3–1.0	q.d.-t.i.d.	5, 10 mg regular tablets 5, 10, 15 mg spansules
Adderall	Mixture of amphetamine salts	0.3–1.0	q.d.-b.i.d.	5, 10, 20, 30 mg scored tablets
Cylert	Magnesium pemoline	1.0–3.0	q.d.-b.i.d.	18.75, 37.5, 75 mg tablets

dose-response relationship is present for both the behavioral and cognitive effects of stimulants when used in children, adolescents, and adults with ADHD. Clinicians face a number of challenges when prescribing stimulants. Since stimulants may decrease appetite in this patient population, it is often useful to administer stimulants during or after meals. Food may even enhance their bioavailability. Stimulant-induced sleep disturbances are common and may diminish their effectiveness. Such disturbances may require alteration of the timing or amount of medication given, or require the administration of a sleep aid. Irritability or dysphoria may occur 1–2 h after administration of stimulants, which suggests an absorption peak phenomenon which may respond to lower, more frequent doses.

2. **Comorbidity. Usually ADHD is comorbid with other disorders which may alter a stimulant's effectiveness.** For instance, patients with ADHD and comorbid mood or anxiety disorders may respond differently to a stimulant, depending on the clinical state of their co-occurring disorders. In addition, stimulants may exacerbate tics, obsessions, or compulsions, although they are frequently used in patients with these conditions.

3. **Tolerance and abuse.** Clinicians are often concerned about growth delays, tolerance, and abuse among stimulant-treated patients. While short-term decreases in weight are often seen in children treated with stimulants, follow-up studies into adulthood have not demonstrated decreases in ultimate height attained. Although tolerance to the effects of stimulants on ADHD symptoms has been debated, **recent data from the NIMH Multimodal Treatment of ADHD demonstrated the persistence of stimulant medication effects.** Dextroamphetamine, Adderall, and Ritalin are schedule II medications that have the potential for abuse. While the rates of substance abuse in patients with ADHD are increased, **the use of sti-mulants does not appear to increase the risk of substance abuse; recent data suggest that successful stimulant treatment of children with ADHD may delay or decrease their risk of substance abuse in adolescence.** Pemoline, a schedule IV medication, has a low potential for abuse.

4. **Narcolepsy and depression in the medically ill.** In the treatment of narcolepsy, both methylphenidate and dextroamphetamine are used in doses of 20–200 mg/day. **Stimulants appear most effective in treating the daytime somnolence and sleep attacks associated with narcolepsy, and less beneficial for cataplexy.** Stimulants **also have a role in the treatment of depressed, apathetic states in the medically ill or elderly, and may rapidly improve mood, interest, medical compliance, and even appetite.** Stimulants may also be **useful in reducing the narcotic requirement of terminally ill patients and diminishing the sedation associated with high doses of narcotics.**

D. **Side Effects**
Stimulants can cause clinically significant anorexia, nausea, difficulty falling asleep, rebound phenomena, anxiety, nightmares, dizziness, irritability, dysphoria, and weight loss. They also are associated with small increases in heart rate and blood pressure which are usually not clinically significant. Occasionally, they may elicit a depressive reaction or psychosis. Stimulant use may exacerbate tics or Tourette's syndrome. Concerns over stimulant-induced growth impairment remain, but have not been borne out. **While a physical withdrawal is not associated with stimulants, patients who have used high doses for a prolonged time may experience fatigue, hypersomnia, hyperphagia, dysphoria, and depression upon discontinuation.** Given the abuse potential of these medications, it is important to inquire about concomitant use of drugs and alcohol.

Long-term use of Pemoline in children has been associated with hepatotoxicity, although reports of this are rare. Patients and parents should be educated regarding the early signs of hepatitis (e.g., change in urine and stool, abdominal discomfort, jaundice) when Pemoline is being prescribed. While the usefulness of routine liver function tests remains unclear, it is prudent to obtain baseline values of serum glutamic-oxalo-acetic transaminase (SGOT) and serum glutamic-pyruvic transaminase (SGPT); the FDA recommends a liver panel every 2 weeks.

E. Drug Interactions

The interactions of stimulants with other prescription and nonprescription medications are generally mild and not a major source of concern. Concomitant use of sympathomimetic agents (e.g., pseudoephedrine) may potentiate the effects of both medications. Concurrent use of antihistamines may diminish the effects of stimulants. Co-administration of monoamine oxidase inhibitors (MAOIs) with stimulants may result in a hypertensive crisis and be potentially life-threatening. Although recent data on the co-administration of stimulants with tricyclic antidepressants (TCAs) suggest little interaction between these compounds, careful monitoring is warranted when prescribing stimulants with either TCAs or anticonvulsants.

II. Beta-Adrenergic Blockers

A. Indications

Beta-blockers have a variety of uses in psychiatry. They are frequently used in the treatment of performance anxiety, lithium-induced tremor, and neuroleptic-induced akathisia. They are also reported to be useful in the control of aggressive outbursts in patients with brain injury, autism, or mental retardation. They have also been used in combination with other agents in the treatment of panic disorder, generalized anxiety disorder (GAD), posttraumatic stress disorder (PTSD), ethanol withdrawal, ADHD, and with severe aggression or impulsivity. Their nonpsychiatric uses include the treatment of hypertension, arrhythmia, neurally mediated hypotension, migraine prophylaxis, glaucoma, symptoms of thyrotoxicosis, and acute myocardial infarction. The beta-blockers most commonly used in psychiatry include propranolol, nadolol, metoprolol, and atenolol (see Tables 50-2 and 50-3).

B. General Effects

Beta-blockers act as competitive antagonists of epinephrine and norepinephrine at postsynaptic beta-adrenergic receptors. Peripherally, epinephrine and norepinephrine modulate control of blood pressure and are released as stress hormones by the adrenal medulla. **Beta-1 receptors are located on the heart; they stimulate it chronotropically and inotropically. Beta-2 receptors are found in the lung and on blood vessels. Beta-2 receptor stimulation produces bronchodilation and vasodilation.** Centrally, the role of epinephrine is limited; however, the noradrenergic system is involved in the regulation of anxiety, mood, hormone release, sleep, pain, and vigilance. In the brain, beta-1 receptors are located on neurons throughout the noradrenergic system, while beta-2 receptors are primarily located on glial cells.

Beta-blockers differ in their selectivity of beta-1 and beta-2 receptor blockade, lipophilicity, route of elimination, and half-life (see Table 50-3). Propranolol and nadolol are nonselective beta-blockers, while metoprolol and atenolol are selective beta-1 receptor antagonists. These medications differ in their lipophilicity, which distinguishes their central and peripheral effects.

Table 50-2. Beta-Adrenergic Blockers: Dosing Schedules

Brand Name	Generic Name	Daily Dose (mg/day)	Dosing Schedule	Preparations Available (mg)
Inderal	Propranolol	10–640	b.i.d.-t.i.d.	10, 20, 40, 60, 80, 90
Inderal-LA	Propranolol-LA	80–320	q.d.	60, 80, 120, 160
Lopressor	Metoprolol	50–450	b.i.d.-t.i.d.	50, 100
Toprol XL	Metoprolol-XL	50–400	q.d.	50, 100, 200
Tenormin	Atenolol	25–100	q.d.	25, 50, 100
Corgard	Nadolol	20–320	q.d.	20, 40, 80, 120, 160

Table 50-3. Beta-Adrenergic Blockers: Pharmacological Properties

Medication	Selectivity	Lipophilicity	Half-life (h)	Route of Elimination
Inderal (propranolol)	Beta-1, beta-2	High	3–6	Liver
Lopressor (metoprolol)	Beta-1	High	3–4	Liver
Tenormin (atenolol)	Beta-1	Low	6–9	Kidney
Corgard (nadolol)	Beta-1, beta-2	Low	14–24	Kidney

Propranolol and metoprolol are highly lipophilic and thus easily cross the blood-brain barrier, whereas atenolol and nadolol have very little central effect. Propranolol and metoprolol are metabolized by hepatic enzymes, whereas atenolol and nadolol are eliminated by the kidneys.

C. Using Beta-Blockers

1. **General guidelines. Beta-blockers should be started at low doses, and gradually titrated up.** Patients should be educated about how to monitor blood pressure and pulse. Side effects (e.g., hypotension, dizziness, bradycardia, and bronchospasm) should be monitored. Doses should be held if blood pressure is less than 90/60 mmHg or the pulse is less than 55 beats/min.

   In adults, propranolol should be started in dosages of 10 mg t.i.d. when using the regular-release preparation, or at 80 mg q.d. for the long-acting (LA) preparation. Propranolol may be titrated up (until the desired therapeutic effect is achieved) with a maximum dose of 640 mg/day of the regular preparation and 320 mg/day of the LA form. In children the dosage range is generally 1–5 mg/kg/day. Metoprolol is usually begun at 50 mg b.i.d., with a maximum dosage of 450 mg/day of the regular-release preparation; the extended-release form is begun at 50 mg q.d. with a maximum of 400 mg/day. Nadolol is started at 20 mg q.d. with a maximum of 320 mg/day. Atenolol is begun at 25 mg q.d. with a maximum of 100 mg/day.

2. **Use in selected conditions. When selecting a beta-blocker, consideration needs to be given to the desired therapeutic effect as well as to the patient's other conditions.**

   a. For **performance anxiety** a single dose of 10–40 mg of propranolol given 30 min prior to the event is often useful. A test dose in an anxiety-provoking environment, but prior to the actual event, is usually indicated to assess tolerability. Since most symptoms of performance anxiety are peripheral, less lipophilic compounds (e.g., nadolol or atenolol) may be equally useful.

   b. **Lithium-induced tremor** often responds to propranolol 20–160 mg/day. Nadolol or atenolol may be as effective, and lessen concern over worsening of depression by beta-blockers.

   c. For **neuroleptic-induced akathisia,** both propranolol (30–80 mg/day) and nadolol (40–80 mg/day) are reported useful.

   d. Atenolol (50–100 mg/day) has utility as an adjunct to benzodiazepines in treatment of **the hyperaroused state associated with ethanol withdrawal.** Beta-blockers are not adequate as a single medicine for detoxification.

   e. In the treatment of **ADHD,** propranolol (in dosages up to 640 mg/day) has been found to be useful in adults with severe temper outbursts. Several clinical reports indicate that combining beta-blockers with stimulants may be useful in improving the tolerability of the stimulants.

   f. There are reports of using high doses of propranolol (range 50–1600 mg/day) to control **aggressive outbursts** in children, and in adults with organic brain dysfunction.

   g. Several open case series describe the utility of propranolol (dosages 2.5 mg/kg/day) in the treatment of children with PTSD.

D. Side Effects

Beta-blockers may have a variety of clinically significant side effects, including hypotension, bradycardia, dizziness, bronchoconstriction (less problematic with selective agents), nausea, diarrhea, constipation, impotence, fatigue, depression, insomnia, vivid dreams, worsening of hypoglycemia in patients with diabetes, and rebound hypertension (if abruptly discontinued). Less frequent reactions include Raynaud's phenomenon, Peyronie's disease, psychosis, and allergies. Beta-blockers may also suppress melatonin, and may potentiate the effects of growth hormone. Beta-blockers have little adverse effect on memory, and they may enhance performance.

E. Drug Interactions

Beta-blockers that are metabolized hepatically (i.e., propranolol and metoprolol) are primarily metabolized by the cytochrome P450 2D6 enzyme. **Thus, medications which inhibit 2D6 activity (e.g.,**

fluoxetine, sertraline, desipramine, clomipramine, haloperidol, fluphenazine, paroxetine, and thioridazine) will increase the levels of these beta-blockers, necessitating a decrease in dosage. Similarly, medication which induces 2D6 activity (e.g., carbamazepine, phenobarbital, phenytoin, and rifampin) may increase the metabolism of these beta-blockers, which results in decreased effects. There have been reports of increased levels of theophylline, thyroxine, and imipramine after the addition of beta-blockers. Propranolol is highly protein-bound; this is an important factor when considering drug interactions.

III. Alpha-Adrenergic Blockers

A. Indications
Clonidine (Catapres) has been used in the treatment of **hypertension** in adults since the 1960s. In psychiatry, clonidine has been used for **opioid withdrawal, nicotine withdrawal, Tourette's syndrome, ADHD, mania, neuroleptic-induced akathisia, behavioral dyscontrol in autism, anxiety disorders, PTSD, and sleep disturbances.** Recently, guanfacine (Tenex) has been used for PTSD, ADHD, Tourette's syndrome, and sleep disorders (see Table 50-4).

B. General Effects
Alpha-2-adrenergic receptors are widely distributed in the brain. Presynaptic alpha-2-adrenergic receptors are located on noradrenergic neurons in the locus coeruleus and the brainstem. These receptors function as inhibitory autoreceptors to suppress cell firing, inhibit release of NE, and downregulate central noradrenergic neurotransmission. Postsynaptic alpha-2-adrenergic receptors modulate neuronal excitability and regulate release of neurotransmitters (e.g., dopamine and serotonin) and hormones (e.g., growth hormone).

Clonidine is an imidazoline derivative with alpha-2-adrenergic agonist properties. Clonidine is almost completely absorbed after oral administration and achieves peak plasma concentrations in 1–3 h. Clonidine's plasma half-life ranges from 8–12 h in children to 12–16 h in adults. Clonidine is highly lipophilic and easily crosses the blood-brain barrier. **While some clonidine is metabolized by the liver, most is excreted unchanged by the kidney.**

Guanfacine is a longer-acting, less sedating, and more selective alpha-2-adrenergic agonist. Guanfacine is eliminated by renal excretion; it has an excretion half-life of 17 h in adults. **Guanfacine appears more selective than clonidine for the alpha-2$_A$-adrenergic receptor.** This characteristic may prove advantageous as these receptors appear to be located primarily in the prefrontal cortex. Thus, guanfacine may have a more selective beneficial effect on attention.

C. Using Clonidine and Guanfacine
When using these medications, it is critical to begin at a low dose and titrate slowly because of sedation and adverse cardiovascular effects. Clonidine is manufactured in tablets of 0.1, 0.2, and 0.3 mg. Depending on the age and size of the patient, clonidine is generally begun at one-half of a 0.1 mg tablet once or twice a day. Titration should proceed slowly and carefully until the desired benefit is reached. The behavioral effects of clonidine seem to last between 3 and 6 h, and thus multiple daily doses are usually required. There is also a transdermal therapeutic system (Catapres-TTS). The patch provides more sustained coverage and eliminates the need for repeated doses. It should be placed on a clean, dry, hairless piece of skin. The patch can be irritating to the skin, and dermatitis can limit its tolerability.

Guanfacine is generally less sedating than is clonidine and is used in the treatment of ADHD, tic disorders, and to some degree in sleep disorders. Two uncontrolled studies noted improvements in hyperactivity, inattention, and immaturity with no effect on mood or aggression. **Guanfacine is one-tenth as potent as clonidine.** It is generally begun with one-half of a 1 mg tablet daily and gradually titrated upwards until the desired benefit is achieved. It is important not to confuse the dosages of clonidine and guanfacine.

Table 50-4. Alpha-Adrenergic Blockers

Brand Name	Generic Name	Daily Dose (mg/day)	Dosing Schedule	Preparations Available
Catapres-TTS	Catapres-TTS	0.1–0.9	One patch per week	0.1, 0.2, 0.3 mg patches
Catapres	Clonidine	0.05–2.4	q.d.-q.i.d.	0.1, 0.2, 0.3 mg tablets
Tenex	Guanfacine	0.5–3	q.d.-t.i.d.	1, 2 mg tablets

D. Side Effects

The alpha-adrenergic agonists may have several clinically significant side effects, including **dry mouth or eyes, sedation, postural hypotension, fatigue, vivid dreams or nightmares, nausea, and depression.** Cardiac side effects, including **dysrhythmia, bradycardia, nonconducted P waves, supraventricular premature complexes, intraventricular conduction delays, and T-wave abnormalities,** have been described. Rare idiosyncratic side effects include hallucinations, rash, pruritus, alopecia, hyperglycemia, gynecomastia, and an increased sensitivity to alcohol. If these medications are abruptly withdrawn, there is a risk (especially when used in doses greater than 0.6 mg/day) of a rebound hypertensive crisis. Symptoms usually begin 18–20 h after the last dose. These medications should be tapered, not abruptly discontinued. Dermatitis may develop if the transdermal patch is used; this may be treated with hydrocortisone cream.

E. Drug Interactions

Clonidine should not be administered concomitantly with beta-blockers since severe adverse reactions have been reported. Recently, concerns have been raised regarding the concomitant administration of clonidine and methylphenidate.

Suggested Readings

Biederman J, Spencer TJ, Wilens TE: Approach to the patient with attention problems or hyperactivity. In Stern TA, Herman JB, Slavin PL (eds): *The MGH Guide to Psychiatry in Primary Care.* McGraw-Hill, New York, 1998:445–453.

Hyman SE, Arana GW, Rosenbaum JF: *Handbook of Psychiatric Drug Therapy*, 3rd ed. Boston: Little Brown, 1995.

Spencer T, Biederman J, Wilens T: Pharmacotherapy of ADHD: a life span perspective. In Oldham J, Riba M (eds): *American Psychiatric Press Review of Psychiatry*, Vol. 18. Washington, DC: American Psychiatric Association, 1997:87–128.

Wilens TE, Biederman J, Spencer TJ: Psychopharmacology for children and adolescents. In Cassem NH, Stern TA, Rosenbaum JF, Jellinek MS (eds): *Massachusetts General Hospital Handbook of General Hospital Psychiatry*, 4th ed. St. Louis: Mosby, 1997:467–486.

Chapter 51

Drug-Drug Interactions in Psychopharmacology

JONATHAN E. ALPERT

I. Introduction

Drug-drug interactions refer to alterations in drug levels and/or drug effects attributed to the administration of two or more prescribed, illicit, or over-the-counter agents in close temporal proximity. While many drug-drug interactions involve drugs administered within minutes to hours of each other, some drugs are implicated in interactions days to weeks after their discontinuation by virtue of their long half-lives and/or long-term impact on the activity of metabolic enzymes. Therefore, **recent as well as current drug use must be considered in the evaluation of potential drug-drug interactions.**

II. Relevance to Clinical Decisions

A. **Drug-drug interactions involving psychotropic medications are ubiquitous,** particularly among patients with treatment-refractory psychiatric disorders and those with comorbid psychiatric or medical illnesses who are likely to require multiple medications.

B. Fortunately, **most drug-drug interactions between psychotropic and other medications do not contraindicate their combined use.** Rather, awareness of such interactions should prompt particularly close attention to dosing, monitoring, and patient education, and should facilitate the timely assessment and treatment of patients who present with unexpected symptomatology or blood levels.

C. The anticipated **clinical significance of drug-drug interactions must be judged in comparison with the influence of other factors** that may alter drug responses, including **age, gender, hepatic or renal disease, smoking, alcohol use, nutritional status, dietary habits, compliance with recommended dosing, and genetic polymorphisms** in the activity of metabolic enzymes. These factors often account for considerable inter-individual variability in the response to medication in the context of which the additional impact of some drug-drug interactions may be small.

D. **Consideration of potential drug-drug interactions is particularly crucial when:**
   1. **Medications** (including **digoxin** [Lanoxin], **warfarin** [Coumadin], **theophylline** [Slo-bid, Theodur], **carbamazepine** [Tegretol], and **lithium** [Eskalith, Lithobid, Lithonate]) **with a low therapeutic index** (i.e., for which the margin between a toxic dose and a therapeutic dose is small) are prescribed.
   2. **Medications,** such as **nortriptyline** (Pamelor), **with a narrow therapeutic margin** (i.e., drugs that are thought to be relatively ineffective at doses below and above a specified therapeutic range), are prescribed.
   3. **Drugs associated with rare but catastrophic drug-drug interactions** (hypertensive crises [**monoamine oxidase inhibitors**—MAOIs] or torsades de pointes [**cisapride** (Propulsid), **astemizole** (Hismanal)]) are used.
   4. **Medications or other substances known to be potent inducers** (e.g., carbamazepine), or inhibitors (e.g., ketoconazole), **of metabolism** are used.

E. **Enhanced surveillance for drug-drug interactions is also important when:**
   1. **A perplexing clinical picture** evolves, including unexplained **mental status changes, clinical deterioration or refractoriness to standard treatment,** or unexpectedly **extreme or erratic drug plasma levels.**
   2. **Clinical states** (including liver and kidney disease, cachexia, gastrectomy, and congestive heart failure) **are present in which drug absorption, serum protein binding, and/or elimination may be markedly altered.**
   3. **Elderly or medically unstable patients** are placed at risk for adverse effects, such as hypotension or urinary retention, that pose particular hazards.
   4. **A drug overdose** has occurred, in which the quantity of drug ingested may lead to significant interactions not typically observed within the usual dose range.

F. **Certain drug-drug interactions may be used to advantage** in clinical settings:
   1. Reversal of central nervous system (CNS) depression following opiate (with naloxone [Narcan]) or benzodiazepine (with flumazenil [Romazicon]) overdose.
   2. **Treatment** of anticholinergic-induced side effects (e.g., urinary retention arising with bethanechol [Urecholine]), or extrapyramidal symptoms associated with antipsychotic medications with benztropine (Cogentin).

3. **Enhancement of drug activity or elimination half-life,** via augmentation of conventional antidepressant medications (with agents such as lithium or buspirone), or inhibition of metabolism of cytochrome P450 isoenzyme substrates (such as cyclosporine), in the presence of specific isoenzyme inhibitors (such as ketoconazole), to reduce the need for high doses and/or to reduce the frequency of administration.

III. Classification

Drug-drug interactions may be described as idiosyncratic, pharmacodynamic, or pharmacokinetic on the basis of the presumed mechanism of interaction.

A. **Idiosyncratic interactions occur unpredictably** in a small number of patients and are **unexpected from the known pharmacokinetic and pharmacological properties** of the drugs involved.

 1. **Evidence for such interactions is often inconclusive** and based upon a small number of case reports concerning complex patients on complicated medical regimens.

 2. Examples include sporadically reported cases of reversible or irreversible neurotoxicity associated with the combined use of **lithium** and **verapamil** (Calan, Isoptin), or the administration of either drug with **carbamazepine** (Tegretol).

B. **Pharmacodynamic interactions involve a known, direct pharmacological effect at biologically active (receptor) sites and do not involve an alteration in drug plasma levels.** These interactions may be additive, synergistic, or antagonistic. They may occur when two or more drugs interact with the same site or when these drugs interact with interrelated sites.

 1. Knowledge about pharmacodynamic interactions is often based upon prediction from basic and preclinical studies and subsequent confirmation in clinical case reports.

 2. Examples of pharmacodynamic drug-drug interactions include:

　a. **CNS depression,** when **alcohol, benzodiazepines,** and/or **barbiturates** are used concurrently.

　b. **Cardiac conduction delays,** when **drugs with quinidine-like effects** (including **low-potency antipsychotics,** such as chlorpromazine [Thorazine], **tricyclic antidepressants** (TCAs) such as amitriptyline [Elavil], and/or **class I antiarrhythmics,** such as disopyramide [Norpace]) are co-administered.

　c. **Anticholinergic toxicity (including ileus, urinary retention, hyperthermia, and delirium)** when drugs sharing antimuscarinic properties (including **TCAs, low-potency antipsychotics, and diphenhydramine** [Benadryl]) are combined.

　d. **Hypotension,** when **drugs associated with alpha-1-adrenergic blockade** (including **atypical and heterocyclic antidepressants, such as trazodone or imipramine, low-potency antipsychotics, and atypical antipsychotics, such as clozapine** [Clozaril] **and olanzapine** [Zyprexa]) are used together.

　e. **The interference with a dopamine agonist or precursor during treatment** of Parkinson's disease or hyperprolactinemia via concurrent administration of **antipsychotic drugs.**

C. **Pharmacokinetic interactions involve a change in the plasma level and/or tissue distribution of drugs, rather than in their pharmacological activity.** Pharmacokinetic interactions are mediated by effects on drug **absorption, distribution, metabolism, or excretion.**

 1. **Drug-drug interactions affecting drug absorption may reduce or enhance the bioavailability of orally administered drugs.** Examples include the effect of drugs that:

　a. **Accelerate gastric emptying (metoclopramide** [Reglan], **cisapride** [Propulsid]) or **diminish intestinal motility** (TCAs, morphine, cannabis), potentially promoting greater contact with and absorption from the mucosal surface of the small intestine.

　b. **Bind to other drugs (cholestyramine** [Questran], **charcoal, kaolin-pectin, nonabsorbable fats)** forming complexes that pass unabsorbed through the intestinal lumen.

　c. **Alter gastric pH** (aluminum hydroxide, magnesium hydroxide, sodium bicarbonate), potentially altering the nonpolar, unionized fraction of drug available for absorption.

　d. **Inhibit metabolic enzymes present in stomach or intestine** (e.g., monoamine oxidase and cytochrome P450 3A4), potentially retarding local degradation of certain drugs or other exogenous substances metabolized by those enzymes (e.g., tyramine), resulting in elevated concentration of these substrates that reach the portal circulation.

 2. **Drug distribution from the systemic circulation to tissue depends upon a variety of factors, including regional blood flow, lipophilicity, amount of drug bound to tissue and plasma proteins, and the adipose to lean body mass ratio of the individual.** Examples of drug-drug interactions that may influence distribution include:

　a. Competition for protein binding sites by two or more drugs that may result in displacement of a previously bound drug (which, in the unbound state, becomes available for pharmacological activity). **Most psychotropic drugs are more than 80% protein-bound and many are more than 90% protein-bound ("highly protein-bound") to albumin, alpha-1-acid glycoproteins, or lipoproteins. Exceptions include lithium, gabapentin** (Neurontin) and **venlafaxine** (Effexor), which are minimally protein-bound, and **citalopram** (Celexa), **fluvoxamine** (Luvox), **molindone** (Moban), **quetiapine** (Seroquel), **lamotrigine** (Lamictal), **and carbamazepine** (Tegretol), which are moderately (60–85%) protein-bound. While **potentially vital to the dosing and monitoring of drugs with a low therapeutic index** (e.g., **warfarin**), the practical significance of protein binding interactions for clinical management is otherwise often small, since the transient rise in plasma concentrations due to displacement of previously bound drug is offset by rapid redistribution of active drug to tissue where it is metabolized and excreted.

   b. **Alterations in regional blood flow** produced by one drug may impede or enhance delivery of other drugs to relevant receptors in tissue.

   c. **Competition for, or other interference with, active transport to tissue** (e.g., across the blood-brain barrier) may hinder access of some agents to relevant receptor sites.

3. Most drugs undergo several types of **metabolism (biotransformation),** usually enzyme-mediated, resulting in metabolites that may or may not be pharmacologically active. Many clinically important pharmacokinetic drug-drug interactions involving psychotropic drugs are based upon interference with this process.

   a. **Phase I metabolic reactions (including oxidation, reduction), and hydrolysis reactions, produce intermediate metabolites which then undergo phase II metabolic reactions (including glucuronidation and acetylation), that result in highly polar, water-soluble metabolites suitable for renal excretion.** Most psychotropic drugs undergo both phase I and phase II reactions. Exceptions include the **3-hydroxy-substituted benzodiazepines (lorazepam [Ativan], oxazepam [Serax], and temazepam [Restoril]) and clonazepam** (Klonopin), **which undergo only phase II reactions** (glucuronidation and acetylation, respectively). **Lithium and gabapentin** (Neurontin) **are excreted by the kidneys without undergoing biotransformation in the liver.**

   b. A growing understanding of metabolic enzymes, particularly the **cytochrome P450 isoenzymes,** has contributed to more rational prediction of drug-drug interactions (see IV). Other enzyme systems (including **flavin-containing monooxygenases [FMOs],** *N*-**acetyltransferase,** and **glucuronyltransferase**) are also critical for the metabolism of a variety of drugs. Many drugs utilize multiple enzyme pathways for metabolism, potentially moderating the impact of drug-drug interactions that affect a single enzyme.

   c. Some drugs are closely associated with metabolic induction or inhibition of other medications and are therefore frequently involved in drug-drug interactions (Tables 51-1 and 51-2). **Introduction of inducing agents results in increased synthesis of metabolic enzymes, thereby producing a slow decline over days to weeks in the blood levels of the co-administered drugs that they metabolize.** The discontinuation of

Table 51-1. Common Inducers of Hepatic Drug Metabolism

Drugs	Other
Carbamazepine	Alcohol, chronic
Phenobarbital	Cigarette smoking
Phenytoin (Dilantin)	Charbroiled meats
Primidone (Myosline)	Cruciferous vegetables (e.g., broccoli)

Table 51-2. Common Inhibitors of Drug Metabolism

- *Antifungals* (ketoconazole [Nizoral], miconazole [Monistat], itraconazole [Sporanox])
- *Macrolide antibiotics* (erythromycin, clarithromycin [Biaxin], troleandomycin [Tao])
- *Fluoroquinolones* (ciprofloxacin, norfloxacin, enoxacin)
- *Antimalarials* (chloroquine, primaquine)
- Isoniazid
- *Protease inhibitors* (ritonavir, saquinavir, indinavir, nelfinavir)
- *Selective serotonin reuptake inhibitors* (except venlafaxine, citalopram)
- *Tricyclic antidepressants*
- *Psychostimulants* (methylphenidate)
- *Phenothiazines*
- Divalproex sodium
- *Beta-blockers, lipophilic* (propranolol, pindolol, timolol, labetalol)
- *Calcium channel blockers* (diltiazem [Cardizem], verapamil [Calan])
- Cimetidine [Tagamet]
- Quinidine
- Disulfiram [Antabuse]
- Alcohol ingestion, acute
- Grapefruit juice

inducing agents is associated with a gradual increase in those levels. **Introduction of agents that inhibit metabolic enzymes results in a typically abrupt elevation over hours to days of blood levels of co-administered drugs whose metabolism they inhibit.** The discontinuation of metabolic inhibitors is associated with a rapid fall in those blood levels.

4. **Drug-drug interactions based upon interference with renal excretion have little relevance to most psychotropic drugs** since the majority of these agents pre-

sent for excretion in the form of inactive metabolites with only a small fraction of parent compound.

a. The principal **exception is lithium, for which drug-drug interactions involving renal excretion may alter lithium levels substantially** (see V.A.1).

b. Drug-drug interactions involving renal excretion are also sometimes utilized in the emergency management of drug overdose. **Acidification of urine** (with agents such as ammonium chloride) **enhances excretion of weak bases** (e.g., phencyclidine [PCP], or amphetamines), **while alkalization** (with agents such as acetazolamide) **promotes excretion of weak acids** (e.g., phenobarbital).

IV. Interactions Involving Cytochrome P450 Isoenzymes

A **subset of important pharmacokinetic drug-drug interactions involve the cytochrome P450 isoenzymes,** a heterogeneous group of over 30 oxidative metabolic enzymes located **predominantly in the endoplasmic reticulum of hepatocytes, as well as in the gastrointestinal tract and the brain.**

A. These enzymes are involved in the **phase I metabolism** of a wide variety of drugs as well as of endogenous substances, such as prostaglandins, fatty acids, and steroids. **The substrates, inhibitors, and inducers of P450 isoenzymes 1A2 and 2D6 and the 3A3/4 and the 2C subfamily have been particularly well characterized** (Table 51-3).

B. **2D6 and 2C19 enzymes exhibit polymorphisms, genetically based differences in enzyme structure (isoforms) that result in altered enzyme activity and a bimodal distribution of efficient or "extensive" metabolizers and of "poor" metabolizers.** Between 7% and 10% of Caucasians are "poor" metabolizers of 2D6 substrates, compared with 1–3% of

---

Table 51-3. Selected Cytochrome P450 Isoenzyme Substrates, Inhibitors, and Inducers

1A2	Substrates	Acetaminophen, aminophylline, caffeine, clozapine, haloperidol, olanzapine (Zyprexa), phenacetin, tacrine (Cognex), tertiary tricyclic antidepressants, theophylline, procarcinogens
	Inhibitors	Fluoroquinolones (ciprofloxacin), fluvoxamine (Luvox), grapefruit juice
	Inducers	Charbroiled meats, cigarette smoking, omeprazole (Prilosec)
2C	Substrates	Barbiturates, diazepam, mephenytoin, NSAIDs, propranolol, tertiary TCAs, THC, tolbutamide, warfarin
	Inhibitors	Fluoxetine, fluvoxamine, ketoconazole, omeprazole (Prilosec), sertraline
	Inducers	Rifampin
2D6	Substrates	Beta-blockers (lipophilic), codeine, debrisoquine, donepezil (Aricept), dextromethorphan, encainide, flecainide, haloperidol, hydroxycodone, mCPP, phenothiazines, risperidone (Risperdal), SSRIs, TCAs, tramadol (Ultram)
	Inhibitors	Antimalarials, fluoxetine, methadone, moclobemide, paroxetine, phenothiazines, protease inhibitors (ritonavir), quinidine, sertraline, TCAs, yohimbine
	Inducers	?
3A3/4	Substrates	Alprazolam (Xanax), amiodarone, astemizole (Hismanal), buspirone (Buspar), calcium channel blockers, carbamazepine, cisapride (Propulsid), clozapine, cyclosporine, diazepam, disopyramide (Norpace), estradiol, HMG-CoA reductase inhibitors (lovastatin, simvastatin), lidocaine, loratadine, methadone, midazolam (Versed), progesterone, propafenone (Rhythmol), quetiapine (Seroquel), quinidine, sildenafil (Viagra), testosterone, tertiary TCAs, triazolam (Halcion), vinblastine, warfarin, zolpidem (Ambien)
	Inhibitors	Antifungals (ketoconazole), calcium channel blockers (verapamil), cimetidine (Tagamet), fluvoxamine (Luvox), grapefruit juice, macrolide antibiotics (erythromycin), nefazodone (Serzone)
	Inducers	Carbamazepine, phenobarbital, phenytoin, rifampin

African-Americans and Asian-Americans. In contrast, 15–20% of African-Americans and Asian-Americans are "poor" metabolizers of 2C19 substrates compared with 1–5% of Caucasians.

C. **"Extensive" metabolizers will be converted, in effect, to "poor" metabolizers in the presence of an inhibitor of the relevant isoenzyme.**

D. **"Poor" metabolizers show higher baseline concentrations of a substrate, lower concentrations of metabolites, and little or no effect from isoenzyme inhibition or induction.**

V. Drug-Drug Interactions According to Psychotropic Drug Class

While drug-drug interactions may be broadly classified in terms of their presumed mechanism, in clinical situations drug-drug interactions are most often discussed according to the particular classes of drugs for which they are relevant, as described below.

A. Mood Stabilizers

The principal mood stabilizers (lithium, valproate, and carbamazepine) are involved in a number of significant drug-drug interactions (Tables 51-4–51-6), particularly by virtue of their **distinctive pharmacokinetic properties.**

1. **Lithium is over 95% eliminated unchanged by the kidney.** It is reabsorbed in the proximal tubules and to a lesser extent in the loop of Henle; both **valproate and carbamazepine are metabolized hepatically.**

2. **Carbamazepine is a potent inducer of metabolism; to a lesser extent, valproate inhibits metabolism.**

3. **Carbamazepine is associated with an active metabolite (carbamazepine-10,11-epoxide)** which has anticonvulsant and possibly other CNS effects.

4. **Lithium is not protein-bound, carbamazepine is only moderately protein-bound, and valproate is moderately to highly protein-bound.**

5. The putative mood-stabilizing anticonvulsant **lamotrigine (Lamictal) is moderately protein-bound and is metabolized by the liver, where its clearance is subject to significant inhibition by valproate** which causes lamotrigine levels to rise dramatically. **Lamotrigine may cause modest metabolic induction of some agents, including valproate.** In contrast, **gabapentin (Neurontin) is excreted largely unchanged by the kidney, is not appreciably protein-bound, and neither inhibits nor induces the metabolism of other agents.**

B. Antidepressants

1. **The selective serotonin reuptake inhibitors (SSRIs) have been implicated in a wide variety of pharmacokinetic interactions (mediated by the cytochrome P450 isoenzymes), as well as in the serotonin syndrome (which involves a pharmacodynamic interaction.** Selected drug-drug interactions involving the SSRIs are presented in Table 51-7.

   a. **The SSRIs, with the exception of venlafaxine (Effexor) and citalopram (Celexa), are moderate to potent inhibitors of P450 isoenzymes.**

Table 51-4. Drug-Drug Interactions Involving Lithium

Increased lithium levels	Thiazide diuretics
	ACE inhibitors (captopril, enalapril, lisinopril)
	NSAIDs (except sulindac, aspirin)
	Metronidazole, spectinomycin, tetracycline
Decreased lithium levels	Aminophylline, theophylline
	Urinary alkalization (acetazolamide, sodium bicarbonate)
	Sodium chloride
	Osmotic diuretics (mannitol, urea)
Increased antithyroid effect	Antithyroid drugs (propylthiouracil, methimazole)
Neurotoxicity (rare)	Antipsychotics, calcium channel blockers, carbamazepine, methyldopa
Prolonged neuromuscular blockade	Neuromuscular blockers (succinylcholine, pancuronium, decamethonium)
Serotonin syndrome (rare)	SSRIs, serotonergic TCAs, tramadol (Ultram), tryptophan, venlafaxine (Effexor)

Table 51-5. Drug-Drug Interactions Involving Valproate

Increased valproate levels	Aspirin (increased unbound fraction)
	Cimetidine
	Erythromycin
	Ibuprofen
	Phenothiazines
Decreased valproate levels	Carbamazepine, phenobarbital, phenytoin
	Rifampin
Inhibited metabolism of co-administered agents	Lorazepam (Ativan), oxazepam (Serax), temazepam (Restoril), diazepam (Valium)
	Carbamazepine (10,11-epoxide) metabolite, lamotrigine (Lamictal), phenobarbital
	Tolbutamide
	Warfarin
	Zidovudine (AZT)
Absence seizures (rare)	Clonazepam (Klonopin)

Table 51-6. Drug-Drug Interactions Involving Carbamazepine

Increased carbamazepine levels	Valproate (active CBZ-E metabolite), P450 3A4 inhibitors, antifungals, macrolide antibiotics, calcium channel blockers, fluvoxamine (Luvox), grapefruit juice, isoniazid, nefazodone (Serzone), protease inhibitors
Decreased carbamazepine levels	Carbamazepine (autoinduction), phenobarbital, phenytoin (Dilantin), primidone (Mysoline)
Induced metabolism of co-administered agents	Anticonvulsants (ethosuximide [Zarontin], phenytoin, lamotrigine, valproate), antidepressants, antipsychotics, benzodiazepines, cyclosporine, glucocorticoids, methadone, oral contraceptives, warfarin

b. **The P450 isoenzyme 1A2, responsible for metabolism of theophylline and clozapine, is inhibited by fluvoxamine** (Luvox).

c. **The 2C isoenzyme subfamily, responsible for metabolism of warfarin and diazepam, is inhibited by fluoxetine, sertraline, and fluvoxamine.**

d. **The 2D6 isoenzyme, responsible for metabolism of TCAs, class IC antiarrhythmics, and codeine, is inhibited by fluoxetine, paroxetine, and, to a lesser extent, sertraline.** Citalopram (Celexa) is a weak, and probably negligible, inhibitor of 2D6 under most circumstances.

e. **The 3A3/4 isoenzymes, responsible for metabolizing astemizole** (Hismanal), **cisapride** (Propulsid), **carbamazepine, and alprazolam** (Xanax), **are inhibited by fluvoxamine** (Luvox), **as well as by the atypical antidepressant nefazodone** (Serzone). Other SSRIs,

particularly fluoxetine and sertraline, appear to be less potent inhibitors of these isoenzymes.

f. The "serotonin syndrome" is a rare but potentially fatal pharmacodynamic complication associated with the combined use of highly serotonergic agents or the contraindicated overlapping use of MAOIs and SSRIs. **Signs and symptoms of the serotonin syndrome include myoclonus, hyperreflexia, nausea, hyperthermia, autonomic instability, agitation, delirium, and coma.**

2. **The TCAs are associated with a broad range of pharmacodynamic drug-drug interactions, and are also subject to drug-drug interactions involving metabolic induction or inhibition.** Significant drug-drug interactions involving TCAs and SSRIs are presented in Table 51-8.

a. **The secondary amine TCAs, including nortriptyline and desipramine, are hydroxylated by P450 2D6. Generally**

Table 51-7. Drug-Drug Interactions Involving Selective Serotonin Reuptake Inhibitors

Inhibited metabolism of co-administered agents	*Antiarrhythmics* metabolized by P450 2D6 and 2C
	Antihistamines metabolized by P450 3A4 (astemizole, loratadine)
	Antipsychotics metabolized by P450 1A2 (clozapine, olanzepine, haloperidol), 2D6 (risperidone, phenothiazines), and 3A4 (quetiapine)
	Benzodiazepines metabolized by P450 2C (diazepam), 3A4 (triazalobenzodiazepines)
	Beta-blockers (lipophilic) metabolized by P450 2C, 2D6
	Calcium channel blockers metabolized by P450 3A4
	Cisapride (Propulsid) metabolized by P450 3A4
	Codeine metabolized by P450 2D6 into active (morphine) metabolite
	Methylxanthines (aminophylline, theophylline) metabolized by P450 1A2
	Secondary amine TCAs metabolized by P450 2D6
	Tertiary amine TCAs metabolized by P450, 1A2, 2C, 2D6, 3A/4
	Warfarin (variable effects)
Serotonin syndrome	*Monoamine oxidase inhibitors* (contraindicated)
	Lithium
	Serotonergic agents

Table 51-8. Drug-Drug Interactions Involving Tricyclic Antidepressants (TCAs)

Increased TCA levels	Antifungals, beta-blockers (lipophilic), calcium channel blockers, cimetidine, macrolide antibiotics, methylphenidate, phenothiazines, quinidine, SSRIs
Decreased TCA levels	Carbamazepine, phenytoin, phenobarbital, primidone, rifampin
Prolonged cardiac conduction	Antiarrhythmics (type I), antipsychotics (low potency), calcium channel blockers
Hypotension	Antihypertensives, antipsychotics (low potency, atypicals), trazodone, MAOIs, vasodilators
Attenuated antihypertensive effects	Clonidine, guanethidine
Anticholinergic toxicity	Antipsychotics (low potency), benztropine (Cogentin), diphenhydramine (Benadryl), mirtazepine (Remeron)

the more sedating tertiary amine TCAs, including amitriptyline and imipramine, are demethylated and hydroxylated by P450 1A2, 2C, 2D6, and 3A4. In addition to serving as substrates for the P450 isoenzymes, the TCAs are also enzyme inhibitors, particularly of P450 2D6.

b. The potential for pharmacodynamic drug-drug interactions is higher for the TCAs than for other antidepressants by virtue of their broad spectrum of activity on muscarinic, histaminic, and alpha-1-adrenergic receptors, and on monoamine reuptake mechanisms and cardiac conduction.

3. Among the psychotropics, the MAOIs are most closely associated with potentially fatal drug-drug interactions.

a. Hypertensive (hyperadrenergic) crisis. Abrupt elevation of blood pressure, severe headache, nausea, vomiting, diaphoresis, cardiac arrhythmias, intracranial hemorrhage, and myocardial infarction can occur when a variety of prescribed and over-the-counter sympathomimetics, particularly indirect sympathomimetics, are used concurrently with MAOIs. Sympathomimetic drugs include: L-dopa, dopamine, cocaine, amphetamines, phenylpropanolamine, oxymetazoline (Afrin),

phentermine, mephentermine, metaraminol, ephedrine, pseudoephedrine, phenylephrine (Neo-Synephrine), **norepinephrine, isoproterenol, and epinephrine.** Safe over-the-counter allergy, cold and cough medications include **plain chlorpheniramine** (Chlor-Trimeton), **brompheniramine** (Dimetane), and **guaifenesin** (Robitussin). The widely available combined preparations that include decongestants or dextromethorphan must be scrupulously avoided. Although **dextromethorphan is not associated with hypertensive crises, its use with MAOIs has been linked to acute confusional states.**

b. **Serotonin syndrome may occur when highly serotonergic agents including the SSRIs and venlafaxine** (Effexor), **clomipramine** (Anafranil), **or tryptophan are combined with the MAOIs.** A minimum wash-out interval of 2 weeks is necessary following discontinuation of MAOIs before the initiation of one of these drugs. Reciprocally, **a minimum of 2 weeks must elapse after discontinuing most serotonergic drugs before starting an MAOI. In the case of fluoxetine, a minimum delay of 5 weeks is necessary because of its long half-life.** Although not associated with a "serotonin syndrome," the combination of buspirone (Buspar) with MAOIs has been associated with reported episodes of blood pressure elevation.

c. **Agitation, convulsions, blood pressure instability, hyperpyrexia, respiratory depression, peripheral vascular collapse, coma, and death may occur when meperidine** (Demerol) **is administered concurrently with the MAOIs.** Their combined use is absolutely contraindicated. Other narcotic analgesics (e.g., codeine, morphine) appear to be safer, although their analgesic and CNS depressant effects may be potentiated and dose adjustments may be necessary.

d. **Cases of adverse, though reversible, events including fever, delirium, convulsions, hypotension, and dyspnea have been reported when MAOIs and TCAs have been combined.** The concurrent use of these two classes of antidepressant is generally contraindicated. However, very cautious addition of an MAOI to an established treatment with a TCA has been carried out successfully in the treatment of exceptionally treatment-resistant depressed patients.

e. The effects of **CNS depressants, insulin, sulfonylurea hypoglycemic drugs, antihypertensive, or vasodilator medications may be potentiated,** with the exception of guanethidine (Esimil, Ismelin) whose antihypertensive effects may be blocked. There have been reported cases of hypertension and bradycardia on beta-blockers, and of hypertension and mental status changes with reserpine and methyldopa. The beta-agonistic effects, including tachycardia, palpitations, and anxiety, of methylxanthines and inhaled bronchodilators may be enhanced. Phenelzine (Nardil) may potentiate neuromuscular blockade on succinylcholine.

4. **The atypical antidepressants are not known to inhibit or induce cytochrome P450 isoenzymes, with the exception of nefazodone (Serzone) which is a moderately potent inhibitor of P450 3A4.** While relatively little is known about interactions of MAOIs with atypical antidepressant drugs, concerns about serious toxicity contraindicate their co-administration.

a. **Mirtazepine (Remeron) is a potent antagonist of the alpha-2-adrenergic receptor; like yohimbine (Yocon), it also blocks the histamine, muscarinic, and alpha-1-adrenergic receptors,** properties shared with many TCA antidepressants and antipsychotic agents. Thus pharmacodynamic interactions with these agents would be expected.

b. **Bupropion (Wellbutrin, Zyban) is metabolized by a distinct P450 isoenzyme, 2B6,** as is nicotine and cyclophosphamide. The metabolism of bupropion **may be inhibited by the muscular relaxant orphenadrine** (Norflex, Noradex), **and may be induced by carbamazepine and phenobarbital.**

C. **Antipsychotics**

Drug-drug interactions involving antipsychotics are presented in Table 51-9.

1. The **lower-potency agents,** such as chlorpromazine, and the **atypical antipsychotics,** are generally more likely than are the high-potency agents, such as haloperidol, to participate in **pharmacodynamic interactions with drugs (such as TCAs) that cause anticholinergic effects, sedation, hypotension, and prolonged cardiac conduction.**

2. **Clozapine, olanzapine (Zyprexa), and haloperidol involve multiple pathways, including P450 1A2.** Their clearance may therefore be **inhibited by fluvoxamine** (Luvox), and **fluoroquinolone antibiotics** (e.g., ciprofloxacin [Cipro]), and may be **induced by omeprazole** (Prilosec), and by **cigarette smoking.**

3. **Phenothiazines** (e.g., perphenazine [Trilafon]) **are both substrates and inhibitors of P450 2D6. Risperidone** (Risperdal) **is also a 2D6 substrate.**

4. **Quetiapine** (Seroquel) **is a P450 3A4 substrate,** whose concentration may be increased by isoenzyme inhibitors (e.g., **erythromycin**), and decreased by inducers (e.g., **carbamazepine** and **rifampin**).

D. **Anxiolytics**

1. **Pharmacodynamic interactions**

a. The most common and potentially serious drug-drug interactions involving benzodiazepines are the **additive CNS depressant effects** that result when these agents are co-administered with **barbiturates, ethanol, narcotics, antihistamines, TCAs, and zolpidem** (Ambien). These effects commonly include sedation and psychomotor impairment. At high doses or in severely compromised patients, fatal respiratory depression may occur.

Table 51-9. Drug-Drug Interactions Involving Antipsychotic Medications

Decreased antipsychotic levels	Beta-blockers (lipophilic), carbamazepine, phenobarbital, phenytoin, rifampin
Interference with antipsychotic drug absorption	Antacids (aluminum, magnesium)
Prolonged cardiac conduction	Calcium channel blockers, TCAs
Hypotension	Antihypertensives, MAOIs, TCAs, trazodone, vasodilators
Anticholinergic toxicity	TCAs, benztropine, diphenydramine, mirtazapine
Interference with dopaminergic effects	Bromocriptine, L-dopa, mirapex
Additive risk of myelosuppression (clozapine)	Carbamazepine, AZT

b. **Flumazenil** (Romazicon) is a **competitive inhibitor of the benzodiazepine receptor;** therefore, it antagonizes benzodiazepine effects. The anticholinesterase **physostigmine also blocks benzodiazepine binding in brain** and can also reverse CNS depression caused by benzodiazepines.

2. **Pharmacokinetic interactions.** While rarely life-threatening, alterations in blood levels of the benzodiazepines may account for the emergence of side effects such as unsteadiness or slurred speech, or for loss of antianxiety or hypnotic efficacy when a new drug is co-administered.

   a. **Antacid suspensions** (aluminum and magnesium hydroxide) **may delay the rate, but less likely the extent, of absorption** of orally administered benzodiazepines, a property **more important for single, as-needed (p.r.n.) dosing rather than for maintenance dosing** of benzodiazepines.

   b. **Inducers of phase I metabolic processes (including carbamazepine, phenobarbital, and rifampin) may reduce the levels of the majority of benzodiazepines, which are subject to oxidative metabolism,** while leaving levels of lorazepam, oxazepam, and temazepam unchanged.

   c. Inhibitors of metabolism account for a variety of drug-drug interactions with benzodiazepines.

      i. **Specific inhibitors of the cytochrome P450 3A3/4 subclass** (Table 51-3) (including the **macrolide antibiotics, antifungals, nefazodone** [Serzone], **fluvoxamine** [Luvox], and **grapefruit juice) may increase plasma levels of the triazalobenzodiazepines (alprazolam** [Xanax], **triazolam** [Halcion], **and midazolam** [Versed]) by interfering with hydroxylation.

      ii. **Specific inhibitors of the cytochrome P450 2C class** (Table 51-1) (including **omeprazole** [Prilosec], as well as **ketoconazole,** and certain SSRIs including **fluoxetine, fluvoxamine** [Luvox], and **sertraline) may increase plasma levels of diazepam** (Valium) by interfering with the *N*-demethylation.

      iii. **Inhibitors of glucuronide conjugation** (phase II metabolism), including **valproate** and **probenecid,** may increase plasma levels of the **3-hydroxy-substituted benzodiazepines (lorazepam, oxazepam, and temazepam)** which are not altered by inhibitors of phase I metabolism.

3. **Idiosyncratic interactions. Absence seizures** have been described in some patients receiving both **valproate** and **clonazepam** (Klonopin), although this drug combination is widely and safely used in many patients with bipolar disorder or seizure disorders.

E. **Miscellaneous**

1. **Zolpidem** (Ambien). Additive CNS-depressant effects are likely to occur when other sedating agents (including **alcohol, barbiturates,** and **benzodiazepines**) are co-administered with zolpidem, which interacts with the $GABA_A$-benzodiazepine complex. The sedative-hypnotic effects of zolpidem are reversed by the benzodiazepine receptor antagonist **flumazenil** (Romazicon). Like the triazalobenzodiazepines, **zolpidem levels are potentially affected by drug-drug interactions involving cytochrome P450 3A4.**

2. **Tacrine** (Cognex) is a **substrate for cytochrome P450 1A2** and may compete with other drugs for this hepatic microsomal isoenzyme. Elevated levels of **theophylline** have been reported in this context. **Donepezil** (Aricept) is a **substrate for 2D6 and 3A4;** its clearance is therefore susceptible to inhibition by such agents as **fluoxetine** and **ketoconazole.** Donepezil (Aricept) is not known to be either an inhibitor or an inducer of the metabolism of other agents. **Cholinergic toxicity is possible when either cholinesterase inhibitor is combined with other cholinomimetic agents** (e.g., **bethanechol** [Urecholine]).

3. **Methadone is a substrate for cytochrome P450 isoenzyme 3A4 and, to a lesser extent, 2D6. It is also a**

2D6 inhibitor which can potentially interfere with the clearance of other 2D6 substrates (e.g., desipramine).

4. **Disulfiram** (Antabuse). **In addition to inhibiting aldehyde dehydrogenase,** thereby resulting in the accumulation of acetaldehyde following ethanol ingestion, **disulfiram inhibits other hepatic microsomal enzymes that interfere with the metabolism of a variety of drugs** (including **warfarin, phenytoin, benzodiazepines, antipsychotics,** and **antidepressants**). The severity of the **disulfiram-alcohol reaction is increased by a variety of agents (including MAOIs, vasodilators, alpha- or beta-adrenergic antagonists, and paraldehyde).** Severe **confusional states may occur when metronidazole has been administered within 2 weeks of disulfiram; therefore, its concurrent use is contraindicated.**

Suggested Readings

Alpert JE, Bernstein JG, Rosenbaum JF: Psychopharmacological issues in the medical setting. In Cassem NH, Stern TA, Rosenbaum JF, Jellinek MS (eds): *Massachusetts General Hospital Handbook of General Hospital Psychiatry*, 4th ed. St. Louis, MO: Mosby, 1997:249–303.

Callahan AM, Marangell LB, Ketter TA: Evaluating the clinical significance of drug interactions: a systematic approach. *Harvard Rev Psychiatry* 1996; 4:153–158.

Ciraulo DA, Shader RI, Greenblatt DJ, et al. (eds): *Drug Interactions in Psychiatry*, 2nd ed. Baltimore: Williams and Wilkins, 1995.

DeVane CL, Nemeroff CB: 1998 guide to psychotropic drug interactions. *Primary Psychiatry* 1998; 5:36–75.

Ereshefsky L: Drug interactions of antidepressants. *Psychiatr Ann* 1996; 26:342–350.

Finley PR, Warner MD, Peabody CA: Clinical relevance of drug interactions with lithium. *Clin Pharmacokinet* 1995; 229:172–191.

Jefferson JW: Drug interactions—friend or foe? *J Clin Psychiatry* 1998; 59 (Suppl. 4):37–47.

Livingston MG, Livingston HM: Monoamine oxidase inhibitors. An update on drug interactions. *Drug Safety* 1997; 14:219–227.

Martin TG: Serotonin syndrome. *Ann Emerg Med* 1996; 28:520–526.

Meyer MC, Baldessarini RJ, Goff DC, Centorrino F: Clinically significant interactions of psychotropic agents with antipsychotic drugs. *Drug Safety* 1996; 15:333–346.

Nemeroff CB, DeVane CL, Pollack BG: Newer antidepressants and the cytochrome P450 system. *Am J Psychiatry* 1996; 153: 311–320.

Spina E, Pisani F, Perucca E: Clinically significant pharmacokinetic drug interactions with carbamazepine: an update. *Clin Pharmacokinet* 1996; 31:198–214.

Chapter 52

Cardiovascular and Other Side Effects of Psychotropic Medications

EDWARD R. NORRIS AND NED H. CASSEM

I. Introduction

Psychiatric illness is regularly complicated by medical symptoms and disorders. The more severe the medical illness, the more frequent is the impact on psychiatric disorders. In a fashion similar to primary psychiatric disorders, proper management of many combined medical and psychiatric disorders requires use of medications. Physicians have long feared the effects of psychotropics in medically ill patients; they continue to be wary of them in severely medically compromised patients. Historically, many psychotropics have been recognized for their potential adverse effects on the cardiovascular (CV) system and on other organ systems. Knowledge of side effects and their prevalence is a requirement for safe and effective treatment of all patients.

II. Management of Side Effects

Safe administration of psychotropics involves management of potential side effects. **Several general principles will enhance safety and compliance.**

A. **Anticipate with the patient the probable side effects;** include a review of the most common side effects. Reassure the patient that there are strategies to minimize the adverse effects of medications.

B. **Select drugs that have the smallest chance of exacerbating current medical problems.**

C. **Use the lowest effective dose and gradually titrate the dose.** This may minimize side effects because side effects are often dose-related. **"Start low, go slow,"** especially in elderly, neurologically impaired, and medically ill patients.

D. **Manage side effects with adjunctive agents** rather than switching to another agent which may delay the therapeutic response.

E. **Reassure the patient;** although this is a temporary treatment of side effects it may allow time for treatment and for side effects to abate.

F. **Educate the patient regularly that psychiatric symptoms often mirror common medication side effects.** Clearly written patient instructions will increase medication compliance. **Symptoms that begin after medication initiation or worsen with dose escalation are likely to be medication-related.**

III. Effects on the Cardiovascular System

A. **Hemodynamic Effects**

1. **Orthostatic hypotension (OH) is correlated to alpha blockade and to alpha-noradrenergic receptor affinity.** OH is of greatest concern for the elderly, for those on antihypertensive medications, and for patients with cardiovascular disease. Many antidepressants, especially tricyclic antidepressants (TCAs) and monoamine oxidase inhibitors (MAOIs), cause OH. Imipramine, desipramine, and amitriptyline are equally likely to produce OH. For TCAs, the incidence of OH in patients with a normal electrocardiogram (ECG) is 7%, with a bundle branch block (BBB) is 32%, and with congestive heart failure (CHF) is 50%. Doxepin and trazodone are also apt to cause OH. **Among the TCAs, nortriptyline is the least likely to induce OH.** A predrug orthostatic fall in blood pressure (BP) increases the risk of OH in patients and predicts response to tricylic antidepressants (TCAs). Unrelated to age or gender, OH occurs before the therapeutic effect of TCAs. Over time, the objective fall in BP will persist, but subjective complaints will diminish.

   MAOI-induced OH is common, but not predicted by a predrug orthostatic fall in BP. Mild OH occurs in 47% of patients, and severe OH occurs in 5–10% of MAOI-treated patients. The maximum effect appears after 3–4 weeks, and OH can subside after 6 weeks. Among other antidepressants, nefazodone and mirtazapine are associated with a low incidence of OH, while fluoxetine, sertraline, paroxetine, citalopram, bupropion, fluvoxamine, and venlafaxine are not associated with OH. However, data indicate that SSRI-treated patients may have as many falls as TCA-treated patients. The mechanism is unknown and the topic is still under debate.

   Low-potency neuroleptics can cause significant OH, especially in patients who are dehydrated or who are taking other BP-lowering agents. While high-potency agents are much less likely to lower BP, clozapine causes significant OH. Therefore, it is recommended that the starting dose be low and that it be titrated slowly. Risperidone, olanzapine, and quetiapine (to a lesser extent) can cause OH.

Benzodiazepines and stimulants rarely cause OH.

2. **Essential hypertension** may arise with use of some medications. Venlafaxine produces a dose-related elevation of supine diastolic BP in 7% of patients taking doses of 200–300 mg/day. It occurs in up to 13% in those with daily doses greater than 300 mg/day. Buspirone in combination with a MAOI or another serotoninergic drug can cause hypertension. Psychostimulants can aggravate hypertension.

3. **The hypertensive crisis, a potentially fatal interaction, is characterized by an elevation of BP, severe headache, nausea, vomiting, and diaphoresis.** It occurs when patients on MAOIs ingest large amounts of tyramine-containing foods. Hypertensive crisis requires immediate medical attention to reduce BP with the alpha-1-adrenergic antagonist phentolamine. Another potentially fatal interaction, serotonin syndrome, produces hypertension, tachycardia, delirium, agitation, and hyperreflexia, and occurs when MAOIs and serotonergic agents, such as SSRIs, clomipramine, or buspirone, are co-administered.

B. Cardiac Conducting System

MAOIs, bupropion, venlafaxine, fluoxetine, sertraline, citalopram, paroxetine, and fluvoxamine appear to have very few or no cardiac conduction effects. Clinically, the low-potency neuroleptics produce more cardiovascular effects than do high-potency neuroleptics. Benzodiazepines have no adverse effects on the heart. Buspirone and naltrexone have no direct effects on the heart.

1. **Heart rate** can be affected by neuroleptics and anticholinergic medications. Tachycardia, arising from anticholinergic vagolytic effects, can pose additional risk to the cardiac patient. While **low-potency neuroleptics and TCAs produce a statistically significant increase in heart rate,** several atypical antipsychotics increase the heart rate as well. Clozapine causes sustained tachycardia of 10–15 beats/min in 25% of all patients, and olanzapine can cause a small amount of tachycardia. **Tachycardia** has occurred in patients using psychostimulants.

2. Although major depression is associated with a higher prevalence of **ventricular arrhythmias,** including ventricular tachycardia and reduced heart rate variability, psychotropic medications often interfere with cardiac conduction. All TCAs appear to prolong both atrial and ventricular depolarization by sodium and potassium channel inhibition. The main effect of TCAs is the prolongation of the conduction in the His-ventricular portion of the His bundle, as occurs with the group IA antiarrhythmic drugs. The hydroxy metabolites of TCAs also prolong conduction. Trazodone, given after myocardial infarction, has been reported to aggravate pre-existing premature ventricular contractions (PVCs). **Although nortriptyline is the least cardiotoxic TCA, all TCAs should be avoided in patients with ventricular arrhythmias.**

All low-potency neuroleptics slow cardiac conduction to the same degree as the TCAs, and high-potency neuroleptics are preferred for patients with conduction disturbances. However, pimozide, risperidone, and clozapine can slow cardiac conduction; clozapine has caused reversible electrocardiographic (ECG) changes. Carbamazepine can produce conduction abnormalities at toxic doses. In patients with pre-existing abnormalities, even therapeutic levels of carbamazepine can result in conduction abnormalities. Prolonged cardiac conduction, caused by TCAs, low-potency neuroleptics, pimozide, clozapine, and risperidone, increases by 3% the risk of death from re-entrant ventricular arrhythmias.

3. The **prolongation of the QT_c interval** can lead to torsades de pointes and sudden death. Patients are at higher risk if their QT_c is greater than 440 msec. Patients with liver dysfunction, those on cisapride, patients on cardioactive drugs, and those who are female are at higher risk for QT_c prolongation. **All TCAs cause prolongation of the QT interval,** especially in combination with neuroleptics. **Antipsychotics can prolong the QT interval,** and low-potency antipsychotics have a higher risk. However, clozapine and risperidone (at higher doses) have been associated with QT prolongation. Intravenous haloperidol at higher doses, often used in emergency situations, carries a risk of QT_c prolongation and torsades de pointes. With lengthening of the QT interval, potassium and magnesium levels need to be checked and repleted prior to treatment.

4. Less severe atrial arrhythmias occur with psychotropics. TCAs, low-potency neuroleptics, and carbamazepine can increase the risk of OH in patients with BBB. Lithium can cause sinus node dysfunction and first-degree atrioventricular block. The elderly are especially prone to the inhibitory effects of lithium on impulse generation within the atrium. Depakote in overdose has been associated with heart block. Amoxapine has been the subject of case reports of atrial flutter and fibrillation.

C. Cardiovascular Disease

1. **TCAs should be used with extreme caution in patients with coronary artery disease (CAD).** TCAs and low-potency antipsychotics increase the risk of angina or myocardial infarction because of tachycardia induced by anticholinergic vagolytic effects. Selective serotonin reuptake inhibitors (SSRIs) have shown vasodilatory effects in healthy coronary arteries, but may cause vasoconstriction in vessels damaged by CAD in rare cases. Disulfiram (Antabuse) is contraindicated in patients with significant CAD. All psychotropics should be used with caution for 4–6 weeks after myocardial infarction.

2. **Congestive heart failure.** TCAs do not appear to exacerbate congestive heart failure (CHF). Low-potency antipsychotics and clozapine should be avoided.

3. **Left ventricular dysfunction.** Even in patients with left ventricular (LV) dysfunction, ejection fraction does not change during imipramine treatment; however, imipramine-treated patients are susceptible to severe OH.

IV. Central Nervous System Effects

A. **A high-frequency tremor can occur as a side effect of TCAs, SSRIs, MAOIs, lithium, valproic acid, carbamazepine, and antipsychotics.** Tremor can be exacerbated by caffeine or by anxiety. The use of low-dose beta-blockers (e.g., propranolol 10 mg t.i.d.) or low-dose benzodiazepines can minimize the tremor.

B. **Increased anxiety and jitteriness may be seen during the initiation of TCAs, SSRIs, venlafaxine, and bupropion.** These symptoms often remit within a few weeks and they can be minimized by starting at low doses or by using benzodiazepines.

C. **Parkinsonism, acute dystonia, and akathisia are common movement disorders caused by use of neuroleptics.** When parkinsonism appears, the dose of medication should be reduced, anticholinergic medication added, or switch to another agent. Acute dystonia is an emergency; treatment involves the use of anticholinergic and antihistaminergic medications. Akathisia is characterized by the subjective feelings of restlessness or the appearance of restlessness. Besides dose reduction or a change of medication, use of beta-adrenergic blocking drugs and benzodiazepines is often helpful. Some patients on SSRIs experience an akathisia-like motor restlessness that may respond to low-dose propranolol or benzodiazepines.

D. **Neuroleptic-induced tardive dyskinesia is a late-appearing disorder of involuntary movements.** The most common movements involve the face, fingers, and toes. Risk factors for tardive dyskinesia include long-term treatment with neuroleptics, female gender, increasing age, and the presence of mood or cognitive disorders.

E. **Neuroleptic malignant syndrome (NMS) is a life-threatening complication of antipsychotic medications.** The symptoms include muscular rigidity with increased creatine phosphokinase (CPK), dystonia, agitation, delirium, and autonomic dysfunction. In addition to supportive medical treatment, dantrolene or bromocriptine can be used.

F. **Fatigue and sedation** can be manifestations of psychiatric symptoms or medication side effects. TCAs, MAOIs, trazodone, nefazodone, mirtazapine, and antipsychotics are each likely to produce sedation. The side effect of sedation can be used to induce sleep in some patients.

G. **Sleep disturbances** can be related to antidepressant treatment and may improve if the medication is moved to earlier in the day. Insomnia can occur with SSRIs, bupropion, venlafaxine, and MAOIs. Reducing caffeine, eliminating daytime naps, and practicing sleep hygiene (e.g., restricting activities in the bedroom to sleep or sexual relations) can be effective.

H. **Hypomania or mania** related to antidepressant use occurs in less than 1% of patients without a history of bipolar disorder. Patients with bipolar disorder who are not on a mood stabilizer are at much higher risk. Switching of mood states can occur with the use of TCAs and are least likely with bupropion.

I. **Seizure threshold** can be reduced in patients taking bupropion.

V. Anticholinergic Effects

A. Anticholinergic activity varies greatly among psychotropics. **It is greatest for the tertiary amine TCAs** (amitriptyline, imipramine, doxepin) **and typical antipsychotics,** and minimal for the newer antidepressants (SSRIs, venlafaxine, bupropion, mirtazapine, nefazodone). Alprazolam and stimulants have essentially no anticholinergic effects. Tolerance often develops to many of the anticholinergic side effects over time.

B. **Dry mouth** (xerostomia) can result in bad breath, stomatitis, and dental caries. Often sugarless gum or hard candy can stimulate salivation. Dry eyes can be treated with artificial tears.

C. **Blurred vision** usually lessens with time, but when persistent can be managed by addition of pilocarpine 1% drops or bethanecol. Patients with

Table 52-1. Side Effects Profiles of Psychotropic Medications

Drug	Sedation	Anticholinergic	Hypotension	Hypertension	Tachycardia	Conduction Slowing
Antidepressants (cyclics)						
Amitriptyline (Elavil)	+++	+++	+++	−	+++	Yes
Amoxapine (Asendin)	+	+	+++	−	+	Yes
Clomipramine (Anafranil)	+++	+++	+++	−	+++	Yes
Desipramine (Norpramin)	+	+	+++	++	+	Yes
Doxepin (Sinequan)	+++	+++	+++	−	+++	Yes
Imipramine (Tofranil)	++	++	+++	−	++	Yes
Maprotiline (Ludiomil)	++	+	++	−	+	Yes
Nortriptyline (Pamelor)	+	+	+	−	+++	Yes
Protriptyline (Vivactil)	+	+++	++	−	+++	Yes
Trimipramine (Surmontil)	+++	++	++	−	++	Yes
Antidepressants (SSRIs)						
Citalopram (Celexa)	+	−	−	−	−	−
Fluoxetine (Prozac)	+	−	−	−	−	−
Fluvoxamine (Luvox)	+	−	−	−	−	−
Paroxetine (Paxil)	+	+	−	−	++	−
Sertraline (Zoloft)	+	−	−	−	−	−
Antidepressants (MAOIs)						
Phenelzine (Nardil)	+	+	+++	+	−	−
Tranylcypromine (Parnate)	+	+	++	++	−	−
Antidepressants (other)						
Bupropion (Wellbutrin)	+	−	−	−	−	−
Nefazodone (Serzone)	++	−	+	−	−	−
Trazodone (Desyrel)	+++	−	++	−	−	Yes
Venlafaxine (Effexor)	+	−	−	++	−	−
Mirtazapine (Remeron)	++	+	+	−	−	−
Antipsychotics (phenothiazines)						
Acetophenazine (Tindal)	++	++	++	−	+++	Yes
Chlorpromazine (Thorazine)	+++	++	+++	−	+++	Yes
Mesoridazine (Serentil)	++	++	++	−	++	Yes
Perphenazine (Trilafon)	+	+	+	−	+	Yes
Thioridazine (Mellaril)	+++	+++	+++	−	+++	Yes

(continued)

Table 52-1. (continued)

Drug	Sedation	Anticholinergic	Hypotension	Hypertension	Tachycardia	Conduction Slowing
Antipsychotics (butyrophenone)						
Droperidol (Inapsine)	+	+	+	–	–	–
Haloperidol (Haldol)	+	+	+	–	–	Yes, with IV form
Antipsychotics (thioxanthene, dibenzazepene, indolone)						
Thiothixene (Navane)	+	+	+	–	+	Yes
Loxapine (Loxitane)	++	++	++	–	++	Yes
Molindone (Moban)	++	++	+	–	++	Yes
Pimozide (Orap)	+	+	+	–	+	Yes
Antipsychotics (atypical)						
Clozapine (Clozaril)	+++	+++	+++	–	+++	Yes
Olanzapine (Zyprexa)	+	+	+++	–	++	–
Quetiapine (Seroquel)	+	+	+	–	+	–
Risperidone (Risperdal)	+	+	++	–	+	Yes
Mood stabilizers						
Valproic acid	+	–	–	–	–	–
Carbamazepine	+	–	++	–	–	Yes
Lithium (Eskalith)	+	–	–	–	–	Yes
Psychostimulants						
Dextroamphetamine (Dexedrine)	–	–	–	+++	++	–
Methylphenidate (Ritalin)	–	–	–	++	++	–

KEY: +, weak; ++, moderate; +++, strong.

narrow-angle glaucoma may experience dangerous elevations of intraocular pressure when anticholinergic medications are used.

D. **Urinary hesitancy and retention** can occur in patients on anticholinergic medications. This can be complicated by urinary tract infection and even renal damage. Elderly patients and those with prostatic hypertrophy or other outflow problems are at higher risk. Severe urinary retention mandates the discontinuation of the antidepressant.

E. **Central nervous system (CNS) anticholinergic toxicity can present with confusion, memory loss, delirium, and psychosis.** Usually this is accompanied by other signs of anticholinergic excess (increased temperature, dry skin, flushing, and urinary retention). Elderly patients, children, and brain-injured patients are at increased risk. Management includes reducing or discontinuing the dose and **physostigmine** 1–2 mg IV push over 2 min. This requires close careful monitoring of vital signs, hemodynamics, and mental status.

VI. Gastrointestinal Adverse Effects

These effects can occur with all psychotropics but usually disappear within a few days or weeks.

A. **Nausea and dyspepsia are common** side effects and can be relieved by the use of divided dosing or dosing with meals. Adjuvant treatment includes over-the-counter antacids, bismuth salicylate, and H_2 blockers. Cisapride should be avoided in patients on fluvoxamine or nefazodone because these agents can significantly increase cisapride levels, risking cardiotoxicity.

B. **Diarrhea** is more commonly seen with use of newer serotonergic antidepressants, such as the SSRIs that lack anticholinergic activity. Management strategies include the use of antidiarrheal agents. For SSRI-induced diarrhea, *Lactobacillus acidophilus* culture and cyproheptadine (a serotonin and histamine antagonist) have been helpful.

C. **Constipation** is common with TCAs but can be seen with all antidepressants. In the elderly, severe constipation and paralytic ileus can be a serious health risk. Hydration and adequate over-the-counter bulk laxatives (Metamucil) or stool softeners may be useful. Bethanecol relieves the constipation caused by anticholinergic antidepressants.

D. **Valproic acid causes dose-dependent rises in liver functions and rarely causes fatal hepatotoxicity.** Carbamazepine causes an idiosyncratic dose-related hepatitis. Antipsychotics have been associated with cholestatic jaundice, which presents with nausea, malaise, fever, pruritus, abdominal pain, and jaundice within the first 2 months of antipsychotic treatment.

VII. Hematological Effects

A. **Agranulocytosis is a potentially life-threatening hematological side effect seen most commonly with clozapine** and rarely with phenothiazines. A white blood count (WBC) drop of 50% or count of less than 3,000 should lead to immediate discontinuation. When agranulocytosis occurs, the causative agent must never be resumed.

B. Carbamazepine is associated with benign and severe hematological toxicities with depression of red blood cells, white blood cells, or platelets. Evaluation of a complete blood count (CBC), closer evaluation of patients with baseline abnormalities, and regular monitoring is required.

C. Valproic acid can cause thrombocytopenia or platelet dysfunction; only rarely is it associated with bleeding problems. Patients on valproic acid should have their platelet count and bleeding time checked before any surgery.

D. Lithium can produce a benign, relative leukocytosis without impairing leukocyte function. The WBC rarely exceeds 15,000 as a result of lithium treatment alone.

VIII. Renal Effects

A. Although lithium commonly causes defects in urine-concentrating ability, it rarely causes renal failure in patients whose lithium levels are maintained in the therapeutic range. The amount of renal damage is higher in those patients who receive lithium in divided doses rather than once-daily dosing.

B. **The most common renal problem due to lithium is polyuria.** This may be partly due to lithium's effect on the renal action of antidiuretic hormone, leading to an inability to concentrate urine. **Polyuria can occur in up to 70% of patients with long-term lithium treatment;** 10% of lithium-treated patients are diagnosed with **nephrogenic diabetes insipidus (DI)**, a urine output of greater than 3 L/day. The treatment includes maintaining the lowest effective lithium level, administering the drug at a single bedtime dose, and using diuretics. **The diuretics amiloride and hydrochlorothiazide markedly reduce urine volume caused by DI.**

C. Lithium also causes an occasional acute rise in serum creatinine, which abates with lithium discontinuation. Lithium-induced nephrotic syndrome has been reported in the literature.

IX. Weight Gain

Weight gain is a common cause of medication noncompliance and is most strongly associated with tertiary amine TCAs (amitriptyline, imipramine, doxepin) and MAOIs (phenelzine). Weight gain may be related to the antihistaminic or serotonergic effects of the agents. The SSRIs, bupropion, venlafaxine, and nefazodone are less likely to cause weight gain. Weight gain is a serious problem with all antipsychotics except molindone (Moban). Phenothiazines have been shown to increase appetite in a dose-related curve. Over 75% of patients on clozapine gain weight, with an average increase of 9–25 lb.

If weight gain occurs, dietary modification and increased exercise are effective countermeasures. There is little experience with the combination of weight loss agents and antidepressants. Package labeling contraindicated the use of D-fenfluramine with SSRIs because of the risk of serotonin syndrome.

X. Dermatological Effects

A. **Up to 10% of patients experience cutaneous reactions to psychotropic medications.** The usual reaction is an erythematous maculopapular rash that tends to occur early in treatment and usually is self-limited with most medications. The decision to continue depends upon the agent used, the level of discomfort, evidence of systemic involvement, and patient history. Rashes that are associated with the mood-stabilizing agents most often require discontinuation of the offending agent.

B. **Systemic involvement (fever, leukocytosis, and elevated liver function) usually indicates a generalized immune response** and discontinuation of the offending medication is necessary. Severe reactions, including generalized urticaria, erythema multiforme, and toxic epidermal necrolysis, may occur.

C. **Cutaneous erythematous plaques with atypical and lymphoid infiltrates and pseudolymphomas have been reported** in some patients on SSRIs and benzodiazepines. The development of severe atypical dermatologic reactions requires discontinuation of the offending agent and dermatologic consultation.

XI. Sexual Side Effects

A. Sexual dysfunction occurs in roughly one-third of patients treated with antidepressants. Sexual dysfunction can occur in up to 60% of all patients on antipsychotic medications. Sexual dysfunction is underreported unless it is specifically asked about. Sexual dysfunction can lead to medication noncompliance if not addressed by the physician.

B. **Decreased libido** can also be a symptom of depression or medication. If it persists after improvement of mood symptoms, a medication effect should be suspected.

C. **Erectile dysfunction** may result from the anticholinergic or anti-alpha-adrenergic effects of medications. **Priapism** can occur with antidepressants or antipsychotics. It is most frequently reported with trazodone use (1 in 1,000 men). All men who receive trazodone should be warned that priapism is a medical emergency which requires evaluation by a urologist.

D. **Delayed orgasm and anorgasmia** may be serotonergically mediated. It is associated with TCAs, MAOIs, SSRIs, and atypical antidepressants.

E. **Treatment of sexual side effects involves use of adjunctive agents or the discontinuation of the offending medication. Yohimbine,** an alpha-2-adrenergic antagonist, can improve erectile and orgasmic dysfunction at doses of 5.4 mg t.i.d. Yohimbine is contraindicated in patients taking MAOIs. Adjunctive use of bupropion can reduce SSRI-induced sexual dysfunction. Cyproheptadine and cholinergic agonists (e.g., bethanechol, 10–80 mg/day) can enhance libido and improve erectile function and ejaculatory problems.

XII. Conclusions

A. Knowledge of the risk of side effects is a requirement to the safe and effective treatment of all patients. **One should anticipate the side effects likely to develop and select drugs that have the smallest chance of exacerbating medical problems. The lowest effective dose should be used and gradually titrated to an effective dose.**

B. Many psychotropics interfere with the CV system, and patients at higher risk for falls or heart disease should be monitored closely. Psychotropic medications with minimal CV effects should be administered.

Suggested Readings

Alpert JE, Bernstein JG, Rosenbaum JF: Psychopharmacologic issues in the medical setting. In Cassem NH, Stern TA, Rosenbaum JF, Jellinek MS (eds): *The Massachusetts General Hospital Handbook of General Hospital Psychiatry*, 4th ed. St. Louis: Mosby, 1997:249–303.

Glassman AH, Rodriguez AI, Shapiro PA: The use of antidepressant drugs in patients with heart disease. *J Clin Psychiatry* 1998; 59 (Suppl. 10):16–21.

Goff DC, Shader RI: Non-neurological side effects of antipsychotic agents. In Hirsch SR, Weinberger DR (eds): *Schizophrenia.* Oxford: Blackwell Science, 1995:566–578.

Grebb JA: General principles of psychopharmacology. In Kaplan HI, Sadock BJ (eds): *Comprehensive Textbook of Psychiatry VI,* 6th ed. Baltimore: Williams and Wilkins, 1995:1895–1915.

Hyman SE, Arana GW, Rosenbaum JF: *Handbook of Psychiatric Drug Therapy,* 3rd ed. Boston: Little, Brown, 1995.

Smoller JA, Pollack MH, Lee DK: Management of antidepressant-induced side effects. In Stern TA, Herman JB, Slavin PS (eds):

The MGH Guide to Psychiatry in Primary Care. New York: McGraw-Hill, 1998:483–496.

Tesar GE: Cardiovascular side effects of psychotropic agents. In Stern TA, Herman JB, Slavin PS (eds): *The MGH Guide to Psychiatry in Primary Care.* New York: McGraw-Hill, 1998: 497–517.

Thapa PB, Gideon P, Cost TW, Milam AB, Ray WA: Antidepressants and the risk of falls among nursing home residents. *N Engl J Med* 1998; 339:875–882.

Chapter 53

Natural Medications in Psychiatry

DAVID MISCHOULON AND ANDREW A. NIERENBERG

I. Introduction

A. Definition
The term **"natural medication,"** as used here, **refers to medications derived from natural products, but not approved by the Food and Drug Administration (FDA)** for their purported indication. **These medications include plants and herbs, hormones and vitamins, fatty acids, amino acid derivatives, homeopathic preparations, as well as other products.**

B. The Popularity of Natural Remedies
Natural medications, in use for thousands of years, are still quite popular in Europe, Asia, and South America. Recently, their use has increased dramatically in the United States. Widely featured on television, in newspapers, books, and internet sites, these agents are now used by the majority of the world's population. The National Institutes of Health (NIH) recently recognized that one-fourth of the people in the United States seek and obtain nontraditional treatments (including natural medications), and **more than 70% of the population worldwide uses nontraditional treatments.** In 1990, more visits were made to alternative practitioners nationwide than to primary care physicians. Unfortunately, traditional medical education has largely neglected the topic of natural remedies in didactic curricula. As psychiatric practitioners, we need to inform ourselves about the topic from medical, scientific, and cultural standpoints.

C. Features that Contribute to Widespread Use of these Agents
1. **A growing dissatisfaction with the medical profession** and with orthodox medicine, which in recent years has been perceived as being more preoccupied with managed care and with profits than with healing.
2. **A recent trend to have patients be more proactive in their treatment**, rather than to assume the traditional "passive" stance when working with a physician.
3. **The ready availability of natural medications without a prescription**, and the heightened sense of independence associated with the ease of access and the ability of patients to "prescribe" for themselves if they wish to bypass the medical establishment.
4. **An increasing number of non-physician practitioners who recommend these medications** without the need to consult with a medical doctor.
5. **Ease of treatment, often at a lower cost.**

II. Problems Associated with Use of Natural Medications

A. Efficacy
Several problems arise when attempting to determine the efficacy of natural medications.
1. **The benefits of natural remedies are not clear.**
2. Manufacturers, suppliers, and the federal government have typically avoided sponsoring clinical research on the benefits of natural remedies.
3. Few systematic studies have addressed whether they are efficacious or whether they are superior to placebo.
4. Most of the data on natural medications are derived from reports, and uncontrolled trials (often with small samples), and not from double-blinded, placebo-controlled studies.

B. Safety
1. **Most people mistakenly believe that "natural" means "safe."**
2. Although relatively few reports of serious adverse effects from these medications exist, some individuals who have taken more than the recommended dosage, or even the recommended dosage, have become toxic.
3. Limited data regarding the safety and efficacy of combining natural medications with conventional medications are available.
4. Natural medications are not regulated by the FDA (although homeopathy is regulated).
5. Systematic study to determine optimal doses, contraindications to use, drug-drug interactions, and potential toxicities is lacking.
6. **A variety of preparations are available; they vary in potency, quality, and purity, and hence in their efficacy.**

C. Cost
1. **Some treatments can be quite expensive; they may even cost more than conventional medications.**

2. Insurance companies generally do not reimburse subscribers for these treatments, so **out-of-pocket payments are required.**

3. Natural remedies may prove less cost-effective in the long run, particularly if they are unhelpful to patients.

III. What Are the Indications for Natural Medications?

Although natural medications are said to help almost any medical problem, **there are relatively few psychiatric disorders for which natural medications are useful.** Psychiatric conditions for which these agents are used include dementia and disorders of mood, anxiety, and sleep, and possibly psychoses. Natural treatments have not been well explored for obsessive-compulsive disorder (OCD).

IV. Natural Antidepressants

A. St. John's Wort (Extract of *Hypericum perforatum* L.)

1. **Efficacy**
   a. Based on results of ten placebo-controlled trials, St. John's Wort has been **shown to be effective for mild-to-moderate depression,** and to be more effective than placebo; roughly two-thirds of patients responded to St. John's Wort.
   b. Shown to be as effective as low-dose tricyclics (imipramine 75 mg, maprotiline 75 mg, or amitriptyline 75 mg) in five active control studies; response rates were about 64% (for hypericum) vs. 59% (for tricyclics). Results against amitriptyline were not as encouraging.
   c. Although St. John's Wort has not yet been compared in head-to-head trials against the newer antidepressants, studies are currently underway.

2. **Presumed active components**
   a. The presumed active components of St. John's Wort are **polycyclic phenols, hypericin, pseudohypericin, and hyperforin.**
   b. Hypericin is generally believed to be the main active component.
   c. However, recent studies of hyperforin suggest this is a key antidepressant component (better results have been obtained with preparations containing 5% vs. 0.5% hyperforin).

3. **Possible mechanisms of action include:**
   a. The inhibition of cytokines (which changes levels of interleukins IL-6, IL-1β, and decreases cortisol).
   b. A decrease in serotonin (5HT) receptor density.
   c. A decrease in reuptake of neurotransmitters.
   d. A result of these components having minimal monoamine oxidase inhibitor (MAOI) activity. [Note: As a result, St. John's Wort should not be combined with a selective serotonin reuptake inhibitor [SSRI], because

of the possibility of development of serotonin syndrome.]
   e. Although the metabolism of St. John's Wort is not well understood, it is presumed to be hepatic, because none has been found in urine.

4. **Suggested dose**
   a. The suggested dose of St. John's Wort is **300 mg t.i.d.** (about 900 μg of hypericin). However, preparations of St. John's Wort differ in the amount of active components.

5. **Adverse effects**
   a. The adverse effects of St. John's Wort may include **dry mouth, dizziness, constipation, and phototoxicity.**
   b. No data are yet available on overdose.
   c. A switch to mania in bipolar patients may be induced by St. John's Wort.

6. **Summary**
   a. St. John's Wort **appears better than placebo, and equivalent to low-dose tricyclics for the treatment of depression. It is apparently safe to use.** More controlled studies are needed.

B. Dehydroepiandrosterone (DHEA)

1. **Characterization of DHEA**
   a. DHEA is **an adrenal steroid**, which is converted to testosterone and estrogen.

2. **Efficacy**
   a. An open treatment study of six middle-aged and elderly depressed patients with 30–90 mg/day of DHEA for 4 weeks resulted in improvement in depressive symptoms, and memory.

3. **Mechanism of action**
   a. Mechanisms of DHEA may include GABA (γ-aminobutyric acid) antagonism, NMDA (N-methyl-D-aspartate) potentiation, increase in brain serotonin and dopamine activity.

4. **Suggested doses**
   a. Suggested doses of DHEA are **5–100 mg/day.**
   b. Over-the-counter strength and purity are not regulated.

5. **Adverse effects**
   a. Side effects **include acne, irritability, insomnia, headaches, menstrual irregularities, increased ocular pressure, and palpitations.**

6. **Summary**
   a. Early data on DHEA are promising, but larger studies are needed. Its role for the treatment of women is unclear.

C. Folate and Vitamin B$_{12}$

1. **Folic acid**
   a. Folic acid is required for the synthesis of S-adenosylmethionine (SAMe), which is needed for synthesis of norepinephrine (NE), dopamine (DA), and serotonin (5HT).
   b. **Between 10% and 30% of depressed patients may have low levels of serum folate.**

c. **Patients with low folate levels respond less well to antidepressants than those with normal folate levels.**

d. The recommended dose of folate is **400 μg/day.**

2. **Vitamin B_{12}**

a. Vitamin B_{12} is converted to methylcobalamin, a substance that is involved in the synthesis of central nervous system (CNS) neurotransmitters.

b. Vitamin B_{12} deficiency may result in an earlier age of onset of depression.

c. The recommended dose of Vitamin B_{12} is **6 μg/day.**

3. **Summary**

a. Physicians should check Vitamin B_{12} and folate in treatment-resistant patients, particularly if they have concurrent medical illness.

b. **Correction of folate and Vitamin B_{12} deficiency may improve depressive symptoms and one's response to antidepressant therapy.**

D. Phenylethylamine (PEA)

1. **Mechanism of action**

a. PEA is **a neurohormone** believed to maintain energy, attention, affect, and courage.

b. PEA's action is probably related to catecholamine release from sympathetic nerves, in a fashion similar to that of amphetamine; it has no tolerance or reinforcement patterns.

c. Deficit in PEA may have a role in development of depression.

2. **Efficacy**

a. Open studies show that **administration of oral PEA in combination with low-dose MAOI is effective in 60% of depressed patients.** [Note: PEA is metabolized by MAO; it is therefore necessary to either give high doses of PEA or concomitant doses of a MAOI].

b. Mood elevation associated with use of PEA may occur in 1–2 days; full remission requires 2 weeks.

3. **Suggested doses**

a. The suggested dose of PEA is **10–60 mg/day**, given along with 5–10 mg of selegiline.

4. **Adverse effects**

a. **Mild anorexia** is the only reported adverse event.

5. **Interactions with other psychotropics**

a. Co-administration of MAOIs, and tricyclic antidepressants (TCAs) can increase PEA levels.

b. Co-administration of lithium may decrease PEA levels.

c. Use of alcohol or marijuana may increase PEA levels.

6. **Manufacturing/distribution issues**

a. PEA is generally not distributed to drug stores.

b. The physician must order powder in bulk from a manufacturer, and enlist a pharmacist to prepare PEA in tablet form; then the patient must buy the medication at that pharmacy.

7. **Summary**

a. While data on the use of PEA are promising, anecdotes about its use are not as encouraging.

b. Logistics of PEA administration and distribution are a limitation to its use.

E. Essential Fatty Acids (EFAs)

1. **Classification**

a. EFAs (primarily omega-3 and omega-6) are **polyunsaturated lipids derived from fish oil.**

2. **Efficacy**

a. The omega-3 EFA docosahexanoic acid (DHA) **may have a protective role against depression and bipolar disorder**, based on lower rates of depression in countries where large amounts of fish are consumed.

b. Omega-3 may also have a role in the treatment of bipolar disorder. One small double-blind, placebo-controlled trial with 30 bipolar disordered patients revealed that, of those who received the omega-3 mix, only one had a recurrence; subjects in this group also had a longer period of remission.

c. Omega-3 and omega-6 mixtures may help alleviate psychotic symptoms. Case reports with EFAs show variable results when used alone or as an adjunct to antipsychotics.

3. **Mechanisms of action**

a. **EFAs may function in a fashion similar to mood stabilizers. They seem to inhibit G-protein signal transduction via reduced hydrolysis of phosphatidylinositol and other membrane phospholipids**, which are precursors to second messengers.

4. **Suggested dosing**

a. Commercially available preparations of omega-3 may have **up to 1000 mg of omega-3 and 120 mg of DHA per capsule.**

b. The suggested dosage is **1–2 capsules/day.**

5. **Adverse effects**

a. Mild dose-related **gastrointestinal distress** appears to be the only side effect associated with use of EFAs.

6. **Summary**

a. Overall, the use of EFAs is promising, particularly in view of the wide variety of illnesses potentially treatable with these substances. However, larger studies are needed.

F. Inositol

1. **Classification**

a. Inositol is **a polyol precursor of second messenger systems** in the brain.

2. **Mechanism of action**

a. Levels of inositol in the cerebrospinal fluid (CSF) may be decreased in the presence of depression.

b. Administration of inositol may reverse the desensitization of serotonin receptors.

3. **Efficacy**

a. Inositol has been studied in a variety of conditions.

i. Depression. In a double-blind, controlled trial of 12 g/day for 4 weeks, inositol was shown to be superior to placebo (28 patients).

ii. Panic disorder. In a double-blind, controlled trial of 12 g/day for 4 weeks, inositol administration

Table 53-1. Natural Medications and their Indications and Usage

Medication	Active Components	Putative Indications	Possible Mechanisms of Action	Suggested Doses	Adverse Events
Black cohosh (*Cimicifuga racemosa*)	Triterpenoids, isoflavones, aglycones	Menopausal symptoms	Suppression of luteinizing hormone	40 mg/day	Gastrointestinal upset, dizziness, headache, weight gain
Chaste tree berry (*Vitex agnus castus*)	Unknown	Premenstrual symptoms	Prolactin inhibition, interaction with dopaminergic receptors	200–400 mg/day	None
Dehydro-epiandrosterone (DHEA)	Adrenal gland steroid hormone	Depression and dementia	GABA antagonism, NMDA potentiation, increase in brain serotonin and dopamine activity	5–100 mg/day in b.i.d.-t.i.d. dosing	Acne, irritability, insomnia, headaches, menstrual irregularities, increased ocular pressure, palpitations
Fatty acids	Essential fatty acids (primarily omega-6 and omega-3)	Depression (docosahexanoic acid—omega-3) Mania (omega-3 fatty acid mix) Psychosis (omega-3 and omega-6)	Inhibition of membrane signal transduction	1000–2000 mg/day	Gastrointestinal upset
Folic acid	Vitamin	Depression	Neurotransmitter synthesis	400 μg/day	None
Ginkgo biloba	Flavonoids, terpene lactones	Dementia	Nerve cell stimulation and protection, membrane/receptor stabilization, free radical scavenging, PAF inhibition	120–240 mg/day in b.i.d.-t.i.d. dose	Mild gastrointestinal upset, headache, irritability, dizziness
Homeopathy	Various herbs and minerals	Various disorders	Unknown	Varies with preparation	Mild transient worsening of target symptoms
Inositol	Second messenger precursor	Depression, panic, OCD	Second messenger synthesis, sensitization of serotonin receptors	12–18 g/day	Mild
Kava (*Piper methysticum*)	Kavapyrones	Anxiety	Central muscle relaxant, anticonvulsant, GABA receptor binding	60–120 mg/day	Gastrointestinal upset, allergic skin reactions, headaches, dizziness, ataxia, hair loss, visual problems, respiratory problems, dermopathy

Table 53-1. (continued)

Medication	Active Components	Putative Indications	Possible Mechanisms of Action	Suggested Doses	Adverse Events
Melatonin	Pineal gland hormone	Insomnia	Circadian rhythm regulation in suprachiasmatic nucleus	0.25–0.3 mg/day	Sedation, confusion, inhibition of fertility, decreased sex drive, hypothermia, retinal damage
Phenylethylamine (PEA)	Neurohormone, amino acid derivative	Depression	Catecholamine release	10–60 mg/day, with 5–10 mg/day of selegiline	Mild anorexia
St. John's Wort (*Hypericum perforatum* L.)	Hypericin, hyperforin, polycyclic phenols, pseudohypericin	Depression	Cytokine production, decreased serotonin receptor density, decreased neurotransmitter reuptake, MAOI activity	900 mg/day in b.i.d.-t.i.d. dosing	Dry mouth, dizziness, constipation, phototoxicity, serotonin syndrome when combined with SSRIs
Valerian (*Valeriana officinalis*)	Valepotriates, sesquiterpenes	Insomnia	Decrease GABA breakdown	450–600 mg/day	Blurry vision, dystonias, hepatotoxicity, mutagenicity?
Vitamin B_{12}	Vitamin	Depression	Neurotransmitter synthesis	6 μg/day	None

resulted in a decrease in frequency and severity of panic attacks and agoraphobia (21 patients).

iii. Obsessive-compulsive disorder (OCD). In a double-blind, controlled trial of 18 mg/day for 6 weeks, inositol resulted in alleviation of symptoms associated with OCD (13 patients).

iv. No effect was apparent in schizophrenia, attention deficit hyperactivity disorder (ADHD), Alzheimer's disease, autism, or electroconvulsive therapy (ECT)-induced cognitive impairment.

4. **Side effects and toxicity**
   a. **No apparent toxicity** has been associated with use of inositol; it has a mild side effect profile.
5. **Summary**
   a. **Overall, inositol is a promising treatment with multiple possible indications.** However, trials so far have been small; larger patient samples are required for a better understanding of this drug's efficacy.

V. Natural Anxiolytics

A. **Valerian (*Valeriana officinalis*)**
   1. **Efficacy**
      a. Valerian is **sedating** and a mild hypnotic.
      b. It is not ideal for acute treatment of insomnia, but it does promote natural sleep after several weeks of use.
      c. Valerian is very popular among Hispanics.
      d. There are only a few (about ten) small, controlled, clinical trials regarding use of valerian. It decreases sleep latency, and improves sleep quality; apparently there is no dependence or daytime drowsiness.
      e. When compared with flunitrazepam in one study, it was found to have the same efficacy, but with fewer side effects.
   2. **Mechanism of action**
      a. Valerian's efficacy is attributed to valepotriates, and sesquiterpenes, but it may function in a fashion similar to benzodiazepines.

b. It decreases GABA breakdown, and causes changes in the electroencephalogram (EEG) during sleep.

c. Its metabolism is not well understood.

3. **Suggested doses**

a. The suggested dose for valerian is **450–600 mg, taken 2 h before bedtime.**

4. **Side effects and toxicity (rare)**

a. Side effects include **blurry vision, dystonias, and hepatotoxicity.**

b. Since Mexican or Indian valerian may pose a mutagenic risk, these preparations should not be used.

5. **Summary**

a. Overall, data on valerian are promising; double-blind trials and trials comparing valerian to more conventional anxiolytic/hypnotics are needed.

b. Unfortunately, the logistics of creating a double-blind trial are complicated by valerian's distinctive and powerful smell (due to isovaleric acid). A placebo with a similar smell will need to be created.

B. **Kava (*Piper methysticum*)**

1. **Origin of kava**

a. Kava originated in the Polynesian Islands. It was originally prepared by virgins of the tribe, who chewed kava roots, placed the mash in a fermenting pot, and then prepared a tea-like drink which was consumed by all tribe members (kava is not prepared this way in the United States!).

2. **Efficacy**

a. Kava is **believed to have a calming and relaxing effect** ("With kava in you, you can't hate"), without altering consciousness.

b. Controlled, double-blind studies (about six trials) suggest it may be helpful for mild anxiety states, including agoraphobia, specific phobias, generalized anxiety disorder (GAD), and adjustment disorder.

3. **Mechanism of action**

a. Kava's mechanism of action is thought to be a result of **kavapyrones.**

b. These agents are central muscle relaxants and anticonvulsants.

c. They are involved with GABA receptor binding, and norepinephrine uptake inhibition.

d. They reduce the excitability of the limbic system, perhaps as well as benzodiazepines do, but they are not associated with either dependence or withdrawal.

e. The half-life of kava varies from 90 min to several hours.

f. Bioavailability can vary up to ten-fold, depending on the preparation.

4. **Suggested doses**

a. The suggested dose of kava is **60–120 mg/day.**

5. **Side effects (mild)**

a. Mild side effects are possible, and **include gastrointestinal upset, allergic skin reactions, headaches, and dizziness.**

6. **Toxic reactions**

a. Toxic reactions may occur with high doses or prolonged use, and **include ataxia, hair loss, visual problems, respiratory problems, and a kava dermopathy** (transient yellowing of the skin, perhaps related to cholesterol metabolism).

b. These toxic effects are reversible if the use of kava is discontinued. Nonetheless, duration of use of kava should not exceed 3 months.

7. **Summary**

a. Kava appears to be **more effective than placebo for mild anxiety states;** studies are needed to compare it with other anxiolytics.

C. **Melatonin**

1. **Definition**

a. Melatonin is **a hormone derived from serotonin;** it is made in the pineal gland.

2. **Efficacy**

a. Melatonin is involved in the organization of circadian rhythms.

b. It is commonly used by travelers to reset their biological clocks when traveling across time zones; this is the main source of melatonin's popularity.

c. It is **believed to be an effective hypnotic;** it works within 1 h of administration, regardless of the time of day it is taken.

d. It may be **more effective for people with insomnia caused by circadian rhythm disturbances.**

3. **Mechanism of action**

a. The effects of melatonin may involve interaction with the suprachiasmatic nucleus.

b. It seems to reset the circadian pacemaker, and attenuates an alerting process.

c. There may also be a direct soporific effect.

4. **Recommended doses**

a. The recommended dose of melatonin for decreasing sleep latency is **0.25–0.30 mg/day.**

b. Many melatonin preparations have as much as 5 mg of melatonin.

5. **Side effects and toxicity**

a. Side effects and toxicity are rare. However, they may **include daytime sleepiness or confusion with high doses, inhibition of fertility, decreased sex drive, hypothermia, and retinal damage.**

6. **Contraindications**

a. Contraindications to use of melatonin **include pregnancy, and an immunocompromised status** (e.g., human immunodeficiency virus (HIV)-positive individuals, or people who take steroids or other immunosuppressant drugs).

7. **Summary**

a. Melatonin is an agent that is promising, and is generally **accepted as safe and effective.**

b. It may also have a potential use in children with sleep disorders.

VI. Medications for Premenstrual/Menopausal Symptoms

A. Black Cohosh (*Cimicifuga racemosa*)
1. **Efficacy**
   a. Black cohosh comes from an herbaceous plant that is used for alleviation of menopausal symptoms (physical and psychological).
   b. Five placebo-controlled studies show black cohosh to be **efficacious,** as measured by changes in various psychometric scales, **in doses of 40 mg/day.**
2. **Active ingredients**
   a. Its active ingredients are **triterpenoids, isoflavones, and aglycones.**
3. **Mechanism**
   a. Its mechanism of action may involve suppression of luteinizing hormone (in the pituitary gland); speculation has been raised that it may also have an anti-breast cancer effect.
4. **Suggested dose**
   a. Its suggested dose is **40 mg/day.**
5. **Side effects (mild)**
   a. Side effects are mild, and **include gastrointestinal upset, headache, dizziness, and weight gain.**
6. **Toxicity**
   a. No specific toxicity has been associated with black cohosh, but data are limited.
7. **Contraindications**
   a. Contraindications to use **include pregnancy, the presence of heart disease, and hypertension.**
8. **Summary**
   a. So far, the use of black cohosh is promising, but further study is needed.
   b. Because of limited data on safety, duration of use is not recommended to exceed 3 months.

B. Chaste Tree Berry
1. **Classification**
   a. The dried fruit of the chaste tree (*Vitex agnus castus*), was reported to help medieval monks keep the vow of chastity (via decreasing their sex drive).
2. **Efficacy**
   a. **Used for the alleviation of premenstrual syndrome (PMS),** based on PTMS scale. One controlled double-blind study (175 mg/day chaste berry vs. pyridoxine) has revealed a decrease in symptoms of PMS.
3. **Mechanism**
   a. Although its clinically active ingredient is not known, its effect may be due to prolactin inhibition (one study of women); its relation to D_2 dopaminergic receptors is under investigation.
4. **Dosing**
   a. Suggested dosing is **200–400 mg/day.**
5. **Adverse effects**
   a. **No adverse events** have been reported.
6. **Summary**
   a. More systematic trials of chaste tree berry are needed.

VII. Cognition-Enhancing Remedies

A. Ginkgo Biloba (Seed from *Ginkgo biloba* Tree)
1. **Efficacy**
   a. Ginkgo biloba has been used in Chinese medicine for over 2000 years, for treatment of cognitive deficits and affective symptoms in organic brain diseases (e.g., Alzheimer's disease and vascular dementias).
      i. **Target symptoms include memory, abstract thinking, and affective symptoms.**
      ii. Ginkgo may also improve learning capacity.
   b. Ginkgo's potential role in the treatment of antidepressant-induced sexual dysfunction is under study.
      i. In males and females on several antidepressants, low-dose ginkgo has resulted in improvement in all aspects of sexual dysfunction (desire, arousal, orgasm, and resolution).
2. **Active components**
   a. The active components of ginkgo **include flavonoids, and terpene lactones.**
3. **Mechanisms of action**
   a. Ginkgo **stimulates still functional nerve cells.**
   b. **It protects them from pathologic effects, such as hypoxia, ischemia, seizures, and peripheral damage.**
   c. A membrane/receptor stabilizer, it appears to be a **free radical scavenger.**
   d. Ginkgolide B **inhibits platelet activating factor;** ginkgo should therefore be avoided in individuals with a bleeding disorder.
4. **Efficacy**
   a. Many double-blind trials have suggested that **symptoms of dementia improve with use of ginkgo** (more than 30 trials).
   b. However, standards for testing the response to treatment have changed over time.
   c. The German Federal Health Agency Mandates of 1991 reported that improvement in dementia *symptoms* (e.g., memory, abstract thinking) is not enough. We also need to see improvement in activities of daily living (ADLs) and a reduced need for care.
   d. Many older studies have therefore been uninformative, as they have not met new methodological criteria.
5. **Recent studies**
   a. A year-long randomized, double-blind study of 309 patients suggests that ginkgo may stabilize and improve cognitive performance and social functioning in demented patients. Changes were modest but significant, and were noticeable by caretakers.
   b. Some studies have compared ginkgo against other nootropics (e.g., ergot alkaloids, nicergoline, and nimodipine).
      i. Studies showed comparable efficacy; ginkgo seems to have had fewer side effects.
      ii. For these reasons, 24–28% of physicians recommend ginkgo.
      iii. Family physicians in particular tend to favor ginkgo over other nootropics.

6. **Suggested dose**
   a. Suggested doses of ginkgo are **120–240 mg/day** (on a b.i.d.-t.i.d. basis).
   b. At least an 8-week course is recommended. The patient should be re-evaluated after 3 months of use; full assessment of effect may require up to 1 year of use.

7. **Side effects**
   a. Side effects **include mild gastrointestinal upset, headache, irritability, and dizziness.**

8. **Summary**
   a. Overall, ginkgo **appears to be effective, with a very low rate of toxicity.** No interactions with other drugs have been detected.
   b. A potential role in the amelioration of antidepressant-induced sexual dysfunction has been studied.
   c. Its full role remains to be clarified.

VIII. Homeopathy

1. **History**
   a. Developed in Germany 200 years ago by Samuel Hahnemann, **homeopathy is the second most utilized health care system worldwide.**
   b. It is **derived from plants and minerals.**
   c. It is regulated by the FDA, and sold over the counter.

2. **Principles and paradoxes of homeopathy**
   a. **Potency is believed to be proportional to the degree of dilution.**
   b. Preparation, therefore, involves dilution to minute quantities.
   c. **Principle of similars**
      i. **Symptoms represent the body's attempt to heal itself.**
      ii. **Therefore, the medication must paradoxically cause the symptoms it intends to alleviate.**
   d. The homeopath obtains a careful history, with the goal of finding the one medication or combination of medications that will help the body heal its symptoms.
      i. Personality, diet, sleep pattern, reaction to temperature, and weather are considered (use of milk products is often an issue).
      ii. Homeopathic remedies are administered orally, and allowed to dissolve on, or under, the tongue.
      iii. **Improvement tends to be gradual, on the order of weeks to months.**
      iv. **A transient aggravation of symptoms may occur early in treatment.**

3. **Mechanism of action**
   a. Its mechanism of action is controversial and **not well understood.** It has drawn on various disciplines to explain it, but none is entirely convincing.
      i. Quantum theory.
      ii. Water clathrate formation (small amounts of crystals can cause lattice change in water, therefore small amounts of medication may cause major changes in disease).

iii. Thalamic neuron theory.

4. **Efficacy**
   a. Most research has focused on physical health rather than on mental health.
   b. One study examined 12 patients with various psychiatric disorders, including social phobia, panic, major depressive disorder (MDD), attention deficit disorder (ADD), and chronic fatigue.
   c. There is also a meta-analysis of 107 trials.
   d. These data suggest that homeopathy may be useful, but most studies are not rigorously designed.

5. **Adverse effects**
   a. Apparently, **side effects are benign, except for the initial worsening of symptoms,** which can often result in discontinuation of treatment.
   b. No known drug interactions or overdose risk have been reported.

6. **Summary**
   a. Homeopathy reveals promising results in some cases, but further studies are needed.
   b. For long-term use of these remedies, many seek assistance from a homeopathic practitioner, in view of the frequent need for combination treatments.

IX. Recommendations for Practitioners

A. **Routinely inquire about patients' use of natural medications,** as many patients will not volunteer information about their use of these remedies.

B. **Monitor patients who are on multiple medications.**

C. **Emphasize to patients that these alternative medications are relatively untested.**

D. **State that it is unclear whether natural medications are appropriate or even preferable to conventional psychotropics.**

X. Candidates for Alternative Treatments

A. Mildly symptomatic patients with a strong interest in natural remedies.

B. Patients who have failed multiple trials of conventional remedies, or who are highly intolerant of side effects.
   1. Keep in mind that these patients are often the most difficult to treat, and alternative agents seem best suited to the mildly ill.

XI. Conclusions

A. Natural medications are a growing field in psychopharmacology, and, in time, they may prove a valuable addition to the pharmacological armamentarium.

B. Early research data and anecdotal reports are promising, particularly with mild-to-moderate illness.

C. To recommend them as effective and safe, we need more systematic, controlled studies on adequate patient samples.

D. The NIH and NIMH have begun to support large-scale studies, and these will hopefully result in more useful guidelines and recommendations for clinicians.

Suggested Readings

Alpert JE, Fava M: Nutrition and depression: the role of folate. *Nutr Rev* 1997; 55:145–149.

Benjamin J, Agam G, Levine J, et al.: Inositol treatment in psychiatry. *Psychopharmacol Bull* 1995; 31:167–175.

Chatterjee SS, Bhattacharya SK, Wonnermann M, et al.: Hyperforin as a possible antidepressant component of hypericum extracts. *Life Sci* 1998; 63:499–510.

Cohen A: Treatment of antidepressant-induced sexual dysfunction: a new scientific study shows benefits of ginkgo biloba. *Healthwatch* 1996; 5(1).

Comas-Diaz L: Culturally relevant issues and treatment implications for Hispanics. In Koslow DR, Salett EP (eds): *Crossing Cultures in Mental Health.* Washington, DC: SIETAR International, 1989:31–48

Crone CC, Wise TN: Use of herbal medicines among consultation-liaison populations. *Psychosomatics* 1998; 39:3–13.

Davidson JR, Morrison RM, Shore J, et al.: Homeopathic treatment of depression and anxiety. *Altern Ther Health Med* 1997; 3:46–49.

Eisenberg DM: Advising patients who seek alternative medical therapies. *Ann Intern Med* 1997; 127:61–69.

Eisenberg DM, Kessler RC, Foster C, et al.: Unconventional medicine in the United States: prevalence, costs, and patterns of use. *N Engl J Med* 1993; 328:246–252.

Ernst E: Harmless herbs? A review of the recent literature. *Am J Med* 1998; 104:170–178.

Farrel RJ, Lamb J: Herbal remedies. *BMJ* 1990; 300:47–48.

Fava M, Borus JS, Alpert JE, et al.: Folate, B12, and homocysteine in major depressive disorder. *Am J Psychiatry* 1997; 154:426–428.

Furnham A, Bhagrath R: A comparison of health beliefs and behaviours of clients of orthodox and complementary medicine. *Br J Clin Psychol* 1993; 32:237–246.

Furnham A, Smith C: Choosing alternative medicine: a comparison of the beliefs of patients visiting a general practitioner and a homeopath. *Soc Sci Med* 1988; 26:685–689.

Itil T, Martorano D: Natural substances in psychiatry (Ginkgo biloba in dementia). *Psychopharmacol Bull* 1995; 31:147–158.

Jenike MA: Hypericum: a novel antidepressant. *J Geriatr Psychiatr Neurol* 1994; 7:S1–S68.

Jonas W, Jacobs J: *Healing with Homeopathy.* New York: Warner, 1996.

Kleijnen J, Knipschild P, ter Riet G: Clinical trials of homeopathy. *BMJ* 1991; 302:316–323.

Krippner S: A cross cultural comparison of four healing models. *Altern Ther Health Med* 1995; 1:21–29.

Laakmann G, Schule C, Baghai T, et al.: St. John's Wort in mild to moderate depression: the relevance of hyperforin for the clinical efficacy. *Pharmacopsychiatry* 1998; 31 (Suppl. 1):54–59.

Leathwood PD, Chauffard F: Aqueous extract of valerian reduces latency to fall asleep in man. *Planta Med* 1985; 2:144–148.

LeBars PL, Katz MM, Berman N, et al.: A placebo-controlled, double-blind, randomized trial of an extract of Ginkgo biloba for dementia. North American EGb Study Group. *J Am Med Assoc* 1997; 278:1327–1332.

Linde K, Ramirez G, Mulrow CD, et al.: St. John's wort for depression—an overview and meta-analysis of randomized clinical trials. *BMJ* 1996; 313:253–258.

MacGregor FB, Abernethy VE, Dahabra S, et al.: Hepatotoxicity of herbal medicines. *BMJ* 1989; 299:1156–1157.

Mathews JD, Riley MD, Fejo L, et al.: Effects of the heavy usage of kava on physical health: summary of a pilot survey in an aboriginal community. *Med J Aust* 1988; 148:548–555.

Matsumoto J: Molecular mechanism of biological responses to homeopathic medicines. *Med Hypotheses* 1995; 45:292–296.

Maurer K, Ihl R, Dierks T, Frolich L: Clinical efficacy of Ginkgo biloba special extract EGb 761 in dementia of the Alzheimer type. *J Psychiatr Res* 1997; 31:645–655.

National Institutes of Health Office of Alternative Medicine: Clinical practice guidelines in complementary and alternative medicine. An analysis of opportunities and obstacles. Practice and Policy Guidelines Panel. *Arch Fam Med* 1997; 6:149–154.

Nierenberg AA: St. John's Wort: a putative over-the-counter herbal antidepressant. *J Depressive Disorders: Index Rev* 1998; III(3):16–17.

Norton SA, Ruze P: Kava dermopathy. *J Am Acad Dermatol* 1994; 31:89–97.

Peet M, Laugharne JD, Mellor J, Ramchand CN: Essential fatty acid deficiency in erythrocyte membranes from chronic schizophrenic patients, and the clinical effects of dietary supplementation. *Prostaglandins Leukotrienes Essential Fatty Acids* 1996; 55: 71–75.

Sabelli H, Fink P, Fawcett J, Tom C: Sustained antidepressant effect of PEA replacement. *J Neuropsychiatry Clin Neurosci* 1996; 8:168–171.

Sack RL, Hughes RJ, Edgar DM, Lewy AJ: Sleep-promoting effects of melatonin: at what dose, in whom, under what conditions, and by what mechanisms? *Sleep* 1997; 20:908–915.

Schulz V, Hänsel R, Tyler VE: *Rational Phytotherapy: A Physicians' Guide to Herbal Medicine*, 3rd ed. Berlin: Springer, 1998.

Schwartz GE, Russek LG: Dynamical energy systems and modern physics: fostering the science and spirit of complementary and alternative medicine. *Altern Ther Health Med* 1997; 3:46–56.

Singh YN: Kava: an overview. *J Ethnopharmacol* 1992; 37:13–45.

Stoppe G, Sandholzer H, Staedt J, et al.: Prescribing practice with cognition enhancers in outpatient care: are there differences regarding type of dementia? Results of a representative survey in lower Saxony, Germany. *Pharmacopsychiatry* 1996; 29:150–155.

Volz HP: Controlled clinical trials of hypericum extracts in depressed patients—an overview. *Pharmacopsychiatry* 1997; 30 (Suppl. 2):72–76.

Wetzel MS, Eisenberg DM, Kaptchuk TJ: Courses involving complementary and alternative medicine at US medical schools. *J Am Med Assoc* 1998; 280:784–787.

Whitmore SM, Leake NB: Complementary therapies: an adjunct to traditional therapies [letter]. *Nurse Pract* 1996; 21:12–13.

Williams LL, Kiecolt-Glaser JK, Horrocks LA, et al.: Quantitative association between altered plasma esterified omega-6 fatty acid proportions and psychological stress. *Prostaglandins Leukotrienes Essential Fatty Acids* 1992; 47:165–70.

Wolkowitz OM, Reus VI, Roberts E, et al.: Dehydroepiandrosterone (DHEA) treatment of depression. *Biol Psychiatry* 1997; 41:311–318.

Chapter 54

Suicide

ROY H. PERLIS AND THEODORE A. STERN

I. Overview

As the **eighth leading cause of death** in the United States, suicide represents a significant public health problem. **Each year, some 31,000 people commit suicide; for every attempt which is successful, roughly 18 will fail.**

Up to two-thirds of those who commit suicide visit a physician in the month prior to making an attempt, though this visit is often not associated with psychiatric complaints. Screening for suicidal ideation and assessing for risk factors provides an opportunity to intervene before an attempt occurs. Such screening is essential in psychiatric populations, as **over 90% of patients who commit suicide carry at least one major psychiatric diagnosis.**

II. Epidemiology (see Table 54-1)

Population-based studies demonstrate that suicide rates vary widely among different demographic groups.

A. **Gender**
   While females attempt suicide at a rate three times that of males, males are up to three times more likely to succeed. This difference has been attributed to the more lethal means often chosen by men.

B. **Age**
   In general, suicide rates increase with age, with the greatest rates seen in those over the age of 60 years. Those age 15–24 years represent an important exception to this trend, as suicide has become the third leading cause of death in this group. Among depressed patients, however, one major study

showed a mean age of 36 years in men and 45 years in women.

C. **Ethnicity**
   In the United States, **suicide rates are highest among Caucasian and Native American populations.**

D. **Individual Factors**
   According to population studies, **individuals who are divorced or widowed, who are unemployed or in financial difficulty, or who live alone, also have higher suicide rates.**

III. Evaluation (see Table 54-2)

Unfortunately, the demographic factors mentioned above are of limited utility in identifying particular patients at risk for suicide. Moreover, people who are contemplating suicide are often reluctant to reveal suicidal thoughts, particularly to clinicians with whom they do not have a long-standing relationship. Thus, suicide risk must be assessed even in those who do not express suicidal ideation.

A. **Survivors of a Suicide Attempt**
   Those patients who have already attempted suicide or inflicted self-harm should be assessed as soon as possible.

B. **Individuals who Express Thoughts of Suicide or Hopelessness**
   Those who openly express suicidal thoughts or hopelessness should be asked specifically about suicidal intention and plans.

Table 54-1. Selected Epidemiologic Risk Factors for Suicide

Demographic
Male gender
Age > 60 years
White or Native American

Personal
Widowed or divorced
Living alone
Unemployed or having current financial difficulties
Recent loss (e.g., of job or close relationship)

Table 54-2. Key Elements of the Suicide Evaluation

- Assess the degree of suicidal ideation
- Inquire about the details of the plan, the access to means, and the possibility of rescue
- Identify the precipitants for suicidal thinking
- Screen for the presence of major psychiatric illness
- Inquire about past suicide attempts
- Screen for risk factors (see Tables 54-1 and 54-3)
- Identify the extent of social supports
- Perform a complete mental status examination

C. Individuals who Exhibit Excessive Risk-Taking
Patients who exhibit excessive risk-taking or who appear accident-prone may be motivated by thoughts of suicide. Frequent automobile accidents or increasing substance use, for example, may presage a suicide attempt.

D. Patients with Psychiatric Illness
Patients with any type of psychiatric illness should be asked directly about suicidal thoughts on multiple occasions.

IV. Approach to the Suicidal Patient

A. General Strategies
1. **Establish rapport first.** A calm, nonjudgmental, empathic approach is usually helpful in this regard. However, it is important to note that **suicidal patients commonly elicit strong feelings** (e.g., anger or anxiety) **in clinicians.** An awareness of these feelings can help to minimize their interference with the evaluation.
2. **Begin with general questions.** When conducting the interview it is often useful to **proceed from asking general questions about suicidal thoughts to asking specific questions about plans and circumstances.** A question such as, "Have you had thoughts that life is not worth living?" can be a useful starting point. Sometimes it will be necessary to rephrase questions or to inquire multiple times, as some patients who initially deny being suicidal may reveal these thoughts once they feel more comfortable during the interview. Inquiring about suicide does not prompt patients to consider the idea for the first time. In fact, some patients are relieved by the opportunity to discuss these feelings.
3. **Gather information from collateral sources.** Since some patients in acute care settings deny being suicidal, **collateral informants** (e.g., family members, friends, or outpatient treaters) **can be essential to the assessment of risk.** Most patients who suicide have communicated their intent to others within 6 months of an attempt.

B. Goals of the Assessment
The goals of assessment include identification of the degree of acute, short-term, and long-term risk for suicide, and determination of ways in which each may be diminished.

C. Specific Elements of History
1. **Determine the nature of suicidal thoughts or attempts.** The intensity, frequency, and duration of suicidal thoughts may reveal acuity and patterns of risk.
2. **Learn the details of the plan,** including when, where and how a patient intends to commit suicide, as they can suggest the potential lethality of a plan

and the possibility of its success. This concept is sometimes quantified as a **risk/rescue ratio,** in which the highest risk is associated with more lethal means and with a small chance for rescue. For example, a patient who plans to drive his truck to a remote country road and shoot himself in the head would have a high risk/rescue ratio. If, instead, he planned to take a few extra capsules of a multivitamin while sitting in his therapist's office, his risk/rescue ratio would be low.

3. **Determine the methods used in attempted suicide.**
   a. **Firearms are used most commonly** as the agent of suicide by both genders; they account for up to 60% of completed suicides.
   b. **Poisoning is the second most common means of suicide for women, compared to hanging for men.**
   c. **Among attempts which do not succeed, drug ingestion is the most common means, used in 70% of failed attempts.** The medications used most commonly include antidepressants, nonnarcotic analgesics, and benzodiazepines; typically these agents are used in combination.

4. **Clarify the expectations of the suicide attempter.** In assessing risk, it is essential to consider a patient's beliefs about a suicide plan, not merely the objective risk that the plan would pose. A patient who genuinely believes that the ten tablets of vitamin C he ingested should have been fatal will still be at significant risk for suicide, even though the objective risk posed by such an "overdose" might be minimal.

5. **Uncover the motivation for actions;** knowledge of these motivations may suggest possible interventions.
   a. **The wish to escape from suffering,** or the wish to be reunited with loved ones, are examples often cited by suicidal patients.
   b. **Hopelessness, or a negative view of the future, is an even stronger predictor of risk than is depression itself.** A patient should be asked about future plans; when one sets affairs in order or says "good-bye," it is often in anticipation of an imminent suicide attempt.
   c. **Recent loss of a relationship** (e.g., through death or divorce) is a risk factor, particularly among substance-abusing patients.
   d. **Manipulative suicide attempts** are common, particularly among patients with personality disorders. However, such attempts must still be addressed seriously, as even chronically suicidal patients may commit suicide.

6. **Perform a careful psychiatric review of systems, which may suggest the presence of major psychiatric illness. Psychiatric illness represents the most powerful risk factor for suicide attempts and for completed suicide.** Among patients who commit suicide the prevalence of psychiatric illness is

greater than 90%; the greatest risk is associated with major depression, substance abuse, anxiety and panic, and psychotic disorders.

7. **Evaluate psychosocial supports** and the patient's ability and willingness to take advantage of them; these factors may help to prevent suicide.

8. **Identify individual risk factors** based upon a detailed history and mental status examination.

V. Risk Factors for Suicide (see Table 54-3)

A. **Psychiatric Disorders**
1. **Major depression is a factor in about 50% of suicides. Patients with major depression have a lifetime risk of suicide of around 15%. Comorbid anhedonia, anxiety or panic attacks, and alcohol abuse** may significantly increase the likelihood of suicide attempts within 1 year after an attempt. The presence of psychotic symptoms also increases risk.
   a. Of note, **suicide rates during depressive episodes are equivalent in unipolar and bipolar depression.**
   b. **Manic states are very rarely associated with suicide;** the risk in mixed states is related to the magnitude of depressive symptoms.
2. **Substance abuse, particularly of alcohol or multiple drugs, is a factor in at least 25% of cases; substance abusers have a lifetime risk of suicide of 15%.** An important associated risk factor is recent personal loss or onset of medical complications; in contrast to depression, suicide among substance abusers often occurs later in the disease course. Even among patients without a long-standing pattern of substance abuse or dependence, substance use greatly increases the risk of suicide. The impaired judgment and impulsivity associated with **acute intoxication play a role in 20% or more of completed suicides.**
3. **Anxiety disorders may play a role in 15–20% of suicides.** The risk posed remains significant even after controlling for comorbid depression and sub-

stance abuse; when anxiety is combined with depression, the risk of suicide may be additive.
4. **Psychosis contributes to 10% or more of suicides, with a lifetime risk among schizophrenics of 15%.**
   a. In contrast to patterns seen in the general population, the schizophrenic patient who commits suicide is most likely to be a young male with high premorbid functioning.
   b. **Akathisia and abrupt neuroleptic discontinuation significantly increase the risk of suicide,** as does onset of depression following the resolution of an acute psychotic episode.
   c. **Command hallucinations for self-harm may signal imminent risk.**
   d. Recently, use of clozapine has been associated with a decreased lifetime risk of suicide.
5. **Having a personality disorder, particularly a borderline personality disorder, contributes to 5% of suicides.** Chronic suicidal ideation, as well as impulsive and often life-threatening manipulative acts, are particularly common in this patient group. Such attempts may "accidentally" succeed and cannot be ignored.

B. **Prior Suicide Attempts**
Prior suicide attempts predispose to suicide; 50% of suicides occur in patients who have made at least one prior attempt. In the year following an attempt, the risk may be up to 100 times that of the general population.

C. **Past Medical History**
Medical disorders can be identified in up to 40% of patients who make suicide attempts; typically, the medical disorder is chronic in nature. In patients over the age of 60 years, up to 70% of suicides are associated with medical illness. Associations have been demonstrated with many illnesses, including acquired immunodeficiency syndrome (AIDS), cancer, and chronic pain.

D. **Family History**
Whether through dynamic or genetic mechanisms, **several elements of family history influence suicidality.** A family history of suicide itself increases risk, as does a history of any psychiatric illness, independent of particular diagnosis. An additional risk is conferred by a "tumultuous" early family environment, which includes abuse of any kind.

E. **Social History**
Epidemiologic data show an association between suicide and marital status; **the greatest risk of suicide occurs in widowed, divorced, or separated individuals.** Both **social isolation** and **living alone** similarly increase the risk of suicide. **Unemployment** and **financial or legal difficulties** are also associated with increased suicide risk. On the other hand,

---

Table 54-3. Clinical Risk Factors for Suicide

- Major depression
- Schizophrenia
- Substance abuse
- History of suicide attempts or ideation
- Hopelessness
- Panic attacks
- Severe anxiety
- Severe anhedonia

suicide rates are lower for parents of children under age 18 years. Statistics aside, the presence or **absence of supports** plays a powerful role in modifying suicide risk. The involvement of family, friends, or outpatient care providers with whom a patient has an alliance may increase the degree of safety.

F. **Abnormal Elements of the Mental Status Examination**
  1. **Gross alterations in attention,** awareness and arousal, such as seen in delirium or acute intoxication, can impair judgment and precipitate a suicide attempt; they require prompt evaluation and intervention.
  2. **Evidence of psychiatric illness** (e.g., **mood, anxiety, or psychotic symptoms**) can compound suicide risk.
  3. **Motor restlessness** may suggest an anxious or agitated depression, or indicate underlying akathisia. Any of these states presents significant risk.
  4. **Impulsivity,** poor judgment and lack of insight may contribute to lethal acts.

VI. Management of the Suicidal Patient

A. **Stabilize Medical Conditions**
  A patient who is treated for a suicide attempt may require concurrent medical evaluation and treatment. At times, a patient who has expressed suicidal ideation will have already taken some action; the examiner needs to maintain a high index of suspicion for unsuspected or unreported drug ingestions.

B. **Ensure Safety**
  1. **Before an evaluation can proceed, both the patient and the examiner must be protected from harm.** A patient may be incredibly resourceful in this regard; almost any setting can be lethal in the right circumstances. Sharp objects may be used to cut; pills or other small objects can be ingested. Falls and hanging are also commonly attempted in hospital settings.
  2. **The least restrictive means necessary to ensure safety should be employed.**
     a. **Frequent supervision** may be adequate for reliable patients who do not appear to be at acute risk.
     b. While **one-to-one supervision** allows for greater patient freedom, it may be inadequate for large or impulsive patients.
  3. **Use of medications** may be extremely helpful for treating anxiety or agitation in suicidal patients.
  4. **Physical restraints** may be required if a patient continues to resist attempts at containment. However, they cannot substitute for supervision, particularly when intoxication is suspected.

C. **Rule Out Intoxication or Withdrawal**
  A patient should be monitored closely for physiological signs of intoxication or for withdrawal reactions; serial mental status exams should be performed. When sober, many patients retract suicidal statements. However, a complete evaluation for safety is still required.

VII. Disposition and Treatment

A. **Make Thoughtful Clinical Decisions**
  The assessment and treatment of suicidal thinking and behavior is fundamentally a question of clinical judgment, guided by an understanding of known risk factors and tailored to the individual patient. By themselves, risk factors alone or in combination have extremely high false positive and false negative rates. Because of the importance of clinical judgment, the **thought process behind clinical decisions should be carefully documented.**

B. **Review Treatment Options**
  1. **Location of treatment.** A number of treatment locales are available for suicidal patients. A general hospital admission may be necessary for a patient who has made an attempt and who requires medical treatment. A patient who is acutely at risk generally requires **hospitalization on a locked psychiatric unit.** An individual who refuses treatment typically requires involuntary commitment. Of note, **the risk of suicide does not subside following admission: 5% of suicides occur among psychiatrically ill inpatients.**
     At times, a patient who requires less containment but is unable to return home may be managed in a partial hospital or in a day-treatment program. Finally, if increased supports may be arranged, a patient may be managed at home.
  2. **Psychosocial treatment.** Psychosocial interventions can be extremely useful while maintaining the safety of a suicidal patient. Involving family and close friends, as well as outpatient treaters, can be particularly helpful.
  3. **Pharmacological interventions**
     a. **Pharmacological interventions depend on the underlying psychiatric illness.** Antidepressants are commonly used, sometimes in combination with anxiolytics. Choice of medications should be guided by a consideration of their lethality in overdose. Thus, selective serotonin reuptake inhibitors (SSRIs) are usually considered as first-line therapy for the depressed patient.
     b. **The impact of medications on the long-term risk of suicide** has recently become a focus of investigation. Among patients with bipolar disorder, **lithium maintenance** has been shown to decrease the risk of suicide.

Among schizophrenic patients, **clozapine** may similarly decrease risk.

C. Complete a Checklist Prior to Discharge

Whatever the disposition, the key factors in decision-making and the plans for maintaining safety should be documented in the medical record. Both the patient and outpatient treaters should participate as much as possible in planning.

While some clinicians utilize **"contracts for safety,"** which represent a verbal or written contract with a suicidal patient, there is **no evidence of their efficacy** in reducing suicide attempts. Moreover, they may be **falsely reassuring** to clinicians, as they cannot substitute for a true alliance.

When planning for hospital discharge clinicians should:

1. Make the potential means of suicide inaccessible.
2. Address the precipitants for suicidal ideation and behavior, if possible.
3. Treat the underlying psychiatric illness, including substance abuse.
4. Develop or enhance outpatient supports.
5. Arrange for close follow-up.

Suggested Readings

Hirschfeld RMA, Russell JM: Assessment and treatment of suicidal patients. *N Engl J Med* 1997; 337:910–915.

Hyman SE: The suicidal patient. In Hyman SE, Tesar GE (eds): *Manual of Psychiatric Emergencies*, 3rd ed. Boston: Little, Brown, 1994:21–27.

Lagomasino IT, Stern TA: Approach to the suicidal patient. In Stern TA, Herman JB, Slavin PL (eds): *The MGH Guide to Psychiatry in Primary Care*. New York: McGraw-Hill, 1998:15–22.

Roy A: Suicide. In Kaplan HI, Sadock BJ (eds): *Comprehensive Textbook of Psychiatry*, 6th ed. Baltimore: Williams and Wilkins, 1995:1739–1752.

Stern TA, Lagomasino IT, Hackett TP: Suicidal patients. In Cassem NH, Stern TA, Rosenbaum JF, Jellinek MS (eds): *Massachusetts General Hospital Handbook of General Hospital Psychiatry*, 4th ed. St. Louis: Mosby, 1997:69–88.

Chapter 55

Psychiatry and the Law I: Informed Consent, Competency, Treatment Refusal, and Civil Commitment

RONALD SCHOUTEN

I. Overview

Psychiatrists interact with the legal system on a regular basis. **Issues related to informed consent, competency to consent to treatment, treatment refusal, and civil commitment are important aspects of daily clinical practice.** These four topics will be reviewed in this chapter. Forensic psychiatry, the subspecialty of psychiatry devoted to the application of clinical principles and practice to the legal system, includes these topics, along with **criminal competencies and criminal responsibility.**

II. Informed Consent

A. **Relevance**
   1. **Case law, also known as common law, prohibits the touching of another person unless consent has been obtained or there is some justification.** In the absence of consent or justification, **the unpermitted touching is a battery and gives rise to a right to sue for damages.**

      Consent can be expressed (the patient explicitly consenting to treatment) **or implied** (e.g., a patient standing in a clearly marked line to get an inoculation). Justification occurs when there is an emergency—i.e., failure to act would likely have an imminent, serious negative effect on the patient's condition.
   2. **Informed consent is an ethical concept** that was made operational by American courts beginning in the 1960s when it began to be converted to a legal duty on the part of physicians. From a clinical and ethical standpoint, informed consent arises from the physician's obligation to respect the **autonomy** of the patient. **Lack of informed consent is a basis for alleging medical malpractice.**

B. **Defining Informed Consent**
   Informed consent is a process through which the physician gets the permission of the patient or a substitute decision-maker to provide treatment to the patient. The decision-maker must be *competent* (i.e., have the capacity to make the decision), must be given enough *information* to make an informed decision, and must make the decision *voluntarily.* The legal requirements of informed consent are likewise information, competency, and voluntariness. Each of these will be described in more detail.
   1. **Information**
      a. **The amount and type of information which must be given to the patient in order to meet the requirements of informed consent varies among jurisdictions.** Three basic standards are used in this area:
         i. **Professional standard:** the amount of information a reasonable professional would provide under similar circumstances.
         ii. **Materiality standard:** what the average patient would require to make a decision under the same circumstances. This is also referred to as a **patient-oriented standard.** In some jurisdictions (e.g., Massachusetts), the concept is extended to require provision of the information that would be material to the particular patient's decision.
         iii. **Combined standard:** requires the information that the reasonable medical practitioner would provide but also examines whether it was "sufficient to insure informed consent."
      b. **Providing the following information to patients will fulfill the information requirements in most jurisdictions.**
         i. **The nature of the condition to be treated and the treatment proposed.**
         ii. **The nature and probability of the risks associated with the treatment.** Minor risks or side effects which occur frequently (e.g., dry mouth), and significant risks that occur infrequently (e.g., hepatic failure secondary to sodium valproate) should be reviewed with the patient.
         iii. **The inability to predict the results of the treatment.**
         iv. **The irreversibility of the procedure, if applicable.**
         v. **The alternative treatments available,** including no treatment. This should include a discussion of the risks and benefits associated with these options.
   2. **Competency.** For a patient to give adequate informed consent, **he or she must have the physical and mental capacity to make informed treatment decisions. How much capacity is required depends upon the nature of the condition and the risks of the proposed treatment.** Less capacity is required for low-risk treatments with high likelihood of a good result (e.g., intravenous fluids for dehydration). A higher level of capacity is required when the treatment is of higher risk or is more invasive, and the results are less likely to be favorable (e.g.,

415

amputation in an elderly diabetic patient with renal failure).

a. Technically, **competency is a legal term not a clinical term,** although these terms tend to be used interchangeably in the clinical setting. **A legal declaration of incompetence strips a person of certain rights and privileges normally accorded to adults** (e.g., making treatment decisions, making contracts, voting, or executing a will).

   i. **All adults are presumed to be competent to make their own treatment decisions in the eyes of the law.**

   ii. **Only a judge can declare a person legally incompetent.** However, **clinical assessments of capacity (competency evaluations) are the first step towards a legal declaration of incompetence** and often indicate the likely outcome of any legal proceedings.

   - Competency evaluations are used as evidence in judicial proceedings on the matter.
   - A competency evaluation which concludes that a patient has the capacity to make treatment decisions can allow treatment to proceed if there are doubts about the patient's mental status.
   - A conclusion that the patient lacks the capacity to give informed consent requires the choice of an alternative decision-maker except in an emergency, or where the patient has a valid advanced directive.

b. **Competence (capacity) can be global or task specific.**

   i. **Global capacity** refers to the ability to undertake and carry out all the normal responsibilities and rights of an adult. A declaration of global incapacity strips an individual of his or her rights as a **legal person.**

   ii. **Specific capacities;** examples:

   - **Testamentary capacity: the capacity to execute a will.** Specific legal standards for testamentary capacity apply in all jurisdictions and may vary. The usual standards require that the person executing the will:

     Know the nature of the document being executed.
     Know the contents of the estate.
     Know the persons who would normally inherit from him or her (the natural objects of his or her bounty).

   - **Testimonial capacity: the capacity to serve as a witness in court.**
   - **Capacity to make treatment decisions.**

c. **Evaluating the capacity to make treatment decisions** (Appelbaum and Grisso, 1988)

   i. Does the patient express a preference?

   ii. Is the patient able to attain a factual understanding of the information provided?

   iii. Is the patient able to appreciate the seriousness of the condition and the consequences of accepting or rejecting treatment?

   iv. Can the patient manipulate the information provided in a rational fashion and come to a decision that follows logically from that information considered in the context of the individual's personal beliefs, experience, and circumstances?

   - It is the process of reaching a decision, not the decision itself, that must be rational. Competent people have a right to make decisions for themselves that may seem irrational to the rest of the world.
   - Disagreement with the treating clinician's recommendations is not a basis, in and of itself, for saying that a patient is irrational.

d. **Consequences of a finding of incapacity**

   i. **Guardianship of the person**

   - The person declared incompetent is the **ward.**
   - The **guardian** is the party appointed by the court to make decisions on behalf of the ward.
   - Depending upon the jurisdiction, the guardian may make decisions based upon the perceived **best interests of the ward** or by means of a **substituted judgment** analysis (what the ward would have decided if he or she were competent to make the decision). In cases involving extraordinary or invasive treatment, the substituted judgment analysis may be carried out by a judge rather than by the guardian.

   ii. Guardianship of the estate (conservatorship).

   iii. Appointment of an agent to act on behalf of the incompetent pursuant to a **durable power of attorney, health care proxy, or other form of advance directive.**

3. **Voluntary**

   a. Simply means free of coercion by those proposing the treatment.

   b. Persuasion by family members does not void informed consent so long as the circumstances do not put the physician on notice that the treatment is being imposed against the patient's will or indicate that the patient is incompetent.

C. Exceptions to the Requirement of Informed Consent

1. **Emergency situations**

   a. When failure to act would result in a serious and imminent deterioration in the patient's condition.

   b. The emergency exception allows for initiation of treatment and stabilization, not for ongoing treatment without obtaining proper consent.

2. **Waivers**

   a. The patient may defer to someone else's judgment.

   b. Waiver may be implied (e.g., presenting oneself to the emergency room after being injured).

3. **Therapeutic privilege**

   a. **Where the process of providing information and obtaining consent would result in a serious risk of deterioration in the patient's condition, that process can be**

deferred until the patient's condition has improved sufficiently.

b. The possibility that providing the information might lead to treatment refusal is not sufficient to invoke therapeutic privilege.

III. Treatment Refusal

A. **All competent people have a right to make their own medical treatment decisions, and all adults are presumed to be competent.**

1. This applies even where the individual is suffering from serious mental illness or is civilly committed.

2. The presumption of competency persists until a court has declared a person to be incompetent, as noted above.

3. When a patient is believed to be incapacitated from making treatment decisions, an alternative decision-maker should be sought rather than relying on the presumption of competence and allowing the patient to continue making treatment decisions.

B. **Individuals who are incompetent still have a right to individual autonomy,** which can be honored by following their preferences for treatment expressed when they were competent or to the extent they can be determined in the absence of prior expression.

C. **The law concerning treatment refusal varies among the states.**

1. States generally draw a distinction between routine and ordinary medical care (e.g., antibiotics, minor surgery), and extraordinary or invasive care (e.g., cancer chemotherapy, coronary artery bypass grafting) when determining what can be done when a patient refuses treatment.

   a. Benzodiazepines and antidepressants are generally considered to be routine, ordinary, and noninvasive.

   b. Antipsychotic medication, electroconvulsive therapy, and psychosurgery are considered to constitute extraordinary, dangerous, and invasive treatments in many states.

2. States differ in terms of what legal steps must be taken before a patient's refusal of treatment can be overridden.

   a. The basic rule in all states is that **competent individuals have a right to make their own treatment decisions, including refusal of treatment that others believe is in the patient's best interest.** Exceptions to this rule exist in matters involving criminal law and the correctional system.

   b. When a patient who appears to lack the capacity to make treatment decisions refuses routine and ordinary care, physicians can generally rely upon family members or significant others who know the patient to make a decision.

   c. When the care to be provided is extraordinary, invasive, or dangerous, many states require that a formal guardian be appointed to make the treatment decisions.

      i. Guardianship is established after a hearing at which family members, treaters, and sometimes the patient, will testify.

      ii. Not all states allow the guardian, once appointed, to make all decisions on behalf of the patient. In some states, extraordinary, invasive, or dangerous care can only be authorized by a judge after a full trial on the issue, with the guardian assigned to monitor the care [Rogers v. Commissioner (Mass. 1983)].

      iii. While some states require full adversarial proceedings and judicial involvement in these matters, others (including federal courts) believe that professional judgment and administrative review satisfy the due process requirements without going to court [Rennie v. Klein (3rd Circuit 1981); U.S. v. Charters (4th Circuit 1988)].

      iv. Refusal of treatment by those awaiting trial or already convicted of a crime has been the subject of considerable judicial attention.

      - Antipsychotic medications may be administered over the refusal of convicted prisoners, competent or incompetent, if an independent review panel agrees that the prisoner suffers from a serious mental illness, is dangerous to himself or others, or is gravely disabled, and the medication proposed is in the prisoner's best interests [Washington v. Harper (U.S. 1990)].

      - Forced administration of antipsychotic medication for the purpose of rendering the inmate competent to be executed violates the Louisiana state constitutional right to privacy and constitutes cruel, excessive, and unusual punishment [Louisiana v. Perry (La. 1992)].

      - Forced administration of antipsychotic medication in order to render a defendant competent to stand trial violated the rights of the defendant under the Sixth and Fourteenth Amendments to the United States Constitution absent a showing by the state that the treatment was both medically necessary and appropriate [Riggins v. Nevada (U.S. 1992)].

IV. Civil Commitment

The process of hospitalizing a person against his or her will is referred to as involuntary civil commitment. Civil commitment statutes are similar in the various jurisdictions, as commitment can only occur when the patient poses a danger to him- or herself or others.

A. Legal Restrictions on Civil Commitment

1. Confinement of an individual against his or her will is considered to be a deprivation of fundamental rights guaranteed under the Constitution of the United States and state constitutions.

   a. Civil commitment is considered to be an act of the state government because it occurs under the authority of the state.

   b. Before a state can deprive someone of their fundamental rights, proper procedural protections (e.g., a court or administrative hearing before a neutral fact finder) must be granted. Such procedures collectively constitute **due process,** which is guaranteed by the Constitution [(Vitek v. Jones, 445 U.S. 480 (U.S. 1980)]. Commitment to a mental hospital entails a massive curtailment of liberty and requires due process protection.

2. **In non-emergencies, the patient is entitled to a full hearing before he or she can be confined.**

3. Lawsuits for deprivation of civil rights, false imprisonment, and negligence can arise from improper civil commitment.

4. **An individual can only be involuntarily committed if he or she is a danger to self or others.** The fact that a patient may demonstrate a clear-cut clinical need for treatment, in the absence of dangerousness, is not sufficient.

   a. A state cannot constitutionally confine a nondangerous individual who is capable of surviving outside the hospital setting on his own or with the help of friends [O'Connor v. Donaldson (U.S. 1974)].

   b. **The standard of proof in civil commitment cases is "clear and convincing" evidence,** more than is required in ordinary civil cases and less than the criminal standard of beyond a reasonable doubt [Addington v. Texas (U.S. 1979)].

B. The details of the commitment process vary among the states.

1. For example, in California an emergency commitment is valid for 72 h, during which time the patient is evaluated to determine whether further commitment is necessary and justified. In Massachusetts, the emergency commitment is for 10 days.

2. States also differ in how mental illness is defined. Some states, for example, do not consider substance abuse and disorders like Alzheimer's disease as mental illnesses for the purpose of civil commitment.

3. Where a patient is offered an opportunity to sign himself into a state hospital voluntarily and does so while lacking the capacity to make an informed decision, he has a constitutional right to due process of law prior to the deprivation of a liberty interest, and the state and its agents can be held liable for a violation of the patient's federal civil rights [Zinermon v. Burch (U.S. 1990)].

C. The Dangerousness Criteria

While the details differ, all states use the criteria of danger to self or others as the basis for involuntary commitment. The danger must be the result of mental illness, rather than ordinary anger or antisocial behavior. For example, a hired killer would not be an appropriate candidate for involuntary commitment to a psychiatric hospital should his murderous intentions become known, absent evidence that a mental illness other than a personality disorder contributed to his dangerousness. However, an individual convicted of a violent crime may be committed to a hospital if it is determined that he poses a danger to himself or others.

1. **Danger to self means attempts at serious self-harm or suicide, or credible threats to cause such self-harm.**

2. **Danger to others generally refers to threats or attempts to cause physical harm to others, or actual harm already inflicted.** In addition, it may include situations in which others are placed in reasonable fear that they will be harmed by the patient.

3. **Individuals may also be involuntarily committed if they pose a substantial risk of harm because they are unable to provide for their own well-being in the community.** In some states, this criterion is referred to as the **gravely disabled** criterion.

   a. Generally, mere difficulty caring for oneself is not enough to meet this criterion. **The risk of harm** (e.g., believing that one is invincible and therefore can walk into traffic) **must be substantial and imminent.** A likelihood of harm in the distant future is not sufficient.

   b. Civil commitment under this criterion, as well as the others, is **permissible only if no less restrictive alternative is available in the community** [Lake v. Cameron (D.C. Cir. 1966)]. Alternatives to civil commitment may include increased outpatient visits, voluntary hospitalization, day hospital programs, custodial care by relatives, or shelters.

D. Civil commitment of criminal defendants and convicted individuals has been the subject of important court decisions.

1. Due process clause requires that the reason for confinement and the nature of the confinement be of reasonable relevance to the purpose of confinement [Jackson v. Indiana (U.S. 1972)].

   a. Jackson was deaf, with limited ability to sign, and had limited intellectual resources. He had been found incompetent to stand trial on charges of shoplifting, and was committed to the state hospital until he was restored to competency, a state which everyone agreed was unattainable under the circumstances.

b. If the state wanted to continue to confine Jackson to a mental institution, he must meet standard criteria for civil commitment.

2. " ... the Constitution permits the Government, on the basis of the insanity judgment, to confine (a defendant) to a mental institution until such time as he has regained his sanity or is no longer a danger to himself or society. This holding accords with the widely and reasonably held view that insanity acquittees should be treated differently from other candidates for civil commitment." [Jones v. United States, 463 U.S. 354 (1983)].

   a. Insanity acquittee may be held as long as he is mentally ill and dangerous, but no longer.

   b. This is a post-Hinckley case arising in DC; many scholars attribute the reasoning to the climate created by the successful insanity plea of attempted presidential assassin John Hinckley.

3. Louisiana statute violated the Due Process Clause of the United States Constitution where it allowed a criminal defendant found not guilty by reason of insanity to be returned to the hospital, even if a hospital review committee found him no longer mentally ill, if he was determined at a court hearing to be dangerous [Foucha v. Louisiana (U.S. 1992)].

   a. Hospital psychiatrist testified that Foucha had recovered from the drug-induced psychosis that had formed the basis for his insanity defense, but also testified that Foucha had been in altercations at the hospital, had an antisocial personality disorder that was not a mental disease and was untreatable, and the psychiatrist would not "feel comfortable in certifying that he would not be a danger to himself or to other people."

   b. Continued confinement in a mental institution is improper without a determination in civil commitment proceedings of current mental illness and dangerousness.

   c. The state's legitimate interest in imprisoning convicted criminals for retribution and deterrence does not exist in the case of an insanity acquittee, who has not been found guilty and cannot be punished.

   d. The state may legitimately detain people who are unable to control their behavior and thereby pose a danger to public safety, provided the confinement takes place pursuant to proper procedures and evidentiary standards.

4. Kansas' Sexually Dangerous Predator Act is not unconstitutional where it establishes procedures for the civil commitment of persons who, due to a "mental abnormality" or "personality disorder," are likely to engage in "predatory acts of sexual violence" [Hendricks v. Kansas (U.S. 1997)].

   a. Involuntary civil confinement, which follows conclusion of criminal sentence if the individual is found to be a sexually dangerous person, did not constitute additional punishment for criminal behavior as it does not have the goals of retribution or deterrence.

   b. Procedures provided by the state, including the right to immediate release when the detainee proves he is no longer sexually dangerous, are adequate.

Suggested Readings

Appelbaum PS, Grisso T: Assessing patients' capacities to consent to treatment. *N Engl J Med* 1988; 319:1635–1638.

Appelbaum PS, Gutheil TG: *Clinical Handbook of Psychiatry and the Law*. Baltimore: Williams and Wilkins, 1991.

Appelbaum PS, Lidz CW, Meisel A: *Informed Consent: Legal Theory and Clinical Practice*. New York: Oxford University Press, 1987.

Grisso T, Appelbaum PS: *Assessing Competence to Consent to Treatment*. New York: Oxford University Press, 1998.

Spring RL, Lacoursiere RB, Weissenberger G: *Patients, Psychiatrists, and Lawyers Law and the Mental Health System*, 2nd ed. Cincinnati: Anderson Publishing Co., 1997.

Winick BJ: *The Right to Refuse Mental Health Treatment*. Washington, DC: American Psychological Association, 1997.

Chapter 56

Psychiatry and the Law II: Criminal Issues and the Role of Psychiatrists in the Legal System

RONALD SCHOUTEN

I. Overview

Psychiatrists play a prominent role in the courts as expert witnesses in both civil and criminal litigation. **This chapter will focus on the subjects of criminal competencies, criminal responsibility, the psychotherapist-patient privilege, and the role of the psychiatrist in court.**

II. Competency in the Criminal System

A. Competency to Stand Trial
1. The basic standard
   a. **Whether the defendant "has sufficient present ability to consult with his lawyer with a reasonable degree of rational understanding, and whether he has a rational as well as a factual understanding of the proceedings against him."** [Dusky v. U.S. (U.S. 1960)].
   b. **This standard applies in all states, the District of Columbia, and federal courts.** States may use their own criteria, so long as those criteria provide as much, or more, protection of the defendant's rights than the federal standard.
   c. **Minimal capacity is required.** In practice, the threshold for competency is low. But see Cooper v. Oklahoma (U.S., 1996) described below, holding that the standard of proof for incompetence is "preponderance of the evidence" and not some higher standard.
2. **The rationale for requiring that the defendant meet basic standards of mental capacity** before he or she can be put on trial [Drope v. Missouri (U.S. 1975)].
   a. The fact-finding portion of the proceedings can only be accurate if the defendant can work with his or her attorney with an understanding of the proceedings.
   b. Only a competent defendant can exercise the constitutional rights to a fair trial and to confront his or her accuser in a meaningful way.
   c. The integrity and dignity of the legal process are preserved by insuring that the defendant is competent to stand trial.
   d. The purposes of retribution and individual deterrence are served only if the convicted defendant was competent to stand trial.
3. **The competency decision**
   a. **The defendant may be ordered by the judge to undergo an evaluation.** This can be done on an outpatient basis, but is more commonly conducted on an inpatient unit with special capabilities to conduct forensic evaluations.
   b. The defendant's consent is not necessary for a competency evaluation; the court can order it over the defendant's objection [U.S. v. Hugenin (1st Circuit 1991)].
   c. The defendant has a right to consult with counsel before the competency evaluation pursuant to the Sixth Amendment, but no right to have counsel present at the evaluation in federal courts. States may provide this right, if they choose [Buchanan v. Kentucky (U.S. 1987)].
   d. **The focus of the competency evaluation is the defendant's mental state at the time of the proceedings, not at the time of the alleged criminal act.**
   e. **The decision whether or not the defendant is competent to stand trial is made by the trial judge.**
   f. If the defendant is found to be incompetent to stand trial, he or she is committed to a state or federal hospital to be treated and restored to competency.
   g. If the defendant cannot be restored to competency, he or she cannot be convicted and must be released from the hospital. However, the defendant can be held in the facility if he or she meets the usual criteria for civil commitment.
4. **Key cases on competency to stand trial**
   a. **The trial judge must raise the issue of competency if either the court's own evidence or that presented by the defense or prosecution raises a bona fide doubt of the defendant's competency** [Pate v. Robinson (U.S. 1966)].
      i. The question of competency can be raised at any point in the trial process.
      ii. The prosecution may raise the question of competency.
   b. **A defendant found incompetent to stand trial and committed to a state facility cannot be held indefinitely if there is no hope of restoration of competency, unless he is committed under the usual civil commitment standards in a regular civil proceeding** [Jackson v. Indiana (U.S. 1972)].
      i. Jackson was deaf, with limited ability to sign, and had limited intellectual resources. He had been found incompetent to stand trial on charges of shoplifting, and was committed to the state hospital until he was restored to competency, a state which everyone agreed was unattainable under the circumstances.

421

ii. If the state wanted to continue to confine Jackson to a mental institution, he had to meet the standard criteria for civil commitment. Otherwise, the continued confinement is in violation of the Due Process clause of the federal constitution.

c. **The defendant's statements made during a competency to stand trial evaluation cannot be used against her in the guilt or sentencing stages of the proceeding** [Estelle v. Smith (U.S. 1981)].

   i. Using the information in that way would violate the Fifth Amendment protection against self-incrimination.

   ii. Limitations on this protection:

- Fifth Amendment rights are not violated if the psychiatrist's testimony is limited to the question of competency to stand trial.
- If the defendant requested the psychiatric evaluation and presents the evidence at trial, the prosecution may use the report of the evaluation to rebut the evidence offered by the defendant [Buchanan v. Kentucky (U.S. 1987)].

d. **If an indigent defendant cannot afford to hire a psychiatric expert to assist in the case, the state must provide "at a minimum … access to a competent psychiatrist who will conduct appropriate examination and assist in evaluation, preparation, presentation of the defense … ."** [Ake v. Oklahoma (U.S. 1985)].

   i. This rule applies whenever a mental health issue may be relevant (e.g., competency, criminal responsibility, aid in sentencing).

   ii. The court may appoint the psychiatrist. The defendant is not constitutionally entitled to select a psychiatrist of his own choosing or to receive funds to hire one of his own.

e. **The standard of proof for competency to stand trial is the preponderance of the evidence,** not the higher standards of clear and convincing evidence or proof beyond a reasonable doubt [Cooper v. Oklahoma (U.S. 1996)].

   i. The defendant exhibited bizarre behavior before and during his trial, including refusing to talk to his attorney, responding to hallucinations, eating his feces, and expressing his belief that his defense counsel had tried to murder him.

   ii. At an initial competency hearing, Cooper was found incompetent and sent to the state hospital for treatment. He was found competent to stand trial at four subsequent hearings where he failed to meet the Oklahoma statutory requirement that the defendant establish lack of competency by "clear and convincing evidence."

   iii. The Due Process clause of the Fourteenth Amendment was violated by the application of a clear and convincing standard of proof because it created the risk that an individual would be forced to stand trial who was more likely than not incompetent.

B. **Competency to Plead Guilty or Serve as One's Own Attorney** [Godinez v. Moran (U.S. 1993)]

1. The defendant, who was taking a number of psychotropic medications, asked to discharge his attorney, to represent himself, and to plead guilty after he was assessed to be competent to stand trial by two psychiatrists.

2. Supreme Court held that **the mental capacity involved in competency for pleading guilty or waiving the right to counsel is the same as for competency to stand trial. No higher standard applies.**

C. **Competency to be Sentenced/Executed**

1. **The standard and rationale**

a. **The standard: whether the convicted individual has an understanding of the nature of the proceedings and an ability to participate in the process.**

b. The rationale for requiring that the convicted individual be competent for the sentencing and punishment phases:

   i. To preserve the integrity of the sentencing and punishment process.

   ii. To insure that the convicted individual will have the ability to contest the decision through all stages of appeal prior to imposition of punishment.

   iii. The deterrent function of punishment is served by only punishing those who have the requisite mental capacity to be sentenced or punished.

2. **The APA position on ethical issues in death penalty cases.** Ethics Committee opinion (1990):

a. **It is unethical for a psychiatrist to participate in executions.**

b. **It is not unethical for a psychiatrist to conduct a competency evaluation in which the prisoner is told of the interview's purpose and the limitations on confidentiality.**

3. **Key cases on competency to be sentenced/executed:**

a. **Estelle v. Smith (U.S. 1982).** Smith's Fifth Amendment right to be free from self-incrimination and Sixth Amendment right to assistance of counsel were denied when the state's psychiatrist, who had examined him solely for the purpose of assessing competency to stand trial, was allowed to testify as to Smith's dangerousness at the penalty phase and **defendant was not informed of the purpose of the evaluation or right to the presence of counsel.**

b. **Barefoot v. Estelle (U.S. 1983). While the state cannot compel a defendant to undergo a psychiatric evaluation, there is no constitutional barrier to allowing psychiatric experts to testify to the defendant's future dangerousness** at the penalty phase based on hypothetical questions.

   i. The APA filed an *amicus curiae* (friend of the court) brief pointing out the unreliability of dangerousness predictions.

   ii. The court rejected the arguments in that brief, holding that such assessments are not so inherently unreliable that they should be excluded totally and that the lack of reliability can be addressed as a credibility issue on cross-examination.

   c. <u>Ford</u> v. <u>Wainwright</u> (U.S. 1986)

     i. Execution of a prisoner who is insane constitutes cruel and unusual punishment in violation of the Eighth Amendment.

     ii. A prisoner is entitled to a full and fair hearing on the issue of competency to be executed.

   d. **<u>Satterwhite</u> v. <u>Texas</u> (U.S. 1988). Admission of testimony based on a psychiatric evaluation conducted without the knowledge of the defendant's attorney constituted a basis for reversal of the conviction,** where it could not be assured that this inadmissible evidence had not influenced the jury.

   e. <u>Penry</u> v. <u>Lynaugh</u> (U.S. 1989)

     i. Imposition of the death penalty upon a mildly or moderately retarded individual is not unconstitutional per se.

     ii. A Texas statute, which did not allow the jury to consider mitigating factors such as a history of mental retardation and child abuse but did allow consideration of aggravating factors, was unconstitutional.

   f. **Forced administration of antipsychotic medication for the purpose of rendering an inmate competent to be executed violates the Louisiana state constitutional right to privacy and constitutes cruel, excessive, and unusual punishment [<u>Louisiana</u> v. <u>Perry</u> (La. 1992)].**

   g. **Forced administration of antipsychotic medication in order to render a defendant competent to stand trial violated the rights of the defendant under the Sixth and Fourteenth Amendments to the United States Constitution,** absent a showing by the state that the treatment was both medically necessary and appropriate [<u>Riggins</u> v. <u>Nevada</u> (U.S. 1992)].

III. Criminal Responsibility

A. In order for an act to be criminal, there must be both a guilty act and guilty intent.

  1. *Actus reus:* the harmful act itself

  2. *Mens rea:* a guilty mind, guilty or wrongful intent

   a. *Mens rea*, in the narrow sense, is the mental state required as an element of a specific crime (e.g., larceny—knowingly taking possession of property that is not yours, for your own use, and with the intent of depriving the true owner of its use).

   b. **In the general sense, *mens rea* refers to blameworthiness or legal liability.** An individual who takes someone else's car for his own use when directed to do so by auditory hallucinations is unlikely to be found blameworthy.

B. The defense of lack of criminal responsibility/not guilty by reason of insanity is based on the concept that some individuals who commit criminal acts should not be held morally blameworthy because they cannot be considered moral agents due to their mental state (Moore, 1984).

C. Voluntary intoxication is not a basis for an insanity defense, although it may provide a basis for a diminished capacity defense. Mental illness caused by substance abuse, exacerbation of an existing mental illness due to intoxication, and pathologic intoxication can all provide a basis for an insanity defense.

D. Evolution of the Standards

  1. **The M'Naghten test** (England, 1843). "To establish a defense on the ground of insanity, it must be clearly proved that, at the time of the committing of the act the party accused was laboring under such a defect of reason, from disease of the mind, as not to <u>know</u> the nature and quality of the act he was doing, or, if he did <u>know</u> it, that he did not <u>know</u> he was doing what was wrong."

   a. It is a cognitive test, focusing only on whether the defendant knew what he was doing or that what he was doing was wrong.

   b. It was adopted after the insanity acquittal of the would-be assassin of Prime Minister Robert Peel, who instead assassinated Peel's secretary.

  2. **Irresistible impulse/loss of control test.** A defendant with a mental disease or defect would be held not responsible for criminal acts, even if he could tell right from wrong, if such disease or defect deprived him of power to choose right from wrong <u>and</u> the alleged crime was so connected with the mental disease as to have been the product of it solely.

   a. The focus is on the existence of a mental illness and on a resulting loss of control over behavior.

   b. The volitional test: a lack of knowledge of wrongfulness is not required.

  3. **The New Hampshire and <u>Durham</u> tests [<u>Durham</u> v. <u>U.S.</u> (DC Circuit 1954)]**

   a. **An accused is not criminally responsible if his unlawful conduct was the product of a mental disease or defect.**

   b. This test is still used in New Hampshire.

  4. **Model Penal Code** (American Law Inst.): combines two older tests: cognitive and volitional.

   a. **A person is not responsible for criminal conduct if at the time of such conduct as a result of mental disease or defect he lacks substantial capacity either to appreciate the criminality (wrongfulness) of his conduct or to conform his conduct to the requirements of the law.**

     As used in this Article, the terms "mental disease or mental defect" do not include an abnormality manifested only by repeated criminal or otherwise antisocial behavior.

   b. Basic elements involve:

     i. A mental disorder (but not Antisocial Personality Disorder).

ii. An impairment in functioning as a result of the disorder; but the impairment need not be complete.

iii. A clear and direct causal connection or relationship between the behavior impairment and the act.

5. **APA/Federal Court test.** It is an affirmative defense to a prosecution under any federal statute that, **at the time of the commission of the acts constituting the offense, the defendant, as a result of a severe mental disease or defect, was unable to appreciate the nature and quality or the wrongfulness of his acts.**

a. This was passed by Congress in response to the insanity acquittal of John Hinckley after his failed assassination attempt on President Reagan.

b. **It requires an <u>inability</u> to appreciate the nature and quality or wrongfulness, not merely a lack of substantial capacity.**

c. **The mental disease or defect must be severe.**

E. Consequences of a Finding of Insanity

1. **An insanity acquittee is remanded to a correctional facility, often a forensic hospital, where there is assessment of dangerousness and the level of security needed.**

2. See Chap. 55 (IV.D) for key cases on continued commitment of insanity acquittees.

F. Guilty but Mentally Ill (GBMI)

1. This category was developed as an alternative to the insanity defense, but it may be offered by a state as an additional option for the trier of fact (judge or jury).

2. **An individual found GBMI is not legally insane and is held responsible for the act, but is acknowledged to have been mentally ill at the time of the act.**

3. It has been adopted in a limited number of states.

G. Diminished Capacity

1. **Diminished capacity can be raised where an individual suffers from a mental illness or cognitive deficit that does not meet the requirements of the insanity defense, but nevertheless provides a basis for not holding the person fully responsible for the behavior.**

2. **The result is usually to reduce the level of the conviction** (e.g., reduction of the finding of guilt from first-degree murder to second-degree murder).

H. Demographics of the Insanity Defense

1. **One-tenth of 1% of felony trials; 2 insanity pleas per 1,000 felony arrests.**

2. Success rate varies by state.

3. Juries hand down only 5%, 40–50% by judges; the rest of the pleas are bargained.

4. Not a "rich man's defense": acquittees tend to be young (20–30 years), white, with on average an 8th grade education, and to be employed as unskilled laborers.

IV. The Role of Psychiatrists in the Legal System

A. The Psychotherapist-Patient Privilege

1. Definition

a. **Psychiatrists have an obligation to keep matters revealed by patients in the course of treatment confidential.** A corollary to confidentiality is the concept of **privilege.** Whereas confidentiality is an ongoing obligation on the part of the physician, **privilege is a right that belongs to the patient that must be raised by the patient before it comes into play. Privilege is the right to have matters revealed to a physician or therapist held in confidence and not revealed against the patient's will, except under certain circumstances.**

b. **Testimonial privilege:** the right of a patient to prevent his or her therapist from testifying in an administrative or judicial proceeding about information revealed during the course of therapy. The privilege belongs to and can only be raised or waived by the patient: if the patient does not raise the privilege, the physician may be compelled to testify.

2. **Exceptions to the privilege**

a. **Expressed waiver by the patient.**

b. Where the patient has put his or her mental status at issue in the course of litigation (e.g., claiming emotional damages in a personal injury suit).

c. Mandated reporting, as in cases of child abuse.

d. Statutory exceptions (e.g., when the patient is involved in billing disputes or malpractice litigation against the physician).

3. Exists in all 50 states, the District of Columbia, and all federal courts [<u>Jaffee</u> v. <u>Redmond</u> (U.S. 1996)].

4. Rationale for the psychotherapist privilege

a. From a societal standpoint, in instances where preservation of the psychotherapist-patient relationship is more important than the information that will be excluded from the trial.

b. The privilege protects the privacy of a special relationship.

B. The Psychiatrist as Forensic Evaluator/Expert Witness

1. **Forensic evaluations: any psychiatric evaluation connected with litigation or for the purpose of providing an expert clinical opinion to assist a deliberative body.**

a. **Not a doctor-patient relationship as there is no clinical care involved.**

b. The Double Agent problem. A treating clinician has a fiduciary obligation to act only in the best interests of the patient; **the forensic evaluator's obligation is to the party requesting the evaluation.**

i. **The client is the attorney, court, agency, etc., that has retained the psychiatrist.**

ii. **Confidentiality is absent in the forensic evaluation. As a result, the forensic evaluator has an ethical**

obligation and, in some states, a legal obligation to obtain informed consent from the evaluee before conducting the examination. This includes warning the evaluee about the limitations on confidentiality.

iii. **No criminal evaluations should be conducted until the defendant has had an opportunity to meet with his or her attorney.**

2. **The expert witness**

   a. **An expert witness is a witness who has knowledge related to the subject matter of the litigation beyond that of the average juror or judge, who can offer information that will be useful to the judge or jury in reaching a decision in the matter.**

   b. Anyone with such additional knowledge can technically be accepted as an expert, although the credibility of the expert may be attacked. For example, a medical student might be accepted as an expert in medicine based on his or her studies, but the credibility of that expert will be attacked based on the lack of experience.

   c. Experts may use any information they would normally use in the course of an evaluation as a basis for testimony, including hearsay (information that they did not obtain first-hand, but rather obtained through the reports of a third party).

3. **The role of the expert witness**

   a. **Provide scientifically and clinically accurate testimony.**

   b. **Provide testimony in an ethically responsible manner.**

   c. **Provide answers to the legal questions raised in the proceeding, to the extent possible.**

   d. **The psychiatrist, once designated as an expert witness, can provide the court with an expert opinion on an issue before the court—e.g., whether the care of a patient was below the standard of care (malpractice), whether the defendant has a mental illness that rendered him unable to conform his behavior to the requirements of the law (criminal responsibility). The fact witness (see below) is not allowed to offer such opinions.**

C. **The Psychiatrist as Fact Witness**

1. **A fact witness is an individual who has information related to the matter being litigated.**

   a. **There are no special requirements to be a fact witness, other than first-hand knowledge relevant to the case.** Anyone, including a child, can be a fact witness.

   b. A fact witness cannot offer an expert opinion or use hearsay.

2. The treating psychiatrist may be called to testify about the mental condition of a patient in a wide variety of settings (e.g., personal injury litigation, workmen's compensation claims, administrative hearings, criminal cases).

3. The rules of the psychotherapist-patient privilege apply, if the patient raises it. The court may decide that the privilege does not apply and order the psychiatrist to testify. **Refusal to testify can lead to a finding of contempt of court, justifying a fine or jail time.**

4. **The rules and exceptions regarding privilege apply.**

   a. If a patient is in litigation related to a motor vehicle claim, but does not raise emotional damages as a claim, the records of the treating physician generally cannot be obtained.

   b. If, in connection with the litigation, the patient claims emotional damages, the records and testimony of the treating physician may be obtained by the other side.

Suggested Readings

Almanzor MC: The effect of intoxication as a "mitigating factor" for murder and manslaughter. *N Engl Law Rev* 1997; 31:1079.

American Medical Association Council on Ethical and Judicial Affairs: *Code of Medical Ethics*, Annotation 2.06. Chicago: AMA, 1997.

Levine AM: Denying the settled insanity defense: another necessary step in dealing with drug and alcohol abuse. *B Univ Law Rev* 1998; 78:75.

Moore MS: *Law and Psychiatry: Rethinking the Relationship.* Cambridge: Cambridge University Press, 1984.

Perlin ML: "The borderline which separated you from me": the insanity defense, the authoritarian spirit, the fear of faking, and the culture of punishment. *Iowa Law Rev* 1997; 82:1375.

Reider L: Toward a new test for the insanity defense: incorporating the discoveries of neuroscience into moral and legal theories. *UCLA Law Rev* 1998; 46:289.

Schouten R: The psychotherapist-patient privilege. *Harvard Rev Psychiatry* 1998; 6:44–48.

Thomason SC: Criminal procedure-crazy as I need to be: the United States Supreme Court's latest addition to the incompetency doctrine. *Univ Arkansas Little Rock Law J* 1998; 20:349.

Chapter 57
Patient Compliance

DOMINIC J. MAXWELL AND JOHN B. HERMAN

I. Overview

Compliance refers to a patient's ability or willingness to carry out his physician's instructions. An often overlooked aspect of medical care, compliance has significant effects on diagnostic and therapeutic interventions; it derives from a patient's personal inner world, and is extremely difficult to study.

Although often thought of as applying only to medication regimens, **compliance refers to any directive** (be it to avoid caffeine, to take daily exercise, or to limit exposure to sunlight) **on the part of the physician.** Compliance with medical instructions begins with clear communication between doctor and patient. Assuming the patient has understood the directive, **the patient must then be willing and able to remember it and then to carry it out.** A break anywhere in this process can result in patient noncompliance. While physicians often blame their patients for noncompliance, the responsibility for ensuring the accurate communication of an instruction and monitoring its execution rests with both parties.

Noncompliance is a significant problem in all branches of clinical medicine. It **is common** (most studies cite noncompliance rates of between 25% and 75%), **and costly,** leading to increased rates of hospitalization, and, among psychiatric patients, to potentially dangerous (suicidal or violent) behaviors. **Noncompliance** exists in many forms, including not showing for appointments, discontinuing medications, and refusing to have blood work drawn.

II. Why Do Patients Fail to Adhere to Treatment Recommendations?

Reasons for noncompliance are varied. No significant differences in compliance rates exist between psychiatric and nonpsychiatric populations. Moreover, no demographic variables (e.g., income, socioeconomic class, occupation, level of education, or type of illness) affect rates of noncompliance to any significant degree. The etiology of the noncompliance may be deliberate or unintentional, and may be conscious or unconscious. **Causes of noncompliance may be subdivided into three categories:**

A. **A genuine misunderstanding between doctor and patient:** clear communication between the two parties is fundamental to compliance.

B. **An inability to comply:** this may be due to economics (the cost of a medication), to a patient's cultural belief system about illness, to family pressures, or to the illness itself. The latter is especially true in psychiatric illness, where hopelessness, psychosis, or memory impairment may make compliance impossible.

C. **Unwillingness to comply:** this may be due to unpleasant effects of prescribed treatments, a need to assert control over the doctor-patient relationship, or a need to retain symptoms.

Regardless of the cause of noncompliance, **it is important to explore the meaning of the patient's unwillingness or inability to carry out his doctor's instructions.** For example, is this simply a case of misunderstanding, is the patient unwittingly communicating feelings of frustration, anger, helplessness, or perhaps both elements are at work? **Noncompliance always conveys important information to the physician, be it about the state of the doctor-patient relationship, the cultural background and belief system of the patient, or the patient's pathology. Recognizing noncompliance and considering its genesis are as important as is working towards correcting it.**

III. What Can You Do about Noncompliance?

The physician's first step when addressing noncompliance is to recognize it. Noncompliance should always consider when a case unexpectedly turns sour, when a stable patient become unstable, or when things just "don't add up." Fostering good compliance is an art, reflecting the dynamic equilibrium between doctor and patient. Fewer patients are willing to take their doctor's word unquestioned, most have a greater need for maintaining or asserting control; with such patients it is important that the caregiver be flexible and open-minded, and that he demonstrate a willingness to elicit and address the patient's concerns. By acknowledging the potential for noncompliance, correction of the behavior is facilitated (e.g., "A lot of patients often miss medication doses from time to time, do you ?"). It is important to encourage a healthy curiosity about decision-making, and, to whatever extent is possible, it is also helpful to share our reasoning with patients.

In the case of medication prescribing, **noncompliance may be thought of as the first barrier to bioavailability. Chronic noncompliance may reflect as much about a patient's pathology as the state of the doctor-patient relationship.** While there is no guarantee to patient compliance, **the following recommendations can help to maximize compliance:**

A. **Give clear simple instructions;** if they can be written, even better. Ask the patient to repeat the instructions to confirm a clear understanding.

B. **Avoid complicated dosing schedules;** be realistic! Instruct the patient and encourage the use of pill boxes and other reminders.

C. **Explain your rationale for treatment** recommendations. Pictures and diagrams are often useful.

D. **Inform the patient of common side effects.**

E. **Inquire about how the patient will pay** for the treatment.

F. **Allow the patient to choose a date and time** when scheduling appointments.

G. **Actively solicit a patient's fears, anxieties, and concerns about the treatment plan.**

In all circumstances, noncompliance provides the clinician with vital data about the patient that need to be recognized and acted upon. When noncompliance is addressed, the result will be improved communication and trust between doctor and patient, and improved care.

Chapter 58
An Overview of the Psychotherapies

Robert S. Abernethy III and Steven C. Schlozman

I. Overview

Psychotherapies are most often categorized by their fundamental theoretical elements. These classifications include treatments (e.g., psychoanalytic psychotherapy, behavioral and cognitive-behavioral therapy, and interpersonal therapy). Other classifications reflect **their duration of treatment** (e.g., brief or short-term psychotherapy), **or the patients in attendance** (e.g., group, couples, or family therapy).

This chapter describes the eight most common forms of psychotherapy: **psychoanalytic or psychodynamic psychotherapy, behavior therapy, cognitive and cognitive-behavioral therapy (CBT), interpersonal therapy, dialectical behavior therapy (DBT), psychoeducational psychotherapy, supportive psychotherapy, and integrative psychotherapy.** Discussion will include which patients are referred for which therapy, and, when possible, to what extent each form of therapy has been studied in terms of efficacy and cost-effectiveness.

II. Psychoanalytical Psychotherapy (Expressive or Psychodynamic Psychotherapy)

A. Overview
1. Psychoanalytic psychotherapy is probably the **most commonly practiced type of psychotherapy in the United States. It is based on the Freudian tradition of uncovering unconscious aspects of a patient's mental life. Unconscious conflicts, repressed feelings, family issues from early in a patient's life, and difficulty with current relationships are the themes commonly addressed in this therapy.** Typically, the therapist takes a **nondirective posture,** paying close attention to **transference, countertransference, resistance, free association, and dreams** as a means of understanding and delineating unconscious conflicts.
   a. **Transference:** the unconscious redirection of feelings and desires retained from the past that are redirected towards the therapist.
   b. **Countertransference:** the unconscious association of feelings or desires from the past that the therapist develops for the patient.
   c. **Resistance:** those forces within the patient, conscious and unconscious, that oppose the purpose of the patient's evaluation and the goals of treatment.
   d. **Free association:** the undirected expression of conscious thoughts and feelings as a means of gaining access to unconscious processes.
2. **Severe and chronic personality disorders, as well as persistent problems in coping with life events, may be approached with psychoanalytic psychotherapy.** Anorexia nervosa also can be managed with long-term psychoanalytic psychotherapy.
3. The length of therapy varies from a **few months to a few years.**
4. Although some **research has supported the efficacy of this form of treatment,** it is important to remember that the nature of psychodynamic psychotherapy makes controlled studies difficult to conduct. Lack of research does not necessarily correlate with lack of efficacy. Based on existing data, cognitive and behavioral therapies (see below) may be more efficient in terms of symptom reduction and length of therapy, and have more rigorous research evidence of effectiveness. Although mood and anxiety disorders may respond to psychoanalytic psychotherapy, combinations of medication and cognitive or behavioral therapy may be more effective and efficient and cost less. Although few insurance programs pay for this type of treatment, many patients pursue and pay out-of-pocket for psychoanalytic psychotherapy because they find it emotionally and intellectually compelling.
5. There are **four principal subtypes of psychoanalytic or dynamic psychotherapy** associated with the following theoreticians:
   a. **Classical psychotherapy: Sigmund Freud**
   b. **Ego psychology: Anna Freud**
   c. **Object relations psychotherapy: Melanie Klein and Donald Winnicott**
      i. Melanie Klein is commonly associated with concepts such as the **depressive, paranoid, and schizoid positions.**
      ii. Donald Winnicott is commonly associated with concepts such as the **transitional object** and the **good enough mother.**
   d. **Self-psychology: Heinz Kohut**
      i. Kohut is commonly associated with the concept of **mirroring.**

429

III. Behavior Therapy

A. Behavior therapy is based on **reducing symptoms by learning relaxation techniques, changing factors that reinforce symptoms, and giving the patient graduated exposure to distressing stimuli. Joseph Wolpe** published the first book on behavior therapy, and **Isaac Mark** demonstrated the effectiveness of behavior therapy on simple phobias.

B. Behavior **therapists usually are directive and encourage homework experimentation. Homework** may involve exposure to a feared situation (e.g., speaking out during a committee meeting). The purpose of this suggestion is to reduce the reinforcing expectation that catastrophe would occur if one speaks out. **Mental imaging** allows the patient to learn how to relax while imagining the feared situation. Behavior therapy equips the patient with **concrete strategies** that can be used after the termination of therapy.

C. Behavior therapy is **generally brief,** requiring **6–20 sessions.**

D. Research evidence has repeatedly demonstrated **efficacy for behavior therapy** for a variety of **anxiety disorders, depression, and some psychosomatic symptoms (e.g., pain).** Behavior therapy is **manual-driven;** each session has a documented direction and goal. **Manual-driven therapies more easily lend themselves to systematic study and research.**

IV. Cognitive Therapy and Cognitive-Behavioral Therapy

A. Cognitive therapy is **based on the assumption that negative thoughts promote depression or anxiety.** Ideally, these negative thoughts are documented by the patient during depressing or anxious experiences that occur between visits, and, during therapy sessions, patients are encouraged to challenge these negative ideas. **Aaron Beck** first described cognitive therapy and demonstrated its effectiveness with controlled research.

B. **Research evidence has demonstrated that cognitive therapy is an effective treatment for depression.** Cognitive therapy is also indicated for **anxiety states** and problems related to **substance abuse. Cognitive-behavioral therapy (CBT)** is the term used to describe the combination of cognitive and behavioral therapies. **CBT is effective for anxiety disorders, such as obsessive-compulsive disorder (OCD), and depression.**

C. Cognitive therapy **generally requires 10–20 sessions.**

D. There is **good research evidence** that cognitive therapy is **effective for depression and some anxiety**

disorders. Cognitive therapy is a **manual-driven psychotherapy.**

V. Interpersonal Psychotherapy

A. Interpersonal psychotherapy addresses **relationships in the "here and now"** that may contribute to depression. Four common interpersonal issues are reviewed to discover the best focus of therapy: **grief, role transition, role dispute, and interpersonal deficits. Gerald Klerman** is credited with the early description and research on interpersonal psychotherapy.

B. Interpersonal psychotherapy has been used **primarily in the treatment of depression.**

C. This is a **brief therapy** with an active focus. The **usual duration is 12 sessions.**

D. There is **good research evidence that this manual-driven psychotherapy is effective.**

VI. Dialectical Behavior Therapy

A. **Dialectical behavior therapy (DBT) is an individual and group program for borderline personality disorder. The main goals of DBT are the reduction of self-injurious behavior and of hospitalizations.** This is a **manual-driven therapy with a psychoeducational focus** on mindfulness, interpersonal effectiveness, emotion regulation, and distress tolerance. **Marsha Linehan** originally described DBT and has demonstrated its effectiveness with borderlines in a controlled research protocol.

B. **DBT was designed especially for borderline personality disorder.**

C. DBT is typically longer than other manual-driven therapies, with a **duration of at least 1 year.**

D. **Controlled research designs** have demonstrated that DBT is **effective with borderline personality disorder at reducing self-injurious behavior and hospitalizations.**

VII. Psychoeducational Therapy

A. This form of **therapy is used to support and educate patients and families** about ways to manage and understand emotional or physical problems.

B. **Psychoeducational therapy has been used with schizophrenic patients and their families to teach** *low expressed emotion* **strategies.**

C. Research has demonstrated the **effectiveness of low-expressed emotions with schizophrenics.**

D. This is usually a **long-term therapy** used for chronic psychiatric problems.

VIII. Supportive Psychotherapy

A. Supportive psychotherapy is usually **brief,** with an **active focus on helping the patient deal with a life crisis.** The therapist offers **advice, sympathy, and support while reinforcing the patient's strengths.**

B. Supportive psychotherapy is anecdotally extremely helpful, but **formal research to demonstrate its effectiveness is lacking.** Supportive psychotherapy appears **especially effective for acute grief reactions.**

IX. Integrative Psychotherapy

A. Integrative psychotherapy represents a **combination of some or all of the therapies described above, and offers a multimodal approach to the patient's problem.** Integrative psychotherapy is widely practiced, but has not been formally researched to demonstrate its effectiveness. **Virtually any psychiatric problem can be treated** with a combination of integrated psychotherapies and appropriate pharmacotherapy. **Arnold Lazarus and Paul Wachtel were early writers on integrative or multimodal psychotherapy.**

B. Integrative psychotherapy **varies in length from brief to long-term.**

X. Brief Psychodynamic Psychotherapies

A number of theorists have developed a variety of brief psychodynamic psychotherapies.

A. **Peter Sifneos:** short-term **anxiety-provoking psychotherapy** that focuses on **unconscious oedipal issues.**

B. **David Malan: time-limited psychotherapy** that focuses on **triangles of conflict** (wish, threat, defense), and on **triangles of insight** (therapist, current, and past relationships).

C. **Habib Davanloo:** intensive short-term dynamic psychotherapy that focuses on **breaking through defenses** to unlock the unconscious.

D. **Lester Luborsky: supportive expressive psychotherapy** that focuses on the core conflictual relationship theme.

E. **James Mann: time-limited psychotherapy** that focuses on **time and loss.**

F. **Hans Strupp: time-limited dynamic psychotherapy** that focuses on **cyclical maladaptive patterns.**

XI. Group Therapies

Group therapy has been used for a **variety of Axis I conditions, such as mood disorders, anxiety disorders, and schizophrenia.** Groups have also been useful in the **long-term management of personality disorders and in grief work.** Some groups comprise patients with different diagnoses, some with the same diagnoses. Groups have been **useful for support and education for patients with medical conditions such as breast cancer and acquired immunodeficiency syndrome (AIDS). David Spiegel's** research has focused on the efficacy of group therapy for women with breast cancer. **Groups can be open-ended, with new patients beginning and other patients terminating over time. Other groups are time-limited, with all patients beginning at the same time and the group terminating at a predetermined date.** Group therapists may address the group as a whole or may focus on individual patients in the group. Finally, groups may embrace any of the theoretical orientations outlined above.

Suggested Readings

Abernethy RS: The integration of therapies. In Rutan S (ed.): *Current Trends in Psychotherapy.* New York: Guilford Press, 1992.

Alonso A, Swiller HI: *Group Therapy in Clinical Practice.* Washington, DC: American Psychiatric Press, 1993.

Basch MF: *Understanding Psychotherapy: The Science behind the Art.* New York: Basic Books, 1988.

Beck AT: *Cognitive Therapy and the Emotional Disorders.* New York: Meridian; 1976.

Hellerstein D, Pinsker H, Rosenthal R, Kee S: Supportive therapy as the treatment model of choice. *J Psychother Pract Res* 1994; 3:300–306.

Klerman G, Weissman M, Rounsaville B, Chevron E: *Interpersonal Psychotherapy of Depression.* New York: Basic Books; 1984.

Linehan MM: *Cognitive-Behavioral Treatment of Borderline Personality Disorder.* New York: Guilford Press, 1993.

Mann J: *Time-Limited Psychotherapy.* Cambridge, MA: Harvard University Press, 1992.

Rutan JS: *Psychotherapy for the 1990s.* New York: Guilford Press, 1992.

Wachtel PL: *Psychoanalysis and Behavior Therapy: Toward an Integration.* New York; Basic Books, 1977.

Chapter 59

Planned Brief Psychotherapy: An Overview

MARK A. BLAIS AND JAMES E. GROVES

I. Overview

Interest in planned brief psychotherapy has grown enormously in the last few decades. Unfortunately, this interest has been fueled more by changing patterns of health care reimbursement than by an appreciation of the clinical value inherent in brief psychotherapy. This chapter provides an overview of an eclectic approach to planned brief psychotherapy. By presenting the important features of brief therapy in a general manner (rather than as a specific school of brief therapy), the essential features of this form of psychotherapy can more easily be assimilated into one's ongoing psychotherapy practice. Still, **to understand even an eclectic version of short-term therapy, one must have a historical context within which to place it.**

II. A Brief History of Brief Psychotherapy

Towards the end of the nineteenth century, **when Breuer and Freud were busy inventing psychoanalysis, hysterical symptoms defined the focus of the work.** These early treatments were brief and symptom-focused, the therapist was active, and, basically, desperate patients selected themselves for the fledgling venture. **In time, free association, exploration of the transference, and dream analysis replaced hypnosis and direct suggestion** as the method of treatment, and the duration of treatment was greatly increased and therapist activity decreased. **Franz Alexander's manipulation of the interval and spacing of sessions was one of the major events in the development of modern short-term therapy. Decreased frequency, irregular spacing, therapeutic holidays, and therapist-dictated scheduling (rather than patient- or symptom-dictated scheduling) all enhanced the reality orientation of therapy.** World War II saw a glut of patients needing treatment for "shell shock" and "battle fatigue." New concepts and theories emerged from treating so many patients so rapidly. **Grinker and Spiegel's treatment of soldiers and Lindemann's work with survivors of the Coconut Grove fire** highlight this period in the development of brief treatment. Finally, **in the early 1960s, Sifneos and Malan independently developed the first theoretically coherent short-term psychotherapies.**

III. The Modern Brief Psychotherapies

Although this chapter focuses on an eclectic approach to brief therapy, it is important to have some sense of the current brief psychotherapy schools. There are basically four schools of brief psychotherapy: psychodynamic, cognitive-behavioral, interpersonal, and eclectic. **All four of these orientations share the essential features of brief therapy: brevity, patient selection, treatment focus, and high levels of therapist activity.**

A. **The psychodynamic short-term therapies** (see Sifneos, 1972; Malan, 1976; Davanloo, 1980) **feature psychoanalytic interpretation of defenses and unconscious conflicts** as their main "curative" agent. **Sifneos' anxiety-provoking therapy** is an ideal example of a brief psychodynamic psychotherapy. This treatment runs for 12–20 sessions and focuses narrowly on issues such as the failure to grieve, fear of success, or triangular, futile love relationships. The therapist serves as a detached, didactic figure who holds to the focus and challenges the patient to relinquish both dependency and intellectualization, while confronting anxiety-producing conflicts. One can think of this method as a classical oedipal level defense analysis with all the lull periods removed. One limiting feature is that it serves only 2–10% of the population, the subgroup able to tolerate its unremitting anxiety.

B. **The cognitive-behavioral brief therapies** (see Beck and Greenberg, 1979) **aim at bringing the patient's "automatic" (preconscious) thoughts into awareness, and demonstrating how these thoughts impact behavior and feelings.** This style of therapy is much more broadly applicable, in terms of both patients and problems. The basic thrust of cognitive therapy, according to Beck, is to get the automatic thoughts more completely into consciousness, to challenge them consciously, and to practice new behaviors that change the picture of the world and the self in it. The patient is actively helped to challenge these automatic thoughts.

C. **Brief interpersonal therapy was developed by Klerman (1984) and is a highly formalized (manualized) treatment. Interpersonal psychotherapy (IPT) focuses not on mental content but on the process of the patient's interaction with others. In IPT,** behavior and communications are taken at face value. IPT was developed primarily to treat patients with depression episodes related to either

433

grief or loss, interpersonal disputes, or interpersonal skill deficits.

D. **The "eclectic" brief therapies are characterized by combinations and integrations of multiple theories and techniques. Budman and Gurman present one very popular version of eclectic brief therapy which focuses on three dimensions of mental life: the interpersonal, the developmental, and the existential.** The model of Budman and Gurman pursues a systematic approach, beginning with the individual's reason for seeking therapy at this time. Major changes in the patient's social support are reviewed. A major feature here is the belief that maximal benefit from therapy occurs early, and the optimal time for change is early in treatment.

IV. The Natural Course of Psychotherapy

Despite the common perception that psychotherapy is a long-term, even timeless, enterprise, most of the existing **data indicate that psychotherapy as it is practiced in the real world has a time-limited course.** For example, using national outpatient psychotherapy utilization data obtained in 1987 (before the nationwide impact of managed care), **Olfson and Pincus found that 70% of psychotherapy users received ten or fewer sessions.** In fact, only 15% of their sample received 21 or more sessions. These data are highly consistent with earlier studies showing a median number of eight sessions for outpatient psychotherapy. Clearly then, in the real world, the majority of patients have a time-limited or brief psychotherapy experience. The material presented in this chapter will help you deliver psychotherapy in a planned and thoughtful manner, which is better matched to psychotherapy's natural course.

V. The Brief Therapy Mind-Set

A certain mind-set needs to be adopted by a therapist hoping to successfully learn and practice brief treatment.

A. **From the start there must be a willing suspension of disbelief and cynicism about brief therapy.** An example of this would be a willingness to consider a quick positive response as something other than a temporary "flight into health."

B. **Therapy must be conceptualized as a time-limited enterprise,** as something that will end at a known planned date. This appears deceptively simple, but in practice it is actually a difficult cognitive change to make and one that has ramifications for all your treatment decisions, particularly your activity level as the therapist. To illustrate, briefly consider how you might approach a new patient if from the start you knew that the therapy would last 14 sessions.

C. **The therapist must expect and accept that patients will return to therapy periodically across their lifespan** (sometimes called intermittent brief therapy across the life-cycle). This relates to the notion of cure and what is an acceptable outcome for treatment. This is often the easiest of the three components to accept.

VI. The Essential Features of Brief Therapy

A. **Patient Evaluation and Selection**
 1. **Initial evaluation. Patient selection is the art of finding the right patient with the right problem for brief psychotherapy** and it starts with the initial evaluation. A **two-session evaluation** format is recommended for determining if a patient is appropriate for brief therapy. This format allows the clinician to conduct a complete psychiatric evaluation and assess the appropriateness of the patient for brief psychotherapy without feeling too much time pressure. To guide you in the selection of patients we present a number of inclusion and exclusion criteria (see Table 59-1). These criteria are fairly general, covering most forms of brief therapy, and restrictive; many patients will be screened out. However, for the new or novice brief therapist the use of these criteria will provide nearly ideal brief therapy patients.
 2. **Exclusion criteria.** Here is a short list of exclusion criteria. **The brief therapy patient should not be actively psychotic, abusing substances, or at significant risk for self-harm.** The actively psychotic patient will not be able to make adequate use of the reality oriented/logical aspects of the brief treatment. Substance-abusing patients should be

---

Table 59-1. Patient Selection Criteria for Brief Therapy

Exclusion criteria

Active psychosis

Substance abuse

A significant risk of self-harm

Inclusion criteria

Moderate emotional distress

A desire for relief

A specific or circumscribed problem

History of positive relationship

Function in one area of life

Ability to commit to treatment

directed to substance abuse treatment prior to undertaking any form of psychotherapy. Patients at significant risk for self-harm are not appropriate for brief therapy due to possible complications with the ending of their treatment at a planned time. These factors should be considered categorical in nature; the presence of any one of them should rule out a patient for brief psychotherapy. This is especially true for a therapist just beginning to learn brief treatment.

3. **Inclusion criteria.** These criteria can be thought of as dimensions, with each patient being rated on how much of each dimension they have. The potential candidate for brief therapy should:

   a. Be in moderate emotional distress, as this provides the motivation for treatment.

   b. Personally want relief from his or her emotional pain; they should not have been sent to therapy reluctantly by a boss or spouse.

   c. Be able to articulate a fairly specific cause of their pain or a circumscribed life problem (or be willing to accept your specific formulation of their difficulty); this helps provide a treatment focus.

   d. Have a history of at least one positive (mutual) interpersonal relationship.

   e. Still be functioning in at least one area of life.

   f. Have the ability to commit to a treatment contract.

   As stated earlier, patients should be rated for their standing on all of these dimensions. The more of these qualities (amount and number) that a patient has, the better the candidate for brief therapy he or she is.

B. Developing a Treatment Focus

Developing a treatment focus is probably the most misunderstood aspect of brief therapy. Many writers talk about "the focus" in a circular and mysterious manner, as if the whole success of the treatment rests on finding *the* one correct focus (Hall et al., 1990). This can be confusing and intimidating to those just learning brief therapy. Rather, **what is needed is the establishment of a focus that both the therapist and patient can agree upon and which fits the therapist's treatment approach.** This can be called **a functional focus.** The main technique for finding a functional focus is the "Why now?" technique developed by Budman and Gurman (1988). **This technique is applied by repeatedly asking the patient "Why did you come for treatment now?"** "Why today rather than last week, tomorrow, etc. . . . ?" (you really need to try this simple technique a few times to see how effective and powerful it can be). The goal is to find out what the triggering event for therapy was, as this might provide an ideal treatment focus.

Budman and Gurman (1988) also describe **four common treatment foci:**

1. **Losses,** past, present, or pending. These can be interpersonal (e.g., the loss of a loved one), intrapersonal (e.g., the loss of a psychological ability, the social loss of a support network), or functional (as in the loss of specific abilities or capacities).

2. **Developmental desynchronies** (being out of step with expected developmental stages). This is often seen in the professional who required extensive periods of education prior to initiating an adult life style.

3. **Interpersonal conflicts,** usually repeated interpersonal disappointments, either with loved ones or bosses.

4. **Symptomatic presentations.** Many patients present for psychotherapy simply with the desire for symptom reduction. It is helpful to memorize these four common foci and review them in your head while conducting an initial evaluation assessment of their relevance to the patient. The most important thing to remember is that you are not finding *the* focus, only *a* focus for the therapy.

C. Completing the Initial Evaluation

By the completion of the second evaluation session you need to:

1. **Decide if the patient is appropriate for brief treatment.**

2. **Select an agreed-upon focus.**

3. **Have a clearly stated treatment contract,** including the number of sessions, how missed appointments will be handled, and how posttermination contact will be handled.

The two-session evaluation format also allows you to see how the patient responds to you and to the therapy. In fact, it can be very enlightening to give the patient some kind of homework to complete between the two sessions. An initial positive response, and feeling a little better in the second session, bodes well (while a strong negative reaction conveys a worse prognosis). A more ambivalent response such as forgetting the task may signal problems with motivation and should be explored.

D. Being an Active Therapist (see Table 59-2)

Conducting a brief (12–16 sessions) psychotherapy requires that the therapist be very active. The therapist performing such therapy must keep the treatment focused and the process of treatment moving forward. Several techniques have been designed to structure and to direct the therapy. These include beginning each session with a summary of the important points raised during the last session, and restating the focus. Assignment and review of homework (out of

Table 59-2. Types of Therapist Activity

- Structuring sessions
- Use of homework
- Developing the working alliance
- Limiting silences
- Clarification of vague responses
- Addressing positive and negative transference quickly
- Limiting psychological regression

session assignments designed to transfer gains from therapy to the patient's life) are tasks that characterize the activity of the therapist. Interventions which focus on the "working alliance" are important, as are timely interventions, which limit silences and deviations from the focus.

The goal of eclectic brief therapy is to restore or improve premorbid adaptation and function. Efforts are made by the therapist to limit and check psychological regressions. **Asking, "What did you think about that?" rather than about feelings and affect (e.g., "How did that make you feel?") can help with the exploration of potentially regressive material.** Limited within-session regression is acceptable and often necessary in brief therapy; however, prolonged regressions accompanied by decreased function are to be avoided.

Clarification is important in brief therapy. Requests for clarification should be made whenever a patient produces vague or incomplete material. This would include asking for examples or for specifics, and empathically pointing out contradictions and inconsistencies.

Transference occurs in all treatments, including brief psychotherapy. **Despite the fact that many aspects of brief therapy are designed to discourage the development of transference, the therapist must be ready to deal with it when it develops.** Two forms of transference are particularly important to recognize quickly: negative and overly positive transferences. Negative transference can be suspected when the patient responds repeatedly with either angry or devaluing statements, or when he or she experiences the therapy as humiliating. Overly positive transference is signaled by repeated and excessively positive comments (e.g., "Oh, you know me better than anyone ever has"). Both of these forms of transference should be dealt with quickly from the perspective of reality. The therapist should review the patient's feelings and reasoning and relate these to the actual interaction. For example, if the therapist was inadvertently

offensive, this should be admitted to, while pointing out that the therapist's motive was to be helpful.

VII. Phases of Planned Brief Therapy

Three traditional phases of psychotherapy as they apply to brief treatment need review.

A. **The initial phase (from the evaluation to session 2 or 3) principally includes evaluation and selection of the patient, selection of the focus, and establishment of a working alliance.** This phase is usually accompanied by some mild reduction in symptoms and a low-grade positive transference, particularly as a working relationship develops. The goal is to set the frame and the structure of the therapy, while also giving the patient hope.

B. **The middle phase** (session 4 to 8 or 9). In the middle phase, the work gets more difficult. **The patient usually becomes concerned about the time limit, feeling that the length of treatment will not be sufficient.** Issues of separation and aloneness come to the fore and compete with the focus for attention. It is important for the therapist to reassure the patient (with words and a calm, understanding demeanor) that the treatment will work, and direct their joint attention back to the agreed-upon focus. The patient often feels worse during this phase and the therapist's faith in the treatment process is often tested.

C. **The termination phase** (session 8 to 12 or 16). In this phase the therapy usually settles down. **The patient accepts the fact that treatment will end as planned and his or her symptoms typically decrease.** In addition to the treatment focus, posttherapy plans and the situational loss of the therapy relationship are explored. At or around the actual termination of treatment it is not unusual for the patient to present some new and often interesting material for discussion. While the therapist may be tempted to explore this new material and thereby extend the treatment, doing so is usually (but not always) a mistake. Interest in the new material should be shown, but, if it is not clinically important, treatment should end as planned.

D. **Posttreatment Contact**
Within the eclectic brief therapy framework it is acceptable for patients to return to therapy at multiple points during their life. When a therapy is completed, a patient should wait about 6 months before considering further therapy. This allows the patient to practice his or her newly learned psychological insights and skills in the real world and time to assess their new level of adaptation and function. In considering posttreatment con-

tact, you should strive to help patients with psychological troubles whenever they develop across the lifespan.

Suggested Readings

Beck S, Greenberg R: Brief cognitive therapies. *Psychiatr Clin North Am* 1979; 2:11–22.

Blais M: Planned brief therapy. In Jacobson J, Jacobson A (eds): *Psychiatric Secrets*. Philadelphia: Hanley & Belfus, 1996.

Budman S, Gurman A: *Theory and Practice of Brief Therapy*. New York: Guilford Press, 1988.

Burk J, White H, Havens L: Which short-term therapy? *Arch Gen Psychiatry* 1979; 36:177–186.

Davanloo H: *Short-Term Dynamic Psychotherapy*. New York: Jason Aronson, 1980.

Groves J: The short-term dynamic psychotherapies: an overview. In Rutan S (ed.): *Psychotherapy for The 90s*. New York: Guilford Press, 1992.

Groves J: *Essential Papers on Short-Term Dynamic Therapy*. New York: New York Universities Press, 1996.

Hall M, Arnold W, Crosby R: Back to basics: the importance of focus selection. *Psychotherapy* 1990; 27:578–584.

Klerman G, Weissman M, Rounsaville B, Chevron E: *Interpersonal Psychotherapy of Depression*. New York: Basic Books, 1984.

Leibovich M: Short-term psychotherapy for the borderline personality disorder. *Psychother Psychosom* 1981; 35:257–264.

Malan D: *The Frontier of Brief Psychotherapy*. New York: Plenum Medical Book Company, 1976.

Mann J: *Time-Limited Psychotherapy*. Cambridge, MA: Harvard University Press, 1973.

Sifneos P: *Short-Term Psychotherapy and Emotional Crisis*. Cambridge, MA: Harvard University Press, 1972.

Sifneos P: *Short-Term Anxiety Provoking Psychotherapy: A Treatment Manual*. USA: Basic Books, 1992.

Chapter 60
Couples Therapy
ANNE K. FISHEL

I. Introduction

Couples therapy is a clinical subspecialty that most clinicians engage in, but few do so with any formal training. **Couples therapy focuses on the pattern of interactions between two people while taking into account the individual history and contribution of each member.**

Clinical work with couples is typically part of child evaluation, ongoing child and adolescent psychotherapy, divorce mediation, crisis work, or child custody evaluation. Couples therapy is also an important component in the treatment of sexual dysfunction, alcoholism and substance abuse, the disclosure of an infidelity, depression and anxiety disorders, infertility, and serious medical illness. Couples therapy is also useful in resolving polarized relational issues, such as the decision to marry or divorce, the choice to have an abortion, or the decision to move to a distant city for one partner's career. The term "couples therapy" rather than "marital therapy" is deliberately used throughout this chapter to include therapy with homosexual couples and unmarried heterosexual couples.

A. Organizing Principles for Couples Therapists

1. **Attraction and mate choice. The couple's therapist often locates the origins of the current dilemma in the nature of the initial attraction.** Two common explanations of attraction are "opposites attract" (elaborated by the psychodynamic construct "projective identification"), and "repetition compulsion."

   a. **Projective identification:** the idea that individuals unconsciously look for something in the other that is difficult and then act to elicit the very behavior in the other that has been disavowed. So, for example, a shy, self-effacing man may be attracted to a self-confident, ambitious woman, but over time complains that she is too self-absorbed. She may initially find his steadiness and calm attractive, only to later criticize him for his cold remove. What is problematic for the self becomes contentious between the couple.

   b. **Repetition compulsion or re-enactment:** the idea that one falls in love with someone who resembles a loving caretaker from childhood, or who resembles an abusive caretaker with whom one wants a second chance to master the abuse. Murray Bowen, a psychodynamic therapist, observed that **individuals at a similar level of psychological functioning tend to marry.**

2. **Contribution from family of origin. Regardless of theoretical orientation, most couple's therapists posit a connection between past family experiences and current marital functioning.** Beginning with the choice of a mate, each member of the couple brings an unconscious template of lover and then proceeds to distort the other to conform with the self's needs. The process of couples therapy is, in large part, one of distinguishing between those distortions based on past familial relationships and the reality of one's actual partner.

3. **Life cycle context. A couple's relationship takes place within the context of changes in each individual and changes in the wider context of family.** Since individuals' psychological growth may take place at different rates, relationships must be able to tolerate divergent growth trajectories, as, for example, when one partner is ready for children, or for retirement, before the other.

   Life-cycle theorists have posited several predictable stages of development for intact middle-class couples with children. Life events, and a particular set of psychological tasks which require change, prompt these stages. It is assumed that **it is in the transition from one stage to another that couples and families are most at risk for divorce and the appearance of individual symptomatology.**

   a. The stages, with the principal concomitant emotional task required, are outlined by Carter and McGoldrick (1989):

      i. Young adults leave home: accepting emotional and financial responsibility for the self.

      ii. Families join through marriage: committing to and forming a new marital system.

      iii. Families have young children: making room for new members in the marital system.

      iv. Families have adolescents: increasing the flexibility of family boundaries to include adolescents' independence as well as grandparents' dependence.

      v. Children get launched and move on: re-evaluating marriage and career issues, as parenting roles diminish.

      vi. Families exist later in life: accepting the shifting of generational roles to care for the older generation and face aging and loss in middle generation.

   b. As the larger social context changes, the parameters of these stages shift as well. At present, for example, couples can expect an average of 20 years from the time their youngest child marries until retirement, as compared to only 2 years for this launching stage at the turn of the century. The lengthening of this stage is due to longer life expectancy and women ending their childbearing at a relatively young age, with fewer children.

4. **Gender.** After decades of overlooking the contribution of gender differences to couples relationships, there has been a burgeoning of writings over the last decade (Luepnitz, 1988; Walters et al., 1988; Tannen, 1990). The influence of gender has been documented in at least two areas:

   a. The effect of marriage and divorce on men's and women's health and well-being. Several researchers have noted that **married men experience better health and greater marital satisfaction than do their female counterparts.** Also, married men achieve greater occupational success than single men, while the opposite is true for married women. Even in dual-career marriages, women continue to do the lion's share of household and childcare tasks, particularly the daily and routine tasks (e.g., cooking and laundry). **The effects of divorce on women are far more devastating than they are on men:** men experience a 42% average rise in their standard of living after divorce, and women experience an average 75% decline in financial resources (Weitzman, 1985).

   b. The effect of gender socialization on communication, roles, and violence. **Boys, in general, are encouraged to be more aggressive and independent, and discouraged from focusing on their emotional worlds. Girls, by contrast, are raised to focus more on their relationships with others and to be concerned with understanding the needs of others. These distinct paths of socialization lead to the creation of two cultures,** making most heterosexual marriages essentially cross-cultural. Tannen (1990) has observed the misunderstandings that can result from this cultural difference, with men arguing and interrupting more and women eager to compromise and capitulate. With the rapid societal changes over the last few decades bringing increasing numbers of mothers into the workplace, and demanding that fathers be more emotionally available in the family than their own fathers were, many couples are experiencing additional stress and confusion about their gender roles.

      The effects of gender socialization can be seen in domestic violence as well. In domestic violence, 95% of all cases are perpetrated by men against women. Goldner et al. (1990) argue that such violence can best be understood in terms of gender socialization. Men who were raised to feel shamed by expressing feelings may defend against perceived feminine threats of dependency and vulnerability by asserting their masculinity through violence.

5. **What is a good relationship?** In recent years, several therapists have grappled with defining healthy marital functioning. In *The Good Marriage,*

Wallerstein and Blakeslee (1995) interviewed 50 happily married couples and concluded that these **couples had dealt successfully with nine tasks:**

   a. They detached emotionally from each member's family of origin.
   b. They built intimacy while preserving a sense of autonomy.
   c. They relaxed the boundaries of the couple's relationship to allow children in while maintaining the emotional richness of marriage.
   d. They confronted the inevitable developmental changes of aging, loss, illness, and came out of crisis with renewed strength.
   e. They safely expressed difference, anger, and conflict without violence or capitulation.
   f. They established a pleasurable sexual relationship that changed in response to the stressors of aging, work, and family life.
   g. They shared laughter and humor.
   h. They provided emotional nurturance and encouragement.
   i. They allowed the marriage to be renewed by the elements of fantasy and attraction that first drew the partners to one another.

6. **Communication. Early models of couples therapy stressed the importance of developing communication skills, sometimes at the expense of other relational dimensions like gender, sex, and family of origin issues.** The emphasis on communication stressed the importance of each partner being able to speak openly and frankly while the other listened with undefensive empathy. In part, this emphasis belies a bias about intimacy: that closeness can be achieved only through the full and open disclosure of each partner's innermost feelings. **More recent interpretations of the role of communication include a wider range of issues: not only talking and listening, but also refraining from making hurtful comments, and focusing on nonverbal action, including acts of affection and sexuality, the giving and receiving of generous acts, and the sharing of mutually enjoyed activities, even if they do not include self-disclosing conversation** (Weingarten, 1990).

II. Conducting an Evaluation

A couple's evaluation should contain an opportunity for the couple to discuss their relationship together and to explore their individual histories separately. The evaluation offers a balance between clinical understanding and empathy on the one hand, and prodding the couple into thinking about their relationship in new, more flexible ways, on the other. Throughout the evaluation, the clinician looks for opportunities to re-establish hope, to point out resources and strengths of the couple, and to provide a forum for each partner's position to be heard without judgment. The clinician will also look for opportunities to transform individual explanations of a problem into systemic, interactive descriptions. **A successful evaluation will determine the motivation of each partner to participate in ongoing treatment and tease out when couples therapy is contraindicated, and when individual, group or no therapy should be recommended instead.**

A. **The First Session** (both members of the couple)
1. **Providing a context of safety and comfort.** The clinician should set a time frame, ask each member to introduce him- or herself separate from the problems that bring them in, and offer certain rules of discourse:
   a. **The "I pass" rule can be introduced.** If anyone is asked a question that feels too intrusive, he or she is encouraged to "pass."
   b. **Setting the expectation that whatever is said in the individual meetings will be shared in the wrap-up meeting.** This guideline prevents the therapist from getting in the untenable position of sharing a secret with one member of the couple about the other.
   c. **Summarizing any contact the therapist has already had with one member of the couple** to demonstrate the therapist's commitment to openness and equity.
2. **Getting each couple member's definition of the problem.** It is essential that the clinician convey that both partners' perspectives will be respected and contained, and that the therapist will not play the role of a judge, arbitrating two adversaries. Each individual should have an opportunity to tell his or her version without interruptions and qualifications by the other.
   a. As an opening question, the clinician might ask: "Often in couples, each member has a different view of the problem and different hopes for change. I'd like to hear from each of you how you see your difficulties."
   b. **It is important to determine whether both parties are engaged in the evaluation process** or whether one member has been dragged, coerced, or threatened by the other. The clinician might ask: "I'd like to hear how you made the decision to give me a call and whose idea it was."
   c. **The therapist will want to know about the larger context** in which the couple lives in order to understand other resources and other stressors. The therapist might ask: "Who else has been concerned and given advice or offered help?" And, "Have there been any other changes in the family in the last year?" (e.g., illnesses, job loss, deaths, moves, infertility, births). Often, a request for couples therapy will coincide with an accumulation of other stressors.
3. **Expanding the couple's view of the problem.** An evaluation should offer the couple ample opportunity to share their working, rehearsed definitions of

the problem as well as a chance to have their ideas challenged and stretched in order to create new strategies for change. Several questions help make the shift from the couple's current view to a more flexible, often interactional definition that paves the way for each member of the couple to change in order to alter the pattern between them rather than the pathology within one. Here are some examples:
   a. **"If you were to be in couples therapy for 6 months and at that point you declared that the therapy had been a wild success, what would I notice that would let me know that your relationship had changed in important ways?** What, for example, would you be talking about or doing with each other or noticing about the other that is not happening now?" (see De Shayzer, 1995). With these questions, the couple is asked to envision a solution and a way of knowing when the therapy would be over.
   b. Since a majority of couples will experience sexual difficulties at some point in their relationship, it is worth asking every couple during an evaluation, even if it is not part of the stated problem: **"Is there anything you would like to change about your sexual relationship?"**
   c. **Since one can often detect the seeds of the current dilemma in the story of the couple's initial attraction to one another, it is useful to ask: "What first attracted you to one another?"** Furthermore, most couples, no matter how upset or angry, will brighten and soften towards one another in answering this question. When there is not a palpable shift towards more positive affect, the therapist may be concerned that there is an absence of affection and friendship to draw on.
   d. Mark Karpel, in *Evaluating Couples*, suggests that the therapist ask each member of the couple: "What is it like being married to you?" **When each member's version of the self matches the partner's view, the therapy is far more straightforward.** When these versions do not match, the therapist will have to attend to the fact that there is no agreement on the relational problem.
   e. **Where is the couple developmentally?** Attending to normative responses to life-cycle changes will alert the therapist to inquire about commonly occurring reactions to these events. For example, if a couple has small children, one will want to ask how their sexual relationship has changed, and do they have fights about the equity of child care and housework.
   f. **"What can you tell me about the family you grew up in that will help me understand your current dilemma?"** This question probes for the themes and issues that each individual brings to the relationship and sets the groundwork for later exploration of projective identification.
   g. **"Tell me about an instance when the problem did not occur." "What did you notice that each of you was doing differently?"** These questions, derived from nar-

rative therapy (White and Epston, 1990), ask the couple to stand apart from their problem and notice the positive examples of their interactions. In addition, such an inquiry guides members to reflect on his or her contribution to the pattern between them.

    h. **Over the course of a marriage, 50% of couples will be unfaithful, so there is a strong possibility that any couple seeking therapy may have an infidelity going on.** It is unlikely, however, that if you ask about a secret affair in the presence of the couple, that you will be told the truth. If you ask in an individual meeting about infidelity, you will more likely hear the truth, but you will be stuck with having a secret that will make you collude with one member and likely enrage the other if the secret comes out. An alternative to asking directly about infidelity is to test the waters by inquiring, "Has fidelity been a challenge for either of you to maintain?" "What has been your understanding about what constitutes infidelity?" **When there is an ongoing affair or, when one member is suspicious of the other's fidelity, these questions will often elicit nonverbal cues of anxiety or anger.**

B. The Two Individual Sessions (one member at each) **These sessions offer an opportunity to get to know the individuals better, and to give them a chance to bring up whatever they want without having to share the time with their partner. In addition it is useful to ask about:**

1. Each individual's current level of commitment to the relationship.
2. Each member's history of, and current use of, drugs and alcohol.
3. Previous and current experiences with therapy and psychiatric hospitalizations.
4. Any history of depression, suicidality, anxiety, or other mental illness.
5. Any history of sexual abuse.
6. Any current medical problems.
7. Particularly with women: "Do you ever feel afraid of your partner? Has your partner ever been violent towards you, your children, or inanimate objects?"

C. The Fourth Wrap-Up, Feedback Session (both members of the couple)
When one partner has been dragged to couples therapy, the evaluation may be the end of the line and the feedback can give the couple ideas to work with even if they forgo further couples therapy.

1. **Comment on positive aspects of the relationship.** Conveying an appreciation of the couple's positive qualities diminishes defensiveness, promotes hopefulness, and places the focus on the relationship. The therapist might note, for example, how intently the couple listened to one another, or how courageous it was for them to come to therapy, or how well they use humor.

2. **Give a reading of the affective temperature of the relationship.** It is crucial that the therapist accurately interpret the couple's level of distress. Is this a couple on the verge of a break-up, in need of a tune-up in a few areas, or in conflict about the extent of the overhaul needed?
3. **Identify the stressors and place the problem in a developmental perspective.**
4. **Offer a relational description of the problem** that includes both perspectives and points to areas of change.
5. **Make recommendations for treatment.**
    a. **When to refer for couples therapy:**
       i. When the therapist and the couple can agree on an interactional definition of the problem.
      ii. When there is irreconcilable disagreement, as with a stalemate about whether to marry, to divorce, or to have children.
     iii. With particular complaints, such as sexual difficulties, chronic fighting, adjustment to serious medical illness in one partner, or the aftermath of the disclosure of an affair.
     iv. When the couple is having difficulty negotiating a life transition; for example, when a couple fears the dissolution of their marriage as they anticipate their oldest child's leave-taking, or when a couple with a newborn feels overwhelmed by the intensity of their fights with one another.
    b. **When to refer for individual therapy:**
       i. If one partner is motivated for therapy and the other is not.
      ii. If an individual symptom requires specialized treatment, as when one member is clinically depressed, has an uncontrolled temper, or is experiencing posttraumatic stress disorder (PTSD).
     iii. If one member is maintaining a secret affair and is conflicted about whether or not to end it and work on the marriage.
    c. **When couples therapy is contraindicated** (note: to recommend against couples therapy is not the same as recommending that a couple separate or divorce):
       i. When only one member can identify a wish to change or make a commitment to working on the relationship.
      ii. When there is ongoing violence and the violent partner is unwilling or unable to negotiate a convincing no-violence contract.
     iii. When there have been repeated failed attempts at couples therapy and a chronic relational problem with a high degree of mistrust and a lack of any positive feelings between them.

III. Treatment Interventions

Each of the interventions listed below belongs to a distinct theoretical orientation. Couples therapists will offer a more

thoughtful, coherent treatment if their interventions derive from theory than if they use an array of techniques in a trial and error fashion. These interventions represent only a sampling of those available.

A. **Interpretation of unconscious processes** that distort the ability of each member of the couple to perceive the other for who she or he really is (**psychodynamic model**). The distortions derive largely from unresolved family-of-origin issues. **Therapeutic work focuses on interpretation of projective identification and transference** (with interpretations made between the members of the couple as well as between the couple and therapist).

B. **Communication Skills Training (Cognitive-Behavioral Model)**
   1. **Active listening.** Each partner practices, both in the session and outside, how to listen with empathy and curiosity to the other. They take turns being speaker and listener, with the latter demonstrating understanding by paraphrasing what was said and asking for confirmation from the speaker.
   2. **Developing a marital quid pro quo.** Each individual makes a list of behaviors that are pleasing to him or her. Then, **the therapist negotiates an increase in pleasing behaviors on the part of each that is contingent on the other emitting comparable behavior.** For example, one spouse may agree to make dinner in return for the other being physically affectionate.
   3. **Learning to fight constructively by following certain rules,** such as sticking to one issue at a time, eliminating name-calling or sarcasm, asking for a specific change, and asking for and giving feedback.

C. **Role-Playing and Other Action-Oriented Techniques (Experiential Model)**
   1. **Psychodrama.** Each member of the couple may enact a present interaction that is repeatedly unsatisfactory or a situation from his or her family of origin that connects to a current marital dilemma. Each member of the couple can then enroll the other in a rewritten enactment that corrects a past injustice. Or, if the husband directs his wife to role-play him, he can show her the way he would like to be responded to.
   2. **Role reversal.** Switching of roles can enhance empathy, increase the behavioral and affective repertoire of each member of the couple, and loosen polarized positions.

D. **Paradoxical Interventions (Strategic Model)**
   These are based on the premise that couples request and shun change simultaneously. To deal with this common dual agenda, strategic therapists offer paradoxical interventions, which mirror the couple's conflicting requests to get out of their mess but without having to change. For example, **with an intervention, known as the "therapeutic double bind," the therapist may tell the symptomatic member not to change because the symptom is accomplishing an important function for the marriage.** If the individual resists the intervention, then change occurs. If he complies, change still occurs, because the symptom will be viewed differently, as being under voluntary control.

E. **Narrative Approaches (Narrative Model)**
   1. **Externalizing the problem. The therapist and couple collaborate on a name for the problem and attribute negative intentions to it.** For example, a couple with chronic fighting might be asked: "Describe the ways that you let your habit of bickering with one another ruin the rest of your relationship."
   2. **Exploring the unique outcome.** There are times when the couple has resisted the problem's pull or when the couple's life was not dominated by the problem. The couple is asked to speculate about what made it possible at those times to resist the usual pattern.
   3. **Using small shifts in language to construct a different view of the problem** that is less constraining and more amenable to solutions.

Suggested References

Bograd M: Values in conflict: challenges to family therapists' thinking. *J Marital Fam Ther* 1992; 18:245–256.

Carter B, McGoldrick M (eds): *The Changing Family Life Cycle: A Framework for Family Therapy*, 2nd ed. Boston: Allyn and Bacon, 1989.

De Shayzer S: *Words Were Originally Magic*. New York: Norton, 1994.

Goldner V, Penn P, Sheinberg M, Walker G: Love and violence: gender paradoxes in volatile attachments. *Fam Process* 1990; 29: 343–364.

Gottman J: *Why Marriages Succeed or Fail*. New York: Simon and Schuster, 1994.

Karpel S: *Evaluating Couples: A Handbook for Practitioners*. New York: Norton, 1994.

LoPiccolo J, LoPiccolo L (eds): *Handbook of Sex Therapy*. New York: Plenum, 1978.

Luepnitz D: *The Family Interpreted*. New York: Basic Books, 1988.

Tannen D: *You Just Don't Understand: Women and Men in Conversation*. New York: William Morrow, 1990.

Wallerstein J, Blakeslee S: *The Good Marriage: How and Why Love Lasts*. Boston: Houghton Mifflin, 1995.

Walters M, Carter B, Papp P, Silverstein O: *The Invisible Web: Gender Patterns in Family Relationships*. New York: Guilford, 1988.

Weingarten K: The discourses of intimacy: adding a social constructionist and feminist view. *Fam Process* 1991; 30:285–305.

Weitzman L: *The Divorce Revolution*. New York: Free Press, 1985.

White M, Epston D: *Narrative Means to Therapeutic Ends*. New York: Norton, 1990.

Chapter 61
Family Therapy
Lois S. Slovik and James L. Griffith

I. Introduction

Family therapy is not new. Originally done by social workers in the late 1800s, what we today call Family (or Systems) Therapy had a resurgence in the late 1940s and evolved from the intersection of societal needs and scientific thinking. The scientific perspective included **Ludwig von Bertalanffy's General Systems Theory and Norbert Wiener's Cybernetic Theory, which had as its focus communication, control, patterning, and the activity of feedback cycles.** From a societal perspective, the sudden reuniting of families at the conclusion of World War II created problems for which the public turned to mental health professionals, and for which individual therapy was insufficient. The focus of the request was interpersonal, and included help with marital discord, divorce, delinquency, and emotional breakdowns in family members. Thus modern-day Family Therapy was reborn.

This chapter will be written from the idea of "drawing distinctions." Human beings punctuate or draw boundaries around particular actions, bring them to the foreground, and give them meanings. **Therapists from each of the "schools" of family therapy have particular distinctions** (like the imprint of a cookie-cutter on rolled-out dough) in mind when they assess or treat a family. **Their theory** (what they think about) **controls what they look for. Once a pattern is "seen," strategies and techniques are used to create change. This chapter is organized as to what therapists from each of the listed schools of family therapy "think about," "look for," and "do."**

II. Psychodynamic Family Therapy

A. What They Think About
1. Strategies and techniques are based upon **object relations and Freudian theory.**
2. **The family is viewed as a system that is composed of individuals embedded within a social context.** They consider an **individual's purposes, feelings, and meanings** as critical factors in the formulation of a family's situation, **with culture being a critical constraint.**
3. The health of the family is considered in the context of its life-cycle, within and across generations.
4. Problems are thought to occur through **multi-generational family failure.**

5. **Interpersonal functioning is tied to attachments to past figures** (incorporation/introjection) from which the family member(s) need to be freed.
6. **Internal processes affect a person's view of the world** and controls his behavior. These can get acted out through the process of **projective identification.**
7. Traumatic events, either on an individual, family, or at a societal level, are associated with intense anxiety and helplessness which often cannot be talked about, but are represented by repetitive patterns of action that are dysfunctional (repetition compulsion).
8. **Pathology is thought to result from a combination of an individual's or a family's developmental arrest, plus stress.**
9. **Change occurs through gaining conscious insight into previously unconscious processes and by reclaiming projections.**

B. What They Look For
1. **Historical information.** It is important to take an extensive history. **Each person has an experiential map (transference) of the world,** which contains meanings for actions and sequences of behaviors, rules of how people are expected to respond, models for being (e.g., a man/woman, husband/wife, mother/father, parent/child). This map develops out of each person's history, and lies embedded in relationships among introjects of important early figures.
2. **Projective identification (PI).** An activity of the ego that modifies the perception of the other (person), and, in a reflexive fashion, alters one's image of the self. This conjoined change in perception influences behavior of the self towards the other (person) (Zinner and Shapiro).
3. **Unresolved loss/grief.** When a family member(s) has not fully grieved the loss of a relationship, a current relationship can become emotionally charged at points where they too closely resemble (or fail to resemble closely enough) the lost relationship. Similar to projective identification, interactions between family members tend to enhance the personality qualities in a living member that resemble the member who has died or has been lost (e.g., a child that may have qualities of the absent parent in a divorce becomes more like that parent).

445

4. **Clarity of ego boundaries.** The lack of clarity of ego boundaries leads to the use of projection, to distortion of reality testing, and to the need for other methods (or defenses) in order to stabilize emotional distance.

C. **What They Do**
   1. **Take a verbal history and/or do a genogram.**
   2. **Clarify communication** process between family members.
   3. **Interpret the transference** (note: family members' transference objects are in the room), and encourage insight.
   4. **Use of psychodramatic techniques,** such as the double or role reversal.

D. **Representative Therapists**
   1. **Nathan Ackerman** (interlocking pathology)
   2. **Norman Paul** (unresolved mourning)
   3. **James Framo** (family of origin)
   4. **Ivan Nagy** (the "family ledger," and contextual family therapy)
   5. **Murray Bowen** (multigenerational transmission through fusion/differentiation and emotional triangles)
   6. **JL Moreno** (psychodrama)

III. Symbolic-Experiential Family Therapy

A. **What They Think About**
   1. Based on early exposure to play therapy and to children's metaphorical, nonanalytical emotional processes, the focus of the therapy is on the **here-and-now. "Learning" takes place spontaneously in the therapy room through the direct effort of the therapist, who sets the context for growth experiences.**
   2. Symbolic/experiential therapists consider themselves to be **"atheoretical."**

B. **What They Look For**
   1. They set out to identify the prominent areas of distress by **experiencing the rigid, repetitive cycling of interaction among family members.**

C. **What They Do**
   1. Use one's self.
   2. Use spontaneity to:
      a. **Disorganize rigid, repetitive cycling of interaction through the use of play and experimentation.**
      b. **Highlight covert family conflicts.**
      c. **Activate and allow constructive anxiety or confusion** in family members other than the symptom-bearer. They tend to increase the focus on others instead of on the scapegoat, and to avoid blame of the caretaking parent (or spouse).
   3. **Redefine the symptoms as efforts for growth.**

4. **Model fantasy alternatives** to real stress, replacing key players in certain conflicts with the therapist. They also tend to encourage and support any new decisions.
5. **Create transgenerational boundaries.** They are known for encouraging extended family reunions.

D. **Representative Therapists**
   1. **Carl Whitaker** (Theater of the Absurd); Whitaker along with Napier is the author of *The Family Crucible.*
   2. **Walter Kempler** (Gestalt).
   3. **Virginia Satir** (Master Communicator) clarified communication and encouraged affect. A physically active therapist, she created a therapy that was both affirming and positively focused. She is known for her book *Conjoint Family Therapy.*
   4. **JL Moreno** (psychodrama).

IV. Behavioral Family Therapy

A. **What They Think About**
   1. Behavior, particularly maladaptive or problematic, is learned through **reinforcement (conditioning) or modeling.** This behavior can be extinguished and replaced by new learned behavior patterns.

B. **What They Look For**
   1. Maladaptive here-and-now behaviors that are reinforced.

C. **What They Do**
   1. Treatment is primarily cognitive, with the use of positive and negative behavioral reinforcement.

D. **Representative Therapists**
   1. **Robert Liberman and Richard Stuart** (behavioral marital therapy/social exchange theory)
   2. **Gerald Patterson** (behavioral parent skills training)
   3. **James Alexander** (functional family therapy)
   4. **Ian Falloon** (expressed emotion [EE])

V. Structural Family Therapy

This therapy evolved out of work with "psychosomatic families" (e.g., those with asthma, diabetes, or anorexia), and multiproblem families, especially those with delinquent children. Structuralists have a relatively fixed image of a normal family with respect to the life-cycle and cultural norm.

A. **What They Think About**
   The **focus for change is the family's "structure,"** which is considered to be a manifestation of the transactional patterns (actions) between the family members.

B. **What They Look For**
   1. Structuralists set out to identify the **"rules" that regulate family relationships** through observing repetitive patterns of behavior. These include:

a. **Boundaries:** who participates in a given activity and how. When a group of people participate in a set of repetitive transactions they form a subsystem. Each subsystem has rules (expectations) for behavior and function; for example, the parental system is in charge of those actions related to nurturance, guidance, and control. The spousal, parental, and child subsystems are the most important. The function of the boundary is to protect the differentiation of the subsystem from interference, allowing for contact between subsystem members and others. Clear boundaries are necessary for proper functioning. Three major types of boundaries exist along a continuum: the disengaged, the permeable, and the enmeshed.

b. **Alignment:** the joining or opposition of a family member in relation to another. These include **alliances** (with another) and **coalitions** (against another).

c. **Power/hierarchy:** this relates to the relative influence of each family member in relation to the others.

2. The following transactional patterns have been identified in psychosomatic and dysfunctional families:

a. **Enmeshment:** poorly differentiated, weak, and easily crossed subsystem boundaries. (Note: this type of boundary would be considered normal between mother and infant, and dysfunctional between parent and adolescent.)

b. **Overprotectiveness:** excessive "nurturance" is constantly elicited and supplied. Family members are hypersensitive to signs of distress in each other. This often occurs at the cost of autonomy and boundary differentiation.

c. **Rigidity:** retaining accustomed ways of interacting when they are no longer appropriate. Here, transactions and rules do not have the flexibility to change when changes in family structure are called for (e.g., during a shift from latency age to adolescence).

d. **Lack of conflict resolution:** problems that are left unresolved consistently reappear and reactivate the system's avoidance circuits. Three types of avoidance mechanisms have been described:

  i. **Triangulation:** a person is caught in a disagreement between two others and is simultaneously asked to side with each.

  ii. **Parent-child coalition:** a child is in a fixed alliance with one parent and against the other parent when needed.

  iii. **Detouring:** a person (often a parent) may detour conflict through their attention to another, often a child.

C. What They Do

1. **The therapist acts as a master director who, in a problem-oriented way, helps change the family's structure (patterns of interaction) through in-session moves and out-of-session tasks.** When pathologic interactions no longer exist, the symptom (seen as a transactional pattern between persons) is no longer needed to stabilize the system.

2. Therapy is done through:

a. **Joining** (relating personally for professional purposes) in order to assess the family's structure (subsystems, boundaries, hierarchy and power).

b. Creation of an in-session **enactment** (asking or provoking family members to act out the problem in the therapy room).

c. **Tracking of sequences** (elucidating individuals' beliefs and repetitive actions that reinforce the stability of the problem).

d. **Goals** are set. This includes the family's overt goal and (often) the therapist's covert goal.

e. Once the above are accomplished, the therapist then sets out to restructure the family's transactions through **reframing** the problem and using in-session **tasks** and out-of-session **homework assignments.**

D. Representative Therapists

1. **Salvador Minuchin** (*Families and Family Therapy, Families of the Slums, Family Therapy Techniques, Psychosomatic Families*)

2. **Stanton and Todd** (drug addiction)

3. **Aponte, Fishman, Montalvo, and Rossman** (multi-problem families, troubled adolescents)

VI. Family Psychoeducational Treatment

Psychoeducational treatment is a strategy for treating disabling, chronic illnesses (e.g., schizophrenia) with functional impairment. The focus of attention is shifted from the etiology of the illness to the determinants of the course of the illness, and to the social processes (e.g., family interactions) which influence it.

A. What They Think About

1. **The central notion is that families and other natural social groups can be trained to create an intentional environment that compensates for, and may partially correct, functional disability in a member of the group.**

2. George Brown, in London, hypothesized that affective factors (**expressed emotion [EE]**) might account for relapse. Expressed emotion consists of both an attitudinal aspect (e.g., highly critical views of the patient), and a behavioral component (e.g., a tendency to be "overinvolved"—highly protective, attentive or reactive) in relation to the patient. He found that, when expressed emotion is high, relapse occurs more frequently.

B. What They Look For

1. **Level of the family expressed emotion.**

2. **Assessment of family structure** (boundaries, alignment, power/hierarchy).

3. **Assessment of communication processes,** especially the presence of blaming, or the ability to make

requests for changes in behavior, to admit vulnerability, to stay on the topic, or to get a consensus on resolution of conflict and problems.

4. **Knowledge** about the illness, and the possession of **coping skills.**

C. **What They Do**

1. **They work both with individual families and with family groups.**

2. **There are four phases of treatment:**

   a. **Engagement** with the family, usually at the time of an acute psychotic episode.

   b. **Education** workshops in which clinicians present information and didactically describe key behavioral guidelines.

   c. A re-entry period, with biweekly sessions focused on stabilizing the patient outside the hospital.

   d. A **rehabilitation** phase that consists of sessions that emphasize the slow and careful raising of the patient's level of functioning.

3. **Work is done directly to decrease the expressed emotion and to help the family resolve conflicts and clarify communication.**

D. **Representative Therapists**

1. **William McFarlane**

2. **Ian Falloon**

3. **Carol Anderson**

VII. Milan Systemic Therapy

The Milan Systemic Therapy began with four Italian psychoanalysts (Selvini-Palazzoli, Boscolo, Cecchin, and Prata). They worked as co-therapy teams, with one team conducting the interview and the other team observing from behind a one-way mirror. In the process, the team behind the mirror noticed ("discovered") the circular pattern of interaction that exists between family members, and between family members and the therapist. They are particularly known for the idea that the therapist is an integral part of the system, and for the development of circular questioning.

A. **What They Think About**

1. The mental significance of any particular behavior or event which may be derived from its social context. Behavioral effects and not intentions are evaluated.

2. **Circular patterns of interaction** exist between family members and between the family and the therapist. **The observer is part of the system being observed.**

3. **Patterns co-evolve** between family members and become redundant. If the family is unable to adopt new patterns of action when change is needed, and instead continue to do more of what they are already doing, they become

"stuck." This intensified redundancy of actions develops into a "symptom."

4. **Change of beliefs leads to behavioral change.**

5. Solutions, and the ability to change, reside within the family, not the therapist.

6. Spontaneous change can occur.

7. There is no one truth (taken from constructivism).

8. The **"team," "family game,"** and **"invariant prescription"** are associated with this school.

B. **What They Look For**

1. **Systemic therapists focus on recursive actions, the circular relationships among the family members, and the beliefs that control the family members' actions.**

C. **What They Do**

1. Milan Systemic therapists are **known for using a team approach, the one-way mirror, and for conducting "long-term brief"** (long sessions with a month between each meeting) **therapy.**

2. Sometime during the session the family therapist(s) stop the interview and confer with the team members behind the mirror. At the end of the interview, a message, composed by the team, is read or sent to the family. This often includes a **paradoxical or positively connoted intervention.**

3. The sessions are noted for **"hypothesizing,"** for **"circularity,"** and for **neutrality** (not allying with the reality of any particular family member).

4. Systemic therapists are particularly known for the use of **"circular questions,"** which move the listener to an observing position.

   a. Circular questions are questions about relationships. They are "circular" because they attempt to make explicit the implicit circular connectedness of actions and of relationships.

   b. This form of questioning allows the physician and family members to experience themselves within the context of their relationships, particularly how they recursively or reciprocally influence each other.

   c. A circular question asks one person to consider the perceptions or beliefs of another person (e.g., family member, peer, medical staff) who is in relationship with the patient or his illness; for example, "What do you think concerns your wife most about your illness?" or "If your illness improves, whose life would change the most? In what way?"

5. Attention is paid to the family's simultaneous and paradoxical request for **change/no change.**

D. **Representative Therapists**

1. **Milan Team (Mara Selvini-Palazzoli, Boscolo, Cecchin, and Prata)**

2. **Peggy Papp and Peggy Penn** (the Greek Chorus)

VIII. Strategic Family Therapy

A. What They Think About

1. The focus of attention is on **problem solving.**
2. **Life-cycle transitions, both predictable (e.g., marriage, birth of a child, adolescence) and unpredictable (e.g., loss of a job, illness, death), demand shifts in how people perceive and relate to each other. At these times, new behavioral ways of relating (solutions for problems) must come into play. If new behaviors don't occur the family becomes "stuck" and a symptom develops.**
3. Problems are perceived as misguided attempts at changing an existing difficulty. **"The solution becomes the problem"** (Watzlawick et al., 1974) when family members persist in trying to change a current difficulty by applying a solution that had worked in other situations, but works poorly for the current problem. The family members' understanding (belief) of "common sense" supports their persistent (behavioral) efforts, even though they are not achieving success. The individual(s) within the family become locked into this (now pathologic) sequence or pattern of behaviors and cannot see a way to alter them (like a tire spinning in the mud).
4. **Strategic therapists believe that an individual can't be expected to change unless the system that sustains his or her symptoms changes.** They believe that problems cannot be considered apart from the context in which they occur and the functions for which they serve. Thus, **a detailed analysis of the current context of the problem is more important than a detailed history of the problem.**
5. The problem is often the result of a **double bind** (a conflict in the content and relationship levels of a message). The person(s) caught in double bind can neither solve the problem nor leave the field.
6. **Pragmatics is important, insight per se is not.**
7. Strategic therapy has been strongly influenced by hypnosis, and the work of **Milton Erikson.**

B. What They Look For

1. Strategic therapists are interested in the here-and-now: **the temporal relationships and repetitive series of actions that maintain the problem.** They are particularly sensitive to the issues of **power** and to those that involve either paradox or a double bind.
2. **Solution-focused strategic therapists** show preferential interest in discovering **"exceptions to the rule"** (when the problem would be expected to occur, but doesn't). Rather than focusing upon an analysis of the behavioral sequences maintaining the problem, they seek to identify naturally occurring behavioral sequences that take place when the problem doesn't happen, and therefore might serve as candidate solutions.

C. What They Do

1. Their **focus is on solving the problem (symptom).** The problem as the family describes it must be changed into a solvable form, one that is co-created by the therapist and the family.
2. Through **questions, enactments, and homework assignments** the therapist tries to discover the "unseen" problem: the family's maladaptive effort to solve what is maintaining the problem. Strategic therapists are interested in who, what, when, where, and in what way, people are involved.
3. Strategies are aimed at **tracking and disrupting the sequences of behavior and meanings** that maintain the problem, and interventions are aimed at **restructuring** the family's transactional sequences in a healthier way.
4. **Psychoeducation and compliance-based directives** are both used.
5. Strategic therapists are best known for their **defiance-based, paradoxical directives.** They include:
   a. **Reframing or relabeling the symptom.** By changing the context of the sequence of actions that constitute the symptom one can change the meaning of the event; e.g., telling an adolescent who consistently comes in past her curfew that she is doing her younger brother a huge favor as her action binds her parents' attention, allowing him to do what he wants without being noticed.
   b. **Prescribing the symptom.** The therapist encourages or instructs the family member(s) to engage in the specific behavior that needs to be eliminated using a "new" rationale that is acceptable in its logic, but makes the old behavior(s) unacceptable; e.g., telling the older sister how wonderful she is to sacrifice herself for her younger brother and to continue her (negative) behavior.
   c. **Restraining the system.** The therapist attempts to discourage or even deny the possibility of change, therefore hoping the family will defy him/her and continue to change.
   d. **Positioning.** The therapist attempts to shift a problematic "position" (usually an assertion that the patient is making about himself, the problem, or another family member), by accepting and exaggerating that position. This is used when one family member's position is considered to be maintained by a complementary or opposite response in the other; e.g., telling the person who is a penny-pincher to be even more frugal because it allows the spendthrift more money to spend.
6. The new **solution-focused strategic therapists focus on identifying, amplifying, and predicting the "exceptions"** to the rule (occasions when the problem or symptom might have been expected to

occur, but doesn't). This allows alternative perceptions, possibilities, and "stories" to be uncovered. The following questions are often used by these therapists:

   a. "Between now and the next time that we meet, I would like you to observe, so that you can describe to us next time, what happens when (e.g.) you would expect John to lie and he doesn't."

   b. **The miracle question:** "Suppose that one night, while you were asleep, there was a miracle and this problem was solved. How would you know? What would be different?" The therapist then negotiates with the family members what part of this new reality they would be willing to implement the next day, as if the miracle had occurred.

D. Representative Therapists

1. The Mental Research Institute (**MRI**) in California (Gregory Bateson, Don Jackson, Jay Haley, Paul Watzlawick, and John Weakland)

2. **J Haley and Cloe Madanes** (paradox and ordeal therapy)

3. **Steve deShazer, Inso Berg, and Michelle Weiner-Davis** (solution-focused strategic therapy)

IX. Narrative Family Therapy

A. What They Think About

Narrative therapists conduct their therapy from a position of "not knowing." That is to say, the therapist does not have any set ideas about what and how change should occur. The therapy is "co-created" by the therapist and family and takes its shape according to the emergent qualities of the conversation that inspires it.

1. The **dominant narratives of an individual's life organizes his/her perceptions and behaviors.**

2. The perceptions that family members have of themselves and others are structured, and limited by the stories, the language, and the metaphors they use.

3. A problem occurs when:

   a. The **narratives available** for guiding perception, cognition, and action **preclude interactions** other than with the ones seen.

   b. Family members lack either the needed emotional vocabulary or narrative skills to make the story of their experience understandable to others.

   c. Family members have become positioned in the relationship where they have stopped talking or listening.

   d. **Therapy provides a context where self-narratives can be told, heard, or expanded in meaning.**

B. What They Look (or Listen) For

1. **Dominant narratives that constrain the relationship.**

2. **Alternative narratives** in unnoticed or forgotten experience.

3. **Through the use of questions that evoke curiosity and reflection, the therapist attempts to understand the way in which the family members' ideas and beliefs are patterned.**

4. Narrative therapists are particularly attentive to listen for **emotionally charged words, and for specific language or metaphors** used in describing the problem. Implicit metaphors serve as maps that are embedded in language—and language always influences the selection of life events that are noticed. The events noticed contain meaning and dictate the selection of behaviors available.

C. What They Do

1. **The therapist and family members work to co-create (jointly develop) new, more useful, life stories.**

2. **Questions are used not to seek information from the listener, but rather to change how the listener processes information.** Karl Tomm introduced the term "interventive interviewing" to describe the use of these questions.

3. **Narrative therapists consider themselves to be collaborative, respectful, and less hierarchical than the earlier family therapists.**

4. Narrative therapists have been known to make use of the **reflecting team** (Tom Andersen). Midway through a family meeting the team behind the one-way mirror changes places with the therapist and family. The family and therapist now observe behind the mirror as the team discusses (reflects on) them. When the reflections are completed, the family and team again change places and the therapist asks the family what they found to be useful. The idea is that family member(s) are only able to take in the new ideas that they are ready to hear.

5. **Externalize the problem.** Michael White and David Epston have created a series of questions that separate the problem from the person. These include:

   a. **Relative influence questions,** which are designed to compare the influence of the problem over the life of the family member(s), and the influence of the family member(s) over the problem. These questions are followed by:

   b. **Unique outcome questions,** which ask for exceptions to the usual descriptions of failure in the struggle with the problem. These exceptions can nearly always be identified, but often go unnoticed when one has accepted a life narrative of failure.

D. Representative Therapists

1. **H. Goolishian and H. Anderson** (the problem-oriented system)

2. **Tom Andersen** and the Tromsø team (reflecting team)

3. **Michael White and David Epston** (externalizing the problem)

4. **Karl Tomm** (interventive interviewing)

X. Conclusion

Family therapy, although still recognizable, is very different now than it was at its inception. The evolution and current integration of theory and clinical need have created a therapy that is more collaborative, respectful, and less hierarchical than earlier forms of family therapy. Therapeutic attention is more focused on strengths and resources and less on pathology. Although the therapist is no longer considered to be the one who holds "the truth," he or she continues to develop ideas and skills useful for healing.

Suggested Readings

Andersen T: Dialogue and meta-dialogue in clinical work. *Fam Process* 1987; 26:415–428.

Aponte H, VanDeusen J: Structural family therapy. In Gurman A, Kniskern D (eds): *Handbook of Family Therapy*. New York: Brunner/Mazel, 1981.

Bodin A: The interactional view: family therapy approaches of the Mental Research Institute. In Gurman A, Kniskern D (eds): *Handbook of Family Therapy*. New York: Brunner/Mazel, 1981.

Bowen M: *Family Therapy in Clinical Practice*. New York: Jason Aronson, 1978.

deShazer S: *Keys to Solution in Brief Therapy*. New York: Norton, 1985.

deShazer S, Berg I, Lipchik E, et al.: Brief therapy: focused solution development. *Fam Process* 1986; 25:207–223.

Goldenberg I, Goldenberg H (eds): *Family Therapy: An Overview*. Monterey, CA: Brooks/Cole, 1980.

Goolishian H, Anderson H: Language systems and therapy: an evolving idea [special issue: Psychotherapy with families]. *Psychotherapy* 1987; 24:529–537.

Hoffman L: Constructing realities: an art of lenses. *Fam Process* 1990; 20:1–13.

Madanes C: *Strategic Family Therapy*. San Francisco, CA: Jossey-Bass, 1981.

Minuchin S: *Families and Family Therapy*. Cambridge, MA: Harvard University Press, 1974.

Penn P: Circular questioning. *Fam Process* 1982; 21:267–280.

Selvini-Palazzoli M, Boscolo L, Cecchin G, Prata G: Hypothesizing-circularity-neutrality: three guidelines for the conductor of the session. *Fam Process* 1980; 19:3–12.

Slovik L, Griffith J: The current face of family therapy. In Rutan S (ed.): *Psychotherapy for the 1990s*. New York: Guilford Publications, 1992.

Stanton MD: Strategic approaches to family therapy. In Gurman A, Kniskern D (eds): *Handbook of Family Therapy*. New York, Brunner/Mazel, 1981.

Tomm K: Interventive interviewing: Part I. Strategizing as a fourth guideline for the therapist. *Fam Process* 1987; 26:3–14.

von Bertalanffy L: *General Systems Theory: Foundation, Development, Applications*. New York: Brazillier, 1968.

Watzlawick P, Weakland J, Fisch R: *Change: Principles of Problem Formation and Problem Resolution*. New York: Norton, 1974.

Weiner A: *Cybernetics*. Cambridge, MA: MIT Press, 1961.

Whitaker C, Napier A: *The Family Crucible*. New York: Harper and Row, 1978.

White M: Negative explanation, restraint, and double description: a template for family therapy. *Fam Process* 1988; 125:169–184.

White M: The process of questioning: a therapy of literary merit. *Dulwich Centre Newsl* 1988; Winter:8–14.

White M: The externalizing of the problem and the re-authoring of lives and relationships. *Dulwich Centre Newsl* 1988/89; Summer.

Zinner J, Shapiro R: Projective identification as a mode of perception and behavior in families and adolescents. *Int J Psychoanal* 1972; 53:523.

Chapter 62

Group Psychotherapy

ANNE ALONSO

I. Introduction

A. Overview

People thrive best in a community that values their participation and protects their dignity. The stresses that impinge on individuals are defined in part by their biology, in part by their family dynamics, and also by the culture in which they live. The integration of mind, body, and social context is vulnerable to assault from problems in any one of these dimensions. **Group psychotherapy offers the opportunity for purposefully created, closely observed, and skillfully guided interpersonal interaction.** Such interactions can positively influence the countless varieties of human distress and malfunction. Distorted perceptions of others, insufficient communications, inadequately discharged affects, stereotyped behaviors, impulsive actions, and alienation can all be addressed and modified within the therapeutic group (see Table 62-1).

B. What Is a Therapy Group?

A therapy group is a collection of patients selected and brought together by the leader for a shared therapeutic goal (see Table 62-1).

C. What Are Common Therapeutic Assumptions?

Group therapy rests on some common assumptions across the whole panoply of therapeutic groups:

1. **A universal and primary need for attachment. The need for attachment is seen as primary** by a whole host of group theorists; the press for belonging is that which yields a sense of cohesion that can help the individual stay with the anxious new moments in a group of strangers.

2. **Contagion. For better and for worse, people who wish to belong to a cohesive community are apt to mimic and identify with the feelings and beliefs of other members of that community.** At its best, this process allows for new interpersonal learning; at its worst, it raises the specter of dangerous mobs.

3. **Amplification. An increasing exposure to feelings, needs, and drives increases the individual's awareness of his or her own passions,** and allows for a more direct and conscious management of those impulses.

4. **Intimate exchanges.** Of necessity **the members of a cohesive group experience their own approaches to intimacy with others and with the self, and receive** immediate feedback on the impact they have on important others in their surround.

D. How Do These Intimate Exchanges Heal?

Close interactions between the members of a group yield beneficent effects **by generating interpersonal situations that:**

1. Reduce isolation.
2. Diminish shame.
3. Evoke early familial interactions and feelings.
4. Expand the individual's emotional and behavioral repertoire.
5. Provide support and empathic confrontation.
6. Help people grieve.

E. What Aspects of Groups Are Therapeutic?

Whatever the model, group therapy rests on the assumptions that there are healing factors that emerge and operate in all groups, and that some of these can be brought into play to allow the individual within the group to grow and develop beyond the constrictions in life that brought that person into treatment. While some group theorists rely on a cluster of factors relevant to their models of the mind and of pathology, all utilize some of the whole group of therapeutic factors identified in Table 62-2.

II. Creation and Goals of Groups

A. How Does the Therapist Plan and Organize a Group?

Before approaching the concrete work of planning and organizing a psychotherapy group, **the goals of the group must be clearly understood and developed by the leader.** These goals in turn will be dependent on the setting, the population, the time available for treatment, and the training and capacity of the leader(s).

B. What Are the Goals of Groups?

Therapists form groups for a whole range of therapeutic purposes. The main ones are to:

1. **Re-establish premorbid levels of functioning. People in acute and immediate distress often find support in groups that have as their main goal a re-establishment of a person's equilibrium.** Patients who have suffered a breakdown of their lives and who have needed hospitalization can utilize groups within the inpatient or partial hospital setting. These

Table 62-1. Comparison of Different Types of Group Psychotherapy

Parameters	Day Hospital/Inpatient Group	Supportive Group Therapy	Psychodynamic Group	Cognitive-Behavioral Group
Frequency	3–5 times/week	Once a week	1–3 times/week	Once a week
Duration	1 week to 6 months	Up to 6 months or more	1–3 + years	Up to 6 months
Indications	Acute or chronic major mental illness	Shared universal dilemmas	Neurotic disorders and borderline states	Phobias, compulsive problems, etc.
Pregroup screening	Sometimes	Usually	Always	Usually
Content focus	Extent and impact of illness; plan for return to baseline	Symptoms, loss, life management	Present and past life situations; intragroup and extragroup relationships	Cognitive distortions, specific symptoms
Transference	Positive institutional transference encouraged	Positive transference encouraged to promote improved functioning	Positive and negative to leader and members, evoked and analyzed	Positive relationship to leader fostered; no examination of transference
Therapist activity	Empathy and reality testing	Strengthen existing defenses by actively giving advice and support	Challenge defenses, reduce shame, interpret unconscious conflict	Create new options, active and directive
Interaction outside of group	Encouraged	Encouraged	Discouraged	Variable
Goals	Reconstitute defenses	Better adaptation to environment	Reconstruction of personality dynamics	Relief of specific psychiatric symptoms

groups have as their primary focus the restructuring of the patient's sensorium, the management of acute distress, and planning for a return to the community. These patients also need help in dealing with the shameful consequences of hospitalization, and with the sometimes elusive process of establishing outpatient treatment that will support them upon discharge. A benevolent inpatient or partial hospital group experience will be of special value with the latter problem, since affordable treatment will be primarily offered in group therapy for the foreseeable future.

Many patients who have been hospitalized after an acute illness, or who attend partial hospitalization programs, need to regain equilibrium, deal with the shame inherent in losing the ability to live independently, and prepare to re-enter the world outside of the therapeutic environment.

2. **Support targeted patient populations.** Since the time that Dr. Pratt offered his "classes" for tubercular patients at the Massachusetts General Hospital in 1905, **people have come together to commiserate with one another around common problems,** to

share information, and to learn how to deal with the impact of those problems on their lives. **Groups have been organized around medical illnesses** (such as cancer, diabetes, and acquired immunodeficiency syndrome [AIDS]), **around psychological problems** (such as bereavement), **and around psychosocial sequelae of trauma** (such as war or natural disasters). The goals of such groups are to provide support and information embedded in a socially accepting environment with people who are in a position to really understand what the others are going through. The treatment may emerge from cognitive-behavioral principles, psychodynamic principles, or psycho-educational ones. Frequently, these groups tend to be time-limited; members often join at the same time and terminate together. The problems addressed in these groups are found in a broad variety of patients, from the very healthy to the more distressed, and cut across other demographic variables, such as age and culture. Increasingly, research data have shown that involvement in these groups can have remarkably positive effects on extending survival

Table 62-2. Some Therapeutic Factors in Group Psychotherapy

Factor	Definition
Acceptance	The feeling of being accepted by other members of the group; differences of opinion are tolerated, and there is an absence of censure.
Altruism	The act of one member's being of help to another; putting another person's need before one's own and learning that there is value in giving to others. The term was originated by August Comte (1798–1957), and Freud believed it was a major factor in establishing group cohesion and community feeling.
Cohesion	The sense that the group is working together toward a common goal; also referred to as a sense of "we-ness"; believed to be the most important factor related to positive therapeutic effects.
Contagion	The process in which the expression of emotion by one member stimulates the awareness of a similar emotion in another member.
Corrective familial experience	The group recreates the family of origin for some members who can work through original conflicts psychologically through group interaction (e.g., sibling rivalry, anger towards parents).
Empathy	A capacity of a group member to put himself or herself into the psychological frame of reference of another group member and thereby understand his or her thinking, feeling, or behavior.
Imitation	The conclusion emulation or modeling of one's behavior after that of another (also called role modeling); also known as spectator therapy, as one patient learns from another.
Insight	Conscious awareness and understanding of one's own psychodynamics and symptoms of maladaptive behavior. Most therapists distinguish two types: (1) intellectual insight—knowledge and awareness without any changes in maladaptive behavior; (2) emotional insight—awareness and understanding leading to positive changes in personality and behavior.
Inspiration	The process of imparting a sense of optimism to group members; the ability to recognize that one has the capacity to overcome problems; also known as instillation of hope.
Interpretation	The process during which the group leader formulates the meaning or significance of a patient's resistance, defenses, and symbols; the result is that the patient develops a cognitive framework within which to understand his or her behavior.
Learning	Patients acquire knowledge about new areas, such as social skills, and sexual behavior; they receive advice, obtain guidance, attempt to influence, and are influenced by, other group members.
Reality testing	Ability of the person to evaluate objectively the world outside the self; includes the capacity to perceive oneself and other group members accurately.
Ventilation	The expression of suppressed feelings, ideas, or events to other group members; the sharing of personal secrets that ameliorate a sense of sin or guilt (also referred to as self-disclosure).

and on the quality of life for the severely ill (e.g., a woman with end-stage breast cancer).

3. **Provide relief for certain symptoms.** Group treatment may target specific symptoms. This approach to psychopathology is congruent with categorical nosological systems, such as the DSM-IV. Diagnosis here is seen as symptomatic rather than developmental; treatment goals include alleviation of symptoms. For example, patients with eating disorders or specific phobias are clustered in groups which can then promote skills for self-mon-

itoring and for replacement of an automatic symptom with a more adaptive set of behaviors and cognitions. These groups may include members with a broad range of intrapsychic development, which is not the primary focus of the group. At the same time, some people who work successfully in these groups may want to continue the work of personality change in open-ended dynamic groups when their symptoms are relieved.

4. **Encourage and stimulate character change. Character difficulties are tenacious for all human**

beings, from the healthiest neurotic to the most regressed patient. For all individuals, character problems are:

a. Outside of the patient's awareness.

b. Syntonic and perceived as "Who I am" when brought into awareness.

c. Resistant to change, even when the patient wants to make such a change.

d. Repeated compulsively until worked through; that is, they are robbed of some of their power with each experience of successful change to better alternatives.

e. Difficult to change without strong motivation to overcome psychological inertia.

The neurotic patient will find intrapsychic conflicts emerging in the interpersonal field of group, and make use of the group's curative factors to overcome the resistances to newer intimacies. Some of the earlier literature on group treatment expressed doubts about the appropriateness of this "uncovering" kind of group for sicker patients. More recently, group theorists have argued that the distributed transferences in a group mitigate an overly threatening regression for such patients. Character problems have a tenacity that is difficult to reorganize in brief treatment. Instead, the process requires frequent regressions in the service of the ego, and attempts to work through the same characterological habits again and again. At the same time, brief analytic and cognitive-behavioral group models have been used to address sectors of the personality difficulties, to good effect.

C. How Should a Therapy Group Be Conducted?
The success of a group depends on the ability of the therapist to provide a safe context and meaning for the therapy group. This is done by designing a contract around the group goal(s) and by carefully selecting members that are suitable for that group. For example, in a symptom-specific group, members should have similar symptoms and concerns; in a more psychodynamic group, members should be selected from a fairly homogeneous level of ego development, although their symptoms and character styles may differ along a wide spectrum.

D. What Are the Roles of the Group Leader?
Before the group begins, the leader must make several decisions that will have major implications for the whole enterprise. Beyond the obvious focus on the kind, duration, and theoretical underpinnings, **the leader must then decide on matters of:**

1. **Membership**
2. **Logistics (e.g., place, time, and fees)**
3. **Whether to work alone, or with a co-therapist.**
4. **Whether patients will be treated in group therapy alone or in some combination of group therapy, individual therapy, pharmacotherapy, or self-help group.**

5. **Managing records, and protecting confidentiality.**
In addition to the logistical decisions listed above, the leader's stance needs to be consistent with the goals of the group. A leader of a psychodynamic open-ended group will probably be more likely to sit back and allow the group's associations to lead the way for the group's work while he or she comments, like a critic at a concert. On the other hand, such a stance makes little sense for the leader of a cognitive-behavioral group, who is engaged in conducting desensitization exercises, and in providing cognitive restructuring, including homework exercises to meet the goals of that therapeutic endeavor.

E. How Should Patients Be Prepared for a Group?
Both anecdotal and empirical evidence shows that investment of significant amounts of time in preparation of a patient for group therapy will improve the chances of a successful entry into a group. In addition to the usual history taking, it is very helpful to examine the patient's fantasies and biases about groups and to collect the history of their participation in all kinds of groups (e.g., family, school, sports, work, friendships). This is the time to discuss the group's agreements and the rationale that underlies them, and to elicit the patient's collaboration in the enterprise by making as much information available as possible. Patients are helped by knowing how the group works, by knowing what the leader's role might be, and by knowing what they might expect for themselves.

A typical agreement includes expectations about constant attendance, duration of the group, the content of the patient's discussions, and the commitment to confidentiality and to financial obligations. Beyond those, each specific group will have more particular expectations; for example, a cognitive-behavioral group may expect "homework" from the members, a more psychodynamic group may encourage dream analysis.

F. How Does the Group Deal with Authority and Group Leadership?
A group leader must exercise authority over each of the above factors if the group is to be safe and containing for its members. Whether a member who is difficult in the group stays or leaves or whether a new member enters must not be left to a vote, just as such decisions are not made within a family. The privilege and burden of administrative and inclusion/exclusion matters is a serious responsibility of the group leader, as is the question of single or co-therapy leadership. It is important to remember that the leader is not a member of the group, despite the ambivalent entreaties of the members to bring the leader into the group. The clearer the

leader is about the boundaries, the safer are the members to indulge their fantasies of wanting to corrupt the process, or overcome the leader's authority.

The fiduciary responsibilities of the leader are better maintained to the extent that the leader exercises restraint and relative neutrality in the sense of nonjudgmental listening and responding to the patients' struggles. By remaining warm and neutral, the leader is in a position to listen nonjudgmentally to all aspects of the whole group's impulses and resistance, without taking sides or carrying the burden of somehow policing the group, and deciding which are good feelings and interactions, and which are not.

G. How Does a Group Deal with the Incorruptibility of the Leader?
In a therapy group, as in any therapeutic work, **the leader must remain as pure as Caesar's wife;** dual roles are unacceptable, no overly familiar incursions into the members' personal lives, nor theirs of the leader are tolerated. No special fee arrangements that are not in the awareness of the group can be tolerated without damaging the integrity of the group boundaries. In short, all group business that cannot be conducted in the group ought not to be conducted at all. This refusal to hold secret any extra-group contacts sets a fine model that says the group is a safe therapeutic agent.

H. How Does One Deal with the Question of Co-therapy?
As in many clinical decisions, **the question of leading alone or with a colleague depends in part on the model, in part on the context and setting, in part on the availability of an appropriate co-therapist, and the system's support,** administrative and otherwise, for committing two professionals to the same task at the same time.

Inpatient or partial hospitalization groups tend to meet several times a week, and, for those groups, co-therapy is a useful way to ensure continuity of leadership. On the other hand, some analytic group leaders avoid co-therapy because of the splitting of the patient-to-leader transferences. There are no rigid rules, but certain caveats must be observed.

Co-therapists work best when:
1. They are truly co-therapists, of relatively equal status and experience. In cases where a student and a supervisor work together, it is useful to acknowledge this reality.
2. They share a common theory base.
3. They are willing to dedicate an hour or so per week to working out their collaborative problems and their perceptions of the group.

4. They are comfortable in sharing the fee.
Failure to observe these agreements may leave the patients low on the priority list of therapeutic concern while the co-therapy pair compete or otherwise undercut one another. On the more positive side, when co-therapy works well, both clinicians and patients have the advantage of two professional heads and hearts working in concert for the benefit of all.

III. Who Should Be Treated in Group Therapy?

A. Indications for Group Treatment
In a psychodynamic group where early developmental conflicts and relationships are assumed to interfere with the here-and-now of the patient's life, it will be important to organize a group that is reasonably homogeneous for the level of ego development and heterogeneous in every other regard. Mixing people of differing gender, cultures, and/or ages can be extremely useful so long as these patients emerge from a similar developmental spectrum. The differences among them can then be addressed and exploited to the advantage of the members in the group. However, when patients diverge sharply in levels of ego development, group cohesion and universality will be compromised. For example, a group of patients who experience severe anxiety around loss consequent to serious abandonment throughout their lives will do well to work together in a group. On the other hand, to mix two or three such patients in a group of people who are conflicted around intimacy and sustained relationships may well result in two subgroups, neither of which has an easy empathic rapport with the other's internal dilemmas. The specific symptom or population designation of other groups points the way by definition to patient selection.

B. Who Should Not Be Treated in Group Therapy?
Some patients are unable to make good use of group therapy without former clinical intervention. For example, the actively manic patient may be more overstimulated than helped in a group. Another category of patients frequently referred to groups includes severely schizoidal people who have really never developed sustained human relationships. To place these patients in a group overrides their capacity and sets them up for early failure. Acutely disturbed patients may need and deserve individual attention prior to entry into an ongoing therapy group. In all of these cases, prior treatment, either psychopharmacological and/or individual supportive therapy, may increase the

likelihood of the patient succeeding in the therapy group.

IV. Combined Therapies

A. **Group Therapy Combined with Individual Therapy**
Occasionally, patients are treated in both individual and group therapy, either by the same therapist or by two different ones. This option is useful for a variety of patients:
1. **The over-intellectualized patient.** For some patients, insight becomes a way to avoid feeling. When it does, it is very useful to place these patients in a therapy group where they can see how they are in the interaction with others who will offer feedback and affective resonance.
2. **The patient who cannot tolerate the dyadic transference of individual treatment.** Dyadic treatment can threaten the fragile ego boundaries of patients who are either very needy, or who are overstimulated by the apparent promises of the individual work. These patients often flee treatment, or regress to terrifying actions that can be life-threatening in what approaches psychotic levels of transference. Adding group therapy can distribute the transferences across the spectrum of all the members of the group and the group leader, and may enable the individual and the group treatment to proceed more safely and more productively.

B. **Collaboration between the Two Therapists**
It is crucial that the two therapists collaborate by frequent phone calls, and by avoiding the patients' likely attempts to split them. In the case where the two therapists do not agree, or do not respect the other's work, then the patient is potentially at great risk of harm, or at least in a stalemate that is iatrogenic in origin.

C. **Combined Treatment with the Same Therapist**
Patients will sometimes be seen in both individual and group therapy with the same therapist. There are many advantages and, as always, some costs to this treatment plan.

It is illuminating to deal with the intrapsychic dimensions of the patient in the individual hour, and then observe the same patient express those internal dilemmas and live them out in the interactions with members of the group. For example, a mild and extremely gentle individual patient might startle his or her therapist by launching a very aggressive attack on one or more members of the group when the shy facade is challenged.

For some patients, however, sharing the therapist's attention can be so distressing that the work of therapy is stalled. It may be far better for that patient to be referred to another leader's group, or to defer group treatment to a more secure time.

D. **Boundaries in Combined Treatment**
Clinicians struggle with how much to preserve the privacy of what they know about the patient from the dyadic hour when the patient enters the group, and how much to disclose. **While there are no hard and fast rules, what matters is consistency, and the prior agreement with the patient about this matter.** Many clinicians opt to protect the information while urging the patient to bring the problems into the group. One major exception is the case where the group or one of its members is at risk; as usual, the rules of confidentiality are suspended when there is any threat to safety of any of the participants. It is very useful to agree that all treaters will be in regular contact with one another in order to work for the patient's advantage.

E. **Is Group Therapy Primary or Adjunctive Treatment?**
As in most treatments that adhere to the biopsychosocial model, psychosocial treatment has an impact on the biology of the patient as well as on the psychology and the social adjustment of that person. In cases of more severe distress, a combination of group treatment, psychopharmacological treatment, and, occasionally, individual treatment, may be ideal. However, **given the cost constraints that delimit most mental health care, group therapy remains a very impressive primary treatment** for a whole host of patient situations and needs.

V. Legal and Ethical Considerations in Group Therapy

A. **The Leader and Confidentiality**
The group leader is bound by the usual rules of confidentiality in the group as in any other clinical encounter with the patient. With the exception of a threat to a person or persons, this confidentiality holds and is usually elaborated in the Code of Ethics of the therapist's professional organization. The same pertains to any conduct of the therapist that violates the code of ethics relative to sexual or other extra-professional contact with a patient.

B. **Group Members and Confidentiality**
The bigger challenge is confidentiality among members. **Aside from stressing the importance of protecting the identities of patients in the group, there is little that the leader can do to ensure compliance, nor is it against the law for members to break confidentiality.** Group therapists worry about whether the group can become a pool of witnesses in the case of a subpoena. Some states extend the same protection to the members that they do to the

leader, namely the patient-therapist privilege, but this has not been tested and may not apply with all professionals across the disciplines.

VI. Research, Outcome, and Evaluation

Research on group therapy has focused mostly on outcomes. More recently, measures have been developed that seek to relate the patient's sense of belonging and feeling valued in the group with the effectiveness of the treatment. Studies continue to support the importance of group cohesion on group effectiveness; feeling valued is seen as a statement of cohesion. Research also indicates greater confidence in the efficacy of group treatment, and shows no appreciable differences between individual, or group therapy, and pharmacotherapy. However, these studies remain problematic, given the problems that bedevil most social science research: it is difficult to control for therapist differences, and attempts to do so by providing manuals for intervention become different models than what happens in real life. Nonspecific factors are elusive, but seem to indicate that patients progress when they feel cared about, when the leader is warm and somewhat structured, when the match with colleagues in the group is appropriate, and when the goal and direction of the group are clear and consistent.

Researchers have moved beyond the question of do groups work, to a finer look at how they work, in what circumstances, and for whom. Proper and careful screening and otherwise preparing a patient to enter a group results in a greater chance of success in entering and staying. Members who are at about the same level of ego development do better in open-ended groups than they do in groups with a large disparity of ego levels of development. Short-term, focused groups are more successful if leaders are structured as to agenda, and time boundaries, and if the patients are more homogeneous with regard to the problem being addressed.

Research instruments are useful for measuring patient satisfaction, and self-reports of increased well-being. The Clinical Outcome Results battery developed by the American Group Psychotherapy Association is but one example; it utilizes such measures as the Symptom Checklist 90-Revised (SCL-90R), The Social Adjustment Scale Self Report (SAS-SR), The Multiple Affect Adjective Check List-Revised (MAACL-R), and the Global Assessment Scale (GAS). More recently, measures such as the Structured Analysis of Social Behavior and the Group Climate Questionnaire (GCQ) have been used extensively by MacKenzie and others who work with patients in structured time-limited groups.

A major shortcoming in group therapy research stems from the pragmatics of conducting research over a long time, and with more amorphous goals. Thus, most of the data emerges from research on time-limited groups, usually within the cognitive-behavioral or interpersonal model. While those findings are very important to secure, they have limited applicability for the more open-ended dynamic models of group treatment. That research remains to be enlarged upon. Of particular interest is the emerging research on recovery from severe physical illness (e.g., women with metastatic breast cancer). Women from that population were found to double their survival time, and to decrease their need for pain medication, if they also participated in group therapy along with their usual oncologic treatments.

VII. Consultation and Supervision for Group Therapy

It is often difficult for group leaders to ask for help, as it is difficult for most professional helpers, once they have gone beyond their formal training years. But failure to find help in conducting a group can increase the strain on the leader exponentially given the number of people in the consultation room, and the multiplicity of countertransference vectors. **A well-running group can look deceptively autonomous of the leader's impact, but the truth is that the leader's calmness and full attention is the platform on which the group grows.** Occasional consultations and/or ongoing peer supervision is a safe, judicious practice. It is also a way for the leader to take advantage of his or her affiliative needs and to avoid using the patient group for dealing with the loneliness of the well-functioning group leader. In addition to departmental faculty with group therapy expertise, there are professional organizations that offer ongoing training and supervision for group leaders at all levels of seniority.

Suggested Readings

Alonso A, Swiller HI (eds): *Group Therapy in Clinical Practice.* Washington, DC: American Psychiatric Press, 1993.

Bion WR: *Experiences in Groups.* London: Tavistock, 1961.

Bloch S, Crouch E: *Therapeutic Factors in Group Psychotherapy.* New York: Oxford University Press, 1985.

Brabender V, Fallon A: *Models of Inpatient Group Psychotherapy.* Washington, DC: American Psychiatric Press, 1993.

Durkin H: *The Group in Depth.* New York: International Universities Press, 1964.

Ezriel H: Psychoanalytic group therapy. In Wolberg LR, Schwartz EK (eds): *Group Therapy: 1973. An Overview.* New York: Intercontinental Medical Book Corp., 1973:183.

Foulkes SH: Group process and the individual in the therapeutic group. *Br J Med Psychol* 1961; 34:23.

Freud S: Group psychology and analysis of the ego. *Standard Edition of the Complete Psychological Works of Sigmund Freud.* London: Hogarth, 1962.

Gans JS: Broaching and exploring the question of combined group and individual therapy. *Int J Group Psychother* 1990; 40:123–137.

Glatzer H: The working alliance in analytic group psychotherapy. *Int J Group Psychother* 1978; 28:147.

Kaplan HI, Sadock BJ (eds): *Comprehensive Group Psychotherapy*, 3rd ed. Baltimore: Williams and Wilkins, 1999.

Kelly JA, Murphy DA, Bahr GR, et al.: Outcome of cognitive-behavioral and support group brief therapies for depressed, HIV-infected persons. *Am J Psychiatry* 1993; 150:1679.

Klein RH, Bernard HS, Singer DL (eds): *Handbook of Contemporary Group Psychotherapy*. Madison, CT: International Universities Press, 1992.

Leszcz M: The interpersonal approach to group psychotherapy. *Int J Group Psychother* 1992; 42:37–62.

MacKenzie KR (ed.): *Classics in Group Psychotherapy*. New York: Guilford Press, 1992.

MacKenzie KR: *Time-Managed Group Psychotherapy*. Washington, DC: American Psychiatric Press, 1997.

Malan DH, Balfour FHG, Hood VG, Shooter AMN: Group psychotherapy: a long-term follow-up study. *Arch Gen Psychiatry* 1976; 33:1303–1315.

Pam A, Kemper S: The captive group: guidelines for group therapists in the inpatient setting. *Int J Group Psychother* 1993; 43:419–438.

Riester AE, Kraft IA (eds): *Child Group Psychotherapy*. Madison, CT: International Universities Press, 1986.

Rutan JS, Stone WS (eds): *Psychodynamic Group Psychotherapy*. New York: Guilford Press, 1993.

Scheidlinger S: On the concept of "mother-group". *Int J Group Psychother* 1974; 24:417.

Spiegel D, Bloom JR, Kraemer HC, et al.: Effect of psychosocial treatment on survival of patients with metastatic breast cancer. *Lancet* 1989; 2(8668):888–891.

Chapter 63

Cognitive-Behavioral Therapy

JOHN MATTHEWS

I. Theoretical Basis

A. **Cognitive-behavioral therapy (CBT) is based on the interplay among cognition, mood, and behavior.** These relationships may be either positive or negative.

B. CBT is derived from numerous schools of thought. Within psychiatry, the major proponent of CBT has been **Aaron Beck,** and his daughter, **Judith Beck.**

C. **CBT assumes that all psychopathology is in part the product of distorted thinking, which in turn has a negative impact on mood and behavior. CBT identifies at least three problematic aspects of cognition:**
   1. **Dysfunctional automatic thoughts.** These thoughts are **spontaneous, unpremeditated misinterpretations of a given situation.**
   2. **Negative core beliefs.** These beliefs are **the product of long-term negative experiences** associated with significant individuals and situations. They form the basis of how individuals view themselves, others, and their environment. Negative core beliefs strongly influence how individuals misinterpret situations in the present; they are the driving forces for the content of dysfunctional automatic thoughts. Core beliefs are generally categorized into three major themes by virtue of whether the patient believes that he or she is lovable, competent, or in control. A patient may have more than one negative core belief, and each belief may be activated at different times and in different combinations depending on the situation.
   3. **Errors in logic.** Errors in logic present in a variety of forms: **dichotomous or all-or-nothing thinking** (events are seen in one of two mutually exclusive categories); **overgeneralization** (a specific event is seen as characteristic of life in general); **mind reading** (an individual assumes that others are reacting negatively without obtaining the necessary evidence); **catastrophic thinking** (negative experiences or events are interpreted as intolerable or in terms of the worst possible outcome); and **personalization** (an individual automatically assumes responsibility for a negative event without considering other possible contributing factors).

D. **The premise of CBT is that core beliefs are learned based on past experience.** The task of CBT is to challenge the validity of maladaptive core beliefs and to replace them with adaptive core beliefs.

E. **CBT addresses not only the impact of cognitions on mood and behavior, but also the impact of mood and behavior on cognition.**
   1. Several studies have demonstrated that mood biases how an individual interprets events and which memories are recalled (a sad mood facilitates recall of sad events, whereas a happy mood facilitates recall of happy events).
   2. An individual's behavior may influence his thoughts by changing the environment and/or by changing other people's reactions to him.
   3. Thus, **there are bidirectional interactions among cognition, mood, and behavior. Beck demonstrates these relationships by describing a triangle with thoughts labeled at the apex, and feelings and behaviors labeled at the two base corners.** Bidirectional arrows join each corner of the triangle indicating the bidirectional relationships of thoughts, feelings, and behaviors.

F. **CBT interventions for symptom reduction may utilize not only cognitive techniques but also techniques that modify mood and behavior.** The clinical state of the individual determines whether cognitive or behavioral techniques are used. A severely depressed patient may not be able to make use of cognitive techniques; thus, behavioral strategies may be used initially to activate him or her.

G. **CBT hypothesizes that, in order to achieve enduring change of problematic emotions and behavior, cognitive techniques must be used to change the individual's maladaptive core belief system.**

II. Principles of Cognitive-Behavioral Therapy (Modified from Judith Beck, 1995)

A. **CBT conceptualizes a patient's negative emotions and problematic behaviors in cognitive terms.** This conceptualization is based on a comprehensive assessment conducted during the first few therapy sessions and is modified, as needed, based on new information. The therapist demonstrates to the patient the relationships among distorted thinking, negative emotions, and problem behaviors, and describes how such faulty thinking perpetuates the patient's distress.

B. **CBT uses a collaborative approach. The therapist and patient work together in determining the goals for therapy, the agenda for each session, the homework assignments, the frequency of meetings, and how long to continue therapy.** The therapist's role is to guide the therapy based on the patient's needs, priorities, and capabilities. The technique used by the therapist to achieve these ends is **"guided discovery." Using "guided discovery," the therapist asks appropriate questions that enable the patient to gain a better understanding of his or her problems, explore possible solutions, and develop strategies to resolve the problems.** It is important that the therapist not be viewed as having the answers or that the therapist impose his or her beliefs on the patient.

C. **CBT requires alliance building.** Although CBT uses a variety of cognitive and behavioral techniques, effective treatment relies on a positive relationship between the therapist and patient. The therapist must be competent, caring, and empathic. Empathy enables the therapist to understand the patient from the patient's point of view, and thus gain insight into the belief systems and rules of logic that determine his or her thoughts, feelings, and behaviors.

D. **CBT is problem- and goal-oriented.** The therapist assists the patient in identifying the specific problems that brought the patient to therapy, prioritizing which problems are most important and most accessible for immediate success, and operationalizing the expected outcome.

E. **CBT initially focuses on the present rather than the past.** Dysfunctional automatic thoughts are generally more accessible to conscious awareness in the here-and-now than are core beliefs, which are a product of past experiences. Thus, the initial task in CBT is to identify patterns of dysfunctional thinking in the present that can provide insight into the underlying core belief. **Once patterns of dysfunctional thinking are identified, the therapist generates hypotheses about possible underlying core beliefs.** The past is addressed later in therapy to help the patient understand how the core beliefs developed.

F. **CBT is generally time-limited.** In treating Axis I disorders, CBT is considered to be "brief psychotherapy," which may include 8–20 sessions. For Axis II disorders, the therapy may last 1–2 years.

G. **CBT sessions are structured.** The therapist and the patient at the beginning of each therapy session set an agenda for that session. **Elements of the agenda include:**
1. **Review of the patient's clinical condition.**
2. **Review of significant events that occurred since the last therapy visit.**
3. **Feedback from the previous session.**
4. **Review of the patient's homework from the previous session.**
5. **Discussion of new problems.**
6. **Development of new homework.**
7. **Feedback from the present session.**

H. **CBT teaches patients a method and skills that will enable them to become their own therapists.** In order to accomplish this task, the therapist first teaches patients about the nature of their disorders and the CBT model. **The therapist teaches the patient the same skills he or she was taught.** By the end of therapy, the patient will possess a strategy and a set of tools to confront problem situations in the future.

I. **CBT uses both cognitive and behavioral techniques to bring about change in thoughts, feelings, and behaviors. The patient is taught to challenge his or her dysfunctional thoughts and beliefs by looking for evidence for and against them.** Behavioral techniques may enable the patient to further test the validity of his or her faulty thoughts or beliefs. The choice of techniques depends on the patient's specific disorder.

J. **CBT teaches relapse prevention.** The last two or three therapy sessions are devoted to relapse prevention. **The therapist encourages the patient to identify potential problem areas that he or she may encounter after therapy and to think of possible solutions** based on knowledge learned from therapy.

K. **CBT is data-based.** CBT treatment techniques have been empirically validated, and the body of research on CBT is large and growing. Also, treatment is driven in large part by patient self-report data, and collected by means of rating scales, diaries, and homework assignments.

III. The Application of Cognitive-Behavioral Therapy

A. **The therapist and patient agree on the goals of treatment based on the therapist's conceptualization of the patient's presenting problems.**

B. To help the patient achieve his or her goals, **the therapist teaches the patient the use of several cognitive and behavioral techniques.**

C. Cognitive techniques (for challenging negative automatic thoughts and core beliefs) **are employed.**

1. **Identification and modification of negative automatic thoughts.**

   a. **Negative shifts in mood provide an excellent opportunity to identify negative automatic thoughts ("(−)ATs").** During the session, the therapist monitors for strong emotional reactions and, once identified, asks the patient, **"What went through your mind just then?"** Patients are generally aware of their intense negative emotions but unaware of the corresponding negative automatic thoughts. According to Beck, "emotion is the royal road to cognition."

   b. **Guided discovery is a technique where the therapist asks the patient a series of inductive questions in an attempt to identify negative automatic thoughts.** The questions also help develop dissonance about the validity of the patient's (−)ATs.

   c. **Examination of the evidence is basic to modifying distorted negative automatic thoughts.** The therapist teaches the patient to treat the (−)ATs as a hypothesis; then they search together for evidence both for and against the hypothesis. The final interpretation is based on the outcome of this "examining-the-evidence" exercise.

   d. **Reattribution techniques are used to help patients reassess their degree of responsibility for the occurrence of problematic events.** A depressed patient, in particular, is more apt to have problems with negatively biased attributions regarding self, the environment, and the future. For example, a depressed patient might take on responsibility for a situation that is only minimally attributable to him or her. The therapist can help the patient recognize that other relevant individuals may have contributed more to the problem. This realization by the patient can help diminish negative emotions, such as guilt and anger.

   e. **The Dysfunctional Thought Record** (DTR) combines many of the techniques noted above. The DTR is used to help the patient identify and modify negative automatic thoughts. **The patient is asked to write down, in three separate columns, a stressful situation and the corresponding negative emotions and negative automatic thoughts. The patient also rates, from 0 to 100, the severity of the negative emotions and the strength of his or her belief in the negative automatic thoughts.** This teaches the patient the relationship between feelings and thoughts. **In a fourth column, the patient records alternative thoughts or evidence against the original negative automatic thoughts.** This technique challenges the original negative automatic thoughts and thus helps the patient gain a more realistic perspective. **In a final fifth column, the patient re-rates his or her belief in the original negative automatic thoughts.** If the alternative thoughts rate high in believability or if the evidence accumulated against the original negative automatic thoughts is convincing, the patient's belief in the original negative automatic thoughts will be diminished, and the intensity of the negative emotions should be correspondingly reduced.

2. **Identification and modification of maladaptive core beliefs.**

   a. Core beliefs are difficult to access since they are often unavailable to conscious awareness. **As the patient identifies a series of negative automatic thoughts, certain patterns of thinking will emerge** that will suggest possible underlying core beliefs.

   b. **Once the patient has identified maladaptive core beliefs, the therapist asks the patient to perform a pro-con analysis using a double column procedure.** In one column, the patient writes down all of the evidence that supports the core belief and, in the other column, all of the evidence that argues against the core belief. This will enable the patient to examine the validity of the core belief.

   c. **Advantages and disadvantages analysis allows the patient to assess the full range of effects of his or her maladaptive core beliefs. On a four-cell grid, the patient writes the advantages and disadvantages of having or not having maladaptive core beliefs.** Some maladaptive core beliefs have few or no advantages (e.g., "I am a loser"), while other maladaptive core beliefs have both positive and negative aspects (e.g., "If I don't do a perfect job, people will think I am incompetent"). In the latter example, doing a perfect job has certain rewards; however, there is a price to pay because of the added effort and stress in doing a perfect job. This analysis will underscore the negative impact of maladaptive core beliefs on the patient's life and thus provide motivation to look for alternative core beliefs.

   d. **Generating alternative core beliefs is facilitated by the therapist through the use of a "brainstorming attitude"** (Wright and Beck, 1994), **guided discovery, role play, and imagery.** The initial goal is to generate more adaptive core beliefs. **This is followed by testing these new core beliefs in the patient's environment and making modifications as needed.** For homework, the patient searches for evidence that supports the new core belief and evidence that contradicts the old maladaptive core belief.

   e. The therapist and patient then address the impact of the revised core beliefs on his or her life. **The patient practices multiple times both in therapy and outside of therapy** in order to reinforce learning the new core belief.

D. Behavioral Techniques

1. **Techniques to identify and modify maladaptive cognitions.**

   a. **Behavioral experiments directly test the validity of automatic thoughts and beliefs.** The therapist and patient clearly identify the belief to be tested and then they collaboratively design an experiment to test the belief. The power of this technique is realized when the patient personally experiences evidence that contradicts the validity of his or her view.

b. **Bibliotherapy is used by the therapist to consolidate certain points during the therapy.** The therapist must monitor the patient's understanding of the material. This technique is consistent with the psychoeducational approach to CBT.

c. **Role play** is effective in helping the patient to identify automatic thoughts, to rationally respond to distorted automatic thoughts, and to modify maladaptive core beliefs. This technique **allows for the activation of specific emotional experiences which may make distressing thoughts and beliefs more accessible to conscious awareness.**

2. **Techniques to change dysfunctional behaviors.**

a. **Graded exposure** is a technique to address the tendency of a patient to become overwhelmed with a task and thus avoid working on it at all. The therapist **helps the patient break down the task into smaller steps and then encourages the patient to focus on the current step rather than the ultimate goal.**

b. **Scheduling activities** is useful for dealing with time-management problems and difficulty with prioritizing tasks. **The therapist has the patient write down on a grid activities for the week. The therapist may ask the patient to write down for each task ratings for mastery, pleasure, and mood.** These ratings provide important data that can be used by the patient and therapist to modify the patient's behavior.

c. **Problem solving** is a technique to assist a patient who did not develop this skill in the process of development. The patient learns to specify a problem, to identify alternative solutions, to examine the pros and cons of each potential solution, to select a solution, to devise a plan for implementation, to implement the plan, and to assess the effectiveness of the results.

IV. The Application of CBT to Specific Disorders

A. Depression

1. Conceptualization. Beck developed CBT out of his clinical interest in depression. According to Beck, a depressed individual views himself, his world, and his future in negative terms. **This "negative cognitive triad" is reflected in the content of the patient's automatic thoughts, which are a product of his or her negative core beliefs. The resulting depressed mood has an impact on the patient's ability to recall positive experiences and successes.** Studies have shown that depressed mood biases recall of past pleasurable and successful experiences. This process prevents the patient from being able to establish perspective and to problem solve, which leads to a worsening of depression and, at times, a sense of hopelessness.

2. **Treatment**

a. **Behavioral techniques**

i. **Activity scheduling.** During the early phase of treatment, a depressed patient may experience significant psychomotor retardation and/or fatigue. This condition may make it difficult for the patient to cooperate with cognitive strategies. **Increasing activity often has a positive effect on improving mood, which, in turn, enables the patient to work more effectively on tasks requiring cognition.**

b. **Cognitive techniques**

i. **Daily thought records.** This technique helps the patient systematically challenge his or her negative views of self, the environment, and the future. **Once the negative automatic thoughts are identified, the patient, in collaboration with the therapist, identifies alternative views and searches for the evidence to support them.**

ii. **Belief work.** Although the correction of negative automatic thoughts is effective in resolving an acute episode of depression, it is crucial to identify and correct the dysfunctional core belief system that is responsible for the distorted views of self, environment, and future. The core beliefs are accessed through the discovery of patterns of negative automatic thoughts in given situations. The therapist, along with the patient, identifies the core beliefs by working backward from the cognitive themes observed in the present. Specific dysfunctional core beliefs tend to generate specific negative automatic thoughts. **Once the dysfunctional core beliefs are identified and corrected, the patient is less likely to relapse in the future.**

3. **Outcome studies**

a. In the acute treatment of mild to moderate major depression, **CBT is comparable to antidepressants in symptom relief.**

b. In preventing relapse, **follow-up studies 1–2 years after termination of treatment demonstrate relapse rates for CBT of between 20% and 30%** in comparison to relapse rates for antidepressants of between 65% and 78%.

B. Panic Disorder

Panic disorder is one type of anxiety disorder. Anxiety is a normal emotional response when an individual is facing a dangerous situation; however, anxiety is an abnormal response if it occurs in the absence of real danger, or if the anxiety response is out of proportion to the dangerousness of the situation. **According to CBT, the thinking of a patient with an anxiety disorder is preoccupied with danger.** The threats of danger may be physical, psychological, or social. **Core beliefs contribute to the interpretation of a situation as being dangerous.** An anxiety disorder patient is more likely to have core beliefs of being inadequate, incompetent, or helpless. According to

Freeman, some of the errors in logic commonly found in an anxious patient include: catastrophization, personalization, overgeneralization, and magnification, and minimization. Perceived danger is maintained by avoidant behaviors and focusing on stimuli, both internal and external, that contribute to the anxiety. **Avoidant behaviors prevent the patient from testing out his or her misinterpretations;** at the same time, the patient tends to focus attention on the stimuli that contribute to anxiety, thus intensifying the anxiety response.

1. **Conceptualization. A patient with panic disorder misinterprets normal anxiety or bodily sensations in a catastrophic way.** Symptoms, including rapid heart rate, shortness of breath, diaphoresis, paresthesias, dizziness, and palpitations, are interpreted as having life-threatening consequences. The triggers for panic attacks can be external (e.g., a crowded shopping mall), or internal (e.g., a physical sensation, an image, or memory of an anxiety-provoking event). Avoidant behavior, such as agoraphobia often develops as a coping strategy when certain external situations tend to trigger panic attacks. According to Clark, panic disorder is maintained by the patient's tendency to become hypervigilant in observing certain bodily sensations and to develop "safety behaviors" as a means of protecting him- or herself from either having a panic attack or experiencing the feared consequence of having a panic attack (e.g., a heart attack). Both the hypervigilance and "safety behaviors" interfere with the patient's opportunity to challenge his or her catastrophic thinking.

2. **Treatment**
   a. The anxiety experienced by a patient with panic disorder is based on his or her belief that certain physical sensations may result in catastrophic medical problems. **Treatment consists of teaching patients coping skills first, then cognitive strategies, to challenge the validity of their catastrophic thinking, and finally developing behavioral experiments to test the validity of their catastrophic thinking.**
   b. Coping skills are particularly helpful in the early phase of the onset of a panic attack.
      i. **Diaphragmatic breathing** is helpful to reduce arousal and to slow down bodily processes, such as heart rate. The patient is instructed to breathe in slowly over 5 sec and then exhale over 10 sec. Each breathing sequence should take about 20 sec.
      ii. **Muscle relaxation** involves tensing and relaxing different muscle groups. One strategy is to begin at the feet and then work up the body to the head. The patient tenses a particular muscle group, holds it, and then releases the tension.

      iii. **Distraction** is a technique to help the patient avoid focusing on his or her physical symptoms, which tends to worsen anxiety. The patient is instructed to focus on external objects and to pay attention to as much detail as possible. This technique should not be viewed as avoiding the problem, but as a means to get more reality focused.
   c. **Cognitive strategies**
      i. **Psychoeducation** about panic attacks is provided early in the treatment. The patient is informed that people do not die from panic attacks, although the experience of a panic attack may feel like a potential seizure or a myocardial infarction.
      ii. **The patient first makes a list of symptoms that occur during a panic attack and then identifies the negative automatic thought associated with each symptom.** Examples of negative automatic thoughts include, "I'll faint," "I'll have a heart attack," "I'll look stupid," and "I'll go crazy." The patient and therapist together challenge the validity of the negative thoughts.
   d. **Behavioral strategies**
      i. **Interoceptive exposure** is a technique that **allows the patient to challenge the feared symptom by having the patient artificially create the symptom in a safe environment and then realize that there is not a catastrophic outcome.** Examples include having the patient spin around in a chair in order to mimic dizziness, hyperventilate to create the sensation of paresthesias, and run up a flight of stairs to generate tachycardia. Each of these induced symptoms can be symptoms of panic disorder.
      ii. **Exposure experiments are important to help the patient resist "safety" and avoidant behaviors,** which are a product of panic attacks and which prevent the patient from learning that his or her symptoms are not dangerous. A patient who has the fear that he or she might have a myocardial infarction might avoid exercise. The therapist would have the patient exercise when the feared sensation was present during a therapy session and then later for homework.

C. **Other Applications**
   1. **Substance abuse. CBT** addresses relapse prevention. It **teaches that cravings and urges to use are the product of addictive beliefs that are triggered by internal (emotions) and external (stresses or situations) cues.** Examples of addictive beliefs include, "I cannot have fun without cocaine," or "The only way I can relax is to have a drink." Cognitive therapists help the patient challenge the validity of these beliefs and identify alternative ways of dealing with the cues that trigger the beliefs. Once the patient experiences cravings and urges to use, permissive beliefs are activated such as, "I deserve a drink for all my stress," or "I can stop after just one drink." The permissive beliefs lead

the patient to start thinking of strategies to get the substance, which results in a lapse or relapse. Each step in the process towards using a substance is an opportunity to intervene either cognitively or behaviorally. Patients are also encouraged to look at the disadvantages of using substances since they tend to focus only on the benefits.

2. **Psychosis. Cognitive therapy addresses** several aspects of the psychotic experience, including: **misunderstandings about the illness and its treatment; noncompliance with treatment; the impact of the illness on self-esteem; challenging the validity of delusions and hallucinations; assisting in the development of better coping strategies; and identifying triggers and early signs of relapse.** Techniques used include psychoeducation, problem solving, stress management, and the identification of evidence that contradicts the psychotic symptoms.

3. **Eating disorders.** The main problem areas include a distorted body image, low weight, and abnormal eating behaviors. **Cognitive techniques address the beliefs that body shape and appearance determine acceptance.** In addition, there is the common belief among these patients that any compromise with the extreme standard of very low weight will result in total loss of control. **Behavioral techniques are used to normalize the eating pattern** (e.g., eating balanced meals at specific times), **and to provide psychoeducation about the medical risks of the abnormal eating behaviors.** Since eating disorders are often seen as a coping strategy to deal with more fundamental belief systems, cognitive therapy may also address the issues of low self-esteem and negative self-image.

4. **Personality disorders.** Beck and others believe that there are four main areas of idiosyncratic cognitions that are unique for each personality disorder: core beliefs; view of self; view of others; and strategies for interpersonal interactions. **Patients with borderline personality disorder may view themselves** as **"defective"** or **"totally undesirable,"** and they view others as rejecting and malevolent. Their social interactions consist of extremes, including idealization and rejection. **Since personality-disordered patients have a predominance of maladaptive core beliefs, therapy tends to be long-term and focus on belief work.**

Suggested Readings

Beck AT, Rush AJ, Shaw BF, Emery G: *Cognitive Therapy of Depression.* New York: Guilford Press, 1979:1–33.

Beck AT, Wright FD, Newman CF, Liese BS: *Cognitive Therapy of Substance Abuse.* New York: Guilford Press, 1993:22–41.

Beck JS: *Cognitive Therapy: Basics and Beyond.* New York: Guilford Press, 1995:1–24.

Beck JS: Cognitive approaches to personality disorders. In Wright JH, Thase ME (eds): *Cognitive Therapy.* Washington, DC: American Psychiatric Press, 1998:73–106.

Blackburn IM: Severely depressed in-patients. In Scott J, Williams JMG, Beck AT (eds): *Cognitive Therapy in Clinical Practice: An Illustrative Case Book.* London: Routledge, 1989:1–24.

Clark DM, Wells A: Cognitive therapy of anxiety disorders. In Wright JH, Thase ME (eds): *Cognitive Therapy.* Washington, DC: American Psychiatric Press, 1998:9–43.

Freeman A, Pretzer J, Fleming B, Simon KM: *Clinical Applications of Cognitive Therapy.* New York: Plenum Press, 1990:3–79.

Kleifield EI, Wagner S, Halmi KA: Cognitive-behavioral treatment of anorexia nervosa. *Psychiatr Clin North Am* 1996; 19(4):715–737.

Mitchell JE, Peterson CB: Cognitive-behavioral treatment of eating disorders. In Wright JH, Thase ME (eds): *Cognitive Therapy.* Washington, DC: American Psychiatric Press, 1998:107–133.

Scott J, Wright JH: Cognitive therapy for chronic and severe mental disorders. In Wright JH, Thase ME (eds): *Cognitive Therapy.* Washington, DC: American Psychiatric Press, 1998:135–170.

Wright JH, Beck AT: Cognitive therapy. In Hales HE, Yudofsky SC, Talbott JA (eds): *The American Psychiatric Press Textbook of Psychiatry*, 3rd ed. Washington, DC: American Psychiatric Press, 1999:1205–1241.

Chapter 64
Hypnosis
SARA KULLESEID AND OWEN S. SURMAN

I. Introduction

Hypnosis is a therapeutic modality that has been used, by one name or another, for thousands of years; however, its popularity, as a technique for the treatment of a wide variety of ailments, has fluctuated. Many have attempted to define hypnosis. It is perhaps best understood as **an event or ritual between a hypnotist and hypnotic subject(s) in which both agree to use suggestion to bring about a change in perception or behavior. Hypnosis depends on several things: the dissociative and imaginative abilities (i.e., hypnotic susceptibility) of the subject(s); the motivation of the subject(s); and the relationship between hypnotist and subject(s) (i.e., demand characteristics).** Multiple clinical applications exist for direct suggestions delivered during hypnosis. Hypnosis has also been used as an adjunct to behavior therapy and for memory retrieval.

II. Historical Background

A. The Pre-Mesmer Era
Suggestive therapies have been used since early civilization. Records of their use date back to 2600 BC; there are even references to a hypnotic process in the Bible. **Through ritual and ceremony, various healers have used suggestion to ease, if not cure, ailments.** The most important element seems to be the intimate connection made between the subject and the healer.

B. Franz Anton Mesmer (1734–1815) and the Marquis de Puysegur (1751–1825)
1. **Mesmer,** working during the Age of Enlightenment, **is thought to be the originator of what later became known as hypnosis. In 1766, he presented his thesis of "universal gravitation" to the** University of Vienna. In it, **he postulated that a fluid contained within all living beings,** as well as in the universe at large, **affected others through gravitational forces.** He called this fluid **"animal magnetism"** and based his model of disease on an imbalance of that fluid in the body. **Mesmer used magnets, literally, to restore equilibrium** to this fluid; later he became convinced that his own animal magnetism could cause fluid movements and therapeutic "crises" in patients. These were distortions in perceptions with a convulsive component, similar to the manifestations of hysteria, that occurred in a hypnotic state. On awakening, many claimed cure. Mesmer saw the importance of the relationship between magnetizer and the patient, and later called this phenomenon, "rapport." In 1784, due to controversy surrounding his work, Mesmer was discredited by an investigative committee of the French Academy of Science which was led by Benjamin Franklin, then a United States Ambassador to France. Ultimately, it was decided that the fluid did not exist and that any effects were due to the forces of suggestion.

2. **De Puysegur,** one of Mesmer's disciples, **also practiced magnetism.** His best known patient, instead of exhibiting a convulsive crisis, fell into a type of sleep that he called "artificial somnambulism." In this state, the patient "confessed" worries without apparent subsequent memory of the encounter. This suggested a different state of consciousness with amnestic barriers. **De Puysegur felt that the magnetizer's belief in his/her own ability to heal was what brought about cure.** Others countered this with the belief that this altered state came from the patient—his/her own ability to be suggestible or to internalize the magnetizer's suggestions.

C. James Braid (1795–1860), Jean Martin Charcot (1825–1893), and Hippolyte Bernheim (1840–1919)
1. Through the work of **James Braid,** hypnosis again became integrated into medical practice. **Braid** is said to **have coined the word "hypnosis," from the Greek, *hypnos*, for sleep.** He believed that magnetism resulted in a type of sleep he called "neurypnology." Braid believed that psychological forces within the individual were critical to the process of magnetism.

2. **Charcot** was a noted nineteenth-century French neurologist; he became interested in hypnosis while working with hysterics and epileptics. **He felt hypnosis was a pathologic neurophysiologic state** akin to hysteria. A student of Charcot's, **Pierre Janet,** furthered this theory. Janet thought that the underlying mechanism was a disconnection or "dissociation" from the conscious state, as occurred in hysteria.

3. **Bernheim** challenged these ideas. He felt that hypnosis was not like hysteria. Rather, Bernheim believed that **hypnosis worked through the power of suggestion** and that the effects of hypnosis

could be achieved in the waking state. Thus, by the beginning of the twentieth century, two prominent theories of hypnosis coexisted.

D. Sigmund Freud (1856–1939), Milton Erikson (1901–1980), to the Present

1. **Freud** was influenced greatly by his work with Charcot. Freud was an experienced hypnotist; however, he moved to psychoanalysis because of what he considered were the limitations in the technique. **Freud felt that hypnosis imposed ideas on a patient which made analysis and critical thinking difficult.**

2. **Erikson,** along with his predecessor, **Clark Hull, contradicted Freud, refuting the need to make unconscious processes conscious to achieve change and relief.** They felt that subtle commands or indirect suggestions could make the patient unconsciously change their behavior.

3. The **Hilgards** in the 1950s and 1960s revisited the dissociative theory of Janet with their **"neodissociation" theory; they furthered the concept that the hypnotic process is involuntary,** is not under conscious control, and involves the notion of altered states of awareness. Other theorists took a **"socio-cognitive"** stance, in which they discussed environmental cues, social expectations, and motivation as key factors for an individual's undergoing hypnosis. The importance of "role," the focus on performance, and expectations were seen as the powers behind hypnosis. As can be seen by this brief history, the debate has, and continues to center around these two camps.

III. Proposed Mechanisms

There is no consensus on how hypnosis works. The psychological debate continues as outlined above between the dissociation/neodissociation theorists and the socio-cognitive theorists. **Whether hypnosis involves an altered state of consciousness or is simply an intense form of role play has been debated.** Hypnosis is viewed by most as idiosyncratic to the individual in a given environmental setting; the ability of subjects to imagine, dissociate, or comply are key to their experience. Indeed, it may be that simpler tasks are due to suggestion and role play, whereas more complex negative hallucinations, such as ignoring pain, probably involve dissociation or a combination of the two.

As intimated above, it is important to note that **not all subjects are hypnotizable. Levels of hypnotizability tend to fall on a bell-shaped curve.** Several scales have been developed to test hypnotizability (e.g., the **Stanford Scale Form C**). A separate measure of subject hypnotic depth is assessed on a numerical scale. Some believe that they can guess a subject's hypnotizability from their capacity

for focused attention or creativity. Symptomatic improvement does not require high levels of hypnotizability. The technique should, however, be shaped to the subject's need and cognitive style.

Multiple observations have been made regarding subjects who undergo hypnosis, **including changes in heart rate, respiratory rhythm, muscle tension, blood pressure, and oxygen consumption,** finding them similar to those that occur in other meditative techniques. Changes on the electroencephalogram (EEG) and in the event-related brain potential (ERP) in the cortex have been recorded. In general, it is unclear what can be made of these observations. It is unclear if these are a consequence of the hypnotic state, or are specific to the arousal, or to the cognitive ability, of subjects.

IV. Applications

There is general agreement that hypnosis is an effective intervention in several areas of medicine, including psychiatry. However, the literature is inconsistent in terms of methodology, scope, and focus. Most clinicians ultimately agree that hypnosis should be used as an adjunctive technique in most situations rather than as the sole therapy. **Some of the more widely used and better studied applications of hypnosis are in the areas of pain, asthma, nausea and vomiting, surgical preparation and procedures, eating disorders, phobic disorders, smoking cessation, habit disorders, and wart removal.** This is by no means an exhaustive list. Forensic uses, such as retrieval of memory, have been highly controversial since memory production is notably inaccurate and subject to subtle influences of the hypnotist.

A. Pain

Pain, one of the most common complaints in primary care and general hospital settings, has a strong psychological component. Several studies have indicated that hypnotic suggestions for analgesia can change the relationship between the degree of noxious stimulation received and the pain reported. In addition, for some patients, hypnosis can help control physiological parameters, such as heart rate and blood pressure, associated with pain. When highly hypnotizable patients are tested, they respond best. Neodissociation theorists would argue that the hypnotized subject's brain blocks out information regarding painful stimuli, and makes it unavailable to consciousness; thus it is capable of being ignored.

Children, often the subjects for pain control studies, have been good candidates for hypnosis, likely due to their ability to imagine and to suspend belief. Adult patients under hypnosis have been more tolerant of anxiety and pain in association with cancer, bone marrow transplantation, colonoscopy, angioplasty, wound debridement, arthritis, interventional radiography, dental procedures, and other conditions.

An area of medicine in which hypnosis has been used widely is the treatment of burn patients, especially where pain is associated with the debridement process.

B. Asthma

Anxious asthmatics often overuse their medications and medical services. Since several studies have shown that respiratory symptoms can be produced with nonbronchoconstricting agents, and that some patients who are known to be reactive to a bronchoconstricting drug develop bronchospasm, clinical studies employed hypnosis. It was found to be superior to relaxation training alone and to medication control in the reduction of symptoms and medication usage.

C. Nausea and Vomiting

Hypnosis has also been studied in the treatment of nausea and vomiting following surgical procedures, in anticipatory nausea and vomiting associated with cancer medications, and in hyperemesis gravidarum.

D. Surgical Preparation and Procedures

Most patients experience moderate to high anxiety while awaiting surgery. Anxiety can interfere with the success of surgery by impairing postoperative mobilization, nutrition, and adherence. Patients treated with hypnosis prior to surgery had diminished anxiety, and required less anesthesia during the procedure, as shown in several studies. Hypnosis has also been useful for those who cannot have local anesthesia due to an allergic response to the anesthesia itself.

E. Habit Disorders

Hypnosis has often been used in the treatment of habit disorders (e.g., smoking, and compulsive overeating). The results for smoking cessation (20% abstinence rates at 1 year) are no better than are attained with other nonspecific techniques. Weight reduction with hypnosis often fails, or proves transient. It has been said that forcing a reluctant patient to change his or her behavior is no more possible for the hypnotist than it is for the physician, the psychotherapist, or a family member.

F. Other Nonpsychiatric Applications

Hypnosis has been used in gastrointestinal procedures, to allay anxiety, as well as with sufferers of irritable bowel syndrome. Obstetric studies indicate that hypnosis may decrease the time of stage 1 labor. Since there is an obvious similarity between the Lamaze method and hypnosis, this may be a technique employed more often in the future. Research on hypnosis in the field of infection and immunity has led to some interesting findings, such as the effective treatment of warts. Cardiac patients have focused much energy on relaxation techniques and their effectiveness in reducing stress and decreasing cardiac events. However, studies using hypnosis in this population are lacking.

G. Psychiatric Applications

Bulimic patients have been noted to be highly hypnotizable, compared with anorectics. It is unclear whether hypnosis will be useful in this population. Hypnosis has been used in the treatment of phobic disorders as sole therapy, and as an adjunct to cognitive behavioral therapy. In forensic psychiatry cases, hypnosis has been used in the retrieval of memories; its value is controversial. Most believe that hypnosis is poor at uncovering memories or as an adjunct to psychodynamic work.

H. Contraindications

The primary contraindication to hypnosis is paranoia; not only are these subjects unwilling to participate, for obvious reasons, but, if a suggestion were made, the patient may forever blame the hypnotist for its presence.

V. Typical Hypnotic Inductions

It is noteworthy that there is no standard induction of hypnosis: it can be done with an individual or a group; in a hospital setting or on a stage; the amount of time can vary; suggestions can be direct or indirect; inductions can be through verbal or nonverbal (prop, e.g., pendulum) means; and there are many different formulations using imagery, counting, breathing, or combinations of these and others. A typical induction might begin by making sure the subject is comfortable, then having them roll their eyes up and focus on a point above them; asking them to take slow, deep breaths, have them think of their eyelids as getting heavy, then closing, continuing to reinforce relaxation and blowing off of tension. At this point, one may ask the subject to imagine a pleasant scene and experience it with as many senses as possible. By raising a hand the subject can indicate they have reached this stage. Using counting (from one to ten, say), the hypnotist can suggest an even deeper state of relaxation, having the subject imagine muscle groups sequentially relaxing. At this point, the hypnotist might indicate that he/she will count to five and the session will end, but that first he/she will give some helpful suggestions. The hypnotist might say that the subject can relax in the future by following this same technique; they will have improved well-being; or other suggestions. The hypnotist may then count to five and have the subject open their eyes, concluding the session.

VI. Conclusions

Hypnosis is a powerful tool, used adjunctively and sometimes solely, for the treatment of a wide variety of medical disorders. It appears that **two types of clinical disorders respond best: those associated with the autonomic nervous system (e.g., anxiety, pain, asthma, possibly irritable bowel), and those related to the principles of classical or operant conditioning (e.g., phobias, nausea, vomiting, and bulimia).** People who are very skilled in hypnosis have found it to be useful in a third class of patients, namely those with dissociative disorders (e.g., multiple personality disorders, and posttraumatic syndromes). Many patients (e.g., those with monosymptomatic phobias) seem to have higher levels of hypnotizability that may contribute to the acquisition and maintenance of their disorder, but conceivably could also be used to cure them.

Physicians have often been wary of using hypnosis in their daily practice. Through exposure and experience to the technique, this could change; if nothing else, it would simply increase physician awareness to the role of suggestion in health care.

Suggested Readings

Covino NA, Frankel FH: Clinical hypnosis. Personal communication, 1998.

Covino NA, Frankel FH: Hypnosis and relaxation in the medically ill. *Psychother Psychosom* 1993; 60:75–90.

Frankel FH: Significant developments in medical hypnosis during the past 25 years. *Int J Clin Exp Hypn* 1987; 35:231–248.

Hilgard ER, Hilgard JR: *Hypnosis in the Relief of Pain.* William Kaufmann, 1975.

Orne MT: The nature of hypnosis: artifact and essence. *J Abnorm Soc Psychol* 1959; 58:277–299.

Riskin JD, Frankel FH: A history of medical hypnosis. *Psychiatr Clin North Am* 1994; 17(3):601–609.

Spanos NP, Stenstrom MA, Johnston JC: Hypnosis, placebo, and suggestion in the treatment of warts. *Psychosom Med* 1988; 50: 245–260.

Surman OS: Postnoxious desensitization: some clinical notes on the combined use of hypnosis and systematic desensitization. *Am J Clin Hypn* 1979; 22:54–60.

Surman OS, Gottlieb SK, Hackett TP, Silverberg EL: Hypnosis in the treatment of warts. *Arch Gen Psychiatry* 1973; 28:439–441.

Weitzenhoffer AM, Hilgard ER: *Stanford Hypnotic Susceptibility Scale, Forms A and B.* Consult Psych Press, 1959.

Chapter 65

Geriatric Psychiatry

M. Cornelia Cremens, Lee E. Goldstein, and Gary L. Gottlieb

I. Introduction

The elderly population is increasing rapidly; coinciding with this increase is a population that requires greater attention to psychiatric and neuropsychiatric problems.

II. Metabolic Changes Associated with Aging

Determining the appropriate medication in older patients is a complex task.

A. **Altered Pharmacokinetics**
   1. **Hepatic function in the elderly is decreased due to reduced blood flow and cardiac output resulting in a decreased first-pass effect.** In addition, enzyme activity is reduced; demethylation and hydroxylation are notably effected.
   2. **Absorption is decreased due to reductions in gastric blood flow, acidity, motility, and surface area.**
   3. **Renal excretion is delayed due to reductions in glomerular filtration rate, tubular excretion, and blood flow.**
   4. **Protein binding and albumin are decreased.**
   5. **The volume of distribution is increased due to reductions in muscle mass, total body water, and cardiac output.** Total body fat increases relative to total body weight and lipophilic drugs will be diluted due to greater distribution in peripheral tissues.

B. **Central Nervous System Changes Associated with Aging**
   The brain demonstrates a remarkable functional compensation for neuronal loss and functional decline. **There is significant age-related loss in neurons, enzymes, neurotransmitters, receptors, dendritic arborization, and compensatory dendritic proliferation.**
   1. **Significant age-related loss of brain-differentiated neurons is permanent;** these cells do not divide or proliferate; by contrast glial cells can divide.
   2. Dendritic arborization and compensatory proliferation allow neuronal pathways to maintain contact despite neuronal loss.
   3. **Neurotransmitters and enzymes levels change with age, resulting in increased monoamine oxidase, decreased acetylcholine, and decreased dopamine.**
   4. Receptors decrease in number with age, and increase in resistance to drug diffusion with age.

5. Approximately 10–60% of neuronal cell loss normally occurs in the neocortex, the cerebellum, and the hippocampus, with less loss in the subcortical areas (with the exception of the locus coeruleus). This loss usually does not affect ordinary functions of living or occupation until after the age of 75 years.

III. Evaluation of the Older Patient

Illnesses often present atypically in older patients, with vague complaints, falls, cognitive deficits, functional losses, and behavioral changes. Patients are often tolerant of symptoms and accept discomfort as a function of aging. Physicians contribute to this myth and poorly document these atypical findings, thereby missing the diagnosis.

Observation of the patient when he/she enters the room is the beginning of the evaluation process. The patient's presentation, interaction with the family, and approach to the physician are critical in the assessment.

A. **Conduct a psychiatric assessment that includes evaluation of affect, behavior, and cognition.**
   1. Many **screening tools are available for the assessment of cognition.**
      a. The most frequently used screen is the **mini-mental state exam** (MMSE) developed by Folstein and associates.
         i. It is quick and can be incorporated within the context of the evaluation process.
         ii. The MMSE is only a screen; it does not fully address the complex neuropsychiatric deficits that can be involved.
      b. Other tools currently available may give a more complete picture.
   2. **Address the symptoms of mood and affect,** which are often subtle in the elderly.
      a. **Sleep** disturbance is either increased or decreased.
      b. **Interests** may be decreased.
      c. **Guilt** is often prominent, as are ruminations.
      d. **Energy** may be reduced.
      e. **Concentration** may be impaired.
      f. **Appetite** and weight loss can occur and be harbingers of dementia, depression, or medical illness.
      g. **Psychomotor** agitation or retardation often occurs and can be confused with the manifestations of neurological illnesses, such as Parkinson's disease.

471

h. **Suicide** is common in the elderly, with the peak age in women of 50–65 years, and 80–90 years in men.
   i. One in nine suicide attempts in the elderly results in death.
   ii. The risk of death by suicide in those over 65 years of age is double that of the United States population at large.
   iii. Statistics report completed suicide and not passive suicides; therefore, suicide in the elderly is probably under-reported.
   iv. Predictors of suicide risk include: advanced age; male sex; being separated, isolated, or divorced; having a debilitating illness; and abusing alcohol.
3. **Psychosis, with hallucinations, paranoia, or delusions, is common** in psychiatric disorders in older patients.
   a. Hallucinations (visual, auditory, olfactory, gustatory, and tactile) are present in a variety of illnesses, not just psychiatric conditions.

B. **Functional Assessment**
1. **Assess activities of daily living (ADLs) and determine if the patient is capable of transferring independently, dressing him- or herself, bathing and maintaining hygiene, feeding him- or herself, toileting and using the bathroom, and maintaining bladder and bowel continence.**
2. **Assess instrumental activities of daily living (IADLs), and determine if the patient can live independently, go shopping for food, cook meals, use the telephone, do light housekeeping, manage medications, handle finances, and arrange transportation.**

C. **Obtain a complete medical history,** and **review the medical records.** Ask the **family** to **summarize the history** of the patient's function over the past several years; if possible have them provide a written summary.
1. History is very important to document.
2. Perform a mental status examination.
3. Conduct a thorough physical examination, and review the records from the primary care physician (PCP).
4. Conduct a neurological examination.
5. Order appropriate imaging study (computed tomography [CT] or magnetic resonance imaging [MRI]) if indicated from history.
6. Obtain an electroencephalogram (EEG) if indicated from the history.
7. Order laboratory testing, after a complete review of records and an evaluation of the patient.

D. **Carefully assess the living situation; determine if the:**
1. **Patient lives alone,** and is **safe at home.**
2. Patient **lives with the family.**
3. Patient **is dependent on the family.**
4. Patient's **family depends on the elder** for money or other financial benefits.

IV. Depression in the Older Patient

A. **Diagnosis**
The diagnosis of depression in the elderly is **not difficult to make,** but often it is overlooked due to impaired cognition, sadness, and confusion, and to a general decline in function or to a failure to thrive. In addition, medical and neurological complications and side effects of medications can obscure the appropriate diagnosis of any psychiatric illness (see Table 65-1).

B. **Impact of Depression**
Depression **lowers life-expectancy** in the elderly. **Suicide rates are higher** in the elderly; only 25% of all suicides in the elderly are reported. Rates increase as isolation increases. Late-onset depression is associated with a higher rate of physical illness; **depression also leads to psychiatric hospitalization in 50% of those afflicted.** Approximately 30% of patients with dementia also have major depression, and those with a history of stroke, Parkinson's disease, or multiple sclerosis are also vulnerable to depression.

C. **Comorbidity**
1. **Grief and loss** also contribute to **depression.**
2. Nearly 60% of depressed patients have **comorbid anxiety.**
3. Roughly **40% of anxious patients have comorbid depression related to medical illness** (e.g., cardiac conditions [such as myocardial infarction—MI], renal failure, cancer, endocrine disturbances, infec-

---

Table 65-1. Common Classes of Drugs Causing Symptoms of Depression

- Analgesics
   Narcotics
   NSAIDS
- Antihypertensives
- Antipsychotics
- Anxiolytics
   Alcohol
   Benzodiazepines
- Chemotherapeutic agents
   Antineoplastics
- Sedative-hypnotic
- Steroids
- Diuretics
   Thiazides
- H_2 blockers

tions), and neurologic illness (e.g., stroke, Parkinson's disease, cerebral neoplasm, multiple sclerosis). <u>**Caveat: undiagnosed medical illness can present as depression.**</u>

D. Epidemiology

Epidemiological studies of the elderly **reveal a 1-month prevalence of all affective disorders of 2.5%.** Depressive symptomatology is recognized in 10–25% of the elderly, but it is rarely diagnosed.

1. According to the Epidemiologic Catchment Area (ECA) study, 1–3% of elderly in the **community** are diagnosed with depression.
   a. A 1-month prevalence of those over 65 years revealed:
      i. Major depression is present in 0.7%.
      ii. Dysthymia occurs in 1.8%.
   b. The 6-month prevalence showed:
      i. Men met criteria 0.5–2.2% of the time.
      ii. Women met criteria 3.1–5.0% of the time.

E. Treatment of Depression in the Elderly (see Table 65-2)

Rapid assessment and treatment of depression is beneficial to prevent onset of a "failure to thrive" syndrome, and progressive deterioration. Factors such as illness, use of medications, and psychosocial problems should be addressed, and treatment initiated.

Polypharmacy is a significant problem in the elderly. Therefore, when considering the use of medications it is important to weigh the risks and benefits while monitoring the interactions with other medications prescribed by other doctors. The addition of one new drug can disrupt the tenuous balance of an established drug regimen.

1. **Begin with a complete review of current medications** and include a review of all drugs, including over-the-counter and homeopathic remedies. Ask the

Table 65-2. Treatments Recommended for Depression in the Elderly

Drugs	Dose Range (mg/day)	Comments
Tricyclic antidepressants		
Nortriptyline	10–150	Reliable blood levels, minimal orthostasis, mildly anticholinergic
Desipramine	10–250	
Monoamine oxidase inhibitors		
Tranylcypromine	10–30	Orthostasis (may be delayed), pedal edema, weakly anticholinergic, dietary restrictions needed
Stimulants		
Dextroamphetamine	2.5–40	Agitation, mild tachycardia
Methylphenidate	2.5–60	
Selective serotonin reuptake inhibitors		
Fluoxetine	5.0–60	Akathisia, headache, agitation, gastrointestinal complaints, diarrhea/constipation
Sertraline	25–200	
Paroxetine	5–40	
Fluvoxamine	25–300	
Citalopram	10–40	
Serotonin/norepinephrine reuptake inhibitors		
Venlafaxine	25–300	Increase in systolic BP, confusion
Alpha-2 antagonist/selective serotonin		
Mirtazapine	15–30	Sedation, weight gain
Atypical antidepressants		
Trazodone	25–250	Sedation, orthostasis, incontinence, hallucinations, priapism
Nefazodone	50–600	Pedal edema, rash
Bupropion	75–450	Seizures, less mania/cycling, headache, nausea

patient or family members to bring all the medication bottles and over-the-counter medications.

2. **Propose an initial diagnostic formulation,** and then proceed to a medication trial. Ensure the **trial is time-limited,** with clearly identified target symptoms. **Re-evaluate often** and give an adequate trial prior to discontinuing a drug. **Avoid drug-drug effects** if possible.

   a. **Start with lowest possible dose of a medication and increase it slowly.** In frail, medically ill, or old-old, "start lower, go slower" as age increases.

      i. In the medically ill patient over 80 years of age, begin even lower and increase medications at longer intervals.

      ii. When side effects appear, discontinue the drug; remember that elimination half-life is longer and can complicate the effects caused by the addition of a second drug.

   b. **Medications for depression**

      i. Evaluate the side effect profile of a drug and use it advantageously—e.g., induce sedation in a patient with insomnia, or weight gain in a patient with significant weight loss.

      ii. Begin one drug at a time, and change one element at a time.

      iii. Treat aggressively when psychosis and suicide are prominent; if depression is life-threatening, consider hospitalization and electroconvulsive therapy (ECT).

3. **Re-evaluate** after a therapeutic trial.

   a. **When symptoms resolve, continue at the current dose for at least 1 year before considering discontinuation of the medication.**

      i. If symptoms have partially resolved, continue and increase dose, or add an adjunctive medication to boost the initial response.

      ii. If there is no response, start another medication, possibly even one within the same class.

      iii. Adjunctive medications can be considered if an initial response was noted.

   b. **The question inevitably arises as to when the medication can be discontinued;** remember that the risk of relapse and recurrence is greater in older patients and a trial off medications may be fraught with complications.

      i. Continue medication for at least 1 year and up to 18 months after treatment response.

      ii. If there is no contraindication, maintain the medication to prevent recurrence.

F. **Psychotherapy is effective alone or in combination with medications.**

1. Structured individual therapies can be successful alone, but are best when in combination with medications.

2. Individual therapies include: supportive, cognitive, behavioral, interpersonal, and psychodynamic. All modalities have been efficacious in the older population.

3. Group therapy:

   a. Specific themes for a group can enable discussion of issues that may be more difficult to identify (e.g., depression, grief, and anxiety).

   b. Support for patient and/or family.

   c. Family:

      i. Dealing with conflict resolution.

      ii. Informative, information gathering.

      iii. Family dynamics.

V. Bipolar Illness

Although not rare, the first onset of symptoms of mania and hypomania is uncommon in the elderly, most patients have had at least one episode earlier in their life. New-onset mania in the elderly should elicit a search for an underlying medical or neurological illness. Complicating the diagnosis of bipolar disorder is a secondary mania due to a medical condition or neurological disorder.

VI. Anxiety

Anxiety is frequently diagnosed in older patients, and symptoms of anxiety are common in 10–20% of older patients. The prevalence is higher in women than in men with a 1-month prevalence of 3.6% in men versus 6.8% in women. Anxiety and depression are often associated with physical illness and may present prior to diagnosis of medical illness. Symptoms of anxiety include: worry, fear, apprehension, concern, foreboding; and somatic complaints of tachycardia, sweating, abdominal distress, and dizziness. **Worries, fears, and concerns center on financial issues, illness, loneliness, dependency, and dementia.** Substances, such as caffeine, ephedrine, and stimulants, can precipitate anxiety in elderly. Withdrawal from benzodiazepines, alcohol, and barbiturates can resemble anxiety and require aggressive treatment.

Treatment of anxiety is similar to younger patients with **medications** and/or therapy. **Cognitive-behavioral therapies** have been incorporated more often over the past several years in order to avoid the side effects of medications. Benzodiazepines have been used extensively for decades, and judicious use of these medications is effective. However, complications of long-term use of these medications are daytime somnolence, confusion or cognitive impairment, unsteady stance or gait, paradoxical effects, memory disturbance, withdrawal, abuse, dependence, and respiratory compromise.

VII. Dementia

Dementia is the most common syndrome of cognitive impairment or decline in the elderly. Dementia involves a chronic and substantial decline in greater than two areas of cognitive functioning.

A. **Age-associated memory impairment (AAMI)** or age-related cognitive decline **is common in elderly.**

1. Although patients and family members worry that symptoms of AAMI may be a harbinger of dementia, these individuals tend not to develop dementia when followed for many years.
   a. **Establishing a baseline of cognitive impairments is of benefit** for two reasons.
      i. Future testing will be compared to the original presentation to assess deterioration in a standardized format.
      ii. Strategize and find useful tools to enhance weaker areas and to implement safety.
   b. **Provide for safety when any memory disorder is present.**

B. **Dementia tends to present with a chronic persistent decline,** albeit subtle, over a period of years. Most dementias have an insidious, slow, and progressive course. Of the approximately 4 million patients occupying half the nursing home beds in the United States, approximately 7% carry the diagnosis of Alzheimer's disease (AD).
   1. **Alzheimer's disease is ultimately a histopathologic diagnosis at autopsy.** The basic criteria are outlined in the NINCDS-ADRDA criteria for clinical diagnosis of probable AD. **The course is slow; over time there is worsening memory and a decline of other cognitive functions with a clear consciousness.** All other reversible causes are ruled out, and a complete neurological evaluation is essential.
      a. A brief synopsis of the **stages of decline** include:
         i. No cognitive decline.
         ii. Very mild.
         iii. Mild, and others now aware of deficits.
         iv. Moderate (with clear deficits); the patient may get lost.
         v. Moderately severe; requires assistance and reorientation.
         vi. Severe; unaware, apathetic, agitated, abulic, violent, with a sketchy memory of the past, and marked personality change.
         vii. Very severe; unable to communicate, incontinent, with focal neurological signs, needs assistance most of the time.
   2. **Lewy body disease (LBD)** is often confused with AD and can complicate the use of medications. **Patients with LBD have more hallucinations and a greater sensitivity to the side effects of neuroleptic medications** than AD patients. LBD is characterized by widespread distribution of Lewy bodies in the brainstem, basal forebrain, and cortex.
      i. Reported as a fairly common form of degenerative dementia.
      ii. Characterized by fluctuating cognitive impairment, transient episodes of marked confusion, prominent behavioral changes, and a high incidence of visual/auditory hallucinations and delusions.
      iii. Extrapyramidal signs are present as is an exquisite sensitivity to neuroleptic medication.

3. **Frontal lobe dementia (FLD)** manifests prominent symptoms of **disinhibition, self-neglect, and self-destructiveness;** patients are often **unaware or unconcerned** that any problem or deficit exists.
4. **Vascular dementia usually presents with a stuttering course,** and the losses are more focal in the territory of the damage.
5. **Alcoholic dementia** gradually damages the area of the dorsal inferior frontal lobe with symptoms similar to frontal lobe lesions. When alcohol use is stopped, cognitive losses should stabilize.

C. **Important issues** should be **discussed with the family members and caretakers;** education around diagnosis of dementia should include:
   1. **Rapid changes in a patient's behavior or cognition**
      a. Consider medical illness.
      b. Consider side effects of medication.
   2. **Incontinence**
      a. Usually presents late in the progression of the disease.
      b. Evaluate for a medical etiology.
      c. Eventually it may involve both urinary and fecal incontinence.
   3. **Driving**
      a. Arrange for alternative transportation.
      b. Hide car keys or disable the vehicle.
   4. **Cooking**
      a. Supervised only.
      b. Remove knobs.
      c. Turn off the gas or electricity.
      d. Hide matches.
   5. **Smoking**
      a. Under close supervision only.
      b. Remove all smoking paraphernalia (e.g., ashtrays, matches).
      c. Do not smoke in front of the patient.
   6. **Firearms**
      a. Remove them from the home.
      b. Keep them locked securely.
   7. **Caregiver support**
      a. Day centers
      b. Help, either during the day or overnight
      c. Visiting Nurse Association
      d. Alzheimer's Association (local or national), even if not AD (Alzheimer's Association, 919 N. Michigan Ave, Suite 1000, Chicago, IL 60611; 1-800-272-3900)
      e. Education with pamphlets, books, and videotapes
      f. Support groups
      g. Legal assistance
         i. Important early in process prior to crisis
         ii. Financial and estate planning
         iii. Future needs, long-term care

VIII. Delirium

Delirium is often under-recognized, under-reported, or inadequately documented by physicians. Signs and symptoms are documented in less than 50% of cases; 10–20% of all hospitalized patients manifest some degree of delirium.

A. Elderly patients are at high risk for delirium.

1. The elderly are at greater risk for delirium due to age-related sensitivity to medications, and to comorbid illnesses.

   a. Life-threatening conditions must be treated swiftly and the underlying cause ameliorated. Medical illness is often the culprit and medications add a second dimension to the problem.

   b. Drug-induced delirium can be precipitated by any medication; close scrutiny of all medications is essential.

2. **Presentation of delirium is variable** and therefore it is difficult to diagnose accurately.

   a. Clinical features of delirium include a prodrome, a rapidly fluctuating course, decreased attention, altered arousal, psychomotor abnormality, sleep-wake cycle disturbance, impaired memory, EEG abnormalities, and affective features of intense anger, fear, sadness, rage, apathy, anxiety, or panic.

   b. **Management of delirium** is complex.
      i. **Accurate diagnosis** is paramount.
      ii. **Treatment of the underlying cause** is required.
      iii. **Elimination of contributing factors** is needed.
      iv. **Supportive care** is helpful, as is maintenance of an adequate fluid balance, nutrition, sedation, rest,

Table 65-3. Neuroleptics Commonly Used in the Elderly

Drug/Dose	Sedation	Anticholinergic Potency	Extrapyramidal Symptoms (Risk)	Equivalency (mg)
Low potency				
Thioridazine (Mellaril) 10–50 mg	High	High	Low	95
Intermediate potency				
Perphenazine (Trilafon) 0.5–5 mg	Medium	Medium	Medium	8
High potency				
Haloperidol (Haldol) 0.25–2 mg	Low	Low	High	2
Thiothixene (Navane) 0.5–4 mg	Low	Low	High	5
Fluphenazine (Prolixin) 0.5–2 mg	Low	Low	High	2
Atypical neuroleptics				
Clozapine (Clozaril) 2.5–100 mg	High	High	Very low	100
Risperidone (Risperdal) 0.5–3 mg	Low	Low	Low-moderate	1–2
Olanzapine (Zyprexa) 5.0–10.0 mg	Moderate	Moderate	Low-moderate	
Quetiapine (Seroquel) 12.5–200 mg	High	Low	Low	

comfort, good nursing care, and encouragement of a family presence, frequent re-orientation, optimal stimulation, a well-lit room, and appropriate use of eyeglasses and hearing aids.

v. **Treatment** includes use of high-potency neuroleptics, with attention paid to target symptoms. **Haloperidol** has been the drug of choice, but newer atypical neuroleptics are being used more frequently (see Table 65-3). The starting dose is always the lowest possible dose. **Haloperidol, used intravenously, has the most rapid effect; start with a low dose and titrate upwards.** Benzodiazepines may be synergistic with neuroleptics, but can disinhibit the patient or cause paradoxical reactions.

vi. **The course and prognosis** need to be watched carefully, as older patients are at a greater risk for death during the illness and for up to 6 months after recovery.

IX. Alcoholism

Alcoholism is often overlooked or minimized in the elderly. The ECA data show that **1% of the elderly have alcoholism.** A life-long pattern of daily use can be a problem and can lead to withdrawal.

A. **Comorbid illness** (psychiatric, neurologic, and medical) **can confound an accurate diagnosis.**

1. A careful history from family, friends, and caretakers is extremely important in this illness characterized by denial.

X. Acute Behavioral Problems

Patients with dementia and delirium can exhibit acute behavioral problems, such as aggression, agitation, rage, wandering, and screaming. These symptoms are difficult to treat; patients are often overmedicated, yet are never successfully relieved of these problems.

XI. Elder Abuse

Elder abuse can present subtly. Family members or caregivers may be overwhelmed. Hotlines are available in every state (Massachusetts 1-800-922-2275).

Suggested Readings

Alexopoulos GS: Affective disorders. In Sadavoy J, Lazarus LW, Jarvik LF, Grossberg GT (eds): *Comprehensive Review of Geriatric Psychiatry-II*, 2nd ed. Washington, DC: APA Press, 1996:536–592.

Almeida OP, Howard RJ, Levy R, David AS. Psychotic states arising in late life. *Br J Psychiatry* 1995; 166:205–214.

Applegate WB, Blass JP, Williams TF. Instruments for the functional assessment of older patients. *N Engl J Med* 1990; 322: 1207–1213.

Cattell H, Jolley DJ. One hundred cases of suicide in elderly people. *Br J Psychiatry* 1995; 166:451–457.

Devanand DP, Jacobs DM, Tang MX, et al.: The course of psychopathologic features in mild to moderate Alzheimer's disease. *Arch Gen Psychiatry* 1997; 54:257–263.

Drevets WC: Geriatric depression: brain imaging correlates and pharmacologic considerations. *J Clin Psychiatry* 1994; 55 (Suppl. 9A):71–81.

Fernandez F, Levy JK, Lachar BL, Small GW: The management of depression and anxiety in the elderly. *J Clin Psychiatry* 1995; 56 (Suppl. 2):20–29.

Jenike MA: *Geriatric Psychiatry and Psychopharmacology: A Clinical Approach.* St. Louis: Mosby, 1989.

Jenike MA, Cremens MC: Geriatric psychopharmacology. *Psychiatr Clin North Am* 1994; 1:125–164.

Jeste DV, Eastham JH, Larcro JP, et al.: Management of late-life psychosis. *J Clin Psychiatry* 1996; 57 (Suppl. 3):39–45.

Lebert F, Pasquier F, Petit H: Behavioral effects of trazodone in Alzheimer's disease. *J Clin Psychiatry* 1994; 55:536–538.

Martin RL (ed.): Geriatric psychiatry: what's new about the old. *Psychiatr Clin North Am* 1997; 20(1):1–268.

McDonald WM, Nemeroff CB: The diagnosis and treatment of mania in the elderly. *Bull Menninger Clin* 1996; 60:174–196.

Newhouse PA: Use of serotonin selective reuptake inhibitors in geriatric depression. *J Clin Psychiatry* 1996; 57 (Suppl. 5):12–22.

NIH Consensus Conference: Diagnosis and treatment of depression in late life. *J Am Med Assoc* 1992; 268:1018–1024.

Oxman TE: Antidepressants and cognitive impairment in the elderly. *J Clin Psychiatry* 1996; 57 (Suppl. 5):38–44.

Pande A, Krugler T, Haskett R: Predictors of response to electroconvulsive therapy in major depressive disorder. *Biol Psychiatry* 1988; 24:91–93.

Pollock BG, Mulsant BH: Behavioral disturbances of dementia. *J Geriatr Psychiatry Neurol* 1998; 11:206–212.

Rothchild AJ: The diagnosis and treatment of late-life depression. *J Clin Psychiatry* 1996; 57 (Suppl. 5):5–11.

Sadavoy J, Lazarus LW, Jarvik LF, Grossberg GT (eds): *Comprehensive Review of Geriatric Psychiatry-II*, 2nd ed. Washington, DC: APA Press, 1996.

Sano M, Ernesto C, Thomas RG, et al.: A controlled trial of selegiline, alpha-tocopherol, or both as treatments for Alzheimer's disease. *N Engl J Med* 1997; 336:1216–1222.

Shorr RI, Robin DW: Rational use of benzodiazepines in the elderly. *Drugs Aging* 1994; 4:9–20.

Tariot PN: Treatment strategies for agitation and psychosis in dementia. *J Clin Psychiatry* 1996; 57:21–29.

Weiss KJ: Management of anxiety and depression syndromes in the elderly. *J Clin Psychiatry* 1994; 55 (Suppl. 2):5–12.

Wilcox SM, Himmelstein DU, Woolhandler S: Inappropriate drug prescribing for the community-dwelling elderly. *J Am Med Assoc* 1994; 272:292–296.

Work Group on Alzheimer's Disease and Related Dementias: Practice guideline for the treatment of patients with Alzheimer's disease and other dementias of late life. *Am J Psychiatry* 1997; 154 (Suppl.):1–39.

Young RC, Klerman GL: Mania in late life: focus on age of onset. *Am J Psychiatry* 1992; 149:867–876.

Zweig RA, Hinrichsen GA: Factors associated with suicide attempts by depressed older adults: a prospective study. *Am J Psychiatry* 1993; 150:1687–1692.

Zyas EM, Grossberg GT: The treatment of psychosis in late life. *J Clin Psychiatry* 1998; 59 (Suppl.):5–10.

SECTION V

Special Topics in Psychiatry

Chapter 66
Psychiatric Epidemiology
ALBERT YEUNG

I. Introduction

Epidemiology is the study of the distribution and determinants of disease frequency in human populations. It is about observing, counting, and comparing the occurrence of disease between different populations at a given time, between subgroups of a population, or between different periods of a population. Since human disease does not occur at random, systematic investigation of the relationship of disease frequency, and of the characteristics of populations, may shed light on the etiology of the disease. **By providing data on the distribution and frequency of diseases, epidemiological studies help to assess service needs in the community or in special institutions, and to describe the natural history of illness.**

To achieve these goals, epidemiological observation studies are conducted with large groups of individuals. The first step is often case recognition. This is especially challenging in psychiatric epidemiology due to the absence of pathognomonic laboratory abnormalities for diagnosing psychiatric disorders.

II. Assessment

A. Case Definition
In 1972, Cooper et al. published the US/UK diagnostic study which demonstrated the variability of diagnosis in psychotic disorders. It highlighted the importance of having explicit operational criteria for case identification. The use of diagnostic criteria as listed in the *Diagnostic and Statistical Manual, Third Edition* (DSM-III) in 1980 represented a great step towards the advancement of the reliability and validity of psychiatric diagnosis.

B. Standardized Instruments for Case Assessment
The clinical interview is generally used to diagnose psychiatric illness. However, differences in personal styles, as well as in theoretical frameworks, may affect the process and the outcome of the psychiatric interview. **To increase inter-rater reliability, a variety of standardized instruments have been used.** The first such instrument was the **Present State Examination (PSE),** which was used in the International Pilot Study of Schizophrenia sponsored by the World Health Organization (WHO). Since the PSE was intended for use by psychiatrists or by experienced clinicians, its use in epidemiologic studies has been limited, due to the high volume

of subjects involved in such studies. Based on other research instruments, including **the Renald Diagnostic Interview (RDI), the St. Louis criteria, and the Schedule for Affective Disorders and Schizophrenia (SADS),** epidemiologists at the National Institute of Mental Health (NIMH) developed the **Diagnostic Interview Schedule (DIS),** a fully structured interview that could be used by non-clinicians to assess large numbers of subjects according to DSM-III criteria. The DIS has been used extensively in the United States and many other countries for surveys of psychiatric illness. Recently, the WHO and the NIMH updated and modified the DIS and developed the **Composite International Diagnostic Interview (CIDI),** which is structurally similar to the DIS and provides both **ICD-10 and DSM-IV** diagnoses.

C. Reliability
Reliability is the degree to which a measurement produces systematic or reproducible results. Use of explicit diagnostic criteria, a structured assessment instrument, and adequate training of raters, each enhance the reliability of making a psychiatric diagnosis. Reliability is a necessary, but not sufficient, condition for a valid diagnosis. **The kappa statistic (κ) is frequently used to measure the reliability between raters** (see Table 66-1). It shows the degree of consistency between raters, with an adjustment of agreement due to chance. An important characteristic of the kappa statistic is that **it is influenced by how common the particular condition is in the study sample. When the frequency of the disorder is very low, kappa statistics will be low despite having a high degree of consistency between raters. Therefore, the kappa statistic is not applicable for measuring the reliability for infrequent disorders.**

$$\kappa = \frac{P_o - P_c}{1 - P_c}$$

where P_o is the observed agreement, P_c is agreement due to chance, $P_o = (a+d)/n$ and $P_c = [(a+c)(a+b) + (b+d)(c+d)]/n^2$.

D. Validity
An instrument is considered valid if the instrument measures what it is intended to measure. Rater or

Table 66-1. Inter-Rater Reliability

Rater B	Rater A		
	Disorder Present	*Disorder Absent*	*Total*
Disorder present	a	b	$a+b$
Disorder absent	c	d	$c+d$
Total	$a+c$	$b+d$	n

instrument validity of a psychiatric diagnosis is ideally done by comparison of the tested rater or instrument with a well-known standard of truth. Unfortunately, in psychiatry, there is no absolute measure of a diagnosis. A criterion instrument (rater) is usually chosen as the truth and is used for comparison with the new instrument (rater) (see Table 66-2).

Sensitivity, specificity, positive predictive power, and negative predictive power are frequently used to express the validity of an instrument. Sensitivity is a measure of the new instrument's ability to detect the true cases of a disorder identified by the criterion instrument. Specificity is a measure of the new instrument's ability to identify the true non-cases identified by the criterion instrument. Higher values of sensitivity and specificity are always desirable. For a given instrument, higher sensitivity is obtained by lowering specificity and vice versa. The only way to improve both sensitivity and specificity without a trade-off is to improve the instrument itself. **Positive predictive power is the proportion of apparent cases, as detected by the new instrument, that are true cases as determined by the criterion instrument. Negative predictive power is the proportion of apparent non-cases, as detected by the new instrument, that are true non-cases as determined by the criterion instrument.**

Sensitivity $= a/(a+c)$

Specificity $= d/(b+d)$

Positive predictive rate $= a/(a+b)$

Negative predictive rate $= d/(c+d)$

III. Measurement of Disease Frequency

A. Prevalence
Prevalence is the proportion of individuals in a population who have a disease at a specific instant; it provides an estimate of the probability that an individual will be ill at any point. Prevalence is determined by the rate at which the disease develops and by the duration of the disease. That is, with the same rate of development, a chronic disease will have a higher prevalence than an acute one. Prevalence rate is more useful for descriptive purposes. It was used to describe the frequency of an illness in a community population. In addition, it reflects service needs:

$$P = \frac{\text{Number of existing cases of a disease at a given point in time}}{\text{Total population}}$$

B. Incidence
Incidence quantifies the number of new events or cases of a disease that develop in a population of individuals at risk during a specified time interval. There are two specific types of incidence measures: cumulative incidence and incidence rate. Cumulative incidence (CI) is the proportion of people who become diseased during a specified period. It is calculated by the equation:

Table 66-2. Validity of a New Instrument

New Instrument	Truth (Criterion Instrument Results)		
	Disorder Present	*Disorder Absent*	*Total*
Disorder present	a	b	$a+b$
Disorder absent	c	d	$c+d$
Total	$a+c$	$b+d$	n

$$CI = \frac{\text{Number of new cases of a disease during a given period}}{\text{Total population at risk}}$$

In real life, some people enter a study at different times, others may become lost during the study and no longer available for follow-up. When a person in the study becomes a case, they stop being at risk and no longer contribute to the denominator. To account for the variable durations for which people are at risk, incidence rate (IR) is used; this is defined as:

$$IR = \frac{\text{Number of new cases of a disease in a year}}{\text{Total person-years of observation}}$$

For example, 100 subjects were studied, two were lost to follow-up at the end of 6 months, and eight developed a disease at the end of the sixth month; 90 subjects were disease-free at the end of 1 year. The person-years of observation was $(90 \times 1 \text{ year}) + (2 \times 0.5 \text{ year}) + (8 \times 0.5 \text{ year}) = 95$ person-years, and $IR = (8 \text{ persons})/(95 \text{ person-years}) = 8.42/100$ person-years of observation.

Incidence rates are more difficult to calculate than prevalence rates, and require more extensive data collection. Unlike prevalence rates, incidence rates are not affected by the duration of the disease. The incidence rate is more precise when measuring disease rate; it is useful in analytical studies of effects of risk factors.

C. **Period Prevalence**
   The period prevalence rate is used to summarize the number of cases of a disorder that exist at any time during a specified time period. Its numerator includes any existing cases at the start of the period plus any new cases that develop during the time period. For a 1-year period, the annual period prevalence rate is approximately equal to the point prevalence rate [(existing cases)/(population at the start)] plus the annual cumulative incidence rate [(new cases in a year)/(population at risk)].

D. **Lifetime Prevalence**
   The lifetime prevalence rate is a measure of persons considered at a point in time who have ever had the illness under study. It is a useful statistic to describe conditions that remit but often recur, such as major depressive disorder.

IV. Study Designs

A. **Descriptive Studies**
   Descriptive studies describe patterns of disease occurrence in relation to selected variables (e.g., person, place, and time). They utilize census data, vital statistic records, and clinical records from hospitals, or national figures on consumption of goods, oil, or other products. **There are three main types of descriptive studies: correlation studies, case reports or case series, and cross-sectional surveys of individuals.** Data from descriptive studies are useful for public health administrators who plan for health care utilization and resource allocation. They are also valuable for formulation of etiologic hypotheses. However, descriptive studies in general cannot be used for testing etiologic hypotheses. For hypothesis testing, analytic design strategies (cohort, case-control, or intervention study) are needed.

B. **Cohort Studies**
   In cohort studies, or follow-up studies, a group of individuals (cohort) is defined on the basis of the presence or absence of exposure to a suspected risk factor for a disease. The rates at which they develop a certain disease or an outcome of interest are measured and compared. By nature of the design, individuals in such a study need to be disease-free at the start of the study. For a prospective cohort study, individuals are followed for a specified period and their outcome is compared. For a retrospective cohort study, information on risk factors is obtained from records collected in the past at the actual time of the exposure, and the information on disease status is obtained at the time of the study.

   Relative risk (RR) is calculated to test for the possible association between exposure and outcome (disease). If the relative risk is greater than 1.0, the exposure is considered to be associated with the disease (see Table 66-3).

$$RR = \frac{a/(a+b)}{c/(c+d)}$$

C. **Case-Control Studies**
   Subjects in case-control studies are selected on the basis of whether they do (cases) or do not (controls) have a particular disease under study. The groups are compared with respect to their proportions of having certain risk factors of interest. A case-control design is usually used for studying rare disorders. **Instead of relative risk, an odds ratio is calculated to detect an association between the risk factor and the disease.** If the odds ratio is greater than 1.0, the risk factor is considered to be associated with caseness (see Table 66-3).

$$\text{Odds ratio} = \frac{ad}{bc}$$

D. **Intervention Studies**
   In an intervention study, the investigator controls the allocation of subjects to different comparison groups and regulates the experimental conditions of each

Table 66-3. Association Between Risk Factors and Disease in Cohort and Case-Control Studies

	New Cases	Non-Cases	Total
Risk factor present	a	b	$a+b$
Risk factor not present	c	d	$c+d$
Total	$a+c$	$b+d$	$a+b+c+d$

group. Study subjects are randomly assigned to comparison groups and followed over time to observe the outcome (e.g., decreased disease frequency or improved clinical condition, of the intervention). Clinical trials are the most common form of intervention studies. To ensure the comparability between groups and to obtain valid results, intervention studies employ three basic research strategies: randomization, placebo-control, and blinding.

E. **Epidemiological Catchment Area (ECA) Study**
   1. **Overview. The ECA study was a multisite, epidemiological study conducted by the National Institute of Mental Health (NIMH) in the 1980s.** Five sites (Yale University, The Johns Hopkins University, Washington University, Duke University, and the University of California in Los Angeles) were selected, which respectively surveyed communities and institutions in New Haven, Baltimore, St. Louis, Durham, and Los Angeles. **It assessed the prevalence, the incidence, and the service-use rates of mental disorders.** The DIS, a fully structured interview administered by lay interviewers, was used to provide current and lifetime diagnoses of many DSM-III disorders. By incorporating the DSM-III diagnostic criteria, the ECA study made a great advance in increasing the precision of case assessment, a precision not previously attained in previous community surveys. Other strengths of the ECA study included its meticulous sampling method, and its high response rate.
   2. **Results. Data from the ECA program revealed that about one-third of adults in the United States report symptoms that meet criteria for one or more psychiatric disorders during their lifetime.** About 20% had an active disorder—i.e., one for which criteria had been met at some time during the past, with at least one symptom (or episode) occurring in the year before the interview. Overall, the ECA data indicated that over their lifetime more men than women met criteria for having a disorder, that younger persons have more disorders than do older persons, that African-Americans are more likely than whites to have a psychiatric disorder,

and that less well-educated individuals have more disorders than do the well-educated. Furthermore, active disorders are more likely to be reported among those who are financially dependent or unemployed, and among those who have a low job status, even if they are employed. Persons who are divorced, separated, or cohabiting also have more active disorders. While men have more lifetime disorders than do women, only two disorders (alcohol abuse, and antisocial personality) showed a sizable male excess. On the other hand, lifetime rates for women exceeded those for men for somatization disorder, obsessive-compulsive disorder, and major depressive episodes.

Phobias and alcohol abuse are the most prevalent disorders in the United States. Over 14% of persons reported a phobia during their lifetime, and nearly 9% reported having a phobia during the past year. Nearly 14% met criteria for alcohol abuse and dependence during their lifetime, and over 6% met criteria during the past year. Other frequently reported disorders include generalized anxiety disorder, major depressive episode, and drug abuse/dependence. **Cognitive impairment, assessed only for an active disorder, occurred in about 5% of individuals. Somatization disorder occurred in about 1 per 1,000 persons** (see Table 66-4).

V. Epidemiology of Major Psychiatric Disorders

A. **Schizophrenia**
   In the United States, the lifetime prevalence of schizophrenia has been reported to range from 1% to 1.5%. In the ECA study, the lifetime prevalence of schizophrenia was 1.3%. About 0.025–0.05% of the total population are treated for schizophrenia in any one year. Genetic loading appears to have a strong influence on the development of schizophrenia (see Table 66-5). The prevalence of schizophrenia in a monozygotic twin of a schizophrenia patient is 47%; with a dizygotic twin it is 12%. The prevalence for a child with two schizophrenic parents is 46.3%; for a child with one schizophrenic parent it is 12.0%. Other risk

Table 66-4. Prevalence Estimates (%) for Specific Disorders

	Lifetime	Active (1 Year)
Phobia	14.3	8.8
Alcohol abuse/dependence	13.8	6.3
Generalized anxiety	8.5	3.8
Major depressive episode	6.4	3.7
Drug abuse/dependence	6.2	2.5
Cognitive impairment (mild or severe)	n/a	5.0
Dysthymia	3.3	n/a
Antisocial personality	2.6	1.2
Obsessive-compulsive	2.6	1.7
Panic	1.6	0.9
Schizophrenia or schizophreniform	1.5	1.0
Manic episode	0.8	0.6
Cognitive impairment: severe	NA	0.9
Somatization	0.1	0.1

n/a, not ascertained.

Table 66-5. Prevalence of Schizophrenia in Specific Populations

Population	Prevalence (%)
General population	1.0
Non-twin sibling of a schizophrenic patient	8.0
Child with one schizophrenic parent	12.0
Dizygotic twin of a schizophrenia patient	12.0
Child of two schizophrenic parents	46.3
Monozygotic twin of a schizophrenic patient	47.0

factors for schizophrenia include being a member of a lower social class, being unmarried, having pregnancy or birth complications, and being born during the winter months. Of note, inhabitants of the Istrian peninsula in former Yugoslavia and on the western coast of Ireland have an unusually high rate of schizophrenia.

B. Bipolar I Disorder
Bipolar I disorder affects men and women equally. It has a lifetime prevalence of 0.4–1.2%. The 1-month prevalence for bipolar disorder is 0.1–0.6%. Bipolar I disorder occurs at much higher rates in first-degree biologic relatives of persons with bipolar I disorder than it does in the general population. **First-degree relatives of those with bipolar I disorder have a 12% chance of having the same disorder over their lifetime.** Another 12% have recurrent major depressive disorder, and roughly 12% more have dysthymia or another mood disorder.

C. Major Depression
The point prevalence for major depressive disorder in Western industrialized nations is 2.3–3.2% for men and 4.5–9.3% for women. The lifetime risk for major depressive disorder is 7–12% for men and 20–25% for women. Prevalence rates are unrelated to race, education, income, or civil status. Risk factors for major depressive disorder include being female, having a history of depressive illness in first-degree relatives, having prior episodes of major depression, having an age of onset under 40 years, being postpartum, having prior suicide attempts, having a medical comorbidity, having lack of social support, experiencing stressful life events, and having a current problem with substance abuse. The point prevalence of major depressive disorder seen in primary care outpatient settings ranges from 4.8% to 8.6%.

D. Panic Disorder
Epidemiological studies have reported lifetime prevalence rates of 1.5–3% for panic disorder and 3–4% for panic attacks. Women are two to three times more likely to be affected than are men, and

the differences among Hispanics, non-Hispanic whites, and blacks are small. The only social factor found to be related to panic disorder is a recent history of divorce or separation. Panic disorder most commonly develops in young adulthood; the mean age of presentation is about 25 years, but both panic disorder and agoraphobia can develop at any age.

E. Alcohol Abuse and Dependence
The ECA study found that 13.8% of all subjects met criteria for a lifetime diagnosis, and that 6.3% met criteria in the year prior to interview. Among psychiatric disorders, alcohol disorders were second only to phobias in prevalence. The mean age of onset was 21 years, and 90% of all subjects experienced their first symptom before the age of 38 years. Alcoholism was correlated with male gender, Hispanic ethnicity, a younger age, being separated or divorced, having a low educational level, and with one's occupational level and income.

Suggested Readings

Agency for Health Care Policy and Research: *Clinical Practice Guideline Number 5, Depression in Primary Care*, Vol. 1. AHCPR Publication No. 93-0551. Rockville, MD: US Department of Health and Human Services, 1993:1–41.

Cooper JE, Kendell RE, Gurland BJ, Sharpe L, Copeland JRM, Simon R: *Psychiatric Diagnosis in New York and London.* London: Oxford University Press, 1972.

Hennekens CH, Buring JE: *Epidemiology in Medicine.* Boston: Little, Brown, 1987:73–100.

Robins LN, Locke BZ, Regier DA: An overview of psychiatric disorders in America. In Robins LN, Regier DA (eds): *Psychiatric Disorders in America.* New York: Free Press, 1991:285–308.

Tsuang MT, Tohen M, Zahner GEP: *Textbook in Psychiatric Epidemiology.* New York: Wiley, 1995:135–156.

Chapter 67

Statistics in Psychiatric Research

Lee Baer

I. History

The word statistics comes from numbers used for the state (i.e., the original statistics were numbers used by rulers of states to better understand their population). Thus, **the first statistics were simply counts of things such as populations of particular towns, or the amount of grain produced by a particular town.**

II. Statistics Relating to an Individual's Score on Some Characteristic ("Psychometrics")

A. Theory

In psychiatry and psychology rarely can we measure directly the characteristics we are really interested in; therefore, we typically rely on a subject's score on either self-report or investigator-administered scales. **Psychometrics is concerned with** how reproducible a subject's score is (i.e., **how reliable is it?**), and how closely it measures the characteristic we are really interested in (i.e., **how valid is it?**).

B. Reliability

1. **Definition. Reliability = dependability (i.e., the dependability of a score),** the degree to which we can be certain that a measurement can be depended upon (i.e., how reproducible is the score?). **For self-rated scales,** such as paper and pencil questionnaires, since there is no rater error to take into account, **the main source of undependability to guard against is differences in the person's self-rating over time.** For example, if a patient completes a depression questionnaire at 3 p.m., how close would his or her score be on the same questionnaire if he/she were to take the same scale at 4 p.m., assuming no change in his/her depression? If the scores were identical, and this were the case for all patients, then the correlation coefficient would be a perfect 1.00 (in this case the correlation coefficient is referred to as the **"reliability coefficient").**

   For scales or measures administered by a rater, the major question is: "Would this patient get the same score on this depression scale if Doctor A rated him, as if Doctor B rated him?" If agreement was perfect for all patients, then the reliability coefficient would be 1.00. If, on the other hand,

there were a random relationship between the scores of the two raters, then the inter-rater reliability would be 0.00.

   Reliability is necessary but not sufficient for a useful scale. Thus, a scale can be perfectly reliable, but have no validity for a particular purpose. For example, every time you ask me my phone number I will give you the same answer (perfect reliability); however, if you attempt to use my phone number to predict my anxiety level you will find a zero correlation (no validity).

2. **Extremes. If a measure has no reliability (i.e., it is not reproducible), then it has zero reliability. If it has perfect reliability, or repeatability, then it has a reliability of 1.00.**

3. **Rules of thumb. For a continuous measure, this is assessed by the correlation coefficient, and a rule of thumb is generally $r = 0.80$ for adequate reliability. For a binary measure** (e.g., the presence or absence of a disease), **this is often assessed by the Kappa coefficient, and a rule of thumb is generally $\kappa = 0.70$.**

4. **Usual notation:** correlation coefficient, r, κ, intraclass correlation coefficient.

C. Validity

1. **Definition. Validity = usefulness (i.e., the degree of usefulness of a score for a particular purpose). The degree to which the test measures what it is supposed to be measuring.** The determination of validity usually requires independent, external criteria of whatever the test is designed to measure. For example, if an investigator develops a single question that he/she purports to be a good screening instrument for clinical depression, then patients' responses to this question should relate well to "gold standard" measures of clinical depression, such as structured interviews and well-established rating scales for depression.

2. **Rules of thumb.** There is no real rule of thumb for validity, since there is no one measure. As a bare minimum, however, **the scale should at least be significantly correlated with gold-standard measures for that characteristic.**

3. **Usual notation:** correlation coefficient, r, or measures of sensitivity and specificity for a screening instrument.

III. Statistics Used to Describe a Group of Two or More Subjects ("Descriptive Statistics")

A. **Theory**

Many human characteristics are distributed "normally"; that is, if subjects' scores are plotted on a histogram, as the number of subjects gets larger, the distribution will look more and more like a "bell-shaped curve," or "Gaussian distribution." This is convenient, since **any normal distribution can be described very well by two measures: its mean indicates its central point, and its standard deviation indicates its spread.** For example, **in a normal distribution, about 95% of all scores fall within 2 standard deviations above or below the mean.**

To make life easier, **researchers usually assume that a characteristic is normally distributed, unless there is strong evidence that this is not true.** For example, gender is a binary (yes/no) variable, so it cannot be normally distributed.

B. **Mean (a measure of the CENTER of the distribution)**

1. **Definition: the average score of a group of individuals.** In a normal distribution, **this is the best single estimate of the "true" score of a group of individuals.** The theory is that the mean of a group of individuals represents the "true" score, and the deviation of each individual's score from the mean is caused by random errors.

2. **Usual notation: mean, X.**

C. **Standard Deviation (a measure of the SPREAD around the mean of the distribution)**

1. **Definition: the average spread of each score from the mean of its group.** Thus, **the smaller the standard deviation, the closer each score is to the mean,** and thus the fewer errors in the scores.

2. **Extremes. If all individuals have the same score, then the standard deviation is zero,** since all scores fall at the mean and there is no error.

3. **Rule of thumb. If the standard deviation is as large or larger than the mean of a group, then there is a large amount of spread in the group, and the mean is probably not an accurate indicator of the group.**

4. **Usual notation: SD, or** (often in tables) **mean $\pm$ SD** (e.g., 14.0 ± 7.0 indicates mean $= 14$, SD $= 7.0$).

D. **Correlation Coefficient (a measure of how two characteristics are related within individuals in the distribution)**

1. **Definition: a single number that summarizes the correlation of two measures in a group of individuals. Technically,** the correlation coefficient is **the slope of the line that best fits a scatter plot of two measures** (in standard scores).

2. **Extremes. If two measures are not related** (i.e., knowing one tells you nothing about the value of the other), **then their correlation is zero. If they are perfectly related, then their correlation is 1.00** (if they both change in the same direction), or -1.00 (if they change in opposite directions).

3. **Rules of thumb. The correlation coefficient squared gives the strength of the relation between the two measures.** For example, a correlation between height and nutrition of 0.70 would mean that 49% (i.e., 0.70×0.70) of a person's height is determined by his or her nutrition, and thus the other 51% must be determined by other factors.

4. **Usual notation: r** (e.g., $r = 0.35$).

5. **Alternatives**

   a. **When very few subjects are available,** or the distributions are markedly different from normality, **the Spearman nonparametric rank correlation test is used to test the association between the ranks of the two groups.**

   b. **When the scores are dichotomous or categorical, the contingency coefficient is used** to test the association between the two groups.

   c. **When we are interested in using one or more measures to PREDICT an individual's score on another measure, multiple linear regression is used (and upper-case "R" is used to represent multiple regression** in place of the lower-case "r" used to represent correlation).

IV. Drawing Inferences from a Group and Generalizing to a Larger Population ("Inferential Statistics")

A. **Theory**

An investigator usually assumes that the subjects are drawn randomly from a population in which the characteristic, which is the outcome measure, is normally distributed. Then, **by computing the difference between the means of two samples, or a correlation coefficient, and knowing the sample size these statistics were computed on, their values in the larger population can be estimated (or "inferred") with varying degrees of confidence. The standard degree of confidence in the behavioral sciences is 95%; hence the "95% confidence interval" around a statistic, and the 0.05 P-value.**

Note: The statistics described below are those used most commonly when the investigator assumes that the characteristic that is the outcome measure (or "dependent variable," or "endpoint") is distributed normally (i.e., in a "bell-shaped curve"). If this is not the case, other statistical methods, called "nonparametric" methods, are available (these do not depend upon the mean and standard deviation of a sample to draw inferences).

B. Null Hypothesis

1. **Definition. An investigator usually begins with the hypothesis that there is a zero** (or "nil") **difference between two means,** or that there is a correlation coefficient of zero (or "nil") between two measures. **Since statistics cannot prove an hypothesis, we usually phrase the "null hypothesis" and present data showing that it is unlikely to be true; the P-value indicates just how "unlikely."**

2. **Usual notation: null hypothesis, H_0.**

3. **Caveat. In ANY very large sample, the null hypothesis is usually rejected.** That is, two groups of individuals rarely have exactly the same mean on any two characteristics; even if they only differ by, say, 0.01 mm, the null hypothesis is not true, and a sample size in the thousands could detect even a tiny difference.

C. t-Test

1. **Definition: test to determine whether the difference between the means of two samples of subjects is likely to be due to chance alone.**

2. **Extremes.** If the difference between two means is zero, the t-statistic will also be zero. If all scores in both groups are the same, they both have standard deviations of zero. In this case, the t-statistic will be infinitely large.

3. **Usual notation: t** [e.g., $t(14) = 5.0$ indicates that the t-statistic with 14 degrees of freedom is 5.0].

4. **Alternatives**
   a. **When very few subjects are available, or the distributions are markedly different from normality, the nonparametric Mann-Whitney U-test is used** to test the difference between the mean ranks of the two groups.
   b. **When the outcome measure is survival at various time points, survival analysis is used to determine whether the survival curves of the two groups are significantly different.**

D. Analysis of Variance

1. **Definition: test to determine whether the difference between the means of TWO OR MORE samples of subjects is likely to be due to chance alone.** The analysis of variance (ANOVA) also tests for interaction effects between factors. For example, if the two factors being tested were drug vs. placebo, and the other factor was young/old, the ANOVA may find that the drug is more effective than the placebo in the young subjects only. **The significance of the analysis of variance is tested by the "F-statistic."**

2. **Extremes.** If the difference between two means is zero, the F-statistic will also be zero. If all scores in both groups are the same, they both have standard deviations of zero. In this case, the F-statistic will be infinitely large (and highly significant).

3. **Usual notation: F** [e.g., $F(1,20) = 5.0$ indicates that the F-statistic with 1 and 20 degrees of freedom is 5.0].

4. **Alternatives**
   a. **When only two groups are being compared, and there are no interactions of concern, the t-test can be used.**
   b. **When the groups differ on some important variable (e.g., age, education, or baseline illness severity), the analysis of covariance (ANCOVA) is used to statistically adjust for these confounding group differences.**

E. Chi-Square Test

1. **Definition: A test to determine whether the frequencies in each cell of a contingency table are different from the proportions expected by chance. It is most commonly used on a 2×2 contingency table, represented as four cells forming a square.**

   A common use is to answer the question: "Is there a difference between the occurrence of a given side effect in the drug vs. placebo group?" In this case the table is arranged with drug vs. placebo as the two rows, and side effect vs. no side effect as the two columns. As the difference between the frequency in each cell gets larger, the chi-square statistic also gets larger, and the more significant the result becomes.

2. **Extremes.** If all cells contain exactly the frequencies that would be expected by chance, then the chi-square statistic is zero. If the frequencies differ greatly from chance, the chi-square statistic gets larger and larger. The size of the chi-square statistic is based on the number of cells in the contingency table.

3. **Usual notation: χ^2** [e.g., $\chi^2(1) = 5.0$ indicates that the chi-square statistic with 1 degree of freedom is 5.0; a 2×2 table has 1 degree of freedom (df)].

F. P-Value

1. **Definition: the chance of a result of statistical test being a false positive (i.e., the probability of a spurious finding).**

2. **Extremes. If a finding is almost certainly a spurious finding, which would not be reproducible in another sample, the P-value will be near 1.00. On the other hand, if the finding almost certainly represents a "true" finding, then the P-value will be near zero (a probability can never reach zero, but small P-values are represented by several zeros after the decimal point (e.g., $P < 0.00001$).**

3. **Rule of thumb. Most journals require ($P < 0.05$ for significance.** If many statistical tests are performed in a study, a more conservative P-value should be used.

4. **Notation: either $P <$ (less exact), or $P =$ (exact and preferable).** Also referred to as alpha (α).

5. **Caution: do not be overly impressed by very low P-values. Remember that all this tells you is the chance that the difference is probably not zero. Also, remember that, given enough subjects, this is very easy to prove.** Thus a very low P-value does not necessarily indicate a large clinical effect, but instead represents that it is a very reliable effect. Check the effect size (the correlation coefficient squared, or the size of the t-statistic) to get an idea of the magnitude of the difference or relation.

G. **Statistical Power**
   1. **Definition: the likelihood of finding a true difference or relation between two or more measures.** Analogous to the sensitivity of a medical test: the higher the sensitivity, the lower the chance of a false negative finding; the chance of not making a type II error (i.e., not finding a false negative). [An analogy: **The power of a telescope (i.e., the magnification) is analogous to the power of a study: both indicate the ability to detect even tiny objects or changes.**]
   2. **Extremes.** If a study had no chance of finding a true difference between two drugs (e.g., with only two subjects per group), the power of the study would be nearly zero. If the study had almost no chance of missing a true difference (e.g., compar-ing the mean height of 10,000 2-year-olds with 10,000 18-year-olds), the power of the study would be nearly 1.00.
   3. **Rule of thumb. Power of 0.80 is usually the minimum suggested by statisticians when designing a study.**
   4. **Usual notation: power, statistical power, $1-\beta$ (where β is the likelihood of finding a false negative).**
   5. **Caution.** Just as any tiny difference can be found to be significant just by having enough subjects, it is possible to find all but huge differences to be non-significant, simply by having few enough subjects! **Be especially wary of false negatives in studies with few subjects, say less than 25 per group.** Several literature reviews have found that the average behavioral science study has a power of only about 40% to detect a medium-sized effect!

Suggested Readings

Anastasi A: *Psychological Testing*, 7th ed. New York: Prentice-Hall, 1996.

Cohen J: *Statistical Power Analysis for the Behavioral Sciences*, 2nd ed. Hillsdale, NJ: Lawrence Erlbaum Associates, 1988.

Fleiss JL: *The Design and Analysis of Clinical Experiments*. New York: John Wiley, 1986.

Chapter 68

Genetics of Psychiatric Disorders

JORDAN SMOLLER AND CANDACE WHITE

I. Basic Principles of Genetics and Gene Mapping

A. The Human Genome

The human genome **encompasses 23 homologous pairs of chromosomes** containing approximately **80,000–100,000 genes.** The larger portion (>95%) of chromosomal DNA comprises noncoding DNA sequences. **The chromosomal location of a DNA sequence is referred to as a genetic locus.**

B. Genotypes and Phenotypes

The sequence of nucleotides that make up a gene or an anonymous genetic marker may differ among individuals. **The different forms of a gene or genetic marker are referred to as alleles.** Allelic differences are also referred to as **polymorphisms** and can be used to distinguish the genotypes of different individuals. **A genotype refers to the combination of alleles at a given locus.** If the two alleles at a locus are the same, an individual is said to be homozygous at the locus; if the alleles differ, the individual is heterozygous. **A phenotype is the manifestation (expression) of a set of alleles, or, more generally, the observable expression of a trait.**

C. Genetic Mapping

For the most part, **gene mapping studies rely on the phenomena of crossing over and recombination** that occur during meiosis. During this process, homologous chromosomes exchange genetic material; thus the gametes formed by meiosis may contain a combination of paternal and maternal chromosomal segments. **To the degree that two loci are physically close together on a chromosome, they are unlikely to be separated when recombination occurs (a violation of Mendel's law of independent assortment). Two loci that are not transmitted independently are genetically linked,** implying that they reside close together on a chromosome.

D. Genetic Linkage

The degree of genetic linkage reflects the proximity of two loci and depends on the frequency of recombination between them. The distance between two loci can be expressed as a genetic distance (in centimorgans) or a physical distance (in base pairs). Loci that are separated by recombination in 1% of meioses are 1 centimorgan (cM) apart; this corresponds roughly to a physical distance of 1 million base pairs.

E. Psychiatric Phenotypes Are "Complex"

A phenotype may be transmitted in a Mendelian fashion (due to the action of a single major gene), or in a "complex" fashion. Mendelian inheritance patterns include dominant, recessive, and X-linked. Neuropsychiatric disorders that are due to single major genes include Huntington's disease (autosomal dominant), Wilson's disease (autosomal recessive), and Fragile X syndrome (X-linked). In the case of Huntington's and Fragile X, the genetic lesion is due to expansion of trinucleotide (triplet) repeat sequences. **Most psychiatric phenotypes, however, are complex traits;** they reflect interactions of genetic and environmental factors that may vary among families. This vastly complicates efforts to identify the genetic basis of psychiatric disorders. The genes involved are often referred to as **"susceptibility genes"** rather than "disease genes" because they **increase risk for a disorder without invariably causing it.**

II. The Tools of Psychiatric Genetics

Genetic epidemiologists and molecular geneticists rely on a well-defined sequence of study designs to determine whether a disorder has a genetic basis, and then to locate the specific genes that may be involved.

A. Family Studies

Family studies address the first question to be answered: does the disorder run in families? **If relatives of affected probands have a higher risk of the disorder than relatives of unaffected probands, the disorder is familial (proband = the individual through whom a family is ascertained).** One index of the strength of familiality is the **recurrence risk ratio for first-degree relatives (λ_1), defined as the ratio of the risk of the disorder in a first-degree relative of an affected individual to the prevalence in the general population.** This ratio can be used to predict the strength of genetic influences on the disorder and the likelihood that gene-mapping studies will have the power to identify the genes involved. **Approximate recurrence risk ratios for a variety of psychiatric disorders** are presented in

Table 68-1. Genetic Epidemiology of Some Psychiatric Disorders

Disorder	Lifetime Population Prevalence (approx. %)	λ_1[a]	Estimated Heritability (Approximate)	Selected Linkage and Association Findings[b]
ADHD	7	2–5	60–90%	Dopamine transporter; DRD4
Alzheimer's disease	10 (>65 years)	2 (late-onset)	60% (late-onset)	Early-onset: presenilin-1, presenilin-2, amyloid precursor protein. Late-onset: ApoE (ε4)
Schizophrenia	1	10	70–89%	Chromosome 6p, 13q, 18p, 22q; $5HT_{2A}$ receptor, DRD3
Bipolar disorder	1	7–10	60%	Chromosome 4p, 18p, 18q, 21q
Unipolar depression	5–17	2–6	33–75%	Tyrosine hydroxylase; Serotonin transporter
Panic disorder	3	7	45%	Adenosine A_{2a} receptor; MAO-A
Alcohol dependence	14	3–7	50–60%	Chromosome 1, 4p, 4q, 7, 11p, 16; alcohol dehydrogenase (ADH)

[a]λ_1, recurrence risk ratio for first-degree relatives: the risk of the disorder in a first-degree relative of an affected individual compared to the general population prevalence of the disorder.

[b]With the exception of the findings for Alzheimer's disease, these findings are tentative and nonreplications of most of these findings have also been reported. This list is illustrative, not exhaustive.

Table 68-1. It is important to bear in mind that the size of these risk ratios depends on both the risk to relatives (numerator) and the base rate of the disorder (denominator). Even when the **relative risk** of a disorder is high, the **absolute risk** to a first-degree relative may be relatively low if the base rate of the disorder is low. For example, siblings of probands with schizophrenia have a roughly 10-fold increased risk of the disorder compared to an individual randomly drawn from the general population. However, because the population prevalence is approximately 1%, the absolute risk of the disorder for the sibling is only about 10% (with a 90% probability of being unaffected). In contrast, the lifetime prevalence of major depression is approximately 15%, so that even a 2-fold increased risk to siblings would be associated with a 30% risk of being affected.

B. Twin and Adoption Studies
It is important to remember that **a disorder may run in families for nongenetic reasons.** For example, shared environmental experiences may produce the disorder in multiple family members. **Twin and adoption studies** can be **used to separate the contribution of genetic and environmental causes of familial aggregation.**
1. **Twin studies compare the concordance rates between monozygotic twins (who are genetically identical)**

and dizygotic twins (who share on average 50% of their alleles). A twin pair is concordant if both co-twins have the phenotype. If we can assume that environmental influences on **monozygotic (MZ) twins** are not different from environmental influences on **dizygotic (DZ) twins** (the "equal environments assumption"), then significantly higher concordance rates in MZ twins reflect the action of genes. Nevertheless, an MZ concordance rate that is less than 100% means that environmental factors influence the phenotype. Twin studies can provide an estimate of the **heritability of the disorder, which refers to the proportion of the phenotypic differences among individuals that can be attributed to genetic factors. Heritability refers to the strength of genetic influences in a population, not a particular individual,** and heritability estimates may differ depending on the population studied. Table 68-1 presents heritability estimates for several disorders.
2. **Adoption studies can disentangle genetic and environmental influences on family resemblance by comparing rates of a disorder in biological family members with those in adoptive family members.** For example, if an adopted child has a genetically influenced disorder, the biological (genetic) parents should have a higher risk of the disorder than the adoptive (environmental) parents. Adoption studies provided the first convincing evidence that

genes play an important role in the development of schizophrenia.

C. Modes of Inheritance

Once genes have been implicated in a disorder, **segregation analysis is sometimes used to determine the mode of inheritance.** This involves fitting various statistical models of inheritance (e.g., **dominant, recessive, multifactorial polygenic**) to the observed pattern of disease in pedigrees and determining which modes of inheritance are consistent, or inconsistent, with the observed data. Information derived from a segregation analysis can be used to guide linkage studies (see II.D.3.a) that actually seek to identify the genes involved in the disorder.

D. Molecular Genetics

Molecular genetic methods are **used to locate and isolate the specific genes that influence a disorder.**

1. The **candidate gene approach examines the inheritance of specific genes which are suspected to be involved in a disorder.** These candidate genes may have been suggested by previous physiologic, pharmacologic or **gene-mapping studies.** For example, the serotonin transporter gene may be considered a candidate gene for mood disorders because serotonergic function has been implicated in the physiology and treatment of these disorders. Because the pathogenesis of most psychiatric disorders is poorly understood, it may be difficult to identify compelling candidate genes for testing.

2. An alternative approach is to perform a **whole genome scan** in which **linkage is tested for genetic markers spaced at intervals along each chromosome. A marker is a polymorphic DNA sequence whose chromosomal location is known;** it may or may not reside within a gene. The **genome scan approach requires no prior knowledge of the function or location of genes involved in the disorder.**

3. Molecular genetic studies of complex phenotypes, such as psychiatric disorders, are complicated for several reasons. **It may be difficult to accurately classify whether an individual is affected with the disease genotype because there may be phenocopies (individuals who have the disorder for nongenetic reasons), incomplete penetrance (individuals with the disease genotype may not manifest the phenotype), variable expression (the disease genotype may produce a spectrum of phenotypes), and genetic heterogeneity (different genes may independently produce the phenotype). Moreover, the boundaries of psychiatric diagnoses are often uncertain and may not capture the phenotypic features that are under genetic influence. In addition, the phenotype may be the result of many genes rather than one**

or a few major genes. For polygenic disorders, each gene may exert only a weak effect.

In general, two types of gene-mapping studies may be performed:

a. **Linkage studies examine whether two or more genetic loci are co-inherited more often than expected by chance. If individuals who are affected with a disorder within a family tend to inherit the same alleles at a marker locus, this implies that the marker locus is linked to (i.e., is physically close to) a gene that influences the disorder.** In classical (parametric) linkage analysis, the **strength of the evidence in favor of linkage is calculated as a LOD (logarithm of the odds) score.** The LOD score compares the likelihood of obtaining the observed genotypes and phenotypes when linkage is present with the likelihood assuming no linkage. Traditionally, **a LOD score of 3 (corresponding to odds of 1000:1 in favor of linkage) has been the threshold for declaring linkage;** but for complex disorders such as psychiatric illnesses, higher thresholds have been recommended. Traditional LOD score linkage analysis has been most successfully applied when a single major gene is involved and the mode of inheritance (e.g., dominant, recessive) is known. Because these assumptions can rarely be used with psychiatric phenotypes, other (nonparametric) methods which do not require knowledge of mode of inheritance are routinely utilized. For example, genome scan linkage analysis may be performed with large numbers of families containing pairs of relatives who are affected. **The affected sibling pair (ASP) method, for example, examines whether affected siblings share alleles at any marker locus significantly more often than would be expected by chance.** If alleles at a locus tend to be shared by affected sibling pairs, this implies that the locus is linked to a disease gene.

b. **Association studies examine whether a particular allele of a candidate gene is significantly more common among individuals with a disorder (cases) than among controls without the disorder.** This method led to the finding that the ApoE-ϵ4 allele is associated with late-onset Alzheimer's disease. Such **case-control association studies can produce false positive results if the ethnic backgrounds of cases and controls differ.** If the case group has a higher proportion of individuals from an ethnic group that happens to have a high frequency of the allele being tested, then that allele will be statistically associated with the disease even though it may play no causal role. **Family-based association studies** avoid this problem by looking at the transmission of alleles within families. However, ascertaining families can be more difficult than ascertaining unrelated cases and controls. With the completion of the Human Genome Project and the identification of all human genes, it may soon be feasible to perform a whole genome scan using alleles of all 100,000 genes as "candidates."

c. **Cytogenetic studies.** A third method for identifying the location of a disease gene involves **cytogenetic studies in which psychiatric phenotypes are shown to be associated with chromosomal abnormalities.** For example, a deletion of material from chromosome 22q can result in velocardiofacial syndrome, which is associated with a wide range of somatic anomalies, as well as learning disabilities, and behavioral/psychiatric symptoms. An excess prevalence of bipolar spectrum disorders and psychotic disorders among patients with this syndrome has been observed, suggesting that a gene influencing these disorders may lie within this region.

III. Genetic Aspects of Psychopathology

Evidence for a genetic component of many psychiatric disorders is growing, and gene-mapping studies have begun to identify the location and identity of some of the relevant loci. Unfortunately, many linkage and association findings have been difficult to replicate, emphasizing the **need for caution in interpreting the results of genetic studies.** Some of these findings have undoubtedly been false positives, but nonreplication can also be due to inadequate power, differences in diagnosis and phenotype definition, and genetic heterogeneity (different genes acting in different samples). The following summary draws largely on data presented in the report of the NIMH Genetics Workgroup (1999). **To date, no specific genes have been definitively shown to influence any of the major psychiatric disorders, with the exception of Alzheimer's disease.**

A. Disorders of Childhood and Adolescence

1. **Attention deficit hyperactivity disorder (ADHD)**

   a. **Family studies. ADHD runs in families, and first-degree relatives (parents and siblings) of ADHD probands have a 2–8-fold higher risk of the disorder than relatives of controls.** Family studies also suggest that ADHD and depression share familial determinants, and that ADHD with conduct or bipolar disorder may be a distinct familial subtype.

   b. **Twin studies and adoption studies. Most heritability estimates for ADHD have ranged from approximately 60% to more than 90%.** Adoption studies have demonstrated that the risk of ADHD is higher among biological relatives than among adoptive relatives of ADHD children.

   c. **Molecular genetic studies.** To date, attention has focused on candidate genes involved in dopaminergic function. Alleles of the dopamine D_2 receptor gene, the dopamine transporter (DAT) gene and the dopamine D_4 receptor (DRD4) gene have been associated with ADHD. The DAT and DRD4 associations have received support in independent studies.

2. **Autism**

   a. **Family studies. The risk of autism to siblings of affected children is approximately 3–4%, which is more than 75-fold higher than the general population prevalence.**

   b. **Twin studies.** Concordance rates for MZ twins are markedly higher than those for DZ twins, and the **heritability has been estimated to exceed 90%.**

   c. **Molecular genetic studies.** Although it appears to be one of the most heritable psychiatric phenotypes, no genetic loci have yet been convincingly linked to, or associated with, autism. Tentative associations with the serotonin transporter gene and the HRAS gene have been reported, and genome scans have provided suggestive evidence of linkage to loci on chromosome 1p and 7q.

3. **Tourette's syndrome**

   a. **Family studies. First-degree relatives of TS probands have an 8.7% risk of the disorder, 174-fold greater than the population prevalence.** There is evidence for variable expression of the genetic liability for TS; for example, relatives of probands with TS have a higher risk of obsessive-compulsive disorder, and chronic motor or vocal tics.

   b. **Twin studies.** In one twin study, MZ concordance rates (53%) exceeded DZ concordance rates (8%).

   c. **Molecular genetic studies.** No genetic loci have been convincingly associated with TS. An association with the DRD4 gene has been reported but not established.

B. Dementia: Alzheimer's Disease

Of the disorders reviewed here, Alzheimer's disease (AD) is the one in which genetic studies have progressed the furthest, and at least four specific genes have been shown to play a role in the disorder.

1. **Family and twin studies.** The familiality of early-onset (before age 60 years) AD has been well established, and three specific genes influencing early-onset AD have been identified (see below). Late-onset AD is far more common and has a more complex etiology. Having a first-degree relative with AD approximately doubles the risk of AD. A large twin study estimated the heritability of late-onset AD to be approximately 60%.

2. **Molecular genetic studies. Mutations in three genes have been shown to produce *early-onset AD* with an autosomal dominant mode of inheritance.** Together, these genes account for roughly half of early-onset cases of AD:

   a. **Amyloid precursor protein gene on chromosome 21**

   b. **Presenilin 1 gene on chromosome 14**

   c. **Presenilin 2 gene on chromosome 1**

   The apolipoprotein E gene (APOE) on chromosome 19 has been associated with *late-onset AD*. There are three common alleles of APOE ($\epsilon2$, $\epsilon3$, and $\epsilon4$) and it is **the $\epsilon4$ allele** which **increases risk for late-onset AD.** (APOE-$\epsilon2$ appears to be associated with a reduced risk of AD.) Unlike the autosomal dominant genes involved in early-onset AD, APOE-$\epsilon4$ is a susceptibility allele which acts as a risk factor for the disease but is neither a necessary nor sufficient cause. **A primary effect of the $\epsilon 4$ allele is to reduce the age of onset of AD;** individuals with two copies of the allele have the earliest age of onset compared to individuals with other APOE genotypes. Other genes are undoubtedly involved in the etiology of late-onset AD; recent studies indicate that a gene residing on chromosome 12 is linked to AD.

C. Psychotic Disorders: Schizophrenia
1. **Family studies.** Family studies of schizophrenia have repeatedly demonstrated that the **disorder is familial.** Compared to the population lifetime risk of approximately 1%, first-degree relatives have an approximately 10% risk. The risk drops to about 4% for second-degree relatives and 2% for third-degree relatives. This pattern of familial risks is consistent with the hypothesis that between two and five interacting genes may be responsible for most of the genetic liability to schizophrenia. There is evidence for variable expression of the genetic diathesis underlying schizophrenia. For example, Cluster A personality traits are more common in the relatives of schizophrenic probands. **A number of neurobiological phenotypes also appear to be more common among nonschizophrenic relatives of individuals with schizophrenia:**
   a. **Smooth-pursuit eye-tracking dysfunction**
   b. **Neuropsychological deficits (in memory, language, and attention tasks)**
   c. **Abnormal P50 auditory-evoked potentials**
   d. **Structural brain abnormalities**
   e. **Reduced hippocampal N-acetyl-D-aspartate (NMDA) levels**

   These phenotypes are sometimes called "intermediate phenotypes" or "endophenotypes" because they may more directly reflect the action of genes than does the clinical phenotype of schizophrenia itself. Incorporating these phenotypes into linkage and association studies may prove critical to unlocking the genetics of schizophrenia.
2. **Twin and adoption studies. The concordance rate for MZ twins ($\sim 46\%$) substantially exceeds that of DZ twins ($\sim 14\%$). The heritability of schizophrenia has been estimated to be 70–89%.** Adoption studies have demonstrated that the prevalence of schizophrenia is significantly higher (approx. 4-fold) in biological relatives than in adoptive relatives.
3. **Molecular genetic studies.** Many linkage and association studies of schizophrenia have been reported and some findings have received support in independent samples. **The strongest evidence to date from genome scan linkage studies has been for a region (spanning about 30 cM) on chromosome 6p (p = short arm; q = long arm).** Other regions which

have been implicated include areas of chromosomes 5q, 8p, 10p, 13q, 18p, and 22q. Some of these regions contain plausible candidate loci. For example, an allele of the serotonin $5HT_{2A}$ receptor, located on chromosome 13q, has been associated with schizophrenia in independent studies. Cytogenetic studies have also pointed to the region on chromosome 22q implicated in linkage studies. Chromosomal microdeletions in this region have been associated with velocardiofacial syndrome, in which affected individuals appear to have an excess risk of schizophrenia and schizoaffective disorder. Other candidate loci that have been associated with schizophrenia include the dopamine D_3 receptor (chromosome 3q), and the G-protein receptor G-olf$_\alpha$ (chromosome 18p). As pointed out earlier, interpreting the results of these studies requires caution; the list of genes with positive associations is expanding but nonreplications are common and none has been firmly established. A promising approach involves the use of intermediate phenotypes directly in linkage and association studies. Among families with schizophrenia, linkage was found between the trait of abnormal P50 auditory-evoked response and a locus on chromosome 15q in the region of the $\alpha 7$-nicotinic receptor gene.

D. Mood Disorders
1. **Bipolar disorder.** As with schizophrenia, studies of bipolar disorder have demonstrated that **genetic factors influence the disorder;** several linkage and association findings have been replicated but not firmly established. It is considered likely that the **inherited susceptibility to bipolar disorder reflects several genes of small effect rather than a single major gene.**
   a. **Family studies. Family studies have consistently demonstrated that there is familial transmission of bipolar disorder. First-degree relatives of individuals with bipolar disorder have an excess risk of both bipolar disorder (7–10-fold) and unipolar depression (2–5-fold) compared to relatives of unaffected controls; relatives of probands with unipolar depression, however, have an excess risk of unipolar depression but not of bipolar disorder.** Among first-degree relatives of bipolar probands, the range of estimates of the risk for bipolar disorder is approximately 5–10%, while the risk for unipolar depression is approximately 10–20%.
   b. **Twin and adoption studies. Concordance rates are substantially higher in MZ twins (33–80%) than in DZ twins (0–8%), and the heritability of bipolar disorder has been estimated to be approximately 59%.** The results of adoption studies have been mixed, although two studies showed higher risk in biological vs. adoptive relatives.

c. **Molecular genetic studies.** Although there have been numerous nonreplications of linkage and association findings for bipolar disorder, some linkage results have received support from independent studies, including regions of chromosomes 4p, 18p, 18q, and 21q. An early report of linkage to 11p among Old Order Amish families was not supported by subsequent analyses, although the tyrosine hydroxylase gene which maps to this region has been associated with bipolar disorder in some studies. Other candidate genes that have received support in some studies include the serotonin transporter, tryptophan hydroxylase and monoamine oxidase A genes. Again, however, nonreplications have been reported for these and other loci that have been associated with bipolar disorder.

2. **Major depression**
   a. **Family studies. Family studies have consistently demonstrated that first-degree relatives of probands with major depression have a higher risk of the disorder (11–18%) than relatives of controls (0.7–7.0%).** The recurrence risk ratio (λ_1) for first-degree relatives has ranged from approximately 2 to 6. **Certain features of major depression in the proband have been associated with increased familial risk: early-onset, recurrent episodes, long duration of episodes, suicidality, and greater levels of impairment.** Relatives of probands with unipolar depression do not have a substantially increased risk of bipolar disorder.
   b. **Twin and adoption studies. Depending on the sample and diagnostic convention used, concordance rates have ranged from 23% to 69% for MZ twins and from 16% to 42% for DZ twins.** Heritability estimates have ranged from 33% to 75%. The results of four available adoption studies have been mixed, providing modest support for a genetic component.
   c. **Molecular genetic studies.** Several small-scale linkage studies have been reported, but no specific loci have been linked to the disorder. Association studies have implicated, but not established, a role for the serotonin transporter and tyrosine hydroxlase genes.

E. **Anxiety Disorders**
   1. **Panic disorder**
      a. **Family studies. The estimated risk of panic disorder to first-degree relatives of affected probands has ranged from 4% to 22%, significantly higher than the risk to relatives of controls (0.8–4.2%). As with several other psychiatric disorders, early onset is associated with increased familial risk.** Overall, the recurrence risk ratio for panic disorder is in the range of 4–10.
      b. **Twin studies. Concordance rates for panic disorder among MZ twins have ranged from 23% to 73%, compared with 0–17% for DZ twins.** In the largest twin study, MZ vs. DZ was 24% vs. 11%, and the **heritability was estimated to be 46%.**
      c. **Molecular genetic studies.** Linkage studies have not identified any loci linked to panic disorder.

Preliminary, unconfirmed associations have been reported for a few candidate genes, including the adenosine A_{2a} receptor, cholecystokinin (CCK), monoamine oxidase A, and the human version of the *Drosophila* "white" gene.

2. **Obsessive-compulsive disorder (OCD)**
   a. **Family studies.** Available family studies have yielded mixed results, although **the risk to first-degree relatives of OCD probands has been higher than the population prevalence of the disorder in several studies.** In one case-control family study, the risk was 10.3% for first-degree relatives of OCD probands compared with 1.9% for relatives of control probands. **Early-onset disorder may be more familial.** The risk of tic disorders (Tourette's syndrome, and chronic tics) is elevated in a subset of families of OCD probands, suggesting that these disorders can share genetic influences. Conversely, studies have also documented an elevated risk of OCD among relatives of probands with Tourette's syndrome.
   b. **Twin studies.** Limited available twin data support the hypothesis that obsessional traits and symptoms are influenced by genetic factors, with heritability estimates ranging from 47% to 68%. The heritability of the DSM diagnosis of OCD itself is unclear.
   c. **Molecular genetic studies.** An association between OCD in males and an allele of the catechol-*O*-methyltransferase gene has been reported in independent samples. Reported associations with the dopamine D_4 receptor, the serotonin transporter, and monoamine oxidase A genes await further replication.

F. **Substance Use Disorders**
   1. **Alcohol dependence**
      a. **Family studies.** An overview of family studies indicates that **first-degree relatives of individuals with alcohol dependence have a 7-fold (range 2.5–20-fold) higher risk of the disorder compared with relatives of unaffected individuals.** Susceptibility to alcohol withdrawal symptoms also appears to be familial.
      b. **Twin and adoption studies.** Most (but not all) twin and adoption studies of alcoholism have supported the role of genetic influences. Heritability estimates have varied depending on the diagnostic criteria applied, but, among studies demonstrating genetic influence, estimated heritability has ranged from approximately 50% to 60%. Several adoption studies have demonstrated an increased risk of alcoholism among adoptees who have an alcoholic biologic parent.
      c. **Molecular genetic studies.** Two genome scans have been reported and provided evidence of linkage to loci on chromosomes 1, 4p (near the $\beta 1$ γ-aminobutyric acid [GABA] receptor gene), chromosome 4q (near the alcohol dehydrogenase gene cluster), chromosomes 7 and 11p (near the DRD4 and tyrosine hydroxylase genes), and chromosome 16. As with other psychiatric disorders (see schizophrenia), efforts have been made to identify endophenotypes underly-

ing the disorder. Differences in P3 event-related brain potentials are heritable and have been associated with alcoholism; a recent linkage study found evidence of linkage to loci on chromosomes 2 and 6 using P3 amplitude as the phenotype of interest. Associations between several candidate genes and alcohol dependence have been reported, including an association between genes affecting alcohol metabolism and reduced risk of alcohol dependence in Asian populations. By altering the rate of alcohol metabolism, certain alleles of the alcohol dehydrogenase (ADH) and aldehyde dehydrogenase (ALDH) genes can produce a build-up of acetaldehyde, causing an endogenous disulfiram-like flushing reaction. By discouraging alcohol consumption, these alleles may be protective against the development of alcoholism. A reported association with an allele of the dopamine D_2 receptor (DRD2) gene has been widely studied but remains controversial. Other unconfirmed associations include the serotonin transporter and GABA receptor subunit genes. More so than with other psychiatric phenotypes, animal models have been used to map genetic loci influencing alcohol consumption, and these should provide crucial clues to the location of homologous human genes.

G. Genetics of Personality and Temperament

An alternative to searching for genes for psychiatric disorders is to identify genes influencing temperament and personality traits. Quantitative variations in these traits reflect individual differences in personality but may also reveal a predisposition to certain Axis I and Axis II disorders. These traits are typically measured with paper-and-pencil tests. **Large twin studies have demonstrated that a variety of personality and temperamental constructs are moderately heritable.** For example, the heritabilities of neuroticism and introversion-extraversion are approximately 40–50%. **An increasing number of gene-mapping studies are reporting evidence of linkage and association between specific loci and personality traits,** but, again, none have been confirmed and nonreplications are common. Widely studied examples include an association of an allele of the DRD4 gene with novelty-seeking, and an association of an allele of the serotonin transporter gene with anxiety-related traits (neuroticism, and harm avoidance).

IV. Implications of Psychiatric Genetics

There is reason to be both optimistic and cautious about progress in psychiatric genetic research. **The benefits of**

identifying and characterizing genes involved in psychiatric phenotypes may include:

1. An improved understanding of the biological basis of psychiatric disorders.
2. An improved understanding of the role of the environment in psychopathology. Genetic studies are a powerful means for dissecting the role of genes, environment, and gene-environment interactions.
3. An improved basis for defining psychiatric disorders. Genetic studies may validate or challenge diagnostic criteria and diagnostic boundaries among disorders.
4. Improved treatment of psychiatric disorders. The growing field of pharmacogenetics aims to identify genetic factors which predict therapeutic response and liability to drug toxicities. An important goal of this work is to target pharmacologic treatment so as to maximize the likelihood of benefit and minimize the risk of adverse drug effects.
5. The possibility of improved prevention efforts. By identifying the role of environment and gene-environment interactions in psychopathology and by identifying individuals at risk, genetic research may facilitate the development of more targeted and effective prevention measures.

On the other hand, **advances in genetic research may well raise important ethical and social challenges for psychiatrists.** For example, **information about genetic susceptibility could have adverse emotional and financial (e.g., insurability) consequences for some individuals and their families.** Increasingly, psychiatrists will need to have an informed understanding of both the potential benefits and limitations of genetic research.

Suggested Readings

Burmeister M: Basic concepts in the study of diseases with complex genetics. *Biol Psychiatry* 1999; 45:522–532.

Faraone S, Tsuang M, Tsuang D: *Genetics of Mental Disorders: A Guide for Students, Clinicians, and Researchers.* New York: Guilford Press, 1999.

Kendler K: Twin studies of psychiatric illness. *Arch Gen Psychiatry* 1993; 50:905–915.

Plomin R, DeFries J, McClearn G, Rutte M: *Behavioral Genetics,* 3rd ed. New York: WH Freeman, 1997.

Report of the NIMH Genetics Workgroup: Genetics and mental disorders. *Biol Psychiatry* 1999: 45:559–602.

Rutter M, Plomin R: Opportunities for psychiatry from genetic findings. *Br J Psychiatry* 1997; 171:209–219.

Chapter 69

Psychiatry and the Law III: Malpractice and Boundary Violations

RONALD SCHOUTEN

I. Overview

The law related to malpractice litigation has had a significant effect on the practice of modern psychiatry. This chapter reviews the legal basics of malpractice litigation, some major topics in malpractice, and the important area of boundary violations.

II. Malpractice Law

A. **Malpractice cases are part of the general field of personal injury or tort law. There are two types of torts:**
   1. **Intentional torts** (e.g., sexual contact with a patient, physical assault on a patient, fraud, or misrepresentation). Malpractice insurance covers intentional torts (e.g., sexual misconduct) only when the intentional act is part of standard practice (e.g., restraint of a patient).
   2. Unintentional torts or negligence. This is the basis for most malpractice claims.

B. **In order to prove a malpractice claim, a plaintiff (the party who claims to have been injured and who is seeking damages) must establish the four elements of a malpractice claim—the 4 Ds:**
   1. **The defendant was derelict in his responsibilities.** This can be established either by showing that the treating clinician departed from or ignored the standard of care, or by establishing that the treating clinician followed the standard of care but did so in an inept fashion.
   2. **The defendant had a specific obligation or duty to the patient.**
      a. **The general duty of physicians is to possess and employ such reasonable skill and care as are commonly had and are exercised by respectable, average physicians in the same or similar community.**
      b. **Specialists are held to a higher standard of performance because they hold themselves out to the community as having special expertise.** A physician who holds him- or herself out as an expert in a specific area will be judged according to this higher standard, regardless of the actual credentials.
      c. **The "school rule." Practice in accordance with the standards of a recognized school of thought or training will be judged according to the standards of that school to which the defendant physician is a member.** For exam-

ple, cognitive behavioral therapists should be judged according to the standard of care for that school of treatment, not according to a psychoanalytic standard of care. However, all clinicians who hold themselves out to the public as being qualified to diagnose and treat illnesses are held to the same basic standard of care with regard to safety, assessment, and conduct. For example, a psychiatrist cannot excuse himself from failing to diagnose his patient's myocardial infarction on the basis that he does not prescribe medication and only does psychotherapy.
      d. **Duty to consult. Physicians have a duty to get consultation when the limits of the physician's knowledge and experience have been exceeded.**
   3. **The dereliction of duty is the direct cause of an injury.** Direct causation has two separate components:
      a. A mechanical notion assessed by the **"but for" rule: "but for" the negligent behavior, the injury would not have occurred.**
      b. **Proximate or legal cause: the harm that occurred was a "reasonably foreseeable" consequence of the negligent action.** In proving causation, a plaintiff may invoke the evidentiary concept of *res ipsa loquitur* (the thing speaks for itself) when the cause of injury to the plaintiff was under the sole control of the defendant and the defendant alone has knowledge of the injurious event. In such cases, the presumption is that the defendant was responsible for the injury and the defendant must rebut that presumption.
   4. **Damages must be proven.** Unless harm is shown to have occurred, the malpractice suit will not succeed, even if there was negligent performance of a duty. **Damages can be of three types:**
      a. **Economic damages** (e.g., lost earnings, cost of medical treatment for the injury)
      b. **Physical damages** (e.g., loss of a bodily function)
      c. **Emotional pain and suffering**

III. Selected Malpractice Issues

A. **Abandonment: the unilateral termination of the doctor-patient relationship, by the doctor, without consent or justification, where the termination results in harm to the patient.**
   1. **Justification can arise in a variety of circumstances;** for example:

499

a. No-show patients

b. Assaultive or abusive patients

c. Noncompliant patients

2. **When it is necessary to terminate the relationship, claims of abandonment can be avoided by providing a referral to another clinician or agency, access to emergency coverage, and medications between the time of termination and the time of the appointment with the new treater.**

3. **Abandonment allegations can arise when the physician is absent for vacation or conferences and fails to provide coverage or provides substandard coverage.** These allegations can be avoided by providing adequate coverage during absences. **The physician is responsible for insuring that the coverage is competent and available.** For example, a physician may be held liable if harm occurs to a patient during his or her absence and he/she knows or should have known that the covering physician was incompetent.

B. **Vicarious liability is the imposition of liability on one party for the negligent acts of another.**

1. **Under the doctrine of** *respondeat superior* **(let the master answer), the "master" (employer) may be held liable for the negligent acts of a second person, the "servant" (employee), committed within the scope of the employment.**

   a. **A master,** for these purposes, **is one who has direct authority over the servant,** as evidenced by the power to hire or fire and veto power over the servant's decisions.

   b. **A consultant is distinguished from a master or employer by being outside the direct line of responsibility for the acts of the second person,** having no direct authority over the second person, and offering advice and direction on a "take it or leave it" basis.

2. This concept applies to the supervision of residents as well as to the supervision of non-physicians.

3. **The physician who signs prescriptions or disability forms for patients who were not evaluated by the physician may be held to the same level of responsibility as if he or she had personally evaluated the patient.**

C. **Confidentiality**

1. **Confidentiality is the physician's duty to hold matters revealed by the patient in the course of treatment in confidence from unauthorized third parties.**

2. There are a number of **exceptions to this general duty,** including:

   a. **Emergency.** This is defined as **a situation when failure to breach confidentiality would result in a serious (e.g., life-threatening) deterioration in the patient's condition.**

   b. **Waiver of the duty by the patient or other appropriate decision-maker.**

   c. **When the patient is temporarily or permanently incompetent,** information may be released about the patient

in order to provide care to the patient. However, when a substitute decision-maker is identified, that individual can insist that the patient's confidence be protected.

   d. Various state and federal laws provide exceptions to confidentiality, such as **releases of information required during civil commitment proceedings, malpractice cases, bill collections, and litigation in which the patient puts his or her mental status at issue.**

   e. **Breaches of confidentiality may be required by statute or case law,** such as obligations to report child abuse or neglect, or the duty to take steps to protect third parties from harm threatened by a patient (see below).

3. **In the normal course of treatment, information about a patient may be shared with a limited group of individuals without getting the express permission of the patient. These are generally held to include the patient, co-treaters, consultants, supervisors, and facilities to which the patient is being admitted or transferred. Before information is released to family members, referring clinicians, lawyers, or law enforcement, the patient's express permission should be obtained.**

4. **In all cases where confidentiality is to be breached, it should be breached to the least extent possible and with the patient being aware.**

D. **The Duty to Protect Third Parties: The Tarasoff Legacy**

1. **Breach of confidentiality is ethically permissible when there is a need to protect the patient or third parties:** "Psychiatrists at times may find it necessary, in order to protect the patient or the community from imminent danger, to reveal confidential information disclosed by the patient." (Principles of Medical Ethics with Annotations Especially Applicable to Psychiatry, Section 4, Annotation 8.)

2. The general concept is that there is a basic duty to protect/warn if a therapist knows or should know of a patient's potential for substantial harm to an identified or readily identifiable individual.

3. The key case in this area is Tarasoff v. Regents of the University of California, 551 P. 2d 334 (1976).

   a. Holding: "When a therapist determines, or pursuant to the standards of his profession should determine, that his patient presents a serious danger of violence to another, he incurs a serious obligation to use reasonable care to protect the intended victim from such danger."

   b. **Implications of the Tarasoff decision**

      i. Psychotherapists and patients have a special relationship which makes the therapist uniquely liable for some actions of the patient.

      ii. It is not necessarily a duty to warn the intended victim or law enforcement, which would require a breach of confidentiality, but a duty to protect which can be fulfilled through a variety of other actions on the part of the treater.

   iii. **The duty that was established by <u>Tarasoff</u> was to an identified victim, although subsequent cases expanded the duty to broader classes of individuals and in some cases to individuals who might be in a "zone of danger" around an intended victim.**

c. While the duty to protect third parties has been rejected by courts and legislatures in several states, the duty saw a rapid expansion in many jurisdictions. As a result, a number of states passed statutes that placed some limitations on the duty. **The American Psychiatric Association (APA) developed a model statute, that provides for liability to third parties for the acts of a patient where there is:**

   i. Communication of an explicit threat to identified victim(s) with apparent intent and ability to carry out the threat, and reasonable steps not taken.

   ii. The patient has a known history of physical violence, and the therapist has a "reasonable basis to believe that there is a clear and present danger that the patient will attempt to kill or inflict serious bodily injury against a reasonably identified victim or victims," and reasonable steps are not taken.

   iii. Reasonable steps are defined as one or more of the following:

- Warn potential victim or victims.
- Notify law enforcement in the area.
- Arrange for voluntary hospitalization.
- Take appropriate steps to commit.

E. The National Practitioner Bank

1. Authorized by **the Health Care Quality Improvement Act of 1986 (HCQIA),** the database applies to physicians, dentists, other health care practitioners.

2. **It requires mandatory reporting of:**
   a. **Payments made to satisfy malpractice claims** (including settlements).
   b. **Adverse privilege actions taken by health care entities.**
   c. **Actions taken on licensure.**

3. The practitioner who is reported must be notified and given an opportunity to respond.

4. Hospitals are required to query the databank for information on each physician, dentist, or other health care practitioner appointed to staff or granted clinical privileges.
   a. Other health care facilities may query.
   b. Malpractice insurers may not directly query.

IV. Boundary Violations

A. An Introduction to Professional Boundaries

1. **Boundaries** between doctors and patients **provide a set of rules and expectations that allow the patient to develop trust in the physician and know what to expect from the relationship.**

   a. **Boundary crossings** involve minor, but potentially important, blurring of the boundaries.

   b. **Boundary violations** involve more clear-cut transgressions of the accepted boundaries between doctor and patient.

2. **What constitutes a boundary crossing or violation is determined both by the nature of the action and by the setting in which it occurs.** For example, in a rural area it might be appropriate for the family doctor to spend time with patients at a social gathering, while the same socializing for a doctor in an urban practice might be considered a boundary crossing.

3. The maintenance of professional boundaries has been the subject of both ethical and legal proscriptions. **The basic principle of these limitations on physician behavior is that physicians have a fiduciary duty to their patients. This duty is to put the best interests of the patient ahead of the physician's interest.**

   a. The Hippocratic Oath includes admonitions about maintaining appropriate boundaries, including maintaining confidences and avoiding sexual relations. **In 1989, the American Medical Association Council on Ethical and Judicial Affairs passed an ethical rule which prohibits physician-patient sexual contact, regardless of specialty.**

   b. **Physician-patient sexual contact, and other forms of physician exploitation of patients, are the basis for discipline by physician registration authorities in all states.**

   c. **The APA** has adopted an ethical guideline which **declares it unethical for a psychiatrist to have a sexual relationship with a former or current patient.**

   d. **A number of states have enacted laws which make it a *criminal offense* for a physician to have a sexual relationship with a patient.**

   i. Statutes vary as to whether they classify doctor-patient sexual contact as a misdemeanor or a felony. Some statutes distinguish between first and repeated offenses.

   ii. While many of the statutes criminalize psychotherapist-patient sexual contact, the term psychotherapy is broadly defined in some statutes as "the professional treatment, assessment, or counseling of a mental or emotional illness, symptom, or condition." Thus, many of these statutes would apply to primary care physicians who treat psychiatric illness.

   iii. Statutes also differ with regard to how they define "patient," and whether and when the prohibition applies.

B. Selected Boundary Issues

1. **Business dealings between doctor and patient**
   a. **The physician-patient relationship is fundamentally a business relationship.** The terms of the contract are that the physician receives a fee in return for helping the patient with medical problems. The arm's-length

nature of the relationship allows the physician to be objective in his or her dealings with the patient.

b. **Involvement in other business dealings can detract from the distance, objectivity, and empathy necessary for the physician-patient relationship to succeed and is prohibited except under special circumstances;** for example, the psychiatrist lives in a small community where the patient operates the only hardware store. Even in this limited situation, the psychiatrist would be well advised to find another store in a neighboring town.

2. **Social (non-sexual) relationships with patients**

 a. In certain settings (e.g., small towns), social contact between physician and patient is unavoidable. Confidentiality and cordiality without undue familiarity can allow these treatment relationships to succeed.

 b. **Close friendships between physician and patient can compromise the physician's objectivity and lead to errors in judgment because of the physician's emotional involvement.** The same principles apply here as apply in the context of physicians treating family members.

3. **Sex in the treatment relationship**

 a. As indicated above, sexual relations with patients has been the subject of great attention in legal and ethical circles. The reasons why physicians get involved in these relationships vary. They include predatory sexual behavior by physicians seeking to take advantage of the patient, as well as infatuation on the part of physicians who are vulnerable because of their own life circumstances. Some patients may be seductive, or at least engage in behavior that may be interpreted by the physician as seductive. Nevertheless, **it is always the physician's responsibility to maintain appropriate boundaries. Failure to do so is always the fault of the physician.**

 b. Sex with patients in the guise of treatment constitutes fraud and misrepresentation, and may provide the basis for criminal prosecution in some states.

 c. Sexual relationships with patients in many cases result from the disparity in power and authority between doctor and patient. Such relationships are inherently coercive and without consent.

 d. Patients who have had sexual relationships with their physicians often suffer significant harm as a result. Such injury becomes a justifiable basis for a lawsuit against the physician. **While involvement in a sexual relationship with a patient constitutes an intentional tort that would ordinarily not be covered by malpractice insurance, courts have held that it represents a mishandling of the transference and countertransference in the treatment relationship, thus putting it within the realm of malpractice.**

Suggested Readings

Bisbing SB, Jorgenson LM, Sutherland PK: *Sexual Abuse by Professionals: A Legal Guide*. Charlottesville, VA: The Michie Company, 1996.

Gabbard GO: *Sexual Misconduct. Psychiatric Update*, Vol. 18. Washington, DC: American Psychiatric Press, 1994.

Gabbard G, Nadelson C: Professional boundaries in the physician-patient relationship. *Forum* 1996; 17(2): 7–8.

Prosser and Keeton on Torts, 5th ed. St. Paul: West Publishing, 1984.

Simon RI: *Clinical Psychiatry and the Law*. Washington, DC: APA Press, 1987.

Chapter 70
Psychiatric Consultation to Medical and Surgical Patients

JOHN QUERQUES, THEODORE A. STERN, AND NED H. CASSEM

I. Overview

A. Functions of Consultation-Liaison (C-L) Psychiatry
C-L psychiatry is a branch of psychiatry that entails:
1. **Consultation to medically and surgically ill hospitalized patients**
2. **Enhancement of nonpsychiatric clinicians' awareness of affective, behavioral, and cognitive disorders**
3. **Education of students and clinicians of all disciplines about the psychosocial and psychiatric aspects of medical care**
4. **Research at the interface of medicine, surgery, neurology, and psychiatry**

B. History of C-L Psychiatry
1. Rooted in psychosomatic medicine and psychobiology, C-L psychiatry has gradually widened its arena from the medical wards of large general hospitals in the 1930s, to critical-care units, to specialized centers that provide care for patients with cancer, human immunodeficiency virus (HIV) infection, and transplanted organs.
2. The mid-1970s marked a growth phase for the field, fueled by the return of the medical model and the provision of grant money by Dr. James Eaton, then the director of the Psychiatric Education Branch of the National Institute of Mental Health, for the establishment of new C-L services and research activities.
3. Whereas in the early 1970s only three-quarters of all psychiatry residency programs even offered an experience in C-L psychiatry, today such rotations are required.
4. Although C-L psychiatry is not recognized by the American Board of Psychiatry and Neurology as a subspecialty, many C-L psychiatrists have fought vigorously for subspecialty recognition. Others contend that the field is more properly considered a supraspecialty.

II. Epidemiology

A. Prevalence of Psychopathology Among the Medically Ill
1. **The frequency of psychopathology in the general-hospital population ranges from 10% to 50%,** depending in large part on the type and severity of underlying medical or surgical illness.
2. Since **psychiatric comorbidity prolongs length of stay, increases costs, and worsens the course of medical illness,** prompt recognition and treatment are essential.

B. Rates of Psychiatric Consultation
1. Despite the high frequency of psychiatric disturbance in general hospitals, in general, **the rate of referral for psychiatric consultation is estimated to be only 3–5%.**
2. Rates of psychiatric consultation vary across institutions based on differences in patient population, length of stay, nature and severity of illness, and personal style of referring physicians and consulting psychiatrists.
3. At the Massachusetts General Hospital (MGH), approximately 6% of all hospital admissions are seen by a psychiatrist.

C. Reasons for Psychiatric Consultation
1. Reasons for which consultation is requested typically **involve affective, behavioral, and cognitive derangements.**
2. Common requests include:
   a. Evaluation of depression and suicidal ideation
   b. Management of patients who have interpersonal difficulties with care providers or who fail to cooperate with the medical-surgical team
   c. Evaluation of decision-making capacity
   d. Evaluation of delirium and dementia

III. Diagnostic Features and Differential Diagnosis

A. Categorization of Psychiatric Problems
Diagnoses assigned by psychiatric consultants fall into one or more of the following categories:
1. **Psychiatric presentations of organic disease or its treatment** (e.g., hypothyroidism with depressive features)
2. **Psychiatric complications of organic disease or its treatment** (e.g., steroid-induced psychosis)
3. **Psychiatric reactions to organic disease or its treatment** (e.g., adjustment disorder after a diagnosis of cancer)
4. **Organic presentations of psychiatric disease** (e.g., depression with multiple somatic complaints)

503

5. **Comorbid independent psychiatric and medical illness** (e.g., schizophrenia and coronary artery disease [CAD])

B. At the MGH, the most common diagnoses are depression, delirium, anxiety, substance abuse, personality disorder, various pain syndromes, and dementia.

IV. Principles of Psychiatric Evaluation of Medical-Surgical Patients

A request for consultation may belie a problem within the patient, among the medical-surgical staff as individuals and as a whole, and/or between patient and staff. An effective consultant recognizes the importance of each of these forces and considers each in an accurate formulation of the problem.

A. **Speak directly with the consultee to define the reason for the consultation and to establish its urgency.**
   1. While the "real" reason for the consultation may not be obvious from the stated request, it may be discerned from a conversation with the consultee.
   2. The consultant is most helpful when he or she understands the consultee's question or concern and then specifically addresses that issue throughout the consultative process.

B. **Review the current and pertinent portions of the old record.**

C. **Review the patient's medications,** including those taken at home and those ordered in the hospital. Be vigilant for recently added and discontinued agents that may bear on the current mental status.

D. **Gather collateral information from family, friends, and staff** without becoming an advocate of these sources' points of view or opinions. Maintain an open mind and avoid premature closure.

E. **Interview the patient and perform a mental status examination (MSE).**
   1. Anticipate:
      a. An atmosphere less formal and rigid than in the outpatient setting
      b. The sights, smells, and sounds of a medical or surgical ward
      c. Frequent interruptions by nurses, other staff, and family
      d. The presence of roommates
      e. The requirement for flexibility in timing and format
      f. The goal to be not only diagnostic but therapeutic
      g. A review of the patient's medical issues early in the interview
      h. An appropriate use of humor
      i. Defense mechanisms activated against fear, anxiety, and mistrust

F. **Do the appropriate physical and neurologic examinations.**

G. **Write a brief, jargon-free note that emphasizes impressions and recommendations and plans for treatment.** Because these sections are the most important to the consultee, it is especially critical to be clear and specific in these sections.
   1. In the medical record, avoid "note wars," criticism of the consultee, and accusations of shoddy work. If the consultee chooses a therapeutic course equally appropriate to the consultant's preferred choice, an indication of agreement in the chart may be more prudent than rigid insistence on the consultant's preference.
   2. The consultation note includes all of the elements of a standard psychiatric note plus:
      a. **A two-sentence summary of the patient's medical and psychiatric history, the reason for admission, and the reason for consultation.** For example:

      This 75-year-old man with a history of CAD, hypertension, and depression was admitted to the medical service yesterday for evaluation of substernal chest pain thought to be secondary to myocardial infarction. Psychiatric consultation is requested to assess the safety of continuing tricyclic antidepressant therapy.

      b. **A brief summary of the present medical illness, test results, and hospital course** that demonstrates a basic appreciation for the medical issues material to the consultation rather than rehashes data already present in earlier notes.
      c. **A brief description of the patient's typical patterns of response to stress and illness**
      d. **Relevant physical and neurologic examinations**
      e. **Relevant current and past laboratory results**
      f. **Differential diagnoses** listed in order of decreasing likelihood. An indication that the patient's symptoms are not attributable to a certain psychiatric disorder may be very helpful.
      g. **Recommendations or plans** listed in order of decreasing importance
         i. **Diagnostics** (laboratory tests, neuroimaging, projective testing, neuropsychological testing)
         ii. **Therapeutics** (biological, psychological, social, behavioral)
            ● (1) For medications, include dose, route of administration, and frequency. The consultee should be able to transcribe recommendations for medications directly onto the order sheet.
            ● (2) Anticipate and address problems that may appear later. For example, for a delirious patient who is currently calm, the consultant may recommend that a neuroleptic agent be given should the patient become agitated in the future.

h. **An indication that the consultant will provide follow-up**
i. **The consultant's printed name and phone or beeper number**

H. **Speak with the consultee, nurses, and other relevant staff about your findings, opinion, and treatment proposal, highlighting the rationale and anticipated outcome of your recommendations.** This step is especially important when diagnoses or recommendations are crucial or controversial (e.g., when a preoperative patient is found to have the capacity to refuse surgery).

V. Treatment

A. **Treatment should proceed along multiple lines: biological, psychological, social, and behavioral.**
   1. **Biological.** When prescribing psychotropic agents for patients who are taking other medications for medical illnesses, the consultant must be vigilant for:
      a. **Drug-drug interactions.** Numerous medicines, including many psychopharmaceuticals, are metabolized in the liver by the cytochrome P450 enzyme system. Many psychiatric medications inhibit this enzymatic pathway and thus raise serum levels of concomitantly administered drugs. (See Chap. 51 for a detailed discussion of these interactions.)
      b. **Protein binding.** Some psychopharmacologic agents are highly protein-bound. These drugs may displace other protein-bound medicines and thus raise their serum concentrations, potentially to dangerous levels. (See Chap. 51 for a detailed discussion of these interactions.)
      c. **Side effects.** Certain adverse effects that medically healthy patients tolerate may be troublesome or dangerous for patients undergoing treatment for active medical illness. These side effects may worsen the medical problem or the side effects of other treatments. For example, the gut-slowing effect of tricyclic antidepressants may worsen postoperative ileus.
   2. **Psychological. Psychotherapy with hospitalized, medically ill patients is brief, present-oriented, and practical.** The consultant's goal is to identify and bolster patients' innate defenses to help them better cope with illness and hospitalization and to explain these coping strategies to the medical-surgical team. To be an effective therapist, the consultant must appreciate the variable stresses that different diseases engender as well as the universality of the experience of (a) **uncertainty** in diagnosis, treatment outcome, and prognosis, and (b) **grief** over disfigurement, disability, or imminent death. Consultants may instruct patients in the use of **relaxation techniques, guided imagery,** and **hypnosis** to quell anxiety and reduce stress.
   3. **Social.** Consultants help the medical-surgical team and patient make decisions about:
      a. End-of-life care (e.g., do-not-resuscitate [DNR] and do-not-intubate [DNI] decisions)
      b. Disposition to an appropriate living situation (e.g., home with visiting nurses, skilled nursing facility, nursing home)
      c. Short-term disability after a protracted illness or hospitalization
   4. **Behavioral. Explanation for the medical-surgical staff of patients' natural coping styles helps the treatment team better understand and care for patients.** For example, an electrical engineer with obsessive-compulsive traits feels out of control when he is admitted to the coronary care unit (CCU) with chest pain. He questions the team frequently because information helps him to feel more in control, even though the team considers his questions bothersome and they begin to avoid him. If the CCU team understands this patient's defensive structure, they will be less hostile toward him, answer his questions appropriately, and provide him with information before he asks for it. The consultant may suggest that the patient decide the times of medication administration or physical therapy (e.g., within an hour or so of the usual time) to help the patient feel more in control. For patients who are agitated or likely to hurt themselves or others, the consultant may recommend physical restraints and/or constant observation.

B. **A key element of effective therapeutics is the provision of periodic (usually daily) follow-up visits** until the patient is psychiatrically stable, is discharged, or dies. This allows the consultant to:
   1. Gather further history from patient, family, friends, previous treaters, and other collateral sources.
   2. Supplement findings of the initial MSE, which provides only a cross-sectional snapshot of a patient's mental functioning at a given time, with longitudinal data.
   3. Refine diagnoses.
   4. Monitor treatment and recommend appropriate changes.
   5. Engage in ongoing dialogue with the consultee and other staff.

C. **"Signing off" of stable cases is acceptable, but the consultant should be prepared to resume follow-up should matters destabilize,** as many neuropsychiatric disturbances wax and wane.

D. **Consultants should be prepared to transfer patients who are psychiatrically unstable to an inpatient psychiatric unit once their medical and surgical issues are resolved.** Patients who require psychiatric follow-up but can safely go home should be referred for outpatient care.

VI. Conclusions

A. The C-L psychiatrist is an expert in the affective, behavioral, and cognitive disturbances of hospitalized, medically or surgically ill patients, with skill in rapid assessment and in biological, psychological, social, and behavioral treatments.

B. First and foremost a competent and thorough physician, the C-L psychiatrist takes a panoramic view of the patient, the disease, and the interrelationships between the two.

C. The effective C-L psychiatrist addresses the needs of both the patient and the medical-surgical team.

D. Accessibility, excellent communication skills, and tolerance for unpredictability are essential attributes.

Suggested Readings

Bronheim HE, Fulop G, Kunkel EJ, et al.: The Academy of Psychosomatic Medicine practice guidelines for psychiatric consultation in the general medical setting. *Psychosomatics* 1998; 39:S8–S30.

Ford CV: Introduction. In Rundell JR, Wise MG (eds): *The American Psychiatric Press Textbook of Consultation-Liaison Psychiatry*. Washington, DC: American Psychiatric Press, 1996:xix–xxi.

Garrick TR, Stotland NL: How to write a psychiatric consultation. *Am J Psychiatry* 1982; 139:849–855.

Goldman L, Lee T, Rudd P: Ten commandments for effective consultations. *Arch Intern Med* 1983; 143:1753–1755.

Hackett TP, Cassem NH, Stern TA, Murray GB: Beginnings: consultation psychiatry in a general hospital. In Cassem NH, Stern TA, Rosenbaum JF, Jellinek MS (eds): *Massachusetts General Hospital Handbook of General Hospital Psychiatry*, 4th ed. St. Louis: Mosby, 1997:1–9.

Kunkel EJS, Thompson TL: The process of consultation and organization of a consultation-liaison psychiatry service. In Rundell JR, Wise MG (eds): *The American Psychiatric Press Textbook of Consultation-Liaison Psychiatry*. Washington, DC: American Psychiatric Press, 1996:13–23.

Lipowski ZJ: Current trends in consultation-liaison psychiatry. *Can J Psychiatry* 1983; 28:329–338.

Lipowski ZJ: History of consultation-liaison psychiatry. In Rundell JR, Wise MG (eds): *The American Psychiatric Press Textbook of Consultation-Liaison Psychiatry*. Washington, DC: American Psychiatric Press, 1996:3–11.

Pasnau RO, Fawzy FI, Skotzko CE, et al.: Surgery and surgical subspecialties. In Rundell JR, Wise MG (eds): *The American Psychiatric Press Textbook of Consultation-Liaison Psychiatry*. Washington, DC: American Psychiatric Press, 1996:609–639.

Popkin MK: Consultation-liaison psychiatry. In Kaplan HI, Sadock BJ (eds): *Comprehensive Textbook of Psychiatry/VI*, 6th ed. Baltimore: Williams and Wilkins, 1995:1592–1605.

Chapter 71
Coping with Medical Illness

HELEN G. KIM AND DONNA B. GREENBERG

I. Introduction

How does one patient with hemophilia become a daredevil sportsman while another fearfully obsesses over the possibility of a fatal bleed? Why does one patient respond to the same disease differently than another? **Psychiatrists are frequently asked to see patients facing medical illness. Whether initiated by overwhelmed staff or by distraught patients, these consultations require careful psychiatric assessment, thoughtful ego lending, timely dynamic interpretation, and support of needed defenses.** Faced with physical illness, patients may feel under siege, betrayed by their bodies, or damned by fate or divine intervention. Psychiatrists can help patients bear these threats to their bodies, mobilize personal and social resources, and overcome maladaptive defenses.

II. Aspects of Coping

A. **Psychological Factors**
   Similar to the elegant feedback loops that maintain physiologic homeostasis, patients also have dynamic and creative mechanisms to maintain psychological balance. Each has a characteristic pattern of cognitive organization and affective response to stressful situations. When confronted by physical illness most patients revert to well-worn patterns of stress response. However, when customary coping mechanisms fail to contain this response, psychic disequilibrium, manifest by anxiety, fear, guilt, despair, or anger, may result. Ultimately a patient achieves a new psychological homeostasis. For some patients, this represents an adaptive progression toward acceptance, mobilization of resources, or sublimation. For others, these crises evolve into maladaptive responses, such as embittered defeat, unyielding denial, help-rejecting attitudes, or treatment noncompliance.
   1. **Coping skills. Individuals defend against losses in subjective ways that can either impede or ease the necessary grieving that accompanies illness. Coping skills may be adaptive in one situation but defeating and self-sabotaging in another.** By classifying these coping mechanisms as "skills," Moos (1977) and others have emphasized that **coping can be taught and used flexibly, and that defenses are not innately pathologic.**

a. **Denying or minimizing the seriousness of one's condition.** An obese woman may welcome an unexplained weight loss and delay medical evaluation rather than interpret it as a possible harbinger of an underlying malignancy. After a teenager is told by her neurosurgeon that her cervical injury has left her paraplegic, she may lament missing her senior prom rather than grieve the loss of ever walking again. Denial protects both patients from intolerable emotions. However, in the first case, denial may delay crucial treatment, while, in the second, denial has less negative consequences and allows her time to gather the necessary resources to assimilate new information.
b. **Isolation of affect** can be highly adaptive in helping a patient overcome immediate challenges posed by physical illness (e.g., keeping appointments or following-through with consultations and tests).
c. **Intellectualization.** Seeking information may help a patient contain the helplessness engendered by disease. The physics professor with prostate cancer may find that focusing on the results of scientific studies is his only means of restoring control. As with other coping skills, intellectualization can be highly adaptive if not used to excess.
d. **Requesting reassurance and support** from family, friends and health care providers can be an important part of countering feelings of isolation and helplessness. While this strategy may seem unfamiliar to the stoical business executive, it could be incredibly liberating and enrich his stagnant relationships. Alternatively, maintenance of defenses which have been adaptive while persevering through financial difficulties may now lead to isolation and alienation of his loved ones.
e. **Learning illness-related procedures** such as checking one's blood pressure and administering insulin may help restore a sense of control and effectiveness. In addition, patients and their relatives may find relief in having concrete means of helping.
f. **Setting concrete limited goals**, such as telling specific individuals of one's diagnosis of HIV (human immunodeficiency virus) infection, attending special events, or fulfilling certain physical tasks (e.g. walking or running a race) can help a patient identify manageable goals amidst seemingly overwhelming obstacles.
g. **Rehearsing alternative outcomes.** Anticipating difficulties and creating alternative strategies can make potentially demoralizing tasks conquerable. For instance, a hard-driving patient might recognize that

Table 71-1. Biopsychosocial Components of Illness Dynamics

Psychological components
Personality traits
Ego mechanisms
Object relatedness
Stage of life during illness
Medical history
Past psychiatric history
Physician-patient relationship

Biological components
Nature and severity of disease process
Physical integrity of the patient
Genetic endowment
Response to pharmacotherapy
Medical history

Social components
Family relationships
Personal history
Family medical history
Cultural factors

SOURCE: Green, 1985.

resuming her hectic work schedule after a myocardial infarction might undermine her recovery. Rather than wait for a resurgence of her angina, she could proactively resume a reduced work schedule with less stressful duties.

h. **Finding meaning.** For one person, a hip fracture following a car accident may seem like punishment from an unjust god. Someone else might be able to appreciate the opportunity to reassess priorities and to redefine life goals. White and Lidden reported that 5–10% of patients who sustained cardiac arrest experienced a "transcendental redirection" of their lives and saw something positive in their illnesses. Whether this outlook improves long-term course remains debatable, but the quality of a patient's mood and relationships will likely benefit.

2. **Character traits** shape the significance of disease for patients. These factors include age, intelligence, cognitive and emotional development, ego strength, object relatedness, and defensive style. In addition, different personality traits can delineate the psychological and personal resources available to a patient coping with disease. For instance, an individual with a poor sense of self may rely more heavily on somatic symptoms, adamantly

deny his symptoms, and depend excessively on health professionals. A more integrated, mature patient might rely more on gathering information to quell fear and anxiety.

3. **The developmental moment** that disease strikes plays an important part in a patient's ability to cope. A back injury in an adolescent male may undermine his developmentally appropriate urge to assert independence and to establish a sexual identity. At this age he may have more limited coping resources than a 60-year-old with the same injury. On the other hand, injury at this later age brings its own challenges; a patient may have to confront threats to self-esteem and awareness of one's mortality, as well as challenges to one's identity as family provider.

4. **Catastrophic fears** evoked by physical illness can become manifest as anxiety, depression, fear, or treatment noncompliance. Directed questions about a patient's greatest fears can identify specific areas of vulnerability. For instance, loss of life may not necessarily be a foremost concern for a patient with terminal illness. Rather, an individual may fear loss of certain faculties, such as sexual function, sight, speech, or continence. The scope of catastrophic fears often includes the following:
   a. Loss of bodily integrity (e.g., colostomy, amputation, hysterectomy)
   b. Loss of power and dignity (e.g., weakness, incontinence)
   c. Abandonment or loss of intimacy (e.g., cognitive or emotional availability to loved ones, sexual function)
   d. Loss of control (e.g., incontinence, dependency on medications for health and survival)
   e. Loss of mental alacrity or memory (e.g., after stroke, dementia)

5. **Grieving**
   a. Coping with physical illness involves a grieving process. Whether one suffers a concrete loss (e.g., blindness or amputation) or a decrease in function (e.g., through weakness), a patient may experience a multitude of losses. While the specific meaning of illness is peculiar to each patient, one should at least expect the patient to mourn his or her previous state of health. Psychiatrists can facilitate a patient's progression to acceptance of new levels of physical functioning and help the individual move through the stages of grief described by Kubler-Ross (1969): denial, anger, bargaining, depression, and acceptance.
   b. **Unresolved grief** following unacceptable losses imposed by illness may leave a patient wallowing in stages of depression, hopelessness, anger, and helplessness. Unresolved feelings may be acted out in ways that affect their psychological, social, and physical well-being. Internalization of these feelings of helplessness and anger may curtail activities and make one

more socially withdrawn and ruminative. Self-imposed limitations may extend far beyond the necessary restrictions of physical illness. In addition, a patient may blindly seek retribution from physicians or family members for impositions caused by their physical illness. For instance, rather than grieve and accept the loss brought on by his illness, an individual may devote himself to baseless malpractice lawsuits, as if money could restore some sense of wholeness in the wake of physical illness. Unresolved grief can also lead to noncompliance with medical treatment. For example, a woman with complete remission of breast cancer after mastectomy and radiation may convince herself that she has conquered her illness and no longer needs her physicians. Such unyielding denial may lead to a Pyrrhic victory over cancer as she misses signs of recurrence that insidiously progress to metastatic disease. Here, denial may be her downfall.

c. Green (1985) characterized the most abnormal psychological responses as denial, anxiety, anger, depression, and dependency. While each of these reflects a normal phase of grief, a patient may interpret illness mainly from the perspective of that emotion. In these cases, rigid defenses may lead to ineffective grieving, psychological stagnation, or regression.

B. Biological and Illness-Related Factors

1. **Symptom meaning.** Patients experience symptoms subjectively. Hand paresthesia can be a minor nuisance for a truck driver, but a devastating threat to self-identity for a concert violinist. Shortness of breath to a man whose father died of lung cancer may induce despair and anger, while resonating with painful feelings of early loss. On the other hand, this same symptom in an aspiring adolescent runner may make him simply question his own physical conditioning. The experience of chest pain to the retired executive 10 years following bypass surgery will understandably differ from the 30-year-old woman with panic disorder. **To determine the significance of a particular symptom, the psychiatrist must appreciate an individual's developmental stage, personal history, and defensive style.**

Different symptoms often have a psychological meaning disproportionate to the actual importance of these symptoms prognostically. For instance, a disfiguring facial burn may have more psychological impact than a chronically progressive disease, such as diabetes. **Different diseases have different impacts, depending on whether they are painful, disfiguring, disabling, or in a body region with special significance (e.g., face, prostate, breast).**

2. **Nature and severity of disease.** HIV infection will probably convey different meaning for a 22-year-old college senior than for a 65-year-old retiree, even if both have the same opportunistic infections,

require the same medications, and have the same viral load. Each has a unique way of perceiving and defending against the loss of health. Each has certain strengths and psychological vulnerabilities that will affect the course of illness. For the college student and retiree their divergent responses to the same disease stage and treatment may make HIV seem like two different illnesses.

3. **Recovery from illness** may impose stress on a patient. After insisting upon discharge, a patient may become overly dependent and fearful when away from the hospital's highly supervised setting. Transfer from the intensive care unit to a general medicine floor may evoke relief in some who interpret it as a sign of recovery or outrage in others who rail against their physician's perceived disregard.

4. **Disease complications** may undermine habitual coping mechanisms. For instance, dementia may hinder a surgeon's defenses of intellectualization and sublimation as he comes to terms with his failing memory and worsening tremor. Physiologic problems (e.g., electrolyte imbalance, anemia, or hypoxia) may also impair cognition and coping.

5. **Psychiatric complications and comorbidity** may accompany physical illness and interfere with recovery and treatment compliance. Despair and anxiety may naturally accompany the psychic damage of physical illness. However, major depression, generalized anxiety disorder, or any Axis I condition should never be dismissed as "appropriate responses to physical illness."

6. **Treatment-related factors. Patients must cope not only with disease but also with medical treatments.** A diabetic patient's response to needing insulin may range from intransigent denial to consuming obsessiveness. Behind such disparate defenses may lie similar fears of disability; however, the first patient's denial may lead to premature blindness and lower extremity amputation while the other's fastidiousness may effect a better long-term course consistent with tightly controlled diabetes.

Special treatment environments (e.g., the dialysis unit, the intensive care unit, or even the doctor's waiting room) may present unique challenges to particular patients. Unfamiliar routines and separation from loved ones may evoke intolerable feelings of inadequacy, doubt, and failure.

The response and attitude of health professionals can influence a patient's ability to cope with illness. A patient may feel intimidated by the power his physician seems to wield. Another stressful aspect of care is the involvement of multiple physicians with no one asserting primary responsibility in what the Balints called a "collusion of anonymity" and Winnicott called the "scatter of responsible agents." Whether a patient asks for a second opinion, pain medication, or a bill, he may shy away from confronting his physician directly for fear he will withdraw care or provide suboptimal treatment.

C. **Social factors** involved in illness dynamics include relationships with family, friends, health care providers, and the wider community. Physical illness can further tax chronically unstable interpersonal relationships, as well as strain empathic, constant ones. Studies have shown that the **quality of social supports can affect a patient's experience of illness as well as his long-term course.**

III. Psychiatric Assessment

A. **Immediate Concerns**
Psychiatrists must consider what has precipitated a patient's seeking consultation in the face of medical illness. Was it her own sense of hopelessness or her physicians' inability to bear the patient's poor prognosis? What troubles the patient most? A wide range of issues (e.g., pain, weakness, separation from family, incarceration in a hospital, and financial strain) may exist. In addition, there may be certain tests or procedures that the patient expects to be particularly problematic, such as an MRI (magnetic resonance imaging) in a claustrophobic patient.

Potential problematic areas for the patient coping with medical illness may include the following:
1. Health and well-being
2. Family responsibilities
3. Marital/sexual relations
4. Job responsibilities
5. Financial problems
6. Religious and cultural demands
7. Self-image
8. Existential issues

B. **Personality Types in Medical Management**
Understanding different personality traits can help psychiatrists anticipate a patient's strengths and vulnerabilities in coping with medical illness. Kahana and Bibring (1964) described the following normal personality types to characterize the basic needs, fears, defenses, and adaptive behaviors which influence the illness experience for individual patients. These simplistic paradigms are presented in modified and extreme form to help the psychiatrist detect subtler versions present in many patients.
1. **The dependent, overdemanding personality.** This patient may unconsciously cling to his physical illness as his only concrete evidence that he deserves love and attention. While the patient may demand

multiple consultations and tests, the victory of getting a diagnosis and receiving extensive medical attention is bittersweet as it is based on the fundamental premise that he is in fact defective. This painfully resonates with the patient's unconscious belief that he is irrevocably damaged and unworthy. His dependency on others for protection and caring speaks to a lack of agency akin to that of the helpless infant he once was, wholly dependent on another (e.g., the mother) for all his needs. His health care providers inevitably fall short of the perfect love of the mother figure, which leaves the patient with feelings of anger, depression, helplessness, and hopelessness. Disappointment and rejection are an inevitable part of this patient's experience of illness as he alienates health care providers with his cloying requests for advice and reassurance.

a. **The illness experience.** The anxiety accompanying illness may reflect this patient's unconscious wish for abundant care, as well as his fear of abandonment and starvation. Illness may provide the regressive pull towards an earlier, secure state of infantile helplessness. The patient's solution to these intense wishes and fears may be to become overly dependent on his physician and unquestioning of any medical recommendations. On the other hand, the patient may resist these unconscious feelings and become overly independent, help-rejecting, depressed, apathetic, withdrawn, or embittered.

b. **Treatment implications.** Health care providers should communicate either implicitly or explicitly their readiness to care for the patient as completely as possible. For the acutely ill patient, tending to the patient's basic physical comfort becomes extremely meaningful in the context of his heightened dependency. The patient's consuming presence and insatiable demands may evoke countertransferential feelings that inspire health care providers to avoid, ignore, or punish the patient. If the patient's demands become excessive, health care providers should offer some concession (e.g., a dietary suggestion) as they set clear, thoughtful limits in order to mitigate the patient's experience of limits as punitive and rejecting.

2. **The orderly, controlled personality.** The orderliness, predictability, and categorical imperatives that organize this patient's world can make him seem admirably disciplined and conscientious, and, at times, annoyingly rigid and obstinate. This heightened insistence on rules and compliance may have its roots in parental intolerance of the child's lack of control over behavior, feelings, or bodily function. An emphasis on thoughts over feelings and behavior leads to the repression of undesirable impulses and the development of inflexible, opposing attitudes. Under stress, this patient may

impress others with his reliance on rational, linear thought, and thorough accumulation of information. However, these attempts at cognitively organizing stressful situations belie this patient's core feelings of ineffectuality and chaos.

a. **The illness experience.** Physical illness threatens the control and self-discipline which define this patient's existence. He may respond with redoubled efforts to suppress intolerable emotions. His health care providers may experience him as opinionated and unyielding in his attitude. The patient's persistence in fact-gathering and educating himself about his illness may come at the expense of dealing with the illness on a more intimate level. Flashes of rage, fear, and despair may break through this patient's rigid defenses only to be readily sequestered by his reflexive and protective self-restraint.

b. **Treatment implications.** Feeding this patient details about his illness will help bind his anxiety. This patient survives by taking in facts and incorporating them into his own understanding of his illness. The goal in treating this patient is to help sustain his cognitive armor by providing information he needs to contain the terrifying loss of control that characterizes his experience of illness. This patient would likely welcome active participation in his treatment (e.g., logging his caloric intake, or changing his own dressings). Acknowledgement of his discernment, rational thinking, and conscientiousness may support his sense of control and bolster his belief that he is doing all he can humanly do to contain the threat of illness.

3. **The dramatizing, emotionally involved, captivating personality.** This patient may strike the physician as charming, fascinating, imaginative, dramatic, flirtatious, or enticing. This patient's intense and engaging interpersonal style stems from his yearning for singular devotion from his health care providers. Often this patient will reject same-sex physicians, who may seem like uncaring, threatening rivals. With opposite-sex physicians, however, this patient can become a caricature of certain gender stereotypes (e.g., the fearless, brute male, or the helpless damsel in distress).

a. **The illness experience.** To this patient, physical illness may feel like a public advertisement that he is in fact defective, weak, and unattractive. The narcissistic injury of physical illness may tap into a male patient's fear of losing power or bodily integrity, or a female patient's fear of losing her unique physical appeal. In striving to quell his anxiety, this patient embarks on dramatic demands for admiration and attention, or at times assumes a nonchalant disregard for the serious implications of their disease. When overt attempts at securing attention and reassurance fail, this patient may also paradoxically become overly glib and concede too readily to procedures or recommendations.

b. **Treatment implications.** Health care providers could offer directed questions about the specific fears driving his anxiety and persistent requests for attention. In addition, consistent encouragement tempered with explicit boundaries are an important part of supporting this patient as he copes with physical illness.

4. **The long-suffering, self-sacrificing patient.** This patient's personal narrative is filled with stories of disappointment, failure, and tragedy. This patient may outwardly lament his misfortune yet precipitate his own misfortune by unconsciously placing himself in harm's way. He may arouse in others uneasy sympathy rather than praise as he flaunts his self-sacrifice and suffering in an exhibitionistic and immodest way. This patient may have experienced a repressed childhood marred by parental intolerance of anger in the child along with corporal punishment, which he may have experienced with both pleasure and pain. As a child he may have found that physical illness prevented his parents from casting aspersions and may have even garnered him more love and attention.

a. **The illness experience.** This patient unconsciously assumes that self-sacrifice and suffering must be the cost for all the love and acceptance he yearned for as a child and now as an adult. The physician may resent this patient's use of his physical illness as unconditionally entitling him to limitless love. The physician may also find the patient intolerable in his disregard of any encouragement or sign of improvement, as well as his focus on only those parts of his physical illness that have not improved.

b. **Treatment implications.** Self-pitying statements are this patient's invitation to others to acknowledge his pain and sacrifices. Countering the patient's defeatism with encouragement may seem dismissive and unempathic. The physician may have to present medical treatment as yet another burden the patient must bear for others rather than as a means to alleviating pain and achieving health.

5. **The guarded, querulous patient.** The world is a lonely place for this patient. He may see himself as the victim of other people's thoughtless disregard or vengeful cruelty. He may feel that tragedy, insult, and injury shadow only him. In his world, disappointment, oppression, and exploitation at the hands of others are inevitable. Self-loathing gets reassigned to others and disclaimed from himself. While he may seemingly free himself of these intolerable feelings, placing them in others fuels his sense of victimization and helplessness.

a. **The illness experience.** Periods of sickness may push him toward the well-oiled pit of paranoia that colors his perceptions and leaves him alone in the world. He may become even more guarded, quarrelsome, and suspicious as he blames others for his medical illness.

b. **Treatment implications.** Clear descriptions of the short- and long-term view of his diagnostic workup and treatment algorithm may mitigate his perception of health care providers as manipulative and reckless. The physician should strive to be courteous without getting either overly involved or distant. Confronting his paranoid and baseless suspicions will further alienate him and may even drive him from treatment. Health care providers could try to empathize with his aloneness in the world and ally with his heightened sense of helplessness and victimization in the setting of physical illness. Rather than reinforcing his suspicions or refuting them outright, one could acknowledge that, for the patient himself, the feelings are very real.

6. **The patient with the feeling of superiority.** Exaggerated self-confidence, arrogance, and condescension shield this patient from his own shame and insecurity. While this patient may come across as smug and condescending to "lesser" treators, his grandiosity may be his only defense.

   a. **The illness experience.** For the patient with narcissistic traits, physical illness may affront his sense of perfection and invulnerability. He may insist on seeing only the most eminent physician, for who else could be worthy of understanding so complex and interesting a person, and who else could sustain his sense of "specialness." No matter how real or inflated his perception of his physician, however, over time he may need to outdo him, dwell on his faults, and belittle his interventions.

   b. **Treatment implications.** Challenging his "specialness" and entitlement may further alienate him. In the service of providing good medical care, one should support his needed defenses by understanding his need to believe in the unique competence of his primary physician.

7. **The patient who seems uninvolved and aloof.** This patient may convey contentedness in his remoteness and disregard for everyday events and interactions with others. Within his solitary world, he may actually use aloofness to defend against his perceived frailty and inner emptiness. He may have an early life marred by repeated disappointments which taught him to avoid investing emotions in any relationships.

   a. **The illness experience.** This patient may experience physical illness as an intrusion on his static and solitary world. Illness may also force him to interact with others (e.g., health care providers) in a way that feels oppressively intimate and leaves him feeling exposed. He may deal with anxieties evoked by illness with renewed denial and familiar defenses of social isolation and emotional distance.

   b. **Treatment implications.** One should try to understand this patient's aloofness and eccentricities as his solution to intolerable fear, anxiety, and vulnerability, rather than as intentional sleights. Health care providers should make limited demands on him for social involvement but insist that he not withdraw completely. It is also important to offer reassurance and support without expecting the gratifying warmth, interest, and indebtedness of other patients.

C. **Coping Capacity**

   Directed, timely and evocative questions can rapidly determine a patient's style of coping, vulnerabilities, adaptive traits, and cognitive flexibility. Weisman described a screening tool to assess a person's coping strengths (Table 71-2). He described good copers as flexible, resourceful, optimistic, practical, and good at identifying pressure points and finding solutions. Bad copers include those that deny the reality of their problems or paradoxically overwhelm their treators with descriptions of their embittered defeat and suffering. Other screening questions include:

   1. What has bothered you most about this illness?
   2. How has it been a problem for you?
   3. What have you done or are you doing about the problem?
   4. What has been the most difficult thing you've had to face until now?
   5. What did you do then?
   6. Whom have you relied on most in the past?
   7. Who do you expect will be most helpful to you now?
   8. In general, how do things usually turn out for you?
   9. What do you dread the most about this illness?

IV. Other Interventions

A. **Judicious and timely provision of medical information** can help shore up a patient's coping strengths.

B. **Psychotherapy (e.g., supportive, psychoeducational, interpersonal, cognitive, or dynamic therapy) can be life- and spirit-saving in the face of medical illness.** Patients can particularly benefit from therapy that addresses **practical issues related to their physical illness** (Moos, 1977). Physicians should introduce these tasks as common concerns to many patients with physical illness:

   1. **Dealing with physical symptoms and incapacitation.**
   2. **Dealing with the hospital environment and special treatment procedures.**
   3. **Developing adequate relationships with professional staff.** Psychiatrists can help their patients advocate for themselves when negotiating confusing health care systems and ambiguous relationships between multiple treators.
   4. **Preserving a reasonable emotional balance.** Physical illness evokes a myriad of distressing feelings, such

Table 71-2. Assessment of Coping Capacity

The problem: What has been the most important problem you've had to face since your illness began? How has your illness affected people closest to you?

The strategy: What did you do about it?

- Seek more information (rationalization/intellectualization)
- Talk with others to relieve distress (shared concern)
- Laugh it off; make light of the situation (reversal of affect)
- Try to forget or put it out of your mind (suppression)
- Do other things to distract yourself (displacement)
- Take firm action based on present understanding (confrontation)
- Accept, but find something favorable to deal with (redefinition)
- Submit, accept the inevitable (fatalism)
- Do something, anything, however reckless or impractical (acting out)
- Negotiate feasible alternatives (if X, then Y)
- Reduce tension by drinking, eating, or taking drugs
- Withdraw into isolation
- Blame someone or something (externalize)
- Seek direction from an authority and go along (compliance)
- Blame yourself, sacrifice, or atone (self-pity/surrender)

The resolution: How did it work for you (or is it working)?

- No resolution or relief
- Uncertain, indefinite, doubtful
- Qualified, limited resolution
- Specific, definite resolution; good relief

SOURCE: Adapted from Weisman, 1978.

as self-blame for not taking care of oneself, anxiety about an uncertain prognosis, alienation from loved ones and friends, resentment at health care providers for not "saving" them. Psychiatrists can help their patients to contain these feelings and to experience them in nondestructive, tolerable aliquots.

5. **Preserving a satisfactory self-image.** Evolving self-identity is a byproduct of coping with medical illness. Patients must incorporate changes in physical functioning and appearance into their self-identity.

The woman who undergoes a hysterectomy for endometrial cancer must grieve the loss of ever bearing children. An obsessive young doctor who contracts genital herpes must contend with feelings of contamination and shame. The corporate lawyer awaiting a heart transplant must contend with the narcissistic injury of illness and dependency. Part of this evolving self-identity includes redefining goals and expectations. For this lawyer, coping with his illness may involve allowing others to assist him and to redefine his work and family role. For the woman with endometrial cancer, coping may include consideration of adoption to complete her family.

6. **Preserving relationships with family and friends.** Psychiatric assessment should include an inventory of relationships which can facilitate or hinder coping. Family and friends may respond to a patient's illness in a way that leaves the patient feeling supported or completely alienated. In addition to redefining one's own self-image, patients must often adapt to changing roles within a family system.

7. **Preparing for an uncertain future**

C. **Behavioral techniques, such as hypnosis**

D. **Family therapy**

E. **Social supports**

F. **Spiritual supports**

G. **Self-help groups**

H. **Financial/legal referrals**

I. **Psychiatric Liaison Roles**
In service to the patient, psychiatrists can inform staff that individuals experience physical illness in highly divergent and subjective ways. Psychiatrists can also help promote collaborative relationships in which countertransference can be normalized, shared, and understood. For instance, some physicians may find that focusing on tests, laboratory values, and clinical signs is more tolerable than addressing unresolved emotions evoked by a patient's illness. Part of the liaison role of psychiatrists involves clarification and containment of such countertransference responses that may compromise patient care.

V. Conclusions

Physical illness can undermine one's identity, family and work role, or effect permanent changes in appearance and bodily function. The personal significance of disease depends on highly subjective factors, such as developmental stage, character traits, and the disease itself. Psychiatrists are uniquely qualified to appreciate the medical aspects of disease while facilitating patient's adaptation to the challenges and uncertainty of illness.

Suggested Readings

Green SA: *Mind and Body: The Psychology of Physical Illness*. Washington, DC: American Psychiatric Press, 1985.

Hamburg P: Bulimia: the construction of a symptom. *J Am Acad Psychoanal* 1989; 17:131–140.

Kahana RJ, Bibring GL: Personality types in medical management. In Zinberg NE (ed.): *Psychiatry and Medical Practice in a General Hospital*. New York: International Universities Press, 1964.

Kubler-Ross E: *On Death and Dying*. New York: Macmillan, 1969.

Lazarus RS, Averill JR, Opton EM: The psychology of coping: issues of research and assessment. In Coelho G, Hamburg DA, Adams JE (eds): *Coping and Adaptation*. New York: Basic Books, 1974.

Moos RH, Tsu VD: The crisis of physical illness. In Moos RH (ed.): *Coping with Physical Illness*. New York: Plenum, 1977.

Weisman AD. Coping with illness. In Hackett TP, Cassem NH (eds): *Massachusetts General Hospital Handbook of General Hospital Psychiatry*. St Louis: Mosby, 1978:264–275.

Chapter 72
Treatment Decisions at the End of Life

Brad Reddick and Ned H. Cassem

I. Introduction

Through the advancement of medical technology and practice, the human lifespan has grown. This has created fertile ground for opportunities and for conflicts. For centuries, medicine as a discipline has followed two age-old credos: **"first do no harm"** (*primum non nocere*), and **"above all relieve suffering."** It is within the final chapter of a person's life that **medicine stands at the crossroads between these two statements** (Cassem, 1999).

At no other point in the care of the patient are the unique skills, knowledge, and nurturance of the physician more important than in the process of a patient's dying. **The physician who has long-term knowledge of the patient and the patient's family can play an important role in increasing the quality of life for the dying patient. The psychiatrist's primary goals are to ensure optimization of palliative care and to assist the patient and the family in the dying process.** This process is one that requires a multidimensional or multiaxial understanding of the patient and his environment and the sometimes complex ethical issues that can arise.

II. The Psychophysiological Process of Dying

As disease pre-empting, death is often that which consumes or destroys the body; **dying patients may interpret even the slightest bodily changes as heralding demise.** Frequently, patients will experience fear with these bodily changes, but more often fear occurs long before these changes take place.

A. **Psychiatric Consultation**
   Requests for **psychiatric consultation at the end of life,** by patients and their caregivers, **occur most commonly for major depression, substance abuse, delirium, organic brain syndromes, personality disorders, pain syndromes refractory to treatment, and difficulties with grieving.** Other common causes for consultation with a psychiatrist include an inability to accept the diagnosis, and/or manifestations of pathological denial.

   In treating the dying patient, **the role of the psychiatrist** is no different than it is with other patients; the aim is to diagnose and to treat. Often the psychiatrist can facilitate treatment, as well as communication between the patient, the family, and caregivers, by modeling qualities most helpful for the patient and sought in caregivers.

B. **Qualities Sought in Caregivers**
   These qualities include being competent, concerned, comforting, cheerful, and consistent. In addition, one should be able to communicate, to have children present, and to facilitate cohesion of the family.

III. Goals for Treatment at the End of Life

The aim is to keep the patients feeling like themselves as long as possible (Saunders, 1978). This goal helps to reconcile and resolve conflicts with loved ones and to pursue remaining hopes (Kubler-Ross, 1969). Kubler-Ross described stages of dying that consisted of denial and isolation, anger, bargaining, and acceptance, which may occur in any order. **Goals for an "appropriate death"** (Hackett and Weisman, 1962) are as follows:
   1. **To be pain free.**
   2. **To operate on as effective a level as possible within the constraints of disability.**
   3. **To satisfy remaining wishes consistent with ego ideals.**
   4. **To recognize and resolve residual conflicts.**
   5. **To yield control to persons who are trusted.**

IV. Hospice Care of the Terminally Ill

Hospice care seeks to allow the dying patient to live to the limit of his or her physical strength, social relationships, and mental and emotional capacity. The average patient is enrolled in hospice care about 1 month before death, with provisions for home nursing, family support, spiritual guidance, pain treatment, medication, as well as medical care.

The World Health Organization (WHO) defines hospice or palliative care as "total care of patients whose disease is not responsive to curative treatments," seeking to aggressively minimize the patient's burdens while maximizing quality of life.

V. Psychiatric Comorbidity and Terminal Illness

A. **Major Depression**
   The more progressively ill a person becomes, the more likely he or she is to develop major depression.

Many have shown the heightened suffering such depression generates when it occurs in the terminally ill. As is true for depression in other stages of life, careful detection and aggressive treatment are essential. When depressed, patients make more restricted advance directives and change them after achieving remission (Ganzini et al., 1994). The wish to end one's life prematurely frequently accompanies depression. Breitbart and coworkers, in a study comparing terminally ill patients with suicidal thoughts with those without suicidal thoughts, found the primary difference to be the presence of depression in those with suicidal thoughts. A similar study by Chochinov et al. (1995) discovered that, of those enrolled in a Winnipeg palliative care unit who wished to hasten death, 62% met diagnostic criteria for major depression. **In the dying patient, suicidal ideation should never be accepted as "understandable"; rather, it demands the same thoughtful examination as when it occurs in any other circumstance.**

A substantial contribution to depression in the terminally ill is made by the physical loss that occurs with declining health, body disfigurement, and loss of social roles. Frequent visits and discussions are essential to facilitate the patient's working through the grieving process.

B. **Anxiety**
Anxiety frequently arises or worsens at the end of life. This anxiety is not limited to the patient, but can occur within the families, friends, and caretakers of those facing death.

The most common fears associated with death are:
1. Death will resemble that of a friend or relative with the same disease.
2. Death will result in a loss of control and helplessness.
3. Death will cause physical pain, injury, or suffocation.
4. Feelings of guilt (being bad) will arise.
5. Death will lead to abandonment.

The anxious patient frequently is unaware of what it is about death that is so frightening, although memories of personal loss and associations to illness may provide clues. Most often anxiety relates to a patient's developmental history; anxiety surfaces as fear of loss of control or helplessness (e.g., unresolved dependency conflicts), or fear of abandonment (e.g., maternal bonding difficulties) arises. It is crucial that the physician explore with the patient fears of isolation, abandonment, anticipated suffering, and separation from loved ones.

C. **Delirium and Dementia**
As terminal illness progresses, cognitive difficulties

are common and interfere with the quality of time spent with family, friends, and caretakers. Diagnosis and treatment of these difficulties are outlined in Chaps. 6, 7, 9, and 36.

D. **Personality Style and Developmental Concerns**
As interpersonal relationships are the most important supporting force for patients at the end of life, **maladaptive personality features and defense mechanisms** associated with personality disorders and mental retardation **can interfere with the patient's ability to attain comfort from these relationships.** Dependency on others, can be especially difficult for the patient at the end of life. Reframing dependency on others, as an opportunity for loved ones to give something back to the patient instead of being a burden, is often helpful. Patients with terminal illness and comorbid narcissistic or borderline character pathology are at great risk for treatment confounds, such as poor communication with caretakers, inadequate pain management, and failure to resolve interpersonal or familial conflicts. This is in part due to the negative feelings aroused in the caretakers of borderline and narcissistic patients as well as the borderline and narcissistic patients' propensity to feel victimized and to distrust those involved in their care. When negative emotions arise in the clinician and/or when the treatment team is divided, a personality disorder should be suspected.

Psychodynamic understanding of the patient's style of coping and personality structure can guide the psychiatrist to convert caretakers' negative countertransference towards the patient into useful data that informs the team as to how they can best help the patient through the process of dying. Close work with family and the many members of the patient's treatment team is essential when working with character-disordered patients.

VI. Psychosocial Considerations

The end of life does not occur in a vacuum; rather, **multiple life and environmental stresses and supports interplay in a way that can both facilitate and complicate treatment at the end of life.**

A. **Family**
The importance of the presence of family in helping patients resolve longstanding conflicts, and providing a context for remembering (and grieving) life and an opportunity to give to younger generations, cannot be emphasized enough. **Psychiatrists can aid both the patient and the family by encouraging reconciliation, by sharing of emotions and memories, and by creation of**

specific plans of the family (e.g., wills, funeral or memorial service, trips), and construction of memorabilia (e.g., photo albums).

B. **Work Relationships**

Similar to family relationships, **relationships at work can help create the sense of a life lived meaningfully.** Mobilization of colleagues and friends can do much toward this aim. Involving those whose relationships centered around recreational activities and participation in self-help groups can be another source for support and personal understanding. The patient's faith and relationship with their religious figure(s) are also essential.

C. **Religion and Faith**

Koenig and colleagues (1995) demonstrated the benefits of reliance on religious faith for coping as a means of reducing cognitive symptoms of depression associated with the end of life. Conversations about death provide the opportunity to explore the patient's beliefs and thoughts about an afterlife. Careful exploration of the patient's attitudes, thoughts, beliefs, and hopes regarding God and religious faith is crucial. Terminally ill patients can benefit from psycho-educational groups; they can improve mood, reduce anxiety, and allow for the use of adaptive coping skills. Significant prolongation of life has been demonstrated in patients with breast cancer and melanoma involved in psycho-educational groups (Spiegel et al., 1989; Fawzy et al., 1993).

VII. Ethical Decisions at the End of Life

As advances in medicine proliferate, so do our abilities to sustain life and to prolong the dying process. Although the potential for increased suffering exists, it is not necessary. **Careful consideration should be given to preserve patient autonomy and to optimize palliative care;** when exercised, suffering can be reduced and the dying process can be facilitated without prematurely ending it. With these advances, **issues pertaining to euthanasia, substituted judgment, and treatment futility remain tender.** In considering management of a patient at the end of life, ethical decisions regarding treatment remain both important and challenging.

A. **Legal Issues**

Several court rulings have provided guidelines for considering ethical issues at the end of life. The Supreme Court's ruling in the case of Nancy Cruzan established several basic tenets, which help to resolve decisions about incurable illness.

1. Competent patients have the right to refuse treatment.

2. Nutrition and hydration are included among medical treatments, such as artificial ventilation and pressor agents, that a competent patient can refuse. In addition to rulings outlined in the Cruzan case, several principles serve as guidelines when considering ethical decision-making at the end of life.

B. **First Do No Harm**

What is in the patient's best interest is the primary aim, and includes limiting treatments that may prolong or intensify suffering in the setting of terminal illness.

C. **The will of the patient, rather than the health of the patient, is the supreme law. Preserving patient autonomy at the bedside is an important role of any care-taker. It involves providing ample information and detail regarding diagnoses, treatments, and the potential outcomes of these treatments.** An autonomous choice is made when a competent informed patient expresses the preferences. Such decision-making is a process, and is made through thoughtful dialogue with the patient, the family, and the primary caretakers. **In communicating facts, physicians should be mindful of how their own feelings about death and dying may influence their interpretation of the medical situation to the patient or family.** The SUPPORT study in 1995 found that less than half of terminally ill patients have had discussions with their physicians about cardiopulmonary resuscitation (CPR). **Physicians are poor at predicting their patient's preferences and underestimate their patient's perceptions of quality of life.** There are many potential confounding factors which may allow for any stated preference to change. **The following is a list of important questions that are raised when assessing a patient's stated preference:**

1. **Are psychiatric issues, such as depression and personality styles, being addressed which may interfere or color a patient's stated preference?**
2. **How is the patient perceiving his or her social supports?**
3. **What is the patient's world view?**
4. **Have the patient's stated reasons for wanting to die been explored?**
5. **Have the dynamics of the patient-doctor relationship been explored?**
6. **Are all symptoms being treated aggressively?**

The 1995 SUPPORT study found that half of the terminally ill patients who died in the hospital were in severe pain. Concomitant substance abuse is a risk factor for the undertreatment of pain.

D. **All decisions involving medical ethics begin with the best facts available. Important facts include the diagnosis, prognosis, treatment options, reversibility**

of the illness, and the potential benefit or harm associated with each treatment. Talking with the patient and family regarding their questions and exploring their concerns is the natural result of sharing these essential facts. **The process of exploration is best accomplished in a quiet room, at a time set aside for this purpose, while sitting down.** Care should be taken not to confront initially when denial is utilized in response to factual information. **When denial is utilized as a defense initially, waiting for the patient's defenses to adapt in the context of repeated interviews is preferred before confronting the patient.** When discussing life-sustaining measures, it is helpful for the family and patient to know that treatments (e.g., mechanical ventilation) may help clarify potential for recovery, and may be tried until it is clear that health can no longer be restored.

E. **When the patient is not competent, treatment decisions rely on either advanced directive or an appointed power of attorney. Competence is a legal concept that is presumed in a patient's exercising choice.** Conditions which may affect competence include medical illnesses producing delirium, mood disorders (e.g., depression), and dysfunction of thought, as occurs in psychotic disorders. **An advanced directive is designed to extend a patient's autonomy; it contains the patient's expressed wishes for what should be done when the patient becomes incompetent or appoints a surrogate (health care proxy) who will express the wishes of the patient as if he or she were competent.** The advanced directive is composed when the patient possesses competence. Hospitals are now required by law to inform and ask patients about advanced directives. Should the patient be alert but incompetent, substituted judgment rather than prior stated wishes should be the guide. In the absence of an advanced directive, both the physician and the patient's close relatives must together provide substituted judgment with the patient's best interest. Should the patient be incompetent but alert (e.g., psychotic depression), guardianship should be considered.

F. **When is treatment limited? The physician should question any treatments that possess risks of burden outweighing potential benefits.** Patients who suffer from an irreversible and progressive illness (e.g., cancer) are particularly at risk for receiving needless burdensome treatments. Competent patients with both irreversible and reversible illness have the right to refuse any treatment, including life-sustaining treatments (e.g., hydration and nutrition). In the setting of irreversible coma, the standard medical recommendation to family would be to stop life-sustaining treatment. In the

event that there is no family available, standard medical practice would be to allow the patient to die, understanding the inevitability of death and the futility of further treatment. When a patient has a functioning brainstem with a loss of cortical function (i.e., is in a permanent vegetative state), the American Academy of Neurology recommends that all life-sustaining treatment be withdrawn due to lack of medical benefit to the patient.

G. **Futile Treatment**
A particular problem arises when, **in the setting of irreversible illness, coma, or a persistent vegetative state, the family wishes that "everything be done,"** but **potential harm of continued life-sustaining measures exists.** Although **a physician is under no obligation to provide futile or harmful treatment,** the definition of *futility* **is under debate and an area of focus for medical ethics.** The approach to such a problem begins with determination of futility. Various ways of examining and enhancing the quality of the communication with the family may lead to at least a partial agreement between the treating physician and the family. To fully appreciate the quality of communication with the family, an honest assessment of the working alliance with the patient and family is important. It is most helpful to review clinical information with the patient and the family in a manner that is free of jargon, is clear, and is open to follow-up questions. **A thoughtful assessment of family dynamics may uncover potential conflicts and issues among family members which confound clear communication** (as is true when faced with any ongoing ethical dilemma). A consultation with an ethics committee or legal counsel can provide further assistance and a fresh perspective.

VIII. Physician-Assisted Suicide and Euthanasia

For many, the topic of physician-assisted suicide is both actively debated and controversial. In struggling with this question it is helpful to review existing policies, standards of practice, and study observations.

The majority of states explicitly outlaw assisted suicide, although there have been two court rulings in the United States striking down such laws. **Most professional organizations,** such as the American Medical Association and the American Geriatric Association, **have issued statements against physician-assisted suicide. Beyond the policy, psychiatrists who are asked to hasten death for the dying patient must seek to understand what underlies the patient's wish to die.** Often careful, gentle questions can illuminate this understanding, and highlight ways in which the physician can improve in caring for the dying patient. Often careful questioning will uncover coexisting depression and disabling anxiety for which active treatment is both available and mandatory. Far too often ongoing despair is related to undertreatment of pain. **Those with concomitant substance abuse and personality disorders are especially at risk for suboptimal pain management.** Aggressive and comprehensive palliative care should make requests for euthanasia rare. Unwillingness on the part of the physician to comply with requests from a patient for euthanasia should not result in the physician's abandoning the patient in treatment. **Ample use of narcotics to treat pain and to promote comfort is not euthanasia; knowing that a patient desires death should never result in withholding pain medication for fear of suicide.**

Suggested Readings

Appelbaum PS, Grisso T: Assessing patient's capacities to consent to treatment. *N Engl J Med* 1988; 319:1635–1638.

Breitbart W, Rosenfeld BD, Passik SD: Interest in physician assisted suicide among ambulatory HIV-infected patients. *Am J Psychiatry* 1996; 153:238–242.

Cassem NH: Depression and anxiety secondary to medical illness. *Psychiatr Clin North Am* 1990; 13(4):597–612.

Cassem NH: The person confronting death. In Nicoli A (ed.): *The Harvard Guide to Psychiatry*, 3rd ed. Cambridge, MA: Harvard University Press, 1999:699–734.

Chochinov HM, Wilson KG, Enns ME, et al.: Desire for death in the terminally ill. *Am J Psychiatry* 1995; 152:1185–1191.

Council on Scientific Affairs, American Medical Association: Good care of the dying patient. *J Am Med Assoc* 1996; 275:474–478.

Fawzy FI, Fawzy NW, Hun CS, et al.: Malignant melanoma. Effects of an early structured psychiatric intervention, coping, and affective state on recurrence and survival 6 years later. *Arch Gen Psychiatry* 1993; 50:681–689.

Ganzini L, Lee MA, Heintz RT, et al.: The effect of depression treatment on elderly patients' preferences for life sustaining medical therapy. *Am J Psychiatry* 1994; 151:1631–1636.

Hackett TP, Weisman AD: The treatment of the dying. *Curr Psychiatr Ther* 1962; 2:121–126.

Kim S, Flather-Morgan A: Treatment decisions at the end of life. In Stern TA, Herman JB, Slavin PL (eds): *The MGH Guide to Psychiatry in Primary Care*. New York: McGraw-Hill, 1998.

Koenig HG, Cohen HJ, Blazer DG, et al.: Religious coping and cognitive symptoms of depression in elderly medical patients. *Psychosomatics* 1995; 36:369–375.

Kubler-Ross E: *On Death and Dying*. New York: Macmillan, 1969.

Report of the Quality Standards Subcommittee of the American Academy of Neurology: Practice parameters: assessment and management of patients in the persistent vegetative state. *Neurology* 1995; 45:1015–1018.

Saunders C (ed.): *The Management of Terminal Illness*. Chicago: Year Book Medical Publishers, 1978.

Spiegel D, Bloom JR, Kraemer HC, et al.: Effect of psychosocial treatment on survival of patients with metastatic breast cancer. *Lancet* 1989; ii:888–891.

SUPPORT Principal Investigators: A controlled trial to improve care for seriously ill hospitalized patients: The study to understand prognoses and preferences for outcomes and risks for treatments (SUPPORT). *J Am Med Assoc* 1995; 274:1591–1598.

World Health Organization: *Cancer Pain Relief and Palliative Care: Report of a WHO Expert Committee*. Geneva: WHO, 1990.

Chapter 73

Organ Transplantation

JOHN K. FINDLEY AND OWEN S. SURMAN

I. Overview

With the advancement of immunosuppressant therapy and the refinement of organ procurement techniques, transplant recipients are living longer. In addition, the types of organs available for transplantation have drastically increased. **This growth in organ transplants has required a teamwork approach to evaluate potential candidates and to provide a comprehensive continuum of care.**

II. Recipient Selection

A. **Ethical Considerations**
   The process by which patients are selected to receive a transplanted organ has been the topic of continuous debate since the first successful kidney transplant (by Murray in 1954) between monozygotic twins achieved excellent long-term function. Since then, three precepts have served as a template to determine which patients should receive a transplant:
   1. A **rights-oriented position**, which advocates the selection of all patients who wish to be included, once the risks and benefits have been determined.
   2. The **utilitarian-oriented position**, which states that recipient selection should include only those patients for whom there is a social advantage.
   3. A **medical necessity-oriented position**, which selects all patients who can physically benefit from the procedure.

B. **Selection Process**
   Once it has been established that a patient could benefit from receiving a transplanted organ, several criteria must be determined:
   1. **Tissue matching. All patients must have the appropriate ABO blood group compatibility** and be without preformed antibodies against the potential organ. However, kidney recipients also require that there be HLA histocompatibility, principally at the Class II locus.
   2. **Medical urgency.** Although prioritization is given for more critically ill patients, sepsis is a contraindication for all forms of single organ transplantation. However, potential lung transplant recipients, unlike other solid organ recipients, are excluded if they are ventilator-dependent.
   3. **Time spent waiting for a donation.** The time and date are recorded when the patient is placed on the transplant list by the surgeon. Therefore, if two patients had an identical tissue match, priority is given to the patient who had been placed on the list first.
   4. **Pediatric considerations.** Pediatric candidates who are waiting for a kidney transplant are given special priority, because potential growth delays secondary to dialysis treatment are problematic.
   5. **Psychiatric exclusion criteria. Although psychiatric exclusion criteria vary among transplant centers, patients with acute psychosis, or suicidal or homicidal ideation, are almost universally excluded,** if unmanageable. **Active substance abuse, dementia, and intractable noncompliance are also considered contraindications.**
   6. **Substance abuse criteria.** All patients require a negative ethanol and urinary drug screening test (UDS) upon admission.
   7. **Infectious disease.** Human immunodeficiency virus (HIV) and hepatitis B virus (HBV) status are determined when the patient is placed on the transplantation list; positive test results may limit or exclude potential recipients.
   8. **American Disabilities Act.** This Act of Congress requires all patients that could medically benefit from an organ transplant be assessed. Reasonable steps (e.g., psychological counseling) to compensate for coexisting disability must be considered.

C. **Predicting Compliance**
   Patient compliance is often difficult to predict accurately. The clinician must recognize potential indicators for noncompliance (e.g., a history of missed medications and clinical visits, or failure to report important symptomatic changes in a timely manner). Other risk factors include prior medical noncompliance, mood disorders, personality disorders, cognitive deficiency, youth, inadequate social supports, and residence at great distances from the transplant center.

III. Psychiatric Screening

A. **Pretransplant Evaluation**
   1. **Procedural factors.** Candidates who meet inclusion criteria, or appear borderline, are referred to a transplantation center for formal evaluation.

Psychological assessment is customarily performed by the team psychiatrist, or, at some centers, by a trained social worker or psychologist. These evaluations should include a social services review and incorporate additional consultative expertise, if required.

2. **Objectives**
   a. **Define the patient's motivation for, and belief system about, organ transplantation** to address misconceptions and to eliminate false expectations.
   b. **Identify all preoperative psychiatric syndromes,** and evaluate the ability to treat them concurrently with the transplant.
   c. **Determine the availability of social supports,** while assessing the patient's pre-existing character style, coping ability, and ego strength.
   d. **Design a treatment plan** to assure that potentially high-risk patients will prove manageable after transplantation, and inform all patients about preoperative psychiatric treatment requirements or treatment options and their availability.

3. **Identification of risk factors**
   a. **The clinician must determine both past and present medical compliance,** as it is paramount to the prediction of future compliance.
   b. **Recognize all Axis I and Axis II disorders,** since these disorders directly influence patient compliance.
   c. **Document all conditions that may contraindicate organ transplantation,** including active suicidal or homicidal ideation, dementia, substance abuse, advanced mental retardation, or intractable noncompliance.

4. **Assessment of risk factors among former substance abusers.** To determine if a former substance abuser has a high potential for relapse, the clinician must recognize if the patient displays any rationalization or denial of their substance abuse history, has previously refused any recommended treatments, lacks social support for maintaining sobriety, or exhibits signs and symptoms of alcohol-related dementia.

B. **Approach to Psychosocially High-Risk Patients**
   1. **Design a practical treatment plan.**
      a. To manage anxiety or depression, patients should be treated with the appropriate psychopharmacological agents. In addition, group or individualized psychotherapy may be indicated.
      b. The clinician should obtain an addiction services consult for transplant candidates with a history of substance abuse.
      c. Provide continued support for the candidate's family or partner.
      d. Observe and document the patient's response to treatment and progress with medical compliance.
      e. Build rapport and encourage identification with transplant goals by fostering a positive relationship between the patient and the transplant team. This

may be aided by encouraging the patient and the family to attend transplant organizations or groups.

IV. Donor Availability: Types of Organ Transplants

A. **Cadaveric Donor Organs**
   1. **Brain death criteria. Cadaveric transplantation is the principal source of donor organs, which relies on brain death criteria for organ availability.** Brain death criteria are based primarily on the clinical criteria of irreversible brainstem damage, determined by fixed and dilated pupils, absent reflexes, unresponsiveness to external stimuli, and the inability to maintain vital functions (e.g., blood pressure, heartbeat, and respiratory rate) without artificial means. The clinical criteria are usually obtained on two examinations, generally separated by 6-h intervals. Documentation of the clinical criteria (which include failure of an apnea test) by a neurologist or neurosurgeon is mandatory. Ancillary laboratory testing, including an electroencephalogram (EEG) or transcranial Doppler, may be appropriate.
   2. **Geographic considerations.** Individual organs vary in their ischemic tolerance. Donor hearts have the lowest tolerance and require that the transplant occur within 4 h from the time of procurement; they have a limited transport of 500 miles. In contrast, kidneys have the greatest ischemic tolerance, and may be transported transcontinentally; they can tolerate 48 h of hypothermic perfusion.

B. **Asystolic Donor Organs**
   In years past, before the development of brain death criteria, asystolic donor organs were the only source of cadaveric grafts. Since the ischemic tolerance of asystolic donor organs is extremely low, these organs are only occasionally used for renal transplantation.

C. **Living-Donor Organs**
   Due to the scarcity of available organs, but also due, in part, to improved and safer surgical techniques, there has been an increase in living-donor organs. Renal transplant recipients occasionally receive living-donor organs, as do patients who receive livers and lungs. Postoperative pain control for the renal donor is often an issue, as a retroperitoneal incision is generally used when laparoscopic techniques are not utilized.

D. **Living-Unrelated Donor Organs**
   These transplants typically require an established relationship between the donor and the recipient. Determination of donor motivation and a review of the risks and consequences are critical.

V. Ethical and Legal Considerations

A. Organ-Sharing Networks
The United Network for Organ Sharing (UNOS) was incorporated to facilitate organ placement throughout the United States on the basis of histocompatibility. It stresses the importance of autonomy and beneficence as guiding principles, as well as the necessity of ruling out coercion or profit.

B. Potential Benefit to Donor
Those **donors with altruistic motives may experience an increased sense of meaning, while friends and family members may benefit indirectly by reducing the recipient's suffering.**

C. Assent to the Risks
The patient, the donor, and the surgeon must agree to the risks.

VI. Donor Assessment: Routine Considerations

The health and motivation of the donor are determined by the transplant team's medical subspecialist and by the donor's primary care physician (PCP). In particular, all potential candidates are evaluated for HIV, HBV, hepatitis C (HCV) and cytomegalovirus (CMV) status. A potential conflict is obviated by the availability of a medical advocate from the team who is not involved in the care of the intended recipient. Psychiatric referral is indicated when:
1. An unrelated living donor is being considered.
2. A psychiatrically impaired or ambivalent patient is being considered.
3. A donor is undergoing a lobectomy or a partial hepatectomy.

VII. Psychological Care of Living Organ Donors

A. **Rule out coercion, attempt resolution of neurotic conflict, and identify a "black sheep" family status.**

B. **Refer donors with reversible psychiatric syndromes for treatment** and re-evaluate them when treatment is satisfactorily completed.

C. **Provide preoperative donor education,** and evaluate for postoperative pain.

D. **Allow ambivalent donors to be excluded by giving them a thoughtful rationale** of nonparticipation.

VIII. Preoperative Psychiatric Considerations

Preoperative management of transplant patients requires recognition of psychological conditions and syndromes common to this population. Informed consent, teaching, and preoperative psychiatric management are essential to medical compliance and to favorable postoperative outcomes.

A. Psychological Conditions and Issues
1. **End organ failure.** End organ failure may result in progressive morbidity, poor treatment decisions, and compliance, the inability to maintain significant relationships, a loss in family-occupational-social role functioning, or a decrease in intellectual activity.
2. **Coping capacity.** Transplant patients vary in terms of their adaptive skills and their social supports. Some may take refuge in spirituality or religious tradition; others maintain a positive expectation of a medical benefit, or avail themselves of a supportive nuclear family or social network. These skills and traits may be evaluated preoperatively by identifying how a patient coped with a serious illness in the past, and by the stability of present interpersonal relationships.
3. **Guilt and denial.** Guilt and denial may affect the acceptance of medical intervention, the acceptance of a cadaveric or live donor organ, their status on the list versus other potential candidates, or even the acknowledgment of progressive end organ failure.

B. Psychiatric Syndromes
1. **Encephalopathy**
   a. **Hepatic encephalopathy,** secondary to liver failure, results from the inability to clear toxins from the gastrointestinal tract. It may result in the putative formation of false neurotransmitters.
   b. **Uremic encephalopathy,** secondary to end-stage renal failure, may result in significant neuroendocrine effects and seizures. In addition, cytosine activation from dialysis membranes may develop, which can potentiate rejection.
   c. **Cardiopulmonary failure** may induce encephalopathy if it results in changes in the cerebral circulation, and adversely alters arterial blood gases. The risk of delirium is significantly increased when intraortic balloon pump treatment is required.
2. **Adjustment disorders** are common to all forms of end-organ failure; these disorders may affect morbidity, coping style, and social supports.
3. **Depression** is associated with an increased risk of perioperative morbidity. It requires knowledge of premorbid depression and familial diatheses, identification, and treatment.
4. **Anxiety** is often increased in patients with cardiac and pulmonary failure. It may be generalized, phobic, or associated with panic.
5. **Personality disorders** are associated with a history of difficult interpersonal relationships. They often have a detrimental impact on medical compliance.

C. Informed Consent

Informed consent may be a useful teaching vehicle to aid patient autonomy and choice. It may also help shape patient expectations and support the therapeutic alliance, thereby decreasing postoperative pain by presenting the operative experience in a constructive and hopeful fashion. In addition, the patient's informed consent may improve compliance by acquainting the patient with the postoperative requirements and with the potential complications of treatment.

D. Preoperative Psychiatric Intervention

1. **Medical management is essential for encephalopathy.** With hepatic encephalopathy, bleeding due to increased prothrombin and partial prothrombin times must be controlled, while at the same time lactulose treatment must be initiated. If uremic encephalopathy is present, dialysis must be instituted. In particular, one must remember to eliminate or reduce the doses of agents that may add to confusion and agitation.

2. **Psychotherapeutic techniques. A variety of psychotherapeutic techniques may be used to enhance motivation, to support family relations, to reduce guilt and anxiety, and to alleviate stress.** They can alleviate guilt by authenticating the sick role status, or proide behavioral treatment for operative phobias. In addition, psychotherapy may enhance interpersonal skills and coping strategies in patients with a history of personality disorder.

3. **Pharmacotherapeutic agents**

   a. **Anxiolytics. Use of short-acting benzodiazepines helps reduce the potential for accumulation of drugs in patients with hepatic or renal failure.** Oxazepam is readily metabolized by the liver. Therefore, dosing must be determined cautiously to prevent obtundation in a patient with hepatic failure.

   b. **Antidepressants**

      i. **Selective serotonin reuptake inhibitors (SSRIs) and bupropion are well tolerated in patients with end-organ failure, but they should be initiated at low doses.**

      ii. Bupropion and methylphenidate are stimulating; therefore they are often preferable in patients with psychomotor slowing.

      iii. Tricyclic antidepressants (TCAs) are helpful with diabetic neuropathy, and may benefit those with insomnia. Start low and follow blood levels.

      iv. Treatment should be initiated for depression, and continued for those requiring chronic maintenance.

      v. Be aware of drug interactions secondary to suppression of the cytochrome P450 enzyme system.

   c. **Neuroleptics.** Haloperidol is preferred in the management of acute delirium. Maintenance therapy should be continued in patients with psychotic disorders.

   d. **Mood stabilizers**

      i. Administer lithium carbonate at low doses after dialysis with bipolar patients and check levels often. Be aware of the increased risk of toxicity with cyclosporine.

      ii. Substitute valproate for patients with lithium-induced side effects and those who are lithium nonresponders.

      iii. Be aware of cytochrome P450 stimulation with valproate and its potential effects on immunosuppressant regimens.

IX. Postoperative Psychological Considerations

Postoperative care of transplant recipients requires recognition of the special complications of immunosuppressant therapy and the need to support patient compliance.

A. Psychological Conditions

1. **Rebirth phenomena. After organ transplantation, patients often experience a rebirth phenomena as a celebration of the chance for renewed life.** It may be associated with an altruistic identification with other transplant patients.

2. **Body image change.** Body image changes are associated with the relationship to allograft incorporation. In addition, significant bodily changes may result from immunosuppressant therapy. In particular, patients often complain of weight gain, hirsutism, acne, diabetes mellitus, and tremor; each is a common side effect of prednisone therapy.

3. **Medical dependence.** Medical dependence involves relinquishing prior medical supports and making the transition to outpatient care. This is often quite stressful, as transplant patients require extensive follow-up and management of medication levels.

4. **Fear of rejection and failed expectation.** Patients often live in fear of organ rejection. This stress may be significant enough to precipitate a psychiatric disorder that has been in remission.

B. Psychiatric Syndromes

1. **Organic brain syndromes. Organ brain syndromes are most commonly caused by medications and anti-rejection drugs (cyclosporine, prednisone, and FK 506).** However, other medications that may induce an organic brain syndrome include anesthetics, analgesics, antiarrhythmics, antihypertensives, and psychoactive agents. Intraoperative changes in cerebral perfusion or a prolonged requirement for bypass (the risk increases when bypass exceeds 4 h) are also common. Finally, these syndromes may be related to rejection or to end-organ failure, as well as an extended postoperative rehabilitation.

2. **Depression.** Several factors may be implicated as causes of postoperative depression (e.g., medications [steroids], rejection, infection, or chronic pain). One must also consider a recurrence of a premorbid psychiatric syndrome.

3. **Anxiety states.** Enhanced postoperative anxiety may be secondary to use of medications. Direct effects are recognized from prednisone, cyclosporine, and FK 506 (which may induce irritability and tremor). Indirect effects may result from altered function or appearance. Enhanced anxiety may be related to actual or anticipated rejection, separation anxiety from medical dependence, or recurrence of premorbid psychiatric syndrome.

4. **Relapse of addictive behavior.**

5. **Noncompliance.** Risk factors for noncompliance include youth, comorbid psychiatric illness, deficient social support, impaired cognition, and substance abuse.

C. **Postoperative Psychiatric Intervention**

1. **Medical strategies.** It is important to emphasize the therapeutic relation and to pay particular attention to medical complaints and worries. One should not hesitate to reach out to individuals at risk for noncompliance. Recognition and treatment of infection are also crucial.

2. **Psychotherapeutic interventions**

   a. Cognitive-behavioral therapy helps reframe patient reactions to postoperative events and reduces postoperative pain. It also may assist in development of strategies for postoperative compliance, and provide additional treatment for anxiety states.

   b. Traditional therapies help with the treatment of transplant patients postoperatively. Supportive psychotherapy is particularly useful in patients at high risk for noncompliance, while individual therapy may benefit those patients with psychiatric disorders. Family and group therapies also provide additional support.

3. **Psychopharmacologic interventions.** These interventions are similar to those used in preoperative management. However, careful examination of possible drug interactions is critical, as is communication of all medical changes to the surgical team.

Suggested Readings

Beresford TP, Turcotte JG, Merion R, et al.: A rational approach to liver transplantation for the alcoholic patient. *Psychosomatics* 1990; 31:241–245.

Brown TM, Brown PUS: Neuropsychiatric consequences of renal failure. *Psychosomatics* 1995; 36:244–251.

Castelao AM, Sabate JM, Grino S, et al.: Cyclosporine-drug interactions. *Transplant Proc* 1988; 20 (Suppl. 6):66–69.

Colon EA, Popkin MK, Matas A, et al.: Overview of noncompliance in renal transplantation. *Transplant Rev* 1991; 5:175–180.

Hibberd PL, Surman OS, Bass M, et al.: Psychiatric disease and cytomegalovirus viremia in renal transplant recipients. *Psychosomatics* 1995; 36:561–563.

Levenson JL, Olbrish ME: Psychosocial evaluation of organ transplant candidates: a comparative survey or process, criteria and outcomes in heart, liver, and kidney transplantation. *Psychosomatics* 1993; 34:314–323.

Schwartz SI, Shires TG, Spencer FC: *Transplantation. Principles of Surgery*, Vol. 10, 6th ed. New York: McGraw-Hill, 1994:377–454.

Surman OS: Psychiatric aspects of organ transplantation. *Am J Psychiatry* 1989; 146:972–982.

Trzepacz PT, DiMartini A, Tringali R: Psychopharmacologic issues in organ transplantation: II. Psychopharmacologic medications. *Psychosomatics* 1993; 34:290–298.

Chapter 74

Chronic Mental Illness

ALICIA POWELL AND DONALD C. GOFF

I. Introduction

A. Definition
Chronic, severe mental illness is characterized by persistent disabling psychiatric symptoms or by severely impaired function. Frequently, this population is labeled as the severely and persistently mentally ill.

B. Scope of the Problem
1. Several events **in the 1950s, including the development of antipsychotic medications and new commitment laws, led to dramatic changes (i.e., deinstitutionalization) in the treatment of the severely and persistently mentally ill. The 1960s brought the Community Mental Health Center Program as an alternative to state hospitalization, as well as new federal programs (Supplementary Security Income [SSI], Social Security Disability Insurance [SSDI], Medicaid, and Medicare health benefits).** Thousands of formerly hospitalized mentally ill persons were discharged to live in the community. Unfortunately, most communities lacked sufficient resources to provide adequate care for these patients.
2. **The prevalence of mental illness is higher in cities and in lower-class neighborhoods.** This is largely due to the drift of chronically ill patients towards urban environments, where aftercare for formerly institutionalized patients has typically been concentrated. Many chronic psychiatric patients experience homelessness at some time during the course of illness.
3. **Direct and indirect costs associated with schizophrenia in the United States were estimated at $33 billion in 1990; treatment of schizophrenia accounted for almost 3% of all health care expenditures.**

C. Demographics
1. **Between 1955 and 1985 the state hospital resident population decreased by 80%, from 559,000 to 110,000.**
2. **The lifetime prevalence of schizophrenia is 0.85%; the incidence of schizophrenia is about 0.4 per 1,000 population per year.**
3. **Roughly one-third to one-half of homeless persons in the United States suffer from schizophrenia, although such estimates remain controversial.**

II. Assessment of the Chronically Mentally Ill

A. Features of the Interview
1. **Be aware of interpersonal space.** Individuals with chronic mental illness, especially when paranoia is present, may require a larger space to feel safe. Be sure to ask the patient whether he or she is comfortable. Do not hesitate to rearrange the seating if you believe it will help put the patient at ease.
2. **Emphasize and clarify issues of confidentiality.** This reassures most patients, especially paranoid or homeless persons who feel disempowered.
3. **Minimize interruptions,** in treatment situations, if possible. The chronically mentally ill patient appreciates promptness and your undivided attention as much as any higher-functioning patient.

B. Special Considerations in History-Taking
1. The chronically mentally ill patient may have difficulty recalling the experience of symptoms, making it necessary to **obtain history from additional sources.** Ask the patient questions such as, "Who else would remember what you were going through before that hospitalization?" or "Who has seen you at your most depressed?" to elicit the best outside sources.
2. **Don't neglect the medical history;** place special emphasis on a history of head injury and seizures. The severely and persistently mentally ill often neglect their medical problems. Therefore, it is important to ask about the patient's last physical examination, and, if necessary, to obtain a review of systems.
3. **Ask about sexual activity,** especially when interviewing a woman of childbearing age. This is important because many psychotropics are teratogenic. Many of these patients underestimate the risks of sexually transmitted disease.
4. **Substance abuse or dependence frequently coexists with severe mental illness.** It is wise to begin your inquiry with questions about more socially accepted addictive substances (e.g., nicotine and caffeine), and then work your way up to other drugs (e.g., alcohol, marijuana, cocaine, opiates, psychostimulants, hallucinogens, barbiturates, benzodiazepines, and inhalants).

5. **The social history of these patients should include information regarding where the patient sleeps at night, who else resides with the patient, what the educational level of the patient is,** whether he or she has served in the armed forces, and what is the major source of the patient's income. **Asking about their history of violence, both as perpetrator and as a victim, is important** for diagnostic, as well as for safety, reasons.

C. **The Mental Status Examination**

1. During the interview, **make mental notes about the patient's hygiene, attire, speech, attitude, and eye contact, as well as any abnormalities of movement, such as tremor, bradykinesia, or odd mannerisms.** At times you can obtain valuable information by asking the patient questions about the patient's attire—e.g., "How did you choose to wear this unusual piece of clothing today?" Be sure to include any noteworthy features in your presentation of the patient.

2. **Use a gradual, gentle approach when asking about psychotic symptoms.** Some patients are relieved to learn that their symptoms can be understood as a result of an extreme form of normal brain activity. For instance, when asking about visual hallucinations, the interviewer might compare them to the experience of "dreaming while you're awake."

3. Since a key concern of board examiners is to determine the candidate's ability to assess a patient's safety, **one should remember to ask the patient about current thoughts of suicide or homicide, or about command hallucinations, thought control by outside forces, a history of violence, and possession of weapons.** Recent evidence suggests that psychiatric patients are more likely to commit violent acts than are those in the general population, and that the prevalence of schizophrenia in samples of murderers is consistently five to 20 times higher than it is in the general population.

III. Diagnostic Issues

A. **Socioeconomic Factors**
Socioeconomic factors often complicate diagnosis. What may be seen as hypervigilance in some is just plain "street smart" for a homeless patient. Paranoia can be complicated by social isolation, or by a lack of a private space due to homelessness.

B. **Negative Symptoms**
Negative symptoms of schizophrenia include apathy, social isolation, poverty of thought or speech, flattening of affect, and neglect of hygiene. Negative symptoms profoundly impair an individual's ability to function and to engage in treatment; these symptoms can also alienate family members and caregivers. The diagnosis of comorbid depression and/or the presence of medication side effects can also be complicated by negative symptoms.

C. **Comorbid Medical Illness**
Since psychotic symptoms can occur in many medical and psychiatric illnesses, **one should inquire about the onset of symptoms in relation to the use of new medications or substances, physical illness, depression, mania, or flashbacks of traumatic experiences.** Be particularly careful to rule out a medical etiology with any new, sudden onset of psychotic symptoms, or when psychotic symptoms begin after the age of 50 years.

IV. Treatment Strategies

A. **Pharmacologic**
1. General considerations to maximize compliance
   a. When choosing medications for this population, remember that **once a day dosing is most convenient for the patient** and is the schedule usually used by these patients.
   b. **Cost of medication is an important consideration.** Although most patients have medication insurance coverage that requires only a small co-payment for each prescription, even this amount may be a burden for a patient, especially when multiple medications are prescribed and the patient is on a fixed income.
   c. Bear in mind that **certain medication side effects (e.g., diarrhea and frequent urination) are problematic in the patient who has limited access to rest-rooms and laundry facilities;** sedation can compromise a patient's need for self-protective vigilance), is very difficult for homeless persons to tolerate, and can lead to discontinuation of treatment.
   d. **If the resources are available, monitored dosing (supervised dosing at the patient's group residence, or daily dosing at the community mental health clinic) can facilitate compliance.**
   e. In patients taking antipsychotics, **consider using a depot preparation of haloperidol or fluphenazine,** if the patient has no contraindications to using these medications. Depot neuroleptics can also be used to "back up" a daily antipsychotic pill regimen.
2. **The atypical antipsychotic clozapine (Clozaril) has been shown effective in the treatment of the disabling negative symptoms of schizophrenia;** effective treatment often enables patients to reach a higher level of functioning.

B. **Nonpharmacologic**
1. **The severely and persistently mentally ill person may be best cared for by an assertive community treatment team,** also known as a Program for Assertive Community Treatment (PACT), or by a Community/Continuous Treatment Team (CTT).

These programs are based upon a model which provides intensive support for a patient by a community-based team available 24 h a day, 7 days a week. Program staff work long-term with patients, families, and agencies in the community to support patients and to help avert hospitalization. Each patient has an identified staff member who coordinates services. When a patient is hospitalized, the team remains directly involved in treatment planning and in discharge preparations. Randomized clinical trials of such programs demonstrated benefits in clinical status, social functioning, medication compliance, employment, and in quality of life, as well as in reduced rates of hospitalizations when compared to conventional outpatient treatment.

2. **The severely and persistently mentally ill patient being treated in the community is often involved with multiple providers,** including case managers, outreach workers, residential staff, social workers, and primary care physicians. Frequent contact between providers may seem time-consuming, but diligent communication enhances treatment and helps to avoid costly and time-consuming hospital stays or other emergency treatment.

3. **Some communities offer respite or short-term crisis management units** that help divert a patient from a prolonged hospitalization when only a brief crisis intervention is necessary. When possible, one should avoid a prolonged, debilitating, and isolating hospitalization to maintain function and connections in the community.

4. **Day treatment also plays an important role in the treatment of the severely and persistently mentally ill;** they provide structure in a safe setting, opportunities to socialize with others, psycho-educa-tional groups, and at times can coordinate vocational training.

5. **While supportive psychotherapy alone is inadequate treatment for schizophrenia, it can be helpful when combined with medications.** Emphasis should be placed on establishing and maintaining an alliance, fostering compliance with medication and other treatment, helping the patient cope with stressors, and assisting with reality testing.

6. Cognitive-behavioral treatments are understudied in the severely and persistently mentally ill, but **recent work with cognitive approaches demonstrates efficacy in teaching social skills and reality testing.**

7. **Education and support for a patient's family has been shown to significantly improve the course of the illness.**

V. Conclusion

Care of the severely and persistently mentally ill is one of the most difficult and costly of all health-related problems in this country. During the second half of the 20th century, the approach of long-term custodial care in state psychiatric hospitals gave way to community mental health models which improved the quality of life for many patients. The future of care for the chronically mentally ill will increasingly incorporate less costly care delivered by a variety of providers. Recent developments of atypical antipsychotics, that have fewer debilitating side effects should aid this population attain a higher level of function.

Suggested Reading

Goff DC, Gudeman JE: The person with chronic mental illness. In Nicholi Jr AM (ed.): *The Harvard Guide to Psychiatry*. Cambridge, MA: The Belknap Press of Harvard University Press, 1999:684–698.

Chapter 75
Domestic Violence

B.J. BECK

I. Introduction

A. Definition
Domestic violence, as used in this chapter, is synonymous with partner violence, spouse abuse, wife beating, battering, and violence in intimate relationships. Domestic violence is the **intentionally violent or controlling behavior of a currently, or previously, intimate partner of the victim.** The goal of the violence is to **coerce, assert power, and maintain control** over the victim. Examples of coercive or violent behaviors include, but are not limited to, any combination of the following:
1. **Actual or threatened physical injury**
2. **Sexual assault**
3. **Psychological or emotional torment**
4. **Economic control**
5. **Social isolation**

B. Overview
Hardly a new problem, **evidence of domestic violence spans the millennia and is seen in all cultures and segments of society.** The public health implications of this endemic problem include injury, physical and mental disability, death, health care costs, lost wages and productivity, and the long-term effects on children who witness violence. Victims' and health care providers' attitudes toward violence are among the barriers to disclosure and detection—the necessary first steps for intervention. That **victims who leave their batterers are at a 75% greater risk (than those who stay) of being murdered by their batterer** underscores the victim's vulnerability, and the complex nature of successful interventions.

II. Epidemiology

A. Prevalence
In the United States, 3–4 million women a year are abused by a partner, or by a former partner. Domestic violence is repetitive, and escalates over time.
1. **Women are six times more likely than men to be victims of partner violence.**
2. 90% of abusive relationships involve men who abuse their female partners. Some women are violent towards their male partners, frequently in self-defense.
3. 30–50% of all married couples experience some episode of physical violence.
4. **Almost 10% of homicides involve a spouse killing a spouse.**
5. Women are more often assaulted, raped, or murdered by current or former partners, than by strangers.
6. Although less well studied, **same-sex couples appear to have similar rates** of domestic violence as those seen in heterosexual couples.
7. **In the medical setting, abused women account for:**
   a. 22–35% of women who present to an emergency room (ER) for any reason
   b. Up to 40% of women in the ER for non-motor-vehicle trauma
   c. 14–28% of women attending general medical clinics
   d. 16–23% of women in routine prenatal care
   e. Over 50% of the mothers of abused children
8. **In the psychiatric setting, abused women account for:**
   a. 25% of women who present for emergency psychiatric services
   b. 33% of women who attempt suicide
   c. 50% of women in psychiatric outpatient services
   d. 64% of women on psychiatric inpatient units

B. Risk Factors for Victims
Although no socioeconomic, educational, professional, ethnic, racial, or religious affiliation bestows immunity to domestic violence, certain women are at greater risk, including those who:
1. Are single, separated, or divorced.
2. Have recently applied for a restraining order.
3. Are between the ages of 17 and 28 years.
4. Are poor.
5. Abuse alcohol or drugs.
6. Have partners who abuse alcohol or drugs.
7. Are pregnant and have been abused before.
8. Have excessively jealous or possessive partners.

C. Risk Factors for Perpetrators
Despite the heterogeneity of abusers, certain men have an increased risk of violence, including those with:
1. Antisocial personality disorder
2. Depression
3. Youth

531

4. Low income
5. Low educational level

III. Clinical Presentation

A. **Victims of domestic violence** represent a broad spectrum of the population. There is no predisposing, or diagnostic, pre-violence personality structure. **The one thing victims have in common is a violent partner.**
   1. Over time, chronic physical and emotional abuse leads to a sense of worthlessness, shame, and incompetence.
   2. **Victims who present to the health care (or legal) setting may appear passive, dependent, unstable, and "somatic."**
      a. **Social isolation, economic control, and threats** (toward the victim, her children, family, or pets) may **render the victim totally dependent** on her abuser. **This is a consequence of the abuse,** not the cause of it.
      b. Victims of domestic violence **may not look abused**—i.e., they may not initially present with injuries or have physical evidence of abuse. They often **present with behavioral or somatic complaints.**
      c. **Addiction, depression, anxiety, posttraumatic stress, and eating disorders are associated with abuse.**
      d. Domestic violence has also been **associated with intractable abdominal pain, chronic headaches, pelvic pain, and musculoskeletal problems.**

B. **Perpetrators of domestic violence** also come from all walks of life. However, perpetrators may **have certain pre-battering cultural or developmental experiences and personality traits in common.** Once the violence has begun, perpetrators often share similar behavioral patterns.
   1. Perpetrators have often **witnessed or experienced violence in their families of origin.**
   2. Violent men have often been **violent in previous relationships.**
   3. They are often **immature, needy, dependent, nonassertive men with fragile self-esteem and intense feelings of inadequacy.**
   4. **"Insanely jealous" and untrusting,** they cannot tolerate even the least hint of autonomy, and **must dominate or control their partners.**
   5. Many perpetrators **abuse alcohol, or alcohol and drugs.** Though they may attribute their violence to the influence of these substances, victims indicate that **violence is not dependent upon the perpetrator's recent substance use or intoxication.**
   6. **Abusers often minimize or deny the violence; they may blame the victim for provoking the violence.**
   7. **Excessively concerned with outward appearances,** perpetrators are **often socially congenial and able to successfully conceal their violence** from friends and professional contacts.
   8. Abusive men often appear **more credible and intact than their victims, whom they portray as prone to exaggeration and emotional instability.**

IV. The Nature of Violent Relationships

A. **The violence does not start at the beginning of the relationship.**
   1. **A nonassaultive prodrome** may include gradual control over the partner's activities, finances, or family, social, or professional contacts.
   2. **Initial overtures may seem caring and exceptionally considerate** (e.g., dropping the partner off at work and picking her up afterwards; multiple phone calls during the day; offering to support the partner or giving her spending money; accompanying her to health care appointments).
   3. A **pattern of control and dependence** gradually develops.
   4. Often a **major event in the couple's life** (e.g., marriage, pregnancy, or the birth of a child) **precipitates actual violence.**
   5. The couple's **response to the initial episode** of violence may be shock and abhorrence, rationalization, and a firm **belief that it is an isolated incident** never to be repeated.

B. **The cycle of violence is repetitive and often predictable.**
   1. **Violence may involve weapons** (guns, knives, clubs), **shoving, punching, kicking, burning, forced sex, or the forced use of drugs or alcohol.**
   2. **Violence escalates over time,** with increased frequency and severity. It may be **life-threatening. Presence of a firearm greatly increases the risk.**
   3. Because **the motivation is to exert control over the victim, physical abuse is often accompanied by emotional abuse, humiliation, intimidation, threats, or coercion.**
      a. **Emotional abuse** includes putting the victim down (especially in front of others), calling her names, playing mind games or making her think she's crazy, making her feel guilty or bad about herself.
      b. **Humiliation** may involve treating her like a servant, making her beg, forcing her to perform degrading or illegal acts.
      c. **Intimidation** encompasses the use of certain looks or gestures to incite fear, the violent destruction of the victim's property, brandishing weapons, reckless driving, or abuse/torture of pets.
      d. **Threats** of violence, murder, suicide, abandonment, loss of children, or harm to a family member may be terrifying.

e. **Coercion** is used to keep the woman in the relationship, to conceal the abuse, or to drop charges. Perpetrators may threaten the victim with psychiatric commitment, deportation, Welfare or legal actions.

4. **Children may witness parental violence,** or be co-opted by the abuser to relay messages. Victims may be made to feel guilty about their children or to fear losing them. Visitation may be used to further torment the victim.

5. **Violence is often followed by a period of extreme contrition and reconciliation.** The remorseful batterer may bestow gifts and affection on the victim, while vowing never to strike her again. In turn, the victim may feel sorry for her assailant, and guilty for having provoked him. **They may both feel hopeful that "this is the last time."**

6. **Remorse is followed by a tension-building phase which inevitably culminates in another outburst of violence.** The anticipation during the tension-building phase may be so stressful that some women seek to induce the violence to get it over with.

C. **Deterrents to leaving a violent relationship** include the consequences of repeated battering, the dynamics of violent relationships, and the reality of inadequate support systems.

1. **Shame, humiliation, and feelings of worthlessness** keep women in abusive relationships. They are repeatedly told, and may begin to believe, that they get what they deserve, and that they cannot expect anything better.

2. **Fear of real and perceived danger** to herself, her children, family, or friends restricts the victim's ability to leave. Batterers may coerce their partners into staying with just such threats. Fear of being homeless, indigent, and unable to care for their children also keeps women from leaving.

3. **Financial dependence** is calculated to keep women in the control of the abuser. She may have no knowledge of, nor access to, family assets. She may have been prevented from working outside the home. The abuser may even have taken control over any money the victim did have.

4. **Isolation** from family, friends, community supports, health care and legal professionals, and educational opportunities make the abuser the victim's single contact with the outside world. She may feel hopeless to find assistance, or even be believed if she tries to escape.

5. **Intermittent reinforcement of apologies, gifts, and affection** give the victim recurrent hope that things will change. Many **victims do not want to end the relationship; they want to end the abuse.**

6. **Unsuccessful prior attempts** are potent deterrents to future attempts. When women have been blamed, not believed, or not supported by family, police, physicians, or social agencies, they have little incentive to risk the real danger of another attempt to leave.

V. Evaluation

A. **Screening for violence should be a routine part of every psychiatric evaluation, and every general medical assessment.** Many patients will not volunteer information, but will respond to empathic, nonjudgmental questioning.

1. Male and female patients should be asked about *their own* violence, as well as whether anyone else is (or has been) hurting them. A simple question (**"Have you been hit, kicked, punched, or otherwise hurt by someone within the past year? If so, by whom?"**) will identify over 70% of women in violent relationships, as detected by lengthier screening tools (Feldhaus et al., 1997). Patients should also be asked about violence in previous relationships, and sexual assault. **Partner rape is often part of domestic violence.**

a. Patients must be asked these questions alone, in private, confidential settings. **Partners, family members, or friends should never be used as interpreters.**

b. Asking about abuse in the presence of a violent partner not only inhibits the patient from responding truthfully, but puts her at increased risk.

2. There are **multiple barriers to screening and detecting domestic violence.**

a. **Provider factors** include **time constraints, lack of training, inadequate supports** (e.g., security, social services, interpreters), **and lack of suspicion or awareness.** Especially when patients are known socially, are highly educated, professional, or of high socioeconomic status, physicians may be **embarrassed, or feel it insulting, to ask about abuse.** They may feel **helpless to "fix" the situation, or frustrated** by a past experience in which the victim would not leave her batterer. They may simply be uncomfortable thinking or talking about violence.

b. **Patient factors** include the effects of chronic abuse: **shame, fear, worthlessness, hopelessness, depression, anxiety, dissociation, or numbness.** Women may **feel they won't be believed or that they will be blamed.** They may **fear not only increased violence, but destitution** if the batterer leaves them, or is jailed.

c. **Certain groups** (e.g., illegal aliens, those addicted to **illegal drugs) are particularly disenfranchised and may fear legal retaliation.** Victims from **certain cultural or ethnic groups** may feel they will shame not only themselves, but their entire extended families. The **chronically mentally ill or cognitively limited** victim may not know how to talk about battering. **Abused men may be especially ashamed** to admit they are victims; they may also **fear counter-allegations** from their partners. **Gay**

and lesbian victims may not feel safe to divulge their sexual orientation, let alone their abuse, to the health care system.

B. **The medical history** may hold clues to previously unsuspected abuse.

1. **Multiple unscheduled, or ER, visits, multiple traumas, "accidents," or unusual injuries** with unlikely explanations are cause for suspicion of abuse. **Multiple, unexplained, somatic complaints** (headaches, abdominal, pelvic, musculoskeletal pains) should also trigger more careful, confidential questioning. **Alcohol and drug addictions** are common sequelae of abuse.

2. **Patients who disclose current or past abuse** should be asked about the **first episode, the worst episode, and the last episode.** If there are children in the family, the **victim should be asked whether the children have witnessed or experienced violence.** Most states have mandatory reporting requirements for physicians who suspect child abuse or neglect, and patients should be advised of this.

C. **A thorough physical examination** should be performed, and carefully documented, by a knowledgeable and empathic general physician. The medical record may become important legal evidence.

1. Care should be taken to **document any injuries, including signs of sexual trauma,** using diagrams, sketches, or photographs. **A screening neurologic examination** should note any focal findings or suggestions of acute or repeated head trauma.

2. The **mental status exam** should be equally thorough. **Thoughts of suicide, or homicide,** should be asked directly. Signs and symptoms of **anxiety, hypervigilance, autonomic arousal, flashbacks, depression, apathy, dissociation, numbness, and psychosis** should be explored and carefully documented.

D. **The psychiatric differential diagnosis of victims of domestic violence** includes **adjustment disorders** (early on), **depression** (with or without psychotic symptoms), **anxiety disorders** (generalized anxiety, panic, posttraumatic stress), **dissociative disorders** (especially in victims with histories of childhood physical or sexual abuse), **eating disorders, substance-related disorders, and mental disorders due to acute or repeated head trauma.**

1. **Repeatedly traumatized patients may** *appear* **personality disordered** (e.g., paranoid, borderline, avoidant, dependent), but **Axis II diagnoses are not appropriate,** unless the clinician has pre-battering knowledge of the victim's personality structure.

2. **Pre-existing or persistent psychiatric disorders** (e.g., bipolar disorder, schizophrenia) **are predictably**

exacerbated in chaotic, violent living situations. If the abuse is not detected, these patients may be assumed to be nonadherent to their medication or treatment programs. Their medications may be inappropriately adjusted.

VI. Treatment Considerations

A. **The detection of violence is the beginning of treatment.**

1. **Physicians should not gauge their success by when or whether the victim leaves the batterer.** Leaving is a very high-risk proposition and needs to be carefully planned out. The patient needs to know the physician's care is not dependent on her leaving. The victim is the best judge of when she is prepared, and it is safe for her, to leave.

2. **It is not the physician's sole responsibility** to intervene, or "fix," the abusive relationship. They should, however, **know appropriate resources** in their area (e.g., hotlines, shelters, advocacy groups, emergency numbers) and be able to refer the patient as necessary.

3. **It is the physician's responsibility to take the patient seriously, to document carefully, and to assert that:**
   a. **Violence is unacceptable, and criminal.**
   b. **The victim does not deserve to be hurt in any way.**
   c. **The victim did not bring this on herself.**
   d. **It is not the victim's fault; the perpetrator is unequivocally responsible for his actions.**

B. **Risk assessment must rely heavily on the victim's own appraisal of the immediate situation** (e.g., how afraid she is right now, what she believes to be the immediate danger). However, **patients may minimize their concerns** to their doctor, or may not think clearly in this stressful situation. They should be asked about the **presence of guns, escalating frequency or severity of threats or violence, or new violence outside the relationship.**

C. **Developing a safety plan** includes an assessment of the patient's social and financial supports, coping strategies in the past, the outcome of any previous attempts to leave or disrupt the violent pattern, the patient's current level of function at home or work, and the status of children in the home. Details of the plan include mobility, phone and car access, safe destination, and timing. Other safety concerns exist for women who are sexually assaulted in their relationships, including prevention, detection, and/or treatment of sexually transmitted diseases or pregnancy.

D. **Treatment of primary psychiatric disorders should avoid the use of benzodiazepines or sedating medications, if at all possible. Victims should not be further dulled, or impaired, in their ability to**

anticipate, flee, or protect themselves (or their children). Iatrogenic addiction is a real, though lesser, concern.

E. **Mandated reporting** of suspected abuse of children, elders (60 years or older), or the disabled should be carefully considered, and carried out in a manner that does not put the victim at greater risk.

VII. Conclusion

A. Domestic violence is common, under-reported, and life-threatening. It escalates over time, and is motivated by the need to exert control over the victim. Although the victims are predominantly women, domestic violence is a public health problem that cuts across all segments of society. Screening for violence should be part of every general medical or psychiatric evaluation. Victims may not voluntarily disclose their abuse, but will often open up to empathic questioning. The physician who detects abuse need not "solve" the problem, but should reframe the violence as unacceptable, document clearly, and make appropriate referrals. There are many deterrents to the victim leaving her batterer, including increased risk of murder. Victims of domestic violence need to know their physicians will respect their decisions and continue to work with them.

B. **RADAR** (Table 75-1) is an acronym designed to remind physicians to screen, recognize, and treat abuse.

Suggested Readings

Alpert EJ: Violence in intimate relationships and the practicing internist: new "disease" or new agenda? *Ann Intern Med* 1995; 123:774–781.

Brookoff D, O'Brien KK, Cook CS, et al.: Characteristics of participants in domestic violence. *J Am Med Assoc* 1997; 277: 1369–1373.

Bullock L, McFarlane J, Bateman LH, Miller V: The prevalence and characteristics of battered women in a primary care setting. *Nurse Pract* 1989; 14:47–56.

Feldhaus KM, Kaziol-McLain J, Amsbury HL, et al.: Accuracy of 3 brief screening questions for detecting partner violence in the emergency department. *J Am Med Assoc* 1997; 227:1357–1361.

Kaplan HI, Sadock BJ, Grebb JA (eds): *Kaplan and Sadock's*

Table 75-1. Use Your RADAR

RADAR[a]

Remember to ask routinely about partner violence in your own practice.

Ask directly about violence with such questions as "At any time, has a partner hit, kicked, or otherwise hurt or frightened you?" Interview your patient in private at all times.

Document information about "suspected domestic violence" or "partner violence" in the patient's chart.

Assess your patient's safety. Is it safe for her to return home? Find out if any weapons are kept in the house, if the children are in danger, and if the violence is escalating.

Review options with your patient. Know about the types of referral options (e.g., shelters, support groups, legal advocates).

[a]The acronym "RADAR" summarizes action steps physicians should take in recognizing and treating victims of partner violence.

SOURCE: Massachusetts Medical Society Committee on Violence, Alpert EJ (chair), 1996.

Synopsis of Psychiatry: Behavioral Sciences, Clinical Psychiatry, 7th ed. Baltimore: Williams and Wilkins, 1994:793.

Karni K: Detecting and managing domestic violence. *Resident Reporter* 1997; 2:29–34.

Massachusetts Medical Society Committee on Violence, Alpert EJ (chair): *Partner Violence, How to Recognize and Treat Victims of Abuse: A Guide for Physicians and Other Health Care Professionals*, 2nd ed. Waltham, MA: Massachusetts Medical Society, 1996.

Reade J: Approach to domestic violence. In Stern TA, Herman JB, Slaven PL (eds): *The MGH Guide to Psychiatry in Primary Care*. New York: McGraw-Hill, 1998:431–436.

Rodriguez MA, Quiroga SS, Bauer HM: Breaking the silence: battered women's perspectives on medical care. *Arch Fam Med* 1996; 5:153–158.

Sugg NK, Inui T: Primary care physicians' response to domestic violence: opening Pandora's box. *J Am Med Assoc* 1992; 267: 3157–3160.

Chapter 76

Abuse and Neglect

ALI KAZIM

I. Overview

The number of reported cases of abuse and neglect in the United States has gradually increased in both children and the elderly. This reflects not only an increase in the incidence of abuse and neglect but also more reporting of these serious social and public health problems. Since the average life-expectancy has risen, the number of geriatric individuals in the population and their issues have become a major concern for the medical and social services fields.

Various national organizations (including the American Psychiatric Association [APA], the National Center on Child Abuse and Neglect [Washington, DC], and Elder Services) have established guidelines and drafted proposals to detect, to monitor, and to recommend interventions for the prevention and treatment of victims of abuse and neglect. In addition, **every state** in the United States **has statutes governing abuse and neglect of children and the elderly.** Laws have been passed at both federal and state levels that include **mandatory reporting of cases by caregivers** (doctors, nurses, therapists, and social workers), police, and others. Although there is some variability in the personnel who are required to report abuse and neglect within the various states, **every state requires physicians to report suspected abuse and neglect.**

II. Types of Abuse and Neglect

Several types of abuse and neglect exist. These include physical abuse, physical neglect, emotional abuse and neglect (psychological maltreatment), and sexual abuse.

A. **Child Abuse**
1. **Definitions.** As with any major psychiatric issue, there has been a continuing debate on the definitions of abuse and neglect. Two major lobbies involved in this issue are the justice system and the mental health system.
   a. **The Federal Juvenile Justice Standards proposed a standard for child physical abuse** that is much stricter than exists in most statutes; intervention is permitted in this context only if "a child has suffered, or there is a substantial risk that a child will imminently suffer, a physical harm, inflicted non-accidentally upon him/her by his/her parents, which causes or creates a substantial risk of causing disfigurement, impairment of bodily functioning or other serious physical injury."

   b. **The Juvenile Justice Standards** added the following **for physical neglect in children:** "[when] a child has suffered, or there is substantial risk that a child will imminently suffer, a physical harm, inflicted non-accidentally upon him/her by his/her parents, which causes or creates a substantial risk of causing disfigurement, impairment of bodily functioning or other serious physical injury as a result of conditions created by his/her parents or by the failure of the parents to adequately supervise or protect him/her."
   c. **The Juvenile Justice Standards** has not defined sexual abuse in children; the definition of the term used is found in state penal codes.
   d. In 1989 the consensus conference of the **National Institute of Child Health and Human Development recommended that maltreatment** be defined as "behavior towards another person, which (a) is outside the norms of conduct, and (b) entails a substantial risk of causing physical or emotional harm. Behaviors included will consist of actions and omissions, ones that are intentional and ones that are unintentional."
   e. **Physical abuse in children has been defined by the Child Abuse Prevention, Adoption and Family Services Act of 1988** (Public Law 100-294) as "the physical injury of a child under 18 years of age by a person who is responsible for the child's welfare, under circumstances which indicate that the child's health or welfare is harmed or threatened thereby, as determined in accordance with regulations prescribed by the Secretary of Health and Human Services."

B. **Emotional Abuse**
   Emotional abuse has been defined by the Study of the National Incidence and Prevalence of Child Abuse and Neglect (1988) **as:**
1. **Close confinement (tying or binding, and other forms):** restriction of movement or confinement of a child to an enclosed area (such as closet) as a form of punishment.
2. **Verbal or emotional assault:** habitual pattern of belittling, scapegoating, rejecting or being overtly hostile or threatening to beat, sexually assaulting, or abandoning the child.
3. **Other unknown abuse:** being overtly punitive, exploitative, or abusive. This also includes attempts at potential physical or sexual abuse, or the deliberate withholding of food, shelter, sleep or other necessities as a form of punishment.

537

A developmental approach has been applied to emotional abuse of children (Garbarino, 1986) and is viewed as a pattern of psychically destructive behavior inflicted by an adult upon a child. This pattern may take five forms: rejecting, isolating, terrorizing, ignoring, and corrupting.

III. Epidemiology of Child Abuse

A. **Incidence of Child Abuse**
1. **The revised 1988 study of the National Incidence of Child Abuse and Neglect of the National Center on Child Abuse and Neglect of the United States Department of Health and Human Services estimated that more than 1,400,000 children in the United States experience abuse and neglect, and 2,000–4,000 deaths occur annually in the United States caused by child abuse and neglect.**
2. The National Center on Child Abuse and Neglect in Washington, DC, also estimated that in the United States **1 million children are maltreated each year and that 1,200–5,000 children die yearly, as in 1988, as a result of maltreatment** (Sedlak, 1991).
3. **Some 150,000–200,000 new cases of child sexual abuse are reported each year.** The actual number of these cases is likely to be higher, as many abused and neglected children still go unrecognized.
4. **The exact incidence of child abuse is unknown secondary to multiple factors, including reporting bias, cultural influences, and utilization of public or private sources of health.** Straus and Geles (1986) found that the rate of physical abuse towards children and adolescents was 19 per 1,000 in children ages 3–17 years. The 1986 National Incidence and Prevalence Study of the National Center on Child Abuse and Neglect estimated that 22.6 per 1,000 (or 1,424,400) children in the United States were maltreated in the study year (Sedlak, 1991). The majority of these cases (64%) involved neglect. The rate of physical abuse reported in this study was 4.9 per 1,000 (or 311,500) children. Females experienced more overall abuse than did males (Sedlak, 1991).

B. **Age of Onset of Child Abuse**
The severity of abuse varies inversely with the age of the child victim (1986 Child Abuse and Neglect Incidence and Prevalence Study). Most fatalities occur in younger children (United States Department of Health and Human Services, 1988). Daro and Mitchel (1990) reported that more than 50% of fatalities involved children less than 1 year old. While child abuse in prepubertal children occurs most often with single parents, ethnic minorities, and those with low income families, the majority of adolescent children who are abused belong to white families, have two parents in the home, and come from families of average income (United States Department of Health and Human Services, 1981).

Fathers are more often the perpetrators of physical abuse of adolescents, while mothers are more often identified as the perpetrators of physical abuse in prepubertal children (Strauss et al., 1980). Most studies report that abuse of adolescent children begins in their adolescence; however, it also could have started in early childhood and continued into adolescence (Libbey and Bybee, 1979).

C. **Risk Factors for Child Abuse**
1. **Parental factors include** mental illness, substance abuse, being a single parent, having young parental age, and having complicated pregnancies.
2. **Child factors include** low birth weight, difficult temperament of the child, and certain developmental stages (toddler, adolescent).
3. **Social factors include** lack of social supports, poverty, being an ethnic minority, lacking acculturation, having four or more children, being exposed to family violence, and being socially isolated.

IV. Clinical Features of Abuse

A. **Psychopathology of Abused Children**
The following have been found to be more prevalent in children and adolescents who have suffered physical abuse and were referred for treatment: **impulsivity and hyperactivity** (Martin and Beezley, 1977), **depression** (Kaplan, 1986), **having a conduct disorder** (Kaplan et al., 1986), **being learning impaired** (Salinger et al., 1984), and **having substance abuse** (Kaplan, 1986).

Kauffman (1991) found that **18% of maltreated children who were abused and/or neglected met criteria for major depression, and 25% met criteria for dysthymia.** Herjanic and Reich (1982) found that abused children and adolescents were more frequently diagnosed as having depression, alcohol abuse, conduct disorders, and attention deficit disorders than were nonmaltreated children and adolescents.

Kaplan (1986) reported that **abused children of psychiatrically ill parents were more often diagnosed as having a psychiatric disorder than were non-abused children** with a psychiatrically disturbed parent.

B. **Findings on the Physical Examination**
1. **The American Medical Association (AMA, 1992) has dictated that every child suspected of being physically abused or neglected should be given a physi-**

cal examination. The AMA Diagnostic and Treatment Guidelines Concerning Child Abuse and Neglect (1985) state: "Characteristically the injuries are more severe than those that could reasonably be attributed to the claimed cause."

2. **Physical signs of abuse include:**
   a. Bruises and welts on the face, lips, mouth, ears, neck, head, trunk, buttocks, thighs, and/or extremities, that form regular patterns or that resemble the shape of the article used to inflict injury (e.g., hand, teeth, belt, or buckle).
   b. Burns inflicted with cigars or cigarettes, especially on the soles, palms, back, or buttocks; immersion burns (stocking- or glove-like on extremities, doughnut-shaped on buttocks or genitals), or patterned burns resembling an electrical appliance.
   c. Fractures of skull, ribs, nose, facial or long bones, frequently with multiple or spiral fractures in various stages of healing.
   d. Lacerations or abrasions.
   e. Rope burns on wrists, ankles, neck, torso, palate, mouth and gums, lips, ears, or external genitalia.
   f. Bruises of the abdominal wall.
   g. Intramural hematomas or perforation of the intestinal tract.
   h. Ruptured liver, spleen, pancreas, kidney, bladder or blood vessels.
   i. Central nervous system (CNS) injuries, including subdural hematomas (often a result of blunt trauma or violent shaking), retinal hemorrhage, or subarachnoid hemorrhage (secondary to violent shaking).

C. **Self-Mutilation and Suicide**
   Self-mutilation is not uncommon in abused children (Green, 1978). Adolescents who attempt suicide have more often been reported as victims of abuse than non-attempters (Deykin, 1985). Child abuse in families of children who have attempted suicide is frequent (Pfeffer, 1986). Parental suicide attempts are known to be major risk factors for adolescent suicide (Shaffer, 1989).

D. **Psychopathology of Abusive Parents**
   Maltreating parents tend to be depressed and aggressive, to have increased somatic concerns, to exhibit an imbalance in the proportion of negative to positive and aversive control behaviors when interacting with the target child, and to have increased arousal and reactivity to any aversive child stimuli when compared to nonmaltreating parents (Kaplan, 1983; Wolfe, 1985; Bland and Orn, 1986). Significantly more psychopathology has been diagnosed in maltreating parents than in nonmaltreating parents (Kaplan, 1996). Mothers in abusive families have more frequently been diagnosed with depression, while perpetrating fathers are more likely to have alcoholism,

antisocial personality, or labile personalities. Substance abuse is more prevalent in maltreating mothers (Kaplan, 1983).

Abuse during childhood makes it more likely that victims will abuse their own offspring. Approximately one-third of those who have been abused will maltreat their offspring (Kaufman and Zigler, 1987).

V. Child Neglect

A. **Definitions**
   While abuse is considered an act of "commission," neglect is considered an act of "omission" (Giovannoni, 1988). Neglect is perpetrated by caregivers of children who fail to fulfill their caretaker obligations to children. **Neglect occurs in the following three situations:**
   1. A parenting problem.
   2. Social deviance of the caretaker that is secondary to the caretaker problems (e.g., substance abuse, mental retardation, mental illness, criminality), or secondary to other problems.
   3. Associated with the physical or sexual abuse of the child.

   This definition of neglect has been further broken down into the following (Kaplan, 1996):
   a. **Physical neglect:** as evidenced by refusal of health care, delay in health care, abandonment, expulsion, custody issues, inadequate supervision, and other physical neglect.
   b. **Educational neglect:** as evidenced by permitted chronic truancy, failure to enroll/other truancy, and inattention to special educational needs.
   c. **Emotional neglect:** as evidenced by "a parent providing inadequate nurturing/affection, exposing a child to chronic or extreme spousal abuse, permitting a child to abuse drugs or alcohol, permitting other maladaptive behavior, or refusing a child psychological care" (National Center on Child Abuse, 1988).

B. **Incidence of Child Neglect**
   The National Incidence and Prevalence of Child Abuse and Neglect Study (1986) indicated that the incidence of neglect was: physical neglect, 8.1 per 1,000 children; educational neglect, 4.5 per 1,000 children; emotional neglect, 3.2 per 1,000 children.

C. **Physical Examination Findings in Neglect**
   1. **Physical neglect:** malnutrition, repeated pica, constant fatigue, poor hygiene, and clothing inappropriate for weather or setting (AMA, 1985).
   2. **Medical neglect:** lack of appropriate medical care for chronic illness, absence of appropriate immunizations or medications, absence of dental care, absence of prostheses (such as eyeglasses or hear-

ing aid), and discharge from treatment against medical advice.

3. **Emotional neglect:** delays in physical development and failure to thrive (AMA, 1985).

D. Psychopathology of Neglected Child

The effects of neglect are less studied than those of abuse. Physically neglected children at 12 months are more likely than nonneglected children to have insecure attachments (Egeland, 1985). At 42 months they are more likely to show low self-esteem and self-assertion, less flexibility and less control, and to have a difficult time dealing with frustration. They are more dependent and exhibit more internalizing behavior and social isolation. Emotionally neglected children are more likely to show declines on cognitive testing, insecure attachments, avoidance of emotional contact, depression, and aggressive behavior (Egeland, 1985).

Children who witness spousal abuse according to child abuse reporting laws are considered to be victims of emotional neglect by virtue of this exposure. Child witnesses of spousal abuse have been described as having separation anxiety, sleep disturbances, psychosomatic symptoms (Wolfe, 1987), generalized fearfulness and withdrawal from conflict, impaired social competence, and conduct disorders (Wolfe et al., 1986). Witnessing spousal abuse increases the risk for becoming either a spouse abuse perpetrator or a spouse abuse victim (Straus et al., 1980).

E. Psychopathology of Neglectful Parents

Neglectful mothers are less verbally responsive than nonneglectful mothers (Aragona and Eyeberg, 1981). The neglectful mothers use more direct commands, less verbal praise, and are more critical than nonneglectful mothers. Substance abuse, depression, and social isolation of parents are risk factors for child neglect.

F. Treatment of Child Abuse and Neglect

1. **Any treatment directed toward victims of child abuse and neglect must incorporate the parents.** As there is a high risk of child and adolescent abuse and neglect associated with parental psychopathology, treatment programs must address treatment for parental mental illness, including substance abuse, as well as treatment for the abused child or adolescent (Kaplan, 1996). In addition to emotional disturbances in parents, other variables, including vulnerability of the child, family dysfunction, and environmental stress factors (e.g., parental unemployment, and social support systems), need to be addressed.

2. **For a treatment program to be effective, a multidimensional approach that addresses the etiology of family violence is needed.** This should include a complete assessment of parental psychopathology, and the ability to make appropriate interventions for possible risk factors. Interventions typically include individual and couples therapy, family therapy, psychopharmacological treatment, and substance abuse treatment. Families who received family therapy for 13–18 months made the most progress (Daro, 1988) and were least likely to have a relapse of child maltreatment requiring re-reporting.

3. Psychotherapy for parents has two primary components. The first is the provision of intense emotional support and positive models of parenting. The tendency of these parents to make unrealistic demands on their children is dealt with directly by teaching them appropriate developmental expectations and effective nonpunitive child-rearing techniques. The second component is aimed at insight and conflict resolution (Kaplan, 1996).

4. **Out-of-home placement of children, because of abuse, low socioeconomic status, older age of child, greater severity of abuse, and/or victim's school behavioral problem, predicted a poor outcome of social services rehabilitative efforts** and the need for permanent out-of-home placement (Barth et al., 1985–1986).

5. **Abused children are at a high risk for serious behavioral and emotional disorders, as well as learning difficulties.** A complete assessment, including detailed history of development, cognitive functioning, and intellectual abilities, is required. A complete medical and neurological evaluation, possibly with neuropsychological testing, should be incorporated in the assessment. Review of school records and relevant data from ancillary sources is essential. Appropriate referral for learning difficulties and special education may be necessary.

6. **Psychopharmacological management for depression, anxiety, and other related disorders should be incorporated in the treatment plan.** Psychotherapy should be directed, not only at the emotional problems related to abuse, but also at facilitation of emotional development in a manner that will overcome the intergenerational cycle of abuse (Kaplan, 1996).

G. Legal Aspects of Abuse and Neglect

1. **All states mandate professionals in the area of health care, social services, law enforcement, and education to report suspected cases of child abuse and neglect. If a mandated reporter fails in his/her duty to report**

suspected cases of child abuse and neglect, various penalties can be imposed on the individual. These vary from state to state.

2. **Twenty percent of cases of suspected child abuse and neglect are involved in court proceedings** (Besharov, 1971). The purpose of these legal proceedings is to determine if abuse or neglect did take place, and to assess the need for custodial care and family rehabilitation.

3. **The Federal Child Abuse Prevention and Treatment Act of 1974 mandated that states provide children with representation independent of their parents, for those children involved in legal proceedings.** Most states have attorneys who are court-appointed guardians for children (termed "guardian ad litem").

H. Prevention involves:
1. **Competency enhancement** (e.g., parent education).
2. **Prevention of the onset of maltreatment**—e.g., through mass media campaigns, crisis hotlines, and community programs for parents.
3. **Targeting of high-risk groups,** including single, adolescent, low socioeconomic status parents, and high-risk pregnant mothers, as well as provision of family support, visiting nurses, or home-visiting parent aides (Rosenberg and Repucci, 1985).

Chapter 77

Aggression and Violence

Robert W. Irvin and Kathy M. Sanders

I. Introduction

Aggression and violence are complex behaviors which occur both inside and outside the realm of psychiatry. When the criminal justice system is not the responsible managing body, it is often left to the medical community, and more specifically to the mental health community, to contain aggressive individuals. The violent patient poses a serious challenge to the psychiatrist, who needs to rapidly and accurately assess the cause of aggressive behaviors.

Much debate has taken place as to whether or not individuals with mental illness are at greater risk for violent behavior than are those in the general population. Current data suggest that people who suffer from mental illness do commit violent acts more often than do individuals with no psychiatric diagnosis. For this reason, the psychiatrist must be familiar with techniques to adequately assess for the risk of violence.

II. Definition and Classification of Aggression

A. Definition

Aggression has been defined in a variety of ways; for the purposes of this text it shall be defined as: a **behavior that is directed by an organism toward a target, resulting in damage** (Renfrew, 1997).

B. Classification

Violent acts and aggression have biological, environmental, and psychological determinants. Because of this, a **classification system to categorize the types and precipitants of aggressive behaviors** was developed (KE Moyer). This schema includes:

1. **Predatory aggression:** seen in animals against their natural prey, as driven by the need for food.
2. **Inter-male aggression:** aggressive acts which occur between males to establish dominance within a hierarchy.
3. **Fear-induced aggression:** when an individual is confined and cannot escape the environs.
4. **Irritable aggression:** often referred to as anger or rage, it can be provoked by a broad range of stressors (e.g., pain, hunger, or sleep deprivation).
5. **Maternal aggression:** aggression exhibited by a mother when her offspring are threatened.
6. **Sex-related aggression:** aggression which occurs in the context of competition for a potential mate.

III. Assessment of the Violent Patient

A. General Considerations

To insure safety for both the patient and those in their immediate environs, the evaluator must act swiftly to provide accurate diagnosis and acute management.

1. **Safety** is the first priority in the assessment of the violent patient. Control of the patient and of the environment must be obtained to prevent harm to the staff and to the individual being assessed. Without proper safety mechanisms, adequate evaluation is impossible.
2. **Diagnosis** of underlying psychopathology, substance abuse, and/or medical conditions guides specific treatment. If there is no condition amenable to medical or psychiatric interventions, then one must consider that the patient's behavior may be more suitably managed by the legal authorities.
3. **Management,** in the form of chemical sedation, with neuroleptics and/or benzodiazepines, and seclusion and restraint, may be required to allow the evaluator to perform a safe and accurate assessment.

B. Interview of the Potentially Violent Patient

1. **Providing a safe environment**
   a. **All potentially dangerous materials should be removed from the patient and from the interview room.** Objects that can be used as weapons (e.g., pens, needles, tourniquets, and phones) should be scrutinized prior to, and during, the interview.
   b. **The interview room should allow for possible escape and should be highly visible.** The ideal room for such an interview should contain an emergency call button; the room should not be lockable from within.
   c. **Pay careful attention to the patient's behavior for signs of imminent danger. Make note of:**
      i. Verbal threats and/or gestures
      ii. Rapid movements, agitation, or pacing
      iii. Furniture that is knocked over, or doors that are slammed
      iv. Invasion of personal space, clenching of the jaw, or signs of muscular tension
   d. If the interviewer's attempts to redirect the patient fail to decrease the patient's level of agitation, **the use of tranquilization and emergency restraints may be necessary** to regain control and to insure safety.

543

2. **Medical history** must be obtained in the initial phases of the interview process to ascertain and to treat any potentially life-threatening medical causes for the patient's agitation or aggressive behavior. **The mnemonic, WWHHHHIMPS,** adapted from Wise (1987), which stands for Withdrawal from barbiturates, Wernicke's encephalopathy, Hypoxia, and Hypoperfusion of the brain, Hypertensive crisis, Hypoglycemia, Hyper/hypothermia, Intracranial bleed/mass, Meningitis/encephalitis, Poisoning, Status epilepticus, **can be used to help rule out life-threatening causes.**

   a. History of head trauma, neurological or seizure disorder may increase the patient's risk for aggressivity as well as guide treatment.

   b. A history of psychiatric illness and substance abuse will be expanded upon later in the chapter.

3. **A history of violence is the most reliable predictor of future violence;** therefore, it is an integral part of the interview.

   a. **Determine the specifics of past violence.**

      i. At what age did violent acts begin? How frequently did those acts occur? What was the most recent act?

      ii. How severe were the actions?

      iii. Has there been a recurring pattern of escalation preceding violence?

      iv. Have there been common precipitants surrounding the acts?

      v. Have any violent actions resulted in legal recourse, or incarceration?

      vi. Has there been a history of recklessness, suicidality, arrests, or impulsivity?

      vii. Does the patient have a family history of violence, abuse, or gang involvement?

   b. **Screening questions:**

      i. Do you ever think of harming anyone else?

      ii. Have you ever seriously injured another human being?

      iii. Tell me the most violent thing that you have ever done.

   c. **Prior evaluations and treatments related to violent behavior, including medical workups, diagnostic tests, and old records, are indicated.**

   d. **Collect information from as many ancillary sources** as possible, including family members, victims, court records, medical records, and previous treatment providers.

C. Examination of the Violent Patient

1. The **mental status examination** of the potentially violent patient begins like a standard examination. However, as has been previously emphasized, careful consideration must be given to safety. If, at any time during the exam, the examiner feels unsafe, the interview should cease until proper measures can be put in place to **insure safety.**

   a. The initial assessment should focus on elements of the mental status (e.g., the sensorium, disordered thought, mood state, cognition, agitation, hallucinations, and evidence of intoxication by drugs or alcohol). Positive symptoms in any of these areas can increase the likelihood of aggressive action and will alert the physician to medical conditions which require further workup or immediate treatment.

   b. **Affective states,** either mania or depression, can impair a patient's judgment and may lead to violence. The impulsivity accompanied by mania can lead to irrational thoughts and aggression. The hopelessness of a depressed individual, combined with psychotic thought, may lead a patient to attempt suicide or to murder.

   c. **Thought disorders,** psychosis with paranoid features, and command hallucinations make for a combination of symptoms which can produce behavior that is dangerous and difficult to predict.

   d. Just as in the evaluation of the suicidal patient, **a patient with violent thoughts toward others must be assessed in terms of their specific plan, the lethality of the plan,** and the possibility of the plan actually being carried out. Determination of the relative risk of violence in this manner helps in the development of a disposition plan (e.g., inpatient vs. outpatient management).

2. **Physical examination**

   a. **As with any patient that presents for evaluation, history and physical exam are mandatory elements of the assessment.** Because of the increased risk for violence in a patient with an organic brain syndrome and acute intoxication, one should focus on elements of the exam that will help to identify these diagnoses.

   b. Based on physical findings and the suspicion from history, **appropriate diagnostic tests should be performed.** These include:

      i. Routine chemistry, blood counts, and serum and/or urine toxicology

      ii. An organic workup for dementia

      iii. Neuroimaging, electroencephalogram (EEG), and other radiologic tests, as indicated

      iv. Neuropsychological and cognitive behavioral testing

D. Psychiatric Differential Diagnosis

1. **General considerations.** The DSM-IV diagnostic system is multiaxial; each of five domains may contribute to aggressive or violent behavior. It is important to make an accurate diagnosis because both acute and chronic management of aggressive behaviors hinges on the diagnosis. The following is an approach to the diagnosis of underlying psychiatric disorders which place an individual at risk for aggression.

   a. **Diagnoses on Axis I**

      i. **Schizophrenia/psychosis NOS (not otherwise specified)**

- The prevalence rate for violent behavior in individuals with schizophrenia is similar to that for those with major depression and bipolar disorder; it is five times higher than individuals with no Axis I diagnosis.
- Individuals who are paranoid, with delusions of persecution, may act violently toward the perceived threat.
- Command hallucinations, associated with violent content toward oneself or others, dramatically increase the potential for violence in those with schizophrenia.
- Disorganized thought and behavior may lead to violence.

ii. **Affective illness**

- Unipolar depression may be accompanied by an increase in hostility and anger attacks (nearly half of the time) that can lead to violent behavior.
- Depression with psychotic features may further increase the chances of violence.
- Bipolar patients with a manic, hypomanic, or mixed presentation often display irritability, anger outbursts, omnipotence, and paranoia, which may lead to impulsive aggression.

iii. **Alcohol and substance abuse**

- **Alcohol abuse/dependence** has been associated with a prevalence of violence which is 12 times that of persons with no diagnosis. In an acutely intoxicated state, patients may be disinhibited and at greater risk for violence. During the withdrawal state, delirium and/or agitation may precipitate violence. Chronic alcohol abuse that causes brain damage or dementia may lead to aggressive behaviors that persist beyond the intoxication or withdrawal state.
- **Psychostimulants** (e.g., cocaine and amphetamine), in both the acutely intoxicated and withdrawal states, can lead to agitation, paranoia, psychosis, and violence.
- **Hallucinogens** (e.g., phencyclidine, and lysergic acid diethylamide [LSD]), may precipitate psychosis and violence.
- **Sedative-hypnotics** (e.g., barbiturates or benzodiazepines) cause disinhibition in some; withdrawal may cause delirium.
- States of **opiate intoxication and withdrawal,** as well as behaviors to obtain these drugs, may increase the risk for violence.
- **Other prescription medications** (e.g., anticholinergics and steroids) may induce aggression.

iv. **Intermittent explosive disorder** is a diagnosis that characterizes individuals who have episodes of dyscontrol, assaultive acts, and extreme aggression that is out of proportion to the precipitating event and is not explained by another Axis I or Axis II disorder.

v. **Attention deficit disorder with (ADHD) or without (ADD) hyperactivity** begins in childhood and can persist into adulthood. The impulsivity, inattentiveness, and behavioral problems that accompany this condition may lead to aggressive acts.

b. **Diagnoses on Axis II**

i. **Antisocial personality disorder** is frequently associated with violent behavior. Individuals with this disorder frequently have criminal records and engage in extremely violent and impulsive actions. Further complicating this is the fact that sociopathic individuals frequently have comorbid substance abuse.

ii. Sufferers from **borderline personality disorder** show aggression as part of their impulsive behaviors.

iii. Individuals with **paranoid personality disorder** react to perceived threats with violent reactions toward that perceived threat.

iv. Those with **mental retardation** and other developmental disorders have poor impulse control; depending on the underlying causes (head trauma) of retardation, these states may lead to violence.

c. **Diagnoses on Axis III**

i. **Organic mental disorders**

- **Primary central nervous system (CNS) disorders** can account for aggressive and violent behavior; in particular, attention should be paid toward **seizure disorders.** Seizure-related aggression involves **ictal** aggression (which is nonpurposeful, stereotyped behavior during the seizure), **postictal** aggression (which is secondary to confusion or agitation), and **interictal** aggression (which may result from subthreshold electrical brain activity) that elicits violence.
- Medical disorders affecting the CNS.

d. **Diagnoses on Axes IV and V. The environmental precipitants are as important as are underlying psychiatric or medical diagnoses when determining a patient's level of dangerousness.** The parameters on Axis IV (occupational, social relationship, educational, housing, economic, and legal problems) can lead to aggression and violence. A patient's current level of functioning (as measured on Axis V) will aid the clinician in predicting the threat of violence in a particular patient. **The more stressors one has on Axis IV and the lower the level of functioning on Axis V, the higher the possibility for violence in those prone to act in a violent manner.**

E. Neurobiology of Aggression and Violence

1. **Neuroanatomy**

a. **While there has never been an identifiable "aggression center" in humans,** many animal studies have implicated several regions that may be involved in the hierarchical control of this complicated set of behaviors. Some of these areas are excitatory when stimulated, while others are inhibitory.

b. The **hypothalamus** regulates the neuroendocrine response through output to the pituitary gland and the autonomic nervous system. Within the hypothalamus, the anterior, lateral, ventromedial, and dorsomedial nuclei are often described as key areas in animal aggression, and are postulated to be involved in the control of this behavior in humans.

c. The **limbic system,** including the amygdala, hippocampus, septum, cingulate, and fornix, has regulatory control of aggressive behaviors in man and animals.

d. The **prefrontal cortex** modulates input from both the limbic system and the hypothalamus; it may have a role in the social context and judgmental aspects of aggression.

2. **Neurochemistry**

a. **Low central serotonin** (5HT) function has been correlated with impulsive aggression. Violent patients have been found to have a low turnover of 5HT as measured by its major metabolite 5HIAA (5-hydroxyindoleacetic acid) in the cerebrospinal fluid (CSF).

b. **Acetylcholine** in the limbic system of animals stimulates aggression; cholinergic pesticides have been cited as provoking violence in humans.

c. γ-**Aminobutyric acid** (GABA) is thought to have inhibitory effects on aggression in both humans and animals.

d. **Norepinephrine** may enhance some types of aggression in animals and could play a role in impulsivity and episodic violence in humans.

e. **Dopamine** increases aggressive behavior in animal models, but its effect in humans is less clear due to its psychotomimetic effects.

3. **Genetics**

a. **There has been no specific chromosomal abnormality associated with an increased risk for aggression; however, tryptophan hydroxylase polymorphisms may be correlated with impulsive aggression.**

b. There has been a questionable relationship between XYY and impulsivity; it remains inconclusive.

4. **Hormonal influences**

a. **Androgens** are often cited as a major factor in aggressive behavior as they may play an organizational role in the development of these behaviors.

b. Some attribute a lower threshold for violence in women during times when **estrogen and progesterone levels fall during the menstrual cycle.**

F. Approach to the Treatment of the Violent Patient

1. Management of the aggressive patient can be divided into **acute management** and **chronic management.** There are no medications targeted specifically at aggressive behavior; the psychiatrist must use some general principles to guide treatment. One should attempt to optimize treatment of the underlying psychiatric illness if present; if that fails it is best to use the most benign treatments in an empirical and systematic way. It is important to assess efficacy by defining parameters that can be observed and measured as a means to determine treatment outcome.

2. In the **acute setting** the goal in treatment of the violent patient should be to reduce the risk of harm to the staff and the patient and to facilitate the diagnostic process. Medications which can be delivered intramuscularly, and have a rapid onset and a favorable side effect profile should be first-line treatments. When the patient is calm and a more thorough assessment can be achieved, one can decide between outpatient management or voluntary vs. involuntary hospitalization.

a. **Benzodiazepines,** given in intramuscular or oral form, can be effective sedatives in the acute care setting.

   i. Alprazolam acts rapidly, but it can only be administered in oral form. The initial dose is generally 0.5 mg and should not in general exceed 4 mg.

   ii. Diazepam (with an initial dose of 5 mg) has a rapid onset of action, can be administered intramuscularly, orally, and intravenously, and has a long half-life. Because of its long half-life (30–100 h), it should be used cautiously in the geriatric population.

   iii. Lorazepam may be given sublingually, orally, intramuscularly, or intravenously. The usual starting dose is 1 mg, and its moderate half-life (10–20 h) makes it an ideal medication for initial treatment.

b. **Antipsychotics,** particularly high-potency agents, are often effective in reducing agitation and associated violence in both the psychotic and nonpsychotic patient.

   i. Haloperidol, a high-potency neuroleptic, is frequently used in this setting because of its side effect profile and safety with regard to its cardiopulmonary side effects. It may be given orally, intramuscularly, or intravenously, and is usually effective in one or two doses of 5 mg IM or IV. Given intravenously, it is less likely to precipitate extrapyramidal side effects; however, regardless of route, one must attend to the risk of *torsades de pointes.*

   ii. Virtually any neuroleptic may diminish aggressivity, but careful consideration should be given to the potency, history of response, side effect profile of the particular medication, and the psychiatric and medical history of the patient.

3. The **long-term management** of the violent patient poses a more complex task to the treating psychiatrist. One should first maximally and appropriately treat any underlying psychiatric disorder using both psychotherapy and pharmacotherapy. Once this has been achieved there are a variety of medications that have been used as ancillary approaches to target specific symptoms.

a. **Atypical antipsychotics** (e.g., clozapine, olanzapine, and risperidone) have been used more in recent years.

b. **Selective serotonin reuptake inhibitors** (SSRIs) have been used with some efficacy in personality-disordered patients, those with dementia, and those with mental retardation. One should be cautious when using any antidepressant in patients with bipolar disorder as this may exacerbate, rather than lessen, symptoms.

c. **Lithium** has been used to reduce aggression in patients with mental retardation, conduct disorder, antisocial personality disorder, and in prison inmates. The target lithium level should be between 0.6 and 0.9 mEq/L.

d. **Anticonvulsants** (e.g., carbamazepine, valproic acid, and phenytoin) have been used with some success in reducing impulsive aggression.

e. **Anxiolytics**

   i. Benzodiazepines may be used in chronic, as well as acute, settings.

   ii. Buspirone, a $5HT_{1A}$ partial agonist, is a non-benzodiazepine anxiolytic that has been used as an adjunct treatment for agitation and aggression.

f. **Beta-adrenergic blockers** have been used in high doses to treat aggression; their effects may not be seen for up to several months. All should be started at a low dose and then titrated to effect and tolerance.

   i. Propranolol may be gradually increased up to 1 g/day; it has been used successfully in patients with dementia and organic brain disorders.

   ii. Nadolol (40–120 mg/day) and metoprolol (200–300 mg/day) may also be used in patients who are chronically aggressive.

g. **Psychostimulants** may be effective in reducing impulsive aggression in children with ADD/ADHD and in adults with residual ADHD.

h. **Psychotherapeutic approaches** (e.g., behavioral techniques, cognitive-behavioral therapy, and group and family therapy) have been used to treat aggression and violence.

4. The **combination of medication and psychotherapy** is the best approach to chronic management of aggression and violence.

Suggested Readings

Alpert JE, Spellman MK: Psychotherapeutic approaches to aggressive and violent patients. *Psychiatr Clin North Am* 1997; 20(2): 453–472.

Fava M: Psychopharmacologic treatment of pathologic aggression. *Psychiatr Clin North Am* 1997; 20(2): 427–451.

Kavoussi R, Armstead P, Coccaro E: The neurobiology of impulsive aggression. *Psychiatr Clin North Am* 1997; 20(2):395–403.

Monahan J: Mental disorder and violent behavior: perceptions and evidence. *Am Psychol* 1992; 47(4):511–521.

Renfrew JW: *Aggression and its Causes: A Biopsychosocial Approach*. New York: Oxford University Press, 1997.

Sanders KM: Approach to the violent patient. In Stern TA, Herman JB, Slavin PL (eds): *The MGH Guide to Psychiatry in Primary Care*. New York: McGraw-Hill, 1998:461–469.

Wise MG: Delirium. In Hales RE, Yudofsky SC (eds): *Textbook of Neuropsychiatry*. Washington, DC: American Psychiatric Press, 1987:89–103.

Chapter 78
Culture and Psychiatry

David C. Henderson

I. Introduction

Sex, race, ethnicity, and culture may have a tremendous impact on the diagnosis, treatment, and outcome for many individuals. While it is impossible to understand every culture, **there are basic principles that must be utilized to minimize culture clashes.** Psychiatric training, in theory, prepares physicians to correctly diagnose and to empathetically treat individuals from all over the world. However, in practice, this is far from the truth. While treating a patient from a different culture, **care must be taken when making observations or applying stereotypes. A clinician must be aware at all times of their own feelings, biases, and stereotypes.** Inter-individual variability is common; a particular individual may not fit into the expectations of their culture. One must probe for cultural clues while remaining flexible enough to recognize that the patient's patterns and behaviors do not necessarily match the clinician's expectations.

II. Culture

A. **Definition**
   Culture is a pattern of beliefs, customs, and behaviors which a people acquire socially and transmit from one generation to another through symbols and shared meanings. It provides the tools by which people of a given society adapt to their physical environment, social environment, and to one another. It is an organized group of ready-made solutions to the problems and challenges which a people face.

B. **Levels of Culture**
   1. **Physical.** Culture (including art, literature, architecture, tools and machines, food and clothing, means of transportation) can be directly observed through the five senses and/or through items collected in a museum or recorded on film. The physical level of culture yields more easily to change and to adaptation than does the ideological level.
   2. **Ideological.** There **are aspects** (including the beliefs and values of the people, the reasons for holding some things sacred and others ordinary, the things and events of which they are proud or ashamed, and the sentiments which underlie patriotism or chauvinism) **of culture which must be observed indirectly, usually through the behavior of people.**

Religion, philosophy, psychology, literature, and the meanings which people give to symbols are all part of the ideological aspect of culture. Without some understanding of the ideological aspect of culture, it is difficult to understand the meaning of things at the physical level.

III. DSM-IV Cultural Formulations

A. **Overview**
   The Diagnostic and Statistical Manual, Fourth Edition (DSM-IV), Appendix I, provides an outline for cultural formulations. **The DSM-IV emphasizes that a clinician must take into account an individual's ethnic and cultural context in the evaluation of each of the DSM-IV axes.** This process, called "cultural formulation," contains the following components:
   1. **Cultural identity.** Ethnic or cultural references and the degree to which an individual is involved with their culture of origin and host culture are important. It is crucial to listen for clues and to ask specific questions concerning a patient's cultural identity. For instance, an Asian-American male who grew up in the southern United States may exhibit patterns, behaviors, and views of the world more consistent with a Caucasian southerner. Also, attention to language abilities and preference must be addressed.
   2. **Cultural explanations.** How an individual understands distress or the need for support is often communicated through symptoms (nerves, possessing spirits, somatic complaints, misfortune); therefore, the meaning and severity of the illness in relation to one's culture, family, and community should be determined. This "explanatory model" may be helpful when developing an interpretation, a diagnosis, and a treatment plan.
   3. **Psychosocial function.** Cultural factors have a significant impact on the psychosocial environment and on function. Cultural interpretations of social stress, support, and one's level of disability and function must be addressed. It is the physician's responsibility to determine the level of disability, and to help the patient and his or her family adjust to the role changes.

4. **The relationship between the clinician and the patient.** Cultural aspects of the relationship between the individual and the clinician need to be considered. Moreover, cultural differences and their impact on the treatment must not be ignored. Language difficulties, difficulty eliciting symptoms or understanding their cultural significance, negotiating the appropriate relationship, and determining whether a behavior is normal or pathological are common barriers.

B. **Cultural Assessment**

How do cultural considerations specifically influence the diagnosis and treatment? Each society determines its own distinctions regarding which forms of behavior are acceptable or abnormal and which represent a medical problem. The overall cultural assessment related to diagnosis and treatment should be included in the formulation. In the oral board examination, presentations are generally opened with identifying data (e.g., Mr. A, a 34-year-old, married, African-American male, ...). Presenters must be prepared to discuss the impact of the African-American culture on the diagnosis and on treatment.

IV. Impact of Ethnicity on Psychiatric Diagnosis

A. **Misdiagnosis**

In the United States, race and ethnicity have a significant impact on psychiatric diagnosis and treatment. People of color are frequently misdiagnosed as having schizophrenia when instead they have bipolar disorder or a psychotic depression. Treatment approaches and responses are often quite different based on the diagnosis.

1. African-American patients also receive higher doses of antipsychotics, have higher rates of involuntary psychiatric hospitalizations, and have a significantly higher rate of seclusion-restraint while in psychiatric hospitals.
2. Biases in psychiatric treatment continue and must be acknowledged.
3. Several studies have confirmed the misdiagnosis of schizophrenia in blacks, Hispanics, and the Amish in the United States.

B. **Differences in Presentation of Illness**

Cultural difference in the presentation of psychiatric illnesses exist. For instance, a Cambodian woman may present with complaints of fatigue and back pain, while she ignores other neurovegetative symptoms and is unable to describe dysphoria.

1. Depression may be easily missed by primary care physicians, while a patient may admit to hearing voices of her ancestors, a feature which is culturally appropriate.
2. In many traditional, non-Western societies, spirits of the deceased are regarded as capable of interacting with and possessing those still alive.
3. Cross-culturally, the evaluation of the meanings of bizarre delusions, hallucinations, and psychotic-like symptoms remains a clinical challenge.
4. It is difficult to determine whether symptoms are bizarre enough to yield a diagnosis of schizophrenia without an adequate understanding of a patient's sociocultural and religious background.

V. Acculturation and Immigration

Recent immigrants arrive in the United States with a host of difficulties and psychosocial problems. A physician must ask about and understand the circumstances surrounding their immigration. An individual may have been a political prisoner, a victim of trauma and torture, or have been lost or separated from family members. Under these circumstances the level of depression and posttraumatic stress disorder (PTSD) experienced may be high. Literature on the contribution of acculturative stresses to the emergence of mental disorder is abundant. The impact of acculturation may also lead to symptoms of depression, "culture shock," and even to PTSD-like symptoms.

VI. Culture-Bound Syndromes

A. **Definition**

Culture-bound syndromes have become popular topics for written board examination questions. **A culture-bound syndrome is a collection of signs and symptoms which is restricted to a limited number of cultures by reason of certain psychosocial features.** Culture-bound syndromes are usually restricted to a specific setting and have a special relationship to that setting. Culture-bound syndromes are classified on the basis of common etiology (magic, evil spells, or angry ancestors), so clinical pictures vary.

B. **Projection**

Projection is a common ego defense mechanism in many non-Western cultures. Guilt and shame are often projected into cultural beliefs and ceremonies.

1. **Guilt and shame** are attributed to other individuals, to groups, or to objects, and may involve acting out, blaming others, and needing to punish others.
2. **Projection** is also seen in magic and supernatural perspectives of existence. This leads to projective ceremonies, and may lead to illness when the ceremonies are not performed.

C. Cultural Psychoses

Cultural psychoses are difficult to define. In cultural syndromes, hallucinations may be viewed as normal variants. Delusions and thought disorder must be re-evaluated within a particular cultural setting. A culture may interpret abnormal behavior as relating to some kind of voodoo or anger, and may regard the symptoms as normal even though symptoms are consistent with schizophrenia.

D. Specific Culture-Bound Syndromes

1. **Sleep paralysis (amafufanyane) is a common symp**tom, which occurs in normal people, in patients with narcolepsy, and in psychiatric syndromes caused by witchcraft (as in young females in the Zulu population of southern Africa; it often contains sexual content and symbols). The somatic symptoms include abdominal pains, paralysis, blindness, hysterical seizures, shouting, sobbing, and amnesia (conversion-dissociation).

2. **Sudden mass assault (amok/benz). Amok is the Malayan word meaning "to engage furiously in battle";** the syndrome is seen in Malaysia, Indonesia, Laos, Philippines, Polynesia (called **cafard or cathard**), Papua New Guinea, Puerto Rico (called **mal de pelea**), and among the Navajo **(itch'aa)**. **It is associated with a sudden, unprovoked outburst of wild rage, causing the person to run madly about with a weapon and attack or kill people and animals before being overpowered or committing suicide.** Amok is often preceded by a period of preoccupation, brooding, and mild depression. Afterwards, the person feels exhausted and amnesic. An attack can last for a few hours, and may be precipitated by magical possessions by demons and evil spirits. Shame and loss of face may also play a role.

3. **Ataque de nervios involves symptoms of distress reported among Latinos from the Caribbean;** it is recognized by many Latin-American and Latin-Mediterranean groups. Reported symptoms include uncontrollable shouting, attacks of crying, trembling, a sense of heat in the chest that migrates to the head, and verbal and physical aggression. Ataque de nervios frequently occurs as a result of a direct event, often related to the family; there is often an associated sense of being out of control. The fact that ataques are associated with a specific event and that there is often an absence of acute fear allows it to be distinguished from panic disorder. Many times individuals experience amnesia and then rapidly return to their usual functioning.

4. **Boufée delirante involves sudden outbursts of agitated and aggressive behavior, confusion, and psychomotor agitation in West Africa and Haiti. It**

may also be accompanied by visual and auditory hallucinations.

5. **Genital retraction (koro). Koro is intense anxiety about the retraction of one's genitals, leading to the attachment of devices to prevent such retraction.** Koro occurs in China and Malaysia. It is difficult to differentiate a delusion from a cultural belief system. Epidemic outbreaks of a koro-like syndrome have also occurred in Thailand. Precipitants may include coitus, cold exposure, fears concerning sexual virility, tales of people dying from the illness, and eating spoiled food.

6. **Startle-matching (Latah) is a syndrome that occurs** in Malaysia and Indonesia. Induced as a startle response, it is characterized by echo phenomena (echolalia, echopraxis). Latah is caused by a sudden stimulus that suspends all normal activity. It triggers unusual motor and verbal manifestations, and a person has no voluntary control. **Latah may be mimetic or an echo reaction—a sudden stimulus triggers compulsion to imitate any action or words. Automatic obedience is common (catatonic).**

7. **Latah involves intense fright reactions involving disorganization of the ego and obliteration of ego boundaries.** It may be brief or chronic, and is related to traditional beliefs in possession states or trance states.

8. **Running (piblokto) is arctic hysteria in Eskimos.** Attacks last 1–2 h, during which the patient screams and tears off clothing, throws himself in snow, or runs wildly about on the ice. **Echo phenomena, hysterical seizures, and amnesia are common.** Broodiness and mutism may precede an attack. It is often attributed to evil spirits.

9. **Falling-out or blacking-out involves a sudden collapse, sometimes preceded by dizziness.** It occurs in the southern United States and Caribbean groups. Afflicted individuals have their eyes open, yet they cannot see. They hear and understand what is going on around them yet cannot respond.

10. **Fright illness** (hexing, voodoo, ghost illness). Hexing and voodoo occur in the Western world. **The dominant symptom is a delusion that one is doomed to die because of a voodoo spell.** It produces a variety of somatic symptoms, often with the belief that one is possessed. Voodoo culture is practiced in **Africa, Brazil, and by native West Indians in Haiti.**

11. **Ghost sickness occurs among Kiowa Apache Indians** in the southern plains, and may be triggered by a death. **The afflicted individual feels that the ghost of a dead person is torturing them.** Symptoms include bad dreams, hallucinations, confusion, fear, anxiety, dizziness, weakness, and loss of consciousness.

12. **"Locura" is a term used by Latinos in the United States and Latin America. It refers to a severe chronic psychosis that is attributed to an inherited vulnerability.** Symptoms include incoherence, agitation, auditory and visual hallucinations, poor social interaction, unpredictability, and the potential for violence.

13. **Mal de ojo** is a term meaning **"evil eye."** It is found in Mediterranean cultures and elsewhere. Children are at highest risk. **Symptoms include crying without a reason, sleeping fitfully, vomiting, and having diarrhea.**

14. **Shenjing shuairo or neuroasthenia.** This is **a condition of physical and mental fatigue, dizziness, headaches, pains, poor concentration, sleep difficulties, and memory loss which occurs in China.** Individuals may also experience nausea, vomiting, diarrhea, sexual dysfunction, irritability, and agitation.

15. **Qi-gong psychotic reaction.** This is **an acute, brief episode of dissociative, paranoid, or other psychotic or nonpsychotic symptoms that occurs during the Chinese practice of qi-gong ("exercise of vital energy").**

16. **Taijin kyofusho. A phobia, in Japan, that refers to an individual's intense fear that his/her body parts/function (appearance, odor, movement, facial expressions) displease, embarrass, or are offensive to others.**

17. **Susto (meaning fright or soul loss). Latinos** in the United States, Mexico, Central America, and South America **attribute this syndrome to a frightening event that causes the soul to leave the body.** Symptoms may appear from days to years after the event has occurred. Symptoms include changes in appetite and sleep, sadness, a lack of interest or motivation, headache, pain, and diarrhea.

VII. Ethnicity and Psychopharmacology

Understanding ethnicity and its impact on psychopharmacology and psychobiology is necessary to ensure that quality care is provided for ethnic minorities.

A. **Nonbiological Issues Affecting Psychopharmacology**

1. **Cultural beliefs.** Culturally shaped beliefs play a major role in determining whether an explanation and treatment plan will make sense to a patient (see explanatory models) (e.g., Hispanic or Asians often expect rapid relief with treatment, and are cautious about potential side effects induced by Western medicine). Concerns about addictive and toxic effects of medications often arise. Since Asians are often prescribed multiple herbal substances, they typically feel polypharmacy is more effective.

2. **Traditional and/or alternative methods.** Asians, Hispanics, and African-Americans continue to use herbal medicines. Some herbal medicines interact with psychotropic medications.

   a. **The Japanese herbs, *Swertia japonica* and Kamikihi-To, and Cuban *Datura candida*, have anticholinergic properties** that may interact with tricyclic antidepressants (TCAs) or low-potency neuroleptics.

   b. **South American holly, *Ilex guayusa*, has a high caffeine content.**

   c. **Nigerian root extract of *Schumanniophyton problematicum*** (which is used to treat psychosis) **is sedating** and may interact with neuroleptics and benzodiazepines.

   d. **The Chinese herbs, *Fructose schizandrae*, *Corydalis bungeana*, *Kopsia officinalis*, *Clausena lansium*, *muscone, ginseng*, and *glycyrrhiza*, increase the metabolism of many psychotropics** by stimulation of cytochrome P450 (CYP) enzymes.

   e. **Oleanolic acid in *Swertia mileensis* and *Ligustrum lucidum* also inhibits P450 enzymes.**

   f. **A herbal weight-loss supplement containing *Ephedra sinica* (Ma-Huang),** which is the main plant source of ephedrine, **has been reported to cause mania and psychosis.**

3. **Patient compliance.** Compliance may be affected by incorrect dosing, medication side effects, and polypharmacy. Other factors include a poor therapeutic alliance, and a lack of community support, money, or transportation, as well as substance abuse or a concern about the addictiveness of a medication.

   a. Beliefs held by a patient regarding illness and treatment should be explored.

   b. Communication difficulties and divergence between a patient and his treaters' "explanatory model" play a role in why an ethnic minority patient is significantly more likely to drop out of treatment.

4. **Social support systems** and the way a family interacts have a significant impact on psychiatric treatment. Hispanics have a greater number of interactions with relatives and may become more demoralized when interactions do not occur. Hispanics and Asians typically have a "closed network," which consists of family members, kin, and intimate friends.

5. **Language issues.** The use of interpreters and a patient's understanding of treatment recommendations significantly impact compliance.

6. **Other factors** affect psychopharmacology. Misdiagnosis of a psychiatric condition, a placebo response, mistrust of the health care system, attention-seeking at a later stage of illness, cultural beliefs and expectation, all may affect drug response and compliance. Often, clinicians do not

take the time to explain the reason for the use of medications and their anticipated side effects.

B. Biological Aspects of Psychopharmacology

1. Pharmacokinetics of medications deal with metabolism, blood levels, absorption, distribution, and excretion. However, other pharmacokinetic variables, such as conjugation, plasma protein binding, and oxidation by the CYP isoenzymes exist. **The activity of liver enzymes is controlled genetically,** although environmental factors can alter activity. Understanding how pharmacokinetics and environmental factors relate to different populations will help to predict side effects, blood levels, and potential drug-drug interactions.

   a. **Pharmacokinetics may be influenced by genetics, age, gender, total body weight, environment, diet, toxins, drugs and alcohol, and other disease states.**

   b. **Environmental factors** include medications, drugs, herbal medicines, steroids, sex hormones, caffeine, alcohol, constituents of tobacco, and dietary factors.

2. CYP 2D6 metabolizes many antidepressants, including the tricyclic and heterocyclic antidepressants, and the selective serotonin reuptake inhibitors (SSRIs).

   a. CYP 2D6 also plays a role in metabolizing antipsychotics, including clozapine, haloperidol, perphenazine, risperidone, thioridazine, and sertindole.

   b. The incidence of poor metabolizers at the CYP 2D6 ranges from 3–10% in Caucasians, 0.5–2.4% in Asians, 4.5% in Hispanics, and approximately 1.9% in African-Americans.

   c. Recently a genetic variation of the extensive metabolizer gene that decreases activity at the CYP 2D6 enzymes ("slow metabolizers") was discovered. This group appear to have enzyme activity levels that are intermediate between poor and extensive metabolizers.

   d. Approximately 18% of Mexican-Americans, and 33% of Asians and African-Americans have this gene variation. This may explain ethnic differences in the pharmacokinetics of neuroleptics and antidepressants.

3. The CYP 2C9 isoenzyme is involved in the metabolism of ibuprofen, naproxen, phenytoin, warfarin, and tolbutamide. Approximately 18–22% of Asians and African-Americans are poor metabolizers of these drugs.

4. CYP 2C19 is involved in the metabolism of diazepam, clomipramine, imipramine, and propranolol; it is inhibited by fluoxetine and sertraline. The rates of poor metabolizers of this enzyme are approximately 3–6% in Caucasians, 4–18% in African-Americans and 18–23% in Asians.

C. Clinical Significance

With the above in mind, some observations have been made concerning the use of psychotropics in different ethnic groups. Keep in mind that significant interindividual variations are prevalent.

1. **Asians tend to require lower doses of TCAs, while African-Americans may respond faster to TCAs and at lower doses,** but with a greater risk of neurotoxicity.

2. **Hispanics may respond to lower doses and experience greater side effects,** although the results of studies have been mixed.

3. **Asians experience extrapyramidal symptoms (EPS) at a greater rate,** followed by African-Americans, Hispanics, and Caucasians.

4. **Asians appear to respond to clozapine at lower doses** and to have greater side effects at the lower doses.

5. **Asians appear to be more sensitive to benzodiazepines,** compared with Caucasians.

6. **Asians respond to lower levels of lithium (0.4–0.8 mEq/L),** while **African-Americans appear to have a greater risk of neurotoxicity** (likely related to a slower lithium-sodium pathway and connected to higher rates of hypertension).

VIII. Oral Boards Recommendations

A. When asked in an oral boards examination, "What dose of the medication would you use?," the wisest approach would be to start low and increase slowly as tolerated and clinically indicated.

B. When encountering a patient of color, one must choose carefully and wisely while understanding the potential dangers of assuming every patient should tolerate the same doses of medications.

C. **Every patient must be asked about the use of herbal medicines,** which has increased dramatically in the United States in the past few years. The potential for drug-herbal medicine interactions exists and should be carefully considered. Many herbal medicines have not been well studied; they may induce side effects or interactions with other medications.

D. **Techniques to Minimize Cultural Clashes and Misdiagnosis**

1. If a diagnosis is unclear or impacted by ethnicity or culture, **consider a structured diagnostic interview** (such as the SCID-DSM-IV), to reduce the possibility of misdiagnosis.

2. For a board examination presentation, a reasonable recommendation would be to **interview the patient with a bilingual, bicultural interpreter.**

3. **Be respectful to all patients and address them formally** (i.e., Mr./Ms./Mrs. . . .).

4. **Acknowledge the need to spend more time with a patient from a different culture.** The relationship will be more complex and take longer to develop trust.
5. **Anticipate that the patient may have frustrations from previous experiences in health care systems.**
6. **Confidentiality may be more important** than usual because of shame.
7. **Pay attention to communication:** nonverbal, expressive styles, and use of meaning of words.
8. **Make use of consultants with cultural knowledge.**

Suggested Readings

American Psychiatric Association: *Diagnostic and Statistical Manual of Mental Disorders, Fourth Edition.* Washington, DC: American Psychiatric Association, 1994.

Herrera JM, Lawson WB, Sramek JJ: *Cross Cultural Psychiatry.* New York: Wiley, 1999.

Lin KM, Poland R, Nakasaki G: *Psychopharmacology and Psychobiology of Ethnicity.* Washington, DC: American Psychiatric Press, 1993.

Mezzich JE, Kleinman A, Fabrega H, Parron DL: *Culture and Psychiatric Diagnosis.* Washington, DC: American Psychiatric Press, 1996.

Chapter 79

Approaches to Collaborative Care and Primary Care Psychiatry

B.J. Beck and Edith S. Geringer

I. Overview

A. **Changes in the health care system have greatly increased the need for new and better approaches to the psychiatric care of patients in the general medical setting.** These changes have been driven by the need to contain health care costs and better manage limited resources, and, to a lesser extent, by advances in medication and technology.

1. **The transition from inpatient to outpatient care,** with shorter medical/surgical hospitalizations and more outpatient procedures (e.g., same day surgery), has moved the locus of psychiatric consultation to the outpatient medical clinic. Shorter psychiatric hospitalizations have also moved the care of more seriously ill psychiatric patients to the community.

2. **Changes in reimbursement** from fee-for-service, to prepaid (e.g., health maintenance organization [HMO]), managed, and capitated health care plans have forced a new awareness of the high cost of untreated (or poorly managed) psychiatric morbidity among high utilizers of medical care.

3. **The primary care provider (PCP) gatekeeper system** has evolved to manage the expense of specialty care. This is both a deterrent to the PCP recognition of psychiatric disorders, as well as an incentive for the PCP to initiate treatment for the more common psychiatric problems in the primary care setting.

4. **The move from patient- to population-based care,** necessitated by the need to allocate limited resources, is among the most painful changes, given our individualistic culture. However, this focus on public, rather than individual, health has highlighted the economic burden of psychiatric disability and the potential cost offset of adequate, timely treatment. The presence of a psychiatric disorder correlates with greater (medical) health care utilization, subjective disability, number of missed work days, unemployment, and mortality.

B. **Epidemiology**

1. **Psychiatric problems in the general population** are prevalent, with about 7% of community residents seeking care in a 6-month period. Of those seeking care for full-criteria mental disorders, less than a quarter see a mental health professional. Most seek care in a medical setting, frequently from their PCP.

2. **Psychiatric problems in primary care** populations have a prevalence of 25–35% when structured diagnostic interviews are used for detection. More than three-fourths of these are depressive syndromes; anxiety accounts for most of the rest.

3. **Recognition of psychiatric problems in primary care** can be difficult. Studies in primary care patients with depressive symptoms suggest that PCPs recognize severely depressed patients. However, a third or more of these patients present subsyndromal symptoms (i.e., symptoms that do not reach full DSM-IV criteria for a diagnosable mental disorder). Primary care patients may present earlier in the course of psychiatric illness, and then primarily with physical complaints, which further complicates the clinical detection of psychiatric problems. The clinical significance of the PCPs' failure to diagnose has not been clearly established.

4. **Outcomes** are generally good in less depressed primary care patients, despite shorter courses of less substantial doses of antidepressant medication. Although research in psychiatric specialty clinics supports the more prolonged use of medication at relatively higher doses, some primary care patients respond to less intensive treatment, and improve without use of medications. This may be because some of the depressive symptoms result from adjustment disorders that clear over a relatively brief time, either with the resolution of the initiating event, or the expressed concern, and the placebo effect of a few days of medication, from their PCP.

C. **Barriers to treatment,** however, go beyond mere recognition. Even when patients are screened and PCPs are informed of the results, treatment may not be initiated. PCP, patient, and systems factors collude to inhibit the necessary discussion to promote treatment ("Don't ask/Don't tell").

1. **Physician factors ("Don't ask")** include the **failure to take a social history or do a mental status examination (MSE).** This has been attributed to deficits in medical school and residency curricula, **time and**

productivity pressures, and **personal defenses** (e.g., identification, denial, isolation of affect). PCPs are more comfortable dealing with their patients' physical complaints, and may **fear patients will leave their practice** if asked about mental health issues. Like many of their patients, the PCP **may not believe treatment will help. Insecurity about what to do** (i.e., how, and whether, to treat or refer) is a major deterrent to identifying the problem within the context of a 15-min primary care visit.

2. **Patient factors ("Don't tell")** include the widespread **stigma** against mental health problems. Patients are often ashamed or embarrassed to bring up what they see as a personal weakness. **They may not know** they have a diagnosable, or treatable, mental disorder. In the primary care setting, patients more frequently **present with physical complaints,** which increases the diagnostic complexity: **medical disorders may simulate psychiatric disorders; psychiatric disorders may lead to physical symptoms; psychiatric and medical disorders may coexist.**

3. **Systems factors have evolved with the financial imperatives to contain cost and increase efficiency.** The necessity to **increase productivity (and documentation)** has excessively shortened the "routine visit," now often less than 15 min. **Mental health carve-outs** have either eliminated, or greatly complicated, the possibility of reimbursing PCP treatment of mental disorders. **Prepaid plans,** such as HMOs, significantly decrease incentives to offer anything "extra."

II. The Goals of Collaboration

A. **Improve Access**
   1. **Patients prefer the primary care setting;** they feel more comfortable there than in the less familiar mental health clinic or psychiatric office.
   2. Receiving mental health care in **the primary care setting is less stigmatizing;** even creating a mental health floor or wing in the primary care setting may decrease patient acceptance.
   3. **Without the onus of referral,** PCPs more readily identify mental disorders.
   4. **PCPs are more likely to initiate appropriate treatment** when there is easy access to a known and trusted consultant.

B. **Improve Treatment**
   1. Without ready consultation, **PCPs often prescribe insufficient doses of older medications** (e.g., amitriptyline 25 mg for major depression); they also **prescribe benzodiazepines more frequently than any other class of psychotropic medication,** even for major depression.

2. Collaboration with the psychiatrist can **improve the choice, dose, and management of psychotropic medications.**

C. **Improve Outcomes**
   1. More **seriously depressed primary care patients have been shown to have better outcomes** with PCP-psychiatrist collaboration.
   2. **Cost offset is difficult to demonstrate** because of the many hidden costs of psychiatric disability. However, some studies have shown a **decrease in total health care spending** when mental health problems are adequately addressed.
   3. Care for the patient's psychiatric problem (e.g., depression) can be **more cost-effective** than the same amount of money spent addressing the, often non-responsive, somatic complaints of high utilizing medical patients.

D. **Improve Communication**
   1. **Collaboration implies communication, an end to the "black box" of psychiatry.**
   2. **Patients must be made aware of the collaboration,** and shared communication, between the PCP and psychiatrist.
   3. Communication should be **written and, whenever possible, verbal.**
   4. Communication is **two-way:**
      a. **PCPs provide pertinent information and state the clinical question.**
      b. **Psychiatrists relate findings, diagnosis, and recommendations.**

III. Collaborative Roles, Relationships, and Expectations

A. **The PCP is responsible for the patient's overall care, and must broker and oversee any specialty services.**

B. **The psychiatrist is a consultant to the PCP, and sometimes a co-treater.**

C. **The patient should clearly understand what to expect from the visit with the psychiatrist when the referral is made by the PCP. Likewise, the consultant should clearly state the parameters of the contact at the beginning of the visit (e.g., a one-time consultation, possibility of medication follow-up, possibility of referral for therapy).** If the patient is seen more than once by the psychiatrist, the relationship between the PCP and psychiatrist may need to be re-stated. This **avoids a sense of abandonment** by the PCP (when the patient is referred to the psychiatrist), or by the psychiatrist (when the patient is returned to the PCP for ongoing psychiatric management).

D. **Collaboration does not breach patient confidentiality, because the PCP and psychiatrist are now within**

the circle of care, and the patient is informed of this relationship. If patients ask that particular details not be placed in their general medical record, and these details do not impact directly on their medical care (e.g., history of childhood incest), it is reasonable to respect this wish. The pertinent information (e.g., patient experienced a childhood trauma) can be expressed in more general terms. However, information that does affect medical treatment (e.g., current or past drug addiction), or safety (e.g., suicidal or homicidal intent), cannot be withheld from the PCP, and the patient should be so informed.

E. **Psychiatric or mental health notes in the general medical record should be color-coded, or otherwise flagged,** so they can be removed when records are copied for general medical release of information. Most states require a specific release for mental health or substance abuse treatment records.

IV. Models of Collaboration

A. **The outpatient consultation model** implies collaboration in so far as the patient is referred to the psychiatrist by the PCP, or the PCP presents the patient to the psychiatrist to obtain expert advice or recommendations. Depending on the setting or the system, there may be one, shared, medical record, or providers may maintain separate records and share pertinent information; patients may be seen in either the psychiatric or primary care setting.

1. **Private psychiatrists** may have established referral sources in the primary care sector, but they **generally do not develop truly collaborative relationships,** with ongoing communication or shared records.

2. **Specialty psychiatric clinics** (e.g., eating disorders clinic), generally maintain separate records, require the patient to be seen in the psychiatric clinic, and must develop some means of ongoing, clinically relevant communication with the PCP. Such clinics are most **often located in teaching hospitals or tertiary care centers.** Patients generally need to have well-defined and recognized problems to get referred; **stigma may interfere with patient adherence to such a referral.** A major advantage of such clinics is the **expert, multidisciplinary approach they provide for patients with complex psychiatric and medical problems.**

3. **Consultation psychiatrists** may render a **one-visit opinion,** most often in the primary care clinic. This model is similar to the consultation model used in the inpatient medical setting. The consultation should be written and placed in the primary care record; **immediate verbal communica-**tion, in person, or by phone or voice mail, greatly **enhances the utility of such consultations.** Treatment is usually not initiated by the consultant, but practical recommendations are made. The role of the PCP, and occurrence in the primary care setting, enhances patient participation and decreases stigma. This model also **promotes opportunities for ongoing informal education between PCP and consultant.**

4. **Psychiatric teleconsultation** is a service with **full-time, experienced, consultation psychiatrists available for immediate telephone consultation to PCPs.** This service, which is not accessible to patients, can provide general **psychiatric information, consultation about pharmacologic or behavioral management, or triage and referral functions.** Computer technology is used to maintain a database, promote timely referrals, and generate follow-up letters to the PCPs. There is currently **no direct third-party reimbursement** for the full-time teleconsultants' services, although increased **capitation may provide a funding source as the cost offset of this timely service is realized.**

B. **The psychiatrist is a member of the medical staff of the primary care clinic. Collaboration and shared care are enhanced in this model.** The psychiatrist may (1) **consult** as a member of the medical team, (2) **evaluate and treat patients** in parallel with the PCP, (3) **alternate visits with the PCP** while treatment is initiated, or (4) **evaluate, stabilize, facilitate referrals to outside mental health providers, and return the patient to the PCP with recommendations** for continued care. This proximity between PCP and consultant promotes communication, formal and informal education, and immediate access to curbside consultation. This arrangement can also provide an **excellent training opportunity for both psychiatric and primary care residents.** Patients appreciate being seen in the more familiar primary care setting, and feel less stigmatized.

1. **Consultations,** as above, are written in the regular medical record. The permanency of the psychiatrist **allows for a more finely tuned consultant-PCP relationship.** For instance, with previously established agreement, the consultant may initiate the recommended treatment. The psychiatrist consultant may **offer clinically relevant suggestions during case conferences** or discussions of more complex patients. The **psychiatrist may also see the patient with the PCP during the primary care visit,** capitalizing on the PCP's extensive knowledge of, and long-term relationship with, the patient, to provide more timely treatment recommendations.

2. If the **psychiatrist assumes the ongoing psychiatric care of patients in parallel with the PCP,** some clinics have separate mental health charts. This requires some overt means of communication to keep all providers informed.

  a. **Some primary care clinics incorporate a mental health unit, or clinic;** to the extent that this is an identifiable, special area within the clinic, it is fraught with the same **problems of stigma** that occur when the clinics are truly separate.

  b. **The psychiatric capacity of primary care clinics** that offer these services **is often inadequate to meet the needs of the total patient population.** This can be problematic, and delay access, since most patients would like to be treated in this setting. **Uniform criteria facilitate the triage of patients for in-house treatment or outside referral,** and include such considerations as **diagnosis, available community resources, language requirements, or payment source.**

    i. Insurances with **mental health carve-outs** may not cover psychiatric care in the same setting in which they do cover medical services.

    ii. **Capitation** will favor treating the patient in-house.

    iii. Patients with **indemnity plans** may have more options for outside referrals.

3. In **collaborative management, the patient alternates visits between the psychiatrist and the PCP, in the primary care setting, during initiation of treatment** (the first 4–6 weeks). The PCP assumes responsibility for patient's continued psychopharmacologic treatment. This model was developed as a research protocol for the treatment of depressed, primary care patients.

  a. **Underlying assumptions of collaborative management:**

    i. **PCPs can initiate appropriate treatment** for depression.

    ii. **PCPs can manage the care of patients stabilized** on antidepressant medications.

    iii. **Collaboration begins with PCP education.**

    iv. **PCPs can better care for more seriously depressed patients with the collaboration of in-house psychiatric consultation.**

  b. **PCPs receive prior training,** and participate in regular teaching conferences.

  c. **Patients are referred by the PCP,** usually after an initial trial of medication has not been effective.

  d. A **psychoeducational module for patients** is an integral part of the treatment.

  e. This intensive program of care has been **cost-effective for more severely depressed, primary care patients.**

4. The **primary care-driven model** evolved from the practical necessity to assist PCPs to provide quality psychiatric care for their own primary care patients, with limited psychiatric resources. This model **incorporates elements of consultation, tele-consultation, and collaborative management,** with the goal of maximizing the treatment of appropriate primary care patients, in the primary care setting. **Established criteria are used for triage; the appropriateness of PCP management is the first consideration. Photocopies of all psychiatric notes and evaluations are sent to the PCP,** as well as being placed in the regular medical record. The clinic provides **psychiatric training for both psychiatric and primary care residents.**

  a. **Underlying assumptions of the primary care-driven model:**

    i. **Collaboration begins with education of PCPs *and* psychiatrists.**

    ii. **Patients' psychiatric needs should be met in the primary care setting when consistent with good care.**

    iii. **PCPs can manage the care of patients stabilized on psychiatric medications.**

    iv. **PCPs can initiate appropriate treatment for some psychiatric disorders.**

    v. **PCPs can better care for the psychiatric needs of more patients with the collaboration of in-house psychiatric consultation.**

    vi. **Some patients and some disorders are unlikely to be stable enough for PCP management.**

    vii. **Responsibility for total care requires communication between the PCP and any other involved care provider or consultant.**

  b. **Request for consultation or referral comes from the PCP, in writing.** It includes the clinical question or problem to be addressed and any medication trials initiated by the PCP. **PCPs are also encouraged to call or stop by the psychiatrist's office, located within the primary care clinical area,** for more general information about diagnoses, medications, psychiatric or behavioral management.

  c. **Mental health services include:**

    i. **Formal evaluation, stabilization over several visits, return of the patient to the PCP's care with recommendations** (e.g., how to follow, how long to continue, when to re-refer).

    ii. **Informal consultation without the patient present** (i.e., "curbside").

    iii. **Brief consultation with the patient and the PCP during the patient's appointment with the PCP.**

    iv. **Behavioral treatment planning for difficult to manage patients.**

    v. **Re-evaluation of patients previously seen when there is a change** (e.g., recurrence of symptoms, new problem, medication side effects, change in medical condition or medications that affects psychiatric symptoms or medications).

    vi. **Facilitation of referral to an outside psychiatrist and/or therapist.**

    vii. **Focused, short-term, goal-oriented, individual or group, therapy with master's level clinicians,** located within the primary care clinical areas they serve.

viii. **Collaborative care management for patients with complicated medical, mental health, and/or addiction problems** who utilize services in multiple settings

d. **Patients not recommended for PCP management** include those with inherently unstable conditions, or complicated medication regimens, who require close monitoring, such as patients with:
  i. **Bipolar disorder**
  ii. **Psychotic disorders**
  iii. **Suicidal ideation**
  iv. **Severe personality disorders**
  v. **Primary substance abuse**

e. **The psychiatrist should help the PCP recognize which patients need ongoing specialty care, and assist with appropriate referral.**

f. **Collaborative care management improves the care of patients with complex medical, psychiatric, and addiction problems, that often require treatment which spans several community agencies.**
  i. After a **comprehensive diagnostic and functional assessment,** necessary releases are signed so that the **care manager serves as a liaison between the PCP and all other care providers.**
  ii. **The care manager involves the patient and all treaters in the development of a comprehensive treatment plan, within a network of services, and tracks the patient from site to site throughout this plan.**
  iii. **As a member of the discharge planning team, the care manager ensures that the patient returns to the appropriate network of services** after care in a hospital, detoxification program, or other residential/institutional setting.

C. **The choice of model** for a given clinical setting depends on a number of factors, including the patient population, payor mix, range of available community resources, and the location, type and size of the practice.

1. Patients with higher **educational or socioeconomic status** may feel less stigmatized and be more able, and willing, to seek, and pay for, outside psychiatric services. Some patients feel more comfortable in private practice settings which allow the greatest possible privacy. **Mental health problems are less acceptable, or even shameful, in some cultures,** which favor a more integrated, "invisible," system of care in the primary care setting.

2. **Capitation will most clearly demonstrate the cost offset and cost-effectiveness of in-house, collaborative models and teleconsultation.**

3. **The primary care-driven model requires adequate community resources** to which patients not appropriate for primary care management can be referred. Suburban or rural **areas that lack these resources are better served by parallel, or shared, care models.**

4. **Small groups or solo practitioners may favor consultation models,** either with a very part-time, but regularly scheduled consultant, or with access to an outside consultant, or teleconsultant, as needed. **Large practices, and especially training facilities, will benefit most from the full range of in-house consultative and collaborative services,** including formal education, case conferences, curbside consultation, and collaborative care management.

V. Summary

The merits of collaboration between psychiatrists and PCPs go beyond the mandates of the changing health care system. These models increase access and improve mental health treatment for patients who would be unable, or unlikely, to receive care outside of the primary care setting. Patient, practice, community, and payor factors help determine the best-fit model for a given setting. The continued evolution of the health care system will require ongoing flexibility, on the part of psychiatrists and PCPs, to incorporate the adaptive changes required to keep models of care viable and cost-effective. Medical, psychiatric, and patient education will need to reflect these changes in caregiver roles and expectations.

Suggested Readings

Barrett JE, Barrett JA, Oxman TE, Gerber PD: The prevalence of psychiatric disorders in a primary care practice. *Arch Gen Psychiatry* 1988; 45:1100–1106.

Carr VJ, Faehrmann C, Lewin TJ, et al.: Determining the effect that consultation-liaison psychiatry in primary care has on family physicians' psychiatric knowledge and practice. *Psychosomatics* 1997; 38:217–229.

Coyne JC, Schwenk TL, Fechner-Bates S: Nondetection of depression by primary care physicians reconsidered. *Gen Hosp Psychiatry* 1995; 17:3–12.

Geringer ES: Approach to collaborative treatment by primary care providers and psychiatrists. In Stern TA, Herman JB, Slaven PL (eds): *The MGH Guide to Psychiatry in Primary Care.* New York: McGraw-Hill; 1998:613–619.

Kates N, Craven MA, Crustolo A, et al.: Sharing care: the psychiatrist in the family physician's office. *Can J Psychiatry* 1997; 42: 960–965.

Katon W: Will improving detection of depression in primary care lead to improved depressive outcomes [editorial]? *Gen Hosp Psychiatry* 1995; 17:1–2.

Katon W, Robinson P, Von Korff M, et al.: A multifaceted intervention to improve treatment of depression in primary care. *Arch Gen Psychiatry* 1996; 53:924–932.

Katon W, Von Korff M, Lin E, et al.: Collaborative management to achieve depression treatment guidelines. *J Clin Psychiatry* 1997; 58 (Suppl. 1):20–23.

Katon W, Von Korff M, Lin E, et al.: Population-based care of depression: effective disease management strategies to decrease prevalence. *Gen Hosp Psychiatry* 1997; 19:169–178.

Shapiro S, Skinner EA, Kessler LG, et al.: Utilization of health and mental health services. *Arch Gen Psychiatry* 1984; 41:971–978.

Simon GE: Can depression be managed appropriately in primary care? *J Clin Psychiatry* 1998; 59 (Suppl. 2):3–8.

Simon G, Ormel J, VonKorff M, Barlow W: Health care costs associated with depressive and anxiety disorders in primary care. *Am J Psychiatry* 1995; 152:352–357.

Simon GE, Walker EA: The consult-liaison psychiatrist in the primary care clinic. In Rundell JR, Wise MG (eds): *Textbook of Consultation-Liaison Psychiatry*. Washington, DC: American Psychiatric Press, 1996:946–955.

Sturm R, Wells K: How can treatment for depression become more cost-effective? *J Am Med Assoc* 1995; 273:51–58.

Chapter 80
Community Psychiatry
B.J. BECK

I. Introduction

A. Overview

Community psychiatry, the "third psychiatric revolution," is best understood as a discipline, or sociopolitical system of care, through an appreciation of its undulant, developmental history. Community psychiatry has, at times, been synonymous with public or population-based psychiatry; at other times it has been more disparate. It has embraced the tenets of public health, prevention, and, at times, social activism, rather than the **patient-focused, psychoanalytic treatments of Freud and his followers (the "second psychiatric revolution").** The history of community psychiatry in America is the history of shifting sources and decreased amounts of financial support, the history of public outrage and reform which has alternated with denial and neglect. Likely no other branch of medicine has had to be as continually creative to fulfill its mandate with such ever-shrinking resources.

B. Terms and Definitions

1. **Social psychiatry:** a theoretical field of research that emphasizes the sociocultural features of mental disorder and treatment; the use of psychiatry and psychological variables to predict, explain, and intervene in social problems.

2. **Community psychiatry:** a clinically applied field of social psychiatry whose various definitions reflect the lack of consensus over its boundaries, appropriate emphasis, general principles, and core services. At the very least, community psychiatry involves work with individuals, groups, and systems, and the development of an optimal system of care, for a defined population, with limited resources.

   a. " ... focusing on the **detection, prevention, early treatment, and rehabilitation** of emotional disorders and social deviance as they develop **in the community** rather than as they are encountered at large, centralized psychiatric facilities" (Stedman, 1982).

   b. " ... responsible for the **comprehensive treatment of the severely mentally ill** in the community at large. All aspects of care—from hospitalization, case management, and crisis intervention, to day treatment, and supportive living arrangements—are included ... " (Kaplan et al., 1994).

   c. " ... subspecialty area in which psychiatrists **deliver mental health services to populations** defined by a common workplace, activity, or geographical area of residence" (Borus, 1988).

3. **Community mental health (CMH): a multidisciplinary system of publicly funded, community-based, mental health services, for all** in need of such services, and residing in a geographically defined area, **regardless of ability to pay;** the vision of the **Community Mental Health Center (CMHC)** Acts of 1963 and 1965.

4. **Public psychiatry:** the **government-funded system of inpatient and outpatient mental health services for those unable to access "private sector"** (e.g., fee-for-service, or third-party insurance) services. Initially conceived to meet the needs of all citizens, the domain of public psychiatry has been **progressively narrowed to the needs of those with severe and persistent mental illness.**

   a. **Privatization:** the request for, and acceptance of, **private sector bids to provide public sector services,** with governmental oversight. The move towards privatization may alter the definition of "public" psychiatry.

5. **Population-based psychiatry: a system of care responsible for the mental health needs of all members of a given group,** as defined by such attributes as geography, workplace, or payor/care system (e.g., health maintenance organization). **Responsibility extends to the defined population, as well as to the individual being treated.**

6. **Catchment:** a geographic, CMH service area with a population of 75,000–200,000. (Taken from sanitation engineering, the term refers to the large cistern into which all the sewage of a given geographic area is dumped.)

7. **Public health models of prevention:**

   a. **Primary prevention:** measures taken to **decrease the incidence (new onset)** of a disease or disorder. Application of the **principles of primary prevention (elimination of causative agents, reduction of risk factors, enhancement of host resistance, and disruption of disease transmission)** has successfully eradicated certain infectious diseases, deficiency states, and toxic exposures, and has contributed to the decrease in heart disease and lung disease. In psychiatry, the effects of primary prevention may be harder to prove since that involves an assumption about what

561

would have happened without an intervention. Examples include **anticipatory guidance** (e.g., for parents with young children), **enrichment and competence building** programs (e.g., Head Start or Outward Bound), **social support or self-help** programs for at-risk individuals (e.g., bereavement or cancer support groups), and **early or crisis intervention** after a traumatic event or experience (e.g., on-site counseling for students after the suicide of a classmate).

b. **Secondary prevention:** measures taken to **decrease the prevalence (number of existing cases in a population at a given point in time) of a disease or disorder, through early recognition (case finding) and prompt treatment. The goals of secondary prevention are to shorten the course and minimize or prevent residual disability.** An example in psychiatry would be community education and screening for postpartum depression.

c. **Tertiary prevention: rehabilitative efforts to minimize the prevalence and severity of residual defect and disability** from a disease or disorder.

8. **Deinstitutionalization:** the policy to discharge long-term inpatients, of public psychiatric hospitals, to live and receive services in the community.

9. **Case, or care, management:** a service, usually provided by a social worker or other mental health clinician, to **assure continuity of care, communication between providers, and the patient's successful negotiation of a complex and fragmented system of agencies, care, and services.**

a. The more numerous and complex the patient's needs, the more intensive the care management needs to be.

b. Care managers use **outreach, support, and advocacy** to engage the patient in appropriate treatment. **A member of the treatment planning team, the care manager follows the patient through all levels** (e.g., inpatient, after-care, residential) and types (e.g., mental health, substance abuse, physical health) of care and services/agencies (e.g., housing, welfare, public entitlements).

c. **There is an inverse relationship between the intensity of care management provided and the allowable size of the care manager's caseload.**

10. **Managed care: organized attempts to control a population's health care costs, and possibly quality, through management and monitoring of allocated services to individuals within that population.**

a. **Managed care organizations (MCOs)** contract to provide this management function for public or private insurers of a given population, sometimes with financial incentives to contain costs within a fixed budget, and/or financial penalties when the service budget is exceeded.

b. **Common cost-containment strategies include pretreatment authorization, primary care referral for specialty services, and concurrent review of treatment (utilization management)** to determine ongoing need and effectiveness of treatment.

c. While cost of care is not a new concern for patients or health care providers, the advent of **managed care has intruded the payor's interests into the doctor-patient relationship** in a way that critics feel impinges on the therapeutic process.

11. **Carve-out:** to separate the benefit management of mental health and substance abuse services from the management of other (physical) health care benefits. **Managed behavioral health organizations (MBHOs)** manage the carve-out, mental health, and substance abuse treatment benefits for public and private insurers.

12. **National Committee for Quality Assurance (NCQA):** the largest single **accrediting body for MCOs, which includes standards for MBHOs or for the behavioral health portion of non-carve-out MCOs.**

a. **NCQA standards attempt to successfully address the critical concerns that managed care is too focused on financial constraints, and not on quality of care. These standards** cover such issues as **accessibility** and **availability** of appropriate, culturally sensitive, services, **coordination** between behavioral and physical health care services, and **communication** between all care providers.

b. MCOs and MBHOs are **required to manage both over- and underutilization** of services to assure that patients receive the care they need and are not denied, or discouraged from accessing care.

c. NCQA also requires a **clear grievance process for patients to appeal the MCO's decisions** about their care.

d. At this writing, only seven MBHOs have achieved NCQA accreditation, while many others are striving to meet their rigorous requirements.

13. **Cost-shifting:** the practice of **shifting the locus of care** either for, or with the effect of, **off-loading the cost of the care to another system** or payment source, without necessarily affecting the quality or overall cost of the care.

a. **State to federal.** Shifting patients from state hospitals to communities makes them eligible for federal subsidies and entitlements, which decreases the financial burden on the individual states.

b. **Public to private.** Privatization transfers the risk of escalating mental health costs from states to MCOs.

c. **Mental health to physical health.** When patients do not access the mental health system, but seek general health services (either for their mental health problems directly, or for somatic complaints), the cost of general and emergency medical care increases.

d. **Mental health to corrections.** Substance abusers, persistently mentally ill, dually diagnosed, and other disenfranchised individuals who do not access appropriate CMH services, may receive their only consistent treatment when they are incarcerated for legal transgressions.

14. **Capitation:** a method of contracting for health care provision, for a given population, based on the up-front payment of a set dollar amount, per member, per month.

   a. **Capitation plans have tended to carve out mental health and substance abuse services,** which set the stage for cost-shifting between mental and physical health capitation pools.

   b. Possibly in response to such cost-shifting, single, or **global, cap programs are now encouraging the development of collaborative and coordinated systems of cost-effective care to provide for the total health of patients, and populations.**

II. Historical Background

A. The Age of Enlightenment (*Reform*)

1. **Late 18th century: Phillipe Pinel, a French alienist (psychiatrist), removed the shackles of mental patients** and promoted the notion that fresh air and work would restore mental health. This was the advent of **"moral treatment," the "first psychiatric revolution."**

2. **Early 19th century: The United States government funded institutions for the mentally ill or behaviorally deviant. Dorothea Dix** advocated for the building of state institutions and **village-type asylums** in which the insane could escape the stresses of everyday life.

3. **Late 19th century: Crowding and serious deterioration** of asylums and state institutions made "moral treatment" an impossible challenge.

   a. **The Industrial Revolution championed productivity and organization** over fresh air and "asylum."

   b. By the end of the century, **burgeoning state hospital populations led to regimented, custodial care (*neglect*), and "scientific" somatic therapies,** most of which, with two notable exceptions, were unproven and not beneficial.

      i. **High malarial fevers were found to cure tertiary neurosyphilis,** leading to the deinstitutionalization of many patients with general paresis.

      ii. Freud and his followers found **psychological understanding of patients useful in the treatment of conversion** and possibly other disorders.

B. Early 20th Century Awareness (*Reform*)

1. **The "mental hygiene" movement: Adolph Meyer** wrote about prevention and the social context in which mental illness occurred. This movement was **parallel to the preventive, public health movement of the time,** fueled by industrialization, urbanization, and the need for sanitation and infection control.

   a. **1905: Clifford Beers published** his first-person report of life and conditions inside the mental institution (*A Mind that Found Itself*).

   b. **1909: Beers, along with Meyer and William James, formed the National Association for Mental Health.**

   c. The movement promoted **smaller hospitals, community-based outpatient evaluation, interdisciplinary training, greater affiliation with medical schools and mainstream medicine, and application of psychodynamic principles.**

   d. **Demonstration outpatient mental health clinics,** focused on evaluation, prevention, and differentiation between chronic and acute disorders; they were **less stigmatizing than state institutions.**

2. **The child guidance movement:** a continuation of the mental hygiene movement.

   a. **Applied psychoanalytic theory in childhood** was thought to result in a **decreased incidence of adult mental disorders.**

   b. **The vague goals and unsubstantiated assumptions** led to disappointment and apathy; the theory remained unmeasurable and unproven.

3. **The Great Depression:** shrinking resources, professional in-fighting, long wait lists, and rigid acceptance criteria led to **disillusionment and abandonment of these programs (*neglect*).**

C. Mid 20th Century Military, Legislative, Pharmacologic, and Epidemiologic Influences (*Reform*)

1. **World War II: Military psychiatrists were prompted to lower screening thresholds for acceptance and move the locus of treatment to the field,** when rejected recruits and psychiatric casualties and evacuees outnumbered the available new armed services recruits.

   a. From this experience, and the post-war optimism, came **three central tenets of community psychiatry:**

      i. **Immediacy:** treatment should not be delayed.

      ii. **Proximity:** treatment should occur "on-site," or close to the patient's usual environment to avoid secondary gain or the development of avoidance.

      iii. **Expectancy:** the system of care should foster the expectation that the patient will improve and return to baseline function.

2. **1946: The National Mental Health Act** provided federal funds **for research and mental health training,** and the **establishment of the National Institute of Mental Health (NIMH), in 1949.**

3. **1954: Chlorpromazine was first used in the United States.**

   a. Decreased psychotic symptoms and behavioral problems exposed the **detrimental effects of long-term, institutional living** (e.g., apathy, poor social and self-care skills).

b. **Patients treated at home with chlorpromazine** were found to have better symptomatic, cognitive, and functional outcomes.

4. **1955: At the height of inpatient custodial care (*neglect*), with 550,000 patients in state hospitals,** public outrage (*reform*) was again kindled by a number of expository works on the overcrowded and dehumanizing conditions.

   a. **The 1955 Mental Health Study Act** created the **Joint Commission on Mental Illness and Health,** and funded its **nationwide assessment of available treatment services for the mentally ill.**

   b. **Late 1950s: deinstitutionalization began,** and eventually decreased the number of state hospital beds to about 100,000. Inadequate community services, limited family supports, and patients' poor advocacy, social, and coping skills, led to a **revolving-door policy, with 80% of patients rehospitalized within 2 years.**

   c. **1961: Report and recommendations of the Joint Commission's nationwide assessment: improve the public hospitals.**
      i. **Decrease their size**
      ii. **Increase their resources**
      iii. **Focus funding on the improvement of treatment for patients with psychosis and major mental illness**

5. **Epidemiologic studies indicated that psychiatric symptoms and mental health functional impairment were exceedingly common** in the general, rural, and urban, populations (Stirling County, 1959 [Leighton, 1959]; Midtown Manhattan, 1962 [Strole et al., 1962]). The New Haven study confirmed that **mental health services were the least available to the population (social class) most in need** (Hollingshead and Redlich, 1958).

D. Birth of the American CMH Movement (*Reform*)

1. **1963: President Kennedy delivered the first presidential message concerning mental illness and retardation to Congress.**

   a. Kennedy invited a "bold new approach," **to successfully treat the majority of the mentally ill in their communities,** where they might resume productive roles.

   b. Kennedy opposed enhancement of the existent institutional system of care, and **called for a "new type of health facility," the community mental health center (CMHC).**

2. Weeks before his assassination, Kennedy signed **the CMHC Act.**

   a. **1963: Provided funds to build the CMHCs.**
   b. **1965: Provided funds to staff the CMHCs.**
   c. **Five essential services** were specified:
      i. **Inpatient care**
      ii. **Partial hospitalization**
      iii. **Outpatient services**
      iv. **24-h emergency care**
      v. **Consultation/education**

3. **Late 1960s: State and federal funds began to decrease (*neglect*).**

   a. **Fewer than projected CMHCs** were built: 800 vs. 2000.
   b. Staff funding was often diminished even as a center was under construction.
   c. The public was critical and conflicted about the appropriate **role of community psychiatrists: social activism vs. treatment.**

4. **Late 1970s: The first grant cycle for staff funds was ending.**

   a. The insurance system was not supporting CMH services.
   b. The decreased state hospital capacity flooded communities with severely mentally ill patients.

5. **1975: Congressional Act was passed** to partially refund and revitalize the CMHCs, **prioritize the care of those who most disturbed the community,** and **increase the mandated essential services** to include:

   a. Specialized programs for **children and elderly**
   b. Direct mental health screening services for the **courts**
   c. Follow-up care and transitional housing for **the deinstitutionalized**
   d. Specialized **drug and alcohol** programs

6. **1977: The President's Commission on Mental Health** was established by President Carter to assess the state of the nation's mental health services.

   a. **Recommendations in the 1980 Mental Health Systems Act (*reform*)**
      i. Fund improved care for the **underserved: the old, the young, the seriously mentally ill, and minorities.**
      ii. Build **new CMHCs.**
      iii. **Improve the coordination of total health care** through linkages between mental and physical health care providers.
      iv. **Fund essential, non-revenue-producing services:** consultation, education, coordination of care, CMHC administration.

7. **1979: National Alliance for the Mentally Ill (NAMI),** started by mothers of mentally ill children, began the **rise of the self-help movement in CMH.**

8. **1981: The Reagan Administration repealed the 1980 Mental Health Systems Act before it was implemented (*neglect*)**

   a. **Thus ended 18 years of categorical federal funding for CMH.**
   b. **Block grants** left the individual states to determine how to spend the inadequate funds for substance abuse and mental health services.

E. Late 20th Century

1. **Early 1980s:** Privatization and exemption from the Diagnosis-Related Groups (DRG) legislation promoted the **growth of for-profit private psychiatric and substance abuse hospitals.**

2. **1984:** Results of the **Epidemiologic Catchment Area (ECA) study:**
   a. More epidemiologic evidence of the prevalence of symptoms and mental disorder in the general population.
   b. **The majority of symptomatic community residents never accessed the mental health system,** but sought care in the **general medical system: the "de facto" mental health system** (Regier et al., 1993).
3. Escalating health care costs, the growth of the private psychiatric hospitals, **the lack of treatment guidelines, standards, or criteria for level or type of care** made mental health an easy **target for managed care,** which was on the rise in private and public sectors.
4. **Carve-out financing and management** of public and private mental health services **promoted cost-shifting strategies. This "pass the buck" avoidance** increased the difficulty of vulnerable populations to access needed services, and **increased the disenfranchisement of the poor, homeless, non-English-speaking, uninsured, and deinstitutionalized.**

III. Underlying Principles of CMH

A. **Population Responsibility**
   The CMHC was conceived to be responsible for **all the mental health needs of all the individuals, and the entire catchmented population,** it served, regardless of ability to pay.
   1. **Geographic catchment areas** serve populations of 75,000–200,000 residents.
   2. **No member of the population can be denied service.**
   3. Responsibility requires **planning for the allocation of limited resources** in the development of the best possible system of care to meet the population's needs.
   4. **Services must match the patient's needs** (e.g., groups should be offered when clinically and culturally appropriate, not as a less costly form of treatment).

B. **Prevention**
   Community psychiatry modeled the public health movement's focus on prevention **to decrease incidence, prevalence, and disability of mental illness or disorders.** Most of the limited treatment resources are now utilized for tertiary prevention—i.e., rehabilitative efforts to limit disability in the seriously mentally ill.

C. **Community-Based Care**
   1. **Services are provided in the patient's community (proximity)** to maintain family and social supports, avoid geographic isolation, and promote the patient's functional roles in that community.

   a. Patients with persistent mental illness also **retain better social and self-care skills** when treated in their own communities.
   b. **An array of services** has evolved to treat and to maintain patients safely in the community, rather than in long-term custodial settings.
   2. **Citizen involvement** dates to the **lay-professional partnership** of Beers and Meyer when they formed the National Association for Mental Health (1909). Citizens are invited to be involved in their community's mental health service system. Community boards work with mental health professionals to **set relevant priorities and formulate general policies.** Involved community members are also **powerful political advocates** for the needed resources to keep the system vital.

D. **Continuity of Care**
   CMHCs were to be "closed systems," encompassing all aspects and levels of treatment, and responsible for both direct service and coordination of all required services. Since this **"circle of care" extended across inpatient, residential, and outpatient settings,** the flow of relevant **information was to follow the patient,** and to facilitate clinical communication between involved providers in the various settings. This total responsibility for the patient's care, regardless of setting, would also **prevent cost-shifting strategies** which have plagued the present, discontinuous system.

IV. Components and Services of CMH Systems

A. **Inpatient Care**
   Not to be confused with the custodial care of the past, hospitalization is **still a needed resource reserved for more seriously and acutely ill patients.** More beds now exist in less stigmatizing, general medical and private psychiatric hospitals for **brief, intense evaluation and treatment, and safe containment.** Many inpatient units are "locked," and require the patient to meet commitment standards (e.g., suicidal, homicidal, or unable to care for self on the basis of mental illness), even to be voluntarily admitted. **The development of less restrictive measures, financial constraints, and legal mandates** to protect the civil liberties of the mentally ill, **have made long-term inpatient care all but nonexistent.** For many of the seriously and persistently mentally ill, **multiple, brief admissions (the revolving door)** have replaced extended hospital stays.

B. **Partial Hospitalization**
   Less expensive, and restrictive, than inpatient hospitalization, "partials" provide structure and

hospital-based treatment programs to patients who transition back to their homes in the community at the end of each day. This gradual resumption of community living, with the extra support of the hospital treatment program, is one attempt to avoid, or decrease the length of, inpatient hospitalization, provide less restrictive care, and combat the revolving door, **for patients with stable living arrangements.**

C. **Outpatient Services**

A broad range of services and service modalities permits the effective treatment of more seriously ill patients in the outpatient setting. These may include:
1. **Medication management**
2. **Individual, group, and family therapies**
3. **Psychoeducation, skills training, and self-help groups**
4. **Day treatment programs**
5. **Transitional housing,** half-way houses, and supervised boarding rooms
6. **Specialized children's services**
7. **Specialized services for the elderly**
8. **Alcohol and drug abuse treatment programs**

D. **24-h Emergency Services**

Crisis teams or crisis clinicians in emergency rooms provide prehospital screening, crisis intervention, and immediate access to care.

E. **Community Consultation/Education**

As federal oversight diminished along with funding, these non-revenue-producing activities have also greatly diminished. However, with the advent of the primary care "gatekeeper" system, community-based psychiatrists are being called upon to consult with primary care providers (PCPs). Many primary care patients present with somatic complaints, mood, anxiety, or addiction problems. As **managed care and global capitation encourage PCPs to treat less complicated mental disorders,** they increasingly look to community psychiatrists to assist them with appropriate diagnosis, treatment, or referral.

F. **Case Management**

The less inclusive nature of CMHCs has made case (or care) management essential to track the patient's progress through a potentially fragmented system of services. Care managers remain the liaison between treators, though appropriate releases are now required to permit this important communication.

G. **Homeless Outreach**

The increasing homeless mentally ill population does not access needed mental health services, either because of poor insight, fear, or previous negative experiences. Flexible outreach workers in non-traditional settings (e.g., public parks, shelters) establish credibility in order to bring services to members of this disenfranchised population.

H. **Disaster or Trauma Response**

The lessons from military psychiatry have prompted some agencies to develop immediate response teams for on-site assessment and treatment of disaster victims, to mitigate posttraumatic syndromes and residual disability.

I. **Evaluation and Research**

Federal mandates notwithstanding, **the real impetus towards program evaluation, or "outcomes research," has been the need to contain cost and to identify cost-effectiveness.** True cost-effectiveness research must span the multiple departments, agencies, and services of the population to determine possible cost-offset from one program to another (e.g., improved, but more costly, mental health services, decrease the overall cost by relatively larger decreases in the expense of general medical care, or increased pharmacy or crisis team expense results in greatly decreased inpatient expense). Just as carve-out management of mental health has been accused of cost-shifting, **global capitation will require total systems research to identify cost-offset.**

V. Trends

A. **Disenfranchisement**

Although the pendulum has swung toward maintaining the seriously mentally ill in the community, and prioritizing the CMH dollar for their care, that dollar and the services it buys continue to shrink, while barriers to access increase. This vulnerable population is increasingly over-represented in the addicted, prison, and homeless populations.

B. **Managed Care: The "Fourth Psychiatric Revolution?"**

Initially charged with cost-shifting ("dumping") and fragmentation of services, the incentives in the more progressive MCOs have shifted from purely financial to issues of quality and cost-effectiveness.
1. When most of the initial savings came from decreased inpatient hospitalization, it was clear that earlier discharge was not sufficient to maintain the persistently mentally ill in the community. What was found to be cost-effective, was to develop a **network of closely affiliated services** that spanned the levels of progressively less intensive and restrictive care, with intensive clinical managers to assist patients through these timely transitions and assure communication between (serial and parallel) treators.

2. **These networks bear a conceptual similarity to the vision of the CMHCs of the 1960s,** and have been developed under some of the same mandates and constraints: to provide coordinated continuity of quality care, for a given population, with finite resources.

3. Also like CMHCs, progressive MCOs invite **input and feedback from members of their lay and provider populations** to insure relevant, culturally appropriate programs and user-friendly service.

4. **MCOs have pushed the public and private sectors to develop alternative levels of care** that were not previously available (or no longer available).

5. The MCOs have gone further. Using data to inform policy, they **have set standards for:**
   a. **Treatment planning, monitoring, and recording**
   b. **Timely access to care**
   c. **Coordination of care**
   d. **Communication with PCPs**
   e. **Relating symptoms and level of function to level of care**

C. **Primary Care**
   The "de facto" system is now, *in fact*, the system encouraged by gatekeeper and global capitation systems, **to care for many of the subsyndromal mental health problems in the community population.** As provider groups assume financial risk for total care of populations, there will be a growing need for innovative programs to integrate and coordinate physical and mental health services.

D. **Creative Solutions**
   Community Treatment Teams (CTT), or Assertive Community Treatment (ACT), are an innovative attempt to engage the persistently mentally ill in community treatment by working with them where they live.
   1. Members of these multidisciplinary teams meet patients in their homes, boarding rooms, or shelters to organize flexibly an array of services, which may include medication management, activities of daily living, and social skills training.
   2. By incorporating the patient's usual setting, family or social supports, into the treatment, patients are monitored more closely, and can be offered more intense services when needed.
   3. ACT has kept these seriously mentally ill patients from falling between the cracks, as evidenced by greatly decreased rates of hospitalization. (Conversely, discontinuation of ACT has resulted in sharply increased rates of admission.)
   4. **A criticism of ACT, and other nontraditional programs, is that they do not fit the usual reimbursement structures.** Flexible community-based programs and clinicians will need the support of flexible administrators to straddle systems and agencies, and maintain a vision of the big picture.

VI. Conclusion

Historical accounts of community psychiatry refer to **three "revolutions": moral treatment, psychoanalysis, and CMH.** The implied **definition of revolution is the overthrow of tradition: radical change.** However, closer scrutiny reveals a complex machine with **multiple revolutions of neglect and reform (defined as cycles or rotations: coming full circle),** and two swinging pendulums of public opinion: one between **focus on the "worried well" versus the persistently mentally ill,** the other between **institutional containment vs. community-based treatment.** History suggests **we are currently in the midst of such repetition,** and provides an opportunity to recognize our gains, hold onto lessons learned, and try not to repeat mistakes. **This will not be the last revolution; systems of care will not only need to be dynamic and responsive, but influential, to meet the needs of their populations.**

Suggested Readings

Borus JF: Community psychiatry. In Nicholi AM (ed.): *The New Harvard Guide to Psychiatry*. Cambridge, MA: Harvard University Press, 1988:780–796.

Duckworth K, Borus JF: Population-based psychiatry in the public sector and managed care. In *The Harvard Guide to Psychiatry*, 3rd ed. Cambridge, MA: Harvard University Press, 1999:778–797.

Hollingshead AB, Redlich FC: *Social Class and Mental Illness*. New York: John Wiley, 1958.

Kaplan HI, Sadock BJ, Grebb JA (eds): *Kaplan and Sadock's Synopsis of Psychiatry: Behavioral Sciences, Clinical Psychiatry*, 7th ed. Baltimore: Williams and Wilkins, 1994:201–206.

Leighton A: *My Name is Legion*. New York: Basic Books, 1959.

Regier DA, et al: The de facto U.S. mental and addictive disorders system. *Arch Gen Psychiatry* 1993; 50:85–94.

Rubin B: Community psychiatry: an evolutionary change in medical psychiatry in the United States. *Arch Gen Psychiatry* 1969; 20:497–507.

Stedman's Medical Dictionary, 24th ed. Baltimore: Williams and Wilkins, 1982:1163.

Strole L, et al: *Mental Health in the Metropolis: The Midtown Manhattan Study*. In Rennie TAC (ed.): *Series in Social Psychiatry*, Vol. 1. New York: McGraw-Hill, 1962.

Talbott JA: Has academic psychiatry abandoned the community? *Acad Psychiatry* 1991; 15:106–114.

Thompson KS: Re-inventing progressive community psychiatry: the use of history. *Commun Mental Health J* 1993; 29:495–508.

Chapter 81

Managed Care and Psychiatry

CARL MARCI, GARY GOTTLIEB, MICHAEL S. JELLINEK, AND PAUL SUMMERGRAD

I. Introduction: Changes in Mental Health Insurance

A. Traditional Indemnity Insurance and the Fee-for-Service Era

1. In the 1970s and 1980s, traditional indemnity (i.e., fee-for-service plans) improved coverage for inpatient services and ushered in an era of expansion for general medicine and psychiatry.

2. Physicians were largely responsible for clinical decisions, and had little regard for costs, such as annual and lifetime limits on hospital days; outpatient visits covered expensive tests and costly care.

3. In 1982, TEFRA retained the cost-based reimbursement structure of psychiatric care, which created an incentive for expansion of general hospital services and freestanding psychiatric units (Kubritsky and Hadley, 1998). As the number of hospitals rose along with per diem costs, more and more inpatient facilities became privately owned by for-profit organizations (Oss and Krizsy, 1991).

4. Length of stays were long, in many cases reflecting the extent of the patient's insurance benefits (Summergrad et al., 1995).

B. Introduction of Managed Care

1. In response to rising costs of health care benefits in the 1980s, employers and government officials began to look for new strategies to contain costs.

2. One of the most effective tools involved a movement away from traditional unrestricted indemnity insurance plans to carefully monitored managed care plans (Kuttner, 1999).

3. Managed care shifted control of resources away from physicians, often to for-profit companies. In addition, through selected contracts, managed care companies shifted care to specific network providers.

C. Health Care in the 1990s

1. In the 1990s, managed care (using utilization control of medical and psychiatric services, as well as financial incentives for physicians and hospitals) is oriented towards cutting costs and generating profits for the managed care companies.

2. Case-management, precertification, and on-going utilization review combine to redirect the care of patients away from extended inpatient stays and intensive utilization.

3. For inpatient psychiatry, this has meant a reduction in the length of stay and a shift in the inpatient standard from comprehensive evaluation and treatment to crisis stabilization and rapid discharge (Sederer, 1992).

4. For outpatient psychiatry, this has meant a shift away from long-term dynamic therapies toward an increased reliance on psychopharmacologic agents and brief psychotherapy, often performed by nonphysician providers.

5. The overall result is an excess capacity in some facilities, a downward pressure on prices, and severe cost competition.

D. The Creation of Behavioral Mental Health Carve-Outs

1. In order to protect themselves from the perceived actuarial unpredictability of mental health, insurers subcapitated behavioral health services to secondary carriers. This resulted in a "carving-out" of mental health risk.

2. The separation of mental health services from primary care was a key step in the control of utilization. Managed care companies took control of all referrals, thereby limiting the influence of the primary care provider (PCP).

3. The carve-out of mental health was facilitated by the disproportionate increase in mental health costs relative to general medicine, by the lack of parity between general medical and psychiatric benefits, and by the stigma associated with mental illness.

4. Carve-out benefits and their direct control of utilization by reviewers, the selection of providers, and the cost-shifting led to increased growth and profit for behavioral managed care companies (Jellinek and Little, 1998).

E. Implementation of Managed Care

While, in general, the widespread implementation of managed care has helped reduce rapid increases in health care costs and led to an overhaul of how medical and mental health care is delivered in the United States, these measures have in many cases left consumers paying more out-of-pocket, reduced the extent of coverage, and disconnected mental health from general medicine, while contributing to an increase in the proportion of Americans without insurance (Walsh, 1997).

II. General Effects of Managed Care on Psychiatry (Summergrad et al., 1995)

A. Change in Clinical Decision-Making Authority

1. In the past, physicians controlled most medical, administrative, and policy decisions.
2. As a result of the rising costs of health care, other professionals (including business leaders, politicians, economists and other non-physician interest groups) have an increasing authority in health care decisions.

B. More Physician Time Spent on Administrative Work

1. In the past, physicians spent more time seeing patients and less time doing paperwork and justifying their practice to anonymous reviewers.
2. Precertification and intrusive utilization review has dramatically increased the amount of non-patient time psychiatrists spend filling out forms and doing other correspondence with insurance companies.

C. Alteration in Referral Patterns and Practice

1. In the past, physicians relied on familiar and trusted colleagues, or on local subspecialists, for telephone referrals or consultations.
2. Mandated and impersonal referral via 1-800 numbers and by selective networks of contracting providers has dramatically changed referral habits and the length of time some patients must wait for an evaluation; in some cases this has led to a reduced access to mental health services.

D. Lower Reimbursement Schedules

1. Lower reimbursement schedules and substitution of non-physician providers have forced some psychiatrists to increase the size of their practice and to see a larger proportion of wealthier patients who can pay out-of-pocket.
2. Lower reimbursement schedules and increased demands on time have decreased incentives for psychiatrists to teach both residents and medical students, thus reducing the amount and quality of psychiatric training.

III. Specific Effects of Managed Care on Psychiatry (Summergrad et al., 1995)

A. Inpatient Services

1. Inpatient length of stays have plummeted (from 40–60 days in the 1980s, to, in many cases, less than 10 days).

2. General hospital units increasingly specialize in the care of patients with combined medical and psychiatric illness to attract elderly and disabled patients with medicare insurance, which still reimburses on a cost basis.
3. Attending physicians are forced to make more rapid treatment plans and to cover more patients; they work longer hours for the same or less wages.
4. Each managed mental health company has its own unique procedures for admissions, for utilization review, and for discharge planning, which further adds to administrative costs.

B. Emergency Services

1. In the past, emergency services served as evaluation centers prior to psychiatric admission. Today, there is increasing pressure to use prolonged emergency care to stabilize patients and to triage care to lower cost and less intense settings.
2. Complete evaluation and precertification procedures demanded by managed care companies have forced reallocation of time away from evaluation and workup to telephone negotiations, reviews, and paperwork.

C. Consultation Services

1. Consultation services in the past traditionally focused on rapid response and on the provision of psychiatric expertise to medically ill inpatients; today, decreased length of stay has frequently moved such consultation to the outpatient setting.
2. As PCPs are increasingly called to diagnose and manage psychiatric illnesses, psychiatrists are being forced to redefine their constituency to include, not only patients, but the continuing education of the PCP.
3. With the carve-out structure of managed care, payments for consultation services often fall between the payers for general medicine and psychiatry.

D. Outpatient Services

1. As managed care has developed, many companies have established selective networks and contracting providers; this strategy often severely limits the number of psychiatrists available for referral.
2. Referrals are now commonly taken by clerks who assign patients to caregivers (often to non-physicians first) based on availability. Given the variable experience of the triage person, the importance of clinical data in provider selection is suspect.
3. Outpatient services are required to develop rapid access to care, effective, nonintrusive, and collaborative review and treatment appeals process with initial evaluation by a psychiatrist for the soundest diagnosis and treatment plan.
4. Some high-quality, busy services cannot meet this standard and are thus not available to patients.

E. Residency Training

1. No major managed care company permits residents to treat their members. This has had a dramatic impact on residency training, as managed care companies have no incentive to support the training mission of academic centers.
2. Shorter length of stays on inpatient units has had a significant impact on the medical student, and resident training environment. No longer are thorough evaluation, longitudinal observation, and intensive psychotherapy possible.
3. In the outpatient setting, the preservation of long-term psychotherapy is jeopardized, as advances in neuroscience, pharmacotherapy, and alternative psychotherapies compete for limited training time.
4. In the emergency room and admitting areas, resident training is undermined by time-consuming and often confrontational precertification procedures.

IV. Specific Issues in Primary Care Medicine Contracting (Summergrad and Jellinek, 1998)

A. Because many mental health and substance abuse services are carved out of general health care contracts, there is an incentive for many PCPs to move care from the primary sector to the mental health sector as soon as problems are diagnosed or become apparent. This may contradict the utilization criteria of the managed care carve-out companies and leave patients between providers and payers.

B. Carving-out mental health services also decreases referrals and utilization since PCPs are a key access point to mental health services.

C. Mental health carve-out companies have little or no incentive to provide mental health services that lower medical costs if it means increasing psychiatric treatment costs.

D. Moreover, the costs of pharmacotherapy provided by the PCP will be the responsibility of the medical managed care company and not the behavioral health carve-out.

V. Ethical Considerations and Reform (Brennan, 1993)

A. Perhaps more than any other profession, medicine, and by extension mental health, is firmly rooted in ethical principles. However, most discussions regarding how to change the current crisis in medicine and mental health are advanced with economic and policy considerations with little concern for ethics, or, more generally, moral philosophy.

B. As a consequence, economic and policy opinions are presented with little perspective on the dual role of health care as a social commitment and an industry.

C. Health care reform often focuses on health insurance reform at the expense of delivery, or ethical considerations, most likely because the current system is too expensive.

D. However, this focus on insurance reform minimizes aspects of the current health care delivery system.

1. Attention to insurance reform and to managed care does not specifically address the source of increasing medical expenses: rising costs of technology and new medications, as well as an aging population.
2. Traditionally, wealthier patients, or those with adequate insurance, subsidized the care of those without benefits. Fragmentation of risk-pools via carve-out behavioral health plans and other mechanisms leaves behind the less well, who must pay higher premiums or accept narrower benefits.
3. This creates the ethical situation in which ability to pay determines the availability and quality of care.

E. Any rational attempt at health care reform must first allow debate on certain foundational issues, including parity between mental health and other health care reimbursements, method of taxation, quality improvement, control of technology, health manpower needs, multiple vs. single payer, nature of benefits, cost control, and financing research and medical education (Jellinek and Nurcombe, 1993).

VI. Strategies for Survival

A. Short-Term Strategies

1. Define your professional standards as to what are reasonable and unreasonable external managed care pressures to conform.
2. Support colleagues who maintain high standards for admission, diagnostic evaluation, and treatment plans.
3. Refuse to participate in any practice that appears dangerous or substandard. Report companies with aberrant behaviors to the appropriate agencies.
4. Learn the rules of appeal and use the process.
5. Inform patients of the constraints within which they and you are operating.

B. Long-Term Strategies

1. Build alliances with other medical colleagues to have them appreciate the value of psychiatry and

to alert them to the potential effects of managed care.

2. Continue to build a scientific basis for treatment based upon methodologically sound outcome studies and rational clinical pathways and protocols.

3. Continue to lobby both state and national agencies, societies, and governments and alert them to the implications of managed care on the practice of mental health.

Suggested Readings

Brennan TA: An ethical perspective on health care insurance reform. *Am J Law Med* 1993; 19:37–74.

Jellinek M, Little M: Supporting child psychiatric services using current managed care approaches: you can't get there from here. *Arch Pediatr Adolesc Med* 1998; 152:321–326.

Jellinek MS, Nurcombe B: Two wrongs don't make a right: managed care, mental health and the marketplace. *J Am Med Assoc* 1993; 270:1737–1739.

Kubritsky C, Hadley T: The managed behavioral healthcare workforce initiative: guidelines, standards and competencies for behavioral health. In Manderscheid RW, Henderson MJ (eds): *Center for Mental Health Services: Mental Health, United States, 1998.* DHHS Pub. No. (SMA) 99-3285. Washington, DC: Supt. of Docs, U.S. Govt. Printing Office, 1998:70–81.

Kuttner R: The American health care system: employer sponsored health coverage. *N Engl J Med* 1999; 340:248–252.

Oss M, Krizsy J: Industry statistics: psychiatric room rates continue to increase faster than average hospital rates. *Open Minds* 1991:16.

Sederer L: Judicial and legislative responses to cost containment. *Am J Psychiatry* 1992; 149:1157–1161.

Summergrad P, Herman JB, Weilburg JB, Jellinek MS. Wagons Ho: Forward on the managed care trail. *Gen Hosp Psychiatry* 1995; 17:251–259.

Summergrad P, Jellinek MS: Dealing with psychiatric issues in an era of managed/capitated care. In Stern TA, Herman JB, Slavin PS (eds): *The MGH Guide to Psychiatry in Primary Care.* New York: McGraw-Hill, 1998:661–666.

Walsh R: Trends in health care coverage and financing and their implications for policy. *N Engl J Med* 1997; 337:1000–1003.

Chapter 82

Coping with the Rigors of Psychiatric Practice

BANDY X. LEE AND EDWARD MESSNER

I. Overview

A. Introduction

Humanitarian ideals that initially inspired the choice of a medical career can later lead to both professional success and stress. Psychiatry is no exception. **Burnout is reaching epidemic proportions in the helping professions** (Grosch and Olsen, 1994). Certain psychological characteristics of physicians can be both adaptive and maladaptive: perfectionism, self-doubt, exaggerated sense of responsibility, and limited capacity for emotional expressiveness (Gabbard and Menninger, 1989). **Medical training further encourages behaviors that contribute to burnout: long work hours with sleep deprivation, repression of feelings, and isolation from ordinary social situations.**

When carried beyond residency and applied to their own personal lives, adaptive mechanisms that once sustained the physician through grueling training can leave one cynical, disillusioned, and unfulfilled at work and at home. Transition from training to career—such as when preparing for the Boards!—is especially stressful (Looney et al., 1980). Understanding the sources of stress and cultivating coping mechanisms can help clinicians identify risks associated with psychiatric practice, and steer them towards preventive or ameliorating interventions.

B. Epidemiology

1. Despite the individual strengths of psychiatrists, many experience depression, substance abuse, and even suicide.
   a. **In the United States, the number of physicians who kill themselves annually would fill an average-size medical school class.**
   b. **Female physicians on average die 10 years earlier than their male counterparts,** the opposite of the gender longevity ratio in the general population.
   c. **Substance abuse often leads to physician impairment.** Up to 12% of resident physicians reported increased use of substances compared with their use before training (Koran and Litt, 1988).

II. Etiologies for Physician Stress and Burnout

A. Dealing with Difficult Clinical Situations and Emotions

1. **Suffering.** Physicians, including psychiatrists, typically receive limited training in the soothing of individuals who are uncomfortable, anxious, and suffering. The obligation to collect clinical information is superimposed on the anxiety of facing emotional nakedness. The all-encompassing and longstanding nature of some psychiatric illnesses, in particular, can place great pressure on the clinician, as the most severely ill also suffer socioeconomic deprivation, neglected by family and society.

2. **Ethical conflicts.** The patient's trust and reliance on the psychiatrist for support and advice raises numerous ethical issues. Within this setting, psychiatrists often find themselves in the difficult position of trying to relieve pain as they initially inflict more through limit-setting or drug side-effects. Furthermore, the psychiatrist may have to institute security measures in the face of violent symptoms (Dubin et al., 1988), or have to restrict patients' freedom in order to proceed with therapy against their will when poor insight presents as part of the illness.

3. **Transference and countertransference.** Transference and countertransference, which can lead to intense feelings between patient and doctor, are a part of every psychiatrist's work experience. Patients may bring expectations or responses based on their past experiences with parents, caregivers, or authority figures that are initially difficult to comprehend. In addition, the clinician's listening to a patient's personal problems, attempting to understand them, and accepting the patient for whom she or he is, can induce powerfully deep, loving, and sometimes dependent attachments to the physician. Dealing on a daily basis with individuals who express or arouse eroticized notions, or who have poor control over their own hostility, paranoid proclivity, or ego boundaries, while maintaining awareness of one's own responses, can pose a great challenge for the therapist.

4. **The perception of failure.** Psychiatrists often counsel patients and families as they struggle with difficult life events, which sometimes involve the psychiatrist intensely (e.g., suicide of a patient). As death is often perceived as a failure of medical intervention by both the caregiver and the patient's relatives, suicide may provoke tormenting feelings of failure, guilt, and self-blame.

B. **Responsibility with Insufficient Authority**
The multifaceted, sometimes intuitive, nature of psychiatry makes it an exciting as well as a pervasively uncertain field. Psychiatrists must often make serious clinical decisions based on incomplete, conflicting, and ambiguous data. These stresses are compounded by other competing demands on psychiatrists as they answer to institutions, insurers, patients, and families. Current health insurance reforms often establish limitations or standards of performance without psychiatrist involvement, which further undermines pride, morale, organizational commitment, and resolve.

C. **Disruption of Social and Marital Relationships**
1. **Social isolation.** Psychiatrists often work in isolation, facing the interpersonal impact of psychopathology alone.
2. **Interpersonal relationships.** Burnout is associated with low satisfaction in relationships with patients, relatives, and staff. Traditional gender roles make women especially vulnerable to burnout and to low job satisfaction, because of family commitments that reduce flexibility in their working hours and impair their career prospects.

D. **Cynicism and Discouragement**
1. **Misanthropy**
   a. Instead of drawing out patients' feelings, psychiatrists frequently find that patients evoke their own feelings of anxiety, defensiveness, and helplessness. Exposure to patients' suffering or hostility—in the form of manipulation, ingratitude, or even physical threats— can produce reactive misanthropy. In response, one may not only lose warmth and concern for patients but can also develop crusty defensiveness or contempt.
   b. Misanthropic attitudes may evolve as a kind of self-protection in the face of the exhaustion and stressful experiences of practice. This kind of emotional isolation may carry over to all patients, so that one no longer recognizes patients who are appreciative, pleasant, and responsive to treatment.
2. **Expansion of antipathy.** In its more malignant forms, the antipathy one develops toward patients may extend to other relationships, including those with fellow psychiatrists, health care professionals, and even friends and family. Such conflict with one's values and intentions can lead to self-punishment, guilt, and feelings of failure.

III. When Coping Strategies Go Awry

A. **How We See Ourselves**
1. **Denial of vulnerability.** As psychiatrists, we wish to see ourselves as immune to emotional impairments. One common way of coping with stress is to work harder and longer, which can ultimately cause even greater damage. Psychiatrists, like other health professionals, may rely on defense mechanisms of repression, rationalization, denial, and reaction formation in the suppression and displacement of emotions. Over time, however, unexamined reactions to stressful situations can undermine relationships, not only with patients, but also with friends and family.
2. **Compromise of familial concerns.** Marital or family concerns may be misjudged as being neither as important nor as urgent as saving lives and relieving pain. Too tired for empathic listening, reasonable conversation, or recreation, clinicians may internalize their own concerns and become self-absorbed. For some, the demands of medical training, the rigors of establishing a practice, and the expectations of colleagues are used as excuses to postpone or avoid emotional intimacy in personal relationships.
3. **Deferment of help-seeking.** Seeking help for personal or family problems is commonly misconstrued as an admission of weakness or personal failure. The stigma of a psychiatric diagnosis also keeps some physicians from seeking appropriate care. While psychiatrists are generally more open to seeking psychotherapy themselves, the possibility of public humiliation and disclosure to colleagues or licensing boards may render asking for assistance difficult. The stress of adopting an omnipotent, directive, and controlling stance can lead to godlike expectations and blame for human fallibility in oneself and in others. This intolerance towards any personal vulnerability can undermine a psychiatrist's well-being, as well as personal and work relationships.

B. **How to Recognize Stress in Oneself**
1. **Signs and symptoms.** Unmanageable stress can lead to clinical states of anxiety or depression that, if left untreated, may have tragic consequences for clinicians, patients, and families. Signals of psychic pain include feelings of overload and exhaustion, apathy, anhedonia, despair, headaches, gastrointestinal disturbances, and verbal incontinence. Other signs include longer and less efficient working hours, poor and irregular sleep and eating

habits, disrupted family relationships, unaccustomed difficulties in memory, concentration, and problem-solving, and multiple suggestions by friends, relatives, or colleagues to seek help.

IV. Interventions

A. "Physician Heal Thyself"

As much as the health care profession requires the giving of oneself, it is necessary to recharge one's own emotional batteries. Each of us has a repertoire of methods for dealing with stressful situations that can be strengthened. Prevention of emotional overload can be achieved through anticipation of, and preparation for, difficulties, rather than through denial of them. Some examples of coping strategies are as follows:

1. **Make a systematic effort to process experiences** (e.g., by talking with a colleague, or through introspection during a long commute). Dealing with the day's stresses can help one refrain from inflicting the emotional effects on family or other cherished relationships. Also, attempting to learn from and to transform tragic events to growth-promoting ones can neutralize some of the misery that they inflict.

2. **Take your own history of responses to past stresses.** Psychiatrists can apply this familiar skill to separate the useful strategies for coping from the counterproductive ones. Under stressful conditions, emotions often go unnoticed until they reach a painful level. Early signs might include unruffled competence at work followed by irritability or explosive anger at home. Clinicians who have not prepared for the stresses of practice may not even recognize the intensity of their needs or the desperation of their impulses.

3. **Make a list of methods that work.** Constructively channeled actions, such as through athletics and prudent sexual engagement, can discharge frustration and anger. Readily available physical expressions include shouting into a bed pillow or running up stairs for release. Stretching or isometric exercises can also reduce muscle tension. A single episode of tearfulness does not indicate emotional instability but may, in fact, represent a restoration of balance.

4. **Maintain a healthy self-regard.** Caring for the mind and body, and the appreciation of one's compassion, honesty, and perseverance, can help individuals cope with stress. Also, the temptation during times of exhaustion to resort to poor eating habits can add weight, reduce fitness, and impair physical appearance, which can undermine attitudes about attractiveness and worth.

5. **Mentally rehearse potential problems** or stressful situations and predict one's emotional reactions to them. Imagining the expression of feelings can decompress intense surges of emotion such as anger, sadness, or fear. Central to the usefulness of such expressive fantasies is the recognition that they are distinct from the corresponding actions; they need not, and usually should not, be enacted.

6. **Engage in directed fantasies** by imagining a scene that is affectively intense. A cruelly manipulative patient can be beaten up by thugs, or a superior might be hit in the face with a cream pie. The more uncivilized the fantasy, the more effective it can be in the management of pent-up emotion. In addition, the more unrealistic the fantasy, the easier it is to maintain the distinction between fantasy and the corresponding enactment.

7. **Dialogue with friends and family regarding anticipated unavailability.** This can help prepare them and sustain relationships. Lovers, spouses, and relatives may respond with anger or withdrawal, which may lead one to feel rejected or punished. On the other hand, as long as communication is maintained, adversity experienced together can lead to intimacy and mutual regard.

8. **Use humor and mutual support** with colleagues to magnify respites, triumphs, and the joy of learning while providing for space to vent your rage and frustration.

9. **Relish mementos of happier times,** recalling previous triumphs and rehearsing original goals. Reassociation with familiar people, places, things, and activities can improve morale. Sustained by recollections of the pinnacles of one's life, the clinician will be in a better position to cope with daily stresses.

10. **Regard patients' behavior as a form of communication.** Collaborative relationships with patients seem to buffer against the worst effects of stress. Patients can evoke in the clinician feelings and attitudes comparable to those of others in the patient's past (complementary identification), and attitudes that the patient experiences (concurrent identification). Difficult behaviors may be a way of saying: "See! Now you know how I feel!" Understanding our own subjective reactions may be a source of clinical data about how to approach patients and recruit their individual strengths.

11. **Learn relaxation techniques and self-hypnosis to relieve stress.** Tension, sleep deprivation, overstimulation, and the dread of returning to work without adequate rest may lure one to benzodiazepines, alcohol, or other sedating agents. Self-prescribed medications should signal caution at the

first dose. As a safe and convenient alternative, autohypnosis can induce sleep and reduce tension. Find a comfortable position and clear the mind of intrusive thoughts. Imagine yourself in pleasant surroundings and then picture your feet relaxing, followed by various segments of the body. Silent, sedating meditation can be brief, depending on skill, practice, and extent of sleep deprivation.

12. **Temporarily suspend the requirement to be logical and relevant.** Observing the contents of one's mind and its spontaneous associations may lead to new insights. Mental experiences other than linear processes can evolve, connect, and merge into one another, and also interplay with our emotions and attitudes. Free association may lead one to ideas, feelings, and perceptions that were formerly outside of one's awareness, inducing delight in their complexity, generativity, and beauty. Poetry, abstract paintings, classical music, or other sources of mindfulness can further increase resiliency and willingness to perceive one's deeper self.

B. **When to Consult**

Professional consultation can add objectivity and expertise when a clinician experiences overwhelming stress or burnout. Burnout is defined as a syndrome of emotional exhaustion, depersonalization towards patients, and reduced sense of personal accomplishment (Martin et al., 1997). An Athenian physician wrote in 2 AD: "These are the duties of a physician: first ... to heal his mind and to give help to himself before giving it to anyone else."

Consider consultation for any of the following:
1. Depression (SIGECAPS mnemonic)
2. Suicidal ideation, including wishes, intentions, plans, or actions
3. Anxiety that interferes with personal or professional enjoyment
4. Alcohol and/or drug abuse
5. Rage and hatred expressed inappropriately
6. Interference with clinical skills or judgment
7. Impulsive or reckless behavior
8. Eating disorder symptoms

C. **Types of Available Professional Help**
1. **Psychotherapy.** Individual psychotherapy involves a commitment to meet with another clinician regularly and provides a unique opportunity for the psychiatrist to experience the other end of the therapeutic relationship. Many psychiatrist-patients find psychotherapy to be a powerful, life-enhancing experience.
2. **Psychopharmacology.** Some physicians may perceive their own need for medication as further admission of personal weakness. On the contrary, failing to treat biologically based psychiatric conditions, as the psychiatrist well knows, is tantamount to denying insulin to the type I diabetic: both omissions can produce fatal consequences.
3. **Couple and family therapy.** Couple therapists and family therapists can be found at most mental health centers, psychiatric clinics, or private group practices. This support can help the psychiatrist's family relationships, which are paradoxically a major source of coping with the stress of medical practice and the first potential casualty of that stress.
4. **Autognosis or "self-knowledge" rounds.** Autognosis rounds allow psychiatrists to share their experiences as they identify their subjective reactions to clinical situations, use this information as diagnostic information, and learn how to minimize potentially harmful effects of reactions to patients (e.g., managing anger towards a patient in a way that does not interfere with her or his care). Autognostic techniques have proved useful to both medicine and psychiatry residents in groups conducted at the Massachusetts General Hospital for three decades (Stern et al., 1993).
5. **Support groups.** Professional support groups outside of the primary work setting can provide opportunities for self-definition and growth.

V. Conclusion

At a Harvard Medical School commencement address, Dr. Ned Cassem charged the graduates with the following: "Fight down your grandiosity: learn to tolerate uncertainty and ... remain more impressed by the mysteries and uniqueness of your patients than by your own expertise. Give yourself a break. Respect your own limits and vulnerabilities." More than warding off impairment and suffering, this makes more accessible the satisfactions and joys of practicing psychiatry.

Selected Readings

Cassem E: Internship, liberty, death and other choices. Harvard Medical School Commencement Address, 1979.

Dubin WR, Wilson SJ, Mercer C: Assaults against psychiatrists in outpatient settings. *J Clin Psychiatry* 1988; 49:338–345.

Gabbard GO, Menninger RW: The psychology of postponement in the medical marriage. *J Am Med Assoc* 1989; 261:2378–2381.

Grosch W, Olsen D: *When Helping Starts to Hurt.* New York: Norton, 1994.

Koran L, Litt I: House staff well-being. *West J Med* 1988; 148:97–101.

Looney JG, Harding RK, Blotcky MJ, Barnhart FD: Psychiatrists' transition from training to career: stress and mastery. *Am J Psychiatry* 1980; 137:32–36.

Martin F, Poyen D, Bouderlique E, et al.: Depression and burnout in hospital health care professionals. *Int J Occup Environ Health*

1997; 3:204–209.

Messner E: *Resilience Enhancement for the Resident Physician.* Durant, OK: Essential Medical Information Systems, 1993.

Stern TA, Prager LM, Cremens MC: Autognosis rounds for medical house staff. *Psychosomatics* 1993; 34:1–7.

Stern TA, Herman JB, Slavin PL: *The MGH Guide to Psychiatry in Primary Care.* New York: McGraw-Hill, 1998.

Chapter 83

Preparing for Psychiatry in the 21st Century

Scott L. Rauch

I. Introduction

If the decade of the brain (the 1990s) is any indication, advancement and change in the new millennium are likely to be unusually swift in comparison to the glacial pace that more typically characterizes shifting trends in medical science and practice. As physicians, we know that prognostication is inexact, that it often relies on extrapolation from change during the recent past to the present, and that our preconceptions about the future tend to actually effect how it unfolds.

In this volume about preparation, **this chapter will be specifically devoted to the future of psychiatry.** After all, apt preparation relies to a large extent on foreseeing what challenges the future holds. I will touch on diverse topics, including the evolution of psychiatric conditions and patterns of care, emerging themes in psychiatric diagnoses, neuroscience research, and new therapies. Such a chapter cannot hope to be comprehensive; instead, **it aspires to be thought-provoking.**

II. Who Will Psychiatrists Treat and What Maladies Will They Battle?

A. Potential for New Diseases

That the face of psychiatric disease will remain entirely stable into the new millennium should not be taken for granted. Given that the acquired immunodeficiency syndrome (AIDS)-dementia complex was nonexistent before the 1980s, **we should expect that new pathogens with ramifications on central nervous system (CNS) function will evolve.** Similarly, as industrial growth and chemical innovation continue around the globe, it stands to reason that **new neurotoxins will likewise emerge.** Further, as new technologies are born and with them the potential for cultural shifts, novel societal contexts are likely. Beyond idiosyncrasies, such as "Y2K-catastrophobia," or anecdotes of "internet addiction," **we may see serious trends towards isolation from human interaction, new forms of peer pressure, and new currencies for self-worth, as well as an inevitable blurring of the line between reality and virtual reality.**

B. Shifting Epidemiological Factors and Market Forces

The above earmarks of our brave new world notwithstanding, **the psychopathology of past centuries will largely carry forward to the next.** In particular, diseases related to advanced age, abuse of substances, and overpopulation are most likely to rise disproportionately. Who psychiatrists treat, however, may change more as a function of medical care models than from epidemiologic imperatives. **Progressively, routine psychiatric intervention will be provided by primary care physicians, and nonphysicians.** Extrapolating from the trends of this past decade, **we will need to refine our consultation skills, and anticipate principally providing direct treatment for patients with more severe or complicated psychiatric illness.** We should hope that political discourse surrounding parity leads to reasonable provisions for humane and effective psychiatric care. Similarly, we should envision that the stigma associated with psychiatric illness will gradually (although incompletely) dissipate, as have the objects of other social prejudices in decades past. Cost-efficient care will, however, doubtless remain a priority, and hence a pressure against extending the duration of human therapeutic contact.

III. What Is the Future of Psychiatric Evaluation and Diagnosis?

A. The Purpose of Diagnosis and the Evolving Psychiatric Classification Scheme

We must keep in mind that **the purpose of diagnosis is not simply to give suffering a name, but to classify illness in a manner that provides an organizing influence for treatment and research.** With the advent of biologically meaningful diagnostic schemes comes information that can guide treatment and educate as to prognosis. In the 21st century, psychiatry will doubtless cross the threshold from a potpourri of syndromic designations, to a diagnostic scheme honed to reflect underlying pathophysiology. This process will largely depend upon advances in psychiatric neuroscience.

B. Evolving Methods of Evaluation

1. **The diagnostic interview. The backbone of clinical evaluation in psychiatry, and in all of medicine, should remain the diagnostic interview.** One can envision that attempts will be made to streamline the process of collecting raw factual historical

information, in the context of automated systems and electronic medical records. Nonetheless, it is difficult to imagine that the role of anamnesis as part history collection, part mental status examination, and part therapeutic process could be usefully replaced in the name of a myopic preoccupation with cost-efficiency. Therefore, we should hope that the diagnostic interview will largely prevail, and further that the skills and art of conducting that enterprise will remain central to the practice of psychiatry. Doubtless, however, the psychiatrist's assessment of clinical presentation and history will be augmented by ancillary data.

2. **Pathophysiology-based nomenclature and neurobiological probes.** In the best tradition of the medical model, **pathophysiology-based diagnostic entities will be ascertained through history and examination, but also ultimately via more direct tests of brain structure and function (e.g., neuroimaging tests), as well as by probes of genotype.** Thus, the diagnostic process and classification system in psychiatry will inevitably evolve in tandem, incorporating contemporary advances in psychiatric neuroscience.

IV. What is the Future of Psychiatric Neuroscience?

A. Evolving Models of Disease

1. **Building on the history of simple models.** During the third quarter of the 20th century, psychiatric neuroscience principally focused on the chemistry and pharmacology of monoaminergic neurotransmitters. The hope that simple deficiencies of one or another transmitter might explain major psychopathologic entities was motivated, in part, by the story of Parkinson's disease, and fueled by early conceptualizations of antidepressant and antipsychotic drug actions. By the early 1990s, the field had matured to appreciate the inadequacy of such models; schizophrenia would not simply be a disease of too much dopamine, nor would depression simply be a disease of insufficient serotonin or norepinephrine. In parallel, the emergence of contemporary neuroimaging techniques has provided a new class of information, allowing for characterization of regional brain activity or chemistry in time and in three dimensions of space. Likewise, growing sophistication in the imaging field has moved us past any reminiscence of phrenology. To the contrary, investigators have quickly come to realize that psychiatric diseases will not simply be reducible to a three-dimensional map of generic regional brain dysfunction. Rather, **neuroimaging will help to characterize pathophysiology in terms of dysfunctional distributed networks, and provide**

for multidimensional assessments of computational deficits at any given locus. These multiple dimensions will potentially include indices of brain activity across a battery of challenge conditions, as well as various parameters of neurochemistry and metabolism.

2. **Defining phenotypes via neuroimaging and molecular biology. Psychiatric neuroscience in the 21st century will continue to rely heavily on neurotransmitter pharmacology,** as well as on the new-found power of neuroimaging methods, to establish phenotypes at the level of brain. However, **there will be a progressive focus on molecular biology, which is necessary to understand the genetic bases of selected vulnerabilities as well as the pre- and postsynaptic processes that mediate neural dysfunction.** Beyond neurotransmitters and their receptors, second messengers as well as other moieties that modulate gene expression are likely to be the critical substrates of psychiatric disease.

B. Integrating Modes of Inquiry

The best of psychiatric neuroscience research will involve integration across modes of inquiry. For instance, factor analysis of clinical phenomena (e.g., symptom dimensions), as measured with standardized instruments, provides means for quantitatively expressing signs and symptoms for use in family genetic studies. Similarly, brain-imaging data can be analyzed to identify neural correlates of symptom dimensions at regional and systems levels. Then, these brain physiology profiles can be modeled in animals at the systems, regional, and, ultimately, cellular and subcellular levels. Finally, investigators can seek to discover genetic and epigenetic factors that are capable of causing these phenotypic profiles spanning the subcellular, cellular, regional, and systemic scales. Enumerating the full range of neuroscience methods to be used in this quest is clearly beyond the scope of this chapter. However, it is worth emphasizing **that contributions will likely come from sophisticated new sequencing methods (including chip technology), by-products of the Human Genome Project, gene knock-out and knock-in techniques, advances in neuroimaging, and electrophysiologic multi-unit recording in freely moving animals, as well as the classic methods of clinical phenomenology.**

V. What is the Future of Psychiatric Treatment?

A. Paradigm Shifts in the Overall Management of Psychiatric Illness

1. **Early diagnosis.** Management, based on early diagnosis, including the potential for prophylactic treatment in the context of identifying at-risk populations or presymptomatic cases, will be an important advance.

2. **Treatment algorithms.** Treatment algorithms will proliferate and be refined. This will lead to more efficient care that is better informed by the cumulative database on psychiatric treatment outcomes. Reciprocally, adherence to treatment algorithms will lead to the rapid accrual of a superior empirical database from which to modify our algorithms. Predictable tensions will exist between the benefits of standardization vs. the pull towards individualized care—in terms both of the individuality of patients and of the individuality of a given practitioner's impressions or instincts.

3. **Predictors of response.** Developing valid and reliable predictors of treatment response will enhance the efficacy of treatment. If such predictors could be gleaned from easily accessible clinical information (e.g., age, gender, constellation of symptoms), this would be most cost-effective. However, **it may be that the most powerful predictors of treatment response will be ascertained via more fine-grained probes of brain function, such as those obtained via neuroimaging.** Already, brain-imaging studies have produced preliminary findings suggesting that particular brain activity profiles predict antidepressant and anti-obsessional responses to medication. Such predictors of treatment response will be most important in the context of candidate treatments that are of long duration, high cost, or great risk (e.g., anti-obsessional medication trials, electroconvulsive therapy [ECT], or neurosurgical treatment). Here it should also be emphasized that reliable predictors of bad outcomes can be just as valuable as reliable predictors of treatment success.

4. **Continuum of care.** There should be a trend toward "filling in the gaps" that exist in our current psychiatric treatment networks. Already there has been expansion in partial hospitalization and residential treatment. Similarly, **there will likely be expansion of long-term care, rehabilitation, and neuropsychiatric facilities.** Moreover, improvement will be necessary in the integration of the various elements that make up these systems, so that patient transfer to the most appropriate setting can be expeditious.

B. New Concepts in Pharmacotherapy

1. **Receptor selectivity and drug development.** Less than a decade ago, the grail of drug development appeared to be agents with maximal affinity, potency, and selectivity. More recently, **it has become clear that some of the most effective agents have modest affinities or selectivities.** For instance, clozapine may be a more effective antipsychotic than conventional neuroleptics despite its modest D_2 receptor binding profile; similarly, clomipramine appears to be as effective an anti-obsessional agent as the newer selective serotonergic reuptake inhibitors (SSRIs). Further, there is now great interest in partial agonists. Consequently, the take-home point should be that the drug development industry is more sophisticated than ever with regard to efficient modeling, synthesis, and evaluation of new agents. Just as important, however, is an evolving open-mindedness about what characteristics might actually lead to an optimal therapeutic profile.

2. **Neuropeptides. Neuropeptides are a popular new target for candidate drug action.** New findings that substance P antagonists might serve as effective antidepressants have just scratched the surface of what will be an explosion in this area during the coming century. Other prime peptidergic targets include elements of the corticosteroid system (i.e., stress hormones), that almost certainly play a role in the genesis and expression of anxiety and affective disorders.

3. **Postreceptor mediated processes. New drugs will be developed to target second messenger systems.** For instance, phosphodiesterase inhibitors are capable of modulating cyclic AMP (cAMP) levels while bypassing receptor systems per se. Such agents will offer a unique profile in comparison to more classic receptor agonists or antagonists. Similarly, inositol and other agents can modulate neurotransmission directly through action at the level of the neural membrane in a non-receptor-mediated manner.

4. **Targeted pharmacotherapy and the "silver bullet."** As we discover the core pathophysiology of particular diseases, **optimal therapies might include a capacity to direct medications to specific cell types or brain regions.** In this way the beneficial effects of medications could be increased and unwanted effects minimized. Techniques for targeted pharmacotherapy of this type are already being developed:

   a. **By attaching a certain chemical moiety to a drug, it is possible to alter its rate of accumulation in specified target cells.**

   b. **By local disruption of the blood-brain barrier, it may be possible to produce regionally disparate concentrations of drug.** For example, first a compound could be designed so that it does not readily penetrate the blood-brain barrier. Then an intervention could be performed to temporarily locally disrupt the blood-brain barrier, thereby producing a regionally elevated brain concentration of the agent. Of note, ultrasound methods are being developed to create such targeted and transient reductions in blood-brain barrier effectiveness.

5. **New preparations and drug delivery systems.** During the 1990s, long-acting preparations and transdermal delivery became popular. In the coming century, **reservoir pump technology may become more commonplace, with physiologic feedback capabilities and exploitation of chip-based technologies.** Such advances will lead to enhanced compliance, as well as more precise dosing capabilities.

C. New Concepts in Somatic Therapies

1. **Gene therapies.** As the genetic basis for psychiatric diseases are discovered, **vector replacement of vulnerability genes could be possible.** Moreover, genetic material can be introduced to modify gene expression, and thereby compensate for epigenetic and acquired disorders as well.

2. **Transplantation.** It is difficult to know whether or not transplantation methods will evolve into useful interventions for psychiatric conditions. To date, this strategy has been adopted as a means to compensate for gross degeneration, such as in the neurologic condition Parkinson's disease.

3. **Neurosurgery.** The psychiatric neurosurgical treatments of today (e.g., stereotactic cingulotomy, and gamma-capsulotomy) are much refined in comparison with the lobotomies of decades past. Still, it seems likely that surgical treatment (in the conventional sense) will remain a relatively crude and blunt method for modulating brain function. Neurosurgical treatments for psychiatric diseases will probably fade in popularity and utility as improved nonsurgical treatment methods evolve.

4. **Transcranial magnetic stimulation (TMS).** Over the next decade, the early promise of TMS as an alternative to ECT will be rigorously tested. While it is appealing to propose that localized brain stimulation could provide advantages in terms of efficacy and adverse effects, this remains an empirical matter. Certainly, advances in our understanding of pathophysiology will help guide the study of this potential treatment modality.

D. Evolving Concepts in Talk Therapies

1. **Telecommunications. The increasing use of telecommunication technologies will challenge the traditional frame of psychotherapy.** Exploiting this strategy may lead to greater cost-efficiency, and serve as a hedge against the market forces which threaten to diminish the use of psychotherapies.

2. **Short-term and group therapies.** Generally, market forces will exert a pressure toward these vs. long-

term individual therapies. There will be much room for innovation, however, such as evidenced by the recent excitement over dialectical behavior therapy for borderline personality disorder. The onus will be on psychiatrists to demonstrate cost-effectiveness for psychotherapies. Consequently, more standardized versions of this type of therapy will likely evolve, in order to help generate an empirical database with which to demonstrate and characterize effectiveness.

3. **Rehabilitation-oriented cognitive therapies.** There has been a recent upswing in interest regarding a role for cognitive rehabilitation in some chronic psychiatric disorders. In fact, insufficient attention has been paid to the morbidity associated with cognitive deficits that accompany the range of chronic psychiatric conditions. For instance, the degree to which cognitive and functional deficits associated with schizophrenia, eating disorders, or obsessive-compulsive disorders resolve with treatment is not well established. It may be that classic treatments which target core symptoms of these disorders actually fail to alleviate the accompanying cognitive deficits. Cognitive rehabilitation may offer a means for treating this aspect of psychiatric conditions as well.

4. **Pharmacologic augmentation of psychotherapy.** If such treatments as desensitization and exposure and response prevention are based on extinction or other forms of learning, it stands to reason that these processes might be accelerated by augmentation with specific pharmacologic agents. Such approaches have never been adequately studied. With a growing emphasis on behavior therapies, this concept of true pharmacologic augmentation is likely to take hold in the next millennium.

VI. Conclusion

These are exciting times in psychiatry. During the next millennium, although our field will face new challenges, these will be overshadowed by the tremendous advances that now seem inevitable. **While the emergence of a few new diseases seems likely, the main challenges that confront psychiatry will be imposed by modest shifts in epidemiology, and by major shifts in health care models.**

We will need to be prepared to help colleagues outside of psychiatry better treat psychiatric conditions, to remind our society about the realities of psychiatric illness, and to provide care ourselves for the most severely ill. We will need to learn more efficient and effective ways to assess patients, that will likely include greater reliance on ancillary data, such as from neuroimaging or serological tests. Simultaneously, we will need to adjust to an evolving diagnostic scheme that will inevitably and progressively become pathophysiology-based in its organization.

We would be well advised to follow neuroscience advances as they relate to the underpinnings of psychiatric diseases. While new techniques for studying brain systems, neurons, and genes will certainly develop, it is the integration of these and existing methods that will lead to the greatest advances in the science of psychiatry.

Finally, our most profound hopes for the future lie in the potential for improved psychiatric treatments, if not prevention, or cure. **As new treatments become available, we will be charged with testing their effectiveness, and ultimately incorporating them judiciously into our armamentarium.** New treatments will include new medications, new forms of psychotherapy, new somatic therapies, and new combinations of interventions. We should perpetually press to insure that we are using the tools at our disposal in the most effective manner possible, while external forces will more than ever prod us to practice efficiently. In this regard, **we will need to lead the process of psychiatric health care system development and education through to the next millennium.**

Suggested Readings

American Psychiatric Association: *Diagnostic and Statistical Manual of Mental Disorders, Fourth Edition*. Washington, DC: American Psychiatric Press, 1994.

Dougherty DD, Rauch SL, Rosenbaum JR (eds): *Contemporary Strategies in Psychiatric Neuroimaging Research*. Washington, DC: American Psychiatric Press, in press.

Duman RS, Heninger GR, Nestler EJ: A molecular and cellular theory of depression. *Arch Gen Psychiatry* 1997; 54:597–606.

George MS (ed.): Transcranial magnetic stimulation. *CNS Spectrums* 1997; 2(1).

Hyman SE, Nestler EJ: *The Molecular Foundations of Psychiatry*. Washington, DC: American Psychiatric Press, 1993.

Jobst KA, Barnetson LP, Shepstone BJ: Accurate prediction of histologically confirmed Alzheimer's disease and the differential diagnosis of dementia: the use of NINCDS-ADRDA and DSM-III-R criteria, SPECT, X-ray CT, and Apo E4 in medial temporal lobe dementias. Oxford Project to Investigate Memory and Aging. *Int Psychogeriatr* 1998; 10:271–302.

Kobak KA, Taylor LH, Dottl SL, et al.: A computer-administered telephone interview to identify mental disorders. *J Am Med Assoc* 1997; 278:905–910.

Kramer MS, Cutler N, Feighner J, et al.: Distinct mechanism for antidepressant activity by blockade of central substance P receptors. *Science* 1998; 281:1640–1645.

Lesch KP: Gene transfer to the brain: emerging therapeutic strategy in psychiatry? *Biol Psychiatry* 1999; 45:247–253.

Mayberg HS, Brannan SK, Mahurin RK, et al.: Cingulate function in depression: a potential predictor of treatment response. *Neuroreport* 1997; 8:1057–1061.

Patrick JT, Nolting MN, Goss SA, et al.: Ultrasound and the blood-brain barrier. *Adv Exp Med Biol* 1990; 267:369–381.

Rauch SL: Advances in neuroimaging research: How might they influence our diagnostic classification scheme? *Harvard Rev Psychiatry* 1996; 4:159–162.

Rauch SL, Dougherty DD, Shin LM, et al.: Neural correlates of factor-analyzed OCD symptom dimensions: a PET study. *CNS Spectrums* 1998; 3:37–43.

Reiman EM, Caselli RJ, Yun LS, et al.: Preclinical evidence of Alzheimer's disease in persons homozygous for the epsilon 4 allele for apolipoprotein E. *N Engl J Med* 1996; 334:752–758.

Swedo SE, Leonard HL, Garvey M, et al.: Pediatric autoimmune neuropsychiatric disorders associated with streptococcal infections: clinical description of the first 50 cases. *Am J Psychiatry* 1998; 155:264–271.

Questions and Answers

Questions

1. All of the following statements about DSM-IV are true EXCEPT

   (A) DSM-IV allows multiple diagnoses to be given to an individual when the symptoms at presentation meet criteria for more than one disorder.
   (B) Clinical judgment is necessary in making diagnostic decisions when the symptoms present difficult diagnostic boundaries.
   (C) DSM-IV addresses etiology and treatment as they relate to the various disorders.
   (D) DSM-IV specifies other disorders that should be considered during the evaluation of criteria for a certain disorder.
   (E) DSM-IV definitions of a mental disorder may involve impairment in more than one function.

2. The process of revising the DSM-III-R to produce the DSM-IV included each of the following EXCEPT

   (A) comprehensive and systematic reviews of the published literature on the various disorders
   (B) re-analysis of data that had already been collected
   (C) development of designated work groups to address each of the diagnostic categories
   (D) surveys of mental health professionals regarding their utilization of previous revisions of the DSM
   (E) extensive issue-focused field trials to evaluate the criteria sets for the various disorder

3. Which of the following are developmentally associated with the preschool years?

   (A) initiative vs. guilt
   (B) egocentricity
   (C) magical thinking
   (D) associative logic
   (E) all of the above

4. According to Erikson, what is the maladaptive function of adolescence?

   (A) despair
   (B) inferiority
   (C) stagnation
   (D) role confusion
   (E) isolation

5. A 2-year-old child is typically capable of all of the following EXCEPT

   (A) climbing stairs
   (B) building an eight-cube tower
   (C) giving his or her first name
   (D) using 50 words
   (E) playing interactive games

6. Risk factors for child abuse include all of the following EXCEPT

   (A) poverty
   (B) low birth weight
   (C) being a handicapped child
   (D) being behaviorally disordered
   (E) having a parent who was abused

7. The concept of conservation develops during which of Piaget's stages?

   (A) pre-operational
   (B) sensorimotor
   (C) formal operations
   (D) concrete operations
   (E) phallic

8. At approximately what age does stranger anxiety develop?

   (A) 6 weeks
   (B) 4 months
   (C) 8 months
   (D) 12 months
   (E) 24 months

9. Each of the following is true about attention deficit hyperactivity disorder (ADHD) EXCEPT

   (A) ADHD is the most common psychiatric disorder in children.
   (B) The disorder does not persist into adulthood.
   (C) Symptoms must be present before the age of 7 years.
   (D) Impairment in functioning must occur in more than one setting.
   (E) Stimulants are the first line of treatment.

10. TRUE or FALSE. A child with Asperger's disorder has a cognitive and language development that falls in the normal range.

11. TRUE or FALSE. Social phobia is the only anxiety disorder listed in the DSM-IV as a childhood disorder.

12. TRUE or FALSE. Children are slower metabolizers of medications than adults and may require half the weight-corrected doses of medications as adults.

13. In addition to memory impairment, each of the following may provide evidence of dementia EXCEPT

   (A) aphasia
   (B) apraxia
   (C) agnosia
   (D) executive dysfunction
   (E) anhedonia

14. In distinguishing delirium from dementia, each of the following characteristics of delirium may be useful EXCEPT

   (A) an acute or subacute onset
   (B) hallucinations
   (C) a fluctuating course
   (D) impaired attention
   (E) an impaired level of consciousness

15. TRUE or FALSE. By DSM-IV criteria, depression cannot be diagnosed in a patient with dementia.

16. Each of the following drugs is commonly associated with impaired cognitive function EXCEPT

    (A) antihypertensives
    (B) narcotics
    (C) benzodiazepines
    (D) SSRIs
    (E) anticholinergics

17. Infectious etiologies associated with dementia include each of the following EXCEPT

    (A) neurosyphilis
    (B) HIV infection
    (C) Creutzfeldt-Jakob disease
    (D) miliary tuberculosis
    (E) *Escherichia coli* in the urinary tract

18. Each of the following blood tests is recommended by the American Academy of Neurology's practice guidelines when screening for dementia EXCEPT

    (A) an ESR
    (B) a vitamin B_{12} level
    (C) a complete blood count
    (D) a thyroid function test
    (E) a syphilis serology

19. TRUE or FALSE. In the early or intermediate stages of Alzheimer's disease, patients may develop impairment of short-term memory, become lost easily, and have difficulty with word-finding.

20. TRUE or FALSE. Delusions and hallucinations are very unusual in Alzheimer's disease.

21. Characteristic features of dementia with Lewy bodies include each of the following EXCEPT

    (A) incontinence
    (B) well-formed visual hallucinations
    (C) parkinsonism
    (D) fluctuating cognitive impairment
    (E) memory impairment

22. Each of the following features are typical of normal pressure hydrocephalus EXCEPT

    (A) magnetic gait
    (B) dementia
    (C) urinary incontinence
    (D) visual hallucinations
    (E) improvement following serial lumbar punctures

23. Drugs which have been shown to have some benefit in Alzheimer's disease include each of these EXCEPT

    (A) tacrine
    (B) donepezil
    (C) vitamin E
    (D) L-dopa
    (E) selegiline

24. Activities of daily living include each of the following EXCEPT

   (A) bathing
   (B) dressing
   (C) using the telephone
   (D) toileting
   (E) feeding

25. The prevalence of mental retardation in the general population is

   (A) 1%
   (B) 2%
   (C) 3%
   (D) 4%
   (E) 5%

26. Which of the following is the most common identified genetic cause of mental retardation?

   (A) Fragile X syndrome
   (B) PKU
   (C) Down's syndrome
   (D) Prader-Willi syndrome
   (E) Lead poisoning

27. The most common identified inherited cause of mental retardation is

   (A) Fragile X syndrome
   (B) PKU
   (C) Down's syndrome
   (D) Williams syndrome
   (E) Lead poisoning

28. The most likely chromosomal abnormality associated with Down's syndrome is

   (A) chromosome 7 deletion
   (B) chromosome 15 deletion
   (C) trisomy 21
   (D) q27, long arm of X chromosome
   (E) trisomy 15

29. The most likely chromosomal abnormality associated with Prader-Willi syndrome is

   (A) chromosome 7 deletion
   (B) chromosome 15 deletion
   (C) trisomy 21
   (D) q27, long arm of X chromosome
   (E) trisomy 15

30. The most likely chromosomal abnormality associated with fragile X syndrome is

   (A) chromosome 7 deletion
   (B) chromosome 15 deletion
   (C) trisomy 21
   (D) q27, long arm of X chromosome
   (E) trisomy 15

31. The most likely chromosomal abnormality associated with Williams syndrome is

    (A) chromosome 7 deletion
    (B) chromosome 15 deletion
    (C) trisomy 21
    (D) q27, long arm of X chromosome
    (E) trisomy 15

32. Individuals with autism/pervasive developmental disorder have mental retardation approximately what percent of the time?

    (A) 10%
    (B) 25%
    (C) 50%
    (D) 75%
    (E) 100%

33. Which of the following is the most common comorbid psychiatric condition with fragile X syndrome?

    (A) OCD
    (B) PTSD
    (C) GAD
    (D) ADHD
    (E) bulimia

34. Individuals with Down's syndrome have a high incidence which of the following?

    (A) multi-infarct dementia
    (B) Alzheimer's dementia
    (C) dementia pugilistica
    (D) NPH
    (E) all of the above

35. Mental disorder due to a general medical condition (DTGMC) should be part of the differential diagnosis for

    (A) any psychiatric syndrome
    (B) a psychiatric syndrome in anyone with no previous psychiatric history
    (C) a psychiatric syndrome accompanied by constitutional signs, such as fever or weight loss
    (D) a psychiatric syndrome that does not meet the criteria for a recognized DSM-IV disorder
    (E) a psychiatric syndrome with persistent symptoms

For the following questions (36–39) one or more of the four suggested responses is correct

    (A) 1, 2, and 3 are correct
    (B) 1 and 3 are correct
    (C) 2 and 4 are correct
    (D) 4 is correct
    (E) All are correct

36. Neurosyphilis, or general paresis

    (1) is seen in 20% of untreated syphilitics, 10 years after primary infection.
    (2) is rare in the postpenicillin era, although it may be on the rise among individuals with AIDS.
    (3) is associated with diffuse, but especially temporal lobe, involvement, with memory and cognitive deficits being the most common early signs.
    (4) when untreated, has classic neurological signs which include tremor, dysarthria, hyperreflexia, hypotonia, and ataxia.

37. Epilepsy is a common neurologic disorder (1% lifetime prevalence) characterized by episodic, disorganized firing of electrical impulses in the cortex of the brain. Which other statements are correct?

    (1) Epilepsy is manifest by nonconvulsive seizures, most commonly partial seizures in 60% of patients; 40% do not show classical focal findings on the EEG.
    (2) Complex partial seizures, often of temporal lobe or other limbic origin, are associated with a 6–12-fold increased risk of psychosis over the general population.
    (3) Depression occurs in more than half of patients with epilepsy, as compared to 30% of matched (medical and neurologic outpatient) controls.
    (4) The suicide rate in patients with epilepsy is five times that of the general public; in patients with temporal lobe epilepsy, the risk may be 25-fold higher than for the general public.

38. The following manifestations of panic attacks help differentiate panic attacks from partial seizures

    (1) They occur "out of the blue."
    (2) They present with hyperarousal, intense fear, perceptual distortion, and dissociative symptoms, such as depersonalization or derealization.
    (3) They respond to benzodiazepines.
    (4) They last 10–20 min with memory of the event intact.

39. In multiple sclerosis

    (1) Psychiatric symptoms may precede physical symptoms.
    (2) Euphoria is the most common mood disturbance.
    (3) Psychiatric symptoms do not clear with remission of physical symptoms.
    (4) Psychiatric symptoms correlate with MRI findings, severity of physical symptoms, and length of illness.

40. TRUE or FALSE. Brain tumors, such as gliomas, multiple metastases, and lymphoma tend to cause diffuse symptoms (e.g., cognitive decline), whereas meningiomas cause more focal, progressive symptoms.

41. TRUE or FALSE. Repeated episodes of hypoglycemia may cause permanent amnesia from hippocampal involvement.

42. The effects of cocaine use during pregnancy include all the following EXCEPT

    (A) fetal growth retardation
    (B) potential brain developmental problems secondary to hyperperfusion of the brain
    (C) rapid transmission of cocaine across the placenta
    (D) the presence of cocaine in breast milk in sufficient amounts to cause observable symptoms, such as increased blood pressure, rapid heart rate, and mydriasis in the newborn
    (E) decreased birth weight and malformations of the urogenital system of the newborn

43. Which of the following statements is TRUE regarding the onset of action and the duration of the high associated with different forms of cocaine?

    (A) For "crack" cocaine the onset of action is 10 sec and the duration of the high is 1–2 min.
    (B) For intranasal cocaine the onset of action is 2–3 min and the duration of the high is 10–15 min.
    (C) For "freebase" cocaine the onset of action is 10 sec and the duration of the high is 5–10 min.
    (D) For intravenous cocaine the onset of action is 10 sec and the duration of the high is 10–20 min.
    (E) For ingestion of coca leaves the onset of action is 20–30 min and the duration of the high is 30–60 min.

44. All of the following are potential medical complications from cocaine EXCEPT

    (A) Cocaine increases the oxygen demand of the heart.
    (B) Although cocaine is measured in breast milk up to 60 h after use, it is not in sufficient quantities to cause physiological effects in the infant.
    (C) Single photon emission computed tomography (SPECT) has demonstrated significant hypoperfusion in the frontal and temporal-parietal areas of the brain. These findings correlate with cognitive impairment.
    (D) A syndrome consisting of fever, shortness of breath, chest pain, and pneumonia is associated with cocaine use.
    (E) Nasal septum necrosis due to vasoconstriction may occur from cocaine use.

45. All of the following statements regarding comorbid psychiatric disorders and opiate use are true EXCEPT

    (A) 80–90% of opiate-dependent individuals carry a lifetime diagnosis of a psychiatric disorder.
    (B) It can be difficult to distinguish between a primary mood disorder and an opiate-dependent mood disorder.
    (C) Except for cigarettes, amphetamine is the most common comorbid substance used by opiate addicts.
    (D) Major depressive disorder and antisocial personality disorder are the two most common comorbid psychiatric disorders in opiate-dependent individuals.
    (E) Children and adolescents with conduct disorder are at greater risk of developing substance abuse problems.

46. Females with schizophrenia tend to have

    (A) a later age of onset than males with schizophrenia
    (B) a poorer course than males with schizophrenia
    (C) a lower lifetime prevalence than males with schizophrenia
    (D) no change in their clinical course after menopause
    (E) the onset of illness before age 30 is found in 50% of cases

47. Negative symptoms of schizophrenia include

    (A) apathy
    (B) angst
    (C) altruism
    (D) hallucinations
    (E) all of the above

48. TRUE or FALSE. Dizygotic twins have a greater concordance rate for schizophrenia than do monozygotic twins.

49. What percentage of the general population will be diagnosed with a manic episode at some point in their lifetime?

    (A) 1%
    (B) 5%
    (C) 10%
    (D) 20%
    (E) 50%

50. A 27-year-old male reports daily depressed mood for 3 months, with decreased sleep, interest, appetite, and energy. He denies any period of euphoric mood in the last few years, but he reports irritable mood for the past month. He denies decreased need for sleep, flight of ideas, or increased talkativeness. His wife reports that he has been spending more money recently. What is the most likely diagnosis?

    (A) bipolar disorder
    (B) cyclothymia
    (C) dysthymia
    (D) unipolar depression
    (E) cocaine intoxication

51. A 35-year-old male reports daily depressed mood for 3 months, with decreased sleep, appetite and energy, and increased guilt and suicidal ideation. He denies any period of euphoric mood in the last few years, but he reports irritable mood for the past month. He denies decreased need for sleep, but reports flight of ideas, increased talkativeness, distractibility, and increased sexual interest. He denies spending sprees. What is the most likely diagnosis?

    (A) a major depressive episode in bipolar disorder
    (B) a hypomanic episode in bipolar disorder
    (C) a manic episode in bipolar disorder
    (D) a mixed episode of bipolar disorder
    (E) cocaine intoxication

52. A 26-year-old female reports daily depressed mood for 6 months with increased sleep and appetite, and decreased interest and concentration. Upon questioning, she denies any periods of euphoric mood but her spouse admits "a few days" of "up" mood "every now and then," with increased energy, decreased need for sleep, increased house cleaning, and increased talkativeness. She denies that those "up" periods interfere with her function; in fact, she functions better during those periods. What is the most likely diagnosis?

    (A) bipolar disorder, type I
    (B) cyclothymia
    (C) dysthymia
    (D) unipolar disorder
    (E) bipolar disorder, type II

53. Ideally, what is the BEST first treatment in a patient with bipolar disorder, type II?

    (A) an antidepressant
    (B) cognitive-behavioral psychotherapy
    (C) lithium
    (D) an anti-anxiety agent
    (E) ECT

54. Which statement best describes an epidemiological feature of bipolar disorder?

    (A) Genetic inheritance in bipolar disorder is mendelian.
    (B) Females more commonly have bipolar disorder than males.
    (C) About one-fifth of persons with bipolar disorder commit suicide.
    (D) The psychosocial outcome of bipolar disorder is invariably poor.
    (E) Most primary mood disorders begin above the age of 40 years.

55. Each of the following are cardinal DSM-IV criteria for mania EXCEPT

    (A) euphoria
    (B) hypersomnia
    (C) irritability
    (D) increased talkativeness
    (E) distractibility

56. A mixed episode of mania and depression could be characterized by all of the following EXCEPT

    (A) depressed mood
    (B) irritable mood
    (C) decreased sleep
    (D) flat affect
    (E) guilt

57. Which of the following is NOT TRUE?

    (A) Distractibility is a central feature of bipolar disorder.
    (B) Psychosis occurs in 50% of lifetime mood episodes in bipolar disorder.
    (C) Rapid-cycling bipolar disorder is characterized by weekly mood episodes.
    (D) The kindling hypothesis predicts more episodes later in the course of bipolar illness.
    (E) Antidepressants can cause mania.

58. Which of the following is TRUE?

    (A) Antidepressants should never be used in bipolar disorder.
    (B) An antidepressant plus a mood stabilizer is good treatment for bipolar depression.
    (C) Antidepressants prevent depressive episodes in bipolar disorder.
    (D) Mood stabilizers have no effect on acute depression in bipolar disorder.
    (E) All antidepressants have the same risk of causing mania.

59. Which agent would be preferable in a patient with bipolar depression?

    (A) imipramine
    (B) fluoxetine
    (C) sertraline
    (D) bupropion
    (E) trazodone

60. What percentage of patients who meet criteria for a psychiatric disorder have a somatic symptom as their chief complaint?

    (A) <2%
    (B) 5–10%
    (C) 10–25%
    (D) 50–75%
    (E) >90%

61. Each of the following should be considered by the physician as a possible cause of a patient's presentation with a somatoform disorder EXCEPT

    (A) to atone unconsciously for a perceived guilt by physical suffering.
    (B) to hold onto a past symptom of their own or that of a loved one to express current distress.
    (C) to unconsciously avoid the social stigma of psychiatric illness.
    (D) to communicate a need or wish to be cared for when the patient does not have access to the proper words due to alexithymia.
    (E) to intentionally make the physician's life miserable.

62. The triad of bodily preoccupation, disease fear, and disease conviction is central to the diagnosis of

    (A) somatization disorder
    (B) pain disorder
    (C) conversion disorder
    (D) hypochondriasis
    (E) factitious illness

63. The disorder marked by many symptoms, some accompanied by pain and some not, spanning different organ systems over a great number of years and marked by inconsistency of symptom recall at each physician follow-up visit is

    (A) somatization disorder
    (B) pain disorder
    (C) conversion disorder
    (D) hypochondriasis
    (E) body dysmorphic disorder

64. The somatoform disorder which classically presents with a pseudoneurologic symptom is

    (A) somatization disorder
    (B) pain disorder
    (C) conversion disorder
    (D) hypochondriasis
    (E) body dysmorphic disorder

65. Each of the following treatments for somatoform disorder have been shown to be helpful EXCEPT

    (A) confronting the patient with the diagnosis
    (B) ordering workups based on objective findings rather than on symptom report
    (C) obtaining a psychiatric consultation
    (D) treatment with SSRIs
    (E) making a referral to group, individual, family, and/or cognitive behavioral therapy

66. Which of the following features has NOT been shown to increase the risk of dissociative episodes?

    (A) younger age
    (B) female gender
    (C) history of childhood trauma
    (D) LSD use
    (E) exposure to a civilian disaster

67. Which of the following features are NOT usually consistent with dissociative identity disorder (DID)?

    (A) internally experienced auditory hallucinations
    (B) complaints by a patient that he or she does not recall a recent behavior
    (C) disorganized speech
    (D) a prevalence that is more common in women
    (E) a dominant personality identity

68. Which of the following statements about the diagnosis of dissociative disorders is FALSE?

    (A) The Dissociative Experience Scale is reliable and cannot be faked.
    (B) Patients who are more hypnotizable are also more likely to experience dissociation.
    (C) The Standardized Clinical Interview for Dissociative Disorders (SCID-D) has achieved face validity only.
    (D) The Minnesota Multiphasic Personality Inventory has not been validated for diagnosing dissociative disorders.
    (E) Patients who are more likely to dissociate are also more easily hypnotized.

69. Which of the following statements regarding dissociative amnesia is TRUE?

    (A) Gender incidence is roughly equal.
    (B) 75% of cases never resolve.
    (C) Amnestic episodes always involve the inability to recall traumatic experiences, but have preserved autobiographical information.
    (D) Recovered patients rarely continue to display a propensity towards future episodes.
    (E) Lost memories are always of a traumatic nature.

70. Dissociative fugue

    (A) is more common during times of peace.
    (B) is more common in men during times of war and peace.
    (C) is commonly caused by illicit substances.
    (D) is sometimes treated with hypnosis or an Amytal interview.
    (E) presents most often in early adolescence.

71. Which of the following statements does NOT apply to dissociative identity disorder (DID)?

    (A) DID was formerly called multiple personality disorder.
    (B) The incidence of reported new cases of DID has been stable over the last two decades.
    (C) DID is more common in patients with a history of trauma.
    (D) Different personality states are sometimes called "alters."
    (E) Somatic complaints may accompany DID.

72. Depersonalization disorder

    (A) is not a formal DSM-IV diagnosis.
    (B) occurs equally in males and females.
    (C) typically lasts from hours to weeks.
    (D) is more common than transient depersonalization.
    (E) is usually easily treated.

73. Feigned dissociative symptoms

    (A) occur in less than 5% of those presenting with dissociative complaints.
    (B) result exclusively from a need to assume the sick role.
    (C) should be suspected when the patient knows little about dissociative diagnoses.
    (D) include the cultural-bound syndrome of Amok.
    (E) should be suspected when the patient appears extremely invested in the diagnosis of a dissociative disorder.

74. Dissociative disorder not otherwise specified might include

    (A) LSD-induced dissociation
    (B) dissociation caused by symptoms of a brain tumor
    (C) patients who complain of paralysis in the absence of a clear medical etiology
    (D) patients who present with two distinct and relatively enduring personality identities
    (E) patients who have been brainwashed

75. Which the following statements is FALSE?

    (A) Amok and Latah are classified as dissociative trance disorders.
    (B) Ganser's syndrome consists of giving partially correct answers to seemingly simple questions.
    (C) Dissociative trance disorder could in the future include patients who feel they are demonically possessed.
    (D) Reports of dissociative disorders increase during times of natural disaster.
    (E) Pierre Janet was instrumental in the early study of dissociation.

76. TRUE or FALSE. The basic physiologic responses of the human body (male and female) to sexual stimulation are widespread vasocongestion and a generalized increase in muscle tension.

77. TRUE or FALSE. Estrogen replacement (with the addition of progesterone in women with a uterus) is the most effective way of reversing vaginal atrophy and improving the sexual well-being in the menopausal woman.

78. TRUE or FALSE. Incest occurs in lower and upper class families with approximately equal frequency.

79. TRUE or FALSE. Menopause appears to have some impact on sexual functioning, but may be less important than other factors, such as physical and mental health, partner limitations, and lifestyle.

For the following two questions answer according to the following format:

(A) 1, 2, and 3 are correct
(B) 1 and 3 are correct
(C) 2 and 4 are correct
(D) 4 is correct
(E) all are correct

80. TRUE statements about premature ejaculation include

(1) Most men experience premature ejaculation at some time in their lives.
(2) Men with chronic premature ejaculation often give a history of withdrawal as a contraceptive technique.
(3) Chronic premature ejaculation often is complicated by subsequent acquired impotence.
(4) The sexual partners of men with premature ejaculation are usually orgasmic.

81. Which of the following statements are TRUE?

(1) Transvestites are usually homosexuals.
(2) Transsexuals usually have underlying psychoses.
(3) Voyeurs and exhibitionists generally have a history of serious psychological, drug, or criminal problems.
(4) A rapist is more likely to seriously physically injure a woman if she offers resistance.

82. TRUE or FALSE. A young woman with anorexia nervosa is 5 feet 4 inches and weighs 85 lb; she is eating some food at each meal, but has been losing 1 pound every 2 weeks. Inpatient care is probably indicated for this patient.

83. TRUE or FALSE. Estrogen replacement therapy can help to prevent bone loss in women with anorexia nervosa.

84. TRUE or FALSE. The majority of individuals with anorexia nervosa can be expected to make a full recovery.

85. TRUE or FALSE. Individuals with anorexia nervosa should generally be given a trial of an SSRI or other antidepressant medication.

86. TRUE or FALSE. Binge-eating disorder is the most prevalent eating disorder.

87. TRUE or FALSE. Medications are more effective in treating the symptoms of bulimia nervosa than is psychotherapy.

88. Which of the following is the more correct sequence for the NREM-REM cycle?

(A) Stage 1, Stage 2, REM, Stage 4, Stage 3, Stage 2
(B) Stage 3, Stage 2, REM, Stage 2, Stage 3, Stage 4
(C) Stage 2, REM, Stage 1, Stage 2, Stage 3, Stage 2
(D) Stage 1, Stage 2, REM, Stage 2, Stage 1, Stage 2
(E) Stage 1, Stage 2, Stage 3, REM, Stage 2, Stage 1

89. All of the following are true about sleep EXCEPT

   (A) Sleep latency is the time from lights out to the first NREM 1.
   (B) Sleep efficiency is the total sleep time divided by the total sleep record time.
   (C) NREM 3 and 4 are most prominent in the first half of the night.
   (D) REM increases over the course of the night.
   (E) REM latency is generally 90–100 min.

90. With regard to sleep in the elderly

   (A) While the total amount of sleep decreases, sleep efficiency increases.
   (B) Total REM time is reduced.
   (C) Sleep latency and REM latency increase.
   (D) NREM 3 and 4 increase, while REM decreases.
   (E) None of the above are true.

91. All of the following are features of narcolepsy EXCEPT

   (A) hypnagogic hallucinations
   (B) onset in late teens to early 20s
   (C) catalepsy
   (D) sleep-onset REM periods (SOREMPs)
   (E) normal total sleep time over a 24-h period

92. Sleep apnea

   (A) Is more common in men than women.
   (B) Is the most common organic disorder of excessive daytime sleepiness.
   (C) Is best treated with continuous positive airway pressure.
   (D) Is less common in premenopausal women than postmenopausal women.
   (E) All of the above are true.

93. All of the following statements are true with regards to periodic limb movements (PLM) and restless leg syndrome (RLS) EXCEPT

   (A) L-dopa can be used in the treatment of both disorders.
   (B) Both disorders are often quite painful.
   (C) Hypersomnia is a common complaint for patients with either disorder.
   (D) RLS affects sleep initiation more than PLM does.
   (E) SSRIs can exacerbate both conditions.

94. Which of the following is TRUE regarding parasomnias?

   (A) Adults are affected more than children.
   (B) Patients often have vivid recall for the events.
   (C) Patients rarely have more than one type.
   (D) REM behavior disorder is perhaps the most common form encountered.
   (E) None of the above are true.

95. Which of the following statements are TRUE with regard to night terrors?

   (A) They consist of terrifying dreams that are remembered by the patient.
   (B) They are a REM phenomenon.
   (C) They have accompanying autonomic arousal and occur early in the night.
   (D) Patients are easily awakened from them.
   (E) None of the above are true.

96. Mr. R, a 71-year-old retired farmer with a history of hypertension and diabetes, presents to a sleep disorder unit with a complaint of "strange things happening" when he sleeps at night. While laughing, he and his wife relate that he often gets out of bed at night, straddles the night stand, and begins shouting "yee haw." When his wife wakes him up, he reports that he was having the "bull riding dream" again. The most likely diagnosis is

    (A) nightmare disorder
    (B) pavor nocturnus
    (C) sleepwalking
    (D) REM behavior disorder
    (E) malingering

97. With regard to REM behavior disorder

    (A) Males are more commonly affected than females.
    (B) There is an association with brainstem pathology.
    (C) The phenomenon occurs due to loss of REM muscle atonia.
    (D) Can be treated with low-dose clonazepam.
    (E) All of the above are true.

98. The following are features of sleep are TRUE in relation to psychosis

    (A) Total sleep time is increased.
    (B) REM is rarely affected.
    (C) Problems with sleep initiation and maintenance are most common.
    (D) REM time is increased.
    (E) All of the above are true.

99. All of the following are TRUE in relation to sleep disturbance and depression EXCEPT

    (A) There is early morning awakening.
    (B) There is increased REM latency.
    (C) There is increased REM density.
    (D) There is increased sleep with atypical depression.
    (E) There are frequent awakenings.

100. Which of the following are TRUE in relation to sleep disturbance and anxiety disorders?

    (A) Anxiety is the most common psychiatric cause of insomnia.
    (B) Sleep initiation is disturbed in anxiety disorder.
    (C) Sleep efficiency is decreased in anxiety disorder.
    (D) Sleep maintenance is poor in anxiety disorder.
    (E) All of the above are true.

101. Which is the correct order of EEG findings as one proceeds from NREM 1 to 4?

    (A) theta waves, sleep spindles, K-complexes, delta waves, alpha waves
    (B) alpha waves, sleep spindles, delta waves, K-complexes, theta waves
    (C) alpha waves, theta waves, sleep spindles, K-complexes, delta waves
    (D) alpha waves, theta waves, delta waves, K-complexes, sleep spindles
    (E) theta waves, alpha waves, sleep spindles, K-complexes, delta waves

102. Impulse control disorders were first defined in DSM-III in 1980; prior to that time, nomenclature considered these disorders as

  (A) monomanias
  (B) personality disorders
  (C) dyscontrol syndromes
  (D) all of the above
  (E) none of the above

103. Of the following impulse control disorders, which is most common?

  (A) pyromania
  (B) pathologic gambling
  (C) kleptomania
  (D) intermittent explosive disorder
  (E) panic disorder

104. Trichotillomania is a relatively new diagnosis that was added to the DSM-III-R in 1987. Correct statements about trichotillomania include all the following EXCEPT

  (A) Sites for hair pulling include scalp, eyelashes, eyebrows, and pubic hair.
  (B) Initially recognized by dermatologists, both dermatologists and psychiatrists recognized the psychogenic origin; yet, few patients reached psychiatric attention.
  (C) The incidence may be as high as 4% with a bimodal onset in childhood and then later in adolescence. The later-onset is predominately female and chronic compared to the early-onset cohort.
  (D) Patients tend to be fully aware of their part in losing hair.
  (E) They seek attention from the medical community for their hair loss.

105. Treatment for the impulse control disorder NOS is very inclusive and unpredictable. Which of the following are NOT useful treatments?

  (A) ECT
  (B) behavioral therapy
  (C) family therapy
  (D) use of SSRIs
  (E) mood stabilizers and atypical neuroleptics

106. Head-injured patients exhibit all of the following impulse control disorders EXCEPT

  (A) kleptomania
  (B) pyromania
  (C) intermittent explosive disorder
  (D) trichotillomania
  (E) pathologic gambling

107. Medical psychiatric conditions associated with intermittent explosive disorder include all of the following EXCEPT

  (A) seizures
  (B) head trauma
  (C) ADHD
  (D) antisocial personality
  (E) HIV seropositivity

108. Which of the following statements is TRUE?

    (A) The process of grieving is uniform across all cultures.
    (B) Denial in the early stages of bereavement is a sign of complicated grief reaction.
    (C) Active suicidality is to be expected in normal bereavement.
    (D) Feelings of anger are a normal part of grieving.
    (E) Acute grief should always be treated with benzodiazepines.

109. During the board examination of a grieving patient it is important to

    (A) Evaluate the severity of neurovegetative symptoms.
    (B) Assess for suicidality.
    (C) Make a brief but sincere expression of sympathy.
    (D) Avoid discouraging a patient's expression of anger at the deceased.
    (E) All of the above are true.

110. Major depression that requires specific intervention may be distinguished from acute grief by

    (A) the presence of insomnia
    (B) the severity of neurovegetative symptoms and disruption of functioning
    (C) the presence of loss of appetite
    (D) the wish to be with the deceased
    (E) guilty feelings

111. Which of the following treatment strategies IS INAPPROPRIATE for a patient with an adjustment disorder?

    (A) individual supportive psychotherapy
    (B) group therapy
    (C) family counseling
    (D) anxiolytic medication
    (E) none of the above

112. The prevalence of premenstrual dysphoric disorder is

    (A) <1%
    (B) 2–5%
    (C) 10–20%
    (D) 20–30%
    (E) 30–40%

113. All of the following are TRUE about psychotropic drug use during pregnancy EXCEPT

    (A) The baseline risk of congenital malformations is 3–4%.
    (B) Misperception of teratogenic risk can lead both physician and patient to terminate otherwise wanted pregnancies or avoid needed pharmacotherapy during pregnancy.
    (C) Prenatal exposure to tricyclic antidepressants does not increase the baseline risk of congenital malformations.
    (D) Carbamazepine is associated with a 20% risk of neural tube defects following first trimester exposure.
    (E) Lithium use during the first trimester has been associated with a 0.05–0.1% risk of Ebstein's anomaly.

114. All of the following are TRUE about hormone replacement therapy (HRT) EXCEPT

    (A) HRT may alleviate mild mood symptoms along with certain physical symptoms, such as vaginal dryness.
    (B) HRT can reduce the risk of osteoporosis and heart disease.
    (C) HRT is associated with an increased risk of uterine cancer.
    (D) HRT has been proven to be an effective monotherapy for major depression.
    (E) HRT can sometimes induce mood or anxiety symptoms.

115. All of the following are TRUE about breastfeeding and psychotropic medications EXCEPT

    (A) All psychotropic medications are secreted in the breast-milk.
    (B) Nursing mothers who require psychotropic medications must balance the risks of infant exposure and the benefits to both the mother and baby.
    (C) For most psychotropic medications, the drug accumulation in the infant's serum is directly proportional to the mother's dose.
    (D) Breastfeeding is associated with decreased incidence of otitis media in infants.
    (E) Women should be cautioned not to breastfeed while taking lithium since infants can develop dangerously high lithium levels, especially if they become dehydrated.

116. All of the following are correct statements about clozapine EXCEPT

    (A) It is a strong dopamine D_2 antagonist.
    (B) It has anticholinergic side effects.
    (C) It may cause agranulocytosis.
    (D) It produces dopamine supersensitivity in the nigrostriatal dopamine neurons.
    (E) It may cause weight gain.

117. Which of the following is TRUE?

    (A) Cigarette smoking may increase neuroleptic blood levels.
    (B) Anticholinergic agents may improve tardive dyskinesia.
    (C) Selective serotonin reuptake inhibitors (SSRIs) may increase neuroleptic blood levels.
    (D) Carbamazepine may increase neuroleptic blood levels.
    (E) Effective lithium blood levels are 1.5–2.5 mEq/L.

118. All of the following may be considered atypical antipsychotic agents EXCEPT

    (A) clozapine
    (B) fluphenazine
    (C) risperidone
    (D) olanzapine
    (E) quetiapine

119. The following statements are TRUE about medication compliance in schizophrenic patients

    (A) 1, 2, and 3 are correct
    (B) 1 and 3 are correct
    (C) 2 and 4 are correct
    (D) 4 is correct
    (E) all are correct

    (1) Monitoring blood levels may be helpful.
    (2) 30–50% of schizophrenic patients do not take their medications as prescribed.
    (3) Carefully assessing and managing side effects may improve compliance.
    (4) Switching to a depot neuroleptic is often not helpful.

120. Which of the following is NOT contraindicated in a patient being treated with tranylcypromine at 30 mg/day?

    (A) buspirone
    (B) bupropion
    (C) fluvoxamine
    (D) clomipramine
    (E) trazodone

121. Which of the following agents may be MOST LIKELY to cause an acute dystonic reaction?

    (A) clomipramine
    (B) amoxapine
    (C) imipramine
    (D) desipramine
    (E) protriptyline

122. Which of the following is MOST LIKELY to treat obsessive-compulsive disorder (OCD)?

    (A) clomipramine
    (B) amoxapine
    (C) imipramine
    (D) nortriptyline
    (E) doxepin

123. Which of the following is a metabolite of imipramine?

    (A) trimipramine
    (B) amoxapine
    (C) maprotiline
    (D) desipramine
    (E) doxepin

124. Which of the following is MOST LIKELY to induce seizures?

    (A) venlafaxine
    (B) bupropion
    (C) sertraline
    (D) phenelzine
    (E) fluoxetine

125. Which of the following has the longest half-life?

    (A) venlafaxine
    (B) paroxetine
    (C) nortriptyline
    (D) protriptyline
    (E) bupropion

126. Which of the following would be the MOST APPROPRIATE first-line treatment for a woman with unipolar major depression, severe, with psychotic features who is 2 months pregnant?

    (A) sertraline
    (B) venlafaxine
    (C) phenelzine
    (D) ECT
    (E) bupropion

127. For a patient taking nefazodone (Serzone), 600 mg q.h.s., which of the following should be avoided?

    (A) orange juice
    (B) grapefruit juice
    (C) milk
    (D) soda water
    (E) tea

128. Lithium is

 (A) metabolized by the liver
 (B) excreted unchanged by the kidney
 (C) metabolized by the liver and excreted by the kidney
 (D) available in a parenteral form
 (E) none of the above

129. Which of the following side effects of lithium is treatable with propranolol?

 (A) weight gain
 (B) sexual dysfunction
 (C) dry mouth
 (D) tremor
 (E) polyuria

130. Which of the following is NOT TRUE?

 (A) Thiazide diuretics raise lithium levels.
 (B) Thiazide diuretics worsen lithium-induced excessive urination.
 (C) ACE inhibitors raise lithium levels.
 (D) Lithium is as effective in pure mania as valproate.
 (E) Lithium levels should be checked 8–12 h after the last dose

131. Which of the following is NOT TRUE?

 (A) Lithium is a serotonergic drug.
 (B) Classic pure mania predicts good lithium response.
 (C) Lithium is less effective in rapid-cycling bipolar disorder than valproate.
 (D) NSAIDS reduce lithium levels.
 (E) Lithium is less effective in mixed mania than carbamazepine.

132. The MOST common cause of lithium noncompliance is/are

 (A) kidney problems
 (B) hypothyroidism
 (C) impaired cognition
 (D) polyuria
 (E) dry mouth

133. Potentially serious medical side effects of lithium include each of the following EXCEPT

 (A) sick sinus syndrome
 (B) hypothyroidism
 (C) diabetes insipidus
 (D) renal failure
 (E) hepatic failure

134. Which of the following is TRUE?

 (A) Anticonvulsants are as effective as lithium in treating mixed mania.
 (B) Lithium is not effective in treating bipolar depression.
 (C) Antidepressants are more effective than lithium in treating bipolar depression.
 (D) Lithium reduces suicide risk more effectively than anticonvulsants.
 (E) Lithium should routinely be dosed thrice daily.

135. Lithium's main mechanism of action involves

    (A) serotonin
    (B) norepinephrine
    (C) dopamine
    (D) G-proteins
    (E) peptides

136. Which of the following is NOT a side effect of lithium?

    (A) nephrotic syndrome
    (B) sick sinus syndrome
    (C) insulin-like effects
    (D) psoriasis
    (E) leukopenia

137. When taken during pregnancy, lithium is typically associated with which of the following?

    (A) neural tube defects
    (B) Ebstein's anomaly
    (C) Trisomy 21
    (D) Tay-Sachs disease
    (E) cleft lip and palate

138. Which of the following medications have been FDA-approved for the maintenance treatment of bipolar disorder?

    (A) carbamazepine
    (B) gabapentin
    (C) lamotrigine
    (D) valproate
    (E) none of the above

139. Carbamazepine has been shown to be useful in the treatment of each of the following conditions EXCEPT

    (A) acute mania
    (B) maintenance treatment for bipolar disorder
    (C) unipolar major depression
    (D) trigeminal neuralgia
    (E) complex partial seizures

140. Common side effects of valproate include each of the following EXCEPT

    (A) alopecia
    (B) weight gain
    (C) thrombocytopenia
    (D) gastrointestinal upset
    (E) elevated transaminases

141. There is good evidence supporting valproate's efficacy (as a single agent) in treating which of the following conditions

    (A) migraine headache
    (B) bipolar depression
    (C) schizoaffective disorder
    (D) social phobia
    (E) heroin dependency

142. Which of the following anticonvulsants has been shown in double-blind, placebo-controlled trials to treat bipolar depression?

    (A) carbamazepine
    (B) gabapentin
    (C) lamotrigine
    (D) valproate
    (E) none of the above

143. Which of the following statement about gabapentin's properties is NOT TRUE?

    (A) Its absorption is linear.
    (B) It is not protein-bound.
    (C) It is excreted unchanged by the kidneys.
    (D) It has a half-life of 6–7 h.
    (E) It has very few drug interactions.

144. Which of is the following is NOT TRUE about clonazepam?

    (A) It is a solo treatment of petit mal seizures.
    (B) It is a treatment for panic disorder.
    (C) It is an adjunctive treatment of depression with SSRIs.
    (D) It treats peripheral neuropathies.
    (E) It is a sole treatment of mania.

145. Lamotrigine

    (A) binds to GABA receptors
    (B) inhibits presynaptic sodium channels
    (C) decreases the release of glutamate
    (D) antagonizes kainate at AMPA receptors
    (E) modulates the GABA transporter

146. Gabapentin

    (A) binds to GABA receptors
    (B) inhibits presynaptic sodium channels
    (C) decreases the release of glutamate
    (D) antagonizes kainate at AMPA receptors
    (E) modulates the GABA transporter

147. Topiramate

    (A) binds to GABA receptors
    (B) inhibits presynaptic sodium channels
    (C) decreases the release of glutamate
    (D) antagonizes kainate at AMPA receptors
    (E) modulates the GABA transporter

148. Carbamazepine

    (A) binds to GABA receptors
    (B) inhibits presynaptic sodium channels
    (C) decreases the release of glutamate
    (D) antagonizes kainate at AMPA receptors
    (E) modulates the GABA transporter

For questions 149–158 choose the correct answer below using the following key.

(A) 1, 2 and 3 are correct
(B) 1 and 3 are correct
(C) 2 and 4 are correct
(D) 4 is correct
(E) All are correct

149. The following are examples of pharmacokinetic drug-drug interactions:

(1) a decline in lithium levels 3 weeks after starting indomethacin
(2) hypotension during the course of combined treatment with clozapine and trazodone
(3) emergence of theophylline toxicity within several days after adding fluvoxamine (Luvox) to a stable regimen of asthma medications
(4) alleviation of urinary retention on clomipramine (Anafranil) following treatment with bethanechol (Urecholine)

150. The following statements concerning pharmacodynamic drug-drug interactions are TRUE

(1) They are usually signaled by a change in serum levels and/or tissue concentrations of drug.
(2) They are mediated through one of four processes including absorption, distribution, metabolism, and excretion.
(3) They are exemplified by competition for protein-binding sites among highly-bound drugs with a low therapeutic index.
(4) They are not influenced by genetic polymorphisms in cytochrome P450 isoenzyme activity.

151. The most accurate pairings of inhibitor or inducer of an enzyme are

(1) paroxetine – P450 2D6
(2) fluvoxamine – P450 1A2
(3) carbamazepine - P450 3A4
(4) valproate - P450 2C19

152. The following drug-drug interactions are UNLIKELY to occur

(1) protein-binding displacement of warfarin by lithium
(2) diminished effectiveness of oral contraception due to carbamazepine
(3) enhanced clearance of desipramine by methylphenidate
(4) severe rash on lamotrigine prescribed in conjunction with valproate

153. Each of the following statements concerning the cytochrome P450 isoenzymes are true EXCEPT

(1) "Poor metabolizers" are expected to show higher concentrations of substrate, lower concentrations of metabolite, and relatively insensitivity to the effects of isoenzyme inhibitors and inducer.
(2) Genetic polymorphisms are known to exist for P450 2D6 and 2C19.
(3) A potential consequence of inhibition of 2D6 would include diminished efficacy of codeine.
(4) Following administration of nefazodone, levels of carbamazepine are likely to fall.

154. All of the following are true regarding monoamine oxidase inhibitors EXCEPT

(1) The "cheese" reaction to tyramine is related to enzyme inhibition in the gut.
(2) Oxymetazoline and guaifenesin are among the only acceptable over-the-counter cold remedies.
(3) Following discontinuation of fluoxetine, 5 weeks should elapse before initiation of an MAOI.
(4) The activity of hypoglycemic agents are likely to be reduced when co-administered with MAOIs.

155. All of the following drug combinations are contraindicated EXCEPT

(1) venlafaxine-phenelzine
(2) lithium-ritonavir
(3) nefazodone-cisapride (Propulsid)
(4) bupropion-cyclosporine

156. All of the following are likely to be inhibit metabolism of co-administered drugs EXCEPT

   (1) macrolide antibiotics
   (2) fluoroquinolone antibiotics
   (3) isoniazid
   (4) rifampin

157. Agents that can result in diminished lithium clearance include

   (1) thiazide diuretics
   (2) ACE inhibitors
   (3) metronidazole
   (4) sodium bicarbonate

158. Plausible drug-drug interactions include ALL of the following EXCEPT

   (1) potentiation of clonidine alpha-2-adrenergic activity by mirtazapine
   (2) diminished clozapine effects when co-administered with fluvoxamine
   (3) antagonism of cardiac conduction delay by calcium channel blockers when co-administered with pimozide
   (4) reversal of CNS depression following benzodiazepine overdose with physostigmine or flumazenil

159. Effective principles to enhance safety and compliance with use of medications include all EXCEPT

   (A) Use the lowest effective dose and slowly titrate the dose.
   (B) Anticipate with the patient the potential side effects.
   (C) When minor side effects occur, switch to another agent.
   (D) Reassure the patient that most side effects abate with time.
   (E) Give clearly written instructions to the patient.

160. Which is the LEAST likely to cause orthostatic hypotension?

   (A) imipramine
   (B) desipramine
   (C) amitriptyline
   (D) nortriptyline
   (E) phenelzine

161. You are called to see a 55-year-old cardiac patient who is on nortriptyline and risperidone. The optimal initial work-up includes all of the following EXCEPT

   (A) an echocardiogram
   (B) a magnesium blood level
   (C) a potassium blood level
   (D) orthostatic blood pressures
   (E) an electrocardiogram

162. Common neurological side effects caused by psychotropic medications are matched with optimal treatment. Which answer is INCORRECT?

   (A) akathisia – low-dose beta-blockers or benzodiazepines
   (B) tremor – low-dose beta-blockers or benzodiazepines
   (C) increased anxiety - benzodiazepines
   (D) acute dystonia - discontinuation of the offending medication
   (E) parkinsonism – dose reduction or anticholinergic medications

163. Neuroleptic malignant syndrome (NMS) is a life-threatening complication of antipsychotic medications. The symptoms include all of the following EXCEPT

(A) an increased creatine phosphokinase
(B) agitation
(C) delirium
(D) autonomic dysfunction
(E) involuntary movements of the face or hands

164. Medications that impair the hematological system include all of the following EXCEPT

(A) clozapine
(B) lithium
(C) carbamazepine
(D) valproic acid
(E) all of the above

165. A 55-year-old patient is recovering from a myocardial infarction. You are consulted for a question of depression and diagnose him with major depression. The LEAST appropriate medication to initiate is

(A) sertraline
(B) nortriptyline
(C) bupropion
(D) venlafaxine
(E) phenelzine

166. A 45-year-old patient with bipolar illness has achieved mood stability with lithium, having failed all other medications. The patient has a urine output of greater than 2 L/day. Which statement is FALSE?

(A) Polyuria can occur in up to 70% of patients with long-term lithium treatment.
(B) The patient has nephrogenic diabetes insipidus.
(C) 10% of lithium-treated patients are diagnosed with nephrogenic diabetes insipidus.
(D) Treatment includes maintaining the lowest effect lithium dose and administering the drug at a single bedtime dose.
(E) Potassium-sparing and thiazide diuretics markedly reduce urine volume caused by nephrogenic diabetes insipidus.

167. Which antipsychotic medication has the LEAST amount of weight gain associated with it?

(A) clozapine (Clozaril)
(B) haloperidol (Haldol)
(C) pimozide (Orap)
(D) quetiapine (Seroquel)
(E) molindone (Moban)

168. A 60-year-old patient on thioridazine presents with delirium, psychosis, an elevated temperature, urinary retention, dry skin, and flushing. Which of the following is the best treatment option?

(A) an anticholinergic medication (diphenhydramine)
(B) a muscle relaxant (dantrolene)
(C) an alpha-1-adrenergic antagonist (phentolamine)
(D) a dopaminergic agent (bromocriptine)
(E) an anticholinesterase (physostigmine)

169. Which of the following features has NOT been shown to be associated with an increased risk for suicide?

   (A) a history of prior attempts
   (B) a history of substance abuse
   (C) a sense of hopelessness
   (D) presence of a terminal illness
   (E) recent travel abroad

170. Which of the following areas of information is NOT useful when assessing the lethality of a prior suicide attempt?

   (A) the method used in attempt
   (B) the likelihood of rescue
   (C) the patient's understanding of how dangerous the method was
   (D) the location of the attempt
   (E) the patient's gender and race

171. Which of the following familial factors does NOT increase risk for suicide?

   (A) a family history of suicide attempt
   (B) a family history of psychiatric illness
   (C) a family history of stroke
   (D) a history of sexual or physical abuse
   (E) the recent death of a family member

172. Which of the following individual factors does NOT increase the risk of suicide?

   (A) having a firearm in the home
   (B) being a parent with young children
   (C) living alone
   (D) having legal difficulties
   (E) being unemployed

173. Which of the following psychiatric illnesses is MOST OFTEN present in patients who commit suicide?

   (A) schizophrenia
   (B) generalized anxiety disorder
   (C) personality disorder
   (D) major depression
   (E) obsessive-compulsive disorder

174. TRUE or FALSE. Akathisia is a risk factor for suicide in psychotic patients.

175. TRUE or FALSE. Patients who express suicidal ideation only when intoxicated are at less risk than those who express suicidal ideation at other times.

176. Which of the following psychiatric illnesses is NOT an independent factor for suicide?

   (A) depression
   (B) substance abuse
   (C) psychosis
   (D) anxiety
   (E) all of these are associated with an increased risk for suicide

177. TRUE or FALSE. Demographic risk factors are of limited utility in predicting suicide risk in individual patients.

178. After medical issues have been addressed, the FIRST step to follow during the assessment of a suicidal patient should be which of the following?

    (A) to perform a complete mental status examination
    (B) to obtain a detailed history
    (C) to gather collateral information
    (D) to take steps to ensure the safety of patient and examiner
    (E) to determine the risk/rescue ratio

179. TRUE or FALSE. Impulsive suicide attempts, such as those sometimes made by borderline patients, may be considered less lethal than planned ones.

180. TRUE or FALSE. Patients may use suicidal threats to manipulate caregivers, but such threats must nonetheless be taken seriously.

181. TRUE or FALSE. Following a suicide attempt, patients who are hospitalized for medical treatment generally do not require further psychiatric care prior to discharge.

182. Following a suicide attempt, which of the following need NOT be established upon discharge from a hospital or an emergency room?

    (A) that the means of suicide have been made inaccessible
    (B) that increased supports have been established
    (C) that a plan for follow-up has been developed
    (D) that reversible risk factors, such as psychiatric illness, have been addressed
    (E) that the patient has signed a written contract pledging not to attempt suicide

183. TRUE or FALSE. No medications have been shown to diminish suicide risk in any population.

184. Which of the following events was historically first?

    (A) Cerletti and Bini's use of electricity to induce a therapeutic seizure
    (B) the use of curare as a muscle relaxant
    (C) the serendipitous discovery of lithium's mood altering effects by John Cade
    (D) Meduna's use of camphor to induce a therapeutic seizure
    (E) Egas Moniz's coinage of the term "psychosurgery" in a paper discussing prefrontal leukotomy

185. Which statement BEST represents the current understanding regarding the mechanism of action of ECT?

    (A) Despite multiple proposed theories the exact mechanism of action of ECT remains unclear.
    (B) ECT fulfills the need for punishment in the self-loathing, depressed patient.
    (C) ECT erases painful memories that led to depression.
    (D) ECT is a dramatic and ritualized procedure, which creates improvement solely via the placebo effect.
    (E) ECT lowers dopamine levels in the CNS.

186. Which of the following is NOT an indication for ECT?

    (A) Major depression
    (B) Bipolar depression
    (C) Catatonia
    (D) Psychotic depression
    (E) Borderline personality disorder

187. Which of the following is an absolute CONTRAINDICATION to the use of ECT?

(A) the presence of an intracranial tumor
(B) pregnancy
(C) previous myocardial infarction
(D) all of the above
(E) none of the above

188. TRUE or FALSE. Since ECT has never been compared with active medication, its use for the treatment of major depression cannot be recommended using evidence-based criteria.

189. You are psychiatrically admitting a delusionally depressed 70-year-old male for a trial of ECT. Which of the following should be routinely included in the admission orders?

(A) NPO after midnight prior to ECT
(B) serum electrolytes
(C) chest X-ray
(D) 12-lead EKG
(E) all of the above

190. d'Elia placement refers to

(A) placement of a blood pressure cuff over a single extremity during the administration of muscle relaxant, allowing observation of seizure duration in the convulsing limb
(B) placement of the patient in a reverse Trendelenburg position to prevent aspiration during the seizure
(C) the old practice of placing a specialized bit guard in the mouth to prevent injury during the convulsion
(D) unilateral placement of electrodes, usually over the nondominant hemisphere
(E) placement of a pulse oximeter on the thumb to monitor oxygen saturation during anesthesia

191. Which of the following may result in an UNSUCCESSFUL course of ECT?

(A) marginally suprathreshold unilateral ECT
(B) consistent seizures of 10 sec in duration
(C) lack of generalization of the seizure
(D) all of the above
(E) none of the above

192. During an informed consent process, the patient asks whether ECT will "wipe out the memory of their childhood." The most accurate response would be

(A) "ECT does not effect memory."
(B) "You may have problems learning new things after the course of ECT, but it won't affect old memories."
(C) "ECT only causes memory loss in patients with underlying dementia."
(D) "Some people do lose memories for events that happened before ECT, but it would be rare for this to extend back beyond a year. ECT does not affect personal identity."
(E) "I thought you wanted to forget that stuff anyway."

193. Which of the following can raise the seizure threshold?

(A) diazepam
(B) valproate
(C) carbamazepine
(D) ECT itself
(E) all of the above

194. Mrs. A is a 70-year-old woman admitted to the surgical service after she fell and fractured her right hip. Three days after surgery, she is confused, disoriented, and inattentive. All of the following are appropriate functions of the C-L psychiatrist consulted in this case EXCEPT

    (A) diagnosis of postoperative delirium and recommendation of appropriate work-up and pharmacotherapy
    (B) criticism of the surgical team for failure to recognize and treat the delirium earlier
    (C) education of the surgical staff about delirium and its possible etiologies in Mrs. A
    (D) suggestion to the nursing staff that they provide orienting cues for Mrs. A
    (E) availability should the patient become acutely agitated

195. All of the following are TRUE about psychiatric epidemiology in the general hospital EXCEPT

    (A) The frequency of psychopathology among medical-surgical patients is 10–50%.
    (B) Prevalence estimates of psychiatric disorders in general hospitals vary based on the nature and severity of the underlying medical or surgical illness.
    (C) One of every ten patients admitted to a general hospital is seen by a C-L psychiatrist.
    (D) Rates of psychiatric consultation vary based on institutional differences.
    (E) Common requests for consultation include evaluations of delirium, dementia, and depression.

196. A C-L psychiatrist may play a helpful role in all of the following situations EXCEPT

    (A) The surgical team questions a 68-year-old demented man's capacity to write his last will and testament while he recuperates from carotid endarterectomy.
    (B) A 72-year-old woman with multiple myeloma is admitted with confusion and lethargy. Serum calcium is 16 mg/dL.
    (C) The medical team tells a 50-year-old man with a 20-pack-year smoking history that his lung biopsy showed adenocarcinoma. While awaiting surgery over the next week, he becomes increasingly withdrawn, apathetic, and anorexic.
    (D) A young woman with bipolar disorder on valproic acid and bupropion is admitted to the medical service for an asthma flare.
    (E) A 40-year-old man is treated with meperidine for pain secondary to acute alcoholic pancreatitis and develops confusion and myoclonus 3 days later.

197. All of the following are TRUE about the approach to the psychiatric consultation EXCEPT

    (A) The need for the consultation may be prompted by a problem within the patient, a doctor or a nurse, and/or the patient-caregiver relationship.
    (B) Communication with the consultee and staff throughout the consultative process is essential.
    (C) Physical and neurologic exams may be necessary.
    (D) The conduct of the interview and the MSE and the preparation of the note are no different in medical-surgical settings than in private venues.
    (E) The note must be brief, jargon-free, and devoid of irrelevant details.

198. All of the following are TRUE about review of the medication history EXCEPT

    (A) A detailed list of a patient's medications—at home, in the present hospital ward, and in previous wards—is an integral part of a thorough consultation.
    (B) Discrepancies between drugs previously taken and those currently administered may explain mental status changes.
    (C) Recent discontinuation of narcotics and neuroleptics may account for withdrawal phenomena.
    (D) Dosage, route, and frequency of administration are key parameters.
    (E) For PRN medications, knowledge of the prescribed frequency is not sufficient; how often the patient actually receives the medication is important to know.

199. All of the following are TRUE about the psychiatric consultation note EXCEPT

   (A) Attention to clear and specific details is especially important in the impressions and recommendations sections of the note.
   (B) The note should be helpful, not critical or adversarial.
   (C) Suggestions for behavioral management of a personality-disordered patient are often very useful.
   (D) The consultant's plan to provide periodic follow-up should be indicated.
   (E) The consultation note should include a detailed psychodynamic formulation of the patient.

200. When recommending medications, the C-L psychiatrist should consider all of the following EXCEPT

   (A) drug-drug interactions
   (B) protein binding
   (C) cytochrome P-450 inhibition
   (D) side effects
   (E) none of the above

201. Mr. N is a middle-aged business executive on the medical service for evaluation of persistent cough. The nurses complain that he refuses to take his medications at prescribed times, demands that his meals be re-heated, and insists that his business partners visit him beyond allotted times. On one occasion, because Mr. N is on the phone when the team makes morning rounds, they leave to see another patient and return to Mr. N 10 min later. He is upset that they did not wait, explaining, "If you had just waited five minutes, I could have chatted with you then." The C-L psychiatrist finds no evidence of Axis-I pathology. In this situation, the psychiatrist should

   (A) Write in the note that there is no severe mental illness, communicate this orally to the team, and then sign-off.
   (B) Explain to the doctors and nurses that Mr. N's behavior is secondary to narcissistic personality disorder.
   (C) Meet with the patient for daily psychotherapy to uncover the roots of his haughty behavior.
   (D) Transfer Mr. N to an inpatient psychiatric unit because the nurses on the medical service are unable to take care of him.
   (E) Explain that underneath Mr. N's narcissistic exterior are fear, anxiety, and stress engendered by undiagnosed medical illness and hospitalization and suggest that the doctors and nurses provide him with adequate reassurance and information to ameliorate these factors.

202. Ms. B is a 20-year-old woman with second-degree burns on both legs. She tells the surgeon that she purposely set her legs on fire so her boyfriend would stay home with her. When the burn surgeon requests that the C-L psychiatrist evaluate Ms. B for suicidality, the surgeon's frustration is obvious. All of the following statements about this situation are TRUE EXCEPT

   (A) The surgeon's frustration is likely a reflection of Ms. B's underlying pathology (e.g., low frustration tolerance).
   (B) The surgeon is likely to be angry with Ms. B for causing her own injuries and may, therefore, treat her differently than he treats patients with accidental burns.
   (C) Ms. B's behavior suggests that she may have borderline personality disorder, and the psychiatrist should probe for further evidence of this disturbance.
   (D) The psychiatrist should explain that the surgeon's countertransference reaction may impair his treatment of Ms. B.
   (E) After excluding suicidal intent, the psychiatrist should explain to the surgeon that Ms. B's behavior is a strategy, albeit maladaptive, for coping with emotional upset.

203. Mr. C is a 28-year-old man with non-Hodgkin's lymphoma on the oncology service for complications of bone-marrow transplantation. Admitted for the third time in as many months, he is well-known by the staff on the unit, and the nurses have become close with his wife and mother. Because he reported a 2-week history of depressed mood and anergia, nefazodone was added to his regimen of cyclosporine and methylprednisolone. Later, a C-L psychiatrist was asked to comment on the appropriateness of antidepressant choice. When the psychiatrist finishes her evaluation, Mr. C's wife asks her about DNR status and disposition plan. All of the following are appropriate steps in the management of this patient EXCEPT

   (A) discussion with Mr. C's wife and mother about resuscitation and intubation decisions
   (B) comment that nefazodone may raise the serum cyclosporine level
   (C) discussion with Mr. C, his family, and the medical team about the appropriateness of hospice care
   (D) focused psychotherapy to help Mr. C cope with the uncertainty of his situation and the probability of death
   (E) willingness to help the staff deal with their own grief reaction to this young man's tragic illness

204. Good copers tend to be

   (A) flexible in their defenses
   (B) optimistic
   (C) practical and resourceful in finding solutions
   (D) insightful about problem areas
   (E) all of the above

205. The liaison role of psychiatrists consulted to help a patient coping with a medical illness includes

   (A) ruling out treatable psychiatric conditions which may be compromising the patient's ability to cope with her illness
   (B) helping the patient advocate for herself in negotiating complex health care systems and dealings with different health care providers
   (C) promoting collaborative relationships with the medical team in which countertransference is clarified, normalized, and contained rather than imposed on the patient
   (D) helping the team understand a difficult patient's coping style
   (E) all of the above

206. Which of the following are signs of a dysfunctional marriage?

   (A) the failure of men to accept influence from their wives
   (B) the presence of blame, withdrawal, contempt, and defensiveness
   (C) the lack of attempts by either partner to repair when there has been a conflict or misunderstanding
   (D) chronic, diffuse, physiological arousal, and immunosuppression
   (E) all of the above

207. What has epidemiological research revealed as the times of greatest risk for divorce?

   (A) after 5 years of marriage
   (B) after 10 years of marriage
   (C) after 16 years of marriage
   (D) A and C
   (E) B and C

208. Which of the following are MYTHS about fidelity?

   (A) Affairs come from bad marriages.
   (B) The affairee is generally a better choice for the person having the affair than is his or her spouse.
   (C) An affair proves that love is gone from the marriage.
   (D) It is more protective of the marriage to keep an affair secret.
   (E) All of the above are correct.

209. Which statement about infertile couples is FALSE?

(A) Both partners tend to place responsibility for the infertility on the woman even when the male is infertile.
(B) When men are infertile, women often collude with their husbands to keep the infertility a secret from friends and family.
(C) During the course of infertility treatment, half of women report that infertility is the most devastating experience of their lives.
(D) Female infertility factors account for more biological explanations of infertility than do male factors.
(E) The only significant rise in infertility over the last 25 years has been in women ages 20–24.

210. Which of the following is TRUE?

(A) 95% of violence is perpetrated by men against women
(B) Almost one-third of all married couples will experience at least one violent episode during the course of their marriage.
(C) The psychological profile of an abuser may feature problems with drugs and alcohol, pathological jealousy, a history of witnessing abuse, and a narcissistic injury, such as a job loss or a wife earning more money.
(D) Abuse may intensify attachments, thus making it hard for the abused partner to leave the relationship.
(E) All of the above are correct.

211. A couples therapist working with gay and lesbian couples should

(A) Know that it is only since 1973 that the American Psychiatric Association (APA) deleted homosexuality from the DSM-II.
(B) Be aware that 25% of lesbian women in committed relationships have experienced physical abuse.
(C) Be gay or lesbian in order to understand first-hand the social stigma associated with homosexuality.
(D) A and C
(E) A and B

212. Which statement about female sexuality is FALSE?

(A) 11–14% of women experience a lifelong lack of orgasm, while for men this rate is very low.
(B) Female orgasm facilitates reproduction.
(C) Low sexual desire is predominantly a dysfunction among women.
(D) When women complain of low sexual drive or inhibited orgasm, a referral for a physiological workup should be made to rule out hormonal and medical factors, before commencing sex therapy.
(E) Among women with sexual dysfunctions, more than one-third were abused sexually as children.

213. The following risk factor(s) has(have) been found to be associated with divorce

(A) The couple meets or marries shortly after a significant loss.
(B) The couple marries before age 25.
(C) The wedding takes place without family or friends.
(D) A and C are correct.
(E) All of the above are correct.

214. Which of the following is NOT associated with psychodynamic family therapy?

(A) problems are thought to occur through a multigenerational family failure plus stress
(B) interpersonal functioning is tied to attachments to past figures
(C) projective identification
(D) psychodrama
(E) Jay Haley

215. TRUE or FALSE. Narrative family therapists narrate a long letter to the family at the end of the session that contains instructions that may contain a paradoxical connotation.

216. TRUE or FALSE. Group therapy is as effective as any other kind of psychotherapy.

217. TRUE or FALSE. Group therapy is a primary treatment as well as an adjunctive one.

218. TRUE or FALSE. Group therapy is not suitable for psychotic patients.

219. TRUE or FALSE. Patients with character disorders are ideally treated in groups.

220. TRUE or FALSE. Patients with serious medical illness are helped by group therapy.

221. TRUE or FALSE. All patients can be treated in group therapy.

222. TRUE or FALSE. Patients in a group need to be homogeneous around treatment goals.

223. All of the following are TRUE about HIV infection EXCEPT

   (A) Dementia is often a late manifestation of HIV infection because the retrovirus does not infect the CNS until late in the course.
   (B) When HIV does infect the CNS, subcortical structures are more damaged than cortical areas.
   (C) Care for many patients with HIV/AIDS may be hampered by clinicians' discomfort with lifestyles they do not share or understand.
   (D) Viruses similar to HIV also cause progressive immunologic and neurologic decline.
   (E) Both CD4 count and presence of complications determine a diagnosis of AIDS.

224. All of the following are TRUE about the epidemiology of HIV/AIDS EXCEPT

   (A) Viral transmission from intravenous drug users (IDUs) to their sexual partners is responsible for a large percentage of AIDS cases among heterosexuals.
   (B) AIDS is increasingly prevalent among minorities and women.
   (C) The prevalence of AIDS has decreased because of the availability of combination antiretroviral therapy.
   (D) AIDS is most prevalent among men who engage in homosexual activity.
   (E) People who are at high risk for HIV infection are also at high risk for psychiatric disorders.

225. All of the following are TRUE about the psychiatric care of HIV/AIDS patients EXCEPT

   (A) At some point during the evaluation, an inquiry about the mode of infection should be made to illuminate who the patient is as a person.
   (B) Psychiatric symptoms should be assumed secondary to HIV CNS infection or systemic disease.
   (C) As a marker for extent of systemic disease, the CD4 count can be used to assess the degree of vulnerability of the CNS.
   (D) Substance-use disorders and side effects of medications used to treat HIV-related illnesses are key considerations when an HIV-infected patient presents with psychiatric symptoms.
   (E) When psychiatric symptoms are secondary to HIV disease or its treatment, therapy with psychotropics is tolerated poorly and wrought with more side effects.

226. All of the following are TRUE about depression and suicide in patients with HIV/AIDS EXCEPT

   (A) Risk of suicide among HIV-infected patients may be most strongly related to concurrent depression.
   (B) The high frequency of depression among patients with HIV/AIDS may be related to the chronicity of illness.
   (C) Because depression in early HIV infection is usually secondary to an HIV-related illness, SSRIs should be started in low doses and increased slowly.
   (D) The differential diagnosis of depression in HIV/AIDS patients includes endocrine disturbances in the adrenal and thyroid glands and in the testes.
   (E) The evaluation of suicide in a patient with HIV/AIDS is no different than in any other patient.

227. All of the following are TRUE about coping with HIV/AIDS EXCEPT

   (A) It requires experience and training, support from others, and brief respites.
   (B) The same people who are at risk for HIV infection are also at risk for poor coping.
   (C) Ineffective coping may present with anxiety, which should raise suspicion for secondary causes in patients with advanced HIV disease.
   (D) Pharmacologic interventions should be reserved for patients in the early stages of retroviral infection.
   (E) Patients with HIV/AIDS face stressors related to symptoms, diagnosis, and treatment of HIV as well as the psychosocial consequences of the disease.

228. All of the following are TRUE about psychosis and delirium in HIV/AIDS patients EXCEPT

   (A) In patients with a CD4 count > 500, symptoms are likely due to use of excitatory substances (e.g., steroids, cocaine).
   (B) Neuroimaging and blood tests are ordered as clinically indicated.
   (C) The incidence of EPS from high-potency neuroleptics is increased in patients with advanced HIV disease.
   (D) Low doses of neuroleptics may be effective in this population because of HIV-related damage to the basal ganglia.
   (E) Neuroleptics are the first line of treatment.

229. All of the following are TRUE about mania in HIV/AIDS patients EXCEPT

   (A) Secondary causes of mania are more likely in advanced disease.
   (B) Combination treatment with lithium and neuroleptics may be poorly tolerated in patients with advanced disease.
   (C) Among anticonvulsants, valproate, which lowers AZT levels, is preferred over carbamazepine, which increases it.
   (D) Volume shifts caused by diarrhea and dehydration may raise serum lithium levels.
   (E) Even when the serum lithium level is within the therapeutic range, HIV-infected patients may experience lithium toxicity.

230. All of the following are TRUE about the neurologic manifestations of HIV/AIDS EXCEPT

   (A) A subcortical process, HIV dementia causes affective, behavioral, cognitive, and motor symptoms and signs.
   (B) Patients with mild neurocognitive deficits inevitably progress to full-blown HIV dementia.
   (C) Toxoplasmosis may be mistaken for CNS lymphoma on neuroimaging studies.
   (D) Toxoplasmosis and cryptococcal meningitis require lifelong suppressive therapy.
   (E) Psychomotor slowing is the hallmark of HIV dementia on neuropsychological testing.

231. All of the following are TRUE about antiretroviral therapy EXCEPT

   (A) Antiretroviral agents include nucleoside and non-nucleoside reverse transcriptase inhibitors and protease inhibitors.
   (B) All of these agents cause neuropsychiatric side effects.
   (C) Non-nucleoside reverse transcriptase inhibitors and protease inhibitors are metabolized by the cytochrome P450 system and inhibit and/or induce this enzymatic pathway.
   (D) SSRIs and TCAs should be avoided in patients on ritonavir and given only in small doses to patients on other protease inhibitors.
   (E) Because they induce P450 enzymes, phenobarbital, carbamazepine, and phenytoin may lower serum levels of protease inhibitors.

232. All of the following are ABNORMAL in HIV/AIDS patients EXCEPT

   (A) amount of lean body mass
   (B) rate of drug metabolism
   (C) sensitivity to drug side effects
   (D) integrity of the blood-brain barrier
   (E) none of the above

233. Which of the following is NOT a risk factor for noncompliance?

(A) youth
(B) deficient social supports
(C) being elderly
(D) having impaired cognition
(E) substance abuse

234. Brain death criteria

(A) are based primarily on clinical criteria of irreversible brainstem damage
(B) require documentation of a neurologist or neurosurgeon
(C) are often determined by two exams performed at 6-h intervals
(D) are partly indicated by failure of an apnea test
(E) all of the above are correct

235. Psychiatric referral is indicated if

(A) an unrelated living kidney donor is considered
(B) a psychiatrically impaired or ambivalent donor is considered
(C) a donor is undergoing a lobectomy
(D) a donor is undergoing a partial hepatectomy
(E) all of the above are correct

236. Which of the following is NOT an objective for pretransplant screening?

(A) To define the patient's motivation for, and beliefs about, transplantation.
(B) To identify preoperative psychiatric syndromes and to evaluate the ability to treat them concurrently with the transplant.
(C) To avoid determining the availability of social supports because they may impede the work of the transplant team social workers.
(D) To design a treatment plan to assure that potentially high-risk patients will prove manageable after transplant.
(E) To inform patients about their perioperative psychiatric treatment requirements or options and their availability.

237. Which of the following is NOT true regarding antidepressants in transplant patients?

(A) SSRIs and bupropion are poorly tolerated in patients with end-organ failure.
(B) Tricyclics are helpful with diabetic neuropathy and may be beneficial for patients with insomnia.
(C) Treatment may be instituted for depression and should be continued for chronic maintenance if required.
(D) One should be aware of all drug interactions secondary to suppression of the cytochrome P450 enzyme system.
(E) Methylphenidate is stimulating and therefore preferable in patients prone to encephalopathy.

238. Which of the following therapies would be classified as manual-driven treatments?

(A) Cognitive-behavioral therapy
(B) Psychoeducational group therapy
(C) Supportive psychotherapy
(D) Psychoanalytic psychotherapy
(E) Expressive psychotherapy

239. Which of the following terms would NOT be associated with psychodynamic psychotherapy?

(A) countertransference
(B) resistance
(C) transitional objects
(D) negative thoughts
(E) dream analysis

240. Which of the following theoreticians is most commonly associated with the term "the Paranoid Position"?

(A) Sigmund Freud
(B) Anna Freud
(C) Habib Davanloo
(D) Heinz Kohut
(E) Melanie Klein

241. A patient presents with a debilitating fear of air travel. Which of the following psychotherapies would be most appropriate?

(A) Supportive psychotherapy
(B) Psychoeducational psychotherapy
(C) Behavior therapy
(D) Couples therapy
(E) Dialectical behavior therapy (DBT)

242. Which of the following patients might best be referred for interpersonal therapy (IPT)?

(A) a young man wishing to explore traumatic memories of childhood abuse
(B) an elderly woman mourning the death of her husband
(C) a middle-aged woman with symptoms of depression who is troubled by difficulties with her husband
(D) a man who has been fired repeatedly from his job for fighting with his employer
(E) a woman who wants to learn more about managing her son, who has recently been diagnosed with schizophrenia

243. Which of the following are the main goals of dialectical behavior therapy (DBT)?

(A) externalization of inwardly directed anger
(B) decreasing self-injurious behavior and hospitalizations
(C) understanding of transference conflicts
(D) reworking of oedipal conflicts
(E) the analysis of unconscious conflicts through regression

244. Which of the following medical conditions have been shown by Spiegel and others to benefit from group psychotherapy?

(A) chronic arthritis
(B) congenital adrenal hyperplasia
(C) posttraumatic stress disorder
(D) breast cancer
(E) blindness

245. Which of the following events or discoveries was NOT important to the development of brief psychotherapy?

(A) Freud's early work with hysteria
(B) Franz Alexander's manipulation of session spacing
(C) World War I
(D) The Coconut Grove fire
(E) Sifneos' development of anxiety-provoking psychotherapy

246. Which of the following is the goal of short-term psychodynamic psychotherapy?

(A) behavior change
(B) a detailed evaluation of the patient's cognitive thought patterns
(C) reviewing the patient's interpersonal relationships and expectations
(D) interpretation of conflict and defenses
(E) demonstrating how thoughts impact behaviors

247. What is the naturally occurring length of psychotherapy?

    (A) Therapy is so variable that there are no good data on its length.
    (B) 70% of patients receive 10 or fewer sessions.
    (C) Successful psychotherapy is measured in years not weeks.
    (D) Most patients receive 21 or more sessions of psychotherapy.
    (E) Longer therapy is always equated with better therapy.

248. When doing brief psychotherapy the therapist's mind-set should NOT include?

    (A) a desire to achieve a total cure
    (B) an openness to the belief that brief therapy can work
    (C) a view of the patient as developing and functioning across a life-cycle
    (D) a focus on time and how it effects the therapy process and activities
    (E) working at being an active therapist

249. What are the essential features of brief psychotherapy?

    (A) patient selection
    (B) brevity
    (C) having a specific focus for the treatment
    (D) being an active therapist
    (E) all of the above are correct

250. TRUE or FALSE. Using a two-session evaluation period is inappropriate for brief therapy.

251. TRUE or FALSE. Selecting a successful treatment focus requires extensive years of clinical experience.

252. Which of the following is NOT an exclusion criteria for selecting patients for brief therapy?

    (A) active psychosis
    (B) unlimited mental health insurance benefits
    (C) substance abuse
    (D) significant risk for self harm
    (E) all the above are correct

253. Which of the following are likely to be potential foci for a brief psychotherapy?

    (A) losses
    (B) developmental desynchronies
    (C) repeated interpersonal conflict
    (D) a patient's symptoms
    (E) all the above are correct

254. TRUE or FALSE. If the patient produces new and meaningful material at the time of termination the therapist should evaluate its clinical implications but generally hold to the termination deadline.

255. TRUE or FALSE. Patients with depression seen in primary care settings respond to lower doses of psychotropic medication compared to those seen in psychiatric settings.

256. TRUE or FALSE. Psychiatric confidentiality requires that the psychiatrist obtain verbal or written consent from the patient before discussing the results of the consultation with the PCP.

257. TRUE or FALSE. In most states, once psychiatric notes become part of the general medical record they can be released with a general medical release of information.

258. Which of the following statements about diagnostic instruments is FALSE?

    (A) They are used primarily in research studies.
    (B) They may be a useful adjunct to the interview in the clinical setting.
    (C) They may allow the quantification of severity of illness.
    (D) They are always self-administered by the patient.
    (E) They help ascertain the degree of response to treatment.

259. Which of the following is a self-administered diagnostic instrument?

    (A) the SCID
    (B) The Hamilton D
    (C) the CGI
    (D) the Beck Depression Inventory
    (E) none of the above

260. Which of the following is a qualitative, nonquantitative diagnostic instrument

    (A) the Hamilton D
    (B) the SCID
    (C) the Beck Depression Inventory
    (D) the Zung SDS
    (E) none of the above

261. The SHORTEST version of the Hamilton-D has how many questions?

    (A) 3
    (B) 4
    (C) 6
    (D) 17
    (E) 31

262. The CGI

    (A) relies only on the clinician's impression
    (B) relies purely on the patient's subjective impression
    (C) measures the severity of depression using only the previous visit as the standard for comparison
    (D) generally requires the use of other diagnostic instruments prior to its administration
    (E) determines only whether or not a patient is depressed, not the degree of severity

263. The SCID

    (A) is probably the most reliable of psychiatric diagnostic instruments
    (B) is used in the clinical setting, as it is easy and fast to administer
    (C) is not very accurate for measuring severity of illness
    (D) answers A, B, and C are all true
    (E) only A and C are true

264. You are in your clinic office assessing a depressed patient with a self-reported history of poor response to medications. You decide to administer a Hamilton D-17 prior to beginning a new antidepressant. Your rationale for this might be explained as follows:

    (A) You suspect that the patient's illness is purely characterological and will probably not respond to antidepressants.
    (B) The Hamilton scores may help you determine the degree of response to the antidepressant at the end of 8 weeks.
    (C) Patients' subjective impression of antidepressant effectiveness is an accurate indicator of the actual effectiveness.
    (D) Because the Hamilton questionnaire is self-rated, it may make the patient feel that he is taking an active role in his treatment
    (E) Patients generally enjoy answering standardized questions, as they help to solidify the treatment alliance.

265. Which of the following instruments may be most helpful for diagnosing a personality disorder?

    (A) the Hamilton D
    (B) the SCID-1
    (C) the SCID-II
    (D) the Zung SDS
    (E) none of the above

266. You are assessing a patient with suspected obsessive-compulsive disorder. Which of the following instruments might be useful for establishing a diagnosis?

    (A) the Hamilton D-17
    (B) the Y-BOCS
    (C) the SCID
    (D) answers B and C only
    (E) all of the above

267. You have been treating a chronic schizophrenic patient with haloperidol for the past 6 months. Which of the following instruments would be most important to administer?

    (A) the SCID
    (B) the BPRS
    (C) the AIMS
    (D) the HAM-A
    (E) the BDI

268. The Community Mental Health Center Act was signed by President

    (A) Kennedy
    (B) Johnson
    (C) Carter
    (D) Reagan
    (E) Truman

269. Most community residents seek help for psychiatric symptoms from

    (A) their community mental health center
    (B) their primary care provider
    (C) a private psychiatrist
    (D) a non-physician mental health provider
    (E) their pharmacist

For questions 270–274 choose the best answer from the key below

    (A) 1, 2, and 3 are correct
    (B) 1 and 3 are correct
    (C) 2 and 4 are correct
    (D) 4 is correct
    (E) all are correct

270. Underlying principles of community mental health include

    (1) continuity of care
    (2) population responsibility
    (3) prevention
    (4) community-based care

271. The "de facto" mental health system refers to

   (1) state psychiatric hospitals
   (2) for-profit private psychiatric hospitals
   (3) community mental health centers
   (4) general medical settings

272. Military psychiatry experience led to the following central tenet(s) of community mental health

   (1) immediacy
   (2) expectancy
   (3) proximity
   (4) quality

273. Consultation/education

   (1) is reimbursed by global capitation
   (2) was mandated by the Community Mental Health Center Act
   (3) decreases the incentive for cost-shifting
   (4) is a non-revenue-producing service of community psychiatrists

274. Currently, the community mental health system in the United States focuses on

   (1) treatment for the seriously and persistently mentally ill
   (2) institutional containment
   (3) community-based treatment
   (4) primary and secondary prevention

275. TRUE or FALSE. Like publicly funded community mental health centers, progressive managed care organizations invite community involvement.

276. Select the BEST completion to the statement. The reliability of diagnosing a psychiatric disorder improves with

   (A) better training of the rater
   (B) using structured diagnostic instruments
   (C) using explicit diagnostic criteria
   (D) having comparable settings for conducting an interview
   (E) all of the above

277. Each of the following is true about the kappa statistic EXCEPT

   (A) It can be used to show reliability between raters.
   (B) It measures whether diagnoses made by raters are valid.
   (C) High values of kappa statistics reflect high reliability.
   (D) It corrects for chance agreement.
   (E) It is inaccurate for measuring reliability of rare diseases.

278. Select the BEST completion to the statement: An instrument for the diagnosis of psychiatric disorders has good validity if

   (A) it has good reliability
   (B) it makes good sense to the investigator
   (C) it has high sensitivity and high specificity
   (D) the items of the instrument contain needed information to make the diagnosis
   (E) all of the above are correct

279. The incidence rate of a disorder is determined by each of the following variables EXCEPT

   (A) the number of persons observed
   (B) the duration of the illness
   (C) the duration of observation
   (D) the number persons who dropped out during study period
   (E) the number of persons who became ill at the end of the study

280. To investigate if an exposure is related to an illness in a case-control study, we calculate

   (A) the odds ratio
   (B) relative risk
   (C) the kappa statistic
   (D) incidence rate
   (E) the Mantel-Haenszel statistic

281. Which was the most prevalent psychiatric disorder recognized in the ECA study?

   (A) panic disorder
   (B) antisocial personality disorder
   (C) major depression
   (D) phobia
   (E) alcohol abuse/dependence

282. The prevalence of schizophrenia in children who have one schizophrenic parent is

   (A) 1%
   (B) 5%
   (C) 15%
   (D) 25%
   (E) 35%

283. Risk factors for depression include

   (A) stressful life events
   (B) female gender
   (C) having prior episodes of depression
   (D) being in the postpartum period
   (E) all of the above

284. The lifetime prevalence of generalized anxiety disorder is

   (A) 1%
   (B) 2%
   (C) 4%
   (D) 8%
   (E) 12%

285. Alcohol abuse is related to each of the following EXCEPT

   (A) low educational level
   (B) male gender
   (C) older age
   (D) divorced status
   (E) low income

286. Which statement about nonparametric statistics is NOT true?

    (A) They are usually used with a small sample size.
    (B) They are used when distribution deviates markedly from normality.
    (C) They are tests are based on means and standard deviations.
    (D) They are tests are based on ranks and frequencies.
    (E) All of the above are correct.

287. "Reliability" is a measure of

    (A) the dependability of a test or measure
    (B) the usefulness of a test
    (C) the sensitivity of a test to clinical change
    (D) none of the above
    (E) all of the above

288. "Interrater reliability" is NOT relevant to

    (A) structured interviews, such as the SCID
    (B) self-report scales, such as the Zung Depression Scale
    (C) clinical diagnoses of personality disorders
    (D) a rater's judgments of tape recorded therapy sessions
    (E) all of the above

289. Which statistical test is most appropriate for comparing the means of three treatment groups?

    (A) t-test
    (B) chi-square test
    (C) multiple linear regression
    (D) analysis of variance
    (E) correlation coefficient

290. "Psychometrics" is the study of

    (A) methods of sampling subjects from a population
    (B) the reliability and validity of a test
    (C) how many subjects are needed to conduct a study
    (D) correlation between two or more symptoms
    (E) MRI-derived volumes of brain structures

291. Which is NOT a measure of the central tendency of a group?

    (A) mean
    (B) median
    (C) variance
    (D) mode
    (E) none of the above

292. Which statistic is NOT a measure of degree of association between two measures?

    (A) confidence interval
    (B) Spearman coefficient
    (C) Pearson coefficient
    (D) r
    (E) none of the above

293. Which change results in an increase of statistical power for a test?

   (A) testing at $P < 0.01$ rather than $P < 0.05$
   (B) using a two-tailed test rather than a one-tailed test
   (C) increasing the number of subjects
   (D) lowering the number of subjects
   (E) all of the above

294. The SENSIVITY of a MEDICAL test is analogous to the _____ of a STATISTICAL test.

   (A) power
   (B) confidence interval
   (C) standard error
   (D) P-value
   (E) significance

295. The SPECIFICITY of a MEDICAL test is analogous to the _____ of a STATISTICAL test.

   (A) standard error
   (B) power
   (C) confidence interval
   (D) P-value
   (E) magnitude

296. Which of the following characteristics is essential for a study to be considered a true experiment?

   (A) The statistics are used to compare the results.
   (B) The subjects are randomly assigned to the various treatments.
   (C) The outcome measures are reliable.
   (D) The outcome measures are valid.
   (E) A placebo is used.

297. Which of the following statements about the genetics of bipolar disorder is TRUE?

   (A) Bipolar disorder is usually transmitted as a recessive rather than dominant disorder.
   (B) Recent studies have shown that environmental factors are not important in the development of bipolar disorder.
   (C) Relatives of individuals with bipolar disorder are more likely to have unipolar depression than bipolar disorder.
   (D) At least two genes have been shown to account for most cases of bipolar disorder.
   (E) A genetic test is now available to aid in the diagnosis of bipolar disorder.

298. For which of the following disorders has a causal role been established for specific genes?

   (A) Obsessive-compulsive disorder
   (B) Bipolar disorder
   (C) Schizophrenia
   (D) Alzheimer's disease
   (E) none of the above

299. The heritability of a disorder refers to

   (A) the proportion of the disorder that is due to genetic factors in an individual
   (B) the probability that a first-degree relative will express the phenotype
   (C) the proportion of the phenotypic variance attributable to genetic factors in a particular population at a particular time
   (D) the concordance rate for monozygotic twins
   (E) none of the above

300. Which of the following statements about the genetics of schizophrenia is TRUE?

(A) First-degree relatives have a three-fold increased risk of the disorder compared to the general population.
(B) Gene-mapping studies have confirmed the role of dopamine receptors in the development of schizophrenia.
(C) Smooth pursuit eye-tracking abnormalities may be an expression of genes that predispose to schizophrenia.
(D) First-degree relatives have a 30% risk of the disorder.
(E) There is no solid evidence that genes play a role in the development of schizophrenia.

301. Expansion of trinucleotide repeat sequences is known to be the cause of which neuropsychiatric disorder?

(A) Huntington's disease
(B) Panic disorder
(C) Alzheimer's disease
(D) Wilson's disease
(E) Korsakoff's syndrome

302. TRUE or FALSE. Linkage to a locus on chromosome 6p has been found in independent genetic studies of schizophrenia.

303. Family studies suggest that in some families there is a genetic connection between Tourette's syndrome and which of the following?

(A) panic disorder
(B) autism
(C) tic douloureux
(D) obsessive-compulsive disorder
(E) none of the above

304. Which of the following statistics indicates the likelihood of linkage between a marker and a disease gene?

(A) the heritability
(B) the lod score
(C) the concordance rate
(D) the relative risk
(E) the family-based association ratio

305. TRUE or FALSE. Family studies can suggest, but not confirm, the role of genetic factors in a disorder.

306. Which of the following phenomena can interfere with gene-mapping studies in psychiatry?

(A) uncertainty about phenotypic boundaries
(B) incomplete penetrance
(C) phenocopies
(D) genetic heterogeneity
(E) all of the above

307. When a psychiatrist notices that she or he is responding to a patient in ways that diverge from her or his usual repertoire, the following are all true EXCEPT

(A) The psychiatrist is not at emotional optimum, as her or his own inner experience is filtering in too powerfully.
(B) The psychiatrist should evaluate the nature of the patient's transference.
(C) The psychiatrist should be vigilant about the patient's hidden agendas.
(D) The psychiatrist should terminate with the particular patient, as she or he is obviously losing control over the therapeutic relationship.
(E) The psychiatrist should give attention to the undercurrents of unspoken feelings between the two.

308. All of the following statements about transference are true EXCEPT

    (A) It is a manifestation of specific psychiatric disorders.
    (B) It may enhance rapport with the caregiver.
    (C) It may diminish rapport with the caregiver.
    (D) It yields important information about the patient.
    (E) It is an unconscious continuation of perceptions and responses that may have developed during childhood.

309. All of the following statements regarding difficult interview situations are true EXCEPT

    (A) It is generally fruitless to try to persuade psychotic patients out of their delusional ideas.
    (B) When a patient becomes hostile, it is best to ignore it so that the patient will move on.
    (C) When a patient threatens violence, providing for physical control is a prerequisite for proceeding with an interview.
    (D) When a patient becomes seductive, the interviewer must clarify that the feelings cannot be acted on.
    (E) Cognitively impaired patients reveal more about their mental status than about their history in an interview.

310. All of the following statements concerning involuntary commitment are true EXCEPT

    (A) Commitment is a decision based on the parens patriae principle.
    (B) Commitment does not have to be to a hospital setting.
    (C) For commitment, courts have set the standard of proof of dangerousness as "clear and convincing."
    (D) Commitment requires the permission of a responsible relative.
    (E) Commitment usually has a time limit.

311. All of the following statements are applicable to informed consent EXCEPT

    (A) The patient is informed of the risks and benefits of the treatment.
    (B) The patient knows of alternative treatments that are possible.
    (C) The patient recognizes that it is a "one-time" procedure.
    (D) The patient understands the consequences of no treatment.
    (E) The patient consents freely and willingly, without coercion.

312. Regarding spousal abuse, all of the following statements are correct EXCEPT

    (A) The abusing spouse is likely to have been abused as a child.
    (B) The abused spouse is likely to have been abused as a child.
    (C) Spousal abuse is often carried out by men who are dependent and nonassertive.
    (D) Abused husbands hide the problem for fear of ridicule.
    (E) Pregnancy usually results in a reduction of abuse.

313. All of the following statements concern men who have been raped EXCEPT

    (A) They often experience sexual dysfunction after the event.
    (B) When attacked by a man, they frequently fear that they will become homosexual.
    (C) Emotional ventilation should be delayed until a clinician of the opposite sex (of the rapist) is available.
    (D) They should be assisted in reporting the assault to the police.
    (E) Recurrent feelings of shame are common.

314. Managed care affects the patient-physician relationship with all the following EXCEPT

    (A) increased physician autonomy
    (B) discontinuity of care
    (C) erosion of confidentiality
    (D) shrinkage of reimbursable service
    (E) experience-rating

315. All of the following statements about medical malpractice are true EXCEPT

    (A) Medical malpractice is defined as negligent care that causes injury.
    (B) Malpractice cases are rarely settled out of court.
    (C) When subpoenaed, the psychiatrist is responsible to testify as to what she or he saw and did and why, rather than to give an expert opinion.
    (D) The plaintiff, or injured patient, must show that the physician's care fell below the "standard of care."
    (E) Doctors "win" most malpractice cases.

316. All of the following are reasonable options for the healthcare professional to help prevent burnout EXCEPT

    (A) anticipating and preparing for difficulties
    (B) seeking psychotherapy
    (C) participating in peer supervision
    (D) joining a professional support group
    (E) gratifying the idealizing transference of patients

317. Which of the following is associated with high levels of treatment success using hypnosis?

    (A) simple phobias
    (B) obsessive-compulsive disorder
    (C) paranoid personality disorder
    (D) bulimia nervosa
    (E) smoking cessation

318. Which characteristic below may help to ascertain someone's hypnotizability?

    (A) motivation
    (B) past successful experience with meditation
    (C) imagination
    (D) ability to focus intently
    (E) all of the above

319. Which of the following is most likely to affect a successful hypnotic intervention?

    (A) the induction process
    (B) the length of induction
    (C) the attitude of the therapist
    (D) the presence or absence of distracting sounds or noises
    (E) the number of subjects being hypnotized

320. Of the following states, which is considered a contraindication to hypnosis?

    (A) hysteria
    (B) paranoia
    (C) obsessive-compulsive states
    (D) amnesia
    (E) acute pain

321. If a patient refuses to come out of a trance, which of the following should be done?

    (A) Call the police.
    (B) Psychiatrically hospitalize the patient.
    (C) Make a loud noise to jar them from the trance.
    (D) Suggest that if they do not come out of the trance, you will not be able to do hypnosis again.
    (E) Kick the patient under the table.

322. TRUE or FALSE. Individuals with mental illness are at no greater risk to commit acts of violence than those who carry no psychiatric diagnosis.

323. TRUE or FALSE. The first step in the assessment of the violent patient involves establishing a safe and secure environment.

324. TRUE or FALSE. Serotonin, in addition to its potential role in depression, has been shown to have a role in the modulation of aggressive behaviors.

325. TRUE or FALSE. Psychotherapy is better at managing aggressive behaviors than is medication.

326. Which of the following structures HAS NOT been implicated in the control of aggression?

    (A) the amygdala
    (B) the ventromedial hypothalamus
    (C) the cerebellum
    (D) the hippocampus
    (E) the prefrontal cortex

327. Which of the following medications has paradoxically increased aggression in patients with brain damage?

    (A) haloperidol
    (B) lorazepam
    (C) propranolol
    (D) droperidol
    (E) lithium

328. Which of the following diagnoses may increase the likelihood of committing an act of violence?

    (A) schizophrenia
    (B) depression
    (C) bipolar disorder
    (D) alcohol abuse
    (E) all of the above

329. TRUE or FALSE. Knowledge of the underlying psychiatric diagnosis does not help guide the management of the patient with chronic aggression.

330. TRUE or FALSE. A history of violence does not help determine the present risk of violence in a given individual.

331. TRUE or FALSE. Among those with a psychiatric diagnosis, schizophrenics have the greatest prevalence of violent acts.

332. "Thought process" is best tested by

    (A) asking the patient to spell WORLD backwards
    (B) having the patient repeat a short phrase
    (C) listening to links between thoughts in spontaneous speech
    (D) asking the patient if they believe someone is "out to get them"
    (E) the Wisconsin Card Sorting Test (WCST)

333. The primary cognitive deficit in the encephalopathic patient is

    (A) expressive aphasia
    (B) receptive aphasia
    (C) disturbance in level of consciousness
    (D) remote memory deficit
    (E) abnormality in visual-spatial processing

334. Mr. Smith presents with right-sided hemiplegia. His speech is mumbled, filled with small words with no clear meaning, and it lacks the normal intonation of speech. He is able to follow simple commands (take off your glasses) and he appropriately nods yes/no to questions. He cannot repeat a simple phrase. Which of the following best describes his presentation?

    (A) fluent aphasia with abnormal comprehension and repetition
    (B) nonfluent aphasia with abnormal comprehension and normal repetition
    (C) fluent aphasia with normal comprehension and repetition
    (D) nonfluent aphasia with normal comprehension and abnormal repetition
    (E) conversion disorder or malingering (description of lesions could not occur together)

335. During a course of ECT for severe depression, Mrs. Jones complains of "memory loss." When asked specifically, she states that the events leading to her admission were now "fuzzy," and she forgot that she attended a niece's wedding the week prior to admission. On exam, she is fully oriented, and is able to recall a short fictitious story after a 3-minute interruption. Her problem is best construed as

    (A) current concentration difficulty due to recent anesthetic
    (B) apathy due to ongoing depression
    (C) adjustment disorder due to recent stressors
    (D) remote (retrograde) memory loss, perhaps as a sequela of ECT
    (E) short-term memory loss

336. Saccades are best tested by

    (A) swinging flashlight test
    (B) having the patient quickly look at the left then the right
    (C) confrontational visual fields
    (D) having the patient track a slow-moving target
    (E) direct funduscopic examination

337. Which of the following is NOT a test of trigeminal nerve function?

    (A) corneal reflex
    (B) pin prick on the forehead
    (C) checking bite strength
    (D) wrinkling the forehead
    (E) palpating the masseter muscle

338. Mr. Schultz presents with acute-onset unilateral facial weakness, with a "drooping" of the right corner of his mouth. There is clear asymmetry of the nasal-labial folds on exam. The weakness seems complete, as he is unable to wrinkle his forehead. These deficits are most consistent with which of the following?

    (A) peripheral facial nerve weakness
    (B) central facial nerve weakness
    (C) sixth nerve palsy
    (D) eighth nerve palsy
    (E) none of the above

339. Which of the following can be screened for by an observation of gait?

    (A) motor strength
    (B) limb coordination
    (C) balance
    (D) proprioception
    (E) all of the above

340. Which of the following is a proprioceptive reflex?

    (A) cremasteric
    (B) ankle jerk
    (C) anal wink
    (D) snout
    (E) Babinski

341. The presence of a grasp reflex would be a normal finding in

    (A) a paraplegic
    (B) an elderly male
    (C) a patient with Pick's disease (frontotemporal dementia)
    (D) a patient with diabetic neuropathy
    (E) an infant

342. The best and safest ancillary test for the further evaluation of the headache patient is

    (A) a lumbar puncture
    (B) a non-contrast head CT
    (C) an EEG
    (D) an MRI scan of the head (with gadolinium)
    (E) laboratory testing including an ESR

343. A 20-year-old woman presents to your clinic with a headache. It is unilateral, pulsating and accompanied by photophobia. She reports that sometimes flashing lights precede the headache. The physical and neurological examination are normal. The headache most consistent with this presentation is

    (A) migraine headache
    (B) tension-type headache
    (C) cluster headache
    (D) headache related to substance use
    (E) pseudotumor cerebri

344. A 40-year-old businessman presents to your clinic with the complaint of a sharp pain behind his eye. Physical examination reveals injected conjunctiva. Neurological examination reveals ptosis. He reports that he just finished a cigarette waiting for you. The headache most consistent with this history is

    (A) migraine headache
    (B) tension-type headache
    (C) cluster headache
    (D) headache related to substance use
    (E) pseudotumor cerebri

345. A 25-year-old woman presents to your clinic with a frontal, band-like pain. She reports that her mother used to get the same headache. She reports that she has been taking her roommate's Valium which relieves the symptoms. Her physical examination is notable only for obesity. Her neurological examination in normal. The headache most consistent with this presentation is

(A) migraine headache
(B) tension-type headache
(C) cluster headache
(D) headache related to substance use
(E) pseudotumor cerebri

346. A 25-year old teacher presents with a dull, generalized headache. She reports that she is worried because her menses are late. She drinks caffeine regularly. Physical examination reveals obesity and papilledema. The headache most consistent with this presentation is

(A) headache secondary to mass lesion
(B) tension-type headache
(C) posttraumatic headache
(D) headache related to substance use
(E) pseudotumor cerebri

347. A 24-year-old male presents to your clinic with brief sharp pains that extend down the right side of his face. The pain is worse with touch as well as with cold liquids. The pain is better at night. The best strategy for this patient is

(A) anesthetic injection in the nerve root
(B) treatment with carbamazepine
(C) MRI with gadolinium
(D) surgical placement of a barrier between the trigeminal nerve
(E) treatment with lithium with a serum level of 0.6 to 1.0 mEq/L

348. A middle-aged patient presents with a severe frontal headache with nuchal rigidity. The patient is so impaired that he arrives by ambulance after a minor traffic accident. He has difficulty giving a history. The LEAST likely causative agent is

(A) meningococcus
(B) pneumococcus
(C) herpes simplex
(D) posttraumatic headache
(E) rupture of cerebral artery

349. The following answers link a headache type with relief treatment. The MISMATCHED headache and treatment is

(A) migraine headache - chocolate
(B) cluster headache - lithium carbonate
(C) tension-type headache - biofeedback
(D) headache due to acetaminophen withdrawal - steroid taper
(E) pseudotumor cerebri - dieting

350. The testing that is NOT helpful in the physical examination of the headache patient is

(A) palpating the skull
(B) auscultation over the temple and eyes
(C) auscultation of the neck for bruits
(D) gait testing
(E) funduscopic examination

351. A 50-year-old male presents with a bilateral, dull headache. The headache has been intermittent for 1 week. His wife notes that he has been a little more irritable this week because he stopped smoking and he is having difficulty with their taxes. His physical examination reveals decreased breath sounds in the left lower lung field. Neurological examination is normal. There is no papilledema. The MOST LIKELY cause of the headache is

(A) migraine headache
(B) tension-type headache
(C) cluster headache
(D) headache related to substance use
(E) headache due to a mass lesion

352. Visual agnosia may be the result of

(A) intoxication with methanol
(B) a glioma in the optic chiasm
(C) bilateral detachment of the retina
(D) bilateral destruction of the parietal lobes
(E) none of the above

For question 353 use the key below to choose the correct answer.

(A) 1, 2, and 3 are correct
(B) 1 and 3 are correct
(C) 2 and 4 are correct
(D) 4 is correct
(E) all are correct

353. Amaurosis fugax (transient monocular blindness) may herald

(1) complete detachment of the retina
(2) permanent blindness from cranial (temporal) arteritis
(3) permanent blindness after methanol poisoning
(4) stroke from carotid artery occulusion

354. Auditory hallucinations of an elementary nature are associated with lesions of the

(A) hypothalamus
(B) cerebellar nuclei
(C) pons
(D) prefrontal cortex
(E) cerebellar cortex

355. Which of the following statements about post-stroke depression is NOT correct?

(A) Males and females are equally affected by post-stroke depression.
(B) Up to 20% of stroke victims suffer from post-stroke depression.
(C) Untreated post-stroke depression has an average duration of 2 months.
(D) Stimulants may be useful for the treatment of post-stroke depression.
(E) Electroconvulsive therapy may be useful for the treatment of post-stroke depression.

356. Occlusion of the anterior cerebral artery may result in

(A) appearance of grasp and suck reflexes
(B) paraplegia
(C) urinary incontinence
(D) sensorimotor deficits in the contralateral lower extremity
(E) all of the above

357. Which of the following statements about eye movements is NOT correct?

   (A) A left pontine lesion may result in gaze deviation to the right.
   (B) A right frontal lesion may result in gaze deviation to the left.
   (C) Internuclear ophthalmoplegia is recognized by inability in adducting to the eye past the midline on the side of the lesion.
   (D) Lesions in the rostral midbrain may affect vertical eye movements.
   (E) Nystagmus may be a manifestation of cerebellar stroke.

358. Which of the following statements about conduction aphasia is NOT correct?

   (A) Word repetition is intact.
   (B) Speech output is fluent.
   (C) Comprehension of written and spoken language is intact.
   (D) Paraphasias are present.
   (E) Lesions of the arcuate fascicle result in a disconnection of Wernickes and Brocas area.

359. Which of the following statements about post-stroke mania is correct?

   (A) Right hemisphere lesions are more often associated with post-stroke mania than left hemisphere lesions.
   (B) Post-stroke mania occurs in 5% of all stroke victims.
   (C) Stroke of the left caudate nucleus is the single most frequent lesion associated with post-stroke mania.
   (D) Lithium is contraindicated for the treatment of post-stroke mania.
   (E) None of the above is correct.

360. Homonymous hemianopia for the left visual field typically results from vascular lesions of the

   (A) left optic nerve
   (B) right hypothalamus
   (C) right parieto-temporal white matter
   (D) left visual cortex
   (E) left lateral geniculate

361. You receive a call from Ms. A, a 50-year-old woman treated with a monoamine oxidase inhibitor for the past 2 years. Ms. A reports that she took earlier in the day an over-the-counter decongestant and that she then experienced, in her own words, "a pounding headache." The pounding headache is now gone, a visiting nurse took Ms. A's blood pressure (140/90 mmHg) and heart rate (85 beats/min) 5 min before the call. Upon further questioning, it becomes apparent that Ms. A has some nausea and also a localized headache centered around the left occiput. Ms. A has experienced left-side headaches several times in her life and reports that "migraine runs in the family." Which of the following is the MOST appropriate response?

   (A) You ask the visiting nurse to check blood pressure every 30 min for the next 2 h.
   (B) You arrange immediate transportation to an emergency department and schedule a non-contrast CT of the head.
   (C) You schedule a diffusion-weighted MRI for the same day in the radiology clinic.
   (D) After ruling out that the ingestion of the decongestant was intended to cause self-harm, you provide reassurance and ask the patient to call you again if the pounding headache reappears.
   (E) You call the primary care physician of Ms. A, in order to discuss the treatment of migraine in this patient.

362. You are asked to opine on a 45-year-old female treated in an ICU setting for fever, tachycardia, dehydration, and intermittent drops in blood pressure. The patient is unresponsive. On physical examination, an increase in muscle tone, intermittent jerks, and intermittent staring at the examiner is noticed. Laboratory abnormalities include leukocytosis and mild hypernatremia. Lithium level is 0.6 mEq/L and CK is within the normal rate. The history is incomplete, but a note from her outpatient psychiatrist indicates that the patient has had a diagnosis since 10 years of age of bipolar I and has been treated with haloperidol and lithium for the past 10 years until the day of this admission. Based on this information, which suggestion is NOT correct?

   (A) discontinue lithium
   (B) discontinue haloperidol
   (C) start lorazepam 2 mg IV
   (D) start Clozaril
   (E) prepare for ECT after a medical and neurological work-up

For questions 363 and 364 choose the correct answer from the key below.

   (A) 1, 2, and 3 are correct
   (B) 1 and 3 are correct
   (C) 2 and 4 are correct
   (D) 4 is correct
   (E) all are correct

363. You diagnosed your patient, a 40-year-old lawyer, with an anxiety disorder with hypochondrical features and start treatment with fluoxetine, 5 mg/day. Two days after you increased the dose to 10 mg/day, the patient presents in your office with a visible, new-onset tremor in the right hand, while the left hand appears to be less affected by the tremor. The patient mentions concerns about having a stroke and becoming crazy. At this time, which of the following measures are the MOST appropriate?

   (1) Explain to the patient the side-effect profile of fluoxetine and reassure the patient that the tremor is best explained in terms of a drug-related tremor.
   (2) Mention to the patient the option to start a beta-blocker or a benzodiazepine.
   (3) Inform the patient that treatment with fluoxetine could be continued and that the tremor may turn out to be of a transitory nature.
   (4) Because of the side preference of the tremor, you refer the patient to a movement disorder clinic.

364. Idiopathic Parkinson's disease is characterized by degeneration of the following neuronal populations

   (1) serotonergic neurons in the raphe nuclei
   (2) tyrosine hydroxylase immunoreactive neurons in the locus ceruleus
   (3) cholinergic neurons in the basal forebrain
   (4) dopaminergic projection neurons in the midbrain

365. Abnormal expansion of trinucleotide repeats is the underlying molecular defect in each of the following degenerative disorders EXCEPT

   (A) fragile X syndrome
   (B) Huntington's chorea
   (C) myotonic dystrophy
   (D) spinal and bulbar muscular atrophy
   (E) dementia with cortical Lewy bodies

For questions 366 and 367 choose the correct answer from the key below.

   (A) 1, 2, and 3 are correct
   (B) 1 and 3 are correct
   (C) 2 and 4 are correct
   (D) 4 is correct
   (E) all are correct

366. Which of the following treatments of major depression in a patient with Parkinson's disease are reasonable as the treatment of choice?

    (1) electroconvulsive therapy for a patient who developed a psychotic depression while being treated with L-dopa
    (2) the monoamine oxidase B inhibitor selegiline for a patient who has not been on anti-parkinsonian drugs in the last 2 months
    (3) L-dopa (given with a peripheral dopa decarboxylase inhibitor) for a patient who never received treatment for Parkinsonian symptoms or depression
    (4) fluoxetine for an elderly depressed patient suspected of having Parkinson's disease and Lewy body dementia

367. The following symptoms may be a manifestation of motor neuron disease

    (1) spasticity in a muscle group of an extremity
    (2) paresis and low tonus of a muscle group of an extremity
    (3) difficulty swallowing
    (4) stool incontinence

368. Which of the following movement disorders is the LEAST likely to be accompanied by psychosis?

    (A) Parkinson's disease
    (B) Huntingtons's disease
    (C) Wilson's disease
    (D) Lou-Gehrig's disease (amyotrophic lateral sclerosis)
    (E) Shy-Drager syndrome

369. Which of the following statements about SSRIs is NOT correct?

    (A) tremor is a potential side-effect
    (B) akathisia is a potential side-effect
    (C) Meigs syndrome may be SSRI-related
    (D) Monitoring for tardive dyskinesia is indicated in patients on long-term maintenance therapy with SSRIs.
    (E) SSRIs may be co-administered with L-dopa in patients with Parkinson's disease and depression.

370. Which of the following statements about tardive dyskinesia is NOT correct?

    (A) women are at increased risk
    (B) children are at increased risk
    (C) rabbit syndrome is defined as perioral tardive dyskinesia
    (D) olanzapine has been associated with tardive dyskinesia
    (E) symptoms of tardive dyskinesia may disappear after changing the dose of the precipitating neuroleptic

371. Which of the following statements about Tourette's disorder is NOT correct?

    (A) Stimulants may worsen motor and verbal tics.
    (B) Stimulants may improve motor and verbal tics.
    (C) Dopamine (D_2) receptor blockers may worsen motor and verbal tics.
    (D) Dopamine (D_2) receptor blockers may improve motor and verbal tics.
    (E) Tic disorders occur are more frequent in families of Tourette's patients, in comparison to controls.

372. Which of the following statements regarding the syndrome of catatonia is TRUE?

    (A) The syndrome is characterized by a small number of behavioral symptoms and most often arises de novo in the absence of neurochemical insults.
    (B) The exact prevalence of catatonia is estimated to be 40% of all psychiatric inpatients.
    (C) Catatonia occurs more often in patients suffering from schizophrenia than mood disorders.
    (D) Its pathophysiology most likely involves the basal ganglia and possibly the prefrontal cortex.
    (E) None of the above

373. Which of the following statements regarding NMS is TRUE?

(A) Mortality rates for patients with NMS have increased from 20% (prior to 1984) to 25.6%, due to the increase in use of neuroleptics.
(B) Just as there are clinical similarities between NMS and malignant hyperthermia (associated with general anesthesia), patients with a history of either NMS or malignant hyperthermia appear to be at increased risk for developing the other.
(C) Lack of uniform diagnostic criteria, concurrent use of other medications, and methodological differences used in epidemiology studies have made estimating the frequency of NMS difficult.
(D) The incidence of NMS is estimated from 2% to 5%.
(E) None of the above

374. Which of the following is NOT a form of reliability?

(A) internal consistency
(B) test re-test reliability
(C) external reliability
(D) Inter-rater reliability
(E) Kappa

375. Which of the following is NOT included in the definition of a psychological test?

(A) standard scoring
(B) standard instructions
(C) normative sample
(D) standard administration
(E) copyright assignment

376. Which of these is NOT a form of validity?

(A) predictive
(B) convergent
(C) divergent
(D) content
(E) projective

377. Which is NOT true. "The MMPI-2"

(A) is a self-report test of psychopathology
(B) is brief
(C) is able to assess test-taking motivation
(D) is computer scored
(E) is able to assess many forms of psychopathology

378. TRUE or FALSE. The history of psychological assessment extends back into ancient times.

379. TRUE or FALSE. Once validated a psychological test is universally valid.

380. Which of the following is NOT true of the Rorschach Inkblot Test?

(A) it contains 10 cards with inkblots on them
(B) it is unreliable
(C) it is less structured than other psychological tests
(D) it provides a good measure of thought quality
(E) none of the above

381. TRUE or FALSE. A clinical psychological consultation should be done "blind" so that non-test data do not influence the findings.

382. TRUE or FALSE. Psychological test reports should focus on reporting the results of each test so that the referring psychiatrist can decide what the findings indicate.

383. TRUE or FALSE. Neuropsychological assessment is the procedure of choice for a definitive diagnosis of attention deficit hyperactivity disorder.

384. The Boston process approach to neuropsychological testing is characterized by

    (A) providing a composite overview of global cognitive strengths or deficits
    (B) having a standardized battery that can be compared across all types of patients or conditions
    (C) varying from patient to patient after establishing baseline intelligence functioning, often testing specific hypothesis generated by referral questions or current performance
    (D) primarily stressing language functions and deficits
    (E) none of the above

385. Neuropsychological exams are NOT germane to diagnosing impairments in

    (A) memory
    (B) attention
    (C) visual spatial construction
    (D) dementia
    (E) none of the above

386. Typically, what pattern of neuropsychological test findings is helpful in differentiating depression from dementia in the elderly?

    (A) memory, with delayed recalled being worse in the demented patients
    (B) attention, with disrupted attention being a hallmark of early dementia
    (C) visual spatial construction indicating weak right hemisphere functioning
    (D) memory, with delayed recall being worse in the depressed patients
    (E) none of the above

387. Which of the following situations would NOT be appropriate for making a neuropsychological assessment referral?

    (A) informing decisions about independent living ability
    (B) adjusting care plans for a patient who has failed multiple psychiatric treatments
    (C) monitoring the course of a progressive neurological condition
    (D) establishing a baseline of cognitive functioning in a recently diagnosed AIDS patient
    (E) none of the above

388. Which of the following tests is NOT likely to be used in a neuropsychological assessment?

    (A) Wechsler IQ test
    (B) memory tests with immediate and delayed recall
    (C) Rorschach inkblot test
    (D) the MMPI-2
    (E) receptive and expressive language tests

389. TRUE or FALSE. If you get an MRI on a patient, you do not need to obtain neuropsychological testing.

390. TRUE or FALSE. The Halstead-Reitan (H-R) test battery is brief and flexible.

391. Which of the following is NOT an important feature of neuropsychological tests?

    (A) a demonstrated relationship to brain functioning
    (B) age and education adjusted norms
    (C) high levels of complexity
    (D) clear instructions
    (E) standard administration

392. What is the number of the affected chromosome in Huntington's disease?

    (A) 2
    (B) 3
    (C) 4
    (D) 5
    (E) 21

393. Which one of these is characteristic for patients with absence seizures?

    (A) spikes, polyspikes, and waves over the temporal region
    (B) 3 Hz spike-wave complexes
    (C) generalized theta activity
    (D) spindle-form complexes
    (E) none of the above

394. Which of these biological markers is decreased in the CSF of patients with suicidal behavior?

    (A) HVA
    (B) 5-HIAA
    (C) serine
    (D) proenkephalin
    (E) none of the above

395. Which one of the following drugs can be detected in the urine after 30 days?

    (A) cocaine
    (B) benzodiazepines
    (C) methadone
    (D) cannabinoids
    (E) none of the above

396. A 76-year-old patient presents to your office with worsening forgetfulness without other psychiatric problems. History and physical are unrevealing. Which of the following tests would NOT be appropriate for initial screening?

    (A) TFTs
    (B) CBC with differential
    (C) CT scan
    (D) PET scan
    (E) CSF analysis

397. Natural medications

    (A) are generally approved and regulated by the FDA for their indications
    (B) offer greater treatment autonomy to patients
    (C) have become less popular because insurers will not cover them
    (D) have well-defined safety profiles
    (E) may be recommended only by medical doctors

398. St. John's Wort

  (A) is currently being compared to SSRIs in clinical trials
  (B) requires a special diet because of its MAOI activity
  (C) never causes a switch to mania in bipolar patients
  (D) may be safely combined with SSRIs in bipolar patients
  (E) has been shown to be more effective than high-dose tricyclics

399. Valerian

  (A) is popular among Hispanic patients
  (B) is recommended for acute treatment of insomnia
  (C) may contain potential carcinogens in some preparations
  (D) A and C only
  (E) A, B and C are correct

400. Which of the following is/are true about kava?

  (A) its use originated in the Polynesian islands
  (B) so far it has shown no evidence of dependence
  (C) It may have anticonvulsant properties.
  (D) It may cause a yellow discoloration of the skin.
  (E) all of the above

Answers

1. The answer is C.
DSM-IV criteria do not address etiology and treatment related to the various disorders.

2. The answer is D.
The process of creating the DSM-IV did not involve surveys of practitioners' practices.

3. The answer is E.
All of the answers are correct.

4. The answer is D.
The challenge for the adolescent is to overcome role confusion.

5. The answer is C.
By age 3 a child is able to give their first and last name.

6. The answer is A.
Although the cases one often hears about are in families of low socioeconomic class, this is not a risk factor for child abuse.

7. The answer is D.
Children develop the ability to understand the concept of conservation between the ages of 7 and 11. At this stage a child is able to understand the concept of the combination of two variables.

8. The answer is C.
Stranger anxiety develops in infants around the age of 8 months.

9. The answer is B.
The disorder persists into adolescence and adulthood in approximately 50% of patients.

10. The answer is True.
This is one of the defining factors of the disorder and it differentiates it from autism.

11. The answer is False.
Separation anxiety disorder is the only anxiety disorder listed in the DSM-IV as a childhood disorder.

12. The answer is False.
Children are more rapid metabolizers and may need two times the weight-corrected dose of medications.

13. The answer is E.
Anhedonia may suggest the presence of depression.

14. The answer is B.
While hallucinations are commonly seen with delirium, they may also be associated with dementia.

15. The answer is False.
Patients with dementia or suspected dementia require careful assessment for depression.

16. The answer is D.
SSRIs may be useful in the treatment of comorbid depression, though almost any drug can be associated with cognitive impairment.

17. The answer is E.
Patients with dementia are, however, particularly susceptible to developing delirium in the presence of any intercurrent infection, including infection of the urinary tract.

18. The answer is A.
An erythrocyte sedimentation rate is not recommended for routine screening, though it may be useful in some cases.

19. The answer is True.
Patients may also develop apraxias (of dressing or eating, for example) and impairment in face recognition.

20. The answer is False.
Psychiatric symptoms are common in Alzheimer's disease; delusions are a feature in up to 50% of cases, while hallucinations are seen in up to 25% of cases.

21. The answer is A.
Incontinence is more commonly associated with other forms of dementia, such as normal pressure hydrocephalus. Answers B-D are particular features of dementia with Lewy bodies; E is typical of any dementia.

22. The answer is D.
Visual hallucinations are more common in other types of dementias.

23. The answer is D.
L-dopa is commonly used to treat Parkinson's disease.

24. The answer is C.
Using the telephone is considered an instrumental activity of daily living.

25. The answer is A.
The generally accepted prevalence of mental retardation is 1%.

26. The answer is C.
Down's syndrome is the most common identified genetic cause of mental retardation.

27. The answer is A.
Fragile X syndrome is the most common identified inherited cause of mental retardation. Up to one-third of female carriers may have mental retardation.

28. The answer is C.
Trisomy 21.

29. The answer is B.
Chromosome 15 deletion (70% of cases).

30. The answer is D.
q27, long arm of X chromosome.

31. The answer is A.
Chromosome 7 deletion.

32. The answer is D.
75–80% of individuals with autism/pervasive development disorder are mentally retarded.

33. The answer is D.
ADHD has been noted to occur in individuals with fragile X syndrome 80% of the time.

34. The answer is B.
Individuals with Down's syndrome have a much higher incidence of Alzheimer's dementia than those in the general population or those with mental retardation in general. They also have a much earlier age of onset of Alzheimer's dementia.

35. The answer is A.
Mental disorder due to a general medical condition (DTGMC) should be part of the differential diagnosis for any psychiatric syndrome. A history of psychiatric symptoms does not rule out the possibility of the current episode being DTGMC. Psychiatric symptoms of some medical conditions may precede physical signs and symptoms, and be indistinguishable from primary psychiatric disorders described in DSM-IV.

36. The answer is C.
General paresis, a form of late (tertiary) syphilis, is seen in less than 10% of untreated syphilitics, 20 years after primary infection. There is diffuse involvement, but the frontal lobes are especially affected; signs and symptoms include personality change, irritability, poor judgment and insight, difficulty with calculations and recent memory, apathy, and decreased personal grooming. Rare in the post-penicillin era, general paresis may be on the rise among individuals with AIDS. Classical neurological signs of untreated tertiary syphilis include tremor, dysarthria, hyperreflexia, hypotonia, ataxia, and Argyll-Robertson pupils.

37. The answer is E.
All of the statements about epilepsy are true. Sixty percent of epileptics in the United States have nonconvulsive seizures, most commonly partial seizures. Complex partial seizures are associated with a 6–12-fold increased risk of psychosis over the general population, with hallucinations, paranoia, and thought disorder (circumstantiality) being the most common symptoms. Depression occurs in more than half of patients with epilepsy, as compared to 30% of matched (medical and neurologic outpatient) controls. Depression may be even more prevalent in patients with partial complex seizures with left hemispheric foci. The suicide rate in patients with epilepsy is five times that of the general public; in patients with temporal lobe epilepsy, the risk may be 25-fold higher than the general public.

38. The answer is D.
Both panic attacks and partial seizures can occur "out of the blue," and present with hyperarousal, intense fear, perceptual distortion, and dissociative symptoms, such as depersonalization or derealization. Long-acting benzodiazepines may be efficacious in both disorders. Automatisms (which involve automatic behaviors such as lip smacking), occur briefly, often with unresponsiveness, in the course of partial seizures, but not with panic attacks. Automatic, catastrophic thoughts (e.g., "I'm going to die, or lose control, or go crazy, or faint.") are more common in panic attacks, and are listed as criteria in the DSM-IV.

Panic attacks typically last longer than partial seizures, with intact memory of the episode, which may lead to agoraphobia, but not confusion. In partial seizures, memory of the episode is usually incomplete, agoraphobia is rare, and post-ictal confusion is common.

39. The answer is B.
In multiple sclerosis, psychiatric symptoms may precede physical symptoms, and may not clear with remission of physical symptoms. Depression and irritability are the most common mood symptoms, with mild mood elevation occurring episodically in about a quarter of patients, and persistent euphoria in less than 10% of patients. Psychiatric symptoms do not correlate with MRI findings, severity of physical symptoms, or length of illness.

40. The answer is True.
Brain tumors, such as gliomas, which account for 50–60% of primary brain tumors, tend to cause diffuse symptoms (e.g., cognitive decline), as they grow slowly and diffusely throughout the cortex. Multiple metastases and lymphoma can also present with this diffuse pattern. Meningiomas, which account for 25% of primary brain tumors, grow extrinsic to the brain and compress a limited area, causing more focal, progressive symptoms.

41. The answer is True.
Hypoglycemic encephalopathy can present with confusion, disorientation, or hallucinations and bizarre behavior. It is often preceded by restlessness and apprehension. Repeated hypoglycemic episodes may cause permanent amnesia from hippocampal involvement.

42. The answer is B.
Cocaine's vasoconstriction properties cause hypoperfusion that results in hypoxia. Another complication from the vasoconstricting properties of cocaine is placental abruption.

43. The answer is C.
Freebase and crack cocaine have the shortest time to onset of effects and the shortest duration of action of any form of cocaine. These properties contribute to their highly addictive nature.

44. The answer is B.
Symptoms observed in infants who ingest cocaine from breast milk include rapid heart rate, increased blood pressure, apnea, diaphoresis, and mydriasis.

45. The answer is C.
Alcohol, benzodiazepines, and cocaine are the most common comorbid substances used by opiate addicts. It is difficult to distinguish between a primary depression from an opioid-induced mood disorder. Therefore, time is required to allow for the effect of the opiate on brain function to clear before making a definitive diagnosis. The diagnosis of antisocial personality disorder is also difficult to make in the context of active opiate-dependence, since one of the complications of opiate addictions is antisocial behavior.

46. The answer is A.
Though the prevalence of schizophrenia is similar in males and females, males typically have a poorer outcome and experience symptoms of schizophrenia in their teens and early twenties while females develop the disorder from their mid-twenties to their mid-forties.

47. The answer is A.
The negative symptoms of schizophrenia include apathy, anhedonia, asociality, affective flattening, alogia, and inattentiveness.

48. The answer is False.
Monozygotic twins have the highest concordance rate (40-50%), as compared to 15% for dizygotic twins.

49. The answer is A.
Most typical epidemiological studies, like the ECA (Epidemiological Catchment Area) study, find a 1% mania lifetime prevalence rate. Studies which include hypomania and milder forms of the bipolar spectrum report higher rates.

50. The answer is D.
He does not meet DIGFAST criteria for mania. Irritability can occur in unipolar depression as well as bipolar disorder. Spending sprees by themselves are insufficient to diagnose bipolar disorder; excessive spending can occur in depression and other conditions. This patient has depressive symptoms in the absence of sufficient criteria for hypomania or mania; thus the diagnosis is unipolar depression.

51. The answer is D.
This patient meets DIGFAST criteria for mania and depressive criteria; hence he is diagnosed with a mixed episode.

52. The answer is E.
Although the patient denied the symptoms, the spouse's report is at least as valid. Thus, this patient meets DIGFAST criteria of hypomania but significant social and occupational dysfunction cannot be established. Since not a single manic episode can be established in the past, and she has experienced at least one major depressive episode and at least one hypomanic episode, the diagnosis is bipolar disorder, type II.

53. The answer is C.
A mood stabilizer is always the best treatment for any patient with bipolar disorder, even with a milder type II condition where depression predominates.

54. The answer is C.
Genetic inheritance is polygenic and non-mendelian. The gender ratio of bipolar disorder is equally male and female. Psychosocial outcome can be excellent, fair or poor. Primary mood disorders begin before the age of 40. The suicide rate in bipolar disorder is about 20%, the highest rate of any axis I disorder.

55. The answer is B.
All of the above criteria are DIGFAST criteria for mania, derived from DSM-IV, except hypersomnia.

Hypersomnia tends to occur in the depressed phase of bipolar disorder, but not in mania. In any case, characteristics of depression are irrelevant to diagnosing bipolar disorder. Since the diagnosis of bipolar disorder is made by identifying only one manic episode, solely manic criteria are relevant.

56. The answer is D.
Mixed episodes are characterized by both depressive and manic symptoms. Flat affect is characteristic of schizophrenia.

57. The answer is C.
Distractibility is a DSM-IV criterion for mania. Psychosis occurs in half of individuals with bipolar disorder, although it is limited to manic or depressive episodes, unlike the course of schizoaffective disorder or schizophrenia. The kindling hypothesis explains a worsening of the illness over time, with more frequent episodes later in the illness. Antidepressant-induced mania is a major problem. Rapid-cycling bipolar disorder is defined by four or more episodes in year; it does not require daily, weekly, or even monthly mood swings.

58. The answer is B.
Antidepressants are appropriately used in severe bipolar depression along with mood stabilizers. However, their benefit is limited to short-term acute improvement of depression; they do not prevent depressive episodes in

bipolar disorder. Some of the newer antidepressants have a lower mania switch-rate than older tricyclic antidepressants.

59. The answer is D.
Imipramine is a tricyclic antidepressant, a class with a high mania switch-rate. The SSRIs, fluoxetine and sertraline, have not been shown to have lower switch rate in type I bipolar disorder, nor has trazodone. Bupropion has been shown to have a lower switch-rate than tricyclic antidepressants in type I bipolar disorder.

60. The answer is D.
Patients with mood and thought disorders often present to their primary care physician with a somatic complaint. Even when speaking to a mental health care professional, patients feel more comfortable using body language to convey distress. "I am tired" or I am in pain" are examples of words that may relate to a patient's physical or emotional state. Recognition of psychiatric symptoms helps prevent further disability of the patient and contains health care costs.

61. The answer is E.
To meet criteria for somatoform disorder, the symptoms cannot be intentionally produced or feigned. This would fall under the category of factitious disorder or malingering. Proposed etiologies of somatoform disorders include learning, psychodynamic, cultural, and biological theories. All are unwittingly produced by the patient. However, the manner in which these patients present, with their long lists of vague and ever-changing complaints, can often make the physician wonder about the intentions of the patient. These patients tend to push the limits of the therapeutic relationship and make caring for them very difficult. Early consideration of the diagnosis and referral for psychiatric consultation can help reduce tension in the therapeutic relationship, reduce further disability of the patient, and lower overall health care costs.

62. The answer is D.
The criteria for hypochondriasis focus on the belief of being ill rather than on any one malady in particular. The actual physical symptoms in hypochondriasis vary from patient to patient; for a given patient, the symptoms may remain constant over time or change. Although the preoccupation persists despite medical evaluation and reassurance, the belief is not so unshakable as is a somatic delusion. Because treatment of hypochondriasis and delusional disorder, somatic type, differs greatly, making the correct diagnosis is crucial.

63. The answer is A.
Somatization disorder is the somatoform disorder which presents as a global recitation of symptoms. All of the following DSM-IV criteria need to be met for the diagnosis of somatization disorder: 1) four pain symptoms each in a different area of the body; 2) two non-pain related gastrointestinal symptoms; 3) one sexual symptom; and, 4) one pseudoneurologic symptom. The symptoms may present at different times in the person's life; an episode can last for 6–9 months and there is often a quiescent period of 9–12 months without any symptoms. Since the patient may present differently at each visit, may not remember earlier complaints, and often sees different physicians, the diagnosis is difficult to make.

64. The answer is C.
Conversion disorder is the most common somatoform disorder. In the DSM-IV criteria, a pseudoneurologic symptom must be present for the diagnosis to be made. Common symptoms include seizures, gait or coordination disturbances, blindness, tunnel vision, and anesthesia. There is often a temporal relationship between the symptoms and a psychologically meaningful precipitant. Although the symptom is not feigned, the patient can sometimes modulate the severity of the symptom. For example, with great concentration, an hysterically blind patient might see more clearly or a patient with astasia-abasia may walk with better control.

65. The answer is A.
Confronting the somatizing patient, especially early on, has not been shown to be helpful. Rather, introduction of psychosocial issues slowly, and use of mind-body language is a better approach. Forcing the patient to "lose face" will only result in humiliation, anger, and a change in physicians. A good relationship with one long-term caring primary care physician has been shown to be most helpful to the patient over time. Allowing the sick role while not encouraging it, scheduling regular follow-up visits of set length, limiting contact outside the visit all must be part of the relationship. Use of a "team approach," calling in other providers such as a psychiatrist or psychotherapist, is often useful.

66. The answer is B.
While many dissociative disorders are more common in women, the tendency to dissociate is roughly equal in men and women.

67. The answer is C.
While patients with DID may experience internally experienced auditory hallucinations, these individuals typically lack evidence for a formal thought disorder and would not be expected to display disorganized speech.

68. The answer is A.
Although the Dissociative Experience Scale has been validated for the diagnosis of dissociative symptoms, it has achieved face validity only. Subjects can purposefully misrepresent their scores, and the results of the DES should therefore be complimented by a careful clinical exam.

69. The answer is A.
75% of cases last between 24 h and 5 days, but most resolve. Amnestic episodes may be either global for all

autobiographical information or for specific memories only. Although memory loss is usually for traumatic experiences, this is not a requirement for the diagnosis.

70. The answer is D.
Dissociative fugue occurs roughly the same in men and women, though the incidence of men suffering from the syndrome increases during wartime, presumably because of the increased number of men experiencing severe trauma. Although fugues may result from drugs or alcohol, these episodes would not be classified as formal dissociative fugues. Dissociative fugue most commonly presents between the second and fourth decades.

71. The answer is B.
There was an increase in reported cases of DID in the 1980s, though the reasons for this increase are controversial.

72. The answer is C.
While transient depersonalization is relatively common in males and females, depersonalization disorder is much rarer and occurs more often in females. Most cases of depersonalization disorder are refractory to treatment.

73. The answer is E.
Patients who are purposefully feigning dissociative symptoms will often be extremely invested in the diagnosis of a dissociative disorder.

74. The answer is E.
Brainwashing and altered states of consciousness resulting from torture are typically classified as dissociative disorder not otherwise specified.

75. The answer is A.
Ganser's syndrome is also sometimes called prison psychosis and is often reported in incarcerated populations. While dissociative trance disorder is not a formal DSM-IV classification, it is intended to include episodes of apparent possession and religious trance states. Pierre Janet was an important figure in the early study of dissociation. Amok and Latah are both usually classified as dissociative disorder not otherwise specified.

76. The answer is True.
The hallmark of vasocongestion (excitement phase) is penile erection in the male and vaginal lubrication in the female. This is followed by increased muscular tension resulting in orgasm (orgasmic phase) in both sexes.

77. The answer is True.
At menopause, with the decline in estrogen levels, external and internal organs change significantly, creating a situation detrimental to sexual functioning. Short-term estrogen replacement therapy (ERT) improves vaginal blood flow, reduces urinary incontinence, and promotes the return of normal pH and bacterial flora.

78. The answer is True.
Incest occurs at every socioeconomic level.

79. The answer is True.
Psychosocial and aging factors are often found to be more important determinants than ovarian function on sexual functioning among middle-aged women. Some of these factors include the availability of a partner, previous sexual behavior and enjoyment, quality of the marital relationship, mental health (including stress), general physical health, expectations, and male partner problems. Marital status has been found to be negatively related to interest (which may be an effect of having a new partner). Cigarette smoking has also been shown to have a negative effect on sexual functioning.

80. The answer is A.
The partners of men with premature ejaculation may not have enough time to build up their erotic response and are often anorgasmic.

81. The answer is D.
Rape is an act of aggression rather than one of sexual expression.

82. The answer is True.
This woman's weight is more than 7% less than the expected 120 lb. for a 5 feet 4 inches woman and she is continuing to lose weight; therefore, inpatient care is probably indicated.

83. The answer is False.
Estrogen replacement therapy has not been proven to prevent bone loss in women with anorexia nervosa. The treatment of choice for bone loss in anorexia nervosa is weight gain. It is also recommended that individuals with anorexia nervosa take 1500 mg of calcium as well as a multivitamin with vitamin D daily. Combination estrogen and progestin treatment may be beneficial in alleviating other symptoms of estrogen deficiency in anorexic women.

84. The answer is False.
Approximately 50% of individuals with anorexia will make a full recovery, whereas 50% make a partial recovery or make no substantial recovery.

85. The answer is False.
There is no medication that is generally useful for the primary symptoms of anorexia nervosa. However, fluoxetine may stabilize recovery for individuals who have recovered their weight to at least 85% of expected weight. Individuals with anorexia nervosa and a comorbid major depression may benefit from an SSRI to target mood symptoms.

86. The answer is True.
Binge-eating disorder occurs in approximately 2.6% of the population, whereas anorexia nervosa occurs in only 0.28% and bulimia nervosa in only 1% of the young adult female population.

87. The answer is False.
Cognitive-behavioral therapy, the best established psychotherapy for bulimia nervosa, has superior efficacy over medication therapy. Reduction of bingeing and purging symptoms with CBT treatment is approximately 70-90%, whereas reduction occurs in only approximately 56% with medication.

88. The answer is B.
The normal NREM-REM cycles are NREM Stage 1, followed by 3 to 4 repeats of 2, 3, 4, 3, 2, REM. In this cycle, Stage 2 is usually proceeded and followed by Stage 3, and REM is entered and exited through Stage 2 sleep.

89. The answer is A.
Sleep latency is the time from lights out to the first NREM 2. It is usually 10–20 min.

90. The answer is B.
REM time decreases as one ages. Total sleep time decreases, as does sleep efficiency, REM latency, and the amounts of NREM 3, 4 and REM. Sleep latency increases.

91. The answer is C.
Catalepsy, which is a condition of maintaining whatever body position one is placed in, is a phenomenon most often seen in catatonia. Cataplexy is the brief attacks of muscular weakness seen in narcolepsy.

92. The answer is E.
All of the statements about sleep apnea are true.

93. The answer is B.
RLS can be irritating, but is rarely painful. Patients with PLM are often unaware of it, and the bed partner is often the first to report it.

94. The answer is E.
Children are affected more than adults. Several parasomnias may occur in the same person. Patients generally have poor recall for the events of a parasomnia when awakened. Sleepwalking, nightmares, and enuresis are by far the most common parasomnias encountered.

95. The answer is C.
Night terror and nightmare disorder are often confused with each other. Night terrors are NREM phenomenon, in which the patient generally screams, flails about in bed, and experiences autonomic activity. Because it occurs in NREM sleep, the episodes are early in the night when NREM is the longest. Patients are often difficult to arouse and amnestic for the content.

96. The answer is D.
With REM behavior disorders, dream content is acted out. Nightmares, while REM-related, have accompanying muscle paralysis. Night terrors and sleepwalking are NREM phenomenon, and patients are often amnestic for events related to them.

97. The answer is E.
Most cases are idiopathic, but there is an association with brainstem pathology and alcoholism.

98. The answer is C.
The findings can be nonspecific, but as a rule, total sleep time is decreased, and REM is affected early in the course.

99. The answer is B.
REM latency is classically decreased in depression.

100. The answer is E.
All of the statements about the relationship of sleep disturbance and anxiety disorder are true.

101. The answer is C.
Alpha waves occur during wakefulness. Theta waves are first seen in NREM 1. Sleep spindles emerge during NREM 2, as do K-complexes. Delta waves are the hallmark of NREM 3 and 4.

102. The answer is D.
In the 1800s monomanias were described as behaviors that were irresistible urges with no apparent motive; they included alcoholism, fire setting, and homicide. In the DSM I and II, these behaviors included passive aggressive, immature, and explosive personality disorders. Menninger and others used the term dyscontrol syndromes, prior to 1980.

103. The answer is B.
It is estimated that 3% of the general population can be diagnosed with pathologic gambling. The epidemiology of pyromania is unknown. True kleptomania is rare (less than 0.6%) an intermittent explosive disorder is a very difficult diagnosis to make. Panic disorder is not considered an impulse control disorder.

104. The answer is D.
Most patients are not aware of their part in the loss of hair; they are generally very distressed by the condition and seek medical help.

105. The answer is A.
There is no evidence that ECT has been useful in this disorder other than to treat comorbid psychiatric conditions.

106. The answer is E.
Pathologic gambling is the only one of these disorders that does not show an increased incidence in the brain-injured population.

107. The answer is E.
HIV seropositivity.

108. The answer is D.
Feelings of anger are a normal part of grieving.

109. The answer is E.
All of the above.

110. The answer is B.
The severity of neurovegetative symptoms and disruption of functioning helps distinguish major depression from acute grief.

111. The answer is E.
None of the above.

112. The answer is B.
While more than 80% of women experience one or two mood or physical symptoms premenstrually, only a small percentage actually meet DSM-IV criteria for PMDD.

113. The answer is D.
First trimester exposure to carbamazepine is associated with a 1% risk of neural tube defects.

114. The answer is D.
There is no evidence to support the use of HRT alone in treating major depression. For major depression during the menopause transition, the treatment of choice remains antidepressants and psychotherapy.

115. The answer is C.
The amount of medication in the infant's serum does not necessarily correspond to maternal drug dose or to the maternal serum level. The accumulation of medication in the infant's serum depends on many complicated variables, including: maternal rate of drug metabolism, maternal volume of distribution, medication dosing schedule, the lipid solubility and extent of protein-binding of the medication, and the breastfeeding schedule.

116. The answer is D.
Clozapine does not appear to produce a dopamine supersensitivity or depolarization in the nigrostriatal neurons. As a result significant EPS are avoided. The nigrostriatal system is associated with EPS.

117. The answer is C.
SSRIs, such as fluoxetine, may increase neuroleptic blood levels secondary to inhibition of cytochrome P450 hepatic enzymes. Of note, fluvoxamine strongly inhibits enzymes that metabolize clozapine (P450 1A2, 3A3/4) which may lead to clozapine toxicity.

118. The answer is B.
Fluphenazine (Prolixin) is a conventional or typical antipsychotic agent. It is a strong dopamine D_2 agent that effects the nigrostriatal pathway leading to EPS and it can elevate serum prolactin levels.

119. The answer is A.
Switching to a depot neuroleptic may be helpful in the noncompliant patient who refuses to take oral medications.

120. The answer is E.
The MAOIs have numerous toxic drug-drug interactions generally classified as the "serotonin syndrome" and "hypertensive crises." The serotonin syndrome, characterized by myoclonus, hypertension, confusion, tachycardia, and fever is brought on by ingestion of serotonergic medications, such as the SSRIs (fluvoxamine and citalopram) and the TCAs, most particularly clomipramine, which has the highest serotonergic uptake inhibition effect among the TCAs. Buspirone also appears to have serotonergic effects. Medications with stimulant properties and dopaminergic agents, such as bupropion, may cause hypertensive crises which are characterized by headache, stroke, pulmonary edema, and cardiac arrhythmias. For insomnia induced by MAOIs, either trazodone, or clonazepam may be safely used to facilitate sleep.

121. The answer is B.
Amoxapine (Asendin) is a metabolite of loxapine and possesses similar neuroleptic activity due to its affinity for the dopamine D_2 receptor. Acute dystonic reactions and parkinsonian symptoms have been noted in patients taking amoxapine at high dosages; even tardive dyskinesia has been observed.

122. The answer is A.
Of the currently available medications, only the SSRIs and clomipramine have been proven to be helpful in treating OCD. The presumed advantage of clomipramine over the other TCAs is derived from its increased affinity for serotonergic receptors and increased serotonergic reuptake blockade.

123. The answer is D.
Imipramine is a tertiary amine TCA. Like all the TCAs it is hepatically metabolized. Its desmethyl metabolite is desipramine, a secondary amine TCA which is less sedating and less anticholinergic than is its parent compound. When imipramine levels are checked, the combined blood levels of imipramine and desipramine must be taken into account.

124. The answer is B.
Though all of the listed medications can induce seizures, bupropion (Wellbutrin) has the highest incidence of seizures, at a rate of 4/1,000. This risk of seizures is increased at higher dosages and for this reason, the maximum recommended dose is 450 mg/day, in divided doses. Comorbid bulimia nervosa or an underlying structural CNS abnormality increases the risk of seizures while taking bupropion. Of the cyclic antidepressants, the tetracyclic antidepressant maprotiline has a higher risk of seizure at therapeutic dosages than other cyclic antidepressants.

125. The answer is D.
The average half-life of protriptyline (Vivactil) is 78 hours, the longest half-life of any of the antidepressants other than fluoxetine ($t_{1/2} = 84$ h). The long half-life of

protriptyline, combined with the TCA side effects, has limited its use for treating depression. The half-life of bupropion is 8–24 h.

126. The answer is D.
Despite extensive clinical usage, the TCAs and SSRIs have not been shown to cause congenital malformations. However, neither has their safety been clearly established. Venlafaxine, phenelzine, and bupropion have not been well studied regarding safety in pregnancy. ECT is known to be safe and efficacious in pregnancy, and is particularly useful in a situation requiring urgent symptom resolution.

127. The answer is B.
Grapefruit juice should be avoided, because it inhibits cytochrome P450 enzymes and raises SSRI levels.

128. The answer is B.
Lithium is not metabolized by the liver; it is simply excreted unchanged by the kidney.

129. The answer is D.
Propranolol treats lithium-induced tremor. Weight gain can be reduced by carbohydrate restriction and exercise. Polyuria is treatable with thiazide diuretics.

130. The answer is B.
Thiazides increase lithium levels because they deplete sodium; lithium is retained by the kidney to replace reduced sodium levels. Since lithium is hydrophilic, water is excreted with it. Since thiazides reduce lithium excretion, they also reduce water outflow. Urinary volume thus declines. ACE inhibitors raise lithium levels. Lithium is less effective than valproic acid in mixed mania but equally effective in pure mania.

131. The answer is D.
Lithium is a mildly serotonergic drug. Lithium response is best in classic pure mania. Rapid-cycling mood disorders are less responsive to lithium. Lithium is less effective in mixed mania than are anticonvulsants, including carbamazepine and valproic acid. NSAIDs increase lithium levels.

132. The answer is C.
Side-effects are the most common cause of lithium noncompliance. Usually impaired cognition is the most difficult to improve and leads to the most impairment in social and occupational function; thus, it leads to medication discontinuation. While kidney and thyroid problems can be serious, they are not extremely common. Polyuria is common but can be tolerated or treated. Dry mouth, while common, is usually not severe and can also be tolerated.

133. The answer is E.
Lithium can cause sick sinus syndrome and impair atrioventricular cardiac conduction. It can cause hypothyroidism, diabetes insipidus (by reducing the kidney's responsiveness to ADH), and renal failure in rare cases after long-term use. Unlike valproic acid, lithium tends not to have significant liver effects.

134. The answer is D.
Anticonvulsants are more effective in mixed episodes than lithium. Lithium can be effective in bipolar depression, and in some studies it was as effective as standard antidepressants. Lithium does not have to be dosed more frequently than once daily. Lithium has been shown to reduce mortality risk by suicide in bipolar disorder, whereas carbamazepine has not.

135. The answer is D.
Lithium has mild serotonergic effects, but these do not account for its mood effects. It has no significant and direct effect on other neurotransmitters. Its main effects are postsynaptic, at the level of G-proteins and second messengers.

136. The answer is E.
Lithium can cause all of the above effects, except leukopenia, which can occur with carbamazepine. Lithium tends to cause the reverse, a temporary leukocytosis, which may be mediated by demargination of circulating leukocytes.

137. The answer is B.
Anticonvulsants are associated with neural tube defects. While chromosomal abnormalities, like trisomy 21, and minor malformations, like cleft lip and palate, can occur with lithium, Ebstein's anomaly is a more typically thought to be a lithium-related fetal malformation.

138. The answer is E.
The only FDA-approved medication for the maintenance treatment of bipolar disorder is lithium. Valproate and lithium are approved for the treatment of acute mania. The other medications are approved only for non-psychiatric indications.

139. The answer is C.
Carbamazepine is FDA-approved for the treatment of partial seizures and trigeminal neuralgia. Though some data are inconsistent, most of the trials indicate carbamazepine's effectiveness in treating mania and as a treatment to prevent relapse in bipolar disorder. In unipolar depression, carbamazepine has been found to be of only marginal benefit.

140. The answer is C.
Thrombocytopenia can occur with valproate but it is rare and usually not life-threatening. Transiently elevated transaminases are common with the initiation of treatment, but are usually of little clinical importance. Alopecia, weight gain, and gastrointestinal upset are common side-effects that often lead to poor patient compliance and to medication discontinuation.

141. The answer is A.
Valproate has been shown to be very effective in the prophylactic treatment of migraine headache; it is FDA-approved for this indication. Though it may play a role in the treatment of bipolar depression and schizo-affective disorder, there is little evidence supporting its role as a single agent. There is open-trial evidence for the efficacy of valproate in treating panic disorder, but there is no evidence for its effect in treating social phobia (gabapentin may be helpful for the treatment of this condition). Valproate may help in benzodiazepine and alcohol withdrawal; its use in heroin dependency is unknown.

142. The answer is C.
A recent study showed that lamotrigine was more effective than placebo for the treatment of bipolar disorder. There are no controlled studies for the effectiveness of gabapentin in the treatment of any phase of bipolar disorder. Carbamazepine and valproate have been shown to be effective in the treatment of mania and the maintenance treatment of bipolar disorder.

143. The answer is A.
Gabapentin is about 60% absorbed from the gut via intestinal amino acid transporters which are saturated at higher doses, making the absorption nonlinear. The other properties are true and make gabapentin a popular drug, especially as an adjunctive therapy.

144. The answer is E.
Clonazepam is FDA-approved for the treatment of childhood epilepsy, including generalized seizures (petit and grand mal) and partial seizures. Multiple studies have demonstrated its effectiveness in panic disorder. A few studies have shown that clonazepam is effective as an adjunctive agent in the early stages of SSRI-treatment and in certain neuropathies. There is little evidence that clonazepam is effective as a single agent for mania, but it is effective as an agent to reduce the need for neuroleptics.

145. The answer is C.
Lamotrigine blocks the release of glutamate and inhibits voltage-sensitive sodium channels.

146. The answer is E.
Gabapentin was designed as a GABA agonist, but it does not bind to GABA sites. Instead, it seems to increase GABA levels by influencing the GABA transporter. Clonazepam binds to the benzodiazepine binding site on the $GABA_A$ receptor.

147. The answer is D.
Topiramate has multiple mechanisms of action but it uniquely prevents kainate inhibition of the AMPA receptor.

148. The answer is B.
Carbamazepine inhibits both pre- and postsynaptic sodium channels.

149. The answer is B.

150. The answer is D.

151. The answer is A.

152. The answer is B.

153. The answer is D.

154. The answer is C.

155. The answer is C.

156. The answer is D.

157. The answer is A.

158. The answer is A.

159. The answer is C.
When minor side effects occur, management with adjunctive agents is often successful and does not delay the therapeutic responses.

160. The answer is D.
TCAs and MAOIs cause orthostatic hypotension (OH). Imipramine, desipramine, and amitriptyline are equally likely to produce OH. Phenelzine, a MAOI, causes mild OH in 47% of patients. Nortriptyline is the least likely of the TCAs to induce OH.

161. The answer is A.
Nortriptyline, a TCA, can prolong the QT_c especially when combined with an antipsychotic. An electrocardiogram should be obtained to check for abnormal conduction and magnesium and potassium levels should be kept in a normal range to minimize the risk of conduction disturbances. Patients on TCAs and neuroleptics are susceptible to OH and to potential falls. An echocardiogram is not useful in the initial evaluation of either OH or conduction disturbances caused by psychotropic medications.

162. The answer is D.
Acute dystonia is an emergency, and treatment requires the use of anticholinergic and antihistaminergic medications. The remaining answers are matched correctly.

163. The answer is E.
The symptoms of NMS include muscular rigidity, an increased creatine phosphokinase (CPK) level, dystonia, agitation, delirium, and autonomic dysfunction. Involuntary movements of the face or hands are consistent with neuroleptic-induced tardive dyskinesia.

164. The answer is B.
Lithium produces a benign, relative leukocytosis without impairing leukocyte function. Clozapine can cause agranulocytosis. Carbamazepine is associated with benign and severe hematological toxicities with depression of red blood cells, white blood cells or platelets. Valproic acid can cause thrombocytopenia or platelet dysfunction.

165. The answer is B.
Nortriptyline, although the safest TCA, can cause tachycardia and conduction disturbances at a higher rate than non-TCA antidepressants. In a patient recovering from a myocardial infarction, the least cardiotoxic medication should be used.

166. The answer is B.
The patient must have a urine output of greater than 3 L/day to be diagnosed with nephrogenic diabetes insipidus.

167. The answer is E.
All antipsychotics except molindone (Moban) cause weight gain.

168. The answer is E.
The patient suffers from an anticholinergic delirium and treatment is with an anticholinesterase (e.g., physostigmine). Dantrolene and bromocriptine are helpful in the treatment of NMS. Phentolamine is used for hypertensive crisis, and diphenhydramine would worsen the anticholinergic delirium.

169. The answer is E.
Hopelessness is an even better predictor of suicide than is depression.

170. The answer is E.
While gender and race represent epidemiologic risk factors, they do not bear on the lethality of a particular attempt.

171. The answer is C.
However, recent death of a family member (e.g., associated with heart disease) could increase one's risk for suicide.

172. The answer is B.
Parents of young children have a lower risk for suicide. However, having young children does not guarantee that an individual will not attempt suicide.

173. The answer is D.
The risk of suicide in bipolar and unipolar patients during a depressive episode is roughly equivalent. Substance abuse is a significant risk factor in its own right, particularly in combination with depression.

174. The answer is True.
The recognition and treatment of akathisia can diminish the risk of suicide significantly.

175. The answer is False.
Many patients who express suicidal ideation when intoxicated retract these statements when sober. However, substance abuse significantly increases the risk of suicide attempts and successful suicide. Impaired judgment and increased impulsivity when intoxicated likely contribute to this risk.

176. The answer is E.
Anxiety remains a risk factor for suicide even after controlling for comorbid depression and substance abuse.

177. The answer is True.
Epidemiologic studies show that the risk of completed suicide is increased among certain populations, including those of Caucasian descent, male gender, and those who are over the age of 60. However, the sensitivity and specificity of these factors is extremely poor. For example, a married 40-year-old woman with small children may still commit suicide.

178. The answer is D.
All of the above factors are important when completing an assessment for suicide, but safety must be established before any of the other elements will be possible.

179. The answer is False.
As with any attempt, details of the plan, taken in the context of knowledge of underlying risk factors, must be considered when determining lethality.

180. The answer is True.
Patients who chronically threaten or attempt suicide may eventually succeed, even if only by accident.

181. The answer is False.
The circumstances that led to the initial attempt are often unchanged immediately after an attempt, and hospitalized patients can and do attempt suicide. Psychiatric consultation can assist in the assessment of appropriate safety measures, as well as in diagnosis and management of psychiatric illness.

182. The answer is E.
"Contracting for safety" has become a popular way to enlist patient cooperation. However, while such a contract may be reassuring for the clinician, it has no demonstrated benefit in preventing suicide. Establishing a true alliance between the treater and the patient is far more important.

183. The answer is False.
While little research has been done in this field, both lithium and clozapine have been shown to reduce the risk of suicide under certain circumstances. In bipolar disorder, lithium maintenance significantly reduces risk of suicide. In schizophrenia, clozapine similarly reduces the risk of suicide.

184. The answer is D.
Ladislaus von Meduna reported his work on the induction of seizures using injections of intramuscular camphor to treat psychiatric illness in 1934. It was 3 years later when Cerletti and Bini first began using electricity to induce a therapeutic convulsion. In the same year (1937) Moniz published his work on prefrontal leukotomy, beginning a trend toward psychosurgery for severe mental illness. A.E. Bennett first used curare as a muscle relaxant in 1940. While lithium had some use during the 19th century, John Cade's work on lithium as an antimanic medication did not come until 1949.

185. The answer is A.
Despite several decades of experience with ECT, the mechanism by which it relieves depression is not clear. The other answers have been proposed as theories, but have largely been debunked with subsequent research.

186. The answer is E.
Despite the presence of affective instability and transient psychosis, borderline personality disorder is not an indication for the use of ECT. The other diagnoses have been shown to respond to ECT and are considered to be well-established indications.

187. The answer is E.
There are no absolute contraindications to the use of ECT. Due to its effects on heart rate, blood pressure and intracerebral pressure, ECT should be used with a high degree of caution in populations with certain medical conditions (vascular disease, intracerebral mass lesions, and pregnancy). Like most procedures, carefully weighing the risks and benefits is critical for the appropriate use.

188. The answer is False.
ECT has been compared with placebo, sham ECT, and several active antidepressant treatments, including TCAs and MAOIs. Response rates are clearly better than placebo and at least equal to (if not better than) other biological treatments for depression. The rate of response for ECT is approximately 75–90%.

189. The answer is E.
Goals for the management of the pre-ECT patient include stabilization of medical illnesses, detection of illness that may complicate ECT and anesthesia, and preparation for the procedure. All of the above are routinely done prior to ECT, usually in conjunction with an anesthesiologist. Depending on this patient's history and exam, other tests or consultations may be necessary.

190. The answer is D.
The d'Elia placement refers to the now-standard positioning of electrodes during the unilateral ECT. This stands in distinction to the bilateral placement of electrodes usually over the frontotemporal areas.

191. The answer is D.
There are several reasons for ECT failure. Improper diagnosis (e.g., personality disorder), premature need to discontinue the series (due to patient request, medical complications, or excessive delirium), and technical features of the ECT administration account for most cases. The answers above may all lead to inadequate treatment, and should be assessed before considering someone an "ECT failure."

192. The answer is D.
ECT can cause both anterograde and retrograde memory loss. This side effect can be significant, and is of great concern to most patients. It is therefore important to include accurate estimations of the type of cognitive deficits expected with ECT in the informed consent process. While underlying dementia can exacerbate the degree of cognitive impairment, memory loss can occur in patients without pre-existing dementia.

193. The answer is E.
Several medications can raise the seizure threshold, increasing the dose of electricity necessary to induce a therapeutic convulsion. Since the increased dose of electricity may contribute to a higher rate of side effects, many of these medications are held (when safe to do so) during a course of ECT. Interestingly, ECT itself leads to an increase in the seizure threshold, a factor thought to be significant in the efficacy of this procedure.

194. The answer is B.
The appropriate role of the C-L psychiatrist is to diagnose, treat, and teach non-psychiatric colleagues about the affective, behavioral, and cognitive derangements that attend medical and surgical conditions. Availability to help the consultee over the long-term is essential to effective consultation, but fault-finding is never an appropriate function.

195. The answer is C.
The rate of referral for psychiatric consultation is only 3–5%.

196. The answer is A.
While a psychiatrist may opine about the etiology of the patient's dementia and about his capacity to make medical decisions, questions regarding legal capacities should be referred to the hospital's attorneys. Choice (B) presents an example of a medical condition (hypercalcemia due to lytic bone lesions) that presents as a psychiatric syndrome (lethargic confusion). The patient described in choice (C) displays signs consistent with an adjustment disorder. Given the presence of apathy and neoplastic disease, the differential diagnosis also includes a frontal-lobe metastasis. In choice (D), independent medical and psychiatric illnesses coexist. Confusion and myoclonus are common signs of normeperidine (the long-acting metabolite of meperidine) toxicity, as described in choice (E).

197. The answer is D.
The need for flexibility, appreciation of the impact of medical-surgical illnesses and their treatments on mental status, and clarity in communication of diagnostic impressions and management recommendations are particularly important in general hospitals.

198. The answer is C.
While benzodiazepines and opiate analgesics are associated with withdrawal syndromes, antipsychotic agents are not. When benzodiazepines and opiates are inadvertently not prescribed when patients are admitted to the hospital or are transferred between different units, patients who are physiologically dependent on them may experience withdrawal syndromes. Insufficient dosages may also result in withdrawal states. An exhaustive review of medication records is essential to diagnose these conditions.

199. The answer is E.
While an understanding of the psychodynamic underpinnings of a case may be important for the consultant, rare is the consultee who will appreciate a detailed psychologic formulation. More important contributions are availability during crises and specific suggestions for managing troublesome and disruptive behaviors.

200. The answer is E.
All of these factors are important to consider.

201. The answer is E.
The absence of severe mental illness in Mr. N does not absolve the psychiatric consultant of responsibility. The psychiatrist's goal is to help the medical team recognize Mr. N's entitled, controlling style as his idiosyncratic expression of fear, anxiety, and stress. Even though the consultant does not have sufficient data to diagnose narcissistic personality disorder, he can still offer strategies to handle narcissistic traits and can defuse the staff's contempt for the patient. In-depth psychotherapy is rarely, if ever, indicated in medically hospitalized patients and would not be useful here. The primary goal is to manage the patient's behavior, not explore its determinants as a psychotherapist would.

202. The answer is D.
The consultant's goal in this case is to explain the patient's self-injurious behavior and thereby lessen the surgeon's hostility for the patient. If the surgeon understands Ms. B's behavior as a manifestation of a psychological vulnerability to frustration (similar to an immunocompromised patient's vulnerability to infection or a cardiac patient's predisposition to heart failure), his visceral reaction of disgust and contempt may abate. While the surgeon's countertransference may very well be problematic, sharing this opinion with the surgeon would not be helpful. Accusation of impaired judgment is likely to raise the surgeon's own defenses and worsen the situation.

203. The answer is A.
Though discussion about end-of-life care (e.g., DNR, DNI, and disposition decisions) is a critical function of a C-L psychiatrist, this discussion should be held with the patient (if he or she has the capacity to make such decisions) not just with the family. The C-L psychiatrist also plays a vital role with the staff, who may struggle with uncertainty, grief, and loss. Addressing the biological aspect of Mr. C's treatment, the psychiatrist should indicate that nefazodone inhibits the cytochrome P450 isoenzyme (3A4) that metabolizes cyclosporine and thus may raise its serum level.

204. The answer is E.

205. The answer is E.

206. The answer is E.
See *Why Marriages Succeed or Fail* (1994) by John Gottman. Simon and Schuster.

207. The answer is D.
Most couples have their first child within the first 4 years of marriage. There is a predictable decline in marital satisfaction that occurs after the birth of children and continuing for 2 years. See Belsky J, Rovine M: Patterns of change across the transition to parenthood: pregnancy to three years postpartum. *Journal of Marriage and the Family* 1990; 52: 5–19. A second low point in marital satisfaction occurs when the first child enters puberty (Silverberg S, Steinberg L: Psychological well being of parents with early adolescent children. *Developmental Psychology* 1990; 26: 658–666).

208. The answer is E.
Frank Pittman, in his book *Private Lies* enumerates several myths including the four listed above. Another myth he disputes is the notion that the affair is the fault of the cuckold and that after an affair, divorce is inevitable.

209. The answer is D.
Diagnostic procedures can now offer physical explanations for all but 10% of infertile couples. Of the 90% diagnosed, 35% are attributable to the female, 35% to the male, and 20% to an interactive factor. See Meyers M, Diamond R, David K, Scharf C, Weinshel M, Rait D: An infertility primer for family therapists: I. Medical, social, and psychological dimensions. *Family Process* 1995; 34: 219–229.

210. The answer is E.
The May-June 1986 issue of the *Family Therapy Networker* features several articles on domestic violence. See Bograd (1992) for a discussion of the complexities involved in conducting couples therapy when one partner is abusing the other. Goldner et al. (1990), in a seminal paper offer an explanation for wife abuse

based on gender socialization and propose a method for treating couples in which abuse is a prominent feature.

211. The answer is E.
See the January/February 1991 *Family Therapy Networker* issue with a special section on gay and lesbian relationships.

212. The answer is C.
While it used to be true that there was a preponderance of women with inhibited sexual desire, in recent years the requests for help with this problem are equally represented by men and women. See LoPiccolo and LoPiccolo (1978).

213. The answer is D.
Other risk factors include: the couple marries before age 20 or after 30; one or both families have a history of divorce and separations; there is an infidelity within the first 2 years of marriage; the couple lives together before being married; the couple has a child within the first year of marriage; the couple has an engagement of more than 3 years; the couple marries after a courtship of less than 6 months; there are religious, educational, class, age or cultural differences; neither partner had opposite-sex siblings; and both partners hold the same birth order position. This list is not meant as a checklist; a higher number of risk factors does not mean a higher chance of divorce. Instead, the list represents several independent research findings. See Carter B, McGoldrick M (eds): *The Changing Family Life Cycle*, 2nd ed. Boston: Allyn and Bacon, 1989.

214. The answer is E.

215. The answer is False.

216. The answer is True.

217. The answer is True

218. The answer is False.

219. The answer is True.

220. The answer is True.

221. The answer is False.

222. The answer is True.

223. The answer is A.
While dementia is more common in advanced HIV disease, the virus is present in certain neural cells early in the course of infection.

224. The answer is C.
Because the availability of combination antiretroviral therapy has improved survival of AIDS patients, the prevalence of AIDS has actually increased in recent years.

225. The answer is B.
While it is important to maintain a high index of suspicion for "organic" causes of psychopathology, such an approach is indicated more in advanced cases (when patients are prone to HIV-related illnesses and take more medications) than in earlier ones.

226. The answer is C.
Any antidepressant, not just SSRIs, should be started in low doses and increased slowly whether the depression is primary, as it usually is in early infection, or secondary, as it usually is in more advanced HIV disease. The suicide evaluation, as in any patient, focuses on determination of patient safety and diagnosis and treatment of underlying disorders.

227. The answer is D.
Ineffective coping should be treated pharmacologically when anxiety is a prominent feature, whether this symptom occurs in early or late stages of HIV/AIDS. Short-term use of benzodiazepines is indicated in this setting.

228. The answer is E.
The first line of treatment is specific therapy for the underlying cause of the delirium or the psychotic state. Neuroleptics are used as first-line agents only for primary psychosis; otherwise they are used empirically and to provide symptomatic control.

229. The answer is C.
Valproate is preferred over carbamazepine but it increases AZT serum level; carbamazepine lowers it.

230. The answer is B.
Some patients with cognitive deficits related to HIV infection follow a stable, nonprogressive course and never meet criteria for full-blown HIV dementia.

231. The answer is D.
SSRIs and TCAs may be given to patients on ritonavir but, as with other protease inhibitors, in small doses. SSRIs and TCAs are not among the many agents to be avoided with ritonavir.

232. The answer is E.
All of these are abnormal in HIV/AIDS patients.

233. The answer is C.

234. The answer is E.

235. The answer is E.

236. The answer is C.

237. The answer is A.

238. The answer is A.
Only cognitive-behavioral therapy is manual driven, though some forms of supportive and psychoeducational therapy may be systematized for research purposes.

239. The answer is D.
Countertransference, resistance, transitional objects, and dream analysis are all aspects of classical psychodynamic theory. Negative thoughts are the presumed etiology of psychiatric illness in the cognitive-behavioral model of psychotherapy.

240. The answer is E.
The concepts of the schizoid, depressive, and paranoid positions are often associated with Melanie Klein. According to Klein, a healthy infant must negotiate the schizoid and paranoid positions before arriving at the more healthy and normal depressive position.

241. The answer is C.
Behavior therapy is often very helpful in the treatment of specific phobias. Typically, the behavior therapist would ask the patient to engage in increasingly anxiety-provoking activities related to flying, and at the same time help the patient to tolerate and modulate the fear that these activities provoke. For example, the patient might first be asked to visualize sitting in an airplane, and near the end of the treatment the patient might actually ride in an airplane.

242. The answer is C.
IPT focuses on current relationships, and is especially useful in the treatment of depression.

243. The answer is B.
DBT was designed for the treatment of borderline personality disorder, with the dual goals of decreasing inpatient hospitalizations and self-injurious behaviors, such as cutting.

244. The answer is D.
Spiegel's work has suggested that in addition to improved psychological well-being, patients with breast cancer who participate in group psychotherapy also frequently improve in terms of the course of the cancer itself.

245. The answer is C.
All other choices played a significant part in the development of modern brief psychotherapy.

246. The answer is D.
As with all psychodynamic psychotherapies, the process of interpretation of unconscious conflict leading to insight is the goal of short-term psychodynamic psychotherapy.

247. The answer is B.
A number of national studies have shown that patients typically receive ten sessions or less of psychotherapy.

248. The answer is A.
The brief therapist needs to be open to the idea that time-limited work can be successful, accept that patients will return across the life-cycle, and understand how time sensitivity changes psychotherapy.

249. The answer is E.
Patient selection, brevity, focus and therapist active are all dimensions which help to define brief therapy.

250. The answer is False.
Because of the importance placed upon patient selection and finding a focus, a two-session initial evaluation is recommended for brief therapy.

251. The answer is False.
There are a number of possible foci for each patient; together the therapist and patient select one relevant focus which they can both agree to work on.

252. The answer is B.
The brief therapy patient should not be psychotic, abusing substances, or at risk for self-harm as these problems disrupt the framework of the treatment.

253. The answer is E.
All the above are listed by Budman and Gurman as likely foci for brief therapy. Keep them in mind as you conduct your evaluation.

254. The answer is True.
This will occur but in general it is best to hold to the termination date unless the new material has significant clinical implications (e.g., suicidal ideation).

255. The answer is True.
Although most patients diagnosed with a particular disorder require the same medication doses regardless of treatment site, outcome studies suggest that primary care patients may respond to lower doses of antidepressants for shorter periods of time with good results. This may be because symptoms are less severe to begin with (subsyndromal disorder), picked up earlier in the course of an illness, or are the result of adjustment disorders rather that major depression.

256. The answer is False.
Once a consultation is initiated, the PCP and psychiatrist are both considered to be part of the patient's "circle of care," and do not require specific releases to discuss medical information. Patients should be informed of this relationship. Psychiatrists should honor patient requests to omit specific details of their psychiatric history from the general medical chart if these details do not directly affect medical treatment.

257. The answer is False.
In most states, a specific release of information is required for both mental health and substance abuse records, whether they are in the general medical chart

or held separately. Institutions should have some means of identification of psychiatric records in general medical charts so they are not inadvertently released.

258. The answer is D.
Diagnostic instruments are used primarily in research studies, but they may be a useful adjunct to the interview in the clinical setting. They may allow the quantification of severity of illness, and help ascertain the degree of response to treatment. Some are self-administered by the patient, and others are administered by the clinician.

259. The answer is D.
The Beck Depression Inventory is a self-rated questionnaire. The others listed are administered by the clinician.

260. The answer is B.
The SCID is a qualitative instrument. It determines the presence or absence of various psychiatric disorders. It does not accurately quantify the degree of severity of illness. The Hamilton D, the BDI, and the Zung SDS provide more accurate information about the severity of depression.

261. The answer is C.
The Hamilton D has several versions, whose number of questions range from 6 to 31.

262. The answer is D.
The CGI relies on both clinician and patient impressions. It measures the severity of depression using the *initial* visit as the standard for comparison. It is generally administered following other diagnostic instruments, as the information from these my facilitate scoring the CGI. The CGI measures presence and degree of severity of depression.

263. The answer is E.
The SCID is the most reliable instrument for determining the presence or a DSM-IV psychiatric disorder. It is used almost exclusively in research studies, as it is lengthy and difficult for the non-researcher to administer. It does not measure the severity of illness very accurately.

264. The answer is B.
A baseline Hamilton D score may be compared with a later one to help determine improvement of depressive symptoms, and may provide more accurate information than relying strictly in the patient's subjective impressions of whether or not the medication "works." Patients with characterological problems may nonetheless experience alleviation of their depressive symptoms when treated with antidepressants. The Hamilton D is administered by the clinician. Some patients may be resistant to standardized questionnaires, as they may make the interview seem impersonal. The clinician should therefore spend a few moments with the patient, clarifying the role of such instruments prior to administering them.

265. The answer is C.
The SCID-II is specifically designed to diagnose personality disorders, although a thorough clinical interview can also accomplish this task. None of the other instruments listed in this question are particularly useful in the diagnosis of personality disorders.

266. The answer is D.
Both the Y-BOCS and the SCID may identify the presence of OCD. The Y-BOCS may quantify the severity of the OCD. The Hamilton D-17 does not inquire about obsessions or compulsions, although some longer versions of the HAM-D include a question about obsessions and compulsions.

267. The answer is C.
The AIMS is important to administer to patients receiving antipsychotics, as a means to monitor for development of tardive dyskinesia or other movement disorders secondary to antipsychotics. The other instruments may yield useful clinical information about comorbid conditions, but they are not as essential in the clinic setting with such a patient.

268. The answer is A.
Shortly before his assassination in 1963, President John F. Kennedy signed the Community Mental Health Center Act which provided funds (in 1963) to build the CMHCs, and funds (in 1965) to staff them.

269. The answer is B.
The 1984 Epidemiologic Catchment Area (ECA) study revealed that psychiatric symptoms in the community are common and that most symptomatic individuals seeking treatment never see any mental health professional; most seek care in the general medical setting, either from their primary care provider, or in emergency rooms.

270. The answer is E.
The underlying principles of CMH include responsibility for an entire catchmented population, prevention, community-based care, and a continuum of inter-related services to provide continuity of care.

271. The answer is D.
The general medical system (e.g., primary care providers, walk-in medical clinics, emergency rooms) has been termed the "de facto" mental health system because the majority of people who seek care for mental health or substance abuse problems initially present to non-mental health professionals in the general medical setting.

272. The answer is A.
The high number of psychiatric casualties and evacuees in the first half of World War II prompted a change in treatment strategy. Immediate treatment in the field, with the expectation of timely return to combat service

was found to greatly improve functional outcome and decrease residual disability. This led to three central tenets of CMH: immediacy, proximity, and expectancy.

273. The answer is C.

Consultation/education was one of five mandated, or "essential," services specified in the 1963 CMHC Act. The other essential services were inpatient, outpatient, partial hospitalization, and 24-h emergency services. With the decreases in federal funding and oversight, non-revenue-producing services, such as consultation/education, have also diminished.

274. The answer is B.

Currently, the community mental health system in the United States prioritizes its limited resources to treat primarily those individuals with serious and persistent mental illness. While the pendulum has historically swung between institutional containment and community-based treatment, the current climate favors community-based treatment. Primary and secondary prevention refer to measures that decrease incidence and prevalence of a disease or disorder, and are rarely the focus of current CMH endeavors.

275. The answer is True.

Like publicly funded community mental health centers, progressive managed care organizations (MCOs) invite community involvement. Similar to community boards of CMHCs, MCOs have advisory panels of providers and community members to help them assess the relevance and cultural appropriateness of their programs.

276. The answer is E.

Reliability is the ability to produce systematic or reproducible results. Being better trained as a rater, using standardized interview settings and structured diagnostic instruments, and having explicit diagnostic criteria improves reliability of psychiatric diagnosis.

277. The answer is B.

The kappa statistic is used to measure reliability of raters and it corrects for chance agreement. Its values range from 0 to 1 and higher values reflect higher reliability. It is inaccurate when the frequency of the disorder is very low. Reliability is a necessary, but not a sufficient condition for validity of a diagnosis.

278. The answer is E.

A valid instrument has face validity, content validity, and criterion validity. An instrument has face validity if it makes good sense to an investigator, and has content validity if its item covers the information for making the diagnosis. High sensitivity and specificity demonstrate that the instrument has criterion validity.

279. The answer is B.

Incidence rates measures the number of new disease that develop in a population of individuals at risk during a specific time interval. It is not affected by the duration of the disease.

280. The answer is A.

Relative risk is for testing the relationship between an exposure and a disease relationship in a cohort study. The kappa statistic is for testing reliability between raters, and Mantel-Haenszel statistic is for pooling relative risks over different strata in cohort and case-control studies.

281. The answer is D.

In the ECA study, the most prevalent psychiatric disorder was phobia, with a lifetime prevalence of 14.3% and one-year prevalence of 8.8%.

282. The answer is C.

The prevalence of schizophrenia for a child with one schizophrenic parent is 15%.

283. The answer is E.

Risks factors for major depression include female gender, a history of depressive illness in first-degree relatives, having prior episodes of major depression, having an age of onset under 40, being in the postpartum period, having prior suicide attempts, having medical comorbidity, having a lack of social support, having stressful life events, and being a current substance abuser.

284. The answer is D.

According to the ECA study, the lifetime prevalence for generalized anxiety disorder is 8.5%.

285. The answer is C.

Alcoholism is correlated with male gender, Hispanic ethnicity, a younger age, being separated or divorced, or having a low educational level, occupational level, or income.

286. The answer is C.

287. The answer is A.

288. The answer is B.

289. The answer is D.

290. The answer is B.

291. The answer is C.

292. The answer is A.

293. The answer is C.

294. The answer is A.

295. The answer is D.

296. The answer is B.

297. The answer is C.

Relatives of individuals with bipolar disorder have an elevated risk of unipolar depression as well as bipolar disorder itself. Although the relative risk of bipolar disorder is higher than for unipolar depression, the absolute risk (probability of being affected) for unipolar depression is higher than it is for bipolar disorder.

298. The answer is D.

At least three specific genes have been shown to produce early-onset AD and one gene, ApoE, is known to be a risk factor for late-onset AD.

299. The answer is C.

300. The answer is C.

Eye-tracking abnormalities and several other biological phenotypes appear to be more common in the relatives of schizophrenic probands.

301. The answer is A.

Trinucleotide repeats in genes can be unstable and expand during DNA replication. Huntington's disease has been shown to be due to expanded CAG repeats. CAG repeats in this gene in the normal population range from 5 to 37, but in individuals with Huntington's disease they range from 37 to 121. Fragile X syndrome, the second most common cause of mental retardation among males, is due to expansion of CGG repeats in the FMR-1 gene on the X chromosome.

302. The answer is True.

303. The answer is D.

Family study data indicate that relatives of probands with Tourette's have an increased risk of OCD and in some families of OCD probands, there appears to be an excess risk of Tourette's.

304. The answer is B.

The LOD score is the $\log_{10}$ of the likelihood of the odds ratio for linkage. A LOD score of 3 or above is usually taken to indicate linkage (although higher thresholds may be necessary for genome scans of complex phenotypes such as psychiatric disorders).

305. The answer is True.

Family studies are an important step in the process of deciding whether genes influence a phenotype. If first-degree relatives of ill probands have a higher prevalence of the trait than first-degree relatives of control probands, the disorder is familial. However, a trait may run in families for primarily environmental rather than genetic reasons. Other types of studies (twin, adoption, molecular genetic) are needed to determine the contribution of genetic factors to familial transmission.

306. The answer is E.

Identifying genes for complex disorders like psychiatric disorders can be complicated by obstacles to classifying accurately whether an individual carries the disease genotype. These obstacles include our uncertainty about how to define psychiatric disorders, incomplete penetrance (having the disease alleles does not always result in expression of the disease phenotype), phenocopies (individuals who have the disease phenotype but do not carry the disease-causing alleles), genetic heterogeneity (different genes or different alleles may cause the phenotype in different families), and variable expression (the disease alleles may result in a variety of phenotypes).

307. The answer is D.

An important skill in psychiatry is to realize that communication occurs on several levels and to learn to listen to oneself and one's reactions to patients. Recognizing in oneself common human drives also allows for understanding of and compassion for a patient. It is important to continually observe not only the content of the conversation but also the process. Countertransference can manifest with negative feelings that may disrupt the patient-doctor relationship or generate disproportionately positive or idealizing reactions.

308. The answer is A.

Emotionally based biases that a patient brings to the patient-doctor relationship are commonly called transference. These include a wide array of positive or negative beliefs, preconceptions, and expectations, which have their origin in persistent experiences with important figures such as parents. Patients may unconsciously and inappropriately distort or displace onto the physician patterns that started in childhood, even before the interview begins. Transference is a quality that is present in people's relationships and is not limited to specific psychiatric disorders.

309. The answer is B.

Hostility during an interview is especially challenging, as it threatens the very formation of a therapeutic alliance. It is best acknowledged and analyzed as much as possible for the interview to proceed; ignoring or undermining the problem is generally not helpful. Alignment, rather than contradiction or persuasion, aids in the rapport with delusional patients. When patients become violent, they are often frightened by their own impulses and desperately desire help to halt loss of control. Management of violent patients is through physical means, such as restraints, with sufficient strength so that there is no contest. The seductive patient's feelings should be acknowledged while being clarified that they cannot be expressed in action.

310. The answer is D.

While most mental health circles agree that patients have a right to receive treatment in "the least restrictive setting," the severity of a person's mental illness may compel ethical and legal reasons for detaining the person against her or his will. Involuntary commitment is based on the principle of *parens patriae* (father of the country) and "police power" of the state, which has the right to intervene and protect an individual when her or his incapacity to make decisions poses danger. For civil commitment, the minimal standard of proof is "clear and convincing," rather than the stricter "beyond a reasonable doubt" for criminal cases. Commitment does not require the permission of a responsible relative, and it usually has a time limit.

311. The answer is C.
The principle of informed consent has developed considerably in the recent decades to involve a more patient-base model that encourages autonomy. It is defined as a *process* through which a physician gets the permission of a patient or substitute decision-maker to provide treatment to that patient, and thus, it may change in the face of a continually evolving clinical picture. In general, informed consent obligates the following criteria: (a) understanding the nature of foreseeable risks and benefits of treatment; (b) knowing of alternative procedures; (c) being aware of the consequences of withholding consent; (d) recognizing that the consent is voluntary; and (e) having the legal capacity to give consent.

312. The answer is E.
Spousal beating occurs in all racial, religious, and socioeconomic groups. Pregnancy is a high-risk period for battering; 15–20% of pregnant women are abused, which frequently results in birth defects. Those who abuse their spouses are generally from violent homes, where they witnessed beating or were beaten themselves as children. The men who batter tend to be immature and fragile, terrified by their dependency needs and enraged at their partners for any sign of autonomy. A large percentage abuse alcohol or drugs. While wife abuse is most common, husbands are also abused, which is underreported due to fear of ridicule.

313. The answer is C.
Rape is predominantly an expression of power and anger. Women who have been raped feel shame, humiliation, confusion, rage, and fear, often lasting for more than a year. Male rape victims often do not seek medical or legal help, but they have strikingly similar feelings or "having been ruined." Homosexual rape is more common in men, and some victims fear that they will become homosexuals after an assault. Effective treatment of a rape victim includes immediate support for the victim to ventilate her or his feelings to sympathetic family members, physicians, and law enforcement officials. Knowing that one has at his disposal a socially acceptable means of recourse, such as arresting and convicting the rapist, can also be therapeutic.

314. The answer is A.
Managed care, broadly defined as patient care determined not solely by the provider, currently focuses on the economic aspects of medical care, with little attention to its effects on the patient-physician relationship. Both patient and physician autonomy is diminished by

managed care. Experience-rating increases premiums for those who need and use care, which contributes to the problem of mental health remaining the only branch of health care with a large public sector system coupled with poor private insurance coverage.

315. The answer is B.
Malpractice claims can pose an unwelcome, taxing burden on the physician. Medical malpractice is defined as injury caused by negligent care, *not* as adverse outcome alone. Since claims have been filed in increasing numbers in recent years, most physicians obtain professional liability insurance. In a claim, the plaintiff, or injured patient, must show that the physician's care fell below the "standard of care," or the level of care that a prudent physician would provide in a similar situation. When subpoenaed, the defendant is a "fact" witness, responsible for testifying only as to what she or he saw and did and why, while experts are "opinion" witnesses called to establish standards of care. Many malpractice cases are dropped by the plaintiff or settled prior to trial, and even when brought to court, result most often in favor of the physician.

316. The answer is E.
Ongoing self-assessment is necessary to recognize early signs of burnout and act on them. Anticipating difficulties, observing oneself through psychotherapy, not working in isolation, and joining groups structured on trust and confidence can provide professionals with the opportunity to get to know themselves as well as themselves-with-others. Gratification of patients' idealizing transference can be tempting when a professional is vulnerable; those who are aware of their weaknesses, including their desire for appreciation and admiration, are less likely to fall into complicated emotional entanglements.

317. The answer is A.

318. The answer is E.

319. The answer is C.

320. The answer is B.

321. The answer is D.

322. The answer is False.
Individuals who have underlying psychiatric illnesses are at a greater risk for acts of violence than those without mental illness. Monahan (1991) has reviewed the literature and Epidemiologic Catchment Area data and has shown that the prevalence of violence is more than five times higher among people who meet criteria for a DSM-III Axis I diagnosis than among people with no diagnosis. Individuals meeting criteria for a diagnosis of substance abuse have a prevalence of violence that is 16 times higher than those with no diagnosis.

323. The answer is True.

In the initial phases of any psychiatric evaluation, the safety of the patient and of those in the immediate environs should be established and maintained. This involves stabilizing the patient medically, clearing the environment of potentially dangerous objects, providing an escape route, and providing seclusion with restraint and chemical sedation if warranted.

324. The answer is True.

Many studies have implicated serotonin as having an inhibitory role in the control of impulsive aggression. Low CSF 5HIAA (a major metabolite of serotonin and a standard measure of central serotonin turnover) has been found in people who are highly violent and suicidal. Some studies have found that SSRIs have reduced impulsive aggression in personality-disordered patients.

325. The answer is False.

There have been no controlled trials to date which have systematically looked at the comparison of medication versus therapy for the treatment of violence. In general, most believe that a combination of therapy and medication is the best treatment for those with chronic aggressive behaviors.

326. The answer is C.

Cerebellum. All of the other structures listed have been shown to have varying influences on the outward manifestation of aggression in both man and animals. The one exception is the cerebellum.

327. The answer is B.

Lorazepam. Benzodiazepines may lead to disinhibition and can lead to aggression or violence in patients with underlying brain damage or dementia.

328. The answer is E.

All of the above. Studies have shown that carrying virtually any diagnosis on Axis I may increase one's risk for committing an act of violence

329. The answer is False.

The psychiatric diagnosis is the primary influence on the treatment of the patient that has chronic problems with outward aggression and violence.

330. The answer is False.

A past history of violence is one of the best predictors of future violence and is a key element in determining present risk.

331. The answer is False.

Patients who carry an Axis I diagnosis of substance abuse have the greatest prevalence of violence and commit violent acts at a prevalence 16 times the rate of violence among individuals with no Axis I diagnosis.

332. The answer is C.

Thought process refers to the manner in which the patient connects and presents individual ideas. Abnormalities lie on a continuum from subtle parenthetical comments to a complete lack of meaningful connection (word salad). The best way to assess for this is simply listening to the patient's spontaneous speech.

333. The answer is C.

The hallmark of encephalopathy (delirium) is an abnormal level of consciousness. This may be severe (coma) or subtle (attentional deficit). It is best tested by having the patient perform a task which requires a maintained focus (serial 7s). Given the high prevalence and morbidity associated with delirium, attention should be tested in all medical inpatients. While other cognitive abnormalities may occur in the encephalopathic patient, they are secondary to the attentional problem.

334. The answer is D.

Asking three simple questions will descriptively communicate the nature of an aphasia without using confusing eponyms. Is the language fluent? Is comprehension normal? Is repetition normal? In this case, the speech does not sound like normal language (non-fluent). While able to receive information, he is unable to repeat simple phrases. This pattern is not uncommon, given evidence of hemiplegia.

335. The answer is D.

This patient reports a loss of recall of previously experienced events shortly after starting ECT. Importantly, she is still able to learn new information, including her current whereabouts. She is unlikely to have abnormalities in concentration or short-term memory (though both can occur during a course of ECT). Her problems cannot be accounted for by apathy or stress. It is best construed as a problem in long-term memory. This type of retrograde amnesia can occur with ECT, but is usually for a brief period of time preceding the treatment. It will occasionally resolve over time.

336. The answer is B.

Saccades are rapid eye movements that allow for brisk transitions in the visual fields. Pursuits are slow voluntary eye movements that allow for smooth tracking of a target. Saccades are best tested by simply observing as the patient glances quickly at one target then another.

337. The answer is D.

The trigeminal nerve supplies sensory innervation to the face, including the cornea and motor innervation to the muscles of mastication (e.g., masseter). The muscles of facial expression, including those that wrinkle the forehead, are innervated by the facial nerve (CrN VII).

338. The answer is A.

Peripheral (Bell's palsy). There is bilateral corticobulbar innervation to the portion of the facial nerve that supplies the forehead; a central (upper motor neuron) lesion will therefore spare the forehead. A palsy of the facial nerve itself will lead to full hemifacial weakness regardless of the corticobulbar input.

339. The answer is E.
A close observation of the patient's gait is essential. The ability to walk requires significant motor strength, coordination of trunk and limbs, and proprioception. Deficits in any of these modalities will impair gait, making it a nonspecific, but sensitive screening test.

340. The answer is B.
Proprioceptive reflexes are based on the reflex arcs activated by tapping on a muscle or tendon. Also known as deep tendon reflexes (DTRs), they are useful in assessing the integrity of corticospinal innervation to these arcs. The ankle jerk is the only proprioceptive reflex listed. The remainder are classified as nociceptive or primitive reflexes.

341. The answer is E.
The grasp reflex, like other primitive reflexes, is present as a normal finding in infancy. Its return during adulthood is never normal.

342. The answer is B.
A non-contrast head CT poses no risk and will demonstrate all important causes of headache. A lumbar puncture is useful when looking for elevated CSF pressure. An EEG is rarely helpful in the evaluation of headache patients. An MRI scan, although more sensitive than a CT scan, is expensive and carries risk to the patient because of the use of gadolinium as a contrast. Return of an elevated ESR is useful when suspicion of temporal arteritis is suspected.

343. The answer is A.
The migraine headache often is unilateral and accompanied by phonophobia or photophobia. An aura, although less common, can precede the headache.

344. The answer is C.
Cluster headaches are more frequent in males than females. The pain is often retro-orbital and sharp. Autonomic dysfunction, including injected conjunctiva, sweating, ptosis, or miosis can accompany the headache. The cluster headache at times is referred to as the "Horton's headache." Tobacco and alcohol can precipitate the headache.

345. The answer is B.
Tension-type headaches are more frequent in females. The pain is often a band-like pain located in the frontal, occipital, or cervical areas. A family history is common. Although benzodiazepines are effective, they should be avoided in tension-type headaches because many less potentially harmful strategies exist.

346. The answer is E.
Pseudotumor cerebri is common in young obese women who often have menstrual irregularities. Papilledema is usually present in these patients. The treatment involves serial lumbar punctures.

347. The answer is C.
Although the patients' symptoms are consistent with trigeminal neuralgia, the age of onset is usually over 60 years old. Occurrence in young people may suggest multiple sclerosis with a plaque involving the trigeminal nerve root. Anesthetic injection, carbamazepine, and surgery are treatment options for trigeminal neuralgia. Lithium is useful in the treatment of cluster headaches.

348. The answer is D.
Posttrauma headaches resemble migraine or tension headaches. Meningococcus or pneumococcus usually cause acute meningitis. Herpes simplex encephalitis can also present as meningitis. A severe headache with nuchal rigidity is the most common symptom of subarachnoid hemorrhage.

349. The answer is A.
Many foods, such as aged cheese, red wines, chocolate and peanuts can precipitate migraine headaches.

350. The answer is C.
Neck bruits, although important in a physical examination, can be caused by carotid stenosis or radiation of a cardiac murmur. They are not useful in the evaluation of headache.

351. The answer is E.
Although there are no abnormal neurologic findings, subtle personality and cognitive changes are usually present with headaches of this type. The smoking history and decreased breath sounds on lung examination suggest a possible lung cancer with metastases to the brain.

352. The answer is E.
Visual agnosia may occur after lesions of the primary visual cortex.

353. The answer is C.

354. The answer is C.

355. The answer is C.

356. The answer is E.

357. The answer is B.

358. The answer is A.

359. The answer is A.

360. The answer is C.

361. The answer is B.
Nausea and localized headache may be signs of cerebellar infarction. In this patient with possible hypertensive crisis after MAOI-decongestant interaction, a hemorrhagic infarction is a likely scenario. Cerebellar hemorrhage may become a neurosurgical emergency. A noncontrast head CT is an excellent test for discovery of hemorrhagic stroke.

362. The answer is D.

363. The answer is A.

364. The answer is E.

365. The answer is E.

366. The answer is E.

367. The answer is A.

368. The answer is D.

369. The answer is D.

370. The answer is C.

371. The answer is C.

372. The answer is D.

373. The answer is C.

374. The answer is C.
Internal consistency is a measure of item reliability, test-retest reliability is a measure of scale stability, and inter-rater reliability (called kappa) is a measure of judge/rater reliability.

375. The answer is E.
A psychological test is a highly standardized method of patient assessment.

376. The answer is E.
Validity data take many forms, including: predicting future behavior based upon a test score (predictive), convergent and divergent association with similar and different tests, and degree to which the test items cover the important aspects of the construct (content).

377. The answer is B.
The MMPI-2 has 567 questions and is one of the longest tests given.

378. The answer is False.
Modern psychological assessment began with the development of the intelligence test by Stanford and Binet in 1905.

379. The answer is False.
The evidence regarding the validity of a test is always evolving and tests are considered valid or not for specific purposes.

380. The answer is B.
With the development of the Comprehensive System the scoring of the Rorschach has become as reliable as that for most other psychological tests.

381. The answer is False.
For a clinical psychological assessment to be most useful all relevant information must be available to the consulting psychologist.

382. The answer is False.
This written test report should integrate all the test findings in a manner which richly describes the patient's strengths and weaknesses.

383. The answer is False.
The definitive diagnosis is made by obtaining a clinical history that is sufficient to meet the symptom criteria for the disorder. Neuropsychological testing can confirm the degree of attentional weakness compared to overall IQ or scholastic achievement. Also, neuropsychological testing can rule out the presence or absence of learning disabilities which are often comorbid with ADHD.

384. The answer is C.
The Boston approach obtains general intellectual data and then assesses all functions that are pertinent to the referral question and information learned by the process of testing; e.g., poor performance on a specific task may influence other tests administered.

385. The answer is E.
Neuropsychological exams are pertinent to all the above disorders. While it is easier to see the relationship with memory, attention, visual spatial construction, and dementia, depression often can have profound effects on cognitive and motor functioning that affects the patients ability to function in their lives.

386. The answer is A.
Neuropsychological assessments of dementia focus heavily upon memory functioning, as poor delayed recall is associated with early dementia.

387. The answer is E.
Neuropsychological assessment is appropriate across a wide range of clinical conditions and situations.

388. The answer is C.
All the above except the Rorschach test would be routinely included in a neuropsychological testing battery.

389. The answer is False.
An MRI reveals structural problems with the brain but provides no information about functional status; neuropsychological testing data can more easily be translated in functional ability.

390. The answer is False.
The H-R assessment battery is time intensive and fixed in length.

391. The answer is C.
As tests become too complex, it is difficult to determine which cognitive functions are being tapped or measure.

392. The answer is C.

393. The answer is B.

394. The answer is B.

395. The answer is E.

396. The answer is D.

397. The answer is B.
Natural remedies are generally not approved by the FDA. They offer greater autonomy to patients, as they are available without a prescription. They are increasingly popular, despite the fact that insurance companies do not cover their costs. Their safety profiles are not well defined. They may be recommended by any practitioner, not just by physicians.

398. The answer is A.
St. John's Wort has been shown to be equally effective to low-dose tricyclics, at least with regard to mild-to-moderate depressions. Clinical trials comparing St. John's Wort to SSRIs are underway. Despite the MAOI activity of some of its components, this activity is minimal, and does not require any dietary restrictions. However, St. John's Wort should not be combined with SSRIs due to risk of serotonin syndrome. There are anecdotes of bipolar patients switching to mania while on St. John's Wort.

399. The answer is D.
Valerian is popular among Hispanic people. It is not recommended for acute treatment of insomnia, but may promote more restful sleep after several weeks of use. Mexican and Indian valerian may contain carcinogenic compounds.

400. The answer is E.
Use of kava originated in the Polynesian islands. It is believed to have anticonvulsant properties. It has shown no evidence of dependence. At high doses or with prolonged use, it may cause kava dermopathy, a transient yellow discoloration of the skin.

Index

The letter t or f following a page number indicates that either a table or a figure is being referenced.

ISBN 0-07-135435-2